NURSING INTERVENTIONS
Effective Nursing Treatments

NURSING INTERVENTIONS
Effective Nursing Treatments

THIRD EDITION

Gloria M. Bulechek, PhD, RN, FAAN
College of Nursing
University of Iowa
Iowa City, Iowa

Joanne C. McCloskey, PhD, RN, FAAN
College of Nursing
University of Iowa
Iowa City, Iowa

W.B. Saunders Company
A Division of Harcourt Brace & Company
Philadelphia London Toronto Montreal Sydney Tokyo

W.B. SAUNDERS COMPANY
A Division of Harcourt Brace & Company

The Curtis Center
Independence Square West
Philadelphia, Pennsylvania 19106

Library of Congress Cataloging-in-Publication Data

Nursing interventions : effective nursing treatments / [edited by] Gloria M. Bulechek,
Joanne C. McCloskey.—3rd ed.

p.   cm.

Includes bibliographical references and index.

ISBN 0–7216–7724–X

1. Nursing.   2. Nursing diagnosis.   3. Nurse and patient.   I. Bulechek,
    Gloria M.   II. McCloskey, Joanne C.
    [DNLM: 1. Nursing Process.   2. Health Promotion–nurses'
    instruction.   3. Nurse-Patient Relations.   4. Therapeutics–nurses'
    instruction.   5. Self-Care–nurses' instruction.   WY 100 N97523 1999]

RT48.N8833   1999

610.73—dc21

DNLM/DLC   98–43443

NURSING INTERVENTIONS: Effective Nursing Treatments   ISBN 0–7216–7724–X

Printed in the United States of America.

Last digit is the print number: 9   8   7   6   5   4   3   2   1

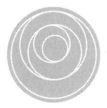

Contributors

Janet D. Allan, PhD, RN, FAAN, CS
Professor and Dean, University of Texas Health Science Center School of Nursing, San Antonio, Texas
Exercise Promotion

Michele A. Alpen, MA, RN, CEN
Trauma Coordinator, University of Iowa Hospitals & Clinics Department of Surgery, Iowa City, Iowa
Airway Management

Ida A. Androwich, PhD, RN, FAAN
Associate Professor, Loyola University, Niehoff School of Nursing, Chicago, Illinois
Telephone Consultation

Mary Lober Aquilino, PhD, RN, FNP
Assistant Professor, University of Iowa College of Nursing, Iowa City, Iowa
Health Education

Mary Kay Bader, MSN, RN, CCRN, CNRN
Neuroscience Clinical Specialist, Mission Hospital Regional Medical Center, Mission Viejo, California
Intracranial Pressure Monitoring

Nancy Bergstrom, PhD, RN, FAAN
Professor, University of Nebraska Medical Center College of Nursing, Omaha, Nebraska
Pressure Ulcer Prevention

Barbara J. Boss, PhD, RN, CS, CANP
Professor, University of Mississippi Medical Center School of Nursing, Jackson, Mississippi
Communication Enhancement: Speech Deficit

Eileen Bourret, MN, RN
Clinical Nurse Specialist, Baycrest Centre for Geriatric Care, Toronto, Ontario, Canada
Constipation/Impaction Management

Barbara J. Braden, PhD, RN, FAAN
Professor and Dean, Creighton University Graduate School, Omaha, Nebraska
Pressure Ulcer Prevention

Pamela J. Brink, PhD, RN, FAAN
Professor of Nursing and Anthropology, University of Alberta, Edmonton, Alberta, Canada
Culture Brokerage

Kathleen C. Buckwalter, PhD, RN, FAAN
Associate Provost for Health Sciences, Professor of Nursing and Psychiatry, University of Iowa, Iowa City, Iowa
Music Therapy; Dementia Management

Gloria M. Bulechek, PhD, RN, FAAN
Professor, University of Iowa College of Nursing,
Iowa City, Iowa
Nursing Diagnoses, Interventions, and Outcomes in Effectiveness Research

Lori Butcher, MS, RN
Assistant Director of Nursing, Horn Memorial
Hospital, Ida Grove, Iowa
Teaching: Preoperative

Lucy Cabico, MScN, RN
Clinical Nurse Specialist, Baycrest Centre for Geriatric Care, Toronto, Ontario, Canada
Constipation/Impaction Management

Norma J. Christman, PhD, RN, FAAN
Associate Professor, University of Kentucky College of Nursing and Department of Behavioral
Medicine, College of Medicine, Lexington, Kentucky
Preparatory Sensory Information

Kathie M. Cole, MN, RN, CCRN
Clinical Nurse Specialist and Director, People–
Animal Connection Program, University of California at Los Angeles Medical Center, Los
Angeles, California
Animal-Assisted Therapy

Perle Slavik Cowen, PhD, RN
Associate Professor, University of Iowa College of
Nursing, Iowa City, Iowa
Abuse Protection: Child

Jeanette Marie Daly, PhD, RN
Research Assistant, Family Practice, University of
Iowa College of Medicine, Iowa City, Iowa
Visitation Facilitation

Mary de Meneses, EdD, RN
Professor and Associate Dean for Educational Services, Southern Illinois University School of Nursing, Edwardsville, Illinois
Sleep Enhancement

Cynthia M. Dougherty, PhD, RN, ARNP
Research Assistant Professor, University of Washington School of Nursing, Seattle, Washington;
Nurse Practitioner, Veterans Administration Puget
Sound Health Care System, Seattle, Washington
Surveillance

Nancy J. Evans-Stoner, MSN, RN, CNSN
Education Manager, Clinical Nutrition Support
Services, University of Pennsylvania Medical Center, Philadelphia, Pennsylvania
Feeding

Rosemary Ferdinand, MS, RN, CNSS
Senior Consultant, Deloitte and Touche, LLC; Psychotherapy Private Practice, Caldwell, New Jersey
Suicide Prevention

Cynthia Finesilver, MSN, RN, C
Assistant Professor, Bellin College of Nursing,
Green Bay, Wisconsin
Positioning

Rita A. Frantz, PhD, RN, FAAN
Professor and Chairperson, Behavioral Area Studies, University of Iowa College of Nursing, Iowa
City, Iowa
Pressure Ulcer Care

Sue Gardner, MA, RN
Doctoral Candidate, University of Iowa College
of Nursing, Iowa City, Iowa
Pressure Ulcer Care

Linda A. Gerdner, PhD, RN
Postdoctoral Fellow, Department of Veterans Affairs, Health Science Research and Development,
The University of Arkansas for Medical Science,
Little Rock, Arkansas
Music Therapy; Dementia Management

Mary E. Godin, MS, RN
Clinical Nurse Specialist, Dartmouth–Hitchcock
Medical Center, Lebanon, New Hampshire
Fall Prevention

Meg Gulanick, PhD, RN
Associate Professor, Loyola University, Niehoff
School of Nursing, Chicago, Illinois
Shock Management

Sheila A. Haas, PhD, RN
Professor and Dean, Loyola University, Niehoff
School of Nursing, Chicago, Illinois
Telephone Consultation

Julia Hagemaster, PhD, RN, ARNP
Assistant Professor, University of Kansas School
of Nursing, Kansas City, Kansas
Substance Use Prevention

Keela A. Herr, PhD, RN
Associate Professor, University of Iowa College of
Nursing, Iowa City, Iowa
Pain Management

Sandra H. Hines, MS, RN, C
Doctoral Student, University of Michigan School
of Nursing, Ann Arbor, Michigan
Pelvic Floor Exercise

Barbara J. Holtzclaw, PhD, RN, FAAN
Hugh Roy Cullen Professor of Nursing and Director of Nursing Research, University of Texas Health Science Center, San Antonio, Texas
Fever Treatment

Juanita K. Hunter, EdD, RN, FAAN
Clinical Associate Professor Emeritus, New York State University, Buffalo, New York
Sustenance Support

Rebecca A. Johnson, PhD, RN
Associate Professor, Northern Illinois University School of Nursing, DeKalb, Illinois
Reminiscence Therapy

Mary Kanak, MA, ARNP, CS
Nurse Clinician, Veterans Affairs Medical Center Department of Psychiatry, Iowa City, Iowa
Mood Management

Virginia Kilpack, PhD, RN
Clinical Nurse Specialist, Dartmouth–Hitchcock Medical Center, Lebanon, New Hampshire
Fall Prevention

Karin T. Kirchhoff, PhD, RN, FAAN
Professor, University of Utah, College of Nursing, Salt Lake City, Utah
Preparatory Sensory Information

Constance A. Koerin, BSN, RN
Senior Research Coordinator, University of Kansas School of Nursing, Kansas City, Kansas
Smoking Cessation Assistance

Vicki L. Kraus, PhD, RN, ARNP, CDE
Advanced Practice Nurse–Diabetes, Department of Nursing and Patient Care Services, University of Iowa Hospitals and Clinics, Iowa City, Iowa
Hypoglycemia Management

Felissa R. Lashley, PhD, RN, FAAN, ACRN
Dean and Professor, Southern Illinois University School of Nursing, Edwardsville, Illinois
Sleep Enhancement

Linda Littlejohns, MSN, RN, CCRN, CNRN
Affiliate/Associate Professor, California State University–Dominguez Hills, Carson, California; Director of Marketing and Clinical Affairs, Neuro Care Group, Camino, San Diego, California
Intracranial Pressure Monitoring

Meridean L. Maas, PhD, RN, FAAN
Professor and Chair of Adult and Gerontology Area Studies, University of Iowa College of Nursing, Iowa City, Iowa
Urinary Catheterization: Intermittent

Joanne C. McCloskey, PhD, RN, FAAN
Distinguished Professor and Chairperson, Organizations, Systems, and Community Area Studies; Director, Center for Nursing Classification, University of Iowa College of Nursing, Iowa City, Iowa
Nursing Diagnoses, Interventions, and Outcomes in Effectiveness Research

Therese Connell Meehan, PhD, RGN, RNT
Lecturer, University College Dublin School of Nursing and Midwifery, National University of Ireland, Dublin, Ireland
Therapeutic Touch

Debbie Metzler, MSN, RN, CCRN
Assistant Professor, Bellin College of Nursing, Green Bay, Wisconsin
Positioning

Paula R. Mobily, PhD, RN
Associate Professor, University of Iowa College of Nursing, Iowa City, Iowa
Pain Management

Theresa Moore, MScN, RN
Nursing Professional Practice Leader, Cognitive Support, Sunnybrook and Women's College Health Sciences Centre, Toronto, Ontario, Canada
Constipation/Impaction Management

Sue Moorhead, PhD, RN
Associate Professor, University of Iowa College of Nursing, Iowa City, Iowa
Patient Rights Protection

Nancy Myers, RN, C
Nurse Clinician, Iowa Veterans Home, Marshalltown, Iowa
Urinary Catheterization: Intermittent

Madeline A. Naegle, PhD, RN, FAAN, CS
Associate Professor, New York University School of Education, Division of Nursing, New York, New York
Medication Management

Marsha G. Oakley, MSN, RN
Private Consultant, Lexington, Kentucky
Preparatory Sensory Information

Kathleen A. O'Connell, PhD, RN, FAAN
Professor, University of Kansas Medical Center School of Nursing, Kansas City, Kansas; Principal Psychologist, Midwest Research Institute, Kansas City, Missouri
Smoking Cessation Assistance

Carol S. Pinkham, BSN, RN
Research Assistant, University of Iowa College of Nursing, Iowa City, Iowa
Culture Brokerage

Alice Poyss, PhD, RN, CRNP, CS
Associate Professor, Hahnemann University School of Nursing, Philadelphia, Pennsylvania
Fluid Management

Carol Ruback, MSN, RN
Clinical Nurse Specialist, Rush Copley Medical Center, Aurora, Illinois
Shock Management

Carolyn M. Sampselle, PhD, RN, C, FAAN
Professor of Nursing and Associate Professor of Medicine and Women's Studies, University of Michigan, Ann Arbor, Michigan
Pelvic Floor Exercise

Debra L. Schutte, MSN, RN
Doctoral Student, University of Iowa College of Nursing, Iowa City, Iowa
Genetic Counseling

Michael R. Sicilia, BSN, RN, CEN
Vice President and Lead Instructor, National Institute of Emergency Care, Philadelphia, Pennsylvania; Staff Nurse, Medical College of Pennsylvania, Philadelphia, Pennsylvania
Conscious Sedation

Margaret R. Simons, MA, RN, CDE
Diabetes Education Coordinator, Veterans Administration Medical Center, Iowa City, Iowa
Patient Contracting

Steven J. Somerson, MS, RN, CRNA, CEN
Senior Instructor, National Institute of Emergency Care, Philadelphia, Pennsylvania
Conscious Sedation

Susan W. Somerson, MSN, RN, FNP, CEN
Adjunct Clinical Professor, Villanova University School of Nursing, Villanova, Pennsylvania; Nurse Practitioner, Frankford Health Care System, Philadelphia, Pennsylvania
Conscious Sedation

Janet P. Specht, PhD, RN
Clinical Associate Professor, University of Iowa College of Nursing, Iowa City, Iowa; Health Science Specialist, Iowa City Veterans Administration Medical Center, Iowa City, Iowa
Urinary Catheterization: Intermittent

Victoria M. Steelman, PhD, RN, CNOR
Advanced Practice Nurse, Intensive Surgical Service, University of Iowa Hospitals and Clinics, Iowa City, Iowa
Latex Precautions

Jacqueline M. Stolley, PhD, RN, CS
Professor, Trinity College of Nursing, Moline, Illinois
Dementia Management

Marita G. Titler, PhD, RN, FAAN
Director, Nursing Research and Quality Management, Department of Nursing and Patient Care Services, University of Iowa Hospitals and Clinics, Iowa City, Iowa
Airway Management

Toni Tripp-Reimer, PhD, RN, FAAN
Professor and Associate Dean for Research, University of Iowa College of Nursing, Iowa City, Iowa
Culture Brokerage

Diane O. Tyler, PhD, RN, CS
Assistant Professor of Clinical Nursing, University of Texas School of Nursing, Austin, Texas
Exercise Promotion

Mary H. Wegenka, MS, RN, OCN
Clinical Nurse Specialist, Hematology/Oncology, University of Alabama, Birmingham, Alabama
Chemotherapy Management

Kay Weiler, MA, RN, JD
Associate Professor, University of Iowa College of Nursing, Iowa City, Iowa
Patient Rights Protection

Sally Willett, BA, RN, C
Nurse Clinician, Iowa Veterans Home, Marshalltown, Iowa
Urinary Catheterization: Intermittent

Janet K. Williams, PhD, RN, CPNP, CGC
Associate Professor, University of Iowa College of Nursing, Iowa City, Iowa
Genetic Counseling

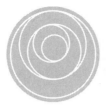

Preface

In 1985 we published the first edition of this book, entitled *Nursing Interventions: Treatments for Nursing Diagnoses.* It included 26 chapters, each on a different nursing intervention. It was a pioneering work developed to fill a void. Until that time, little attention had been paid to the conceptualization and identification of nursing interventions. Although nurses had done treatments for patients for decades, the idea of discussing nursing interventions as concepts was new. Our text and another that year were the first to focus on independent nursing interventions.

The second edition in 1992, *Nursing Interventions: Essential Nursing Treatments,* featured an expanded definition of nursing interventions to capture both the autonomous and the collaborative roles of the nurse. It featured 45 essential interventions that were more clinically focused than in the first edition. The chapter authors covered the research base for the interventions and defined a clinical protocol to carry out the intervention. Case studies were included to illustrate the use of the content.

Much has happened in nursing and health care since the second edition. With the increase in computerization, the need to contain costs, and the emphasis on establishing quality care, nursing leaders and policymakers recognize that we need to document and evaluate the effects of nursing care. In order to do that, we must systematically label and define those things that nurses do so that nursing can be included in information system databases. The first comprehensive standardized language to describe nursing treatments appeared in 1992. The Nursing Interventions Classification (NIC) was developed by a research team that we founded at the University of Iowa. The first edition contained 336 interventions composed of a naming label, a definition, a set of activities for implementation, and a list of background readings. The chapters from the previous editions of this book provided the background for many of the interventions in the NIC. The second edition of the NIC was published in 1996. It contains 433 interventions organized in a coded taxonomic structure. The development of the NIC made the need for a parallel classification of patient outcomes obvious; in order to evaluate the effectiveness of nursing interventions, outcomes must be identified. In 1997, the Nursing Outcomes Classification (NOC), describing 190 outcomes sensitive to nursing interventions, was published. The NOC was produced by another research team at the University of Iowa, so we have been able to coordinate the development of the two classifications.

The NIC and the NOC have been recognized by the American Nurses Association (ANA) Database Steering Committee. The ANA has also recognized other classifications and databases, including the North American Nursing Diagnosis Association (NANDA); the Omaha System; and the Georgetown Home Healthcare Classification. All five classifications have been incorporated in the Metathesaurus for a Unified Medical Language by the National Library of Medicine, which is bringing visibility to nursing as part of the health care team. The ANA uses these classifications to describe nursing and to lobby for the inclusion of nursing elements in national databases and in the forthcoming computerized patient record.

NEW FEATURES OF THE THIRD EDITION

The third edition of *Nursing Interventions* (now subtitled *Effective Nursing Treatments*) has several new features:

1. The NIC taxonomy is the organizing framework for the book. The five sections of the book—Physiological: Basic Interventions; Physiological: Complex Interventions; Behavioral Interventions; Safety Interventions; and Health System Interventions—represent five of the six domains of the NIC taxonomy. We did not include interventions in the sixth domain, Family, because this edition continues to focus on the adult individual. We selected only a small portion of the interventions in the NIC to include in this book. Interventions with a known research base were targeted, and a knowledgeable author was invited to prepare each chapter. The overviews to each section highlight the material in each of the 43 chapters and can be used to select individual chapters for reading.

2. This edition is based on the NIC definition of a nursing intervention. This definition has been incorporated into the 1995 revision of *Nursing's Social Policy Statement* by the ANA.

   A nursing intervention is: *Any treatment based upon clinical judgment and knowledge, that a nurse performs to enhance patient/client outcomes.* Nursing interventions include both direct and indirect care; both nurse-initiated, physician-initiated, and other provider-initiated treatments (McCloskey & Bulechek, 1996, p. xvii).

3. This edition contains chapters on 15 interventions not included in either the first or the second edition. The remaining 28 chapters all contain new material. Each chapter describes the research and use of one intervention. A table contains the intervention name, definition, and activities as they appear in the NIC. The author reviews the research base and tells how to implement the intervention. One or more case studies illustrate how to use the intervention. The authors were asked to identify the associated NANDA diagnoses and NOC outcomes for each intervention. All chapters

use terms from three classifications: NANDA, NIC, and NOC. We salute our authors for the effort made to incorporate all three of the standardized languages. The pioneering aspect of this edition is that it is one of the first textbooks to feature application of NANDA, NIC, and NOC.

4. The introductory chapter has been revised to update content on diagnoses, interventions, and outcomes. Information is given about the three classification systems featured in this edition. A model for clinical data management that shows the benefits of implementing standardized language is featured. Systematic collection of clinical data is a prerequisite to effectiveness research.

5. Three appendices include alphabetical listings of NANDA diagnoses, NIC interventions, and NOC outcomes.

WHO SHOULD USE THIS BOOK

This book is useful for several audiences. Although the book was chiefly written with graduate students in mind, it will be useful in both undergraduate and graduate programs. The book can be used as a text in graduate courses that focus on interventions. It can be a supplementary text in a theory course when an instructor desires to provide illustrations of nursing's developing theory or in an informatics course that deals with how to capture clinical data. Undergraduate programs might want to use the book across the curriculum, assigning sections of the book or individual chapters appropriate to the course content. The book is very helpful in showing how a research base guides the application of an intervention. Researchers developing studies in any of these areas will find the content here an excellent starting point. The book could be particularly useful in RN to BSN/MSN programs, where nurses can approach familiar activities from a conceptual perspective, having already been exposed to them through basic education and clinical practice. All practicing nurses can find help in how to use standardized language in nursing practice from these chapters.

Gloria M. Bulechek
Joanne C. McCloskey

References

American Nurses Association. (1995). *Nursing's social policy statement.* Washington, DC: American Nurses Publishing.

Bulechek, G. M., and McCloskey, J. C. (Eds.) (1985). *Nursing interventions: Treatments for nursing diagnoses.* Philadelphia: W. B. Saunders.

Bulechek, G. M., and McCloskey, J. C. (Eds.) (1992). *Nursing interventions: Essential nursing treatments* (2nd ed.). Philadelphia: W. B. Saunders.

McCloskey, J. C., and Bulechek, G. M. (Eds.) (1992). *Nursing interventions classification (NIC).* St. Louis: Mosby–Year Book.

McCloskey, J. C., and Bulechek, G. M. (Eds.) (1996). *Nursing interventions classification (NIC)* (2nd ed.). St. Louis: Mosby–Year Book.

Johnson, M., and Maas, M. (Eds.) (1997). *Nursing outcomes classification (NOC).* St. Louis: Mosby–Year Book.

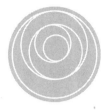

Acknowledgments

The success of this book is a result of the combined efforts of many people. We are grateful to all the contributors. They worked diligently to get the most up-to-date literature for their chapters and to incorporate the three standardized languages. Several commented that they wanted to help because they use this book in their courses.

We thank the readers and users of the book for your continued support. We were able to publish this third edition because you found the previous editions helpful. We thank our international colleagues for the interest they have demonstrated in the second edition.

We thank our colleagues at the University of Iowa who are engaged in the classification projects. This book has benefited from our continuing dialogue with them.

Several individuals deserve special thanks. Our editor at W.B. Saunders, Thomas Eoyang, provided timely and helpful comments. We particularly appreciate Thomas' continued support of this book and his recognition and appreciation of its contribution to the knowledge base of nursing. We also thank Jennifer Clougherty and Kara Logsden, who provided administrative and secretarial support for the book.

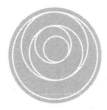

Contents

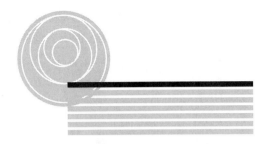

Nursing Diagnoses, Interventions, and Outcomes in Effectiveness Research

Gloria M. Bulechek and Joanne C. McCloskey

The key to an autonomous profession is a clearly defined base of knowledge. Certainly nursing will continue to use knowledge from other disciplines, but it must define what it is that nurses do and whether what they do makes a difference. In the late 1960s, the nursing process movement, a systematic problem-solving methodology used to describe the process of delivering patient care, initiated work in this area. More recently it is being recognized that there are also products resulting from the nursing process movement; these are the classifications that have evolved to describe nursing diagnoses, interventions, and outcomes. These classifications are providing the building blocks for a base of knowledge that is uniquely nursing and are the essential elements for effectiveness research in nursing.

This chapter provides an overview of the classification of nursing diagnoses produced by the North American Nursing Diagnosis Association (NANDA); the Nursing Interventions Classification (NIC) produced at the University of Iowa; and the Nursing Outcomes Classification (NOC) produced at the University of Iowa. This chapter, as well as the 43 chapters that follow, shows the reader how to select an intervention and use the three classifications. This chapter also presents a model that illustrates how nursing practice data (diagnoses, interventions, and outcomes) incorporated in nursing information systems can be used at the individual and aggregate levels, particularly in determining the effectiveness of nursing interventions.

BACKGROUND

Organized nursing has come to recognize that classifications of nursing knowledge are essential in making explicit the nature of nursing. The value of nursing care cannot be universally recognized until we have standardized databases that provide ongoing evaluation of nursing's effectiveness. Consensus has emerged that standardized language is needed in the areas of diagnoses, interventions, and outcomes (American Nurses Association [ANA], 1989; International Council of Nurses [ICN], 1996; Lang, 1994; Nursing Information and Data Set Evaluation Center [NIDSEC], 1997). There are five purposes for classification systems of nursing practice.

Purpose 1: To link knowledge about diagnoses, treatments, and outcomes.

Guidelines are recommendations for patient management based on scientific knowledge and expert opinion. An ad hoc advisory panel of nurses to the Agency for Health Care Policy and Research (AHCPR) concluded that the purpose of guidelines "is to guide practice by providing linkages among diagnoses, treatments, and outcomes, and by describing the alternatives available for each patient" (AHCPR, 1990, September). Practice guidelines are needed to help practitioners determine which of several courses of action are best given a particular set of circumstances. That is, we need to determine what interventions, based on research, are most effective for patients with a particular diagnosis or set of diagnoses.

The development of guidelines is occurring in many arenas. The American Nurses Association (ANA) has prepared a manual on the development of guidelines to bring some consistency to the field in the definition and format of guidelines (Marek, 1995). Specialty nursing organizations are working on guidelines for the diagnoses that are central to their specialty practice. Many nurses are using the 18 interdisciplinary guidelines that have been completed by the AHCPR in their practice. We need to implement the standardized language in the areas of diagnoses, interventions, and outcomes and then use this language in information systems to determine the linkages among the variables. When we have standardized documentation by nurses about the diagnoses of their patients, the treatments they have performed, and the resulting patient outcomes, we will be able to determine the best interventions for a given population. As nursing's ability to link diagnoses, interventions, and outcomes grows, middle-range theories for nursing practice will evolve (Blegen & Tripp-Reimer, 1997).

Purpose 2: To facilitate the development of nursing and health care information systems.

In 1983, at a conference in nursing information systems, it was pointed out that even though nurses spend much of their time documenting their patient care, this documentation has not been systematically organized to advance nursing knowledge, to develop nursing practice, or to improve patient care (Study Group on Nursing Information Systems, 1983). In 1984, Zielstroff asserted that the major impediment to the development of computerized nursing information systems is the deficiencies in nursing's knowledge base:

Those who work in the design and development of nursing information systems constantly bemoan the fact that there are so few clinical problems in nursing for which the etiology, symptoms, treatments, and expected outcomes are known. There are no known probability estimates for prevalence or incidence of common nursing problems; or for relating symptoms to diagnosis, or treatment to outcomes. Indeed, there is neither a standard terminology nor a widely accepted format for data gathering. It is impossible to derive hard and fast rules for computer assistance in decision making with such an ill-defined data base. (1984, p. 9)

At the January 1988 Conference on Research Priorities in Nursing Science, the National Center for Nursing Research (NCNR) identified as a high priority the development of nursing information systems (Hinshaw, 1988). An expert panel was convened by the NCNR to identify the research priorities in informatics, with development of nomenclature being one of the recommended areas for funding (Ozbolt, 1992). The Iowa research teams received funding from the National Institute for Nursing Research (NINR) to help develop NIC and NOC, producing much-needed nomenclature in the areas of interventions and outcomes.

Responding to the growing use of computerized information systems in health care and the need for standards in this area, the ANA in 1996 established the Nursing Information and Data Set Evaluation Center (NIDSEC). NIDSEC (1997) has developed standards pertaining to the automated information systems that nurses use to document nursing care. The standards evaluate the completeness, accuracy, and appropriateness of four dimensions of nursing data sets and the systems that contain them: (1) nomenclature, (2) clinical content, (3) clinical data repository, and (4) general system characteristics. The standards pertaining to nomenclature require the use of ANA-recognized vocabularies. NANDA, NIC, and NOC have been endorsed as ANA-recognized languages. The purpose of NIDSEC standards is to help vendors develop information systems that accurately reflect nursing's vital contributions to patient outcomes and to help purchasers of such systems to be informed about nursing information system requirements. A voluntary accreditation process is available to the vendors.

Purpose 3: To facilitate teaching of decision making to nursing students.

Clinical judgment has been defined by Tanner (1987) as the use of knowledge in making one or more of several kinds of decisions: (1) the decision of which observations should be made in a particular situation, (2) the decision of what the observed data mean with the recognition of patterns, and (3) the selection of actions to be taken on behalf of the patient. There are two important aspects of clinical judgment: first, the knowledge used for the judgment; and second, the thinking process used by the nurse in making the judgment (Tanner, 1989).

In the past, we taught students from medical-surgical and specialty textbooks based mostly on medical knowledge; from nursing process books based mostly on untested nursing theory; and from audiocassettes, films, and skills manuals based mostly on tradition (McCloskey, 1988). We have students practice technical skills in a laboratory before they try them with patients, but at present they have little opportunity to practice more difficult decision-making skills. Some help is available in case-study books and some computer patient simulations. There are, however, increasing numbers of texts based on nursing diagnoses, and new editions are beginning to incorporate NIC and NOC. Now that the concepts describing clinical practice in the NANDA, NIC, and NOC classifications are available, students and teachers can spend more effort on decision making and clinical judgment and less time on concept development. As nursing information systems that meet the NIDSEC standards become more widely available, databases from actual clinical practice can be used to enhance clinical judgment abilities. The addition of nursing's standardized languages to the metathesaurus for a unified medical language by the National Library of Medicine (NIDSEC, 1997) and the index of the

Cumulative Index to Nursing and Allied Health Literature (CINAHL) makes the retrieval of nursing clinical practice literature easier for all users.

Purpose 4: To help determine the costs of services provided by nurses.

There have been multiple efforts reported in the literature to "cost out" nursing. Most of the studies had small sample sizes, were conducted in one institution, and used patient classification systems without much regard to their validity and reliability (McCloskey, Gardner, & Johnson, 1987). The wide variety and nonstandardization of patient classification systems is, in fact, a key reason for the difficulty of obtaining large data sets for comparison of nursing costs. The determination of costs based on interventions performed would be a great improvement. We now have a standardized list of interventions in the form of NIC to use in this effort. The model presented later in this chapter indicates a way to determine costs of nursing service based on the interventions delivered.

Indeed, reimbursement to nurses is a key issue in the reduction of health care costs. Physicians bill for their services based on the codes in the *Physician's Current Procedural Terminology* (CPT), a manual published by the American Medical Association (AMA) (1993). Griffith, Thomas, and Griffith (1991) have shown that nurses often perform some of the procedures for which physicians are paid. Henry et al. (1997) compared the frequency with which 21,366 nursing activity terms could be categorized using NIC and the CPT. The data set of nursing activities was collected for the years 1989 through 1992 from patient interviews, nurse interviews, intershift reports, care plans, flow sheets, and kardexes for 201 patients with acquired immunodeficiency syndrome (AIDS). The activities were categorized into 80 NIC interventions and 15 CPT codes. NIC was able to capture 100% of the activities for all six of the data sources, whereas the CPT captured only 1.3% (care plan) to 16.4% (intershift report) of the activities. Nursing clearly needs acceptance of a coding system that captures nursing treatments for reimbursement to nurses by third-party payers.

Purpose 5: To articulate with the classification systems of other health care providers.

The federal government, insurance companies, and the medical community have been collecting standardized health information for a number of years to direct reimbursement, guide research priorities, and develop health policy. Several health data sets have been developed under the auspices of the National Committee on Vital and Health Statistics, including the Uniform Hospital Discharge Data Set (UHDDS), the Ambulatory Medical Care Minimum Data Set, and the Long-term Health Care Minimum Data Set. These data sets collect information about the patient and the physician and the medical diagnoses and procedures, but no information is included about nursing diagnoses or interventions. The major systems for classification of the medical diagnoses and procedure are the *International Classification of Diseases* (ICD), the CPT, the *Diagnostic and Statistical Manual of Mental Disorders* (DSM), and the *Systematized Nomenclature of Medicine* (SNOMED). Overviews of these classifications are presented elsewhere (Gebbie, 1989; McCloskey & Bulechek, 1996).

These data sets and coding classifications are not representative of nursing practice. The nursing community has recognized the need to have nursing variables included in these and other data sets. Werley and colleagues have published extensively on the need for a unified Nursing Minimum Data Set (NMDS) that would be collected systematically in all agencies (Devine & Werley, 1988; Werley & Lang, 1988; Werley, Lang, & Westlake, 1986). The nursing care variables identified for inclusion in the NMDS are diagnoses, interventions, outcomes, and acuity. The ANA's Steering Committee on Databases to Support Clinical Nursing Practice is working to put forth nursing's classifications in federal databases and the forthcoming computerized patient record.

In summary, the existing data sets and classification systems that are currently used for determining United States health care policies do not include nursing data. As a result, nursing is invisible in its impact on patient care or health care costs. We must document our practice in the areas of diagnoses, interventions, and outcomes with the standardized language classifications (NANDA, NIC, NOC) that are now available and get these data included in the federal and state databases.

NURSING DIAGNOSES

The profession's acceptance of making nursing diagnoses came in 1980 when the ANA published *Nursing: A Social Policy Statement,* which stated that "nursing is the diagnosis and treatment of human responses to actual or potential health problems" (1980, p. 9). The 1995 update retains this statement and further elaborates that "diagnoses facilitate communication among health care providers and the recipients of care and provide for initial direction in choice of treatments and subsequent evaluation of the outcomes of care" (ANA, 1995, p. 9). Nursing diagnoses are an integral part of the standards of nursing practice (ANA, 1992). These standards were jointly developed by ANA and more than 15 specialty organizations.

NANDA has taken the lead in developing the standardized language for the human responses that nurses treat. This group was formulated in the early 1970s as the National Conference Group for the Classification of Nursing Diagnoses at St. Louis University. Through a series of invitational conferences the group began the work of identifying nursing diagnoses (Gebbie, 1975; Gebbie & Lavin, 1975; Kim, McFarland, & McLane, 1984; Kim & Moritz, 1982). In work sessions, the participants developed, reviewed, and grouped diagnoses based on their expertise and experience. By 1982 they had produced an alphabetical list of 50 nursing diagnoses accepted for clinical testing. During this period there was a great deal of discussion about a conceptual framework that would provide a classification schema for the diagnoses, and a group of nurse theorists assisted with analyzing the various levels of abstractions in the list and proposed various ways of clustering the diagnoses.

In 1985, a taxonomy committee was appointed. This was the first conference open to all nurses and the first held under the bylaws of the new organization, NANDA (Hurley, 1986). At the next conference, the taxonomy committee proposed Taxonomy I based on nine human response patterns: Exchanging, Communicating, Relating, Valuing, Choosing, Moving, Perceiving, Knowing, and Feeling. The membership endorsed Taxonomy I for development and testing and approved 21 new diagnoses (McLane, 1987). Guidelines for classification were developed to incorporate new diagnoses as they evolved. New diagnoses were accepted at the eighth conference (Carroll-Johnson, 1989) and the ninth conference (Carroll-Johnson, 1991). In 1989 Taxonomy I was submitted to the

World Health Organization for inclusion in the 10th version of the ICD, although it was not accepted (Fitzpatrick et al., 1989).

At the 1990 conference a proposed Taxonomy II was presented, which sparked much subsequent debate about the organizing framework for the diagnoses (Jenny, 1995). At the 10th, 11th, and 12th conferences, debate about the taxonomy structure continued, and there was discussion about linkages with other classifications. There was also discussion of how to expand the number of diagnoses, and a staging method for evaluation of candidate diagnoses has now been put in place (NANDA, 1997). A collaborative agreement for a joint venture between a research team at the University of Iowa College of Nursing and NANDA was reached to extend the NANDA work. The goal is to improve the comprehensiveness, scope, and clinical usefulness of the NANDA taxonomy (Craft-Rosenberg & Delaney, 1997). Methods for validation of diagnoses have been developed (Fehring, 1986; Hoskins, 1997; NANDA, 1989), and validation studies have become a major part of the biannual conferences and of *Nursing Diagnosis,* the NANDA journal. The most current version of the classification, Taxonomy I 1997–1998, was used in the preparation of this book. The labels and definitions from this version appear in Appendix A. One example from the classification, Altered Oral Mucous Membrane, appears in Table 1.

Although the profession has accepted the making of a diagnosis as part of a nurse's role and has developed Taxonomy I, debate continues about the nature of a nursing diagnosis. The NANDA struggle with operationalizing a definition is recounted by Mills (1991). At the ninth conference the following definition was accepted after floor debate and revision: "A nursing diagnosis is a clinical judgment about individual, family or community responses to actual or potential health problems/life processes. Nursing diagnoses provide the basis for selection of nursing interventions to achieve outcomes for which the nurse is accountable" (Carroll-Johnson, 1991, p. 50).

Developing the definition has been difficult because the definition is predicated on the scope of nursing. Should nursing diagnoses guide both independent and interdependent aspects of nursing care? Gordon (1987) has taken the position that nursing diagnoses should be used only if independent interventions are needed. Carpenito (1987) also recommends use of nursing diagnoses to guide

Table 1 NANDA Nursing Diagnosis Example

1.6.2.1.1 Altered Oral Mucous Membrane

DEFINITION

The state in which an individual experiences disruptions in the tissue layers of the oral cavity.

DEFINING CHARACTERISTICS

Oral pain/discomfort; coated tongue; xerostomia (dry mouth); stomatitis; oral lesions or ulcers; lack of or decreased salivation; leukoplakia; edema; hyperemia; oral plaque; desquamation; vesicles; hemorrhagic gingivitis; carious teeth; halitosis.

RELATED FACTORS

Pathological conditions—oral cavity (radiation to head or neck); dehydration; trauma (chemical, e.g., acidic foods, drugs, noxious agents, alcohol; mechanical, e.g., ill-fitting dentures, braces, tubes [endotracheal/nasogastric], surgery in oral cavity); NPO (nothing by mouth) for more than 24 hours; ineffective oral hygiene; mouth breathing; malnutrition; infection; lack of or decreased salivation; medication.

Source: North American Nursing Diagnosis Association. (1996). *Nursing diagnoses: Definitions and classification 1997–1998.* Philadelphia: Author.

independent interventions but suggests the use of collaborative problems to guide interdependent interventions. In viewing health status, nursing has a tradition of holism that takes into account the physiological, psychological, sociological, cultural, and spiritual aspects of health. This focus makes it difficult to divide nursing care into independent and interdependent realms.

Two issues have been the subject of recurrent debate in regard to the nature of nursing diagnoses. First, there has been continuing controversy surrounding the use of physiology and pathophysiology in the nursing diagnostic process. Should physiological diagnoses be included in the taxonomy? Can nurses collect the data to determine such diagnoses, or are the needed laboratory tests physician controlled? Does an autonomous practitioner use protocols? Kim (1984) and Cassmeyer (1989) present convincing arguments that nursing does need to reemphasize the biologic sciences in the diagnostic process. The primary concern for nurses in critical care and many chronic care situations is alterations in the physiological aspects of health. Two sections of this book, Section I on Physiological: Basic Interventions and Section II on Physiological: Complex Interventions include several interventions for physiological nursing diagnoses. There is need for more physiological diagnoses to direct some of these interventions, as the chapter authors point out.

The second issue concerns how the wellness perspective of nursing can be incorporated into the nursing diagnosis movement. Should wellness diagnoses be represented in the taxonomy? The problem orientation has dominated the nursing diagnosis development. Yet nursing claims health promotion as a philosophic basis for practice. Popkess-Vawter (1991) reviews the literature that supports wellness nursing diagnoses and advocates their incorporation in the taxonomy. We reaffirm our previous statement (Bulechek & McCloskey, 1989) that wellness diagnoses are not necessary. We believe that nurses work to enhance client strengths through interventions to treat actual diagnoses or in redirection of risk factors for potential diagnoses. In our view, most of the examples of wellness diagnoses (e.g., increased activity tolerance, effective airway clearance, effective breastfeeding, health seeking behaviors) are outcome statements, not diagnoses. Both diagnostic and outcome terms describe client states. Much care is delivered in an episodic rather than in a longitudinal time frame. It is often the time of measurement that determines which classification will be used, and one often sees the success of another provider's intervention when doing an assessment.

The question "What is a nursing diagnosis?" will continue to be revisited. In our own words, a nursing diagnosis is the identification of a patient's problem that the nurse can treat. Some patients have many nursing diagnoses, some only one or two, and some none at all. Nursing diagnoses change more frequently than do medical diagnoses, and some patients with no nursing diagnoses one day may have several a few days later as a result of medical intervention. Nursing diagnoses are more fluid, varying, and episodic than medical diagnoses (ANA, 1980). Diagnoses describe a client state, and more than one discipline may identify the client state. One emerging issue in this area is whether diagnostic terminology should be consistent across the classifications of the various disciplines.

In order to classify and standardize nursing diagnoses and treatments, it is necessary to accompany a diagnosis with the signs, symptoms, and etiology that led to the making of it. Several formats exist for stating a nursing diagnosis: PES (problem-etiology-signs/symptoms) format, related to format, supporting data format, and POR (problem-oriented record) format. Examples of diagnoses made in each format are in Table 2. The basic elements of each format are the diagnosis (problem), its etiology (related factor), and its characteristics (signs and symptoms). Whatever the format, supporting data (etiology and characteristics) are important because they give clues as to how to treat the problem. This will not always be necessary; at some point in the future a nursing diagnosis will mean, just as a medical diagnosis means now, a precise set of signs and symptoms and etiology that will call for certain treatments.

NURSING INTERVENTIONS

In the past, multiple terms have been used to label the intervention and treatment portion of the nursing process, including action, activity, intervention, treatment, therapeutics, order, and implementation. The following are typical of interventions listed in current textbooks: measure intake and output; measure central venous pressure; help patient with personal hygiene; watch for signs and symptoms of infection; have patient turn, cough, and breathe deeply. From these examples, it can be seen that interventions are often viewed as discrete actions with little conceptualization of how the actions fit together. Nurses perform many activities to benefit the client. The focus of concern with nursing intervention is nurse behavior—those things that nurses do to assist client status or behavior to move toward a desired outcome. This differs from nursing diagnosis

Table 2 Nursing Diagnoses Expressed in Four Different Formats

PES (PROBLEM-ETIOLOGY-SIGNS/SYMPTOMS) FORMAT

Problem:	Impaired Reality Testing (Acute)
Etiology:	Psychosis
Signs and Symptoms:	1. Impaired perception
	2. Impaired attention span
	3. Impaired decision making (Bruce, 1979)

RELATED TO FORMAT

Anxiety related to impending surgery as characterized by verbalization.
Knowledge deficit related to diabetes as characterized by inability to give self insulin, inadequate diet, and poor hygiene.

SUPPORTING DATA FORMAT

Knowledge deficit

Supporting data: Newly diagnosed diabetic. Does not know how to give daily insulin injections. Daily intake list for past week reveals diet not followed, although instructed by dietitian 7/1. Overweight. Poor hygiene practices. Believes diabetes will go away in a few years.

POR (PROBLEM-ORIENTED RECORD) FORMAT

S. Believes diabetes will go away in a few years. Says does not know how to give daily insulin.
O. Newly diagnosed diabetic. Daily intake for past week reveals does not follow diet although was instructed by dietitian 7/1.

Weight 180. Ht./wt. chart puts desirable weight at 144.

Nails dirty and large toenails ingrown.

A. Knowledge deficit related to diabetes.
P. List above diagnosis as problem #3 on patient's problem list.

Teach patient and wife about diabetes, complications, and insulin.

Stress need for foot care, diet, and urine testing. Referral to visiting nurse for postdischarge evaluation.

and nursing outcomes where the focus of concern is client behavior (McCloskey et al., 1990).

The first edition of this book, *Nursing Interventions: Treatments for Nursing Diagnoses,* and Snyder's book, *Independent Nursing Interventions,* both published in 1985, were the first to propose nursing interventions as symbolic concepts that require a series of actions for implementation. These two classic texts were the first to describe nurse-initiated treatments that were done in response to a nursing diagnosis. The second edition of this text, *Nursing Interventions: Essential Nursing Treatments,* featured an expanded definition of nursing interventions to capture both the autonomous and the collaborative roles of the nurse. It featured 45 essential interventions that were more clinically focused than those in the first edition. The first volume of comprehensive standardized language to describe nursing treatments, the *Nursing Interventions Classification (NIC),* was developed by a research team at the University of Iowa led by McCloskey and Bulechek. The first edition, published in 1992, contained 336 interventions made up of a naming label, a definition, a set of activities for implementation, and a list of background readings. It featured nurse-initiated and physician-initiated interventions, and the chapters from the previous editions of this book provided the background for several of the interventions. The second edition of *Nursing Interventions Classification (NIC)* was published in 1996 and included both direct and indirect care interventions as well as nurse-initiated and physician-initiated interventions. The definitions of terms that NIC and this book are based on appear in Table 3. The definition of an intervention that appears in Table 3 has been incorporated into the 1995 revision of *Nursing: A Social Policy Statement* by ANA.

Description of NIC

NIC is a comprehensive list of 433 nursing interventions performed by nurses in all specialties and all practice settings. Each intervention as it appears in the classification includes a label name, a definition, a set of activities integral to its performance, and background readings. An example of one intervention with each of these components, Oral Health Restoration, appears in Table 4. The alphabetical list of the 433 NIC intervention labels with accompanying definitions appears in Appendix B.

The portions of the intervention that are standardized (i.e., no changes can be made in terminology; suggestions for change go through a peer review process and are included in the next edition) are the label and the definition. With standardization, all providers are using the same terms to mean the same interventions. This enhances communication and continuity of care among different providers. Care can be individualized through the activities. The nurse can select the specific activities that apply to a particular patient's plan of care, modify activities to fit the local setting, and add additional activities if needed. All modifications in activities should be congruent with the definition of the intervention.

NIC interventions include both the physiological (e.g., Acid-Base Management, Airway Suctioning, Pressure Ulcer Care) and the psychosocial (e.g., Anxiety Reduction, Preparatory Sensory Information, Home Maintenance Assistance). There are interventions for illness treatment (e.g., Hyperglycemia Management, Ostomy Care, Shock Management), illness prevention (e.g., Fall Prevention, Infection Protection, Immunization/Vaccination Administration), and health promotion (e.g., Exercise Promotion, Nutrition Management, Smoking Cessation

Table 3   Nursing Interventions Classification (NIC) Definition of Terms

NURSING INTERVENTION

Any treatment, based upon clinical judgment and knowledge, that a nurse performs to enhance patient/client outcomes. Nursing interventions include both direct and indirect care; both nurse-initiated, physician-initiated, and other provider-initiated treatments.

A *direct care intervention* is a treatment performed through interaction with the patient(s). Direct care interventions include both physiological and psychosocial nursing actions; both the "laying on of hands" actions and those that are more supportive and counseling in nature.

An *indirect care intervention* is a treatment performed away from the patient but on behalf of a patient or group of patients. Indirect care interventions include nursing actions aimed at management of the patient care environment and interdisciplinary collaboration. These actions support the effectiveness of the direct care interventions.

A *nurse-initiated treatment* is an intervention initiated by the nurse in response to a nursing diagnosis; an autonomous action based on scientific rationale that is executed to benefit the client in a predicted way related to the nursing diagnosis and projected outcomes. Such actions would include those treatments initiated by advanced nurse practitioners.

A *physician-initiated treatment* is an intervention initiated by a physician in response to a medical diagnosis but carried out by a nurse in response to a "doctor's order." Nurse may also carry out treatments initiated by other providers, such as pharmacists, respiratory therapists, or physician assistants.

NURSING ACTIVITIES

The specific behaviors or actions that nurses do to implement an intervention and that assist patients/clients to move toward a desired outcome. Nursing activities are at the concrete level of action. A series of activities is necessary to implement an intervention.

TAXONOMY OF NURSING INTERVENTIONS

A systematic organization of the intervention labels based upon similarities into what can be considered a conceptual framework. The NIC taxonomy structure has three levels: domains, classes, and interventions.

Source: McCloskey, J. C., and Bulechek, G. M. (Eds.). (1996). *Nursing interventions classification (NIC)* (2nd ed., p. xvii). St. Louis: Mosby-Year Book.

Assistance). Interventions are for individuals or for families (e.g., Family Integrity Promotion, Family Support). Indirect care interventions (e.g., Emergency Cart Checking, Supply Management) and some interventions for communities (e.g., Environmental Management: Community) are also included.

The interventions are grouped into 27 classes and six domains for ease of use (Table 5). Each domain (1–6) and class (A-Y, a and b) is coded, and each NIC intervention has a unique number (e.g., 1730 for Oral Health Restoration; see Table 4) that can facilitate computerization. NIC interventions have been linked with NANDA nursing diagnoses, the Omaha System problems, and NOC outcomes. There is a form and review system for submitting suggestions for new or modified interventions.

Development of NIC

The ongoing research to maintain NIC is part of the Center for Nursing Classification at the University of Iowa College of Nursing. NIC was developed by a large research team representing multiple areas of clinical and methodological expertise. The work has received 7 years of funding from the National Institutes of Health, National Institute of Nursing Research. Support has also been received from the Rockefeller Foundation and the University of Iowa.

Table 4 An Example from Nursing Interventions Classification (NIC): Oral Health Restoration

DEFINITION: Promotion of healing for a patient who has an oral mucosa or dental lesion.

ACTIVITIES:

Remove dentures in case of severe stomatitis

Use a soft toothbrush for removal of dental debris

Use toothettes or disposable foam swabs to stimulate gums and clean oral cavity

Encourage flossing between teeth twice daily with unwaxed dental floss if platelet levels are above $50,000/mm^3$

Encourage frequent rinsing of the mouth with any of the following: sodium bicarbonate solution, warm saline, or hydrogen peroxide solution

Discourage smoking and alcohol consumption

Monitor lips, tongue, mucous membranes, tonsillar fossae, and gums for moisture, color, texture, presence of debris, and infection, using good lighting and a tongue blade

Determine the patient's perception of changes in taste, swallowing, quality of voice, and comfort

Reinforce oral hygiene regimen as part of discharge teaching

Instruct patient to avoid commercial mouthwashes

Instruct patient to report signs of infection to physician immediately

Monitor for therapeutic effects of topical anesthetics, oral protective pastes, and topical or systemic analgesics as appropriate

Instruct and assist patient to perform oral hygiene after eating and as often as needed

Monitor patient every shift for dryness of the oral mucosa

Assist patient to select soft, bland, and non-acidic foods

Increase mouth care to every 2 hours and twice at night if stomatitis is not controlled

Monitor for signs and symptoms of glossitis and stomatitis

Consult physician if signs and symptoms of glossitis and stomatitis persist or worsen

Plan small, frequent meals, select soft foods, and serve chilled or room temperature foods

Avoid use of lemon-glycerin swabs

Increase liquids on the meal tray

Apply topical anesthetics, oral protective pastes, and topical or systemic analgesics as needed

Source: McCloskey, J. C., and Bulechek, G. M. (Eds.). (1996). *Nursing interventions classification (NIC)* (2nd ed., p. 407). St. Louis: Mosby–Year Book.

The research, which began in 1987, has progressed through three phases:

Phase I—Construction of the Classification
Phase II—Construction of the Taxonomy
Phase III—Clinical Testing and Refinement

Multiple research methods have been used. An inductive approach was used in phase I to build the classification based on existing practice. Original sources were current textbooks, care planning guides, and nursing information systems. Content analysis, focus group review, and questionnaires to experts in specialty areas of practice were used to augment the clinical practice expertise of team members. Phase II was characterized by more quantitative methods including similarity analysis, hierarchical clustering, and multidimensional scaling. In the clinical field testing of phase III, steps for implementation were developed and tested, and the need for linkages between NANDA, NIC, and NOC were identified. More than 1,000 nurses have completed questionnaires, and approximately 50 professional associations have provided input about the classification. All this development work is reported in detail in the beginning chapters of *Nursing*

Table 5 NIC Taxonomy Structure

	Domain 1	Domain 2	Domain 3	Domain 4	Domain 5	Domain 6
Level 1 *Domains*	1. *PHYSIOLOGICAL: BASIC* Care that supports physical functioning	2. *PHYSIOLOGICAL: COMPLEX* Care that supports homeostatic regulation	3. *BEHAVIORAL* Care that supports psychosocial functioning and facilitates lifestyle changes	4. *SAFETY* Care that supports protection against harm	5. *FAMILY* Care that supports the family unit	6. *HEALTH SYSTEM* Care that supports effective use of the health care delivery system
Level 2 *Classes*	A *Activity and Exercise Management:* Interventions to organize or assist with physical activity and energy conservation and expenditure B *Elimination Management:* Interventions to establish and maintain regular bowel and urinary elimination patterns and manage complications due to altered patterns C *Immobility Management:* Interventions to manage restricted body movement and the sequelae D *Nutrition Support:* Interventions to modify or maintain nutritional status E *Physical Comfort Promotion:* Interventions to promote comfort using physical techniques F *Self-Care Facilitation:* Interventions to provide or assist with routine activities of daily living	G *Electrolyte and Acid Base Management:* Interventions to regulate electrolyte/acid base balance and prevent complications H *Drug Management:* Interventions to facilitate desired effects of pharmacologic agents I *Neurologic Management:* Interventions to optimize neurologic function J *Perioperative Care:* Interventions to provide care prior to, during, and immediately after surgery K *Respiratory Management:* Interventions to promote airway patency and gas exchange L *Skin/Wound Management:* Interventions to maintain or restore tissue integrity M *Thermoregulation:* Interventions to maintain body temperature within a normal range N *Tissue Perfusion Management:* Interventions to optimize circulation of blood and fluids to the tissue	O *Behavior Therapy:* Interventions to reinforce or promote desirable behaviors or alter undesirable behaviors P *Cognitive Therapy:* Interventions to reinforce or promote desirable cognitive functioning or alter undesirable cognitive functioning Q *Communication Enhancement:* Interventions to facilitate delivering and receiving verbal and nonverbal messages R *Coping Assistance:* Interventions to assist another to build on own strengths, to adapt to a change in function, or achieve a higher level of function S *Patient Education:* Interventions to facilitate learning T *Psychological Comfort Promotion:* Interventions to promote comfort using psychological techniques	U *Crisis Management:* Interventions to provide immediate short-term help in both psychological and physiological crises V *Risk Management:* Interventions to initiate risk reduction activities and continue monitoring risks over time	W *Childbearing Care:* Interventions to assist in understanding and coping with the psychological and physiological changes during the childbearing period X *Life Span Care:* Interventions to facilitate family unit functioning and promote the health and welfare of family members throughout the life span	Y *Health System Mediation:* Interventions to facilitate the interface between patient/family and the health care system a *Health System Management:* Interventions to provide and enhance support services for the delivery of care b *Information Management:* Interventions to facilitate communication among health care providers

Source: McCloskey, J. C., and Bulechek, G. M. (Eds.). (1996). *Nursing interventions classification (NIC)* (2nd ed., pp. 56–57). St. Louis: Mosby-Year Book.

Interventions Classification (NIC) (McCloskey & Bulechek, 1996) as well as in numerous articles and chapters. Current information is available on the Center for Nursing Classification's Web page: http://www.nursing.uiowa.edu/cnc.

Each of the chapters in this book is based on one intervention from the NIC classification. A table displays the definition of the intervention and the associated practice activities. The chapter author reviews the research base for the intervention and provides direction on how to implement the intervention. Each chapter includes lists of NANDA diagnoses and NOC outcomes that could be linked with the intervention to provide help to the reader with use of the three standardized languages. Further help is provided in the illustrative case studies.

NURSING OUTCOMES

Patient outcomes, which should be specified before an intervention is chosen, serve as the criteria against which to judge the success of a nursing intervention. Outcomes describe behaviors, responses, and feelings of the patient in response to the care provided.

Many variables influence outcomes, including the interventions prescribed by the health care providers, the health care providers themselves, the environment in which care is received, the patient's own motivation and genetic structure, and the patient's significant others. The task for nursing is to define which patient outcomes are sensitive to nursing care—that is, to identify for each patient the expected and attainable results of nursing interventions.

Since the 1960s, there has been considerable effort expended on developing outcome measures useful for evaluating nursing practice (Donabedian, 1980; Horn & Swain, 1978; Marek, 1989; Martin & Scheet, 1992; McCormick, 1991; Waltz & Strickland, 1988). The Medical Outcomes Study (MOS), which attempted to evaluate the impact of physician practice on patient outcomes (Tarlov et al., 1989), has received wide attention among health service researchers and has implications for the development of nursing models. As a part of its mandate to develop a research agenda for outcomes and effectiveness research, AHCPR, in cooperation with the Health Care Financing Administration (HCFA), sponsored an April 1991 conference mandated by Congress to develop agendas for future research in 10 different areas of outcomes and effectiveness research. There was general agreement that there is much need for standardization of language in this area and that instruments need to be validated.

The efforts by AHCPR are paralleled in nursing by efforts by the NINR. A major nursing initiative on outcomes research was begun in May 1990 when an expert planning group discussed strategies concerning patient outcomes and nursing research. This group coined the term *nursing-sensitive outcomes,* meaning those patient outcomes that are sensitive to nursing intervention. A follow-up state-of-the-science conference about nursing-sensitive patient outcomes research occurred in the fall of 1991.

In 1991 a research team, led by Marion Johnson and Meridean Maas, was formed at the University of Iowa to develop a classification of patient outcomes sensitive to nursing care. With subsequent funding support from Sigma Theta International and the NINR, a large team has completed a series of research steps similar to those used to produce NIC. The *Nursing Outcomes Classification (NOC)* (Johnson & Maas, 1997) contains 190 outcomes sensitive to nursing treatments. (See Appendix C for outcome labels and definitions.) The NOC contains outcomes for individual patients and family caregivers that are representative for all settings and clinical specialties and describes patient states at a conceptual level with indicators expected to be responsive to nursing intervention. The definitions of NOC terms appear in Table 6. The outcomes and indicators are variable concepts. This allows measurement of the outcome states at any point on a continuum from most negative to most positive at different points in time. Rather than the limited information provided by the measurement of whether a goal is met, NOC outcomes can be used to monitor the extent of progress, or lack of progress, throughout an episode of care and across different care settings. The NOC outcome Oral Health is displayed in Table 7 to show the label, definition, indicators, and measuring scale. NOC outcomes have been linked to NANDA diagnoses, and the linkages appear in the back of the NOC book. Since the publication of the first edition, a NOC taxonomy and coding structure have been developed and additional outcomes have been prepared. Additional funding from NINR has been awarded to work on measurement of the indicators. Current information can be found at http://www.nursing. uiowa.edu/cnc.

SELECTION OF A NURSING INTERVENTION

The selection of a nursing intervention depends on several factors. We have identified six: (1) the desired patient outcome; (2) the characteristics of the nursing diagnosis; (3) the research base associated with the intervention; (4) the feasibility of successfully implementing the intervention; (5) the acceptability of the intervention to the client; and (6) the capability of the nurse. Each of these factors is enumerated more fully in the following paragraphs showing application of the NANDA, NIC, and NOC terms related to the health concerns of oral hygiene.

Table 6 Nursing Outcomes Classification (NOC) Definition of Terms

---

NURSING-SENSITIVE PATIENT OUTCOME

A measurable patient or family caregiver state, behavior, or perception that is conceptualized as a variable and is largely influenced by and sensitive to nursing interventions. A nursing-sensitive patient outcome is at the conceptual level. To be measured, an outcome requires identification of a series of more specific indicators. Nursing-sensitive patient outcomes define the general patient state, behavior, or perception resulting from nursing interventions.

NURSING-SENSITIVE PATIENT OUTCOME INDICATOR

A specific variable referent of a nursing-sensitive patient outcome that is sensitive to nursing interventions. An indicator is an observable patient state, behavior, or self-reported perception or evaluation. Nursing-sensitive patient outcome indicators characterize a patient state at the concrete level. Examples of indicators are: "describes reasons why medication must be taken according to prescribed dose and schedule," "notifies caregiver when needs to urinate."

NURSING-SENSITIVE OUTCOME MEASURES

The operations or activities that describe precisely what outcome indicator is to be measured, how it is to be measured, and how it will be quantified. Quantification will reflect a continuum, such as 1 = toilets self independently; 2 = requires some assistance with clothing for toileting; 3 = requires assistance with transfer for toileting; and 4 = requires total assistance for toileting.

Source: Johnson, M., and Maas, M. (Eds.). (1997). *Nursing outcomes classification (NOC)* (p. 22). St. Louis: Mosby-Year Book.

Table 7 An Example from Nursing Outcomes Classification (NOC)

Oral Health—1100

DEFINITION: Condition of the mouth, teeth, gums, and tongue

Oral Health	Extremely Compromised	Substantially Compromised	Moderately Compromised	Mildly Compromised	Not Compromised
Cleanliness of mouth	1	2	3	4	5
Cleanliness of teeth	1	2	3	4	5
Cleanliness of gums	1	2	3	4	5
Cleanliness of tongue	1	2	3	4	5
Cleanliness of dentures	1	2	3	4	5
Cleanliness of dental appliances	1	2	3	4	5
Fit of dentures	1	2	3	4	5
Fit of dental appliances	1	2	3	4	5
Moistness of lips	1	2	3	4	5
Moisture of oral mucosa and tongue	1	2	3	4	5
Color of mucosa membranes	1	2	3	4	5
Oral mucosa integrity	1	2	3	4	5
Tongue integrity	1	2	3	4	5
Gum integrity	1	2	3	4	5
Tooth integrity	1	2	3	4	5
Breath odor	1	2	3	4	5
Breath free of halitosis	1	2	3	4	5
Other _____ Specify	1	2	3	4	5

Source: Johnson, M., and Maas, M. (Eds.). (1997). *Nursing outcomes classification (NOC)* (p. 223). St. Louis: Mosby-Year Book.

1. Desired patient outcome: The primary consideration in selecting a nursing intervention is to identify one that will help the client move toward one or more desired outcomes. This action has traditionally been referred to as the planning portion of the nursing process. After completing a patient assessment, the nurse can rate the patient on the selected NOC outcome scale and identify the desired rating to be achieved following the intervention. For example, indicators for the outcome Oral Health (see Table 7) may be rated *extremely compromised,* and the goal for a 5-day hospital stay might be to move to *moderately compromised.* The goal for a home visit 1 week after discharge might be a rating of *not compromised.* NOC outcomes measured along a continuum allow the nurse to evaluate the amount of progress or lack of progress for individual patients. The nurse may choose all the indicators or only those pertinent to an individual patient, or the nurse may use only the scale with the overall outcome to determine patient status.

2. Characteristics of the nursing diagnosis: A second consideration in selecting a nursing intervention is the characteristics of the nursing diagnosis. The intent is to direct the intervention toward altering the related factors (etiology) associated with the diagnosis. If the etiology is correctly identified during the nursing assessment and if the intervention is successful in altering the etiology, the client's status can be expected to improve. This improvement can be measured by a change in the outcome indicators associated with the diagnosis.

The diagnosis Altered Oral Mucous Membrane (see Table 1) has a number of related factors. Table 8 displays a number of outcomes and interventions linked with the diagnosis Altered Oral Mucous Membrane through the related factors. If the related factor is ineffective oral hygiene, it would be appropriate to select the outcome Oral Health and select from the NIC interventions Oral Health Maintenance, Oral Health Promotion, or Oral Health Restoration. The related factor of dehydration would be associated with the outcome of Hydration and

Table 8 One Example: Linkage of NANDA, NIC, and NOC Terms

NANDA Diagnosis
ALTERED ORAL MUCOUS MEMBRANE: The state in which an individual experiences disruptions in the tissue layers of the oral cavity.

NANDA Related Factors	NOC Outcomes	NIC Interventions
Ineffective Oral Hygiene	Oral Health	Oral Health Maintenance Oral Health Promotion Oral Health Restoration
Dehydration	Hydration	Fever Treatment √ Fluid/Electrolyte Management Fluid Management √ Intravenous (IV) Therapy
Infection	Infection Status	Infection Control Infection Protection Medication Administration Medication Administration: Topical
Malnutrition	Nutritional Status	Nutrition Management Nutrition Therapy Nutrition Monitoring Nutritional Counseling Teaching: Prescribed Diet
Malnutrition	Nutritional Status: Food & Fluid Intake	Feeding √ Fluid Management √ Nutrition Management Self-Care Assistance: Feeding TPN Administration Bottle Feeding IV Therapy Sustenance Support √
Self Care Deficit	Self-Care: Oral Hygiene	Self-Care Assistance: Bathing/Hygiene Self-Care Assistance: Feeding Health Education √
Pathological Conditions	Tissue Integrity: Skin & Mucous Membrane	Chemotherapy Management √ Health Screening Health Education √ Infection Protection Incision Site Care Wound Care

√ See the Table of Contents to locate the chapter describing this intervention.

the listed NIC interventions related to fluids. The related factor of infection would be associated with the outcome of Infection Status and the NIC interventions related to infection. The related factor of malnutrition would be associated with the outcomes Nutritional Status and Nutritional Status: Food and Fluid Intake. There are a number of NIC interventions related to feeding and teaching about nutrition. The patient who cannot perform self-care requires assistance, and there are a number of associated NIC interventions listed in Table 8.

Although the prognosis of successfully treating a nursing diagnosis is better if the related factors can be changed, this is not always possible. In some instances, factors related to a pathologic condition cannot be altered and it is necessary to treat the signs and symptoms. In such instances it may be possible to achieve the desirable outcome criteria for a finite period of time. Referring again to the diagnosis of Altered Oral Mucous Membrane, we may be working with a patient who is receiving chemotherapy or radiation to the head and neck. This patient may be initially rated *not compromised* on the outcome Tissue Integrity: Skin and Mucous Membrane. An appropriate goal might be to keep the rating at *moderately compromised* or above through use of the associated NIC interventions listed at the end of Table 8 throughout the medical therapy.

Nurses also treat clients with potential health problems. These clients display known risk factors that are predictive of future development of a health problem. NANDA has identified several such diagnoses and has included the phrase *potential for* in the diagnostic label. In these diagnoses, the risk factors are viewed as the etiology; the preventive intervention is aimed at altering or eliminating the risk factors. Examples of such health promotion/disease prevention interventions include Exercise Promotion (see Chapter 7), Smoking Cessation Assistance (see Chapter 27), Health Education (see Chapter 29), and Substance Use Prevention (see Chapter 30).

3. Research base associated with the intervention: A third consideration when selecting an intervention is the research base associated with it. Since the early 1960s, the profession has been working to produce clinical research that will give direction to nursing practice. Dumas and Leonard's (1963) classic study on preoperative preparation demonstrated that it is possible to test nursing interventions in the natural setting. Subsequently, many clinical studies have been produced by faculty members, graduate students, and clinical specialists. The results of these studies were slow to appear in practice for many reasons that have been well described by other authors (Aydelotte, 1976; Jacox, 1974; Martinson, 1976; Smoyak, 1976), but in the past decade there is encouraging evidence that the gap between research and practice is diminishing (Weiler, Buckwalter, & Titler, 1994).

In the mid-1970s, the Michigan Nurses' Association undertook a statewide federally funded project to bridge the gap between research and practice. The Conduct and Utilization of Research in Nursing Project (CURN Project) developed and tested a model to facilitate the use of scientific nursing knowledge in clinical practice settings. Three categories of criteria were established for selecting research that was sufficiently developed to merit utilization in practice (Haller, Reynolds, & Horsley, 1979). The first category pertained to evaluating the research base of the studies and included criteria on replication, scientific merit, and risk. The second category dealt with relevance to practice. Criteria included clinical significance, nursing control, feasibility, and cost. The third category dealt with potential for clinical evaluation by clinicians. Through application of these criteria, the CURN Project developed and field tested 10 research-based practice protocols.

Brett (1987) identified 14 innovations ready for implementation in clinical practice. She found that the majority of nurses in her samples were aware of the 14 innovations but that use of the innovations had no relationship to hospital policies or procedures. In a subsequent study (Brett, 1989) it was found that in small hospitals a higher level of integration was related to increased nurse innovation adoptions, whereas in large hospitals the reverse occurred. Goode, Lovett, Hayes, and Butcher (1987) have reported on the implementation of research-based practice in a rural community hospital. With the leadership of a master's prepared nurse administrator, staff nurses learned to critique research, identify a research base, and translate the findings into clinical innovations. This project built on the CURN Project and emphasized the interaction between organizational commitment, change agents, planned change process, and the outcomes of research-based practice (Goode & Bulechek, 1992). Titler et al. (1994) described the Iowa model for research-based practice to promote quality care. Developed for use in an academic center, changes in practice can be initiated by problem-focused triggers or knowledge-focused triggers. After synthesis of the research base, a decision is made to utilize research if sufficient knowledge is available or to conduct research if there is inconclusive evidence. These research models and others have emphasized that research-based practice requires organizational commitment and support when nurses work in groups in bureaucratic settings. Curriculums are including more content and experience with research utilization for all levels of nursing students.

More research is being conducted, and there are more vehicles for dissemination. New journals, such as *Applied Nursing Research* and *Clinical Nursing Research*, have emerged that focus on the clinical implications of nursing research. Most specialty journals print original research for a portion of their articles. The *Annual Review of Nursing Research* is well into its second decade, and an *Encyclopedia of Nursing Research* (Fitzpatrick, 1998) has been created. A number of meta-analyses have been conducted related to nursing interventions, and some of these have been incorporated by the chapter authors in this book.

4. Feasibility of successfully implementing the intervention: Many factors contribute to concerns about feasibility when a nursing intervention is selected. Most patients have several nursing diagnoses, and the order or priority in which to treat them must be decided. There may also be several medical diagnoses. There are likely to be other health professionals in addition to the nurse working with the client. Therefore, it is necessary to think about the total plan of care for the client. Consideration must be given to interaction of the nursing interventions with treatments being provided by other health professionals. Such interactions may be either beneficial or detrimental for the client. A concerted effort by everyone involved is needed to achieve a successful client outcome; at times the health team must establish a priority ranking of treatments to avoid overwhelming the client.

Cost and time are other feasibility concerns. Will there be third-party reimbursement for the intervention? Is there a critical path associated with the condition or a related procedure? Will the intervention be conducted in the hospital, clinic, or home? Can both the client and the nurse give the amount of time required for the intervention? Today's consumer expects quality health care but is also concerned about the cost.

5. Acceptability of the intervention to the client: Each client comes for health care with a perception of the problem and a notion of what should be done about it. Whatever the nurse assesses, diagnoses, and treats is going to be interpreted by the client within his or her own frame of reference. The treatment plan must be congruent with the client's reality, or it is doomed to failure. If the nurse has established rapport during the assessment, the client should be ready to participate in the selection of outcomes. Whenever possible, it is important for the client to participate in outcome selection. The nurse is frequently able to recommend a choice of nursing interventions to assist in reaching the outcome. For each intervention, the client should be given information about the conduct of the intervention and how he or she is expected to participate to help make an informed choice. The client's values, beliefs, and culture must be considered when selecting a nursing intervention.

6. Capability of the nurse: To successfully implement an intervention, a nurse must have (1) knowledge of the scientific rationale for the intervention, (2) the necessary psychomotor and interpersonal skills, and (3) the ability to function within the setting to effectively use health care resources. As our profession matures, we are becoming comfortable with the notion that all nurses are not alike. Each has unique knowledge with skills developed through education and experience. It is important for each nurse to differentiate the clients and nursing diagnoses he or she can treat from those who should be referred to other nurses or health professionals.

This consideration (capability of the provider) is becoming increasingly important as some health care agencies increase the use of unlicensed assistants. Although the assistant may have the necessary skill and the permission to use resources in the setting, he or she may not have the educational background to enable knowledge of the scientific rationales. In some cases, interventions—or specific activities related to an intervention—may safely be delegated to less-prepared personnel, but decisions to delegate must be made wisely based on knowledge of the capability of the assistant.

NURSING PRACTICE DATA

The use of standardized language to document care via a nursing information system allows for creation of a nursing database that can be linked with other databases and is useful for many purposes. A model developed by the Iowa Intervention Research Team illustrates how nursing practice data (diagnoses, interventions, and outcomes) can be used at three levels: individual, unit/ organizational, and network/state/country (Figure 1). (Note: The model and its explanation are also published in other places.) A reader interested in knowing more about this is referred to the Iowa Intervention Project (1997a, 1997b).

At the model's *individual level* each nurse uses standardized language (e.g., NANDA, NIC, NOC) in the areas of diagnoses, interventions, and outcomes to communicate patient care plans and to document care delivered. An individual nurse working with a patient or group of patients asks herself or himself several questions according to the steps of the nursing process. What are the patient's nursing diagnoses? What are the patient outcomes that I am trying to achieve? What interventions do I use to obtain these outcomes? The identified diagnoses, outcomes, and interventions are then documented using the standardized language in these areas.

At the *unit/organizational level*, the information about individual patients is

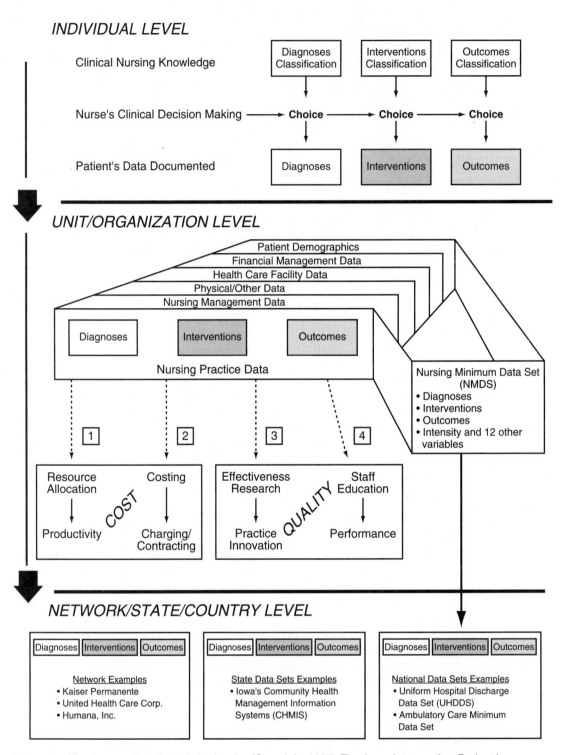

Figure I   Nursing practice data: three levels. (Copyright 1997, The Iowa Intervention Project.)

aggregated for all the patients in the unit and, in turn, in the entire facility. This aggregated nursing practice data can then be linked to information contained in the nursing management database. The management database includes data about the nurses and others who provide care and the means of care delivery. The conceptualization of a Nursing Management Minimum Data Set (NMMDS) (Delaney & Huber, 1996) brings the profession closer to standardization in this important area. The NMMDS defines and proposes standardized measures for 17 variables, including the type of nursing unit or service, the method of care delivery, the staff demographic profile, and the unit or service budget. These two databases (nursing practice and nursing management) compose the nursing information system. In turn the nursing practice and management data can be linked with data about the treatments made by physicians and other providers, facility information, patient information, and financial data. Most of these data, with the exception of data about treatments of providers other than physicians are already collected in a uniform way and available for use.

The model illustrates how the clinical practice data linked with other data in the agency's information system can be used to determine both *cost* and *quality* of nursing care. The *cost side of the model* addresses resource allocation and costing out of nursing services; the *quality side of the model* addresses effectiveness research and staff education. The use of standardized language to plan and document care does not automatically result in knowledge about cost and quality but provides the potential for data for decision making in these areas. The four paths do not mean to imply that these are mutually exclusive. The two sides of the model are interactive; cost and quality should always be considered hand in hand.

The *network/state/country level* involves the "sending forward" of nursing data, (i.e., the Nursing Minimum Data Set [NMDS]) (Werley & Lang, 1988) to be included in large databases that are used for benchmarking for determination of quality and for health policymaking. Examples of two national databases and one state database are listed on the model. In addition, there are a growing number of networks of care providers (the model lists three) who are also constructing databases. Nursing has remained essentially invisible in these clinical and administrative databases because we have not had standardized languages to describe our work. The ramifications of the invisibility of nursing in the databases are that we cannot (1) describe the nursing care received by patients, (2) describe the effects of nursing practice on patient outcomes, (3) compare nursing care across settings, (4) identify what nurses do so that they may be reimbursed, and (5) compare patient care delivered by nurses with patient care delivered by physicians (Jacox, 1995).

EFFECTIVENESS RESEARCH

One of the paths in the model is about effectiveness research, which has also been called outcomes research. According to Guadagnoli and McNeil (1994), outcomes research can be thought of as having two components: (1) identifying the links between the care given and the outcomes achieved and (2) determining which providers or systems of care deliver better-quality care than others. The essential effectiveness question is "What works best for which patients?" Nursing outcomes research, then, is about studying the effects of nursing interventions.

In the future, databases concerning nursing practice information generated from care actually delivered will become available. Questions concerning which interventions work best for which patients and at what cost can readily be studied from the existing sources of data. Nursing will be able to participate in benchmarking types of research to evaluate care from one region of the country to another. When new technologies are introduced, the databases will contain baseline information for comparison of effectiveness. The progress of nursing science should move more quickly when existing data can be used rather than each researcher having to collect new data each time a research question or hypothesis is proposed.

With the help of these databases, we will be able to determine which nursing interventions work best for a given population. We will be able to address research questions such as the following:

1. What interventions work best for the achievement of a specific outcome?

Documentation of care with standardized classifications allows for the integration of research and practice. Researchers will use the data collected by practitioners in different settings and will be able to address more complex research questions. Through the analysis of large clinical practice databases, the effects of specific interventions can be studied. This research information can then be used by practitioners in their prescriptions for care with particular patients.

2. What interventions are typically used together?

When we systematically collect information about the treatments we perform, we will be able to identify clusters of interventions that typically occur together for certain types of patients. We need to begin to identify interventions that are frequently used together for certain types of patients so that we can study their interactive effects. This information will also be useful in the construction of critical paths, in determining costs of services, and in planning for resource allocation.

3. What interventions are typically used in certain areas or specialties?

The development and implementation of a standardized list of nursing treatments make it now possible to compare interventions used in one setting with those used in another. No particular group of nurses is expected to use all the interventions in NIC. Determining the interventions used most frequently on a specific type of unit/agency will help determine which interventions should be on that unit's nursing information system. It will also help in the selection of personnel to staff that unit and in the structuring of the continuing education provided to the personnel on these units.

The identification of research questions to address is what Guadagnoli and McNeil (1994) call the "effectiveness space." That is, what are the variables in addition to diagnoses, interventions, and outcomes that are needed to conduct nursing effectiveness research, and what level within each variable is of interest to evaluate effectiveness? Guadagnoli and McNeil point out that specificity is necessary in effectiveness research but that with every increase in specificity, the amount of data required is increased. When the nursing community begins to drown in data, then our thinking about what is clinically meaningful becomes bogged down. The nursing community has only begun to wrestle with this issue—that of how much data to collect.

As one example of nursing's effectiveness space, the following variables should be collected to answer the previous three questions: the *patient's* identity number (to allow linking of information), age, sex, race/ethnicity (these three to provide some demographic information), episode admission or encounter date, discharge or termination date, disposition (where the patient went after discharge), and outcomes (both expected and achieved); the *physician's* diagnoses and interventions; the *nurse's* diagnoses and interventions, including the specific medications administered (in order to control for the medications' effects in relationship to other nursing interventions); and the *work unit's* type, staff mix, average patient acuity, and workload (also necessary as controls). Each of these variables needs a standardized definition and measure. (See the chapter by the Iowa Intervention Project [1997b] for the definitions and measures of 24 variables proposed for the basis of a nursing database.)

Our work with the identification and measurement of variables necessary for the conduction of effectiveness research demonstrates that the profession still needs to grapple with several issues related to the collection of standardized data. For example, the collection and coding of medications in easily retrievable form is not yet available in most facilities. Although nursing effectiveness research can be done without knowledge of medications, many of the outcomes that are achieved by nurses are also influenced by certain drugs, and so the control for medication effect is desirable. Also, at the present time there is no unique number that identifies the primary nurse. Consequently, it is not currently possible to attribute clinical interventions or outcomes to particular nurses based on documentation data. Additionally, health care facilities do not yet collect the unit data in a standardized way.

An additional challenge is having a measure of the "dose" of the intervention. Maintaining the integrity of the intervention across participants and settings is important in effectiveness research, as inconsistent intervention delivery may result in variability in the outcomes achieved (Braden & Braden, 1998; Carter, Moorhead, McCloskey, & Bulechek, 1995). Using NIC, this means that a substantial number of the activities listed for a particular intervention should be done and that all activities that are done should be consistent with the definition of the intervention. It is important that the activities be tailored for individual care, but they must not vary so much that the intervention is no longer the same. In experimental research, when a particular intervention is studied under controlled conditions (called efficacy research), the consistent delivery of the intervention is possible, but these ideal conditions rarely happen in actual practice, so effectiveness research (what actually happens in practice) is imperative. At the present time, there is no solution to the issue of "dose" of the intervention. A proxy measure, such as the amount of time a practitioner uses when doing the intervention, is helpful and may suffice as a measure of "dose" in some studies. But the best solution is to know the number and extent of the specific activities that are done. Some of the databases that are being developed by individual agencies and vendors include this information, but others do not have the memory storage required for large data sets and have chosen not to document this level of detail. Although the documentation of the intervention label is most important for comparison of data across sites, it is also important to have a way to ascertain the consistent implementation of the intervention. This can be done by an agency's adoption of a standard protocol for the delivery of the intervention, by the collection of the time spent for intervention delivery, or by documentation of the activities related to the intervention. A simple way to collect data about the number and extent of implementation of intervention activities is shown in Figure 2.

Despite the remaining challenges, we have made enormous progress in our ability to engage in effectiveness research. The chapters in this book discuss

Name of Intervention:

Definition:

<u>No Use</u>:

_____ The intervention was not used for this patient.

<u>Use</u>:

Insert the NIC activities here; add any additional ones that are appropriate for this patient but not included in NIC.

For each activity, give a number:

0 = not applicable for this patient
1 = applicable but not implemented
2 = implemented somewhat
3 = implemented a moderate amount
4 = throughly implemented

<u>Scoring</u>:   Total the numbers and divide by the number of items that were rated 1 or more.

Figure 2   Scale to measure the degree of implementation (dose) of an intervention. (Copyright 1998, The Iowa Intervention Project.)

what is known about the interventions, mostly through case study and efficacy research methods. With the development of standardized language that can be used for documentation of actual clinical practice, we can now add effectiveness methods to our ability to study the impact of our interventions. New, more complicated questions can now be asked and answered. The journey for the discovery of nursing knowledge continues.

References

Agency for Health Care Policy and Research (AHCPR). (1990 September). *Nursing advisory panel for guideline development: Summary* (program note). Washington, DC: US Department of Health and Human Services, Public Health Service, AHCPR.

American Medical Association. (1993). *Physicians current procedures terminology* (CPT-93). Chicago: Author.

American Nurses Association. (1980). *Nursing: A social policy statement.* Kansas City: Author.

American Nurses Association. (1989). *Classification systems for describing nursing practice: Working papers* (Publication NP-74). Kansas City: Author.

American Nurses Association. (1992). *Standards of nursing practice.* Kansas City: Author.

American Nurses Association. (1995). *Nursing: A social policy statement.* Washington, DC: Author.

Aydelotte, M. K. (1976). Nursing research in clinical settings: Problems and issues. *Reflections, 2,* 3–6.

Blegen, M. A., and Tripp-Reimer, T. (1997). Implications of nursing taxonomies for middle-range theory development. *Advances in Nursing Science, 19*(3), 37–49.

Braden, S., and Braden, C. J. (1998). *Evaluating nursing interventions: A theory-driven approach.* Thousand Oaks, CA: Sage Publications.

Brett, J. L. (1987). Use of nursing practice research findings. *Nursing Research, 36*(6), 344–349.

Brett, J. L. (1989). Organizational integrative mechanisms and adoption of innovations by nurses. *Nursing Research, 38*(2), 105–110.

Bruce, J. (1979). Implementation of nursing diagnoses: A nursing administrator's perspective. *Nursing Clinics of North America, 14*(3), 509–515.

Bulechek, G. M., and McCloskey, J. C. (Eds.). (1985). *Nursing interventions: Treatments for nursing diagnoses.* Philadelphia: W.B. Saunders.

Bulechek, G. M., and McCloskey, J. C. (1989). Nursing interventions: Treatments for potential nursing diagnoses. In R. M. Carroll-Johnson (Ed.), *Classification of nursing diagnoses* (pp. 23–30). Philadelphia: J. B. Lippincott.

Bulechek, G. M., and McCloskey, J. C. (Eds.). (1992). *Nursing interventions: Essential nursing treatments.* Philadelphia: W.B. Saunders.

Carpenito, L. J. (1987). *Nursing diagnosis: Process and application* (2nd ed.). Philadelphia: J.B. Lippincott.

Carroll-Johnson, R. M. (Ed.). (1989). *Classification of nursing diagnoses: Proceedings of the eighth conference.* Philadelphia: J.B. Lippincott.

Carroll-Johnson, R. M. (Ed.). (1991). *Classification of nursing diagnoses: Proceedings of the ninth conference.* Philadelphia: J.B. Lippincott.

Carter, J. J., Moorhead, S. A., McCloskey, J. C., and Bulechek, G. M. (1995). Using the Nursing Interventions Classification to implement Agency for Health Care Policy and Research guidelines. *Journal of Nursing Care Quality, 9*(2), 76–86.

Cassmeyer, V. L. (1989). Using physiology and pathophysiology in the nursing diagnostic process. *Journal of Advanced Medical Surgical Nursing, 1*(3), 1–10.

Craft-Rosenberg, M., and Delaney, C. (1997). Nursing diagnosis extension and classification (NDEC). In M. Rantz and P. LeMone (Eds.), *Classification of nursing diagnoses: Proceedings of the twelfth conference* (pp. 26–31). Glendale, CA: Cumulative Index to Nursing and Allied Health Literature.

Delaney, C., and Huber, D. (1996). *A nursing management minimum data set (NMMDS): A report of an invitational conference.* Chicago: American Organization of Nurse Executives.

Devine, E. C., and Werley, H. H. (1988). Test of the nursing minimum data set: Availability of data and reliability. *Research in Nursing and Health, 11*(3), 97–104.

Donabedian, A. (1980). *The definition of quality and approaches to its assessment.* Ann Arbor, MI: Health Administration Press.

Dumas, R. G., and Leonard, R. C. (1963). The effect of nursing on the incidence of post operative vomiting. *Nursing Research, 12,* 12–15.

Fehring, R. (1986). Validating diagnostic labels: Standardized methodology. In E. Hurley (Ed.), *Classification of nursing diagnoses: Proceedings of the sixth conference* (pp. 183–190). St. Louis: Mosby-Year Book.

Fitzpatrick, J. (Ed.). (1998). *Encyclopedia of nursing research.* New York: Springer.

Fitzpatrick, J. J., Kerr, M. E., Saba, V. K., Hoskins, L. M., Hurley, M. E., Mills, W. C., Rottkamp, B. C., Warren, J. J., and Carpenito, L. J. (1989). Translating nursing diagnosis into ICD code. *American Journal of Nursing, 89*(12), 493–495.

Gebbie, K. M. (1975). *Classification of nursing diagnoses: Proceedings of the second national conference.* St. Louis: Clearinghouse for Nursing Diagnosis.

Gebbie, K. M. (1989). Major classification systems in health care and their use. In staff, *Classification systems for describing nursing practice: Working papers* (pp. 48–49). Kansas City: American Nurses Association.

Gebbie, K. M., and Lavin, M. A. (Eds.). (1975). *Classification of nursing diagnoses: Proceedings of the first national conference.* St. Louis: C.V. Mosby.

Goode, C., and Bulechek, G. M. (1992). Research utilization: An organizational process that enhances quality care. *Journal of Nursing Care Quality,* Special Report, 27–35.

Goode, C. M., Lovett, M., Hayes, J., and Butcher, L. (1987). Use of research based knowledge in clinical practice. *Journal of Nursing Administration, 17*(12), 11–18.

Gordon, M. (1987). *Nursing diagnosis: Process and application* (2nd ed.). New York: McGraw-Hill.

Griffith, H. M., Thomas, N., and Griffith, L. (1991). MDs bill for these routine nursing tasks. *American Journal of Nursing, 91*(1), 22–27.

Guadagnoli, E., and McNeil, B. J. (1994). Outcomes research: Hope for the future or the latest rage? *Inquiry, 31*(1), 14–24.

Haller, K. B., Reynolds, M. A., and Horsley, J. A. (1979). Developing research based innovation protocols: Process, criteria and issues. *Research in Nursing and Health, 2,* 45–51.

Henry, S. B., Holzemer, W. L., Randell, C., Hsieh, S., Miller, T. J., and Reilly, C. A. (1997). Comparison of Nursing Interventions Classification and Current Procedural Terminology codes for categorizing nursing activities. *Image: Journal of Nursing Scholarship, 29*(2), 133–138.

Hinshaw, A. S. (1988). The new national center for nursing research: Patient care research programs. *Applied Nursing Research, 1*(1), 2–4.

Horn, B. J., and Swain, M. A. (1978). *Criterion measures of nursing care* (DHEW Pub. No. PHS78-3187). Hyattsville, MD: National Center for Health Services Research.

Hoskins, L. (1997). How to do a validation study. In M. Rantz and P. LeMone (Eds.), *Classification of nursing diagnoses: Proceedings of the twelfth conference* (pp. 79–86). Glendale, CA: Cumulative Index to Nursing and Allied Health Literature.

Hurley, M. (Ed.). (1986). *Classification of nursing diagnoses: Proceedings of the sixth national conference.* St. Louis: C. V. Mosby.

International Council of Nurses. (1996). *The international classification for nursing practice: A unifying framework.* Geneva: International Council of Nurses.

Iowa Intervention Project. (1997a). Defining nursing's effectiveness: Diagnoses, interventions and outcomes. In M. Rantz and P. LeMone (Eds.), *Classification of nursing diagnoses: Proceedings of the twelfth conference* (pp. 293–303). Glendale, CA: Cumulative Index to Nursing and Allied Health Literature.

Iowa Intervention Project. (1997b). Proposal to bring nursing into the information age. *Image: Journal of Nursing Scholarship, 29*(3), 275–281.

Jacox, A. (1974). Nursing research and the clinician. *Nursing Outlook, 22,* 382.

Jacox, A. (1995). Practice and policy implications of clinical and administrative databases. In N. M. Lang (Ed.), *Nursing data systems: The emerging framework* (pp. 161–165). Washington, DC: American Nurses Association.

Jenny, J. (1995). Advancing the science of nursing. In M. Rantz and P. LeMone (Eds.), *Classification of nursing diagnoses: Proceedings of the eleventh conference* (pp. 73–81). Glendale, CA: Cumulative Index to Nursing and Allied Health Literature.

Johnson, M., and Maas, M. (Eds.). (1997). *Nursing outcomes classification (NOC).* St. Louis: Mosby-Year Book.

Kim, M., and Moritz, D. A. (1982). *Classification of nursing diagnoses: Proceedings of the third and fourth national conferences.* New York: McGraw-Hill.

Kim, M. J. (1984). Physiologic nursing diagnosis: Its role and place in nursing taxonomy. In M. J. Kim, G. K. McFarland, and A. M. McLane (Eds.), *Classification of nursing diagnoses: Proceedings of the fifth national conference* (pp. 60–72). St. Louis: C.V. Mosby.

Kim, M. J., McFarland, G. K., and McLane, A. M. (Eds.). (1984). *Classification of nursing diagnoses: Proceedings of the fifth national conference.* St. Louis: C.V. Mosby.

Lang, N. M. (Ed.). (1994). *An emerging framework: Data system advances for clinical nursing practice.* Washington, DC: American Nurses Publishing.

Marek, K. (1995). *Manual to develop guidelines.* Washington, DC: American Nurses Association.

Marek, K. D. (1989). Outcome measurement in nursing. *Journal of Nursing Quality Assurance, 4*(1), 1–9.

Martin, K. S., and Scheet, N. J. (1992). *The Omaha system: Applications for community health nursing* (pp. 90–98). Philadelphia: W.B. Saunders.

Martinson, I. M. (1976). Nursing research: Obstacles and challenges. *Image: Journal of Nursing Scholarship, 8*(1), 3–5.

McCloskey, J. C. (1988). The nursing minimum data set: Benefits and implications for nurse educators. In *Perspectives in Nursing 1987–1989* (Pub. No. 41-2199) (pp. 119–126). National League for Nursing Press.

McCloskey, J. C., and Bulechek, G. M. (Eds.). (1992). *Nursing interventions classification (NIC)*. St. Louis: Mosby-Year Book.

McCloskey, J. C., and Bulechek, G. M. (Eds.). (1996). *Nursing interventions classification (NIC)* (2nd ed.). St. Louis: Mosby-Year Book.

McCloskey, J. C., Bulechek, G. M., Cohen, M. Z., Craft, M. J., Crossley, J. D., Denehy, J. A., Glick, O. J., Kruckeberg, T., Maas, M., Prophet, C. M., and Tripp-Reimer, T. (1990). Classification of nursing interventions. *Journal of Professional Nursing, 6*(3), 151–157.

McCloskey, J. C., Gardner, D., and Johnson, M. (1987). Costing out nursing services: An annotated bibliography. *Nursing Economics, 5*(5), 245–253.

McCormick, K. A. (1991). Future data needs for quality of care monitoring, DRG considerations, reimbursement and outcome measurement. *Image: Journal of Nursing Scholarship, 23*(1), 29–32.

McLane, A. M. (Ed.). (1987). *Classification of nursing diagnoses: Proceedings of the seventh national conference*. St. Louis: C.V. Mosby.

Mills, W. C. (1991). Nursing diagnosis: The importance of a definition. *Nursing Diagnosis, 2*(1), 3–8.

North American Nursing Diagnosis Association. (1989). Monograph of the invitational conference on research methods for validating nursing diagnoses. St. Louis: Author.

North American Nursing Diagnosis Association. (1996). *Nursing diagnosis: Definitions and classification 1997–1998*. Philadelphia: Author.

North American Nursing Diagnosis Association. (1997). Guidelines for nursing diagnosis submission. In M. Rantz and P. LeMone (Eds.), *Classification of nursing diagnoses: Proceedings of the twelfth conference* (pp. 489–492). Glendale, CA: Cumulative Index to Nursing and Allied Health Literature.

Nursing Information and Data Set Evaluation Center (NIDSEC). (1997). *Standards and scoring guidelines*. Washington, DC: American Nurses Publishing.

Ozbolt, J. G. (Ed.). (1992). *Nursing informatics: Enhancing patient care. A report of the priority expert panel on nursing informatics*. Bethesda, MD: National Institutes of Health, National Center for Nursing Research.

Popkess-Vawter, S. (1991). Wellness nursing diagnoses: To be or not to be? *Nursing Diagnosis, 2*(1), 19–25.

Smoyak, S. A. (1976). Is practice responding to research? *American Journal of Nursing, 76*, 1146–1150.

Snyder, M. (1985). *Independent nursing interventions*. New York: John Wiley.

Study Group on Nursing Information Systems. (1983). Computerized nursing information systems: An urgent need. *Research in Nursing and Health, 6* (Special Report), 101–105.

Tanner, C. A. (1987). Teaching clinical judgment. In J. J. Fitzpatrick and R. L. Taunton (Eds.), *Annual review of nursing research* (pp. 153–173) (Vol. 5). New York: Springer.

Tanner, C. A. (1989, August). Research needs and priorities related to clinical decision making in nursing. Unpublished paper commissioned by National Center for Nursing Research.

Tarlov, A. R., Ware, J. E., Greenfield, S., Nelson, E. C., Perrin, E., and Zubkoff, M. (1989). The medical outcomes study: An application of methods for monitoring the results of medical care. *Journal of the American Medical Association, 262*(7), 925–930.

Titler, M. G., Kleiber, C., Steelman, V., Goode, C., Rakel, B., Barry-Walker, J., Small, S., and Buckwalter, K. (1994). Infusing research into practice to promote quality care. *Nursing Research, 43*(5), 307–313.

Waltz, C. F., and Strickland, O. L. (1988). *Measurement of nursing outcomes: Measuring client outcomes* (Vol. 1). New York: Springer.

Weiler, K., Buckwalter, K., and Titler, M. (1994). Is nursing research used in practice? In J. McCloskey and H. Grace (Eds.), *Current issues in nursing* (4th ed., pp. 61–75). St. Louis: Mosby-Year Book.

Werley, H. H., and Lang, N. M. (Eds.). (1988). *Identification of the nursing minimum data set*. New York: Springer.

Werley, H. H., Lang, N. M., and Westlake, S. K. (1986). The nursing minimum data set conference: Executive summary. *Journal of Professional Nursing, 2*, 117–224.

Zielstroff, R. D. (1984). Why aren't there more significant automated nursing information systems? *Journal of Nursing Administration, 14*(1), 7–10.

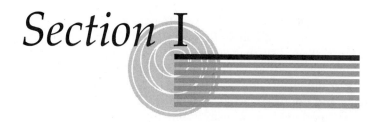

Section I

Physiological: Basic Interventions

Overview: Care That Supports Physical Functioning

Gloria M. Bulechek

Joanne C. McCloskey

The basics of nursing care include those activities necessary for normal life function. Usually people do these activities for themselves, but when illness or disability prevents this, the tasks fall to the nurse or the family. The interventions in this section are basic treatments that nurses perform to support physical functioning. These interventions are at the core of nursing and represent the nursing philosophical belief that nurses assist individuals in caring for themselves. These interventions are usually taught in the first course in a nursing curriculum. Sometimes we take these interventions for granted; given the frequency of their use by nurses, however, it is important that we understand the research base for the interventions.

Food is a basic need of everyone, and feeding those who cannot do this for themselves is not as simple as it sounds. In Chapter 1, **Feeding,** Nancy J. Evans-Stoner discusses the components of Feeding and the clinical implications of malnutrition. The ultimate goal of Feeding is to provide adequate nutrients to prevent malnutrition. A secondary goal is to restore the patient's independence in this basic self-care area. Evans-Stoner outlines several high-risk situations that may indicate a feeding problem, including individuals with neuromuscular impairment, anorexia, cognitive deficits, and sensory perceptual deficits. The nursing diagnosis most appropriate for the intervention of feeding is Self Care Deficit: Feeding. The author discusses multiple activities and strategies that a nurse must use to feed a patient successfully. A case study illustrates use of the intervention. Although Feeding is a basic and, at times, simple nursing intervention, at other times getting a person to eat is challenging. At all times, nurses must have a "strong theoretical knowledge base regarding the physiological and psychological components of nutrient intake."

Sleep is also a basic need, but many individuals suffer from some type of sleep deprivation. In the next chapter, Felissa R. Lashley and Mary de Meneses first overview the causes of sleep disturbances and then address the assessment that is needed to determine the specific cause for an individual patient. The intervention of **Sleep Enhancement** is addressed through a review of the research on pharmacologic and nonpharmacologic activities. Related nursing diagnoses and outcomes are identified. A case study illustrates some of the information contained in the chapter.

The basics also include assisting with urine and bowel elimination. Janet P. Specht, Meridean L. Maas, Sally Willett, and Nancy Myers discuss the intervention **Urinary Catheterization: Intermittent.** Incontinence is a major problem, affecting approximately 30% of the elderly who live in the community and 50% of those in nursing homes. The authors say that too frequently health providers, including nurses, assume that nothing can be done and resort to disposable pads or indwelling catheters. In Chapter 3 the authors review the strong research base for intermittent catheterization, which was first introduced as a bladder-training technique for paraplegic patients after World War II. They discuss the pros and cons of sterile versus clean technique and recommend the clean procedure, which has the advantages of flexibility, convenience, and low cost. They also recommend that more research comparing the two methods be done. The intervention is appropriate for the diagnoses of reflex incontinence, urge incontinence, and overflow incontinence for clients of all ages. Two case studies illustrate the use of the intervention, and procedures for catheterization of a male and a female are included. The authors urge nurses to use this intervention more often and publish the results in the literature.

Another intervention that can be used for treatment of incontinence is **Pelvic Floor Exercise,** also known as pelvic muscle exercise or Kegel's exercise. In the next chapter, Carolyn M. Sampselle and Sandra H. Hines explain the physiology of urinary continence and the relationship of exercise of the pelvic muscle to improved continence. The purpose of the intervention is to strengthen the voluntary muscles of the pelvic floor so that the muscles are better able to support the urethra in times of increased intra-abdominal pressure and better able to counter increased pressure within the bladder. The authors review a good deal of research that has demonstrated the effectiveness of Pelvic Floor Exercise in decreasing symptoms of urinary incontinence in women of all ages, in postpartum women, and in men following prostatectomy. The specific intervention protocol is individualized based on the patient's neurological function, the adequacy of pelvic support, and the severity of the incontinence. Two case studies illustrate use of the intervention, which has positive outcomes for both the client and the caregivers.

In Chapter 5, Theresa Moore, Eileen Bourret, and Lucy Cabico discuss the intervention **Constipation/Impaction Management.** They begin the chapter by pointing out that there is no agreed-upon definition of constipation, which makes recognition and treatment of the problem difficult. Nursing actions for the problem are discussed in the categories of nonpharmacologic management and pharmacologic management. Nonpharmacologic activities include intake of fluids, fiber supplementation, exercise, and toileting. Pharmacologic activities include appropriate use of laxatives, suppositories, and enemas. The authors include an excellent overview of different types of laxatives: bulk forming, emollient, saline, hyperosmotic, and stimulant. They summarize the use of their excellent review of the literature in the form of guidelines for nonpharmacologic prevention and management of constipation, guidelines for pharmacologic management for acute constipation/impaction, and guidelines for pharmacologic management of chronic constipation. The chapter concludes with a case study.

When a person is immobilized and unable to move in bed, assistance with turning and positioning is very important. Debbie Metzler and Cynthia Finesilver discuss the intervention of **Positioning,** which helps prevent the complications of immobility, promotes comfort, and facilitates healing. The authors structure the chapter by first discussing the research base for specific activities in the NIC intervention. They then suggest additional activities that should be included based on their excellent and comprehensive literature review. The second half of the chapter addresses the literature related to differing positions: supine, lateral, prone, and Trendelenburg. They also include sections on Positioning for clients with altered respiratory function, for clients with altered neurological function, and for the elderly. NOC outcomes that can be affected by the intervention of Positioning are identified. The chapter concludes with a case study that identifies NANDA diagnoses, NOC outcomes, and specific NIC positioning activities individualized for the particular patient.

Although the need for exercise is recognized, most adults do not exercise enough. The intervention of **Exercise Promotion** is discussed in Chapter 7 by Janet D. Allan and Diane O. Tyler. The focus of their chapter is "helping adults incorporate sufficient exercise into their lives in order to improve health." The chapter is applicable to a variety of patient populations. The authors provide a comprehensive literature review of the benefits of exercise, discuss ways that exercise can be quantified, provide an assessment guide for taking an exercise health history, and discuss ways to tailor the Exercise Promotion intervention to the needs of the individual. They discuss the design of an exercise program, ways to prevent common injuries, and strategies to help an individual maintain the exercise program. One of the biggest challenges in the implementation of this intervention is maintenance, with more than 50% of participants dropping out of all exercise programs in the first months. Nursing diagnoses and patient outcomes related to this intervention are identified. A case study of a 40-year-old man who is disease free with a nursing diagnosis of Altered Health Maintenance related to sedentary lifestyle is included. As Americans and, indeed, adults from an increasing number of other countries lead more sedentary lifestyles, nurses in all countries will find this chapter helpful in improving the health of people worldwide.

Pain is a problem that nurses frequently encounter, and techniques to decrease and prevent pain are part of basic nursing care. The last two chapters in the section discuss interventions that promote comfort. One of the interventions is a traditional nursing intervention, Pain Management, and the other, Therapeutic Touch, is increasingly used but controversial.

Chapter 8, by Keela A. Herr and Paula R. Mobily, discusses the intervention of **Pain Management** as well as several more specific pain management interventions. The authors point out that although there have been several federal guidelines on the clinical management of both acute and chronic pain, research continues to document inadequate care of persons with pain. To assist the nurse in more accurately determining the level of pain, the authors discuss the available pain assessment instruments for both children and adults. Examples are included of a visual analogue scale, a numeric rating scale, and a verbal descriptor scale. The authors also discuss the misbeliefs that may influence the patient's receptivity of different pain intervention strategies. They believe that incorporating both pharmacologic and nonpharmacologic strategies is the most effective approach to managing pain. Factors to take into consideration when choosing specific strategies include the individual's past experience with pain, knowledge of strategies, personal preferences, and willingness and ability to participate in particular strategies. The authors point out that many of the non-pharmacologic strategies require assistance; thus, the inclusion of a supportive person in the teaching aspects of the intervention may be important. They discuss three classes of analgesic drugs and some approaches to the use of analgesics. Nursing diagnoses and patient outcomes associated with the intervention of Pain Management are identified, and a case study of a person suffering severe pain in her knee illustrates many of the points made in the chapter.

In the last chapter of the section, Therese Connell Meehan does a thorough job of describing the controversial intervention of **Therapeutic Touch.** Developed by Dora Kunz and Delores Krieger in the early 1970s, Therapeutic Touch is viewed as an energy field interaction. Meehan reviews the theoretical basis for the intervention and the practice and research literature. Although nurse use of Therapeutic Touch has been documented in a growing body of literature, the research on the intervention has a wide range of methodologic problems. Meehan does an excellent job of discussing both the limitations of the research and the controversy surrounding the intervention. She ends her chapter with a brief overview of two intervention tools, detailed comments on the current NIC intervention, and a case study. Her suggestions for change will be incorporated in the next edition of NIC and will update the intervention to reflect current knowledge of the experts.

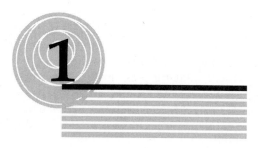

Feeding

Nancy Evans Stoner

Every careful observer of the sick will agree in this that thousands of patients are annually starved in the midst of plenty, from want of attention to the ways which alone make it possible for them to take food.

Florence Nightingale (1859)

The word *nutrition* derives from the Latin for to nurse, feed, or care for. Taylor (1988) describes nutrition as an art as well as a science but suggests that modern medicine and modern society attach more value to nutrition as a science. Gavan, Hastings-Tolsma, and Troyan (1988) state that "little is as basic to the human experience as nutrition and many of our earliest memories are embedded within the context of feeding." Eating and maintaining a sense of well-being are basic human instincts. Professional nurses have always been concerned about human responses, focusing on health care maintenance, recovery from illness, and promotion of well-being (Leininger, 1988). Nutritional well-being of patients has been a constant concern of nurses.

The complexity of health care today demands that nursing practice be based on sound theory. However, this demand is tempered by the suggestion that no amount of scientific theory ever got food into a patient and that nurses should be encouraged to value the humanistic skills that result in patients being fed (Taylor, 1988). There is no denying the technological advances of modern medicine that allow nutrients to be given to patients in a mechanized, highly technical way. Enteral and parenteral nutrition have added a new meaning to the word *feeding* and are lifesaving therapies for patients who are unable or unwilling to take in food orally. Caregivers should not use these therapies for individuals with a functional gastrointestinal tract who might ordinarily eat if given the opportunity and the proper assistance. This chapter describes the components of feeding, identifies settings in which Feeding is a critical intervention, and suggests useful strategies to maximize nutrient intake and prevent the occurrence of malnutrition.

LITERATURE REVIEW

Feeding, as defined by Webster, is giving food or supplying nourishment. Feeding can be described as a set of specific actions taken by oneself or a caregiver to ensure adequate nutrient intake to sustain life. The nursing intervention of Feeding in the Nursing Interventions Classification (NIC) is defined as "providing nutritional intake for patient who is unable to feed self" (McCloskey & Bulechek, 1996, p. 286) (Table 1–1). The success of Feeding is influenced by physiological and psychological factors. The ability to take in nutrients is dependent on complex neuromuscular coordination as well as individual cognitive abilities. The desire for food determines the quantity and quality of food intake and is not entirely dependent on physiological need.

Components of Feeding

Hunger is a familiar set of sensations stimulated by the depletion of nutrient stores. It can be viewed as a protective mechanism. Hunger is associated with

Table 1–1   Feeding

DEFINITION: Providing nutritional intake for patient who is unable to feed self.

ACTIVITIES:

Identify prescribed diet

Set food tray and table attractively

Create a pleasant environment during mealtime (e.g., put bedpans, urinals, and suctioning equipment out of sight)

Provide for adequate pain relief before meals, as appropriate

Provide for oral hygiene before meals

Identify presence of swallowing reflex, if necessary

Sit down while feeding to convey pleasure and relaxation

Offer opportunity to smell foods to stimulate appetite

Ask patient preference for order of eating

Fix foods as patient prefers

Maintain in an upright position, with head and neck flexed slightly forward during feeding

Place food in the unaffected side of the mouth, as appropriate

Follow feedings with water, if needed

Protect with a bib, as appropriate

Ask the patient to indicate when finished, as appropriate

Record intake, if appropriate

Avoid disguising drugs in food

Provide a drinking straw, as needed or desired

Provide finger foods, as appropriate

Provide foods at most appetizing temperature

Avoid distracting patient during swallowing

Feed unhurriedly/slowly

Postpone feeding, if patient is fatigued

Encourage parents/family to feed patient

Source: McCloskey, J. C., and Bulechek, G. M.(1996). *Nursing interventions classification (NIC)* (p. 286). St. Louis: Mosby–Year Book.

the physiological need to eat and is accompanied by various physical responses including rhythmic contractions of the stomach, tight or gnawing feelings in the stomach, and vague feelings of tension or restlessness (Guyton, 1991). The lateral hypothalamus is described as the hunger center (Vick, 1984).

The experience of hunger may be disrupted by situations that distract or reduce an individual's mental awareness (Anderson, 1982). For example, the stress of illness, injury, surgery, or emotional distress may disrupt the hunger response. Many patients may be alert to feelings of hunger but are unwilling or unable to respond. For example, aphasic or cognitively impaired patients may be unable to communicate verbally and may not eat unless the caregiver is sensitive to their nonverbal cues.

Appetite is the psychological desire to ingest food that usually accompanies hunger (Vick, 1984). It is an affective state, associated with pleasure rather than physiological need. Although the term is often used interchangeably with hunger, appetite is defined as a desire for a specific type of food. This desire for food is shaped by an individual's past experience, cultural traditions, and economic situation (Donoghue, Nunnally, & Yasko, 1982). The appetite center, located in the hypothalamus, receives messages from the cerebral cortex pertaining to vision, smell, taste, and touch, and is therefore subject to some degree of conscious control.

Physical ability determines whether a patient can independently complete the task of feeding. It requires smooth, well-coordinated motions of the arms and hands. The activity requires energy; a 70 kg man expends up to 2.5 kcal/min during eating (Caldwell & Kennedy-Caldwell, 1981).

Mechanical aspects of food ingestion also determine the success of feeding patients. Once food is made available to an individual, the success of safe nutrient intake is largely dependent on the effectiveness of chewing and swallowing. Mastication is necessary to prepare foods for digestion. It is controlled by muscles that are innervated by the motor branch of the fifth cranial nerve (Guyton, 1991). The condition of the oral mucosa is critical to the ability to take in food. The oral mucosa must be moist, with adequate saliva production to facilitate and aid in the digestion of food. The oral mucosa may be altered by infection, medications, chemotherapy, radiation, and surgical procedures.

The swallowing mechanism is a complex set of precisely timed movements that result in the safe passage of food into the stomach. Table 1–2 describes the three stages in the swallowing mechanism: (1) voluntary stage, (2) pharyngeal stage, and (3) esophageal state. Both chewing and swallowing are controlled by

Table 1–2 Stages of the Swallowing Mechanism

Stage	Function
Voluntary	• Food is moved into the pharynx by action of the tongue against the palate

Pharyngeal	• Presence of food in the pharynx stimulates swallowing receptors:
	    trachea closes
	    esophagus opens
	    peristaltic wave carries food into esophagus

Esophageal	• Esophagus accepts food from pharynx • Esophagus transports food bolus by peristaltic action into the stomach

Source: Guyton, A. C. (1991). *Textbook of medical physiology.* Philadelphia: W. B. Saunders.

Table 1–3 Cranial Nerve Function in the Chewing and Swallowing Mechanism

Cranial Nerve	Name	Function	Outcome Loss
5th	Trigeminal	Controls muscles of mastication; provides sensation of face, teeth, gums, and tongue	Loss of sensation; inability to move mandible
7th	Facial	Provides the sense of taste; controls the muscles of the face	Increased salivation; pouching of food in cheeks
9th	Glossopharyngeal	Transmits sensation to the tongue, pharynx, and soft palate; influences sense of taste, production of saliva, and swallowing	Decreased sensation of taste and salivation; diminished or inhibited gag reflex
10th	Vagus	Controls sensation in larynx, base of tongue, pharynx, and palate and their muscles	Increased difficulty swallowing; nasal regurgitation; reduced or lost gag reflex
12th	Hypoglossal	Controls the extrinsic and intrinsic muscles of the tongue	Inability to position food for chewing, resulting in pouching

Source: Donahue, P. A. (1990). When it's hard to swallow. Feeding techniques for dysphagia management. *Journal of Gerontological Nursing, 16*(4), 9.

an intricate neuromuscular network, and damage to the cranial nerves that control this system results in specific loss of function (Table 1–3).

Identification of High-Risk Situations

Metabolic demands of hospitalized patients are increased owing to the stress of illness. Nurses must be able to identify patients who cannot meet these demands independently. Deficits occur in the physical ability to coordinate muscles to bring food to the mouth, the mechanics of chewing and swallowing, or the ability to understand the task of feeding. Table 1–4 lists some common high-risk situations that require a more focused assessment.

Anorexia is a well-documented problem in cancer patients (Sigal & Daly,

Table 1–4 High-Risk Situations

Neuromuscular Impairment	Cognitive Deficits
Cerebral vascular accident	Psychiatric illness
Myasthenia gravis	Confusion state
Multiple sclerosis	Dementia
Amyotrophic dystrophy	Organic brain syndrome
Parkinson's disease	**Sensory Perceptual Deficits**
Immobility	Age
Trauma to upper extremities	Medications
Spinal cord injury	Cerebral vascular accident
Anorexia	
Chronic illness: cancer, chronic obstructive pulmonary disease	
Treatment: chemotherapy, radiation therapy	
Depression	

1990). Possible pathophysiological causes include sustained stimulation of receptors in the gastrointestinal (GI) tract resulting in early satiety, release of tumor byproducts, difficulty swallowing, or fatigue (Knox, 1983). Treatment-related causes of anorexia in cancer patients occur because of alterations in taste, oral inflammation, nausea and vomiting, infection, and fatigue. Other causes can be anxiety and depression associated with the diagnosis of cancer.

Decreased appetite is common in patients with chronic lung diseases (Openbrier & Covey, 1987). Although the etiology is unclear, anorexia may be caused by dyspnea, fatigue, coughing, increased sputum production, and side effects of medications (Dougherty, 1988).

The frail elderly are particularly at risk for impaired feeding. They may not have the manual dexterity, energy, or ability to feed themselves. Conditions that affect their ability to eat include arthritis, recurrent strokes, neurological disorders, sensory perceptual deficits, fractures, and poor oral conditions. Clinically significant swallowing abnormalities are more common in the elderly. For example, Siebens et al. (1986) found the incidence of swallowing abnormalities in a group of elderly nursing home patients to range from 30% to 40%. Anatomical changes that occur in the very old may also affect oral intake. These changes include the following: (1) decreased ability to swallow related to decreased saliva and dehydration; (2) dilated esophagus; (3) decreased peristalsis in the esophagus; (4) decreased secretion of acid in the stomach; and (5) hiatal hernia, which is common in obese elderly women (Ergun & Miskovitz, 1992; Hogstel & Robinson, 1989).

The context in which Feeding takes place can affect nutrient intake. Like many nursing interventions, Feeding is influenced by the development of a therapeutic relationship. Norberg et al. (1988) observed feelings of anxiety in the caregiver when a patient refused to eat. It is an extremely stressful situation for a caregiver when a patient is refusing to eat, because it is difficult to discern whether the patient is refusing or simply unable to eat. This study observed how caregivers in 24 Swedish nursing homes conceptualized food refusal and how they treated patients who refused food. In the 143 nursing interviews there were 138 accounts of food refusal. Interviewees were able to describe an event of patient refusing food during a Feeding intervention more than 50% of the time. The reasons for food refusal included physical reasons, such as the patient was too ill or could not perform the eating activities or had GI complaints. Interviewees also described psychological reasons; some caregivers felt the patient wished to die or did not understand the situation. Finally, they described cultural reasons, which included food taboos and lack of acquaintance with certain types of food presented. The investigators identified the lack of a therapeutic nurse-patient relationship and suggested a more consistent patient care assignment so that caregivers were more familiar with individual patient responses and more confident in interpreting the behavior.

Backstrom, Norberg, & Norberg (1987) studied feeding difficulties in chronically ill patients at 24 Swedish nursing homes. The aim of the nursing care for patients with eating problems was to help maintain or regain independence in feeding. Over a 4-week period there was a median of 16 to 20 feeders for each patient. The average duration of feeding in totally dependent patients was 20 minutes, and difficulty in feeding was reported in 81% of the feeding encounters. Caregivers described the process of feeding as dependent on the psychosocial aspects of the feeding situation. Dealing with impairments of sensory perception and cognition resulting in feeding problems requires a detailed knowledge of the patient and his or her disease as well as continuity of care.

Patients with eating problems can create such anxiety that caregivers often rotate these assignments to reduce the stress level. Athlin and Norberg (1987) described the development of the interaction between the patient and the caregiver in the patient assignment system by observing six severely demented women and five caregivers. Feeding problems were described as impaired reflexes and lack of purposeful behavior. Caregivers documented impaired communicative behavior and verbalized overwhelming concern in interpreting the patient's behavior. Very often the caregivers were not sure if the patients could understand their attempts to communicate.

Clinical Implications

Malnutrition starts when patients do not eat enough to meet their needs (Jeejeebhoy, 1990). If patients are unable or unwilling to eat, nurses must quickly intervene to prevent the rapid depletion of the body's protein and energy reserves. Nurses must appreciate the deleterious outcomes that can result when patients are not fed.

Malnutrition in the hospital setting is well documented. When questioned, almost any clinician will support the importance of nutrition, yet the prevalence of malnutrition in hospitalized patients has been reported to vary from 30% to 50% (Bistrian, Blackburn, & Hallowell, 1974; Bistrian, Blackburn, & Vitale, 1976). A more recent study of hospitalized patients documented malnutrition on admission to the hospital in several different groups of patients: 46% of general medical patients, 45% of patients with respiratory disease, and 43% of elderly patients (McWhirter & Pennington, 1994). Malnutrition is associated with increased morbidity and mortality (Buzby et al., 1980; Studley, 1936).

The result of inadequate intake from either total or partial starvation is a mobilization of the body's available energy stores. The quick energy sources available in muscle and liver glycogen supply only 24 to 48 hours of fuel. Adipose tissue provides a more abundant source of fuel for the body and in normal-weight individuals can supply energy for about 2 months (Cahill et al., 1988). Total unstressed starvation will result in a weight loss of 15% over a 3-week period. In stressed starvation, a patient will sustain weight losses similar to those of total unstressed starvation when receiving as much as 50% of calories needed (Hill & Beddoe, 1988). In early unstressed starvation, a great deal of muscle protein is catabolized daily to provide fuel; however, within a few days the body is able to reduce the amount of muscle catabolism and ketoadapt in order to maintain muscle mass. In stressed starvation, this regulatory function is impaired, and skeletal muscle will continue to be catabolized, resulting in further depletion of protein stores. The cost of unrelenting negative protein-energy balance is evident in organ dysfunction and negative clinical outcomes (Table 1–5).

The relationship between nutritional status and patient outcome is evaluated in terms of morbidity and mortality. To define this relationship, one must be sure that objective measures accurately predict nutritional status. Mullen et al. (1979) developed a prognostic nutritional index (PNI). The equation incorporated four measurements (albumin, transferrin, triceps skinfold, and delayed hypersensitivity) to calculate relative risk of mortality and morbidity. This model accurately predicted 89% of patients who developed complications after major GI surgery.

Table 1–5 Consequences of Malnutrition

Organ System	Pathophysiology	Clinical Outcome
CARDIAC	Decreased cardiac muscle mass	No evidence of cardiovascular disturbance
PULMONARY	Decreased diaphragm weight Decreased respiratory strength Decreased endurance	Inability to clear secretions; decreased tolerance; inability to wean from ventilator
IMMUNE FUNCTION	Decreased cell-mediated immunity Delayed cutaneous hypersensitivity	Increased incidence and severity of infection
WOUND HEALING	Decreased collagen synthesis	Delayed wound healing
SKELETAL MUSCLE STRENGTH	Alterations in muscle contraction Relaxation response Decreased muscle endurance	Fatigue; inability to perform activities of daily living

Source: Data from Kinney, J. M., Jeejeebhoy, K. N., Hill, G. L., and Owen, O. E. (Eds.). 1988. Nutrition and metabolism in patient care. Philadelphia: W.B. Saunders.

NURSING DIAGNOSIS AND CLIENT GROUPS

The nursing diagnosis most appropriate for the intervention of Feeding is Feeding, Self Care Deficit, *or* Self Care Deficit: Feeding, as described by the North American Nursing Diagnosis Association (NANDA) (1997). The diagnosis Feeding, Self Care Deficit characterizes the individual with impaired motor function or cognitive function, which causes a decreased ability to feed oneself (Carpenito, 1983). Neuromuscular impairments such as Parkinson's disease, muscular dystrophy, myasthenia, muscular weakness, and central nervous system tumors are contributing factors. Visual disorders can occur with glaucoma, cataracts, or cerebrovascular accidents. Situational factors are immobility, trauma, and the placement of external fixating devices that restrict arm movement. The elderly may experience decreased visual and motor abilities as well as muscle weakness and changes in taste and appetite.

Other nursing diagnoses in which the nursing intervention Feeding plays an important role include the four Sensory/Perceptual Alteration diagnoses in the NANDA taxonomy: Sensory/Perceptual Alteration: Gustatory, Sensory/Perceptual Alteration: Olfactory, Sensory/Perceptual Alteration: Tactile, and Sensory/Perceptual Alteration: Visual, as well as Altered Nutrition: Less than Body Requirements.

PROTOCOL FOR INTERVENTION

Feeding, an independent nursing intervention, has been a cornerstone of nursing practice since the days of Florence Nightingale. Nurses are involved in the day-to-day care of patients and are highly aware of feeding difficulties. They are present during mealtimes and are able to assess what patients are able to eat and to try to discern any problem with eating. A successful Feeding intervention ensures that the patient safely takes in adequate nutrients to meet metabolic demands (see Table 1).

Feeding as an intervention requires a specific plan that targets the deficit or cause of impairment. The ultimate goal is to provide adequate nutrients to prevent malnutrition. A secondary goal is to restore the patient's independence in this basic self-care activity. Assessment of the individual for a feeding plan should include a nursing history and physical examination. A thorough nursing history will determine the presence of risk factors and guide the clinician in a more focused assessment of the specific feeding impairment.

Assessment of Feeding Impairment

There is often a great deal of anxiety related to assessing why the patient will not eat. It can be difficult to identify whether the problem is physical or psychological. Emotional problems may be related to the patient's feelings about not eating. In the hospital setting, where patients have a lack of control over their environment, eating may be one area where they feel they can exercise some decision-making power (Ross, 1987). Furthermore, they may be angry at their diagnosis and displace their anger onto eating behavior. Additionally, the depression or despair related to a situational event can take the appetite away.

It is important to explore the patient's feelings about not eating. A subjective assessment should include the patient's own description of hunger and appetite.

Assessing patient level of consciousness will alert the nurse to those patients at risk for aspiration. Patients who were obtunded are obviously in danger of aspiration. Patients' cognitive abilities must be assessed, because this will affect their ability to understand and complete the task of feeding independently. Demented, disoriented, or confused patients, although alert, are at risk for feeding problems because of a lack of understanding of the importance of eating and the propensity for being distracted during the task.

Assessing the patient's physical ability to feed and identifying those patients with impairments is imperative for planning a successful intervention. Table 1–6 reviews key assessment criteria and suggests possible causes for deficits. Assessing the time it takes to eat may reveal patients who are slow. The pace of eating varies among individuals; however, patients who routinely take longer than 60 minutes to complete a meal may be partially dependent feeders and require assistance. In some patients, the ability to bring food to the mouth may be inconsistent. They often start out feeding themselves without problems but quickly tire. Poor coordination can result in food landing on a patient's bed, meal tray, or floor but never reaching the patient's mouth. Patients who are not

Table 1–6   Assessing the Patient's Ability to Eat

Assessment Criteria	Possible Cause of Impairment
Time it takes to eat	Dysphagia, fatigue, fear of choking
Ability to bring food to the mouth	Neuromuscular impairments, decreased endurance, fatigue
Ability to see all food on tray	Visual field cuts: cerebrovascular accident (CVA), glaucoma, cataracts, diabetic retinopathy
Ability to handle eating utensils	CVA, neuromuscular impairment, immobility, missing limbs, external devices, casts
Ability to chew food	Ill-fitting dentures, oral infections, poor oral hygiene, trauma, surgery to oral cavity
Ability to swallow food	Neurological impairment, cranial nerve damage

Source: Data from Buelow, J. M., and Jamieson, P. (1990). Potential for altered nutritional status in the stroke patient. *Rehabilitation Nursing, 15*(5), 260.

able to see the tray may leave various foods untouched. Patients who cannot handle utensils will eat those foods on the tray that can be easily picked up with the fingers and leave behind foods that require utensils. If chewing is a problem and proper menu selection has not occurred, patients will favor liquids and soft foods.

Identifying those patients at risk for swallowing difficulties and recognizing those with abnormal swallowing are critical pieces of assessing feeding problems. Ensuring the safety of patients by preventing potential aspirations is critical.

Signs of abnormal swallowing include

1. Packing food in the cheeks

2. Drooling

3. Throat clearing during a meal

4. Frequent coughing during a meal

5. Fluid leaking from the nose after swallowing demands

Implementation of Feeding Intervention

General strategies to improve nutritional intake relate to choices of menu and the accessibility of dietitians and food service personnel who can evaluate likes and dislikes and assist in meal planning. Patients should have a choice of menu to avoid food monotony. Dietitians should be accessible on the units during mealtimes to help assess individual preferences. Kitchen facilities should be available at the unit level to increase patient choices. Dedicated refrigeration and microwave supplies for patients encourage patients' families to bring foods that are appealing to patients and allow more flexible mealtimes.

Appetite is often impaired in a hospital setting for a variety of reasons, which obstructs the desire for food intake. Several strategies can be used to maximize or enhance an individual's appetite. First, the nurse can create a pleasant environment during mealtime. This can be done by clearing the area of unsightly bedpans, urinals, suctioning equipment, or dressing supplies. Reducing other noxious stimuli includes adequate pain relief before meals and avoidance of invasive procedures immediately prior to a meal.

Appetite can be enhanced by taste, smell, and vision. Taste alterations can occur as a result of radiation to the oral cavity, surgical resection to the tongue, medication, and oral infections. Oral hygiene is important to support the optimal function of taste buds. Routine mouth care should include the following:

1. Cleansing the mouth after each meal and at bedtime

2. Using a soft-bristle toothbrush

3. Rinsing with warm saltwater

4. Avoiding alcohol-containing mouthwash

5. Avoiding glycerine and lemon juice

The ability to smell prepared foods also stimulates the appetite. Although patients cannot participate in food preparation, offering them a chance to smell food before meals may stimulate appetite. Nurses can also reduce all noxious odors that might negatively affect appetite, allow patients to see the food to help stimulate their appetite, position the food so that it is visible, and describe the different foods. Description is especially important for patients with visual impairment.

Eating is ordinarily a time for social interaction (Sanders, 1990), yet patients are usually given meals in their own rooms. Creating social contact by feeding patients in a central area may be one option, as is encouraging family and friends to visit during mealtimes. Patients' care assignments should be designed so that patients requiring Feeding can be assigned to the same caregiver as much as possible. As the patient and caregiver develop a therapeutic relationship, the Feeding will become a more pleasurable and successful experience for both.

Patients with sensory or perceptual deficits require specific nursing actions to ensure adequate food intake. The nurse should be sure any corrective lenses are on and properly fitted and should describe the food and its location on the tray. The use of different color trays and dishes is helpful to patients with these deficits. Arranging the food in a clocklike pattern is an easy way to orient the patient to the position of various foods on the tray. Describing the position of foods is imperative for patients with visual field cuts. Food should not be placed on the blind side.

Cognitive impairments can result in the patient's misunderstanding the task of eating or being unable to complete the task because of a short attention span. Such patients require frequent cuing and close supervision. The following nursing actions are useful steps in feeding patients with cognitive impairments:

1. Create a quiet unhurried environment.

2. Explain the procedure.

3. Orient the patient to the purpose of feeding equipment.

4. Provide frequent cuing to the patient (e.g., "Mrs. S, pick up the toast," or "Mr. S, chew the food in your mouth").

5. Provide several small meals for patients with short attention spans.

Various neuromuscular impairments can make the seemingly simple activity of Feeding difficult or impossible. The occupational therapy department can be consulted for assistance in planning the Feeding intervention and the correct use of assistive devices. Patients with physical impairment should be allowed privacy and adequate time for eating, be positioned at a 90-degree angle with the meal tray at elbow height, and be provided with assistive devices (e.g., plate guards, built-up spoons).

Another physical factor that can affect patients' ability to feed themselves is endurance. They may be able to start the task but are quickly fatigued and cannot complete the task. The individual's ability to maintain a level of performance is related to the functioning of the cardiovascular, respiratory, neurological, and musculoskeletal systems. Creative planning by the nurse can provide rest periods before mealtimes. Rest periods should be scheduled before meals and after activities such as physical therapy and ambulation. Assisting in meal setup by opening packages and cutting food enables patients to conserve energy for eating.

Chewing and swallowing dysfunction are frequent additional reasons for difficulties in eating. Dysphagia accompanies various neurological insults. A team approach has been described in the literature for the successful management of patients with swallowing impairments (Emick-Herring & Wood, 1990). Speech pathologists can be helpful in localizing the impairment and suggesting useful strategies. The nurse must also understand the complexity of normal swallowing mechanisms in order to plan appropriate interventions.

The following four steps should be taken prior to Feeding to assess patient readiness:

1. Assess the level of consciousness; the patient must be alert.

2. Assess the patient's gag reflex by tickling the back of the throat.

3. Have the patient produce an audible cough.

4. Have the patient produce a voluntary swallow.

Feeding should take place in a calm, adequately supervised environment. Patients should be positioned in a normal eating position with the feeder clearly visible. Some patients may have difficulty moving the food bolus from the front to the back of the mouth. Food should be placed in the unaffected side of the mouth. If the tongue is damaged or impaired, assistive devices such as adapted feeding syringes will move food toward the pharynx, where the swallowing reflex (if intact) takes over. Once the food bolus makes it to the pharynx, the patient should tilt the chin down, to decrease the risk of aspiration. Massaging the throat on the affected side helps stimulate the tactile areas that initiate the swallowing reflex. Patients who have difficulty coordinating chewing, breathing, and swallowing should be instructed to hold the head forward and to hold their breath before swallowing. After the food is put in the mouth, the nurse should watch the thyroid cartilage to see whether the patient has swallowed and inspect the mouth before introducing more food into the oral cavity. Allowing sufficient time between each mouthful ensures that patients adequately chew and swallow the food. Nurses must be alert for signs that the patient is becoming fatigued, restless, or agitated. Suction equipment should always be available in case of an emergency, and nurses should know how to perform the Heimlich maneuver.

Evaluation of the Intervention

The intervention of Feeding is used to maintain or improve the nutritional status of patients. The nurses design creative strategies to assist or support the individual's ability to take in nutrition. One aspect of evaluation may be the achievement of independence in feeding. The Nursing Outcomes Classification (NOC) outcome of Self Care: Eating can be used to assist in the evaluation (Johnson & Maas, 1997). Evaluation of the success of the intervention must also include objective measures of nutritional assessment.

A comprehensive nutritional assessment must be completed initially to establish a baseline and evaluated serially to document the success of the nursing intervention. A comprehensive nutrition assessment allows the practitioner to diagnose the presence of malnutrition and identify the severity of malnutrition (Curtas, Chapman, & Meguid, 1989). Assessment should consist of the following:

1. Medical/surgical history

2. Physical examination: Height, weight, skinfold thickness, somatic muscle mass

3. Visceral protein status: Albumin, prealbumin, transferrin

4. Energy expenditure: Estimated/measured

5. Nitrogen balance

The most important piece of the nutritional history is a carefully chronicled description of weight change. This should include a history of weight loss or weight gain and the duration of change. Ask the patient the highest weight and the lowest weight achieved and determine whether the weight change was intentional or unintentional. It is often helpful to ask patients at what weight they considered themselves healthy.

Dietary history is an important component of a nutritional assessment and includes the type, consistency, and quantity of dietary intake. For example, a patient unable to take solid foods and dependent on liquids may not get adequate protein intake. Another with specific food aversions may have a deficient intake of certain vitamins or minerals. Elderly patients with limited financial resources or impairments in ability to buy or cook food typically eat diets high in carbohydrates and low in protein. Even a well-balanced diet in an insufficient quantity can result in a nutritional deficit. It is important to accurately document the duration of change of any alterations in dietary habits that patients describe.

Muscle and fat depletion is often obvious during physical examination of patients who are moderately to severely depleted. They appear cachectic, with wasting of fat stores. Bony prominences are obvious in the ribs and scapulae, and the arms and legs appear spindly. The waist is pinched in, and there is temporal wasting. Determination of height and weight will indicate whether a patient is at or below the ideal or usual body weight. Skinfold thickness and mid-arm circumference indicate the degree of fat and somatic muscle depletion. Biochemical levels define the presence and severity of visceral protein depletion. Table 1–7 identifies common nutritional assessment parameters used to determine the presence and severity of malnutrition. Downward trends in these measures should alert the nurse to reevaluate the nursing care plan.

Energy expenditure defines the caloric needs of individuals. It can be estimated by using the Harris-Benedict (1919) equation:

$$\text{Basal energy expenditure (male)} = 66.47 + (13.75 \times \text{weight}) + (5.0 \times \text{height}) - (6.76 \times \text{age})$$

$$\text{Basal energy expenditure (female)} = 65.10 + (9.56 \times \text{weight}) + (1.85 \times \text{height}) - (4.68 \times \text{age})$$

Energy expenditure can also be measured by using indirect calorimetry, a more accurate way to determine the energy requirements of patients (Feurer,

Table 1–7 Degree of Malnutrition

Indicator	Normal	Mild	Moderate	Severe
Albumin (g/dL)	>3.5	3.0–3.5	2.4–2.9	<2.4
Transferrin (mg/dL)	>200	150–200	100–150	<100
Prealbumin (mg/dL)	>20	10–15	5–10	<5
Weight (%IBW)*	90–120	80–90	70–80	<70
Weight (% UBW)†	96–120	85–95	75–84	<75

*% ideal body weight = [current weight/ideal weight] × 100
†% usual body weight = [current weight/usual weight] × 100
Source: Data from Curtas, S. (1988). Nutritional assessment. In C. Kennedy-Caldwell and P. Guenter (Eds.), *Nutrition support nursing core curriculum* (2nd ed., pp. 29–41). Silver Spring, MD: Aspen.

Crosby, & Mullen, 1984). Nitrogen balance evaluates the degree of catabolism and the adequacy of protein intake. In normally nourished individuals, the nitrogen balance should be 0; however, in many disease states and catabolic conditions, increased losses and decreased intake disrupt this equilibrium, resulting in a negative nitrogen balance (Mullen, 1981). Calorie counts document intake and compare it with the documented protein and energy needs.

The purpose of conducting a nutritional assessment is to make a nutritional diagnosis. Marasmus is defined as the wasting of body fat and skeletal muscle with a sparing of the visceral protein stores. This is often seen in patients suffering from prolonged starvation, chronic illness, or anorexia and in elderly patients (Grant, 1981). Overall dietary intake may be poor, but despite this low intake, there is a relatively adequate protein-to-calorie ratio. These patients appear malnourished on physical examination. Kwashiorkor is defined as the wasting of visceral proteins with a preservation of fat and somatic muscle. This is often seen in periods of acute illness when there is a decreased protein intake and a catabolism of skeletal muscle. Affected patients can have normal or above-normal anthropometric measures, but their serum proteins are depleted. They usually have increased extracellular water, pitting edema, and, in severe depletion states, ascites and anasarca. Some patients have a mixed marasmus-kwashiorkor, with aspects of both. This combination is associated with the highest risk of morbidity and mortality.

Interestingly, malnutrition assessed by a more subjective approach is often consistent with diagnoses made using traditional objective parameters. Various researchers have found approximately 80% agreement between the subjective global assessment (SGA) and the more traditional objective measures such as anthropometrics and serum proteins (Baker et al., 1982; Hirsch et al., 1991). They do suggest that the accuracy of the assessment may be related to the level of clinical expertise and the degree of malnutrition.

A second more recently studied method to assess nutrition risk is the nutritional risk classification designed as an admission nutrition screening tool for nurses (Kovacevich et al., 1997). Table 1–8 outlines the categories in the nutritional risk classification, which include diagnosis, nutrition intake history, ideal body weight standards, and weight history. This tool uses a combination of subjective and objective parameters to classify a patient as *at low nutritional risk* or *at nutritional risk*. The investigators found high interobserver agreement between the nurse and the nutritionist using the tool and a high degree of sensitivity (84.6%). The screening tool does not diagnose malnutrition but identifies those at risk who require further evaluation and early intervention.

SUMMARY

Providing nutrition, or Feeding, is deeply rooted in our culture as a symbol of caring and compassion (Knox, 1993). It is a basic need that evokes a great deal of emotion and sense of moral duty. Yet this usually pleasurable experience can become painful, humiliating, and even dangerous for some patients. Nurses using Feeding as an intervention must have a strong theoretical knowledge base regarding the physiological and psychological components of nutrient intake. This theoretical knowledge must be combined with the art of nursing to design active patient care plans.

Table 1–8 Features of the Admission Nutrition Screening Tool

A. Diagnosis

If the patient has at least ONE of the following diagnoses, circle and proceed to section E to consider the patient AT NUTRITIONAL RISK and stop here.

Anorexia nervosa/bulimia nervosa

Malabsorption (celiac sprue, ulcerative colitis, Crohn's disease, short-bowel syndrome)

Multiple trauma (closed-head injury, penetrating trauma, multiple fractures)

Decubitus ulcers

Major gastrointestinal surgery within the past year

Cachexia (temporal wasting, muscle wasting, cancer, cardiac)

Coma

Diabetes

End-stage liver disease

End-stage renal disease

Nonhealing wounds

B. Nutrition Intake History

If the patient has at least ONE of the following symptoms, circle and proceed to section E to consider the patient AT NUTRITIONAL RISK and stop here.

Diarrhea (>500 mL × 2 days)

Vomiting (>5 days)

Reduced intake (<½ normal intake for >5 days)

C. Ideal Body Weight Standards

Compare the patient's current weight for height to the ideal body weight chart.

If at <80% of ideal body weight, proceed to section E to consider the patient AT NUTRITIONAL RISK and stop here.

D. Weight History

Any recent unplanned weight loss? No _____ Yes _____ Amount (lb or kg) _____

If yes, within the past _____ weeks or _____ months

Current weight (lb or kg) _____

Usual weight (lb or kg) _____

Height (ft, inch, or cm) _____

Find percentage of weight loss: $\dfrac{\text{usual wt} - \text{current wt}}{\text{usual wt}} \times 100 = \%$ wt loss

Compare the % wt loss with the chart values and circle appropriate value

Length of time	Significant (%)	Severe (%)
1 week	1–2	>2
2–3 weeks	2–3	>3
1 month	4–5	>5
3 months	7–8	>8
5+ months	10	>10

If the patient has experienced a significant or severe weight loss, proceed to section E and consider the patient AT NUTRITIONAL RISK.

E. Nurse Assessment

Using the above criteria, what is this patient's nutritional risk?

_____ LOW NUTRITIONAL RISK

_____ AT NUTRITIONAL RISK

Source: Kovacevich, D. S., Boney, A. R., Braunschweig, C. L., Perez, A., and Stevens, M. (1997). Nutrition risk classification: A reproducible and valid tool for nurses. *Nutrition in Clinical Practice, 12,* 22.

CASE STUDY

RT, a 79-year-old female, was admitted to the hospital because of mild dehydration and malnutrition. She has a history of chronic organic brain syndrome/dementia and arthritis.

RT lives alone in an apartment and has no living relatives nearby. She has been homebound for the last 6 months because of increasing pain in her hands, back, and knees. RT's case is followed by a local visiting nurse, who has been providing Meals-on-Wheels and homemaker services.

RT appears thin but not wasted. She is 5 feet, 4 inches tall; her current weight is 108 pounds—86% of her ideal body weight and less than her usual 125 pounds. RT is alert and oriented to person. Serum protein values are as follows: albumin 2.9 mg/dL, prealbumin 9 mg/dL, and transferrin 120 mg/dL.

RT states that she has no appetite because of severe pain in her joints (8 on a scale of 1 to 10). The nurse's aide reports that RT takes no initiative in feeding herself. Assessment of RT's mouth reveals poor oral hygiene. Her gag reflex is intact, and she can produce an audible cough and a voluntary swallow. The nursing diagnoses are Al-tered Nutrition: Less Than Body Requirements; Feeding, Self Care Deficit; and Impaired Physical Mobility, secondary to joint pain.

The first step in the Feeding intervention is treating RT's pain, which is contributing to her anorexia. Pain management should be timed so that she is comfortable during mealtimes. The nurse has documented that the patient can safely swallow; however, RT is unable to feed herself because of limited mobility in her upper extremities. She is a partially dependent feeder and will need assistance in meal setup (opening cartons, cutting meats). Each meal should be supervised, and the environment should be calm and unhurried, with no distractions. The nurse should provide frequent cuing and simple commands to direct RT in the task.

Later evaluation reveals that RT describes an increased appetite. Objective measures of nutritional status are improved. With close supervision and frequent commands, she can now feed herself. Because of limited social support at home, RT is being evaluated by social services for placement in a nursing home.

References

Anderson, J. (1982). The significance of hunger to nursing. In C. Norris (Ed.), *Concept clarification in nursing* (pp. 192–222). Rockville, MD: Aspen Publications.

Athlin, E., and Norberg, A. (1987). Caregivers' attitudes to and interpretations of the behavior of severely demented patients during feeding in a patient assignment care system. *International Journal of Nursing Studies, 24*(2), 145–153.

Backstrom, A., Norberg, A. and Norberg, B. (1987). Feeding difficulties in long-stay patients at nursing homes. Caregiver turnover and caregivers' assessments of duration and difficulty of assisted feeding and amounts of food received by the patient. *International Journal of Nursing Studies, 24*(1), 69–76.

Baker, J. P., Detsky, A. S., Wesson, D., Wolman, S., Stewart, S., Whitewell, J., Langer, B., and Jeejeebhoy, K. N. (1982). Nutritional assessment. A comparison of clinical judgment and objective measurement. *New England Journal of Medicine, 306*(16), 969–972.

Bistrian, B. R., Blackburn, G. L., and Hallowell, E. (1974). Protein status of general surgical patients. *Journal of the American Medical Association, 230*, 858–860.

Bistrian, B. R., Blackburn, G. I., and Vital, J. (1976). Prevalence of malnutrition in general medical patients. *Journal of the American Medical Association, 235*, 1567–1570.

Buzby, G. R., Mullen, J. L., Matthews, D. C., Hobbs, C. L., Rosato, E. F. (1980). Prognostic nutritional index in gastrointestinal surgery. *American Journal of Surgery, 139*, 160–167.

Cahill, G. E., Jeejeebhoy, K. N., Hill, G. I., and Owen, O. E. (1988). Starvation: Some biological aspects. In J. M. Kinney (Ed.), *Nutrition and metabolism in patient care* (pp. 193–204). Philadelphia: W.B. Saunders.

Caldwell, M., and Kennedy-Caldwell, C. (1981). Normal nutritional requirements. *Surgical Clinics of North America, 61*(3), 489–507.

Carpenito, J. L. (1983). *Nursing diagnosis: Application to clinical practice.* Philadelphia: JB Lippincott.

Curtas, S., Chapman, G., and Meguid, M. (1989). Evaluation of nutritional status. *Nursing Clinics of North America, 24*(2), 301–313.

Donoghue, M., Nunnally, C., and Yasko, J. (1982). *Nutritional aspects of cancer care.* Reston, VA: Reston Publishing.

Dougherty, S. (1988). The malnourished respiratory patient. *Critical Care Nursing, 8*(4):13–22.

Emick-Herring, B., and Wood, P. (1990). A team approach to neurologically based swallowing disorders. *Rehabilitation Nursing, 15*(3), 126–132.

Ergun, G. A., and Miskovitz, P. F. (1992). Aging and the esophagus: Common pathologic conditions and their effect upon swallowing in the geriatric population. *Dysphagia, 7*, 58–63.

Feurer, I. D., Crosby, L. O., and Mullen, I. L. (1984). Measured and predicted resting energy expenditure in clinically stable patients. *Clinical Nutrition, 3*, 27–34.

Gavan, C. A., Hastings-Tolsma, M. T., and Troyan, P. J.

(1988). Explication of Newman's model: A holistic systems approach to nutrition for health promotion in the life process. *Holistic Nurse Practice, 3*(1), 26–38.

Grant, J. (1981). Current techniques of nutritional assessment. *Surgical Clinics of North America, 61*(3), 437–464.

Guyton, A. C. (Ed.). (1991). *Textbook of medical physiology* (8th ed). Philadelphia: W.B. Saunders.

Harris, J. L., and Benedict, F. G. (1919). *A biometric study of basal metabolism in man* (Publication 279). Washington, DC: Carnegie Institute.

Hill, G. L., and Beddoe, A. H. (1988). Dimensions of the human body and its compartments. In J. M. Kinney, K. N. Jeejeebhoy, G. L. Hill, and O. E. Owens (Eds.), *Nutrition and metabolism in patient care* (pp. 89–118) Philadelphia: W.B. Saunders.

Hirsch, S., deObaldice, N., Peterman, M., Rojo, P., Barrientos, C., Iturriaga, H., and Bunout, D. (1991). Subjective global assessment of nutritional status: Further validation. *Nutrition, 7*(1), 35–38.

Hogstel, M. D., and Robinson, H. B. (1989). Feeding the frail elderly. *Journal of Gerontological Nursing, 15*(3), 16–20.

Jeejeebhoy, K. N. (1990). Assessment of nutritional status. In J. Rombeau and M. Caldwell (Eds.), *Clinical nutrition, enteral and tube feeding* (2nd ed., pp. 123–127). Philadelphia: W.B. Saunders.

Johnson, M., and Maas, M. (Eds.). (1997). *Nursing outcomes classification (NOC)*. St. Louis: Mosby-Year Book.

Knox, L. S. (1983). Nutrition and cancer. *Nursing Clinics of North America, 18*(1), 97–110.

Knox, L. (1993). Ethics and nutrition support in the intensive care unit. *Critical Care Nursing Clinics of North America, 5*(1), 17–21.

Kovacevich, D. S., Boney, A. R., Braunschweig, C. L., Perez, A., and Stevens, M. (1997). Nutrition risk classification: A reproducible and valid tool for nurses. *Nutrition Clinical Practice, 12*, 20–25.

Leininger, M. M. (1988). Transcultural eating patterns and nutrition: Transcultural nursing and anthropological perspectives. *Holistic Nursing Practices, 3*(1), 16–25.

McCloskey, J. C., and Bulechek, G. M. (Eds.). (1996). *Nursing interventions classification (NIC)* (2nd ed.). St. Louis: Mosby-Year Book.

McWhirter, J. P., and Pennington, C. R. (1994). Incidence and recognition of malnutrition in hospital. *British Medical Journal, 308*, 945–948.

Mullen, J. L. (1981). Consequences of malnutrition in the surgical patient. *Surgical Clinics of North America, 61*(3), 465–487.

Mullen, J. L., Buzby, G., Waldman, M., Gertner, M., Hobbs, C., and Rosato, E. (1979). Prediction of operative morbidity and mortality by preoperative nutritional assessment. *Surgical Forum, 30*, 80–82.

Nightingale, F. (1859). *Notes on nursing: What it is and what it is not.* London: Harrison & Sons.

Norberg, A., Backstrom, A., Athlin, E., and Norberg, B. (1988). Food refusal amongst nursing home patients as conceptualized by nurses aides and enrolled nurses: An interview study. *Journal of Advanced Nursing, 13*, 478–483.

North American Nursing Diagnosis Association (NANDA). (1997). *Nursing diagnoses: definitions and classification.* Philadelphia: Author.

Openbrier, D. R., and Covey, M. (1987). Ineffective breathing pattern related to malnutrition. *Nursing Clinics of North America, 22*(1), 225–247.

Ross, B. (1987). Helping the patient who won't eat. *Nursing, 17*(4), 29.

Sanders, H. N. (1990). Feeding dependent eaters among geriatric patients. *Journal of Nutrition for the Elderly, 9*(3), 69–74.

Siebens, H., Trupe, E., Siebens, A., Cook, F., Anshen, S., Hanauer, R., and Oster, G. (1986). Correlates and consequences of eating dependency in the institutionalized elderly. *Journal of the American Geriatric Society, 34*, 192–198.

Sigal, L. K., and Daly, J. M. (1990). Enteral nutrition and the cancer patient. In J. Rombeau and M. Caldwell (Eds.), *Clinical nutrition, enteral and tube feeding.* (2nd ed., pp. 263–280). Philadelphia: W. B. Saunders.

Studley, H. O. (1936). Percentage of weight loss: A basic indicator of surgical risk in patients with chronic peptic ulcer. *Journal of the American Medical Association, 106*, 458.

Taylor, M. (1988). Food glorious food. *Nursing Times, 84*(13), 28–30.

Vick, R. L. (1984). *Contemporary medical physiology.* Reading, MA: Addison-Wesley.

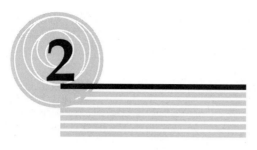

Sleep Enhancement

Felissa R. Lashley and Mary de Meneses

Disturbed sleep and the alteration of sleep patterns are prevalent complaints among both clients who have a specific illness and those considered healthy. The actual prevalence depends on the population surveyed and other methodological factors. Some type of sleep deprivation probably affects about 40% of the U.S. population at some time (Kryger, Roth, & Dement, 1994). Sleep alterations arise from a variety of causes. The spectrum of causes has been reflected in the International Classification of Sleep Disorders, developed by the American Sleep Disorders Association (Diagnostic Classification Steering Committee, 1990) (Table 2–1). Dyssomnias, the first major category of sleep disorders, include intrinsic sleep disorders in which the primary cause originates within the body. Examples are narcolepsy and obstructive sleep apnea syndrome. Extrinsic sleep disorders and circadian rhythm disorders are also classified under dyssomnias. In extrinsic sleep disorders, the cause is considered to be outside the body, such as in environmental sleep disorder or hypnotic-dependent sleep disorder. The second major category is parasomnias. Parasomnias are undesirable physical phenomena that can occur during sleep, arousal, or in the transition between sleep and arousal or vice versa. These include conditions such as sleepwalking and teeth grinding (bruxism). The third category consists of sleep disorders that are associated with medical/psychiatric disorders such as psychoses, alcoholism, and diseases such as peptic ulcer disease. The final category, called proposed sleep disorders, includes pregnancy-associated sleep disorder.

There is a good deal of variation in the length of sleep a normal person gets during the night due to age and gender—variables not subject to change by the nurse. In general, sleep is sufficient if there is no subjective complaint and no disruption of daytime (or waking time) performance. The range in hours for

Table 2–1 Classification of Sleep Disorders

Classification	Examples
DYSSOMNIAS	
Intrinsic sleep disorders	Narcolepsy, central sleep apnea syndrome
Extrinsic sleep disorders	Inadequate sleep hygiene, hypnotic-dependent sleep disorder
Circadian rhythm disorders	Disorders of the sleep-wake schedule such as time-zone change syndrome
PARASOMNIAS	
Arousal disorders	Sleepwalking
Sleep-wake transition disorders	Nocturnal leg cramps
Parasomnias usually associated with rapid eye movement (REM) sleep	Nightmares
Other parasomnias	Sleep bruxism, sleep enuresis
SLEEP DISORDERS ASSOCIATED WITH MEDICAL/PSYCHIATRIC DISORDERS	
Associated with mental disorders	Mood disorders
Associated with neurological disorders	Epilepsy, Parkinson's disease
Associated with other medical disorders	Fibrositis
PROPOSED SLEEP DISORDERS	
Pregnancy-associated sleep disorders	

Source: Adapted from Diagnostic Classification Steering Committee, 1990.

"normal" sleep in adults is 5.5 to 10 hours, with 7 to 9 hours being most usual (Kryger et al., 1994). The elderly have increased complaints of sleep problems; about 50% of those 65 years and older complain of these (Ancoli-Israel, 1997). The most common sleep problems seen in the elderly are sleep apnea, advanced sleep phase syndrome, periodic leg movement syndrome (affecting about 44% of the elderly), medical illnesses, and medication use in addition to poor sleep habits (Ancoli-Israel, 1997). Elderly people tend to sleep less soundly, wake more frequently and for longer times than when they were younger, and awaken earlier in the morning. There may be an increase in daytime napping (Asplund, 1996; Spiegel, 1981).

Whatever the cause, disruption of nighttime sleep due to insomnia is a common complaint or symptom but not a specific disease in itself. It may arise from a variety of causes. For example, it may be seen in a disorder of excessive sleepiness such as narcolepsy in which the affected person is sleepy during the day but has disrupted nocturnal sleep (Cohen, 1988). It may result from such diverse causes as schedule change, jet lag, acute stress (including hospitalization), grief, illness, anxiety, depression, drug or alcohol dependency, environmental factors such as noise, physical symptoms or problems such as pain or gastroesophageal reflux, poor sleep environment or habits and prescribed medications. Disturbed nighttime sleep may include difficulty in falling asleep, sleep fragmentation or awakening during the night one or more times with or without difficulty in returning to sleep, disturbing dreams, early morning awakening and inability to return to sleep, and feelings of not being rested upon awakening (Kryger et al., 1994; Kupfer & Reynolds, 1997). Consequences of a poor night's sleep in addition to sleepiness and fatigue include decreased performance levels, the propensity for accidents, cognitive and mood changes, and other effects.

This is particularly dangerous for persons such as truck drivers and those using dangerous machinery (Mitler, Miller, Lipsitz, Walsh, & Wylie, 1997).

The sleep disturbance most frequently encountered by nurses is insomnia, which can be caused by primary sleep disorders, medical or psychiatric illnesses, medications, pregnancy, or chronobiological problems. Insomnia has been reported to be a risk factor for the later development of depression and is one of the features of major depression (American Psychiatric Association, 1994; Chang, Ford, Mead, Cooper-Patrick, & Klag, 1997). The most common primary sleep disorders are narcolepsy and the sleep apneas. Narcolepsy is a central nervous system disorder with the following characteristic symptoms: excessive daytime sleepiness with sleep attacks, cataplexy, sleep paralysis (loss of muscle tone between awakening and falling asleep), hypnagogic hallucinations (vivid, terrifying hallucinations often occurring during sleep paralysis), and other visual and sleep-related disturbances (Aldrich, 1992; Baker, 1985; Cohen, 1988; Green & Stillman, 1998). Sleep apnea is defined as cessation of airflow for more than 10 seconds that may occur multiple times a night (National Center on Sleep Disorders Research, 1995). Sleep apneas are classified as obstructive, central, peripheral, or mixed. Symptoms of obstructive sleep apnea (the most common type) include excessive daytime sleepiness, sleep attacks, nocturnal breath cessation, and snoring, snorting, and gasping sounds. Nighttime sleep is disrupted and restless. Symptoms are usually noticed before age 40, and many of these patients are obese, hypertensive males. It is a potentially life-threatening disorder (Kales, Vela-Bueno, & Kales, 1987). In central apnea, cessation of respiratory movement accompanies airflow cessation. This type may be associated with neurological or neuromuscular disorders. In mixed apnea, there is typically a central apnea component followed by an obstructive component (Thorpy & Yager, 1991).

Insomnia must be assessed in terms of duration, severity, and nature. The major consensus statement on insomnia from 1984 is still used today, although the International Classification of Sleep Disorders categorizes insomnia by cause. Acute or transient insomnia lasts for several days and is seen in previously normal sleepers experiencing a stress such as schedule change, jet lag, or personal problems or an acute stress such as hospitalization. Short-term insomnia lasts for 1 to 3 weeks and may be associated with situational problems at work or with the family, or it may be due to illness. It can be precipitated by such events as grief, illness, or anxiety. Careful management using sleep hygiene techniques (discussed later) is critical in order to prevent persistent or chronic insomnia. Persistent or chronic insomnia is insomnia that has continued for more than 3 weeks or even for months or years and may be due to psychiatric, medical, or environmental conditions that include conditioned insomnia and drug or alcohol dependency ("Drugs and Insomnia," 1984). Hospitalized patients may be victims of sleep deprivation due to endogenous causes such as illness, stress, or drugs and also to exogenous causes such as environmental disturbances and frequent awakening. Hospitalization often results in transient or short-term insomnia (Erman, 1985). Severity of the insomnia is measured not only by the degree of sleeplessness experienced but also by the degree of impaired daytime performance and sleepiness that occurs.

ASSESSMENT

Before initiating the intervention of Sleep Enhancement (Table 2–2) aimed at restoring a comfortable pattern of sleep for individual patients, assessment of the problem is necessary. Assessment of sleep disturbances includes both objec-

Table 2–2 Sleep Enhancement

DEFINITION: Facilitation of regular sleep/wake cycles.

ACTIVITIES:

Determine patient's sleep/activity pattern

Approximate patient's regular sleep/wake cycle in planning care

Explain the importance of adequate sleep during pregnancy, illness, psychosocial stresses, etc.

Determine the effects of the patient's medications on sleep pattern

Monitor/record patient's sleep pattern and number of sleep hours

Monitor patient's sleep pattern, and note physical (e.g., sleep apnea, obstructed airway, pain/discomfort, and urinary frequency) and/or psychological (e.g., fear or anxiety) circumstances that interrupt sleep

Monitor participation in fatigue-producing activities during wakefulness to prevent overtiredness

Adjust environment (e.g., light, noise, temperature, mattress, and bed) to promote sleep

Encourage patient to establish a bedtime routine to facilitate transition from wakefulness to sleep

Facilitate maintenance of patient's usual bedtime routines, presleep cues/props, and familiar objects (e.g., for children, a favorite blanket/toy, rocking, pacifier, or story; for adults, a book to read, etc., as appropriate)

Assist to eliminate stressful situations before bedtime

Monitor bedtime food and beverage intake for items that facilitate or interfere with sleep

Instruct patient to avoid bedtime foods and beverages that interfere with sleep

Assist patient to limit daytime sleep by providing activity that promotes wakefulness, as appropriate

Instruct patient how to perform autogenic muscle relaxation or other nonpharmacologic forms of sleep inducement

Initiate/implement comfort measures of massage, positioning, and affective touch

Promote an increase in number of hours of sleep, if needed

Provide for naps during the day, if indicated, to meet sleep requirements

Group care activities to minimize number of awakenings; allow for sleep cycles of at least 90 minutes

Adjust medication administration schedule to support patient's sleep/wake cycle

Instruct the patient and significant others about factors (e.g., physiological, psychological, life-style, frequent work shift changes, rapid time zone changes, excessively long work hours, and other environmental factors) that contribute to sleep pattern disturbances

Encourage use of sleep medications that do not contain REM sleep suppressor(s)

Regulate environmental stimuli to maintain normal day-night cycles

Discuss with patient and family comfort measures, sleep-promoting techniques, and life-study changes that can contribute to optimal sleep

Source: McCloskey, J. C., and Bulechek, G. M. (Eds.). (1996). *Nursing interventions classification (NIC)* (2nd ed.). St. Louis: Mosby–Year Book.

tive and subjective measures. These may include family, medical, and social histories, sleep history, sleep diary, paper-pencil measures of sleepiness, and physical examination. Sleep laboratory data including polysomnography and the multiple sleep latency test may be necessary to make a definitive medical diagnosis (Cohen, 1997; Kryger et al., 1994). Polysomnography generally is performed in a sleep laboratory and consists of overnight measurement of, at a minimum, electroencephalogram, electrocardiogram, electromyogram, electrooculogram, and measurement of respiratory parameters plus other measurements suited to the diagnostic problem. The multiple sleep latency test consists of polygraphic monitoring of these same measurements that is usually done the day after polysomnography with nap opportunities given at 2-hour intervals five times a day. The parameter of interest is usually time to sleep onset and time of appearance of rapid-eye-movement (REM) sleep (Kryger et al., 1994). Home ambulatory recording may be used. The actigraph is a small device that records movement, based on the fact that fewer limb movements occur during sleep than during wakefulness (Hauri & Wisbey, 1992). Because sleep disruption, particularly of a persistent nature, is often associated with psychiatric disorders, psychiatric evaluation may be necessary for a complete assessment and treatment of the problem. In the final analysis, only the affected person can indicate his or her satisfaction with sleep (Closs, 1988).

If the patient is a regular client of the nurse or has a history on record, some components of the assessment may be obtained from the chart or existing records. Medication use should be assessed. Some medications known to contribute to sleep difficulties include adrenergic and dopaminergic agonists, steroids, thyroid hormone, antihypertensives, anticonvulsants, narcotics, cancer chemotherapeutic agents, antidepressants, theophylline derivatives, antipsychotics, central nervous system depressants, and stimulants. Alcohol, tobacco, and caffeine consumption also can cause sleep disturbances (Gregory, Simmon, & Berger, 1988; Kupfer & Reynolds, 1997). Paradoxically, some medications used to induce sleep can cause rebound insomnia after long-term use (Kupfer & Reynolds, 1997; *Physicians' Desk Reference*, 1998).

A full description of the sleep complaint is important to assess. Patients should be asked to describe their sleep problem—the duration, the circumstances under which it developed, factors that precipitate or accentuate it, previous treatment, and what the impact of the problem is on their lives and family (Gregory et al., 1988). If the patient says that he or she is not sleeping well, a first step is to clarify what is meant by that statement. Is it that the patient has trouble falling asleep or remaining asleep, or is it the quality of the sleep that is a problem? If they are awakening during the night, how many times do they awaken? Can they describe what it is that wakes them up? Items to assess directly related to the sleep history are shown in Table 2–3. It is helpful to question the patient's bed partner or roommate in order to get information on snoring, gasping, or apneic periods or the apparent presence of bad dreams, restlessness, leg movements, or sleepwalking ("An Office Work-up," 1986; Cohen, 1988; Kales, Soldatos, & Kales, 1980). Because the sleep environment is also important, a description of the room and surroundings in which the patient usually sleeps should be obtained (Table 2–4).

Other factors should be examined. Find out whether patients take daytime

Table 2–3 Assessment of Sleep

- Usual bedtime
- Usual "lights out" time
- Time patient falls asleep or how long it takes to fall asleep
- Tired when patient goes to bed
- Usual bedtime routine
- How often patient has difficulty in falling asleep
- Medications to sleep, and how often taken
- If patient wakes up at night and the reason
- How often patient wakes up at night
- Presence of parasomnias such as sleepwalking, bruxism, etc.
- Does the patient associate any event or reason for awakening?
- How long it takes to fall back to sleep
- What helps patient fall back to sleep
- If patient gets out of bed when he or she wakes up during the night. If so, what patient does
- Dreaming during the night. If so, were the dreams disturbing?
- Quality of sleep
- What time patient awakens in the morning
- Whether it is difficult to awaken in morning
- Whether patient takes any daytime naps. If so, number and length
- Body movements during deep sleep
- Snoring
- How patient feels upon morning awakening

Sources: Cohen (1988); Cohen, Ferrans, Vizgirda, et al. (1996); Lashley (1998).

Table 2–4 Assessing the Sleep Environment

- **Lighting:** Is the bedroom dark? Is a night light used?
- **Bedding:** How many and what type of pillow is preferred? Any special bedding? How many and type of blankets?
- **Temperature:** What is the preferred temperature of the bedroom?
- **Noise:** Is the bedroom usually quiet? Is quiet required to facilitate sleep?
- **Ventilation:** Does the patient like to sleep with window or door open or closed?
- **Positioning:** What is the usual sleep position?
- **Behavioral:** Does the patient usually sleep alone?

Sources: Cohen (1988); Cohen, Ferrans, Vizgirda, et al. (1996); Lashley (1998).

concerns such as those related to their job to bed with them. Probe to determine whether or not this is related to some specific recent change (e.g., a job layoff). Are there other emotional concerns such as those related to interpersonal or family relationships or financial problems that can be contributing to disrupted sleep? Are disturbing dreams or nightmares a cause of awakening, or is the anticipation of them keeping the patient from falling asleep? ("An Office Work-up," 1986; Cohen, 1988).

Physical symptoms are a frequent cause of sleep disruption, and sleep problems due to specific symptoms need to be addressed and relieved if possible. The sleep problem secondary to the symptom may then be resolved. For example, in a study of patients infected with the human immunodeficiency virus (HIV), the most common reason for sleep disruption was getting up at night to use the bathroom (Cohen, Ferrans, Vizgirda, Kunkle, & Cloninger, 1996). Thus the nurse must look at the role of such symptoms or disease manifestations. Does the person have to get out of bed because of the need to use the bathroom? Is the person having trouble falling or staying asleep because of pain, cramping, or other physical symptoms? Such symptoms as heartburn or gastric pain may cause difficulty when the person lies down. Respiratory symptoms such as shortness of breath or wheezing may contribute to problems. Patients may recall awakening because of choking or difficulty in breathing or because of their own snoring. Does the person complain of discomfort in the feet and legs that is relieved by getting up and walking around (restless legs syndrome)?

For longer or chronic sleep disturbances, it is often helpful for the patient to keep a sleep diary. This can be of assistance in establishing the sleep patterns for that particular individual and triggering events that disturb sleep. For the person with long-standing sleep pattern disturbances, this record should be maintained over a period of several weeks. It should include actual napping periods, the time the person gets into bed, the approximate time of falling asleep, the time of awakening in the morning, medication use and times taken, exercise patterns, mealtimes, cigarettes smoked, alcohol use, quality of sleep, and any feelings of emotional upset such as worry or stresses. Are the sleep problems of which the patient complains relatively constant or are they episodic? How does the person feel the next morning—tired, fatigued, excessively sleepy, or alert? Does the person have periods of falling asleep during the day? What other symptoms are experienced? The nurse should inquire about symptoms that are known to often accompany complaints of excessive daytime sleepiness such as losing muscular control, nighttime snoring, or sleep attacks ("An Office Work-up," 1986; Cohen, 1988; Cohen, Nehring, & Cloninger, 1996; Rall, 1990). For those experiencing sleep disturbances due to altered sleep-wake cycles, it is important to separate out short- versus long-term alterations (e.g., rapid time zone transitions like jet lag versus chronic shift rotation).

SLEEP ENHANCEMENT

Sleep Enhancement is defined by McCloskey & Bulechek as "facilitation of regular sleep/wake cycles" (1996, p. 513). Activities to implement the intervention fall into two basic categories: pharmacologic and nonpharmacologic. Often activities from one or both of these categories are used together to create a plan for Sleep Enhancement that addresses the needs of the individual client. The nurse is involved in all of these depending on his or her level of education, skill, and job. Research into nonpharmacologic approaches to Sleep Enhancement have been frequent in nursing. One of the major limitations common to many of these studies is the frequent choice of subjective, author-designed, nonstandardized measures for collecting data rather than use of questionnaires that have been more standardized or use of objective measures such as polysomnography. Many nursing research findings from 1987 through 1992 are summarized by Jensen and Herr (1993). Questionnaires for aspects of sleep disturbance most widely used include the Stanford Sleepiness Scale, the Epworth Sleepiness Scale, the Pittsburgh Sleep Quality Index, the St. Mary's Hospital Sleep Questionnaire, the Sleep Dysfunction Scale, the Sleep Disorders Questionnaire, and the General Sleep Disturbance Scale. Instruments to measure sleep may be found in the reference by Cohen (1997).

Pharmacologic Activities

There is a vast amount of literature on research into Sleep Enhancement pharmacologic activities and drug therapy to initiate or enhance sleep. Advanced practice nurses may prescribe such medications for patients with insomnia. Nurses in other roles are involved in pharmacologic management in other ways.

Drug therapy is indicated for certain types of sleep disruption, particularly for short-term insomnia. It is also useful to treat narcolepsy, one of the primary sleep disorders. In narcolepsy, it is important to note that large doses of central stimulants such as methylphenidate and methamphetamines are often necessary to achieve alertness. Frequently such patients are erroneously suspected of drug abuse.

There have been an assortment of drugs used to treat insomnia, including barbiturates, chloral hydrate, antidepressant medications, hypnotics, melatonin, over-the-counter medications, and others (Kryger et al., 1994). Sedative and hypnotic agents are most frequently used for the treatment of insomnia. They are generally central nervous system depressants, with the exception of the benzodiazepines. Currently, the benzodiazepines are widely used in the treatment of situational insomnia. Their effects as a group include sedation, hypnosis, decreased anxiety, muscle relaxation, and anticonvulsant activity. The major drugs of choice for short-term use are sedative-hypnotics, such as the benzodiazepines, cyclopyrrolines, and imidazopyridines. Examples of currently recommended hypnotics are estazolam (ProSom), flurazepam (Dalmane), lorazepam (Ativan), quazepam (Doral), temazepam (Restoril), triazolam (Halcion), zolpidem (Ambien), and zopiclone. Short-acting hypnotics (such as triazolam) may be used for those who have difficulty getting to sleep but who stay asleep once they do.

Thus, determining whether the problem is one of getting to sleep or of staying asleep is important in selecting the appropriate drug to give ("Drugs and Insomnia," 1984; Kryger et al., 1994; Kupfer & Reynolds, 1997; Maczaj, 1993). Relatively common side effects of these drugs as a group include weakness, lightheadedness, impairment of mental and psychomotor skills, memory difficulties (often occurring the next day), headache, blurred vision, dizziness, and gastrointestinal effects. Depending on what time the patient takes the medication, and depending on the duration of action, effects such as drowsiness, memory problems, and diminished coordination can occur in the morning. Generally, drugs are most useful for situational insomnia on a short-term basis of a few days. Often they are discontinued after acceptable sleep has occurred for one or two nights. Gradual discontinuation may be necessary ("Drugs and Insomnia," 1984; Kryger et al., 1994; Kupfer & Reynolds, 1997; Maczaj, 1993; *Physicians' Desk Reference*, 1998). On a long-term basis, hypnotic agents tend to produce rebound insomnia, and decreasing benefit is derived. Increases in nightmares may be found for a time after withdrawal. Caution is needed for use of hypnotic agents with the elderly. Major patient information and nursing measures to consider in the administration of the hypnotic drugs are listed in Table 2–5.

Nonpharmacologic Activities

Included in this category are sleep hygiene measures and environmental adjustments. Sleep hygiene measures include educational and behavioral approaches to Sleep Enhancement such as adjusting the environment to promote sleep. Application of sleep hygiene techniques is useful for improvement in sleep and prevention of chronic insomnia. These techniques can be rather easily implemented to at least some extent by the nurse in whatever setting the patient is located.

Manipulation of the environment to enhance sleep may be used in the hospital or at home. Many nursing research studies have demonstrated that hospital disruption, particularly noise, and nighttime awakenings disturb the sleep of hospitalized patients. Within the hospital, sharing a room with strangers, not being able to control temperature or lighting, and difficulty with sleep position are all potential sleep inhibitors. Topf, Bookman, and Arand (1996) found that well subjects exposed to sounds of the critical care unit in the laboratory had

Table 2–5 Information Related to Use of Hypnotic Drugs to Promote Sleep Enhancement

- Usually use for 7 to 10 days or less.
- Alert patient to report any unusual or disturbing thoughts or hallucinations and look for behavior such as agitation, confusion, or suicidal thoughts.
- Find out whether female patient is planning pregnancy or nursing infant.
- Do not use in pregnancy.
- Warn patient not to use alcohol or antidepressants with hypnotic drugs.
- Warn patient not to drive car or operate dangerous machinery until it is known if sleepiness or lightheadedness will occur.
- Let patient know he or she may experience rebound insomnia the first few nights after discontinuing medication.
- Patients should not increase or discontinue drug on their own.
- Take right before bedtime as instructed.
- A type of amnesia occurring in the period within several hours of taking the drug is possible; usually the person will be asleep but if traveling, this can be problematic.

Sources: Ashton, 1994; Maczaj, 1993; *Physicians' Desk Reference*, 1998.

poorer subjective sleep than those who were not exposed to these sounds. This nursing role was identified as environmental activist by Topf (1994), because the nurse enhances the person-environment compatibility. In Nursing Interventions Classification (NIC), the intervention is called Environmental Management: Comfort and is defined as "manipulation of the patient's surroundings for promotion of optimal comfort" (McCloskey & Bulechek, 1996, p. 257).

For persistent insomnia caused by disturbances of the sleep-wake cycle due to shift work, other changes may be needed. For example, the person who works 12 AM to 8 AM might plan to sleep on returning home in the morning, or later in the afternoon. Different eating and sleeping patterns can be tried for the most optimal results. Short naps may be useful. Work schedules can be adjusted so that forward rotation (moving from days to evenings to nights) occurs. Timed exposures to special bright artificial light and darkness over 2 to 3 days can be useful in resetting the biological clock. Depending on the degree of perceived difficulties, the person may choose to change his or her working schedule. Some people may feel that they need "permission" to do this.

Chronotherapy may be used for advanced and delayed sleep phase syndromes. In advanced sleep phase, sleep onset is early (from 8 PM to 9 PM) with early morning awakening (from 3 AM to 5 AM). Systematic advancement of bedtime can be used until the desired bedtime is reached. For elderly patients with advanced sleep phase disruption, Ancoli-Israel (1997) suggests using more exposure to bright light, particularly in the late afternoon and early evening. In delayed sleep phase syndrome, in which sleep onset is delayed until 3 AM to 6 AM with natural arousal at 11 AM to 2 PM, bedtime is delayed by 3-hour increments each day, establishing a 27-hour day until the desired bedtime is reached. Then the 24-hour day is reestablished (Kryger et al., 1994). Nonpharmacological sleep enhancement activities are included in the NIC intervention (see Table 2–2) and the reference by Hauri (1998). Various combinations of these may be used depending on assessment results.

ASSOCIATED NURSING DIAGNOSES

Sleep Pattern Disturbance is a broad nursing diagnosis that can apply when people experience a primary or secondary sleep disorder (McFarland & McFarlane, 1989). Sleep Enhancement is an appropriate intervention for this diagnosis (McCloskey & Bulechek, 1996; North American Nursing Diagnosis Association, 1995–1996). Because usual sleep patterns are individual, data collected through a comprehensive assessment as described in this chapter are needed to determine the cause of the disturbance for each person. Responses to sleep disturbances are also individual, and people may exhibit a variety of other related problems.

Pain, Fear, and Anxiety may be exhibited by people who have concurrent medical conditions that underlie the sleep disturbance. Fatigue and Altered Role Performance are likely to be present regardless of the reason for the disturbance, because of the lack of restful nocturnal sleep. Risk for Injury exists if people who are excessively fatigued continue to participate in their usual activities such as driving a car or working with heavy machinery. When people are deprived of sleep over an extended period of time, behavior indicating Sensory/Perceptual Alterations and Altered Thought Processes is often exhibited. Sleep Enhancement is also a nursing intervention for the Environmental Interpretation Syndrome, Impaired. Research into the effects of the intensive care unit environment on sleep deprivation has demonstrated that many patients who received less than 50% of their usual sleep time hallucinated and became disoriented, combative, paranoid, and delusional (Theland, Davie, & Urden, 1990). Ineffective Individual Coping and Knowledge Deficit may be present when individuals resort to chronic use of hypnotics and sedatives and over-the-counter medications to control a sleep disturbance. People with a primary sleep disorder that is chronic (e.g., narcolepsy) may experience Ineffective Family Coping and Altered Family Processes, especially if the family members have a difficult time believing that symptoms such as excessive daytime sleepiness and sleep attacks cannot be voluntarily controlled by the individual experiencing these symptoms. People with one of the sleep apnea syndromes experience Impaired Gas Exchange and Ineffective Breathing Patterns that may require extensive medical and nursing therapies. In infants, sleep disruption may contribute to Infant Behavior Disorganization, and Sleep Enhancement can be used in approaches to Infant Behavior, Potential for Enhanced, Organized that lead to integration. The reader is referred to other chapters in this book that may provide assistance in dealing with the variety of concurrent nursing problems that can occur when people experience a sleep pattern disturbance.

Outcomes

The central outcomes for this patient population are Sleep and Rest, defined in the Nursing Outcomes Classification (NOC) (Johnson & Maas, 1997) as extent and pattern of sleep and diminished activity for mental and physical rejuvenation. Other outcomes that may apply to individuals who experience a sleep pattern disturbance are

Adherence Behavior—Self-initiated action taken to promote wellness, recovery, and rehabilitation

Anxiety Control—Ability to eliminate or reduce feelings of apprehension and tension from an unidentifiable source

Comfort Level—Feelings of physical and psychological ease

Compliance Behavior—Actions taken on the basis of professional advice to promote wellness, recovery, and rehabilitation

Coping—Actions to manage stressors that tax an individual's resources

Knowledge: Treatment Regimen—Extent of understanding and skills conveyed about a specific treatment regimen

Pain: Disruptive Effects—Observed or reported disruptive effects of pain or emotions and behavior

Physical Aging Status—Physical changes that occur with adult aging

Quality of Life—An individual's expressed satisfaction with current life circumstances

Risk Control: Alcohol Use—Actions to eliminate or reduce alcohol use that poses a threat to health

Risk Control: Drug Use—Actions to eliminate or reduce drug use that poses a threat to health

Well-Being—An individual's expressed satisfaction with health status

CASE STUDY

Maudie, a 77-year-old woman, came to a neighborhood clinic with complaints of restless sleep during the night and daytime fatigue and sleepiness. She noticed these symptoms had been worsening over the past 5 to 10 years. When interviewed, Maudie described difficulty in falling asleep, frequent awakenings throughout the night, and difficulty returning to sleep. Sleep onset was problematic because she found herself ruminating about events of the day and because she had trouble finding a comfortable position for her legs. She spoke of an "inner sense of restlessness" relieved only by getting out of bed and walking for a few minutes. Once she was asleep, her sleep was not sound.

Her husband, Albert, confirmed that her sleep was restless. Three years ago, he decided to sleep in a separate bed in another room because Maudie snored loudly. One night Albert noticed that Maudie's legs twitched in a recurrent pattern. He was not sure if she stopped breathing for short periods during her sleep because they had not slept in the same room for several years.

When Maudie awoke in the morning, she described low energy, fatigue, and sleepiness—as if she had been fighting all night long. If she was active throughout the daytime, she would not fall asleep. However, if she was not in a stimulating situation, such as watching news on television, she would drift off to sleep. Maudie denied cataplexy, hypnagogic hallucinations, or sleep paralysis. She said she had some difficulty concentrating during the daytime, as well as memory difficulties. On two occasions, she fell asleep briefly while driving. She was so frightened by these incidents, she asked family members to drive when possible.

Initial Assessment

Maudie's physician wanted to determine whether she had sleep apnea syndrome, which occurs in elderly people who complain of daytime sleepiness and heavy snoring. He also wanted to evaluate Maudie for restless legs syndrome or periodic limb movements disorder, which occur on retiring to bed.

Further diagnostic testing was appropriate to clarify Maudie's diagnosis and to guide the physician's treatment plan.

Diagnostic Work-up

Routine admission diagnostic tests
Sleep laboratory studies, including polysomnography
Audiovisual recordings of sleep-related behaviors

The sleep study confirmed severe sleep disturbance at night, evidenced by disruptions in sleep continuity and sleep staging. Sleep apnea was confirmed by frequent apneic events and associated oxyhemoglobin desaturation. Clinical complaints of restless legs before onset of sleep confirmed the diagnosis of restless legs syndrome and periodic limb movements disorder. REM-sleep disorder was ruled out, as was any complex behavioral disturbance.

Treatment Plan

The initial step in Maudie's treatment was to address the sleep apnea syndrome. Nasal continuous positive airway pressure (CPAP) was successful in maintaining airway patency and thus preventing airway collapse, which leads to apnea. Positive outcomes documented included reduced frequency in apneic events during sleep and maintenance of oxyhemoglobin saturations at above 85% for most of the night.

The second step in treatment was easing both restless legs syndrome and periodic limb movements disorder with medication (clonazepam). Maudie was monitored by polysomnographic recording when this drug was first begun, because a benzodiazepine may exacerbate sleep apnea. Positive outcomes documented included a reduction in periodic leg movements and significant improvement in sleep continuity.

With the combination of these two treatments, Maudie noticed a marked improvement in her ability to fall asleep, sleep continuity, daytime alertness, and ability to perform her daily tasks. She also commented on not having as many frightening nightmares and on how well she felt since beginning treatments.

After her physician completed his instructions, a nurse met with Maudie to review some sleep hygiene measures that would help her get a good night's sleep. They discussed inexpensive ways to make her bedroom into a quiet, peaceful, and relaxed place where her chances of getting restful sleep were greater. The nurse helped Maudie identify some bedtime "habits" that she would enjoy trying on a regular basis. Maudie decided to go to bed at the same time each night (11 PM) and to rise at the same time each morning (7 AM). Although staying out of her bed except to sleep was not a significant problem for Maudie, she agreed to go to bed only for the number of hours she needed for a restful night's sleep (7 to 9 hours). On days Maudie had to set her alarm clock to make sure she got up on time, she decided to place the clock underneath her bed to minimize distractions. Also, she decided she would keep an interesting book on her bedside table because she learned that reading or watching television may lead to drowsiness. After the nurse finished discussing sleep hygiene measures, Maudie thought of other changes she could make: she and her husband could take their evening walk earlier (right after they ate—around 7:00 PM); she would change from taking a 10-minute shower to a relaxing hot tub bath around 10:00

PM; and before she went to bed, she would eat two graham cracker squares and drink a glass of warm milk.

Maudie was encouraged to keep her follow-up visits to the clinic, because continued use of the prescribed medication may help only temporarily. Her medication may need to be changed to another if her body adapts to the effects of clonazepam.

References

Aldrich, M. S. (1992). Narcolepsy. *Neurology, 42*(7 Suppl 6):34–43.

American Psychiatric Association. (1994). *Diagnostic and statistical manual of mental disorders: DSM-IV* (4th ed.). Washington, DC: Author.

An office work-up for sleep disorders. (1986). *Patient Care, 20*(2), 20–38.

Ancoli-Israel, S. (1997). Sleep problems in older adults: Putting myths to bed. *Geriatrics, 52,* 20–30.

Ashton, H. (1994). Guidelines for the rational use of benzodiazepines. *Drugs, 48,* 25–40.

Asplund, R. (1996). Daytime sleepiness and napping amongst the elderly in relation to somatic health and medical treatment. *Journal of Internal Medicine, 239,* 261–267.

Baker, T. L. (1985). Introduction to sleep and sleep disorders. *Medical Clinics of North America, 69,* 1123–1152.

Chang, P. P., Ford, D. E., Mead, L. A., Cooper-Patrick, L., and Klag, M.J. (1997). Insomnia in young men and subsequent depression. *American Journal of Epidemiology, 146,* 105–114.

Closs, S. J. (1988). Assessment of sleep in hospital patients: A review of methods. *Journal of Advanced Nursing, 13,* 501–510.

Cohen, F. L. (1988). Narcolepsy: Review of a common life-long sleep disorder. *Journal of Advanced Nursing, 13*(50), 546–556.

Cohen, F. L. (1997). Measuring sleep. In M. Frank-Stromborg and S. Olsen (Eds.), *Instruments for clinical health care research* (2nd ed., pp. 264–285). Sudbury, MA: Jones & Bartlett Publishers.

Cohen, F. L., Ferrans, C.E., Vizgirda, V., Kunkle, V., and Cloninger, L. (1996). Sleep in men and women infected with human immunodeficiency virus. *Holistic Nursing Practice, 10*(4), 33–43.

Cohen, F. L., Nehring, W. N., and Cloninger, L. (1996). Symptom description and management in narcolepsy. *Holistic Nursing Practice, 10*(4), 44–53.

Diagnostic Classification Steering Committee (Thorpy, M. J., Chairman). (1990). *International classification of sleep disorders* (Diagnostic and coding manual). Rochester, MN: American Sleep Disorders Association.

Drugs and insomnia. (1984). *Journal of the American Medical Association, 251,* 2410–2414.

Erman, M. K. (1985). Insomnia management. *Journal of Enterostomal Therapy, 12,* 210–213.

Green, P. M., and Stillman, M. J. (1998). Narcolepsy. Signs, symptoms, differential diagnosis, and management. *Archives of Family Medicine, 7,* 472–478.

Gregory, J. G., Simmons, E. C., and Berger, B. R. (1988).

Approaches to insomnia. *North Carolina Medical Journal, 49,* 502–504.

Hauri, P. J. (1998). Insomnia. *Clinics in Chest Medicine, 19*(1), 157–168.

Hauri, P. J., and Wisbey, J. (1992). Wrist actigraphy in insomnia. *Sleep, 15,* 293–301.

Jensen, D. P., and Herr, K. A. (1993). Sleeplessness. *Nursing Clinics of North America, 28*(2), 355–405.

Johnson, M., and Maas, M. (Eds.). (1997). *Nursing Outcomes Classification (NOC).* St. Louis Mosby-Year Book.

Kales, A., Soldatos, C. R., and Kales, J. D. (1980). Taking a sleep history. *American Family Physician, 22,* 101–107.

Kales, A., Vela-Bueno, A., and Kales, J. D. (1987). Sleep disorders: Sleep apnea and narcolepsy. *Annals of Internal Medicine, 106,* 434–443.

Kryger, M. H., Roth, T., and Dement, W. C. (Eds.). (1994). *Principles and practice of sleep medicine* (2nd ed.). Philadelphia: W.B. Saunders.

Kupfer, D. J., and Reynolds, C. F., III. (1997). Management of insomnia. *New England Journal of Medicine, 336*(5), 341–346.

Lashley, F. R. (1998). Sleep alterations. In M. Ropka and A. Williams (Eds.), *Handbook of HIV nursing* (pp. 471–483). Sudbury, MA: Jones & Bartlett Publishers.

Maczaj, M. (1993). Pharmacological treatment of insomnia. *Drugs, 45*(1), 44–55.

McCloskey, J. C., and Bulecheck, G. M. (Eds.). (1996). *Nursing interventions classification (NIC)* (2nd ed.). St. Louis: Mosby-Year Book.

McFarland, G. K., and McFarlane, E. A. (1989). *Nursing diagnosis & intervention: Planning for patient care.* St. Louis: C. V. Mosby.

Mitler, M. M., Miller, J. C., Lipsitz, J. J., Walsh, J. K., and Wylie, C. D. (1997). The sleep of long-haul drivers. *New England Journal of Medicine, 337,* 755–761.

National Center on Sleep Disorders Research. (1995, September). Sleep apnea: is your patient at risk? (NIH Publication No. 95-3803). Bethesda, MD: National Institutes of Health, National Heart, Lung, and Blood Institute.

North American Nursing Diagnosis Association (NANDA) (1995–1996.) *NANDA nursing diagnoses: Definition and classification, 1995–1996.* Philadelphia: Author.

Physicians' desk reference (52nd ed.). (1998). Montvale, NJ: Medical Economics.

Rall, T. W. (1990). Hypnotics and sedatives: Ethanol. In A. G. Gilman, T. W. Rall, A. S. Nies, and P. Taylor

(Eds.), *Goodman and Gilman's the pharmacological basis of therapeutics* (8th ed, pp. 345–379). New York: Pergamon Press.

Spiegel, R. (1981). *Sleep and sleeplessness in advanced age.* New York: S. P. Medical Books.

Theland, L. A., Davie, J. K., and Urden, L. D. (1990). *Textbook of critical care nursing: Diagnosis and management.* St. Louis: C. V. Mosby.

Thorpy, M. J., and Yager, J. (1991). *The encyclopedia of sleep and sleep disorders.* New York: Facts on File.

Topf, M. (1994). Theoretical considerations for research on environmental stress and health. *Image: Journal of Nursing Scholarship, 26,* 289–293.

Topf, M., Bookman, M., and Arand, D. (1996). Effects of critical care unit noise on the subjective quality of sleep. *Journal of Advanced Nursing, 24,* 545–551.

Urinary Catheterization: Intermittent

Janet P. Specht, Meridean L. Maas,

Sally Willett, and Nancy Myers

Intermittent Catheterization is regular periodic use of a catheter to empty the bladder (McCloskey & Bulechek, 1996), leaving the client catheter free. Intermittent Catheterization is performed by the client or a caregiver and can be used by clients in their homes or in institutions. The catheterization can be done using clean or sterile procedures. The clean procedure is referred to as Clean Intermittent Catheterization (CIC) and is the one most often recommended, especially for persons living in their own homes (Grose, Brooman, & O'Reilly, 1995). The purposes of Intermittent Catheterization are to (1) eliminate residual urine in the bladder, (2) reduce urinary infections by reducing residual urine, (3) prevent incontinent episodes, (4) regain bladder tone, (5) achieve dilatation of the urethra (Grose et al., 1995), (6) increase client control of urinary elimination, and (7) facilitate self-care. Intermittent Catheterization is an intervention for specific types of urinary incontinence and for persistent urinary infections that also may cause incontinence. Intermittent Catheterization is an effective nursing intervention for Overflow Incontinence, Reflex Incontinence, and Urge Incontinence secondary to infection and inflammation of the bladder.

Nurses are frequently the health professionals who discover and assume responsibility for treating and managing the problem. Yet more than half of Americans with urinary incontinence have had no evaluation or treatment (National Institutes of Health, 1990). It has been estimated that health care providers are aware of only half of incontinent cases (Yarnell & St. Leger, 1979) because of the reluctance to report this intimate and embarrassing problem to physicians or nurses.

Incontinence is a regularly occurring problem, with about one third of persons afflicted reporting daily or weekly episodes of wetness (Burgio, Matthews, &

x

OK

x

OK

x

OK

OK

OK

OK

OK

Engel, 1991). Approximately 13 million Americans are affected by urinary incontinence, with the highest incidence among both noninstitutionalized and institutionalized elderly (Fantl et al., 1996). Although the incidence of incontinence in the elderly
is known to be substantially higher than the 4% incidence identified in the general
population, studies of prevalence vary widely in their findings. Approximately 30%
of community-resident elderly and at least one half of all nursing home residents
have urinary incontinence (Smith & Newman, 1990). In acute care settings, the
incidence of incontinence varies from 5.5% to 48% (Palmer, 1988), with settings
reporting higher incontinence rates having a higher proportion of elderly patients.
In a study of 18,084 patients of general physician practitioners in Great Britain—one
of the few studies including children—Thomas et al. (1980) found a 6% incidence
of incontinence among children 5 to 14 years, a 5% incidence in patients 15 to 64
years, and a 10% incidence among patients 65 years and older. The seriousness of
the problem for the elderly is underscored by the finding that elderly people who
are incontinent suffer the problem for an average of 9 years (Jeter & Wagner, 1990).
Further, there are an estimated 1 million nursing home residents incontinent of
urine, many of whom could be successfully treated if those afflicted, health care
providers, and families did not view treatment as futile (Palmer, 1994).

The nursing intervention Urinary Catheterization: Intermittent, as described in
the Nursing Interventions Classification (NIC) (McCloskey & Bulechek, 1996)
(Table 3–1), is evaluated in this chapter. The research base for the intervention is
summarized, and its use by nurses to treat incontinence is discussed. Despite its
potential to promote continence and to provide an alternative to indwelling
catheters or disposable pads, Intermittent Catheterization has received little attention in the nursing literature as a nursing intervention. The inclusion of Intermittent Catheterization in NIC emphasizes its importance as a nursing intervention.

Too frequently persons with urinary incontinence, families, and health care
providers, including nurses, assume that nothing can be done and too quickly
resort to disposable pads or indwelling catheters as the solution. In a survey of
three Massachusetts nursing homes, Ribeiro and Smith (1985) found that 40% of
the 412 residents had an indwelling urinary catheter. Getliffe (1997) reports a
prevalence rate of 10.75% for long-term catheterization from an unpublished
study conducted in three nursing homes in Great Britain. Although the use of
indwelling catheters in nursing homes is decreasing since the Omnibus Budget
Reconciliation Act (1987) mandated standardized assessment and reporting of
urinary incontinence and use of indwelling catheters, some use continues.

Indwelling catheters and disposable pads are frequently used in nursing homes
as the only interventions for incontinence. Although serious side effects, including
urinary tract infections and severe fistulas, can result from indwelling catheters,
and disposable pads are costly and offer no active intervention for incontinence,
indwelling catheters are used in approximately 16% to 28% of incontinent individuals living in long-term care institutions (Kunin, Chin, & Chambers, 1987; Ouslander,
Greengold, & Chen, 1987) and disposable pads are used in almost all nursing
homes. Disposable pads are the most common method of managing urinary incontinence (Herzog et al., 1989). The extent of use of disposable absorbent pads is
reflected by the growth in the market of the product, which increased from $9
million in 1972 to $496 million in 1987 (Urinary Incontinence Guideline Panel, 1992).

LITERATURE REVIEW

Intermittent Catheterization was first introduced after World War II as a bladder-
training technique for paraplegic and quadriplegic patients (Champion, 1976).

Table 3–1 Urinary Catheterization: Intermittent

DEFINITION: Regular periodic use of a catheter to empty the bladder.

ACTIVITIES:

Perform a comprehensive urinary assessment, focusing on causes of incontinence (e.g., urinary output, urinary voiding pattern, cognitive function, and preexistent urinary problems)

Teach patient/family purpose, supplies, method, and rationale of intermittent catheterization

Teach patient/family clean intermittent catheterization technique

Teach designated staff at child's daycare/school how to perform intermittent catheterization, as appropriate

Monitor technique of staff who perform intermittent catheterization in daycare/school settings and document as required by state regulations

Instruct designated staff how to monitor and support child performing self catheterization at school

Provide quiet, private room for procedure

Provide child a private place at school to store catheterization supplies and a school bag or other carrying case that is acceptable to child

Monitor child performing self catheterization on a regular basis, and provide continued instruction and support as needed

Demonstrate procedure and have a return demonstration as appropriate

Assemble appropriate catheterization equipment

Use clean or sterile technique for catheterization

Determine catheterization schedule based on a comprehensive urinary assessment

Adjust frequency of catheterization to maintain output of 300 cc. or less for adults

Maintain patient on prophylactic antibacterial therapy for 2 to 3 wk at initiation of Intermittent Catheterization as appropriate

Complete a urinalysis about every 2 wk to 1 mo

Establish a catheterization schedule based on individual needs

Maintain a detailed record of catheterization schedule, fluid intake, and output

Teach patient/family signs and symptoms of urinary tract infection

Monitor color, odor, and clarity of urine

Source: McCoskey, J. C., and Bulechek, G. M. (Eds.). (1966). *Nursing interventions classification (NIC)* (2nd ed.). St. Louis: Mosby–Year Book.

At that time Intermittent Catheterization was conducted only under sterile conditions by a physician. Patients were catheterized at frequent intervals throughout the day. The procedure worked much like a bladder drill. Thus, the rationale for Intermittent Catheterization was to train the bladder, prevent inhibition of the detrusor muscle by an indwelling catheter, and promote bladder muscle tone (Comarr, 1972). Early studies showed that patients trained in such a manner for about 7 weeks were able to void normally (Guttman & Frankel, 1966). Guttman and Frankel published results of an 11-year study of 476 paraplegic and quadriplegic patients for whom sterile intermittent catheterization was used and demonstrated that 62% of patients remained infection free and most patients regained normal voiding. In addition, there was low incidence of hydronephrosis, vesicoureteral reflux, and calculosis. Studies by Bors (1967), Walsh (1967), and Lindan and Bellomy (1971) also demonstrated a high percentage of sterile urine, a lack of complications, and success with regaining continence without continued catheterization. Only Pelosof, David, and Carter (1973) reported any negative findings using Intermittent Catheterization. They found two cases of hydronephrosis and recommended that renal function tests be performed before initiation of intermittent catheterization.

The introduction of Intermittent Catheterization was the biggest single advance in the management of neurogenic urinary elimination difficulties, because it allows regular emptying of the bladder and the ability to remain catheter free (Hasan et al., 1995; Oliver, 1990). The Intermittent Catheterization procedure was modified based on studies by Lapides, Diokno, Silber, and Lowe (1972) and Champion (1976) and is now taught as a clean, not sterile, self-catheterization used for bladder training as well as for clients for whom nerve supply to the bladder is disrupted.

Clean Intermittent Catheterization (CIC) is a clean, not sterile technique in which patients self-catheterize or are catheterized by caregivers at regular intervals. CIC is recommended for use in clients with urinary retention related to a weak or atonic detrusor muscle (as in neuropathy in persons with diabetes or in children with spina bifida), overflow incontinence related to blockage of the urethra (as in benign prostatic hypertrophy), or reflex incontinence related to spinal cord injury (Lapides, Diokno, Gould et al., 1976; Ouslander et al., 1985; Ouslander & Uman, 1985). The technique of CIC has been widely adopted for the long-term management of people with persistent large residual urine volumes (Oliver, 1990).

The rationale for CIC is based on the assumption that the blood supply to the bladder must be maintained in order to promote the bladder's ability to fight infection. The emphasis is not on maintaining sterility, but on frequent emptying of the bladder to prevent ischemia. Bladder overdistention slows bladder circulation, predisposes the bladder to infection, and prevents normal bladder muscle contraction. Thus, frequent clean catheterization of the bladder prevents overdistention, allows the bladder to fight infection, and promotes reestablishment of bladder muscle tone (Horsley, Crane, & Haller, 1982). The technique has been shown to reduce the incidence of complications associated with indwelling catheter use (Ouslander et al., 1995).

Lapides et al. (1976) reported a review of 218 patients who were taught CIC. The subjects' ages ranged from 4 to 84 years, with 145 subjects between 21 and 84 years of age. A number of different diagnoses related to voiding difficulties and incontinence were represented in the sample. The results of the survey were that for clients experiencing Reflex Incontinence or Overflow Incontinence, CIC combined with anticholinergic and alpha-adrenergic medication alleviated incontinence as well as chronic perineal dermatitis (Lapides et al., 1976). Confirming the findings of Lapides et al., Champion (1976) followed up seven patients for 1 year who used CIC and who had previously been managed with sterile intermittent catheterization. Urine specimens and renal function remained unchanged after use of clean compared with sterile intermittent catheterization for all the patients. In summary, the studies of Lapides and others (Champion, 1976; Hasham et al., 1975; Kass, McHugh, & Diokno, 1979; Lapides et al., 1975; Lapides et al., 1976; Lapides et al., 1973; Lapides et al., 1972) provide support for the use of the CIC intervention for treatment of reflex, overflow, and urge incontinence due to infection without complications of exacerbated urinary tract infection or compromised renal function, as long as catheterizations are frequent enough to maintain 300 mL or less urine volume in the bladder.

Most work with children has been done with those suffering from spina bifida (Kaye & Van Blerk, 1981) and spinal injury patients (Pearman, 1976). More recently CIC has been used for all categories of children with incomplete bladder emptying. CIC has dramatically improved bladder and renal function, greatly enhancing the duration and quality of life in children with these problems (McLaughlin, Murray, & Van Zandt, 1996). Altshuler, Meyer, and Butz (1977) instituted a clean intermittent self-catheterization program in 1973 with pediatric patients with spinal cord injuries and myelomeningocele patients, aged 2 to 17 years, at the University of Wisconsin Hospitals. Parents of young children were taught the procedure, and older children learned self-catheterization. Criteria for inclusion in the study were (1) a bladder capacity of more than 50 mL, (2) some anal sphincter tone, and (3) grossly undamaged kidneys and ureters. Although the children did not always regain continence without use of the intermittent catheter, all were able to remain dry between catheterizations. The clean intermittent self-catheterization intervention did provide a means for the children to manage their own urinary elimination. Most were able to learn quickly, the intervention allowed them to avoid wet clothing, and they were spared the embarrassment of accidents and odors that usually accompany incontinence. Further, the children were able to participate in more activities characteristic of their age groups, the intervention was not expensive, and the equipment needed was minimal and nonrestrictive of activities and socialization.

Other studies in children (Hasham et al., 1975; Kass, McHugh, & Diokno, 1979) indicate that age is not a contraindication for the use of the CIC intervention, although the equipment and techniques may be somewhat different. Wyndaele and Maes (1990) taught children aged 8 to 9 years old, who were previously catheterized by a parent, to self-catheterize intermittently. The 8- to 9-year olds were part of a sample of 75 patients who had bladder dysfunction for 1 to 16 years prior to the intervention and who performed CIC for an average of 7 years. Most of the patients had neuropathic bladder dysfunction. The majority of the patients regained continence, and 92% were continent at the end of the study period, although some were also assisted by medication. Sixty-two percent of the patients were able to remain dry with catheterization every 4 hours. Fourteen of 19 patients who started the study with hydronephrosis returned to normal following CIC. Fifteen of the patients experienced complications, but most were found to be due to inappropriate technique, and complications did not occur until after 5 years of using the procedure. Males, however, were found to be more susceptible to urethral wall damage and stricture from repeated catheterization. No recurrent infections were found in persons who were free of infection at the start of the study, and most of the patients who started the study with an infection improved. Based on their research, Kuhn and Zaech (1991) conclude that CIC can be of great help, with infection rates greatly reduced, in neurogenic bladder rehabilitation, provided persons are properly selected, motivated, trained, and monitored over time.

As found by Binard et al. (1996), who evaluated 246 consecutive time-directed catheterizations with spinal cord injured patients, there is often a high rate of "too early" and "too late" catheterizations, increasing the risk of urethral trauma and infections. Ultrasound bladder volume measuring devices, such as the PCI 5000 or the Bladder Manager developed by Diagnostic Ultrasound of Seattle, are useful for these patients in determining the appropriate bladder volume for initiating catheterization. Volume-directed catheterization is recommended to avoid unnecessary catheterization, particularly among spinal cord injured persons (Binard et al., 1996).

Specht et al. (1991) reported good success in restoring continence with the use of CIC in a state long-term care veterans' home with clients who had atonic bladders. However, they point out the need for further testing in the elderly, because much of the research with the intervention has been done with children and young adults. It is unclear whether complications might be more common in a geriatric population (Ouslander et al., 1985). Palmer (1990) advocates the use of CIC when surgical or pharmacologic intervention is inappropriate or unsuccessful for the voiding dysfunction with large volumes of postmicturition residual urine that becomes increasingly common with advancing age. If CIC will keep the older adult continent, whether in an institutional setting or in the community, every effort should be made to ensure that this is done (Palmer, 1990). Older persons often require Intermittent Catheterization less often than younger people with voiding problems, because residual urine accumulates more slowly in the older bladder (Oliver, 1990).

Nurses are often skeptical of the technique of CIC, fearing it will lead to infections or cause trauma to the urinary tract. There are mixed recommendations about the use of clean versus sterile technique for Intermittent Catheterization, particularly if the client is institutionalized or not performing self-catheterization. Nurses particularly struggle with the idea of clean versus sterile technique. Some sources recommend that while patients are in institutions the sterile procedure be used to prevent cross-contamination (Long, 1991). However, no studies have been reported that compared the use of the two forms of the Intermittent Catheterization intervention in institutions, making this comparison an important area for systematic nursing research.

Clearly, there is a strong research base for the use of CIC by nurses to treat reflex and overflow incontinence, to prevent urge incontinence resulting from urinary tract infection, and to avoid the use of indwelling catheters. The research base provides strong support for the CIC nursing intervention, which has the added advantages of flexibility, convenience, and low cost for clients across settings. These advantages also are important for use by nurses who are more apt to prescribe and implement the intervention when it is not costly and requires a minimum of equipment and time.

NURSING DIAGNOSES AND CLIENT GROUPS

The nursing intervention Intermittent Catheterization is proposed to treat specific nursing diagnoses of urinary incontinence as classified by the North American Nursing Diagnosis Association (NANDA) (1997). Assessment and diagnosis of the specific urinary incontinence diagnosis is essential for the appropriate prescription of intermittent catheterization. There are six urinary incontinence diagnoses in the NANDA taxonomy: Reflex Incontinence, Urge Incontinence, Overflow Incontinence, Stress Incontinence, Functional Incontinence, and Total Incontinence (NANDA, 1997). Specht et al. (1991) proposed a seventh diagnosis, Iatrogenic Incontinence. Although it results in one of the six NANDA diagnoses, it is useful to identify Iatrogenic Incontinence as a distinct diagnosis to encourage early detection and correction, which is most often discontinuation of the offending nursing or medical treatment. Intermittent Catheterization is usually effective in the treatment of Overflow Incontinence, Reflex Incontinence, and Urge Incontinence due to urinary tract infection and inflammation, and in Iatrogenic Incontinence when retention and bladder overflow are manifested. All these diagnoses can be observed in clients of all age groups; however, Overflow, Urge, and Iatrogenic Incontinence are most common among elderly clients, and Reflex Incontinence is most common among younger adults and children, who are more prone to spinal cord damage due to accidents or congenital anomalies.

Overflow Incontinence occurs when the bladder becomes sufficiently overdistended that voiding attempts result in frequent, small amounts of urine, often in the form of dribbling (NANDA, 1997). The causes of Overflow Incontinence are bladder hypotonia due to impaired bladder neuromusculature and bladder outlet obstruction. Large amounts of residual urine, hesitancy, slow stream, passage of infrequent small volumes of urine (dribbling), a feeling of incomplete bladder emptying, sudden leakage of urine related to bending or turning, dysuria, and a palpable full bladder are common signs and symptoms seen with all causes of Overflow Incontinence.

Urge Incontinence is involuntary urination that occurs soon after a strong sense of urgency to void (NANDA, 1997). Heightened urgency results from bladder irritation, reduced bladder capacity, or overdistention of the bladder. The irritation of the bladder stretch receptors causes spasms and emptying. The common signs and symptoms for Urge Incontinence are the ability to identify the urge to void and precipitancy. Urine loss is larger and more prolonged than with Stress Incontinence.

Reflex Incontinence is the involuntary loss of urine caused by completion of the spinal cord reflex arc (bladder contraction) in the absence of higher neural control (NANDA, 1997). Bladder filling or perineal or lower abdominal stimuli precipitate reflex bladder contraction. Voiding is observed when a specific and predictable volume is reached with no reported sensation of urgency or voiding (Wheatley, 1982).

Iatrogenic Incontinence results from physician- and/or nurse-controlled factors, such as restraints, medications, fluid limitations, bed rest, and intravenous fluids (Specht & Mass, in press). Without the treatment the client would be continent; thus assessment data for the diagnosis include onset of incontinence coincident with the initiation of medical or nursing treatments that can influence control of urine.

PROTOCOL FOR INTERVENTION

The first step of the intervention protocol is to perform a comprehensive assessment of the client in order to determine the specific nursing diagnoses of urinary incontinence and to focus on causes (McCloskey & Bulechek, 1996; Specht & Mass, in press) (Table 3–2). The NIC intervention includes this step as the first activity listed. The activity, however, does not note the importance of identifying a specific incontinence diagnosis. Although the activities included in the NIC intervention are appropriate, they too often refer only to children. The NIC intervention should be revised to state the need for the nurse to identify the specific incontinence diagnosis(es) of the patient and to include activities that apply to all age groups, especially the elderly. Detailed discussion and tools for assessment are reported by Specht and Maas (in press). Many clients, particularly the elderly, have two or more specific incontinence diagnoses. Thus, Intermittent Catheterization is often prescribed along with another nursing intervention (e.g., Kegel's exercises for Stress Incontinence).

The next step of the intervention protocol is to teach the client, family, or staff caregivers the basic rationale for Intermittent Catheterization as a nursing intervention to treat the specific nursing diagnosis of incontinence. The basic rationale is that overdistention of the bladder (150 mL for clients 1 to 5 years, 240 mL for clients 6 to 9 years, and >300 mL for clients 9 years and older) (Lowe, 1982) causes bladder wall ischemia and interferes with the bladder's ability to fight infection and its muscle contractility. Thus, if the bladder volume is kept equal to or less than 300 mL in older children and adults, continence is

Table 3–2 Linkage of Urinary Catheterization: Intermittent with NANDA
Diagnoses and NOC Outcomes

DIAGNOSES	OUTCOMES
Reflex Incontinence	Knowledge: Treatment Regimen
Urge Incontinence	Urinary Continence
Urinary Retention (Overflow Incontinence)	Urinary Elimination
	ASSOCIATED OUTCOMES
Urinary Elimination: Altered	Infection Status
ASSOCIATED DIAGNOSES	Self-Care: Toileting
Altered Sexuality Patterns	Self-Esteem
Impaired Social Interaction	Social Involvement
Risk for Impaired Skin Integrity	Tissue Integrity: Skin and Mucous
Risk for Infection	Membranes
Self-Care Deficit: Toileting	Well-Being
Self Esteem Disturbance	

Sources: Johnson, M. R., and Maas, M. L. (Eds.). (1997). *Nursing outcomes classification (NOC)*. St. Louis: Mosby–
Year Book; North American Nursing Diagnosis Association. (1997). *Nursing diagnoses: Definitions and classification*.
Philadelphia: Author.

promoted by preventing urinary tract infection, kidney damage due to reflux of
urine up the ureters, and the ineffectiveness of detrusor muscle contractions to
empty the bladder. Recent research has revised the 300 mL volume to 400 mL
(Bakke & Vollset, 1993), and success of the revised volume is reported in practice
(Newman, Smith, & Goetz, 1992). Clients, family members, and/or staff are
also taught to not force fluids, because increased fluids contribute to bladder
overdistention and thus to incomplete bladder emptying, although it is important that persons have at least 1,000 mL of fluid in 24 hours.

Assessment for clients who will benefit from Intermittent Catheterization will
also include (1) manual and mental ability to perform the catheterization procedure or availability of a family member or staff caregiver who can perform the
procedure, (2) willingness of the client to do self-catheterization at regular
intervals or to have someone else do it, (3) 100 mL or greater bladder capacity
of the client to prevent too-frequent catheterization, and (4) an intact and unobstructed urethra (Lapides et al., 1976).

Next, the abilities of the client to perform self-catheterization are assessed,
along with the setting within which the client resides and the availability of
family or staff to perform the Intermittent Catheterization if the client is unable.
A candidate for self-CIC must have the manual dexterity to manipulate the
catheter and must be motivated to perform the technique frequently throughout
the day (usually when the bladder has distended with approximately 300 mL of
fluid) and in any number of settings. Caregivers must possess these same
qualities. A determination must be made whether to use clean or sterile Intermittent Catheterization, although outside a health care institution this is not debat-
able; the intervention is CIC. Although there is an insufficient research base to
evaluate the potential untoward effects of CIC in all settings, we believe that the
use of the clean technique enhances the maintenance of the needed frequency of
catheterizations and that it is more cost-effective and more convenient in all
settings. The advantages of frequent emptying of the bladder using the clean
technique are expected to more than offset any increased risk of infection.

Bacteria carried into the bladder will be quickly inactivated by the healthy bladder tissue (Lapides et al., 1975). Therefore, the use of CIC is recommended.

The person (client or other) who will be doing the catheterization must be taught catheterization technique along with care of the equipment (Grose et al., 1995). A step-by-step training procedure is the most proven method (Lin-Dyken et al., 1992). Detailed instructions for a catheterization procedure are provided in Table 3–3. The person should successfully demonstrate his or her skill to the prescribing nurse. For self-catheterization, having a full bladder while practicing the technique will help the person learn more quickly. Providing privacy for the client is important to avoid embarrassment. Before attempting the procedure, the client, family member, or staff person needs to be familiar with the equipment and body structures. For women doing self-catheterization, it is often helpful to use a mirror to visualize the vulva, labia, and meatus. A device known

Table 3–3   Procedure for Clean Self-Catheterization

Male	Female
Items Needed	Items Needed
Red rubber catheter	Red rubber catheter
Prepared container with Alconox and water (1 tablespoon Alconox to 1 gallon water)	Prepared container with Alconox and water (1 tablespoon Alconox to 1 gallon water)
Lubafax	Lubafax (optional)
Large container for urine collection—calibrated	Large container for urine collection—calibrated
	Mirror
Procedure	Procedure
1. Place 1 gallon water in a container large enough to hold catheters. Add 1 tablespoon Alconox.	1. Place 1 gallon water in a container large enough to hold catheters. Add 1 tablespoon Alconox.
2. Place catheters in Alconox solution and allow catheters to soak at least ½ hour.	2. Place catheters in Alconox solution, and allow catheters to soak at least ½ hour.
3. Wash hands well.	3. Wash hands well.
4. Remove catheter from Alconox solution and rinse well with tap water. Place in a convenient clean place.	4. Remove catheter from Alconox solution and rinse well with tap water. Place in a convenient clean place.
5. Squirt a small amount of Lubafax on tip of catheter.	5. Assume position with legs separated, mirror in place so meatus can be easily seen.
6. Pick up penis with left hand, and with right hand insert tip of catheter into penis. (Right hand will be used to pick up penis if you are left-handed.) Continue to advance catheter until urine starts to flow. From this point advance catheter approximately 1 inch more. Because a small catheter is used, it may be necessary to perform Credé's maneuver on bladder while catheter is in place.	6. Take catheter in right hand (left if left-handed), and separate labia with left hand. Lubafax may be squirted on catheter if desired. Insert tip of catheter into urethra. Continue to advance catheter until urine starts to flow. From this point, advance catheter approximately 1 inch more. Because catheter may be small, perform Credé's maneuver on bladder while catheter is in place.
7. Continue until urine stops flowing	7. When bladder is empty, remove catheter slowly, pausing at any point where urine starts to flow again. After catheter is completely removed, wash and set aside to be placed in Alconox.
8. When bladder is empty, remove catheter slowly, pausing at any point where urine starts to flow again. After catheter is completely removed, wash and place in Alconox solution.	8. If you wish to take catheter outside the home, rinse catheter, which has soaked in Alconox solution, and wrap in Saran Wrap. Be sure catheter is rinsed well in tap water so that no Alconox solution remains.
9. If you wish to take catheters outside the home, rinse catheter well in tap water after it has soaked in Alconox for at least ½ hour. Wrap catheter in Saran Wrap.	

as the Autocath can assist the patient in locating the urinary meatus, and foam or other devices can be used to help the person grip or manipulate the catheter more easily (Newman et al., 1992). For quadriplegics, however, an umbilical appendicovesicostomy procedure has been used to create a catheterizable channel and has been successful in enabling independent living for these patients (Sylora et al., 1997). Catheter size is dependent on the age of the client. A 12 to 14 catheter is recommended for adults. Red rubber catheters are more flexible and cause less trauma but may become brittle and difficult to clean. For this reason, some clinicians recommend plastic catheters (Newman et al., 1992). Lubrication (water-soluble gel) should be used when catheterizing males. For persons who complain of discomfort with catheterization, Xylocaine gel can be used as a lubricant. The patient should be monitored for urethral trauma from repeated catheterization, although the recent introduction of a disposable, hydrophilic, low-friction catheter (LoFric) promises to reduce these complications (Diokno et al., 1995; Waller et al., 1995).

It is important to monitor performance of the self-catheterization periodically after the individual has demonstrated proficiency and is performing the procedure independently. Some clients, particularly children and the elderly, often need ongoing instruction and support. Staff who perform Intermittent Catheterization for the client must also be monitored to determine that they are using the appropriate catheterization technique for the client, including persons in schools and in long-term care institutions.

Patients are frequently maintained on antibacterial medication for a period of 2 to 3 weeks, as well as on anticholinergic or cholinergic medications to assist bladder control (Horsley et al., 1982). Sterilization of the urine with antibacterial chemotherapy (e.g., nitrofurantoin, ampicillin, sulfamethoxazole) when the Intermittent Catheterization begins has been recommended (Lapides et al., 1976). However, more recent recommendations are to not use antibacterial chemotherapy when bladder infection is present and emphasize the importance of more frequent catheterization to maintain a volume of less than 400 mL of urine in the bladder (Bakke, Digranes, & Hoisaeter, 1997). In a study of 302 patients using CIC, bacteriuria was found equally among men and women, but clinical urinary tract infection (UTI) was significantly higher among women. Patients using anti-infective agents had fewer episodes of bacteriuria but significantly more clinical UTIs compared with nonusers (Bakke & Vollset, 1993).

Anticholinergics (e.g., oxybutynin, propantheline bromide) are prescribed for patients with uncontrolled bladder contractions as evidenced by incontinent episodes between catheterizations. The cholinergics (e.g., bethenechol) are used for persons who have atonic and partial motor paralytic bladders. The nurse should discuss the assessment data of the client's incontinence problem and the plan for treatment with the client's advanced practice nurse (APN) or physician to obtain the needed supportive medical therapy.

Prescribing the frequency of catheterization is the crucial step in the Intermittent Catheterization protocol. Catheterization every 3 hours and once during the night is recommended for most adults. However, the frequency of catheterization is determined by the amount of urine obtained at each catheterization. The frequency must be adjusted so that the volume of urine obtained is 300 to 400 mL or less for adults. If more than 400 mL is obtained, the interval between catheterizations must be shortened. Likewise, if the volume of urine is substantially less than 300 mL, the interval can be lengthened.

Urinalysis and renal function tests are performed prior to initiation of the Intermittent Catheterization intervention. Urinalysis should be repeated after 3 days of catheterizations, 5 days after the discontinuation of antibacterial medication, and every 2 weeks to 1 month thereafter. Renal function tests should be done every 6 months. Finally, the effectiveness of the Intermittent Catheterization must be continuously evaluated. A detailed record must be kept of the catheterization schedule, fluid input, and amount of urine obtained with each catheterization. Any voidings by the client must also be recorded, including the time and amount of urine voided. The nurse must closely monitor these data along with medications and the client's attitude and motivation regarding the catheterization intervention. Thus, if the individual is doing self-catheterization independently, it is important that the nurse teach the person to maintain a daily detailed record of the catheterization schedule, fluid intake, and fluid output. The desired outcomes of no incontinence episodes, absence of urinary tract infections, social enhancement, and voiding without incontinence are also monitored (see Table 3–3). This will require that the nurse teach the person or family the signs and symptoms of UTI and to monitor the color, odor, and clarity of the urine.

CASE STUDIES

Two case studies are presented to illustrate the use of the intervention with different diagnoses of urinary incontinence, the types of information that are needed to evaluate the intervention, and the problems that might be encountered.

Case Study I

Mr. DS is a 70-year-old man, separated from his wife, who has been living in a long-term care facility for the past 7 years. Mr. DS is alert and oriented but suffers from a number of chronic conditions. He has degenerative joint disease, with the left knee most affected, has left residual paresis from a cerebrovascular accident (CVA) suffered in 1979, chronic obstructive lung disease, hypertension, diabetes, and a history of alcoholism. He is 5 feet 10 inches tall and weighs 290 pounds. From April 1992 to January 1997 Mr. DS has had urinary symptoms the majority of the time. Symptoms included difficulty starting a stream, dribbling, and voiding in small amounts with recurrent bladder infections. In 1986 he complained of increased dribbling to the point of needing to regularly change his clothes because of wetting. In January 1994, a transurethral prostatic resection was performed for benign prostatic hypertrophy with bladder neck obstruction, found to be the cause of the recurrent urinary tract infections. In April 1994 he was still having some problems with dribbling, but it seemed improved. January through September 1995, Mr. DS had no urinary tract infections and little dribbling or incontinence. In October 1995 the dribbling increased; Mr. DS believed the increase was a result of his diuretic. Exasperated with the continued dribbling and wetness and the difficulty in maintaining his hygiene, Mr. DS demanded an indwelling catheter so he could remain dry. Whenever he had an indwelling catheter placed, he had increased difficulties with UTIs. Because he wanted to remain mobile, he wanted a leg bag on in the daytime, making it impossible to maintain a closed system of drainage and increasing his risk for infection. He had an indwelling catheter intermittently until September 1996, when he had an indwelling catheter continuously until January 1997. Evaluations at the Genitourinary (GU) Clinic at the Veterans Administration Medical Center (VAMC) recommended removal of the catheter, but Mr. DS refused to be without the catheter if he was always to be wet.

At the time of his evaluation at the GU Clinic at the VAMC in November 1996, he was diagnosed with hyperspastic bladder/hypertonic neurogenic bladder. A cystoscopy and cystometrogram were done, which showed mild hypertrophy of the prostate, inflamed bladder, and a small-capacity bladder with uninhibited contractions. His bladder capacity was 120 mL, and his first detrusor contraction was at 70 mL of urine volume in the bladder. He was told at the clinic that nothing could be done about the dribbling and that he should not use an indwelling catheter. Mr. DS returned to the long-term care facility where he resided. He was unable to wear the condom catheter recommended at the VAMC because of his small penis and obesity. He again insisted that he have an indwelling catheter. Following a comprehensive assessment of his presenting signs and symptoms, his primary nurse made the following nursing diagnoses: Urge Incontinence due to chronic infection and inflammation, and small, hyperactive bladder; Overflow Incontinence due to a mildly enlarged prostate; and Reflex Incontinence due to sacral nerve damage secondary to CVA. The outcomes selected to be monitored by the nurse and Mr. DS were (1) Urinary Continence, focusing specifically on the indicators of "free of urine leakage between voidings," "absence of post void residual greater than 100-200 cc," "absence of urinary tract infections (less than 100,000 WBC)," and "fluid intake of 2500 cc or less"; (2) Urinary Elimination, monitoring indicators of "BUN within normal limits (WNL)" and "creatinine WNL"; and (3) Well-Being, particularly measuring "satisfaction with social interaction" (Johnson & Maas, 1997).

Mr. DS's nurse determined to use the intervention of Intermittent Catheterization to treat the three problems by targeting the causes of recurrent UTIs and bladder neck obstruction and to control premature reflex bladder emptying. A urinalysis was obtained showing 1+ *Escherichia coli* bacteria. His blood urea nitrogen (BUN) and creatinine levels were within normal limits. Mr. DS was agreeable to trying anything that might help. He had a large urine output, usually 1,000 to 2,000 mL every 8 hours. He was asked to restrict his fluid intake to 2,500 mL in 24 hours, a substantial reduction for him. In consultation with the physician, a 2-week series of Macrodantin 50 mg b.i.d. was initiated, and Ditropan two times per day was initiated to help control the uninhibited bladder contractions. Clean, rather than sterile, Intermittent Catheterization was used to enhance compliance with the frequent catheterizations required and to decrease the time required to carry out the procedure. Because Mr. DS's obesity and limited range of motion made it impossible for him to perform the procedure himself, the procedure was done by licensed nurses.

Before initiating the Intermittent Catheterization activities and to form the basis for the schedule of catheterizations-voidings, a 3-day urinary elimination record was completed to determine the number and frequency of incontinence episodes; number, frequency, and amounts of voidings; and Mr. DS's fluid intake. Because he was nearly al-

ways wet from the constant dribbling, the Intermittent Catheterization schedule was initially set up for every 2 hours with a protocol to have him void immediately prior to each catheterization. Instructions on the nursing prescription sheet were as follows:

1. Wash hands before beginning the catheterization.
2. Remove catheter from the Betadine solution and rinse with tap water. Place catheter on a clean paper towel.
3. Position resident comfortably supine.
4. Put on disposable gloves.
5. Lubricate tip of catheter.
6. Insert catheter and allow bladder to drain until urine stops flowing. Remove the catheter slowly when the bladder is empty.
7. After the catheterization is done, cleanse the meatus with soap and water.
8. Record urine output.

Instructions for care of the catheter between uses were as follows:

1. Wash the catheter with baby shampoo and water. Rinse with running water.
2. Place the catheter in a covered pan containing Betadine solution until the next use.
3. Change Betadine solution daily and change the pan weekly.
4. Use 10 mL of Betadine to 100 mL of tap water.

The amounts of voiding, the amount of urine obtained with catheterization, and the number of times Mr. DS was incontinent or wet during the 2-hour intervals were recorded. The procedure was implemented on January 16, 1997, at midday. During the first 2 days of the intervention, 300 mL of urine was obtained in one catheterization. Mr. DS had only two incontinent episodes; they occurred when he was absent from the unit and did not return for the catheterization. The positive results were shared with the staff and Mr. DS, and the schedule was changed to 3-hour intervals.

For the next 10 days, the 3-hour interval was used, with more than 300 mL obtained from only one catheterization. Many catheterizations resulted in no urine or in volumes of less than 50 mL. There were no incidents of incontinence, and Mr. DS's voidings steadily increased in volume. The schedule was then changed to every 6 hours. Amounts of Mr. DS's voidings continued to increase, and during the next 2 weeks he had only three incontinent episodes, all occurring during the day when he drank large amounts of fluid and delayed toileting because of social activities. On February 19, the Intermittent Catheterization procedure was discontinued. Monitoring of incontinent episodes continued through March 10 with no further incidents of incontinence observed. In March, his BUN and creatinine levels remained within normal limits, and a urinalysis result was negative. Mr. DS regained continence and voided on his own with no symptoms of urinary infection or dribbling. Mr. DS and the nursing staff were pleased with the outcome.

Case Study 2

Mr. JL is a 71-year-old widower who has lived in a long-term care facility for the past 3 years. He had a fracture of the sixth thoracic vertebrae of the spine with paraplegia following a fall from a roof in 1987. He also has a history of rectal ulceration, chronic obstructive lung disease, and cardiac arrhythmias. Since he was taught at a Veterans Administration Rehabilitation Center following his fall, Mr. JL has been doing CIC to manage Reflex Incontinence. Nursing-sensitive outcomes identified by the nurse and Mr. JL to be monitored and recorded every 3 months included (1) Knowledge: Treatment Regimen and indicators "description of rationale," "description of self-care responsibilities for ongoing treatment," "performance of treatment procedure," and "performance of self-monitoring techniques"

and (2) Urinary Elimination with indicators "urinary continence," "urine odor," "urine clarity," "urine microscopic findings WNL," "BUN WNL," and "serum creatinine WNL" (Johnson & Maas, 1997). Mr. JL performs the catheterization every 6 hours. He has enough upper-body control to carry out the procedure independently. However, during the past several months, he has had continuous, asymptomatic UTIs. More frequent (biweekly) monitoring of the outcomes and indicators was ordered by the primary nurse to evaluate whether the correct catheter cleansing technique cleared his UTIs. On investigation, it was found that he was doing inadequate cleansing of the catheter between catheterizations, causing the recurrent UTIs. Mr. JL's BUN and creatinine levels were within normal limits. The UTIs persisted, but monitoring of the amounts of urine obtained with each catheterization as part of his performance of self-monitoring revealed a pattern of large amounts of urine in the bladder, causing pressure in the bladder and eliminating the infection-controlling effect of adequate blood flow to the bladder wall. The interval between CICs was changed to every 4 hours. Mr. JL has no incontinent episodes between catheterizations and values the control that CIC gives him. This case study illustrates the use of CIC to manage Reflex Incontinence when it is not anticipated that the client will always need to manage urinary elimination with catheterization. It also illustrates the need for continued follow-up and evaluation to ensure that the procedure is carried out correctly with the desired outcomes achieved.

SUMMARY
■

Intermittent Catheterization is a nursing intervention for the nursing diagnoses Reflex Incontinence, Overflow Incontinence, and Urge Incontinence secondary to bladder infections and inflammation and Iatrogenic Incontinence that is often a cause for the other diagnoses. It is a versatile intervention that can be used across settings and can be performed by the client, family members, and other caregivers. The intervention can be used by clients across all age ranges, including young children and the elderly. The intervention is an alternative to indwelling catheters and disposable pads and can result in correction of long-term incontinence. We recommend the clean procedure, although the effects of its use, compared with sterile procedure, need more clinical research. One of the hardest obstacles to overcome with this intervention is the resistance to the required frequency to maintain a urine volume of less than 300 to 400 mL of urine in the bladder. Because of convenience, clients and caregivers are eager to do the procedure less often. The use of the clean procedure helps ameliorate this problem to some extent because less equipment and time are required to perform the procedure. Some clients are clearly opposed to catheterizations even for collection of data needed to diagnose the incontinence problem. Intermittent Catheterization may not be a viable option for these persons. Evaluation of the effectiveness of Intermittent Catheterization by monitoring the amounts of urine voided, the amounts obtained with catheterization, the number of incontinent episodes, urinary infections, urethral patency, and renal function is essential to ensure that the desired results are obtained, to provide feedback and encouragement to the client and caregivers, and to monitor for untoward effects.

A research base is developing for the use of Intermittent Catheterization by nurses to treat specific types of urinary incontinence. Nurses need to use the intervention more and share the results of clinical use in the literature. The CIC nursing intervention needs to be tested further with clients of all ages and in all settings. Continued nursing research is needed to test the nursing intervention Intermittent Catheterization to build the clinical knowledge required for nurses to treat the devastating condition of incontinence.

References

Altshuler, A., Meyer, J., and Butz, K. J. (1977). Even children can learn to do clean self-catheterization. *American Journal of Nursing, 77*(1), 97–101.

Bakke, A., Digranes, A., and Hoisaeter, P. A. (1997). Physical predictors of infection in patients treated with clean intermittent catheterization: A prospective 7-year study. *British Journal of Urology, 79*, 85–90.

Bakke, A., and Vollset, S. E. (1993). Risk factors for bacteriuria and clinical urinary tract infection in patients treated with clean intermittent catheterization. *Journal of Urology, 149*, 527–531.

Binard, J. E., Persky, L., Lockhart, J. L., and Kelley, B. (1996). Intermittent catheterization the right way! (volume vs. time-directed). *Journal of Spinal Cord Medicine, 19*(3), 194–196.

Bors, E. (1967). Intermittent catheterization in paraplegic patients. *Urologia Internationalis, 22*, 236–249.

Burgio, K., Matthews, K. A., and Engel, B. T. (1991). Prevalence, incidence and correlates of urinary incontinence in healthy, middle-aged women. *Journal of Urology, 146*, 1255–1259.

Champion, V. (1976). Clean technique for intermittent self-catheterization. *Nursing Research, 25*(1), 13–18.

Comarr, A. E. (1972). Intermittent catheterization for the traumatic cord bladder patient. *Journal of Urology, 107*(5), 762–765.

Diokno, A. C., Mitchell, B. A., Nash, A. J., and Kimbrough, J. A. (1995). Patient satisfaction and the Lo-Fric catheter for clean intermittent catheterization. *Journal of Urology, 153*, 349–351.

Fantl, J., Newman, D., Colling, J., DeLancey, J., Keeys, C., Loughery, R., McDowell, B., Norton, P., Ouslander, J., Schnelle, J., Stasken, D., Thes, J., Urich, V., Vitousee, S., Weiss, B., and Whitmore, K. (1996). *Urinary incontinence in adults: Acute and chronic management* (Clinical practice guideline no. 2, 1996 update. AHCPR Publication No. 96-0692). Rockville, MD: Agency for Health Care Policy and Research, Public Health Service, U.S. Department of Health and Human Services.

Getliffe, K. (1997). Catheters and catheterization. In K. Getliffe and M. Dolman (Eds.), *Promoting continence: A clinical and research source* (pp. 281–341). London: Balliere Tindall.

Grose, K., Brooman, P. J., and O'Reilly, P. H. (1995). Urological community nursing: A new concept in the delivery of urological care. *British Journal of Urology 76*, 440–442.

Guttman, L., and Frankel, H. (1966). The value of intermittent catheterization in the early management of traumatic paraplegia and tetraplegia. *Paraplegia, 4*, 63–84.

Hasan, S. T., Marshall, C., Robson, W. A., and Neal, D. E. (1995). Clinical outcome and quality of life following enterocystoplasty for idiopathic detrusor instability and neurogenic bladder dysfunction. *British Journal of Urology, 76*, 551–557.

Hasham, A. I., Meyer, J., Altshuler, A., Butz, M., Norderhaug, K., and Uehling, D. T. (1975). Clean intermittent catheterization for myelomeningocele. *Wisconsin Medical Journal, 74*, 117–118.

Herzog, A. R., Fultz, N. H., Normolle, D. P., Brock, B. M., and Diokno, A. C. (1989). Methods used to manage urinary incontinence by older adults in the community. *Journal of the American Geriatrics Society, 37*, 339–347.

Horsley, J. A., Crane, J., and Haller, K. B. (1982). *Intermittent catheterization: CURN Project, Michigan Nurses Association.* Philadelphia: Grune & Stratton.

Jeter, K., and Wagner, D. (1990). Incontinence in the American home: A survey of 36,500 people. *Journal of the American Geriatrics Society, 38*, 379–383.

Johnson, M. R., and Maas, M. L. (Eds.). (1997). *Nursing outcomes classification (NOC)*. St. Louis: Mosby–Year Book.

Kass, E. J., McHugh, T., and Diokno, A. C. (1979). Intermittent catheterization in children less than six years old. *Journal of Urology, 121*, 792–793.

Kaye, K., and Van Blerk, P. H. (1981). Urinary continence in children with neurogenic bladders. *British Journal of Urology, 53*, 241.

Kuhn, W., and Zaech, G. A. (1991). Intermittent urethral self-catheterization: Long term results (bacteriological, evolution, continence, acceptance, complications). *Paraplegia, 29*, 222–232.

Kunin, C. M., Chin, Q. F., and Chambers, S. (1987). Indwelling catheters in the elderly: Relation of catheter life to formation of encrustations in patients with and without blocked catheters. *American Journal of Medicine, 82,* 405–411.

Lapides, J., Diokno, A. C., Gould, F. R., and Lowe, B. S. (1976). Further observation of self catheterization. *Journal of Urology, 116*(2), 169–171.

Lapides, J., Diokno, A. C., Gould, F. R., and Lowe, B. S. (1976). Urinary tract infection in women: Part 2. *Journal of Practical Nursing, 26,* 25–27.

Lapides, J., Diokno, A. C., Lowe, B. S., and Kalish, M. D. (1973). Followup on unsterile, intermittent, self catheterization. *Transactions of the American Association of Genito-Urinary Surgeons, 65,* 44–47.

Lapides, J., Diokno, A. C., Silber, S. J., and Lowe, B. S. (1972). Clean, intermittent, selfcatheterization and treatment of urinary tract disease. *Journal of Urology, 107,* 458.

Lin-Dyken, D. C., Wolraich, M. L., Hawtry, C. E., and Doja, M. S. (1992). Followup of clean intermittent catheterization for children with neurogenic bladders. *Urology, 40,* 525–529.

Lindan, R., and Bellomy, V. (1971). The use of intermittent catheterization in a bladder training program. *Journal of Chronic Disease, 24*(12), 727–735.

Long, M. (1991). Managing urinary incontinence. In W. C. Chenitz, J. T. Stone, and S. A. Salisbury (Eds.), *Clinical gerontological nursing: A guide to advanced practice* (pp. 203–215). Philadelphia: W.B. Saunders.

Lowe, B. S. (1982). Intermittent catheterization procedure. In Section of Urology, Department of Surgery. Ann Arbor, MI: University of Michigan Medical Center.

McLaughlin, J. F., Murray, M., Van Zandt, K., and Carr, M. (1996). Clean intermittent catheterization. *Developmental Medicine and Child Neurology, 38,* 446–454.

McCloskey, J. C., and Bulechek, G. M. (Eds.). (1996). *Nursing interventions classification (NIC)* (2nd ed.). St. Louis: Mosby-Year Book.

National Institutes of Health. (1990). Urinary incontinence in adults. National Institutes of Health Consensus Development Conference. *Journal of the American Geriatrics Society, 38,* 265–272.

Newman, D. K., Smith, D. A., and Goetz, G. (1992). Neurogenic bladder dysfunction causing urinary retention. *Journal of Home Health Practice, 4*(4), 45–60.

North American Nursing Diagnosis Association (NANDA). (1997). *Nursing diagnoses: Definitions and classification.* Philadelphia: Author.

Oliver, L. (1990). The neurogenic bladder. In K. Jeter, N. Faller, and C. Norton (Eds.), *Nursing for continence* (pp. 169–184). Philadelphia: W.B. Saunders.

Omnibus Budget Reconciliation Act, Nursing Home Reform Amendments, Pub L. N. 100–203. (1987).

Ouslander, J. G., Greengold, B., and Chen, S. (1987). Complications of chronic indwelling catheters among male nursing home patients: A prospective study. *Journal of Urology, 138,* 1191–1195.

Ouslander, J., Kane, R., Vollmer, S. L., et al. (1985). Technologies for managing urinary incontinence (Health Care Technology Case Study 33). Washington, DC: U.S. Congress, Office of Technology Assessment.

Ouslander, J., and Uman, G. (1985). Urinary incontinence: Opportunities for research, education, and improvements in medical care in nursing homes. In E. L. Schneider (Ed.). *The teaching nursing home* (pp. 173–197). New York: Raven Press.

Palmer, M. H. (1988). Incontinence: The magnitude of the problem. *Nursing Clinics of North America, 23*(139), 139–157.

Palmer, M. H. (1990). Incontinence in the elderly. In K. Jeter, N. Faller, and C. Norton (Eds.), *Nursing for continence* (pp. 139–158). Philadelphia: W.B. Saunders.

Palmer, M. H. (1994). Basic assessment in management of urinary incontinence in nursing homes. *Nurse Practitioner Forum, 5*(3), 152–157.

Pearman, J. W. (1976). Urological followup of ninety nine spinal-cord injured patients initially managed by intermittent catheterization. *British Journal of Urology, 48,* 297.

Pelosof, H. V., David, F. R., and Carter, R. E. (1973). Hydronephrosis: Silent hazard of intermittent catheterization. *Journal of Urology, 110,* 375.

Ribeiro, B., and Smith, S. (1985). Evaluation of urinary catheterization and urinary incontinence in a general nursing home population. *Journal of the American Geriatrics Society, 33,* 479–481.

Smith, D. A., and Newman, D. E. (1990). Urinary incontinence: A problem not often assessed or treated. *Focus on Geriatric Care and Rehabilitation, 3*(10), 1–9.

Specht, J. P., and Maas, M. L. (in press). Urinary Incontinence. In M. L. Maas, K. Buckwalter, M. Hardy, T. Tripp-Reimer, and M. Titler (Eds.), *Gerontological nursing: Integrating diagnoses, interventions and outcomes.* St. Louis: Mosby.

Specht, J., Tunink, P., Maas, M., and Bulechek, G. (1991). Urinary incontinence. In M. Maas, K. Buckwalter, and M. Hardy (Eds.), *Nursing diagnoses and interventions for the elderly.* Redwood City, CA: Addison-Wesley.

Sylora, J. A., Gonzalez, R., Vaughn, M., and Reinberg, Y. (1997). Intermittent self-catheterization by quadriplegic patients via a catheterizable Mitrofanoff channel. *Journal of Urology, 157,* 48–50.

Thomas, T., Plymat, K., Blannin, J., and Meade, T. W. (1980). Prevalence of urinary incontinence. *British Medical Journal, 281,* 1243–1245.

Urinary Incontinence Guideline Panel. (1992). Clinical practice guideline: Urinary incontinence in adults (AHCPR Publication No. 92-0038). Rockville, MD: Agency for Health Care Policy and Research, Public Health Service, U.S. Department of Health and Human Services.

Waller, L., Jonsson, O., Norlen, L., and Sullivan, L. (1995). Clean intermittent catheterization in spinal cord injury patients: Long-term followup of a hydrophilic low friction technique. *Journal of Urology, 153,* 345–348.

Walsh, J. J. (1967). Further experience with intermittent catheterization. *Proceedings of the Annual Clinical Spinal Cord Injury Conference, 17,* 134–140.

Wheatley, J. (1982). Bladder incontinence: Four types and their control. *Postgraduate Medicine, 7,* 75–82.

Wyndaele, J., and Maes, D. (1990). Clean intermittent self-catheterization: A 12-year followup. *Journal of Urology, 43,* 906–908.

Yarnell, J., and St. Leger, A. (1979). The prevalence, severity, and factors associated with urinary incontinence in a random sample of the elderly. *Age and Ageing, 8*(2), 81–85.

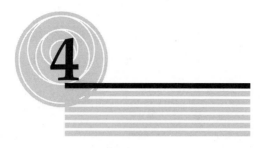

Pelvic Floor Exercise

Carolyn M. Sampselle and Sandra H. Hines

U rinary incontinence is defined by the International Continence Society as the involuntary loss of urine that results in a social or hygienic problem and is objectively demonstrable (Bates et al., 1979). There are four major classifications or types: (1) urge, associated with a strong sense of urgency; (2) stress, associated with activities that increase intra-abdominal pressure such as coughing, sneezing, laughing, lifting, brisk walking, or jogging; (3) mixed, which is a combination of urge and stress incontinence; and (4) overflow, associated with overdistention of the bladder. Types 1, 2, and 3 are most commonly found in women, whereas type 4 is most often found in men. In recent years, substantial federal resources have been allocated to the study of incontinence. This has generated a body of research results that provides a strong evidence base for nursing practice (Fantl et al., 1996).

Some of the most convincing evidence is for the value of Pelvic Floor Exercise, a method for strengthening the supportive muscles of the pelvic floor. In the Nursing Interventions Classification (NIC), Pelvic Floor Exercise is defined as "strengthening the pubococcygeal muscles through voluntary, repetitive contraction to decrease stress or urge incontinence" (McCloskey & Bulechek, 1996) (Table 4–1). The technique is also referred to as Kegel's exercise, in recognition of the physician who originally recommended its use in the United States (Kegel, 1948). Pelvic Floor Exercise is a self-care technique, effectively taught by nurses, that has demonstrated the ability to reduce or cure stress incontinence; the practice is also useful in conjunction with bladder training for the treatment of urge incontinence (Sampselle et al., 1997a). Although Pelvic Floor Exercise was developed to address the types of incontinence most often found in women, the practice also benefits conditions affecting males that will be identified.

Table 4–1 Pelvic Floor Exercise

DEFINITION: Strengthening the pubococcygeal muscles through voluntary, repetitive contraction to decrease stress or urge incontinence.

ACTIVITIES:

Determine ability to recognize urge to void

Instruct patient to tighten, then relax, the ring of muscle around urethra and anus, as if trying to prevent urination or bowel movement

Instruct patient to avoid contracting the abdomen, thighs, and buttocks or holding breath during the exercise

Instruct female patient to identify the pubococcygeal muscle by placing a finger in the vagina and squeezing

Teach patient to stop and start urine flow

Write instructions for patient to perform muscle tightening and urine stop exercises for 50 to 100 repetitions each day, holding the contractions for 10 seconds each

Teach patient that it takes 6 to 12 weeks for exercises to be effective

Provide positive feedback for doing exercises as prescribed

Use biofeedback to assist patient to know correct muscles are contracting and strength of muscle contractions

Discuss daily record of continence with client to provide reinforcement

Source: McCloskey, J. C., and Bulechek, G. M. (1996). *Nursing interventions classification (NIC)* (2nd ed.). St. Louis: Mosby–Year Book.

PREVALENCE AND SIGNIFICANCE OF URINARY INCONTINENCE

Approximately 20% of women between the ages of 25 and 64 years report urinary incontinence (Herzog & Fultz, 1990). This figure probably underestimates the true prevalence of the condition because of client reluctance in reporting. Lifestyle and developmental stages associated with the development of urinary incontinence include athletic and fitness activities, pregnancy and the postpartum period, perimenopause, and advanced age. A survey of women with an average age of 38.5 years revealed that 33% of those who exercised experienced incontinence; exercise that involved repetitive bouncing, such as running or high-impact aerobics, was associated with greater severity (Nygaard, DeLancey, Arnsdorf, & Murphy, 1990). Symptoms of urinary incontinence are common during pregnancy, as reported by more than half of all pregnant women (Dimpfl, Hesse, & Schussler, 1992; Sampselle, DeLancey, & Ashton-Miller, 1996). Following vaginal birth, approximately 8% of women who did not have objectively demonstrable symptoms of incontinence during pregnancy show leakage that persists through 12 months post partum (Sampselle, DeLancey, Ashton-Miller, & Antonakos, 1997b). History of vaginal birth is a significant predictor of incontinence across the life span. Women who have had even one vaginal birth are more than two and a half times as likely to report incontinence as are their nulliparous counterparts (Jolleys, 1988; Sommer et al., 1990). Incontinence increases in the perimenopausal years, when 31% of women report episodes at least once per month (Burgio, Matthews, & Engel, 1991). Lagace, Hansen, and Hickner (1993) documented increases in overall incontinence and in more severe or bothersome levels of accidental urine leakage among women in their forties and fifties. Among older women who reside in the community, 38% of those aged 60 years and older reported symptoms of urinary incontinence (Diokno, Brock, Brown, & Herzog, 1986). From these prevalence figures it is clear that incontinence affects large numbers of adult women at various points across the life span.

Many people consider urinary incontinence an inevitable and untreatable condition. Fewer than 50% of affected women seek advice from health care providers about the problem (Burgio et al., 1991). Therefore, it is essential that providers routinely screen clients for urinary incontinence when they present for health care.

Urinary incontinence exerts a tremendous impact on health, quality of life, and economics. In decisions that have direct bearing on physical health, incontinent women often elect to restrict their fluid intake (Brink, Wells, & Diokno, 1987) or discontinue a fitness activity that causes leakage (Nygaard et al., 1990). Emotional and social consequences of incontinence revolve around loss of self-esteem and diminished capability for an independent lifestyle. Documented difficulties include concern about visiting places where restroom location is unknown, problems if travel time exceeds 30 minutes, and fear of embarrassment (Wyman, Harkins, Choi, Taylor, & Fantl, 1987). There are also direct financial implications associated with the personal management of urinary incontinence. For those with limited income, the cost of absorbent protection may impose a financial burden. At the national level, Hu (1994) has estimated the direct cost of care for incontinent individuals living in the community at $11.2 billion annually. Moreover, incontinence is a major factor in the decision of family care providers to institutionalize a family member, with the additional economic drain on health care resources of an estimated $5.2 billion annually (Hu, 1994).

The Agency for Health Care Policy and Research (AHCPR) organized an interdisciplinary panel to review the existing research base on adult incontinence. A comprehensive literature search and critical evaluation rating the strength of the evidence resulted in publication of the *Clinical Practice Guideline: Urinary Incontinence in Adults* (Fantl et al., 1996). Convergent research support, based on the results of well-designed and implemented controlled trials, gave rise to the panel conclusion that: "Pelvic muscle exercises are strongly recommended for women with stress urinary incontinence" (Fantl et al., 1996, p. 36). Moreover, as pelvic muscle contraction is an integral component of bladder training, this self-care practice is important in the nursing management of Stress, Urge, and Mixed incontinence. The following sections discuss the related literature, intervention protocols, and associated nursing diagnoses and outcomes. The evidence base was derived from a search of literature available in Medline, CINAHL (Nursing and Allied Health), and the Wilson Index through May 1997.

REVIEW OF RELATED LITERATURE

The mechanism for the effectiveness of Pelvic Floor Exercise is not fully understood. The generally accepted explanation for the improved continence status is increased muscle strength (Miller, Kasper, & Sampselle, 1994). The pubococcygeal muscle is commonly believed to be the target of Pelvic Floor Exercise, but the entire levator ani, a complex muscle that includes the pubococcygeus, and the urogenital muscles are the actual exercise focus (DeLancey, 1994). Moreover, simple knowledge of the muscle function and conscious contraction are also important factors (Miller, Ashton-Miller, & DeLancey, 1998).

Functional Dynamics of Urinary Continence

Research has greatly expanded our understanding of the relationships between specific structures of the pelvic floor and how they function to maintain urinary continence (DeLancey, 1994; Gosling, 1985; Oelrich, 1983; Smith, Hosker, & Warrell, 1989a, 1989b). Effective function of the continence system depends on the interaction of several components or dynamics: (1) functional muscle attachments to the levator ani maintain a high position on the vesical neck, (2) the fascial attachments to the arcus tendineus contribute to the vesical neck support provided by the levator ani, (3) the internal urethral sphincter, at the level of the vesical neck, maintains urethral closure at rest, and (4) the more distal external urethral sphincter exerts urethral closure force at midurethra. These components are shown in Figure 4–1.

The first two components, attachments of muscle and fascia, are important to the maintenance of functional vesical neck support. In the presence of an abdominal pressure increase (e.g., during coughing, laughing, or bearing down), the urethra must be kept closed with pressure that is greater than that exerted on the bladder or leakage will occur. Supportive structures to the vesical neck and the urethra are necessary to achieve sufficient closure pressure. Intact connective tissue attachments of the suburethral fascia to the fascia of the arcus tendineus and to the levator ani muscles allow contraction of the muscles to produce a firm shelf or platform that remains relatively stable in the face of force generated by a cough or sneeze. The downward force exerted by the increased abdominal pressure encounters this firm platform, and as the downward force is halted, the urethra is compressed. A good analogy for understanding these pressure dynamics is a very flexible garden hose with water running through. If the hose is resting on solid ground and is stepped on, the water stops because the hose is compressed against the firm "shelf" of ground. On the other hand, if the hose rests on soft mud, when stepped on it just sinks into the mud and the water keeps flowing.

The third element of the continence system is the internal urethral sphincter at the level of the vesical neck. The involuntary, smooth muscle of the vesical neck operates in concert with the striated support to keep the proximal urethra closed. An open vesical neck allows urine to flow into the proximal urethra where, with the added load of increased abdominal pressure, it will escape before urethral compression can be accomplished. The importance of the internal urethral sphincter is readily seen when women with myelodysplasia are considered. The neuropathology of myelodysplasia includes an internal sphincter that

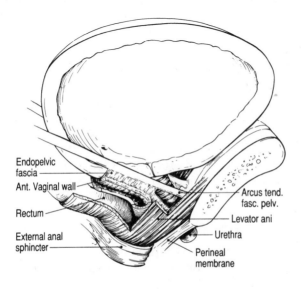

Figure 4–1   Lateral view of pelvic floor structures. (From DeLancey, J.O.L. [1994]. Structural support of the urethra as it relates to stress urinary incontinence: The hammock hypothesis. *American Journal of Obstetrics and Gynecology, 170,* 1713–1720.)

Endopelvic fascia
Ant. Vaginal wall
Rectum
External anal sphincter
Arcus tend. fasc. pelv.
Levator ani
Urethra
Perineal membrane

remains open at rest. Despite the presence of an otherwise intact and healthy pelvic floor, myelodysplastic women typically develop urinary incontinence (Wall, Norton, & DeLancey, 1993).

The fourth component is the external urethral sphincter. Its most important function is during a cough or other activity that raises abdominal pressure. During a sudden increase in abdominal pressure, resting pressure is not sufficient to maintain continence. At this point active events such as the extraurethral factors of fascial support, levator ani function, and the activity of the external urethra assume greater importance. In the presence of a sudden increase in abdominal pressure, the musculature must also provide additional force at the level of the external sphincter. This pressure supplements the resting urethral pressure and increases the urethral closure pressure. The supplemental forces must be brought to bear on the urethra if continence is to be maintained.

The complementary functions of the striated midlevel muscles and levator ani muscles are accomplished through the respective activity of type I and type II muscle fibers (Gilpin, Gosling, Smith, & Warrell, 1989). Type I (slow) fibers generate less intense, sustained contractions and provide postural stability over time. More specific to urinary continence, the continuous, although lower-intensity, contraction maintains a general level of support and resting urethral pressure. Type II (fast) fibers, on the other hand, produce a strong, rapid contraction. It is the action of type II fibers that is called into play when intra-abdominal pressure increases. Without the supplemental opposing force supplied by type II fibers, the increased abdominal pressure causes urine leakage. Type II fibers decrease with inactivity, innervation damage, and aging (Koelbl, Strassegger, Riss, & Gruber, 1989). It is noteworthy that in women with stress urinary incontinence, Gilpin et al. (1989) found that the percentage of type II fibers in the levator ani ranged from 0% to 10% as compared with 22% in asymptomatic women.

Research done using microtip pressure transducers to record pressure events in the bladder and the urethra demonstrates the role of the external urethral sphincter (DeLancey, Kyu-Jung, Ashton-Miller, & Stohbehn, 1996). The argument is as follows: If passive pressure transmission from the intra-abdominal to the extra-abdominal urethra was the only force determining continence, then it is logical to expect the greatest recording of force generated by a cough or sneeze to occur in the proximal urethra, because this is the area that is most proximal to the source of the pressure increase. Moreover, even if perfectly transmitted, this passive force in the distal urethra could not exceed 100%. In fact, microtransducer study reveals that the greatest area of force is *not* located in the bladder or proximal urethra. Rather, the highest level of force during a cough is exerted in the midurethra, where the external sphincter is located. In addition, the pressure elevation at midurethra is typically greater than 100% of the pressure recorded within the bladder. That is, the pressure in the distal urethra exceeds the level of abdominal pressure originally generated by the cough. Finally, the rise in urethral pressure precedes the intravesical rise, suggesting that some aspect of the event that increases abdominal pressure activates and prepares the pelvic musculature to counteract the imminent pressure. Clearly, this evidence documents an active role of the pelvic floor in the presence of increased abdominal pressure, a response that augments resting urethral pressure to deter urine leakage.

Up to this point we have focused on the integrity of the musculofascial structures, but it is also important to consider the role of innervation in muscle contraction. There is evidence of denervation in the form of slower conduction time and increased myofiber density. (Increased myofiber density occurs when increasing numbers of muscle fibers rely on innervation from a single motor axon.) In women with stress urinary incontinence, increased myofiber density has been demonstrated in the perineal branch of the pudendal nerve and in the striated muscle of the urethrovaginal sphincters (Snooks, Swash, Mathers, & Henry, 1990; Snooks, Swash, Sechell, & Henry, 1984).

Other investigators have demonstrated that women with stress urinary incontinence have significantly longer conduction times both to the striated urethral muscle and to the levator ani in comparison with their continent counterparts; for example, a woman with a pudendal nerve conduction time to the urethral sphincter of greater than 2.4 ms has a 97% chance of experiencing stress urinary incontinence (Smith et al., 1989a). In longitudinal studies of motor unit potential before and post birth, urinary incontinence developed in those women who had the greatest increase in motor unit potential (Smith et al., 1989b).

Taken together, the above evidence underlines the importance of the interrelationships among the various elements of the continence system. Although it is possible for a strong element to compensate for weakness in another aspect of the system, the most functional circumstance is for all elements to operate in concert to establish a dynamic response to any increase in abdominal pressure. Pelvic Floor Exercise obviously cannot restore disrupted musculofascial attachments, nor can it benefit the smooth muscle of the internal urethral sphincter. Rather, Pelvic Floor Exercise is designed to improve the functional capability of the levator ani and external urethral sphincter, both of which are composed of striated voluntary muscle.

Principles of Exercise Physiology

A review of exercise physiology reveals that when striated muscle is repeatedly contracted at maximum intensity, the cross-sectional diameter and the ability to exert force are enhanced (Goldberg, Etlinger, Goldspink, & Jablecki, 1975; Gonyea, 1980). In order for the desired improvement to occur, it is essential that the correct or target muscle be trained. This is particularly problematic with respect to Pelvic Floor Exercise. Many women are not aware of these muscles, hidden as they are within the pelvis, and do not understand their function.

Maximum or near maximum intensity of contraction is necessary in order to recruit those muscle fibers that are specialized to exert force (type II) rather than to endure over time (type I). It is estimated that approximately 70% of the muscle fibers in the pelvic floor are slow-twitch (i.e., specialized to maintain posture) (Gilpin et al., 1989). The fast-twitch fibers (i.e., those specialized to exert force) are drawn into use only after the majority of slow-twitch fibers have been recruited. Thus, the intensity of contraction must be greater than 70% if strength training is the goal.

Evidence-based Outcomes of Pelvic Floor Exercise

As originally conceptualized, Pelvic Floor Exercise was thought to be specific for stress urinary incontinence because the expected outcome of strengthened pelvic musculature was increased urethral closure pressure. Indeed, Pelvic Floor Exercise has demonstrated its effectiveness in treating stress incontinence, but it has also shown benefits for urge and mixed types of incontinence.

With regard to demonstrated stress incontinence, programs of Pelvic Floor Exercise increase muscle strength and reduce incontinent urine loss. Klarskov et al. (1986) found significant reductions in incontinence episodes with Pelvic Floor Exercise, with 42% of the participants so satisfied with their improved status that they did not desire surgical intervention. Similarly, significant improvement of nearly 50% was found in number of incontinent episodes and amount of urine lost among women who practiced Pelvic Floor Exercise (Nygaard, Kreder, Lepic, Fountain, & Rhomberg, 1996). In a randomized clinical trial, Burns et al. (1993) showed reductions in urine leakage for women with moderate and severe urine leakage who were assigned to a pelvic muscle training group (biofeedback-assisted Pelvic Floor Exercise) but not for those in a nontreatment group; moreover, 23% of the biofeedback group and 16% of the Pelvic Floor Exercise group experienced complete remission of incontinence symptoms. Dougherty, Bishop, Mooney, Gimotty, & Williams (1993) showed significant improvement in force and duration of muscle contraction and significant reductions of 62% in the amount of urine leakage and reported episodes of incontinence following a 16-week course of Pelvic Muscle Exercise.

Women with urge and mixed types of incontinence also benefit from Pelvic Floor Exercise. Among women who completed a 3-month program of Pelvic Floor Exercise, Nygaard et al. (1996) reported a greater than 80% decrease in incontinence episodes for those with urge type incontinence and a decrease of nearly 50% for those with mixed incontinence. In a group of older women, mean age 76 years, Flynn, Cell, and Luisi (1994) showed significant decreases of 82% in the number of incontinent episodes.

Long-term follow-up studies suggest that the positive effects of Pelvic Floor Exercise are maintained over time. In a 5-year follow-up of women who were taught Pelvic Floor Exercise, pelvic floor muscle strength increases were maintained and 70% of the women not treated surgically were satisfied with their present status (i.e., they did not desire more extensive treatment) (Bo & Talseth, 1996). Subsequent to a Pelvic Floor Exercise program, a survey at 2 to 7 years follow-up revealed that 11% were symptom free and another 44% continued to be improved (Hahn, Wilson, Fall, & Ekelund, 1993).

The intervention of Pelvic Floor Exercise is often recommended to minimize childbirth-related incontinence based, in part, on the convincing evidence of its benefit for symptomatic women. Dougherty, Bishop, Abrams, Batich, & Gimotty (1989) randomized postpartum women into two Pelvic Floor Exercise groups and one control group. No significant increases in pelvic muscle strength were found in any group, although those in the Pelvic Floor Exercise groups showed a pattern of greater strength at each time point. Postpartum women who participated in a specially designed 8-week Pelvic Floor Exercise protocol had significantly greater pelvic muscle strength at 8 and 16 weeks post partum than did their control counterparts (Morkved & Bo, 1996). Sampselle et al. (1998) randomized primiparae into a treatment group that received systematic instruction in Pelvic Floor Exercise or a noninstructed control group; as compared with their counterparts, women in the exercise group demonstrated a pattern of accelerated pelvic floor muscle restitution and significantly diminished incontinence symptoms at 35 weeks' gestation and 6 weeks and 6 months post partum.

Even before sufficient time has elapsed for the development of stronger muscle fibers, women who are practicing Pelvic Floor Exercise have reported decreases in frequency and amount of urine loss. This phenomenon demonstrates that awareness of pelvic musculature function and the conscious use of precisely timed contraction prior to events known to result in leakage can deter urine loss. For example, women can consciously tighten the pelvic muscles before and during coughing. A significant reduction in urine loss has been documented in incontinent women who learn Pelvic Floor Exercise and consciously use this "knack" to initiate the contraction in advance of increased intra-abdominal pressure in order to develop opposing force at the level of the urethra (Miller et al., 1998).

Although research on Pelvic Floor Exercise has been done with women, there is also limited support for the benefit of pelvic floor exercise to treat conditions in men. Erectile dysfunction with demonstrated venous leakage was significantly improved in men randomized to either Pelvic Floor Exercise or surgery (i.e., both treatments were equally effective); after 12 months, greater numbers in the Pelvic Floor Exercise group reported a positive response as compared with those who had surgery (Claes & Baert, 1993). Following prostatectomy, men with persistent incontinence treated with biofeedback-assisted Pelvic Floor Exercise demonstrated an average decrease of 81% in urge incontinence and 78% in stress incontinence (Burgio, Stutzman, & Engel, 1989). A significant decrease in number of incontinent episodes was documented for 57% of men after prostatectomy, with those who had transurethral and perineal procedures showing the greatest improvement at 74% and 61%, respectively (Meaglia, Joseph, Chang, & Schmidt, 1990).

Research on the use of Pelvic Floor Exercise in the disabled population is limited. Fried, Goetz, Potts-Nulty, Cioschi, & Staas (1995) used biofeedback-assisted Pelvic Floor Exercise along with adjustment in bowel program, caffeine intake, fluid intake, toileting schedule, transfer training, and medications. In 54 male and female patients with diverse disabilities who were able to void voluntarily and could contract their pelvic muscles, the decrease in the average number of incontinent episodes per day was statistically significant. The daily episodes decreased from 3.6 before intervention to 0.8 after intervention. In patients who were unable to quantify incontinent episodes, the number of pads used per day decreased from 3.5 to 1.9.

In summary, Pelvic Floor Exercise has demonstrated its effectiveness in decreasing symptoms of urinary incontinence in women across the life span, in postpartum women, and in men following prostatectomy. There is strong and convergent support for this technique to be incorporated into practice. Health care providers should incorporate the teaching of Pelvic Floor Exercise into the care plan for appropriate clients.

INTERVENTION PROTOCOLS

Before initiating a Pelvic Floor Exercise protocol, it is important to rule out conditions that can cause incontinence in otherwise continent individuals. Atrophic vaginitis/urethritis, retention of urine, constipation, irritable bowel syndrome, urinary tract infection, and hematuria should be ruled out or treated before the Pelvic Floor Exercise intervention is instituted. Current prescription and over-the-counter medications should be evaluated. Diuretics and caffeine can cause urgency, frequency, and incontinence; anticholinergics can impair detrusor contractility, resulting in overflow incontinence; alpha-adrenergic blockers can cause incontinence through lowering of urethral tone (Fantl et al., 1996).

In order to incorporate Pelvic Floor Exercise into the care plan, clinicians must develop the diagnostic and intervention skills that are presented in this section. Three categories of pelvic floor testing techniques that are applicable in the clinical setting are reviewed: neurological function, adequacy of pelvic support, and severity of identified urinary incontinence. Following this, correct Pelvic

Floor Exercise technique, recommended frequency, and effective teaching strategies are discussed.

Neurology Assessment

Because an intact neurological axis is necessary for physiological function of the continence system, a brief neurological assessment should be incorporated into the physical examination. It is important to rule out any neurological condition and to refer clients with identified conditions for specialized work-up before developing a treatment plan for incontinence. Some fairly common neuropathies are associated with incontinence, such as spinal cord trauma, multiple sclerosis, central lumbar disc prolapse, pelvic surgery or irradiation, and benign spinal cord tumor. Thus, the following general screening procedures for identification of neurological pathology should be conducted: observation of gait and balance, presence and bilateral equality of deep tendon reflexes, palpation of the lumbosacral spine for lesions or deformity, evaluation of bilateral equality of muscle strength in legs (and pelvic floor), and examination of ability to abduct the toes. (The ability to spread the toes laterally is derived directly from intact sacral 3 efferent fibers.)

A general evaluation of neurological intactness can be accomplished by observing perineal movement during a pelvic muscle contraction. The clitoris should descend toward the vagina and the anus should draw upward and inward. (During this maneuver the anus is similar in appearance to the pursed lips of someone drinking through a straw.) If there is any reason to suspect neurological pathology, more extensive assessment can be conducted.

Alterations in perineal sensation or reflexes can signal dysfunction of sacral 2, 3, or 4. Reflexes that demonstrate intact sacral 2 through 4 pathways are the anal "wink," the bulbocavernosus, and the cough reflex. The anal "wink" is elicited by lightly stroking the skin just lateral to the anus with a cotton swab and observing for a drawing-in response. The intact bulbocavernosus reflex yields a similar anal response and is elicited by a light tap to the clitoris. (Obviously, both of these procedures should be preceded by an explanation to the woman.) A strong voluntary cough should result in reflex contraction of the pelvic floor. Women with normal neurological axes may have asymmetry or absence of one or more reflexes. However, the presence of these signs in the context of other neuropathological evidence, such as history of diabetes mellitus or pelvic surgery, calls for a neurology referral.

Pelvic Support Adequacy

Assessment of the integrity of the pelvic floor musculofascia is accomplished through a pelvic examination. Prior to any palpation of pelvic support, a general external inspection of the vulva should be conducted. Specific lesions, including excoriation secondary to scratching and skin breakdown secondary to contact with urine, should be noted. Urogenital atrophy, a condition often readily resolved with topical estrogen, is also an important factor in urinary incontinence. Prior to palpation, having the woman strain down forcefully will bring out any problems with pelvic organ support.

Digital strength score and time required to interrupt urine flow, as described later, provide ways for clinicians to quantify baseline status of pelvic floor strength. Tracking these measures over time is a way to document strength changes during a Pelvic Floor Exercise protocol and to provide feedback to the client about progress.

A basic digital assessment of pelvic muscle tone as well as symmetry of contraction can be obtained by asking women clients to maximally contract the pelvic floor. During the contraction the provider can evaluate strength and make bilateral comparisons by pressing with a single finger approximately 5 cm inside the vaginal introitus in the areas of 5 and 7 o'clock (Wall et al., 1993). Strength can be quantified on a scale of 0 (no visible or palpable contraction), 1 (very weak contraction often barely perceived as a "flick"), 2 (a weak, but clearly perceived contraction), 3 (well-perceived contraction, but not maintained when moderate finger pressure is applied), 4 (good force of contraction, but not maintained when intense finger pressure is applied), or 5 (maximum strength contraction with strong resistance to oppositional pressure).

This simple digital assessment can be augmented by specific attention to the characteristics of pressure, displacement, and duration of the muscle contraction. Scoring guidelines for each of the characteristics of pelvic muscle contraction are provided in Table 4–2. This expanded digital measure is conducted with the examiner's index and middle fingers inserted 6 to 8 cm (Brink, Wells, Sampselle, Root Tallie, & Mayer, 1994; Sampselle, Brink, & Wells, 1989). In addition to providing specific data about the various elements of pelvic muscle contraction and quantifying the muscle strength for the purpose of ongoing monitoring, this procedure is useful in teaching correct pelvic muscle contraction technique (Sampselle & Miller, 1996).

Health care providers should assess pelvic muscle strength as a routine part of a pelvic examination. Such systematic evaluation expands the clinician's understanding of the range of pelvic muscle function and, with appropriate client education, can increase women's awareness of the location and purpose of these muscles.

A further clinical test of pelvic muscle strength can be obtained with the standardized Urine Stream Interruption Test (Sampselle, 1993; Sampselle & De-Lancey, 1992). This test is based on the premise that the stronger the pelvic musculature, the more quickly a woman will be able to interrupt the stream of urine during micturition. The test does, in fact, correlate strongly and positively with other measures of pelvic muscle strength. The procedure is done as follows: (1) confirm that the woman has a bladder sufficiently full that she would normally empty (a volume of at least 150 mL is desirable to ensure that the pelvic floor has been adequately tested); (2) position for uroflowmetry measurement if a visual record of the test is desired or on a standard commode with a collector hat in place; (3) instruct that after she begins to void she will be given a command to stop the flow and that at that time she should contract the pelvic floor in an attempt to interrupt the flow of urine; (4) give the signal to stop 5 seconds after flow is initiated. The test score is derived from the time from the signal to interrupt to the point of cessation of flow.

In the past, women were erroneously advised to train the pelvic muscle by starting and stopping the urine flow with each void. This practice interferes with physiological micturition and is not recommended. However, women can use their ability to interrupt urine stream to self-monitor increasing pelvic muscle strength accomplished during a pelvic muscle rehabilitation schedule. For self-monitoring purposes, it is recommended that the procedure be done no more frequently than once a week.

Severity of Incontinence

To quantify the severity of urinary incontinence, the standing cough stress test and the leak point pressure are useful techniques. Each test elaborates on the

Table 4–2 Scoring Pelvic Muscle Contraction Characteristics with Digital Examination

Characteristic of Contraction	Criteria for Scoring					
	0	1	2	3	4	5	6
PRESSURE	None, no pressure perceived by examiner's finger(s)	Flick at only one point along finger(s)	More than one flick at same time at different points along finger(s)	Weak pressure all around finger(s)	Snug pressure all around finger(s)	Finger(s) compressed	Finger(s) override (only used if two-finger examination is conducted)
DISPLACEMENT	None, no displacement of examiner's finger(s) occurs	Base of finger(s) lifts	Base to middle of finger(s) lifts	Total length of finger(s) lifts	Total length of finger(s) lifts with additional lift at tip of finger(s)	Finger(s) drawn into vagina	
DURATION	Number of seconds up to 10 that contraction is maintained. Instruct to contract on the count of three and time (stopwatch) from initial pressure of contraction to first fading.						

practice of clinically evaluating urine leakage during a cough. The tests have the further advantage of being conducted with the client in the standing position, the position in which leakage typically occurs.

Results of the cough stress test and the leak point pressure are dependent on the amount of urine in the bladder, because volume influences the load placed on the continence system. When urodynamic testing is conducted, the amount of fluid in the bladder is standardized by filling the bladder through the urethra to a known volume. In contrast, the results presented here were obtained in women whose bladders filled physiologically. The volume was determined after the test through measurement of the total void. A minimum of 150 mL was required for the test to be considered valid.

The standing cough stress test or paper towel test is a refinement of the test already done by clinicians in which the urinary meatus is observed for leakage during a cough while the woman is in a supine or standing position. Miller refined the procedure and developed a method to quantify the amount of urine loss. With the presence of a clinically full bladder confirmed, the woman is asked to stand with her feet approximately 14 inches apart. The perineum is blotted to remove any artifact due to vaginal secretions, and the woman is asked to cough deeply with a folded paper towel held at the perineum (Miller et al., 1998). Any leakage appears as a wet spot on the paper towel and is measured in millimeters. The product of the maximum width and length of the area is documented for future reference.

Quantification of leak point pressure requires the use of a pressure transducer so that an index of abdominal pressure is available. Women are asked to cough with increasing forcefulness until urine loss is observed or the intra-abdominal pressure reaches 150 cm H_2O. This technique allows precise quantification of the pressure at which incontinence occurs. The lower the pressure with first evidence of incontinence, the more severe the condition. Although standard urodynamic practice uses urethral catheterization to locate transducers intravesically and intraurethrally, study suggests that the vagina may be the preferred site for a single pressure transducer (Miklos, Sze, & Karram, 1995). Bearing down and cough leak point pressures have been shown to be significantly lower when measured with an intravaginal catheter as opposed to a transurethral-intravesical catheter.

The standing cough stress test and the leak point pressure provide indices for the severity of incontinence. Over time, they can also be used to evaluate improvement or deterioration of the continence status.

Pelvic Floor Exercise Technique

Basic information that underlies a successful Pelvic Floor Exercise intervention includes client understanding of the purpose of the muscle training, the anatomy of the pelvic floor, and the characteristics of both effective and ineffective contractions. The purpose of pelvic muscle training is to strengthen the voluntary muscles of the pelvic floor so that the musculature is better able to support the urethra in times of increased intra-abdominal pressure and better able to exert periurethral force to counter the increased pressure that arises within the bladder during activities that increase intra-abdominal pressure. As noted earlier, pelvic muscle contraction is also an effective strategy in suppressing symptoms of urgency. Explanations of pelvic floor anatomy are effectively provided with a simplified illustration such as those available in the National Institute of Diabetes and Digestive and Kidney Diseases (NIDDK) publication *Bladder Control for*

Women (NIDDK, 1997). The three different levels of pelvic floor musculature (superficial, mid-level or urogenital diaphragm, and pelvic diaphragm, which provides the most proximal support to the urethra) can be pointed out and linked to the need to contract all three levels. These are the muscles that are targeted for training, but because they are not visible nor routinely used, many women are unaware of their existence and of the voluntary control that can be exerted on them. Thus, clients must be taught how to isolate the target muscles and to contract them correctly.

The characteristics of an ideal pelvic muscle contraction are listed in Table 4–3. Correct Pelvic Floor Exercise technique features three positive and three negative attributes. The positive attributes include descent of the clitoris toward the introitus, upward and inward motion of the anus, and lifting of the examining fingers by three distinct perivaginal muscle layers. Undesirable attributes, which should be absent in an ideal contraction, are straining downward, thigh contraction, and gluteal contraction. The most undesirable behavior is a straining or bearing-down effort, which is the opposite of the recommended upward and inward contraction. This maneuver imposes force on the pelvic structures that can exacerbate urinary incontinence.

Bump, Hurt, Fantl, & Wyman (1991) found that 25% of women who received only written instructions mistakenly executed a bearing-down or straining effort. To help a female patient avoid this common mistake, the nurse should first talk her through a bearing-down effort (i.e., instruct her to take a deep breath, hold it, and bear down, and encourage her to note the bulging of the perineum). Women should be advised that if they notice this sort of an effect during their practice of pelvic muscle contraction, they should discontinue the exercise program until they can seek one-to-one feedback from a qualified health care provider during a pelvic examination. In addition to avoiding straining down, women can be encouraged to use a mirror and observe the perineum for evidence of correct technique (i.e., downward movement of the clitoris toward the vaginal introitus and pulling inward and upward of the rectum).

Women who execute a bearing-down effort may be helped to avoid this if their attention is drawn to the outward thrust of the perineum that occurs with such straining and the need to perform the motion in the opposite direction is emphasized. Avoiding breath holding by gently exhaling and keeping the mouth open during Pelvic Floor Exercise helps women reverse the direction of their effort.

As discussed earlier, to gain the highest level of benefit, each contraction should be at maximum or near maximum intensity. This requires sufficient relaxation (at least 10 seconds) between each contraction. Thus, women should pay attention to their body's readiness to exert a maximum contraction and rest

Table 4–3 Characteristics of Ideal Pelvic Muscle Contraction

Characteristics of Pelvic Muscle Contraction	Present	Absent
Clitoris descends toward vaginal introitus	X	
Anus lifts upward and pulls inward	X	
Examining fingers are lifted by three muscle layers	X	
Straining or bearing down effort		X
Thigh muscle contraction		X
Gluteal muscle contraction		X

until that readiness is apparent. Finally, women should be alerted to the need to do Pelvic Floor Exercise for several weeks before improvements are seen. For older women, the time period is even longer.

Contraction Frequency

A wide array of Pelvic Floor Exercise protocols have demonstrated desired outcomes, as is shown in Table 4–4. Although the Clinical Practice Guidelines (Fantl et al., 1996) recommend a frequency of 30 to 80 pelvic muscle contractions per day, positive results can be achieved using the lower level of this range (Dougherty et al., 1993; Sampselle et al., 1998). Because it is more likely that women will initiate and maintain a program of exercise that requires fewer, rather than more, repetitions, providers should initially prescribe frequencies that build to a regular regimen of 30 to 50 contractions per day, adding repetitions only if improvement does not occur.

Once women have learned how to do a correct pelvic muscle contraction, the carefully timed use of this technique may diminish urine leakage even before muscle strength has increased (Miller et al., 1998). Nurses can help women identify what events are most likely to result in urine leakage (e.g., coughing, heavy lifting). Women can then consciously contract the pelvic muscles when they approach an activity that is likely to cause urinary incontinence. This application of pelvic muscle contraction often results in an immediate improvement in symptoms.

Effective Teaching Strategies

In addition to learning the correct Pelvic Floor Exercise technique and regimen, clients need counseling about how to incorporate a new self-care practice into their daily lives. During the initial learning period for Pelvic Floor Exercise it is advisable to set aside dedicated times each day for its practice. This contradicts the recommendations of many women's magazines, which suggest that the exercises can be performed anywhere, any time. In our experience, it is best to practice Pelvic Floor Exercise in the absence of outside distraction; most women are surprised to discover that proper execution requires considerable concentration.

Women who are initiating this program of self-care should also be aware that results may not become apparent for 6 to 12 weeks. Older women may need to perform Pelvic Floor Exercise consistently for 2 months or longer before they notice any reduction in urine leakage.

Because any new exercise program involves a lifestyle change, clients should be encouraged to identify strategies that will foster success. Sessions should be planned to fit into the usual daily routine—preferably linked to something that will serve as a reminder, a reward, and/or a long-term incentive for monitoring progress. We have used stickers and magnets placed where they can serve as a reminder to do Pelvic Floor Exercise. Choosing a particular time of day for the practice of Pelvic Floor Exercise (e.g., before arising, before sleep, during a daily television program) can help ingrain the habit. Rewards should be selected by the client (e.g., allowing oneself to call a favorite relative only after pelvic floor exercise has been accomplished for the day, buying flowers after 10 or 30 days of consistent Pelvic Floor Exercise practice).

A number of audiotapes and videotapes are available to assist in the incorporation of Pelvic Floor Exercise into daily life. The client can be helped to plan

Table 4–4 Comparison of Pelvic Floor Exercise Protocols

Study	Pelvic Floor Exercise Protocol	Statistically Significant Improvement In
Benvenuti, Caputo, Bandinelli, et al. (1987)		
• 22 female outpatients, age 36–65 with genuine stress incontinence. Pretest/posttest; no control.	• Contract pubococcygeal muscles for the count of 5 initially and progressively working up to the count of 30. • Repeat as frequently as possible; at least 10 times an hour. • 3-month study period.	• Reduction/absence of incontinent episodes per voiding diaries, and daily micturition frequency. • Increased functional urethral profile length and maximal urethral closure pressure at rest, and during maximal voluntary contraction of pelvic floor muscles.
Burgio, Stutzman, & Engel (1989)		
• 20 men with persistent postprostatectomy incontinence. 2 weeks' timed voiding followed by 1–5 biofeedback training sessions. Pretest/posttest; no control.	• Sustained 10-second contractions with 10-second periods of relaxation. • 51 sphincter exercises daily done in sets of 17 repetitions, 3 times daily. • 1–5 biofeedback sessions	• Decreased frequency of stress incontinence and urge incontinence.
Bo, Hagen, Kvarstein, et al. (1990)		
• 52 women aged 24–64 years with stress urinary incontinence randomized to one of two Pelvic Floor Exercise groups; either home exercise group (HE) or intensive exercise with instructor group (IE)	• 8–12 maximal pelvic floor muscle contractions 3 times a day for 6 months. • Intensive exercise (IE) group also exercised intensively for 45 minutes once a week, performing long-lasting contractions with the supplement of 3–4 fast contractions at the end of each long-lasting contraction.	• Continence or near continence for IE group. • Decreased urinary leakage and pad test in IE group. • Improved maximum resting urethral closure pressure in IE group. • Increased maximum pelvic floor muscle (MPFM) strength after 1 month.
Wells, Brink, Diokno, et al. (1991)		
• (n = 157) Community-living women aged 55 to 90 with stress urinary incontinence. Randomly assigned treatment with Pelvic Floor Exercise or phenylpropanolamine hydrochloride.	• 6 months of active pelvic muscle exercise. Daily goal of 90–160 exercise units daily (10-second contraction/10-second rest). • Exercises distributed throughout the day.	• Digital test for pelvic muscle strength in the Pelvic Floor Exercise group. • Otherwise no statistically significant difference between groups.
Burns, Pranikoff, Nochajski, et al. (1993)		
• Community-dwelling women (n = 35) randomized in a single-blind trial to biofeedback, Pelvic Floor Exercise, or control groups.	• Treatment period 8 weeks. Pelvic Floor Exercise beginning with 4 sets of 20 repetitions (10 quick/10 sustained). • Increase to a daily maximum of 200 exercises.	• Self-reported urine loss in Pelvic Floor Exercise and biofeedback groups. • Maintenance of reduced urine loss for at least 6 months in Pelvic Floor Exercise and biofeedback groups.

Table continued on following page

Table 4–4 Comparison of Pelvic Floor Exercise Protocols *Continued*

Study	Pelvic Floor Exercise Protocol	Statistically Significant Improvement In
Dougherty, Bishop, Mooney, et al. (1993) • (n = 65) Parous women aged 35–75 years with mild to moderate stress urinary incontinence.	• 16 weeks. Starting with 15 Pelvic Floor Exercise repetitions (10 seconds/15-second rest) every other day. • Increased to 45 repetitions every other day by the 16th week.	• Urine loss on the 24-hour pad test. • Decreased episodes of urine loss. • Increase in pressure of pelvic muscles
Hahn, Milsom, Fall, & Ekelund (1993) • Women with genuine stress urinary incontinence (n = 170) participated in a Pelvic Floor Exercise program. 27 women awaiting surgery served as a control group.	• Instructed to practice pelvic floor squeeze in provocative situations. • Home training program: women instructed to use the exercise program 6–8 times per day. • Visited physiotherapist once weekly for 4–5 weeks, then monthly until improvement achieved (range 1–18 months).	• Cure/reduction of stress urinary incontinence by report. • Provocation test scores improved. • Digital palpation of pelvic muscle strength improved.
Flynn, Cell, & Luisi (1994) • 32 community-residing men and women aged 58–92, referred to Continence Program (urge and mixed incontinence).	• Contract for 10 seconds and relax for 10 seconds. • Recommended 25 repetitions twice daily.	• Reduced number of incontinent episodes. • Increased length of time between voiding.
Nygaard, Kreder, Lepic, et al. (1996) • 55 women aged 25–81 (stress, urge, and mixed) randomly assigned to exercise with or without audiotaped music and verbal cues.	• Instructed to exercise in two 5-minute daily sessions, beginning with 4 count contractions and progressing to 8 counts. • Study period was 3 months.	• Decreased number of incontinent episodes per day in all three diagnostic categories.
Berghmans, et al. (1996) • 40 women aged 18–70 years (mild to moderate stress incontinence) randomized to Pelvic Floor Exercise and biofeedback or Pelvic Floor Exercise only groups.	• Twelve treatments 3 times weekly, 25–35 minutes per visit. • Pelvic Floor Exercise performed in supine position, followed in the side, standing, and crawling positions. Contraction duration varied from 3–30 seconds, frequency varied from 10–30. Began with 4 sets of 10 (5 quick/5 sustained) and increased by 10 per set until 30 times per set were realized. • Functional training (Pelvic Floor Exercise combined with coughing, climbing stairs, lifting, and jumping) completed the exercise program.	• Group with biofeedback reached significantly greater improvement after 6 treatment sessions. No significance after 12 treatment sessions.
Sampselle, Miller, Mims, et al. (1998) • 46 primigravidas, 37 with vaginal births, enrolled at 20 weeks' gestation and followed to 12 months post partum.	• 30 pelvic muscle contractions per day at maximum or near maximum intensity.	• Decreased urinary incontinence at 35 weeks' gestation, 6 weeks post partum and 6 months post partum.

these aids into the pattern of a normal day (e.g., keeping the audiocassette in the car so that Pelvic Floor Exercise can be done on the drive to and from work). There is scant research and mixed results to support the value of such "cues to action." Gallo and Staskin (1997) taught a group of stress-incontinent women to do Pelvic Floor Exercise and then randomized them into a treatment group who received an audiotape and a control group who did not. Four to 6 weeks later, 65% of the control group reported practice of the Pelvic Floor Exercise protocol once a day as compared with 100% of the treatment group. Significantly, more of those who received the tape were practicing Pelvic Floor Exercise twice a day (83%), in comparison to 12% of their control counterparts. Other findings were reported by Nygaard et al. (1996) in a prospective randomized trial looking at the use of an audiotape in 71 women with stress, urge, and mixed incontinence being treated with Pelvic Floor Exercise. After 3 months, 56% of enrollees who completed the treatment course had at least a 50% improvement in the number of incontinent episodes per day. There was no difference in the dropout rate or the efficacy measures of incontinent episodes per day, pad weight, muscle strength, or leakage index score between the women who received the audiotape and those who did not. Given current mixed findings, there may be value in offering an audiotape and allowing the client to determine whether it would be a helpful strategy.

As in any new self-care endeavor, some lapses are common and expected. It is useful to alert the client to the fact that there will be times when she will forget to do Pelvic Floor Exercise. Such anticipatory guidance can contribute to self-efficacy, a key factor in predicting planned behavior (Ajzen & Madden, 1986) such as establishment of a Pelvic Floor Exercise self-care program. Lapses are most likely during a deviation from normal routine (e.g., a weekend excursion or a longer vacation). Educating the client about the normality of this phenomenon can serve to "inoculate" her against failure (Meichenbaum, 1985). This concept is similar to anticipatory guidance. Clients should be advised to simply resume the Pelvic Floor Exercise protocol when they realize that a lapse has occurred. It is also important to counsel clients not to try to "make up for lost time" by overexercising. Excessive Pelvic Floor Exercise has resulted in myalgia, requiring a period of rest before soreness subsides (DeLancey, Sampselle, & Punch, 1993).

An alternative teaching strategy that may be more cost-effective than individual patient teaching is to provide classes for groups of up to 15 to teach the purpose of Pelvic Floor Exercise, pelvic floor anatomy and physiology, Pelvic Floor Exercise technique, recommended protocol, and lifestyle change (Sampselle, Miller, Herzog, & Diokno, 1996). The information can be effectively taught in a group session of about 1 to 2 hours. It is recommended that women receive individual verification of technique in a follow-up pelvic examination. This verification can be readily incorporated into a routine annual pelvic examination.

Specialty Incontinence Care

Some women are not able to perform even a weak pelvic muscle contraction. When this situation occurs, there are mechanical and electronic devices available to augment learning Pelvic Floor Exercise. A set of vaginal cones of increasing weight is available (Moore & Metcalfe, 1992). A selected weight is inserted into the vagina and retained via pelvic muscle contraction at specific times each day. Women with stress incontinence who used vaginal cones were more aware of and able to contract the pelvic floor muscles; the result was effective exercise and decreased urine leakage (Peattie, Plevnik, & Stanton, 1988).

A variety of electrical biofeedback equipment is available. The supplemental stimuli of simple biofeedback provides the client with visual and/or auditory feedback about the force exerted during Pelvic Floor Exercise (Burgio, Robinson, & Engel, 1986). Electrical stimulation of the pelvic muscles is a technique that contracts the muscle despite lack of voluntary control (Plevnik, Janez, & Vodusek, 1991). A small randomized trial of electrical (or neurotropic) stimulation demonstrated that incontinent women who received the treatment had a significant reduction in leakage as compared with the untreated controls (Blowman et al., 1991).

The use of biofeedback and electrical stimulation requires specialized training. Some providers, often nurse practitioners, specialize in the care of individuals with incontinence and are skilled in the use of this equipment. A directory of health care providers in various regions of the United States is maintained by the National Association for Continence (800-252-3337).

ASSOCIATED NURSING DIAGNOSES AND APPROPRIATE CLIENT GROUPS

The intervention of Pelvic Floor Exercise is most frequently used with the nursing diagnoses of Urge Incontinence, Stress Incontinence, and Bowel Incontinence. Outcome data on Pelvic Floor Exercise for bowel incontinence are limited, but some investigators have reported decreased fecal incontinence with biofeedback (Cerulli, Nikoomanesh, & Schuster, 1979) or Pelvic Floor Exercise (McIntosh, Frahm, Mallett, & Richardson, 1993).

Any type of incontinence not adequately controlled may lead to Impaired Skin Integrity. Persons experiencing incontinence may also experience psychosocial disturbances including Self Esteem Disturbance and Body Image Disturbance. Individuals practicing Pelvic Floor Exercise to correct incontinence are appropriately diagnosed with Health Seeking Behaviors and, if improvement is realized, with Effective Management of Therapeutic Regimen.

Caregiver Role Strain may occur in families caring for individuals with incontinence because of additional time and burden for the caregiver. Intervention with Pelvic Floor Exercise may also result in the diagnosis of Coping: Potential for Growth (i.e., the family member may provide support and encouragement about the Pelvic Floor Exercise regimen as well as reminders to practice). Willingness to continue in the caregiver role may be influenced by improved continence resulting from the intervention.

Both men and women may suffer incontinence, especially those with physical disabilities, men who have had a prostatectomy, and pregnant, postpartum, and peri- and postmenopausal women.

NURSING-SENSITIVE OUTCOMES

Outcomes of Pelvic Floor Exercise that are sensitive to the quality of nursing intervention include adherence behavior and continence of urine as shown in Figure 4–2. The continence outcomes can be further broken down into individual effects as well as positive and negative caregiver effects.

Urinary incontinence creates negative effects on family members caring for an individual by increasing Caregiver Lifestyle Disruption and Caregiver Stressors. Successful treatment or reduction of urinary incontinence by Pelvic Floor Exer-

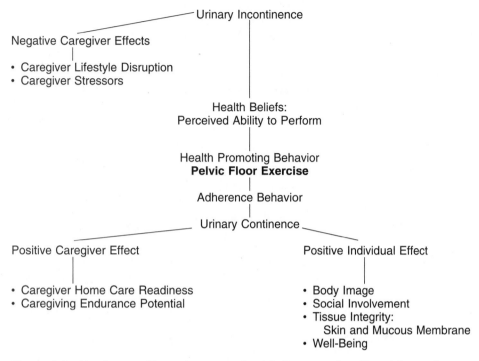

Figure 4–2 Nursing-sensitive outcomes and pelvic floor exercise. (See Johnson & Maas, 1997.)

cise promotes positive effects on the individual experiencing the problem. These effects include positive Body Image, improved Social Involvement, promotion of Tissue Integrity: Skin and Mucous Membrane, and overall well-being. Also, if a family member is acting as caregiver, improvement is seen in Caregiver Home Care Readiness and Caregiving Endurance Potential.

CASE STUDIES

Case Study I

LL is a 53-year-old woman who is referred for mixed urinary incontinence. She has had three vaginal deliveries. LL is the human resources director at a manufacturing facility. She reports loss of urine with coughing and exercise for 10 years that has become progressively worse. She also experiences frequent sudden urges to urinate with loss of small amounts of urine when she is unable to get to the bathroom in time; often these episodes occur as she gets home from work, while unlocking the door to her house. Her health and cognition are very good, and her history is negative for stroke, vaginal surgery, neurological disease, or cancer; she is 5 feet 4 inches tall and weighs 158 pounds. LL's urinalysis findings, glucose level, and blood pressure are normal; postvoid residual urine is 30 mL. Medications include estrogen and progestin taken on a continuous regimen; she also takes a daily multivitamin and calcium supplement. The urine loss has negatively affected her body image. She wears an absorbent pad at all times while awake and must always empty her bladder prior to any physical exercise, regardless of the amount of time that has passed since previously emptying. Currently, she uses two to four maxi-pads per day. She attended an aerobics class until recently, when she stopped because of urinary leakage during the class; she has also stopped playing golf because of loss of urine when she swings the club. LL describes the urinary loss as severely restricting the activities she has enjoyed and her general sense of well-being. She does not consider herself incontinent and considers loss of urine a normal part of aging for women. For this reason, she has not previously discussed urine loss at annual examinations.

LL is evaluated for pelvic muscle strength and vaginal relaxation. Physical examination reveals that she has a mild cystocele, no rectocele, and no uterine prolapse. Bimanual examination is normal. Written instructions for Pelvic Floor Exercise are given and reviewed with LL, and she is instructed to contract the muscles used to stop urine flow or avoid passing gas. Digital examination shows that she is able to perform the exercises correctly without the use of abdominal, buttocks, or thigh muscles. When asked to contract her pelvic muscles, she is able to contract enough so that loose pressure is felt the full circumference of two fingers placed in the vagina, there is no displacement of the fingers, and duration of the contraction is 4 seconds.

LL is given a voiding diary and asked to keep track of frequency of voiding during waking hours and frequency and amount of accidental urine loss for 3 consecutive days. She is instructed to practice the exercises. Fast repetitions are done holding each strong contraction for 3 seconds followed by a 10-second rest period. Slow repetitions are done holding the contraction for 10 seconds and separating each exercise with a 10-second rest. She is instructed to perform 5 fast repetitions followed by 10 slow repetitions twice daily every day during the first week. The second week she should add 5 slow repetitions to the regimen. She is reassured that if she cannot hold the long contractions for 10 seconds, she should hold them as long as possible and slowly increase the length of the contractions to 10 seconds. Planning for fitting the exercises into her daily schedule is discussed. She decides to do them during her lunch period and just before going to bed. LL is encouraged to keep track of the times she is doing Pelvic Floor Exercise and to reward herself for excellent compliance.

LL will return to the clinic in 2 weeks with her completed voiding diary to assess that she is continuing to perform the pelvic muscle exercises correctly. Any questions or problems will be answered and discussed. At that time she will be instructed to add 5 slow contractions per session per week until she is doing 5 fast contractions and 20 slow contractions twice daily and to con-

tinue at that level. Evaluation of the effectiveness of fitting the pelvic muscle exercises into her daily schedule will be discussed, with problem solving done as necessary. The possibility of poor adherence to the exercise regimen will be discussed, along with encouragement to continue the exercises for 12 weeks, at which time she should complete another 3-day voiding diary and return for a follow-up evaluation to determine whether Pelvic Floor Exercise has helped with the urinary incontinence. If the improvement is satisfactory, she will be encouraged to continue performing the regimen at least three to four times weekly for maintenance. If improvement is unsatisfactory and she has not adhered to the regimen, her interest in continuing the regimen with plans to improve adherence will be discussed in addition to alternative treatment options. If LL has adhered to the regimen but improvement is unsatisfactory, she will be given the option to continue the exercises for an extended amount of time or to try alternative treatments of medication, surgery, or various continence appliances. All these actions are to promote LL's health beliefs: perceived ability to perform.

Case Study 2

JL is a primigravida; she is 28 years old and at 22 weeks' gestation. The pregnancy is without complications, and overall JL is of good health and cognition. She expresses concern about the possibility of urinary incontinence after the delivery of the baby. Her sister has recently delivered a baby and is experiencing problems with urinary incontinence post partum.

She is informed that women with increased pelvic muscle strength tend to experience fewer symptoms of urinary incontinence both during the third trimester of pregnancy and post partum. She is also informed that some decrease in pelvic muscle strength should be expected post partum, especially after a vaginal delivery. Although the postpartum follow-up examination is scheduled for 6 weeks after delivery, her pelvic muscles will probably not return to normal strength until 6 to 12 months post partum. The rationale is presented that increasing the strength of her pelvic muscles during the pregnancy will also help accelerate their rehabilitation post partum and help reduce symptoms of urinary incontinence. This may promote adherence behavior in JL's health promoting behavior.

The results of JL's urinalysis are normal, and she has had no experience of urinary incontinence to date. Vaginal examination reveals no vaginal relaxation. Digital examination of pelvic muscle strength reveals that she is able to isolate the pelvic muscles for a contraction that produces snug pressure the full circumference of two fingers with lifting of the entire length of the fingers, gentle lift at the fingertips. She is able to maintain the muscle contraction for 8 seconds. Written instructions for Pelvic Floor Exercise are given and reviewed with JL. The muscles used for Pelvic Floor Exercise are described as the muscles she would use to stop urine flow or avoid passing gas. Initially, she tightens the gluteal and thigh muscles with pelvic muscle contraction but is able to correctly isolate the pelvic muscles after instruction by the nurse. She is instructed to perform 30 pelvic muscle contractions at moderate to maximum intensity, working up to a hold of 10 seconds per contraction. She is told to rest 10 seconds between contractions. Recommended minimum time for Pelvic Floor Exercise is 10 minutes daily, 5 days each week. JL is also taught to check her own pelvic muscle strength by placing two fingers or the thumb into the vagina and contracting the muscles. She is encouraged to continue doing the exercises throughout the rest of the pregnancy and also during the postpartum period. She can also verify that she is using the right muscles by attempting to stop urine flow once a week while voiding. If she can stop or slow the urine flow, she is using the right muscles.

JL should be questioned at each prenatal visit about her ability to incorporate Pelvic Floor Exercise into her daily schedule and encouraged to continue practicing even if she cannot exercise every day. She should be questioned about symptoms of urinary incontinence and reassured that urine loss in the third trimester and postpartum period is normal. This will facilitate a sense of well-being. Should urine loss occur, she should be evaluated and given a regimen of lower intensity if needed. At the 6-week postpartum visit, she should also be reevaluated and placed on a regimen that best utilizes the pelvic muscle strength she has. At the postpartum visit, JL should be asked about symptoms of urinary incontinence. If the symptoms are present, results of urinalysis and urine culture are negative, and physical examination is normal, she should be evaluated for graduated strength training and taught the recommended level at which to practice Pelvic Floor Exercise along with the correct progression.

SUMMARY

Pelvic Floor Exercise is a self-care strategy that should be taught to women (or men with appropriate conditions) as a first step in managing urinary incontinence. Nurses are well qualified to provide Pelvic Floor Exercise instruction. Moreover, use of this technique as a first-line intervention in no way jeopardizes future therapy should it be needed at a later date. The many individuals who have reported complete cure of urinary incontinence with the use of Pelvic Floor Exercise and the many others who are satisfied with the significant decrease in symptoms that they have been able to attain through Pelvic Floor Exercise underline the validity of educating clients about this noninvasive intervention.

References

Ajzen, I., and Madden, T. J. (1986). Prediction of goal-directed behavior: Attitudes, intentions, and perceived behavioral control. *Journal of Experimental Social Psychology, 22,* 453–474.

Bates, P., Bradley, W., Glen, E., Griffiths, D., Melchior, H., Rowan, D., Sterling, A., Zinner, N., and Hald, T. (1979). The standardization of terminology of lower urinary tract function. *Journal of Urology, 121,* 551–554.

Blowman, C., Pickles, C., Emery, S., Creates, V., Towell, L., Blackburn, N., Doylc, N., and Walkden, B. (1991). Prospective double blind controlled trial of intensive physiotherapy with and without stimulation of the pelvic floor in treatment of genuine stress incontinence. *Physiotherapy, 77*(10), 661–664.

Bo, K., and Talseth, T. (1996). Long term effect of pelvic floor muscle exercise 5 years after cessation of organized training. *Obstetrics and Gynecology, 87*(2), 261–265.

Brink, C., Wells, J. J., and Diokno, A. C. (1987). Urinary incontinence in women. *Public Health Nurse, 4*(2) 114–119.

Brink, C. A., Wells, T. J., Sampselle, C. M., Root Tallie, E., and Mayer, R. (1994). A digital test for pelvic muscle strength in women with urinary incontinence. *Nursing Research, 43*(6), 352–356.

Bump, R. C., Hurt, W. G., Fantl, J. A., and Wyman, J. F. (1991). Assessment of Kegel pelvic muscle exercise performance after brief verbal instruction. *American Journal of Obstetrics and Gynecology, 165,* 322–329.

Burgio, K. L., Matthews, K. A., and Engel, B. T. (1991). Prevalence, incidence, and correlates of urinary incontinence in healthy, middle-aged women. *Journal of Urology, 146,* 1255–1259.

Burgio, K. L., Robinson, C. J., and Engel, B. T. (1986). The role of biofeedback in Kegel exercise training for stress urinary incontinence. *American Journal of Obstetrics and Gynecology, 154,* 58–64.

Burgio, K. L., Stutzman, R. E., and Engel, B. T. (1989). Behavioral training for post prostatectomy urinary incontinence. *The Journal of Urology, 141,* 303–306.

Burns, P. A., Pranikoff, K., Nochajski, T. H., Hadley, E. C., Levy, K. J., and Ory, M. G. (1993). A comparison of effectiveness of biofeedback and pelvic muscle exercise treatment of stress incontinence in older community-dwelling women. *Journal of Gerontology, 48*(4) M167–M174.

Cerulli, M. A., Nikoomanesh, P., and Schuster, M. M. (1979). Progress in biofeedback conditioning for fecal incontinence. *Gastroenterology 76*(4), 742–746.

Claes, H., and Baert, L. (1993). Pelvic floor exercises versus surgery in the treatment of impotence. *British Journal of Urology, 71,* 52–57.

DeLancey, J. O. L. (1994). Structural support of the urethra as it relates to stress urinary incontinence: The hammock hypothesis. *American Journal of Obstetrics and Gynecology, 170,* 1713–1720.

DeLancey, J. O. L, Kyu-Jung, K., Ashton-Miller, J., and Stohbehn, K. (1996). Relative contribution of resting urethral pressure and transmission ratio in determining pressure equalization [Abstract]. *Neurourology and Urodynamics, 15*(4), 301–302.

DeLancey, J. O. L., Sampselle, C. M., and Punch, M. R. (1993). Kegel dyspareunia: Levator ani myalgia caused by overexertion. *Obstetrics and Gynecology, 82*(4), 658–659.

Dimpfl, T., Hesse, U., and Schussler, B. (1992). Incidence and cause of postpartum urinary stress incontinence. *European Journal of Obstetrics, Gynecology, and Reproductive Biology, 43,* 29–33.

Diokno, A. C., Brock, B. M., Brown, H. B., and Herzog, A. R. (1986). Prevalence of urinary incontinence and other urologic symptoms in the non-institutionalized elderly. *Journal of Urology, 136,* 1022–1025.

Dougherty, M., Bishop, K., Mooney, R., Gimotty, P., and Williams, B. (1993). Graded pelvic muscle exercise. Effect on stress urinary incontinence. *Journal of Reproductive Medicine, 39*(9), 684–691.

Dougherty, M. C., Bishop, K. R., Abrams, R. M., Batich, C. D., and Gimotty, P. A. (1989). The effect of exercise on the circumvaginal muscles in postpartum women. *Journal of Nurse-Midwifery, 34*(1), 8–14.

Fantl, J. A., Newman, D. K., Colling, J., DeLancey, J. O. L., Keeys, C., Loughery, R., McDowell, B. J., Norton, P., Ouslander, J., Schnelle, J., Staskin, D., Tries, J., Urich, V., Vitousek, S. H., Weiss, B. D., and Whitmore, K. *Urinary incontinence in adults: Acute & chronic management.* (Clinical Practice Guideline, No. 2, 1996 Update) (AHCPR Publication No. 96-0682). Rockville, MD: U.S. Department of Health and Human Services.

Flynn, L., Cell, P., and Luisi, E. (1994). Effectiveness of pelvic muscle exercises in reducing urge incontinence. *Journal of Gerontological Nursing, 20*(5), 23–27.

Fried, G. W., Goetz, G., Potts-Nulty, S., Cioschi, H. M., and Staas, W. E., Jr. (1995). A behavioral approach to the treatment of urinary incontinence in a disabled population. *Archives of Physical Medicine and Rehabilitation, 76,* 1120–1124.

Gallo, M. L., and Staskin, D. R. (1997). Cues to action: Pelvic floor muscle exercise compliance in women with stress urinary incontinence. *Neurourology and Urodynamics, 16,* 167–177.

Gilpin, S. A., Gosling, J. A., Smith, A. R. B., Warrell, D. W. (1989). The pathogenesis of genitourinary prolapse and stress incontinence of urine. A histological and histochemical study. *British Journal of Obstetrics and Gynaecology, 96,* 15–23.

Goldberg, A., Etlinger, J., Goldspink, D., and Jablecki, C. (1975). Mechanism of work-induced hypertrophy of skeletal muscle. *Medicine and Science in Sport and Exercise, 7,* 248–261.

Gonyea, W. J. (1980). Role of exercise in inducing increases in skeletal muscle fiber number. *Journal of Applied Physiology, 48,* 421–426.

Gosling, J. A. (1985). The structure of the female lower urinary tract and pelvic floor. *Urology Clinics of North America, 12,* 207.

Hahn, I., Milsom, I., Fall, M., and Ekelund, P. (1993). Long-term results of pelvic floor training in female stress urinary incontinence. *British Journal of Urology, 72,* 421–427.

Herzog, A. R., and Fultz, N. H. (1990). Prevalence and incidence of urinary incontinence in community-dwelling populations. *Journal of the American Geriatrics Society, 38,* 273–281.

Hu, T. (1994, January). *The cost impact of urinary incontinence on health care services.* Paper presented at the National Multi-Specialty Nursing Conference on Urinary Continence, Phoenix, AZ.

Johnson, M., and Maas, M. (Eds.). (1997). *Nursing outcomes classification (NOC).* St. Louis: Mosby-Year Book.

Jolleys, J. V. (1988). Reported prevalence of urinary incontinence in women in a general practice. *British Medical Journal, 296,* 1300–1302.

Kegel, A. H. (1948). Progressive resistance in the functional restoration of the perineal muscles. *American Journal of Obstetrics and Gynecology, 56,* 238–248.

Klarskov, P., Belving, D., Bischoff, N., Dorph, S., Gerstenberg, T., Okholm, B., Pedersen, P. H., Tikjob, G., Wormslev, M., and Hald, T. (1986). Pelvic floor exercise versus surgery for female urinary stress incontinence. *Urology, 41,* 129–132.

Koelbl, H., Strassegger, H., Riss, P. A., and Gruber, H. (1989). Morphologic and functional aspects of pelvic floor muscles in patients with pelvic relaxation and genuine stress incontinence. *Obstetrics and Gynecology, 74*(5), 789–795.

Lagace, E. A., Hansen, W., and Hickner, J. M. (1993). Prevalence and severity of urinary incontinence in ambulatory adults: An UPRNet study. *Journal of Family Practice, 36*(6), 610–614.

McCloskey, J. C., and Bulechek, G. M. (Eds.). (1996). *Nursing interventions classification (NIC)* (2nd ed.). St. Louis: Mosby-Year Book.

McIntosh, L. J., Frahm, J. D., Mallett, V. T., and Richardson, D. A. (1993). Pelvic floor rehabilitation in the treatment of incontinence. *Journal of Reproductive Medicine, 38,* 662–666.

Meaglia, J. P., Joseph, A. C., Chang, M., and Schmidt, J. D. (1990). Post-prostatectomy urinary incontinence: Response to behavioral training. *Journal of Urology, 144,* 674–676.

Meichenbaum, D. (1985). *Stress inoculation training.* New York: Pergamon Press.

Miklos, J. R., Sze, E. H. M., and Karram, M. M. (1995). A critical appraisal of the methods of measuring leak-point pressures in women with stress incontinence. *Obstetrics and Gynecology, 86*(3), 349–352.

Miller, J. A., Ashton-Miller, J. A., and DeLancey, J. O. L. (1998). A pelvic muscle precontraction can reduce cough-related urine loss in selected women with mild SUI. *Journal of the American Geriatrics Society, 46*, 870–874.

Miller, J. A., Kasper, C., and Sampselle, C. M. (1994). Review of muscle physiology with application to pelvic muscle exercise. *Urologic Nursing, 14*(3), 92–97.

Moore, K., and Metcalfe, J. B. (1992). Effectiveness of vaginal cones in treatment of urinary incontinence. *Urologic Nursing, 12*(2), 69–72.

Morkved, S., and Bo, K. (1996). The effect of post natal exercises to strengthen the pelvic floor muscles. *Acta Obstetrics and Gynecology Scandinavia, 75*, 382–385.

National Institute of Diabetes and Digestive and Kidney Diseases (NIDDK), National Institutes of Health. (1997). Bladder control for women (NIH Publication Nos. 97-4186, 97-4189, 97-4190). Washington, DC: U.S. Government Printing Office.

Nygaard, I. E., DeLancey, J., Arnsdorf, L., and Murphy, E. (1990). Exercise and incontinence. *Obstetrics and Gynecology, 75*(5), 848–851.

Nygaard, I. E., Kreder, K. J., Lepic, M. M., Fountain, K. A., and Rhomberg, A. T. (1996). Efficacy of pelvic floor muscle exercises in women with stress, urge and mixed urinary incontinence. *American Journal of Obstetrics and Gynecology, 174*(1), 120–125.

Oelrich, T. M. (1983). The striated urogenital sphincter muscle in the female. *Anatomical Record, 205*, 223–232.

Peattie, A. B., Plevnik, S., and Stanton, S. L. (1988). Vaginal cones: A conservative method of treating genuine stress incontinence. *British Journal of Obstetrics and Gynaecology, 95*(10), 1049–1053.

Plevnik, S., Janez, J., and Vodusek, D. B. (1991). Electrical stimulation. In R. J. Krane and M. B. Siroky (Eds.), *Clinical neuro-urology* (2nd ed., pp. 559–572). Boston: Little, Brown.

Sampselle, C. (1993). The urine stream interruption test: Using a stopwatch to assess pelvic muscle strength. *The Nurse Practitioner: American Journal of Primary Health Care, 18*, 14–20.

Sampselle, C. M., Brink, C., and Wells, T. (1989). Digital measurement of pelvic muscle strength in childbearing women. *Nursing Research, 38*(3), 198–202.

Sampselle, C. M., Burns, P. A., Dougherty, M. C., Newman, D. K., Thomas, K. K., and Wyman, J. F. (1997a). Continence for women: Evidence-based practice.

Journal of Obstetric, Gynecologic and Neonatal Nursing, 26(4), 375–385.

Sampselle, C., and DeLancey, J. O. L. (1992). The urine stream interruption test and pelvic muscle function. *Nursing Research, 41*(2), 73–77.

Sampselle, C. M., DeLancey, J. O. L., and Ashton-Miller, J. (1996). Urinary incontinence in pregnancy and postpartum [Abstract]. *Neurourology and Urodynamics, 15*(4), 329–330.

Sampselle, C. M., DeLancey, J. O., Ashton-Miller, J. A., and Antonakos, C. L. (1997b, September). Objectively demonstrable de novo stress urinary incontinence in primiparas. *Neurourology and Urodynamics, 16*, 382–384.

Sampselle, C. M., and Miller, J. M. (1996). Pelvic muscle exercise: Effective patient teaching. *The Female Patient, 21*, 29–36.

Sampselle, C. M., Miller, J. M., Herzog, A. R., and Diokno, A. C. (1996). Behavioral modification: Group teaching outcomes. *Urologic Nursing, 16*(2), 59–63.

Sampselle, C. M., Miller, J. M., Mims, B. L., DeLancey, J. O. L., Ashton-Miller, J. A., and Antonakos, C. L. (1998). Postpartum pelvic muscle exercise outcomes: Earlier return of urinary continence. *Obstetrics and Gynecology, 91*, 406–412.

Smith, A. R., Hosker, G. L., and Warrell, D. W. (1989a). The role of partial denervation of the pelvic floor in the aetiology of genitourinary prolapse and stress incontinence of urine. A neurophysiological study. *British Journal of Obstetrics and Gynaecology, 96*, 24–28.

Smith, A. R., Hosker, G. L., and Warrell, D. W. (1989b). The role of pudendal nerve damage in the aetiology of genuine stress incontinence in women. *British Journal of Obstetrics and Gynaecology, 96*, 29–39.

Snooks, S. J., Swash, M., Mathers, S. E., and Henry, M. M. (1990). Effect of vaginal delivery on the pelvic floor: A 5-year follow-up. *British Journal of Surgery, 77*, 1358–1360.

Snooks, S. J., Swash, M., Sechell, M., and Henry, M. M. (1984). Injury to innervation of pelvic floor sphincter musculature in childbirth. *The Lancet, 2*(8402), 546–550.

Sommer, P., Bauer, T., Nielsen, K. K., Kristensen, G. G., Hermann, K. S., and Nordling, J. (1990). Voiding patterns and prevalence of incontinence in women. A questionnaire survey. *British Journal of Urology, 66*, 12–15.

Wall, L., Norton, P., and DeLancey, J. O. L. (1993). *Practical urogynecology.* Baltimore: Williams and Wilkins.

Wyman, J. F., Harkins, S. W., Choi, S. C., Taylor, J. R., and Fantl, J. A. (1987). Psychosocial impact of urinary incontinence in women. *Obstetrics and Gynecology, 70*, 378–381.

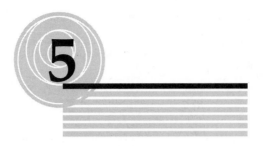

Constipation/Impaction Management

Theresa Moore, Eileen Bourret,

and Lucy Cabico

Despite the prevalence of constipation among persons of all ages, there is no agreed-upon definition of constipation. Towers et al. (1994) summarized the many epidemiological studies that have been conducted to define normal bowel habits, noting that in large population surveys 99% of all adults have bowel movement frequencies that range from three per day to three per week. These results were similar for adults older than 60 years of age. Despite this, 30% to 50% of older adults use laxatives. Thus, the definition of constipation for older adults may not correlate with frequency of bowel movements. The Diagnostic Review Committee of the North American Nursing Diagnosis Association (NANDA) at the Seventh Conference defined constipation as a "state in which an individual experiences a change in normal bowel habits characterized by a decrease in frequency and/or passage of hard dry stool" (Carroll-Johnson, 1989).

ASSESSMENT

A comprehensive bowel function history should be conducted with the patient that encompasses a determination of the patient's usual bowel pattern. This includes documenting the usual frequency of bowel movements, observation of stools (shape, volume, and color), toileting routines, and beliefs and values related to bowel function (e.g., how often does the person believe he or she should have a bowel movement?). Research suggests that there may be a discrepancy between the recall of bowel movements and their actual occurrence (Orr, Johnson, & Yates, 1997); thus it is important to complete a bowel function record for at least 2 weeks to determine the patient's bowel function pattern.

Many factors contribute to constipation, so additional data should be collected related to the patient's cognition and affect; nutritional status, including any dysphagia, state of dentition, diet, and fluid intake; level of mobility; and laxative use and current medications, with particular attention paid to those medications associated with constipation (Baycrest Centre for Geriatric Care, 1990; Gibson, Opalka, Moore, Brady, & Mion, 1995; Karam & Nies, 1994; Read, Celik, & Katsinelos, 1995; Towers et al., 1994; Wald, 1993; Williams & Rae, 1995) (Table 5–1). A review of the patient's diet (e.g., completion of a 3-day calorie count) should be done to evaluate the diet for nutritional content. No literature was found that recommends weighing patients to assess for presence of constipation or to evaluate the effectiveness of interventions. However, Preston and Lennard-Jones (1986) suggest that anorexia and nausea associated with constipation lead to decreased intake. Therefore, weighing the patient at regular intervals may provide further corroboration of the adequacy of the patient's nutritional intake. Identification of predisposing disease states, such as neurogenic disorders and metabolic or endocrine diseases, is also important.

A physical examination should be performed as part of the assessment for constipation. Particular attention should be paid to the abdominal examination (including inspection, auscultation of bowel sounds, percussion, and palpation of the abdomen) to assess for impaction, presence of abdominal masses, tenderness, and/or rigidity. A digital rectal examination is used to assess anal sphincter tone and to detect hemorrhoids, fissures, rectal prolapse, feces, and rectal masses. Individuals with chronic constipation may also require a barium enema, colonoscopy, defecography, anorectal motility, or colonic transit studies (Orr et al., 1997). A physician should be consulted if there is an increase or decrease in the frequency of the patient's bowel sounds, if the patient has signs or symptoms of bowel rupture and/or peritonitis (e.g., fever, rigid abdomen, persistent abdominal pain), or if the patient's constipation or fecal impaction persists after nonpharmacological and pharmacological interventions.

A nursing diagnosis can be made based on the assessment findings. The nursing diagnoses associated with the Nursing Interventions Classification (NIC) intervention of Constipation/Impaction Management include Bowel Incontinence, Constipation, Colonic Constipation, and Perceived Constipation (NANDA, 1992). Constipation is characterized by bowel movements that are more infrequent than usual for the patient, bowel evacuation that may be difficult or painful, and/or a digital rectal examination that indicates the pres-

Table 5–1   Drugs Associated with Constipation

Analgesics (particularly opiate analgesics)	Neurally Active Agents
Anticholinergics	Opiates
Antispasmodics	Antihypertensives
Antidepressants (particularly tricyclic antidepressants)	Ganglionic blockers
Antipsychotics	Vinca alkaloids
Antiparkinsonians	Anticonvulsants
Cation–Containing Agents	Calcium channel blockers
Iron supplements	Laxatives (when abused)
Aluminum (e.g., antacids)	
Calcium (e.g., antacids, supplements)	

Source: Adapted from Wald (1993).

ence of stool in the rectum that may be hard and dry or soft and puttylike. The assessment may also reveal fecal impaction, which is characterized by decreased appetite, nausea, vomiting, and abdominal pain and distention. There may be paradoxic "diarrhea" as liquid stool leaks around the impacted fecal mass (Tierney, McPhee, & Papadakis, 1997). Depending on the location of the impaction, there may be feces in the rectum (hard or soft and puttylike) on digital rectal examination. Other diagnoses that may be associated with constipation/ impaction are Impaired Mobility, Pain, and Knowledge Deficit (NANDA, 1992).

Some patient groups are more likely to experience constipation. Constipation is prevalent among elderly persons for a variety of reasons. The aging bowel has anatomical changes (e.g., presence of diverticula that contribute to uncoordinated colonic muscle contraction) and pathophysiological changes (e.g., diminished contractile muscle tone and loss of neuronal sensitivity) that make defecation more difficult (Yakabowich, 1990). The elderly person who has faulty eating habits, decreased food intake, or delayed response to the urge to defecate is also at greater risk for constipation.

Other groups at risk for constipation are those suffering from endocrine and metabolic diseases (e.g., diabetes mellitus, hypothyroidism, hypercalcemia), Parkinson's disease, neurogenic disorders, stroke, dementia, colonic obstruction, and spinal cord injury (Read et al., 1995; Wald, 1993).

NONPHARMACOLOGICAL ACTIVITIES

NIC (McCloskey & Bulechek, 1996) outlines nursing activities for the prevention and alleviation of constipation/impaction (Table 5–2).

These activities can be classified as nonpharmacological or pharmacological. The nonpharmacological NIC activities are (1) encourage increased fluid intake, unless contraindicated; (2) instruct patient/family on high-fiber diet, as appropriate; and (3) instruct patient/family on the relationship of diet, exercise, and fluid intake to constipation/impaction. The research and general literature pertaining to these activities are discussed in turn. Specific details about how to use the activities are outlined in the guidelines for nonpharmacological prevention and management of constipation (Table 5–3).

An increase in fluid, typically to a minimum of 1,500 mL/day, is often advocated to prevent constipation, facilitate fiber action, and prevent obstruction during fiber supplementation. However, the benefits of additional fluid in normally hydrated persons has been questioned from several perspectives. First, it has been suggested that the addition of hundreds of milliliters of fluid would not be significant in these individuals and would likely be excreted by the kidneys (Klauser & Muller-Lissner, 1993; Ziegenhagen, Tewinkel, Kruis, & Hermann, 1991) because 7 to 10 L of fluid is secreted into the gastrointestinal tract daily (Porth, 1986; Ziegenhagen et al., 1991). Second, community studies have not found a strong association between constipation and fluid intake (Donald, Smith, Cruikshank, Elton, & Stoddart, 1985; Towers et al., 1994; Whitehead, Drinkwater, Cheskin, Heller, & Schuster, 1989). Third, a small study of healthy subjects ingesting bran found that acceleration of gastric emptying was the only significant effect of adding 600 mL of fluid to a baseline intake of 1,000 to 1,200 mL (Ziegenhagen et al., 1991). Finally, bran has been administered without any adverse effects to persons in the community and institutions who consumed only 1 L of fluid per day (Mantle, 1992; Ziegenhagen et al., 1991). On the other hand, actual dehydration has many adverse effects, including significant decreases in stool frequency and weight (Klauser, Beck, Schindlbeck, & Muller-

Table 5–2   Constipation/Impaction Management

DEFINITION: Prevention and alleviation of constipation/impaction.

ACTIVITIES:

Monitor for signs and symptoms of constipation

Monitor for signs and symptoms of impaction

Monitor bowel movements including frequency, consistency, shape, volume, and color as appropriate

Monitor bowel sounds

Consult with physician about a decrease/increase in frequency of bowel sounds

Monitor for signs and symptoms of bowel rupture and/or peritonitis

Explain etiology of problem and rationale for actions to patient

Identify factors (e.g., medications, bed rest, diet) that may cause or contribute to constipation

Encourage increased fluid intake unless contraindicated

Evaluate medication profile for gastrointestinal side effects

Instruct patient/family to record color, volume, frequency, and consistency of stools

Teach patient/family how to keep a food diary

Instruct patient/family on high-fiber diet as appropriate

Instruct patient/family on appropriate use of laxatives

Instruct patient/family on the relationship of diet, exercise, and fluid intake to constipation/impaction

Evaluate recorded intake for nutritional content

Consult physician if signs and symptoms of constipation or impaction persist

Administer laxative or enema as appropriate

Inform patient of procedure for manual removal of stool if necessary

Remove the fecal impaction manually if necessary

Administer enema or irrigation as appropriate

Weigh patient regularly

Source: McCloskey, J. C., and Bulechek, G. M. (Eds.) (1996). *Nursing interventions classification (NIC)* (2nd ed.). St. Louis: Mosby–Year Book.

Lissner, 1990). Although a minimum daily intake of 1,000 to 1,500 mL can be established as a goal, it is more important to assess for signs of dehydration, recognizing that these can be unreliable in elderly persons (Chidester & Spangler, 1997; Turner & Turner, 1987), and to intervene with those persons at risk.

Although the primary activity is promotion of fluid intake, difficulties in achieving this have been identified by several researchers (Beverley & Travis, 1992; Goldstein, Melnick Brown, Holt, Gallagher, & Hutner Winograd, 1989; Ouellet, Turner, Pond, McLaughlin, & Knorr, 1996). Strategies to promote fluid intake include providing a full glass of fluid with medications and toileting, serving juice during recreational activities, using a symbol to alert staff to patients who are at risk for low intake, involving housekeepers in offering fluids (Hagberg, Fines, & Doyle, 1987), offering small amounts frequently (Haight & Burggraf, 1991), and educating patients. Techniques proven to improve protein and calorie intake, such as touch and verbal cuing (Eaton, Mitchell-Bonair, & Friedmann, 1986; Lange-Alberts & Shott, 1994), may also prove valuable.

Fiber supplementation is another dietary activity frequently recommended to prevent constipation. The fiber in bran can decrease intestinal transit time by adding nonnutritive bulk to the stool. Fiber also binds with water to form a

Table 5–3 Guidelines for Nonpharmacological Prevention and Management of Constipation

Use assessment findings, including patient's routines, to choose and/or prioritize actions.

Fluids and Fiber

1. Assess for signs of dehydration and encourage fluids (minimum 1,000–1,500 mL) to maintain normal hydration status.
2. Promote high-fiber menu choices.
3. Consider fiber supplements if fluid intake is greater than 1,000 mL/day.

Exercise

1. Encourage independently mobile patients to walk three times a day to a distance as tolerated.
2. Assist weak patient with ambulation at least daily (preferably to toilet after breakfast).
3. Work with physiotherapy to (a) inrease mobility and (b) teach family techniques.

Toileting

1. Toilet after a meal based on patient's pattern (breakfast usually most effective use of gastrocolic reflex).
2. If on bed rest, assist patient into high Fowler's position on bedpan if possible.
3. Use toilet or commode if possible with patient's trunk forward and feet supported.
4. Promote visual, olfactory, and auditory privacy.

Patient/Family Education

Provide information as needed about (a) myths surrounding "normal" bowel habits; (b) recording of stools and reporting symptoms of constipation; (c) fluid, fiber, exercise, and toileting; (d) appropriate use of laxatives and constipating medications; and (e) techniques for use of suppositories, enemas, or disimpaction.

sticky gelatinous substance that acts to inhibit resorption of water by the intestinal wall (Rodrigues-Fisher, Bourguignon, & Vonthron-Good, 1993). Studies examining the effectiveness of high fiber have been conducted in the community (Badiali et al., 1995; Groth, 1988; Neal, 1995; Valle-Jones, 1985; Voderholzer et al., 1997), acute care (Graham, Moser, & Estes, 1982; Kochen, Wegscheider, & Abholz, 1985; Ouellet et al., 1996; Rajala, Salminen, Seppanen, & Vapaatalo, 1988; Read et al., 1995; Schmelzer, 1990), and long-term care settings (Battle & Hanna, 1980; Beverley & Travis, 1992; Brown & Everett, 1990; Cameron, Nyulasi, Collier, & Brown, 1996; Finlay, 1988; Gibson et al., 1995; Hankey et al., 1992; Hope & Down, 1986; Hull, Greco, & Brooks, 1980; Mantle, 1992; Pringle, Pennington, Pennington, & Ritchie, 1984; Rodrigues-Fisher et al., 1993; Snustad et al., 1991; Stewart, Moore, Stat, Marks, & Hale, 1992). The type and dose of fiber supplements vary greatly among the studies. Most intervention protocols also include a minimum fluid intake of 1,500 mL, and several specify exercise and toileting regimens. The most common outcomes measured by the researchers are bowel frequency and/or laxative use; less commonly reported outcomes include cost, stool weight, transit time, and patient symptoms. The majority of studies have found one or more positive effects from fiber supplementation. However, positive findings have not been universal, and a number of parameters remain unclear, hampering the practical application of this recommendation to practice:

1. Patients often find fiber supplements unpalatable and consume less than the prescribed amount (Hankey et al., 1992; Kochen et al., 1985; Ouellet et al., 1996; Schmelzer, 1990). Further study is needed on more comprehensive diet changes.

2. There is no consensus on the amount of fiber that is desirable, feasible, and effective (Goldstein et al., 1989).

3. There is no consensus on the best form of dietary fiber as evidenced by the great variety of supplements that have been evaluated. The various forms of fiber have different effects on the gastrointestinal tract (Battle & Hanna, 1980; Edwards, Tomlin, & Read, 1988; Groth, 1988) influenced by characteristics such as solubility and particle size (Jenkins, Peterson, Thorne, & Ferguson, 1987). Furthermore, questions have arisen about the safety of such commonly used fiber supplement ingredients as prune juice, which is purported to distort the colon and cause atonia with long-term use (Kinnunen, 1991; Neal, 1995).

4. Fiber may not be effective with certain conditions, including right colonic stasis, outlet obstruction (Chaussade et al., 1989), and spinal cord injury (Cameron et al., 1996).

Exercise is another activity commonly recommended for constipation. The proposed mechanisms for a relationship between inactivity and constipation include lack of stimulus to cause mass propulsion, loss of normal reflexes when response to rectal distention is delayed, dilation of the rectum (Brocklehurst, 1980), increased transit time, reduced visceral blood flow, and loss of assistance from gravity (Oettle, 1991). Research on the relationship between exercise and constipation has focused on community populations and, with one exception (Stewart et al., 1992), has found that inactivity is associated with self-reported constipation (Donald et al., 1985; Everhart et al., 1989; Kinnunen, 1991; Levy et al., 1993; Sandler, Jordan, & Shelton, 1990). Studies of the effects of exercise on colonic motility have involved only small samples of healthy persons, and results have been contradictory (Bingham & Cummings, 1989; Coenen et al., 1992; Cordain, Latin, & Behnke, 1986; Oettle, 1991; Robertson et al., 1993).

Numerous recommendations for types of exercise are found in the literature, including walking (Baycrest Centre for Geriatric Care, 1990; Hogstel & Nelson, 1992; Karam & Nies, 1994; Sunnybrook Health Science Centre, 1992, 1994), rolling (Hogstel & Nelson, 1992; Wright & Staats, 1986), encouraging self-propulsion of the wheelchair, hip flexion (Baycrest Centre for Geriatric Care, 1990; Sunnybrook Health Science Centre, 1992), pelvic tilt, leg lifts, trunk rotation (Richards et al., 1995), leg kicks, abduction, Kegel's exercises, stomach pulls, and stationary bicycling (Karam & Nies, 1994). However, no studies have isolated the contribution of exercise to constipation management, and only three studies have included exercise in their comprehensive bowel management protocols (Gibson et al., 1995; Karam & Nies, 1994; Richards Hall, Rakel, Karstens, Swanson, & Davidson, 1995). Of note, two of these studies (Karam & Nies, 1994; Richards Hall et al., 1995) identified problems with patient or staff compliance with the prescribed exercise. Although there is no research evidence to provide direction for choosing among these interventions for managing constipation, there is general acceptance that exercise is an important component of patient care that can prevent deterioration of health and hasten recovery from illness. Feasibility and patient preference are important considerations in selecting specific exercises.

In addition to the aforementioned nonpharmacological measures for Constipation/Impaction Management, toileting is proposed for inclusion in the NIC activities. Richards Hall et al. (1995) assert that "the availability of adequate toilet facilities, privacy, and the time necessary to defecate are as important to normal bowel function as an intact gastrointestinal tract." Others note that prolonged inhibition can result in progressive ineffectiveness of the defecation reflex (Maas & Specht, 1991).

As was the case with exercise, several studies have examined the effectiveness of toileting activities in combination with other interventions (Gibson et al., 1995; Karam & Nies, 1994; Read et al., 1995; Stewart, Innes, Mackenzie, & Downie, 1997), but its contribution has not been isolated. Specific toileting recommendations included in the guidelines for nonpharmacological prevention and treatment (Table 5–3) were adapted from the unpublished protocols from the authors' facilities (Baycrest Centre for Geriatric Care, 1990; Sunnybrook Health Science Centre, 1992, 1994), which are feasible and consistent with anecdotal recommendations found in the literature.

Finally, the role of education in management of constipation has also not been isolated in research to date. However, it is important to educate patients and families about the risk factors identified during assessment and the recommended activities. Education about medications may include constipating side effects of medications, appropriate use of laxatives, and techniques for administering suppositories and enemas. In addition, it is useful to identify and correct any false beliefs (such as the need for daily bowel movements) and to teach patients and families to monitor and report the frequency and characteristics of bowel movements and any symptoms of constipation.

PHARMACOLOGICAL ACTIVITIES

Pharmacological NIC activities are (1) instruct patient/family on appropriate use of laxatives; (2) administer laxative or enema, as appropriate; and (3) administer enema or irrigation, as appropriate. There is very limited research on these activities and specific pharmacological agents. The few laxative trials that are available vary widely in the definition of constipation used, patient population studied, and outcomes measured (Harari, Gurwitz, & Minaker, 1993). However, it is important for the nurse to understand the different types of laxatives, their mechanisms of action, indications, and interactions with other medications.

Laxatives may be classified as bulk-forming, emollient or softener, saline, hyperosmotic, stimulant, suppositories, and enemas (deRond, 1991; Hutchison, 1978; Tedesco & DiPiro, 1985; Wald, 1993). The actions, precautions, and research support for each of these drug categories are discussed in turn. General considerations in laxative selection are then identified, followed by guidelines for pharmacological management of acute constipation/impaction and chronic constipation, including specific indications for the various laxatives.

Bulk-forming Laxatives

Bulk laxatives such as psyllium, methylcellulose, and polycarbophil increase the frequency of bowel movements and soften stools by holding water in the stool (Ashraf, Park, Lof, & Quigley, 1995; Yakabowich, 1990). They should be taken with at least 250 mL of water to minimize the risk of impaction or intestinal obstruction and should be avoided in patients with intestinal obstruction, low fluid intake, or swallowing difficulty (Baycrest Centre for Geriatric Care Formulary, 1995; Sunnybrook Health Science Centre Formulary, 1996). Psyllium should also be used with caution with hypertensive and sodium-restricted patients because it contains large amounts of sodium (Yakabowich, 1990). Cramping, flatulence, and bloating can occur during the first week of bulk laxative use but can be minimized by gradual introduction. Bulk laxatives can also bind with and decrease the absorption of many drugs, including warfarin, cardiac glycosides, salicylates, and nitrofurantoin (Judd, Wong, & Preece, 1982).

In their summary of the literature, Harari et al. (1993) concluded that (1) synthetic bulking agents and natural fibers are equally effective in increasing stool frequency and volume; and (2) bulk laxatives have been shown to reduce constipation in bedridden elderly patients, reduce abdominal pain in patients with irritable bowel syndrome, and relieve painful defecation in patients with hemorrhoids. The results of a more recent study comparing psyllium with placebo (Cheskin et al., 1995) were equivocal. Subjects receiving psyllium had significantly reduced transit time, but the underlying abnormality of pelvic dyssynergia was not corrected.

Emollient (Lubricant) Laxatives

Emollient laxatives include mineral oil and docusate salts. Mineral oil given orally or rectally lubricates the mucosa and softens the stool. Because oral mineral oil may decrease the absorption of fat-soluble vitamins, it should be administered between meals (Wald, 1993). It should be avoided in persons with swallowing difficulties because aspiration of mineral oil may result in lipid pneumonia, localized granuloma, and pulmonary fibrosis (Wald, 1993; Yakabowich, 1990). Docusate salts are anionic surfactants that promote water retention in the fecal mass, thus softening the stool. Docusate salts should not be used in combination with mineral oil because they increase absorption of mineral oil. Although docusate is frequently prescribed as a laxative, its main action is fecal softening and its efficacy as a laxative has been questioned. A randomized double-blind study found no significant qualitative or quantitative differences in bowel movements between patients receiving placebo and those receiving docusate (Castle, Cantrell, Israel, & Samuelson, 1991).

Saline Laxatives

Saline laxatives, such as magnesium citrate, magnesium hydroxide, magnesium sulfate, and sodium phosphate, attract water osmotically into the lumen of the intestines. Fluid accumulation alters stool consistency and distends the bowel, inducing peristaltic movements (Smith, 1987; Yakabowich, 1990). Magnesium hydroxide should be used with caution in patients with renal insufficiency because of the danger of magnesium intoxication (Tedesco & DiPiro, 1985; Wald, 1993; Yakabowich, 1990). Magnesium salts have a rapid onset of action and may also cause abdominal cramping and watery stools, which can precipitate dehydration and fecal incontinence, particularly with elderly persons (Harari et al., 1993). Although magnesium hydroxide is among the most common laxatives used in hospital and community settings, there is a lack of quality data on its efficacy and safety (Harari et al., 1993).

Hyperosmotic Laxatives

Hyperosmotic agents include polyethylene glycol, lactulose, sorbitol, and glycerol. These agents draw fluid into the bowel and soften stool. The dose should be adjusted to minimize adverse effects (e.g., bloating, flatulence, diarrhea) and modulate defecation. Although lactulose has been called the drug of choice for treatment of chronic constipation in elderly persons and has been shown to be safe and effective (Bass & Dennis, 1981; Rousseau, 1988; Sanders, 1978; Wesselius-Descasparis, Braadbaart, van der Bergh-Bohlken, & Mimica, 1968), use of this agent has been limited by its cost (Tedesco & DiPiro, 1985). Several studies have identified less expensive alternatives, such as sorbitol (Lederle, Busch, Mattox, West, & Aske, 1990), senna (Sykes, 1996), and senna combined with fiber (Passmore, Wilson-Davies, Stroker, & Scott, 1993) or metamucil (Kinnunen, Winbald, Koistinen, & Salokannel, 1993), which were all comparable in efficacy and safety. Polyethylene glycol (GoLYTELY) is a more potent hyperosmotic laxative usually prescribed for bowel cleansing prior to colonoscopy, but a controlled study found that 225 to 450 g (250 to 500 mL) daily is effective in the treatment of chronic constipation (Andorsky & Goldner, 1990).

Stimulant Laxatives

Stimulant laxatives include castor oil, anthraquinones (e.g., cascara sagrada, senna), and diphenylmethanes (e.g., phenolphthalein, bisacodyl) with varied mechanisms of action (Wald, 1993). Patients should be monitored for dose-dependent side effects of cramping, diarrhea, and dehydration (Harari et al., 1993; Wald, 1993). Chronic use may result in laxative-dependent bowel, fluid and electrolyte imbalance, and melanosis coli. In addition, bisacodyl is a gastric irritant, and enteric-coated tablets should not be crushed or chewed nor given with antacids or milk of magnesia (Yakabowich, 1990). Excessive use of bisacodyl may also induce osteomalacia secondary to impaired absorption of vitamin D and calcium (Yakabowich, 1990). One study found senna comparable to lactulose in maintaining normal bowel function; however, the subjects receiving senna experienced significantly more adverse effects, mainly abdominal pain (Sykes, 1996).

Laxative Suppositories

Laxative suppositories include glycerin, which draws water into the feces, and the stimulant bisacodyl. Because suppositories are invasive and irritate the mucosa, they are generally recommended only when oral laxatives have failed or when prompt and thorough cleansing of the bowel is desired. However, the less irritating glycerin can be useful for bowel-retraining programs (Sunnybrook Health Science Centre Formulary, 1996). Effectiveness of suppositories can be enhanced by administering them after breakfast, avoiding use with hard dry stool, and ensuring that the suppository is placed against the rectal mucosa beyond the internal and external sphincters (Harari et al., 1993; Sunnybrook Health Science Centre Formulary, 1996; Yakabowich, 1990).

Enemas

Enemas containing sodium phosphate, mineral oil, tap water, or soapsuds induce evacuation as a response to mechanical distention of the distal colon (Harari et al., 1993). Enemas should not be used routinely because they are highly invasive and frequent use may damage the mucosa. Incorrect use can lead to fluid and electrolyte imbalances and sometimes even colonic perforation (Yakabowich, 1990). Enemas should be used only in the presence of impaction or when oral laxatives and suppositories have failed. Mineral oil may be chosen when stool is very hard; tap-water enemas are useful with very high or large impactions (Harari et al., 1993). Soapsuds enemas should not be used because they cause discomfort, disrupt homeostasis, and damage the mucosa (Harari et al., 1993; Sunnybrook Health Science Centre Formulary, 1996).

SELECTION OF SPECIFIC PHARMACOLOGICAL AGENTS

Selection of specific pharmacological agents should be made after considering the following:

1. The factors contributing to the individual's constipation, including concurrent illnesses

2. Side effects of the agents, including drug interactions

3. The patient's home bowel management pattern and plan (pharmacological and nonpharmacological measures)

4. Opportunities to enhance nonpharmacological measures

5. Research evidence on the effectiveness of the drug

6. Invasiveness of the agent

7. Provider and patient preference

Several step-wise approaches to the pharmacological treatment of constipation and impaction have been developed (deRond, 1991; Harari et al., 1993; Hutchison, 1978; Preece & Judd, 1982; Sunnybrook Health Science Centre, 1994; Tedesco & DiPiro, 1985). The most commonly accepted pharmacological approaches to Constipation/Impaction Management from these sources are outlined in Tables 5–4 and 5–5. Table 5–6 identifies considerations for disimpaction, a procedure that may be necessary when acute constipation is not relieved by pharmacological agents.

Table 5–4 Guidelines for Pharmacological Management of Acute Constipation/Impaction

If absent or inadequate bowel movements for 3–5 days:

Option 1: (For Patients Who Accept Rectal Therapy and Require Urgent Relief)	Option 2: (For Patients Who Refuse Rectal Therapy or Urgent Relief Is Not Required)
• Glycerin suppository • If ineffective in 30 min, give Fleet enema • If ineffective in 30 min, repeat Fleet enema • May repeat regimen to clear excess stool	• Milk of magnesia 30 mL at bedtime for 1–2 nights

For constipation lasting >5 days:

Option 1:	Option 2:
• Fleet enema. May repeat in 30 min.	• Mineral oil enema • Follow in 1 hr by Fleet enema if needed

If ineffective, select one of the following clean out regimens (options 1 or 2 preferred):

Option 1:	Option 2:	Option 3:
• Sodium phosphate oral solution 45 mL by mouth, repeat in 5 hr	• Gastrointestinal lavage solution, GoLYTELY, up to 4 L by mouth	• Mineral oil 30 mL by mouth q 2 hr while awake until one large or multiple small oily bowel movements occur
(Usually effective within 12 hr)	(Usually effective within 12 hr)	(May take several days to produce an effect)

• If ineffective, consider disimpaction (see Table 5–6) or gastroenterology consult.

• Once constipation/impaction relieved, maximize nonpharmacological measures and request orders for laxatives to prevent recurrence (see selection of specific pharmacological agents).

Table 5–5   Guidelines for Pharmacological Management of Chronic Constipation

Chronic constipation is indicated by history of premorbid constipation; hard, dry stools; difficult or incomplete evacuation; or infrequent stool compared with the person's usual pattern.

Implement appropriate nonpharmacological interventions (see Table 5–3):

If Constipation Is Relieved:	If Constipation Is Not Relieved, Add:	
• Continue nonpharmacological measures • Use Guidelines for Acute Constipation as needed.	Option 1: Docusate calcium 240–480 mg daily	Option 2: Psyllium 5–20 g daily at breakfast or supper Divide doses if >10 g daily

If Effective:	If Ineffective, Add:	
• Continue all interventions prophylactically • Consider reducing dose or discontinuing laxative if stool becomes too soft or diarrhea occurs	Option 1: Milk of magnesia at bedtime in an amount to produce 1–3 normal bowel movements (up to 60 mL)	Option 2: Senokot 1–4 tablets at bedtime to produce 1–3 normal bowel movements
	If Ineffective, Add a Local Agent:	
	• Glycerin suppository after breakfast • If ineffective in 30 min, give bisacodyl suppository (can repeat × 1) • If ineffective in 30 min, give Fleet enema • Continue with nonpharmacological measures, using acute constipation guidelines as needed. • Reduce laxatives to minimum amount required in order to maintain bowel function.	

EVALUATION

The same assessment activities outlined at the beginning of this chapter can be used to evaluate the effectiveness of nursing actions to treat constipation/impaction. Several patient outcomes from the Nursing Outcomes Classification

Table 5–6   Considerations for Disimpaction

1. Determine whether disimpaction is indicated (i.e., hard stool is present, patient is acutely distressed, and pharmacological measures have been ineffective).
2. Determine whether any contraindications exist (i.e., recent rectal, gynecological, or prostate surgery; increased intracranial pressure; active rectal bleeding; neutropenia; platelets less than 20,000 μL; or acute myocardial infarction).
3. Explain procedure to patient and ask patient to report any dizziness, chest pain, severe cramps, rectal bleeding, or other discomfort.
4. Consider administering mild analgesics or topical anesthetics prior to disimpaction.
5. Position patient on the left side (proper position if enemas have to be given immediately after disimpaction).
6. Gently insert a gloved, lubricated finger into the rectum and remove any smaller particles of stool before attempting to remove very hard stool. Insert two fingers to break stool into smaller fragments.
7. Remind patient to exhale when bearing down (prevents unnecessary straining).
8. Pause frequently to monitor patient response and provide rest and reassurance.
9. Administer a small retention enema (Fleet) to stimulate complete evacuation.
10. If patient is unable to retain enema, insert a bisacodyl suppository to stimulate peristalsis.

Source: Adapted from Mager-O'Connor, 1984; Sunnybrook Health Science Centre, 1994.

(NOC) may be affected (Johnson & Maas, 1997). The specific nursing actions that are selected based on the assessment findings will determine which outcomes are influenced. Those outcomes most likely to be affected by the intervention include the following:

Bowel Continence
Bowel Elimination
Comfort Level
Hydration
Immobility Consequences: Physiological
Knowledge: Diet, Medications, and Prescribed Activity
Nutritional Status: Food and Fluid Intake
Self-Care: Toileting

CASE STUDY

Mrs. D, an 84-year-old widow, lived alone in a seniors' apartment. She was independent in most of her activities of daily living but needed assistance from her children for shopping and banking. Homemakers provided housecleaning and cooking assistance. Mrs. D had urinary incontinence and bilateral total hip replacements. Mrs. D ate bran flakes every morning to maintain her bowel function. She had a soft bowel movement every 2 days after breakfast. Medications taken regularly included docusate sodium 1 capsule od, indomethacin 25 mg po bid, and oxybutynin HCl (Ditropan) 5 mg po tid.

One day Mrs. D fell in her apartment and was unable to get up to summon help. She lay on the floor for 36 hours before her sister discovered her. Assessment at the nearest hospital revealed a right Colles' fracture and an undisplaced subtrochanteric crack fracture of the right hip.

Mrs. D was admitted to the hospital. A cast was placed on her right arm. Surgery was not done on her hip (because of the previously inserted prosthesis), but Buck's traction was applied to the right lower extremity and an indwelling catheter was inserted. In addition to her regular medications, a number of as-needed (prn) medications were ordered, including meperidine, acetaminophen with codeine, dimenhydrinate, and lorazepam. She received meperidine intramuscularly for 4 days and then received acetaminophen with codeine regularly.

Three days after admission to the hospital, Mrs. D informed the nursing staff that she was constipated. Abdominal examination revealed a moderately distended abdomen. A mass was palpable in the left lower quadrant. There was no abdominal tenderness. Findings of a rectal examination were negative except for the presence of a large mass of impacted stool. A tentative diagnosis of colonic constipation was made.

Guidelines for management of acute constipation/impaction were followed. Mrs. D was given a glycerin suppository. This was not effective within 1 hour, so she was then given a Fleet enema, which was effective. Thereafter, magnesium hydroxide 30 mL po was given daily at bedtime. In addition, selected nonpharmacological activities were instituted. Mrs. D was encouraged to drink 1,500 mL per day and was monitored for signs of dehydration. She received bran flakes every morning, simulating her home routine. She was placed on a fracture bedpan daily after breakfast until the traction was removed. Once the traction was removed, Mrs. D was toileted on a bedside commode. When ambulation was increased, she was toileted in the bathroom. With this combination of pharmacological and nonpharmacological activities, Mrs. D was able to maintain her usual bowel function. Because Mrs. D was no longer able to manage independently in her apartment, she was transferred to a nursing home. The bowel regimen established for Mrs. D was communicated to the receiving facility.

References

Andorsky, R., and Goldner, F. (1990). Colonic lavage solution (polyethylene glycol electrolyte lavage solution) as a treatment for chronic constipation: A double blind, placebo controlled study. *American Journal of Gastroenterology, 85,* 261–265.

Ashraf, W., Park, E., Lof, J., and Quigley, E. (1995). The effects of psyllium therapy on stool characteristics, colon transit and anorectal function in chronic idiopathic constipation. *Alimentary Pharmacology and Therapeutics, 9,* 639–647.

Badiali, D., Corazziare, E., Fortunee, I. H., Tomei, E., Bausano, G., Magrini, P., Anzini, F., and Torsoli, A. (1995). Effect of wheat bran in treatment of chronic nonorganic constipation. A double-blind controlled trial. *Digestive Diseases and Sciences, 40,* 349–356.

Bass, P., and Dennis, S. (1981). The laxative effect of lactulose in normal and constipated subjects. *Journal of Clinical Gastroenterology, 3*(Suppl. 1), 23–28.

Battle, E., and Hanna, C. (1980). Evaluation of a dietary regimen for chronic constipation: Report of a pilot study. *Journal of Gerontological Nursing, 6,* 527–532.

Baycrest Centre for Geriatric Care (Toronto, Canada). (1990). *Bowel management protocol.* Unpublished document.

Baycrest Centre for Geriatric Care Formulary (Toronto, Canada). (1995).

Beverley, L., and Travis, I. (1992). Constipation: Proposed natural laxative mixtures. *Journal of Gerontological Nursing, 18*(10), 5–12.

Bingham, S. A., and Cummings, J. (1989). Effect of exercise and physical fitness on large intestinal function. *Gastroenterology, 97,* 1389–1399.

Brocklehurst, J. C. (1980). Disorders of the lower bowel in old age. *Geriatrics, 35,* 49–54.

Brown, M. K., and Everett, I. (1990). Gentler bowel fitness with fiber. *Geriatric Nursing, 11,* 26–27.

Cameron, K. J., Nyulasi, I. B., Collier, G. R., and Brown, D. J. (1996). Assessment of the effect of increased dietary fibre intake on bowel function in patients with spinal cord injury. *Spinal Cord, 34,* 277–283.

Carroll-Johnson, R. (Ed.). (1989). *Classification of nursing diagnoses: Proceedings of the eighth conference.* Philadelphia: J. B. Lippincott.

Castle, S., Cantrell, M., Israel, D., and Samuelson, M. (1991). Constipation prevention: Empiric use of stool softeners questioned. *Geriatrics, 46,* 84–86.

Chaussade, S., Abdallah, K., Roche, H., Garret, M., Gaudric, M., Couturier, D., and Guerre, J. (1989). Determination of total and segmental colonic transit time in constipated patients. *Digestive Diseases and Sciences, 34,* 1168–1172.

Cheskin, L., Kamal, N., Crowel, M., Schuster, M., and Whitehead, W. (1995). Mechanisms of constipation in older persons and effects of fiber compared with placebo. *Journal of the American Geriatrics Society, 43,* 666–669.

Chidester, J. C., and Spangler, A. A. (1997). Fluid intake in the institutionalized elderly. *Journal of the American Dietetic Association, 97*(1), 23–30.

Coenen, C., Wegener, M., Wedmann, B., Schmidt, G., and Hoffmann, S. (1992). Does physical exercise influence bowel transit time in healthy young men? *American Journal of Gastroenterology, 87,* 292–295.

Cordain, L., Latin, R. W., and Behnke, J. J. (1986). The effects of an aerobic running program on bowel transit time. *Journal of Sports Medicine, 26,* 101–104.

deRond, D. (1991). Constipation: Treatment with laxatives. *On Continuing Practice, 18*(4), 35–39.

Donald, I. P., Smith, R. G., Cruikshank, J. G., Elton, R., and Stoddart, M. (1985). A study of constipation in the elderly living at home. *Gerontology, 31,* 112–118.

Eaton, M., Mitchell-Bonair, I. L., and Friedmann, E. (1986). The effect of touch on nutritional intake of chronic organic brain syndrome patients. *Journal of Gerontology, 41,* 611–616.

Edwards, C. A., Tomlin, J., and Read, N. W. (1988). Fibre and constipation. *British Journal of Clinical Practice, 42*(1), 26–32.

Everhart, J. E., Go, V., Johannes, R., Fitzsimmons, S., Roth, H., and White, L. (1989). A longitudinal survey of self-reported bowel habits in the United States. *Digestive Diseases and Sciences, 34,* 1153–1162.

Finlay, M. (1988). The use of dietary fibre in a long-stay geriatric ward. *Journal of Nutrition for the Elderly, 8*(1), 19–30.

Gibson, C., Opalka, P., Moore, C., Brady, R., and Mion, L. (1995). Effectiveness of bran supplement on the bowel management of elderly rehabilitation patients. *Journal of Gerontological Nursing, 21*(10), 21–30.

Goldstein, M. K., Melnick Brown, E., Holt, P., Gallagher, D., and Hutner Winograd, C. (1989). Fecal incontinence in an elderly man. *Journal of the American Geriatrics Society, 37,* 991–1002.

Graham, D., Moser, S., and Estes, M. (1982). The effect of bran on bowel function in constipation. *American Journal of Gastroenterology, 77,* 599–603.

Groth, F. (1988). Effects of wheat bran in the diet of postsurgical orthopaedic patients to prevent constipation. *Orthopaedic Nursing, 7*(4), 41–46.

Hagberg, R., Fines, M., and Doyle, B. (1987). A fiber-supplemented dietary regimen to treat or prevent constipation in one nursing home. *Nursing Homes, 36,* 28–33.

Haight, B., and Burggraf, V. (1991). Tips on promoting food and fluid intake in the elderly. *Journal of Gerontological Nursing, 17*(11), 44–46.

Hankey, C., Cullen, A., Wynne, H., Death, J., and Kenny, R. A. (1992). Non-starch polysaccharide / dietary fibre supplementation using small meals in long-stay frail elderly patients. *European Journal of Clinical Nutrition, 4,* 521–523.

Harari, D., Gurwitz, J., and Minaker, K. (1993). Constipation in the elderly. *Journal of the American Geriatrics Society, 41,* 1130–1140.

Hogstel, M., and Nelson, M. (1992). Anticipation and early detection can reduce bowel elimination complications. *Geriatric Nursing, 13,* 28–33.

Hope, A., and Down, E. (1986). Dietary fibre and fluid in the control of constipation in a nursing home population. *Medical Journal of Australia, 144,* 306–307.

Hull, C., Greco, R., and Brooks, D. (1980). Alleviation of constipation in the elderly by dietary fiber supplementation. *Journal of the American Geriatrics Society, 28,* 410–414.

Hutchison, B. (1978). Constipation in the elderly. *Canadian Family Physician, 24,* 1218–1222.

Jenkins, D., Peterson, D., Thorne, M., and Ferguson, P. (1987). Wheat fiber and laxation: Dose response and equilibration time. *American Journal of Gastroenterology, 82,* 1259–1263.

Johnson, M., and Maas, M. (Eds.) (1997). *Nursing outcomes classification.* St Louis: Mosby–Year Book.

Judd, C., Wong, H., and Preece, C. (1982). Stepwise

treatment of constipation. *Canadian Pharmaceutic Journal, 115*(6), 228.

Karam, S., and Nies, D. (1994). Student/staff collaboration: A pilot bowel management program. *Journal of Gerontological Nursing, 20*(3), 32–40.

Kinnunen, O. (1991). Study of constipation in a geriatric hospital, day hospital, old people's home and at home. *Aging, 3*(2), 161–170.

Kinnunen, O., Winbald, I., Koistinen, P., and Salokannel, J. (1993). Safety and efficacy of a bulk laxative containing senna versus lactulose in the treatment of constipation in geriatric patients. *Pharmacology, 47*(Suppl. 1), 253–255.

Klauser, A. G., Beck, A., Schindlbeck, N. E., and Muller-Lissner, S. A. (1990). Low fluid intake lowers stool output in healthy male volunteers [Abstract]. *Zeitschrift fur Gastroenterologie, 28*, 606–609.

Klauser, A. G., and Muller-Lissner, S. A. (1993). How effective is nonlaxative treatment of constipation? *Pharmacology, 47*(Suppl. 1), 256–260.

Kochen, M., Wegscheider, K., and Abholz, H. (1985). Prophylaxis of constipation by wheat bran: A randomized study in hospitalized patiients. *Digestion, 31*, 220–224.

Lange-Alberts, M., and Shott, S. (1994). Nutritional intake: Use of touch and verbal cuing. *Journal of Gerontological Nursing, 20*(2), 36–40.

Lederle, E., Busch, D., Mattox, K., West, M., and Aske, D. (1990). Cost effective treatment of constipation in the elderly: A randomized double blind comparison of sorbitol and lactulose. *American Journal of Medicine, 89*, 597–601.

Levy, N., Stermer, E., Steiner, Z., Epstein, L., and Tamir, A. (1993). Bowel habits in Israel: A cohort study. *Journal of Clinical Gastroenterology, 16*, 295–299.

Maas, M., and Specht, J. (1991). Bowel incontinence. In M. Maas, K. C. Buckwalter, and M. Hardy (Eds.), *Nursing diagnoses and interventions for the elderly* (p. 171). Redwood City, California: Addison-Wesley.

Mager-O'Connor, E. (1984). How to identify and remove fecal impactions. *Geriatric Nursing, 5*, 158–161.

Mantle, J. (1992). Research and serendipitous secondary findings. *The Canadian Nurse, 88*, 15–18.

McCloskey, J. C., and Bulechek, G. M. (Eds.) (1996). *Nursing interventions classification (NIC)* (2nd ed.). St. Louis: Mosby-Year Book.

Neal, L. J. (1995). "Power Pudding" natural laxative therapy for the elderly who are homebound. *Home Healthcare Nurse, 13*(3), 66–71.

North American Nursing Diagnosis Association (NANDA). (1992). *Proceedings of the 10th conference.* St. Louis: Author.

Oettle, G. J. (1991). Effect of moderate exercise on bowel habit. *Gut, 32*, 941–945.

Orr, W. C., Johnson, P., and Yates, C. (1997). Chronic constipation: A clinical conundrum. *Journal of the American Geriatrics Society, 45*, 652–653.

Ouellet, L. L., Turner, T. R., Pond, S., McLaughlin, H., and Knorr, S. (1996). Dietary fiber and laxation in postop orthopedic patients. *Clinical Nursing Research, 5*, 428–440.

Passmore, A., Wilson-Davies, K., Stroker, C., and Scott, M. (1993). Chronic constipation in long stay elderly patients: A comparison of lactulose and senna fibre combination. *British Medical Journal, 307*, 769–771.

Porth, C. M. (1986). *Pathophysiology: Concepts of altered health states.* Philadelphia: J. B. Lippincott.

Preece, C., and Judd, C. (1982). Constipation in the elderly: Are drugs the only alternative to irregularity? *Canadian Pharmaceutical Journal, 115*, 136–139.

Preston, D. M., and Lennard-Jones, J. E. (1986). Severe chronic constipation of young women: 'Idiopathic slow transit constipation.' *Gut, 27*, 41–48.

Pringle, R., Pennington, M. J., Pennington, C. R., and Ritchie, T. (1984). A study of the influence of a fibre biscuit on bowel function in the elderly. *Age and Ageing, 13*, 175–178.

Rajala, S. A., Salminen, S. J., Seppanen, J. H., and Vapaatalo, H. (1988). Treatment of chronic constipation with lactitol sweetened yoghurt supplemented with guar gum and wheat bran in elderly hospital in-patients. *Comprehensive Gerontology, 2*, 83–86.

Read, N., Celik, A., and Katsinelos, P. (1995). Constipation and incontinence in the elderly. *Journal of Clinical Gastroenterology, 20*(1), 61–70.

Richards Hall, G., Rakel, B., Karstens, M., Swanson, E., and Davidson, A. (1995). Managing constipation using a research-based protocol. *Medsurg Nursing, 4*(1), 11–20.

Robertson, G., Meshkinpour, H., Vandenberg, K., James, N., Cohen, A., and Wilson, A. (1993). Effects of exercise on total and segmental colon transit. *Journal of Clinical Gastroenterology, 16*, 300–303.

Rodrigues-Fisher, L., Bourguignon, C., and Vonthron-Good, B. (1993). Dietary fiber nursing intervention. *Clinical Nursing Research, 2*, 464–477.

Ross, D. (1990). Constipation among hospitalized elders. *Orthopaedic Nursing, 9*, 73–77.

Rousseau, P. (1988). Treatment of constipation in the elderly. *Postgraduate Medicine, 84*, 339–349.

Sanders, J. (1978). Lactulose syrup assessed in a double blind study of elderly constipated patients. *Journal of the American Geriatrics Society, 26*, 236–239.

Sandler, R., Jordan, M. C., and Shelton, B. J. (1990). Demographic and dietary determinants of constipation in the US population. *American Journal of Public Health, 80*(2), 185–189.

Schmelzer, M. (1990). Effectiveness of wheat bran in preventing constipation of hospitalized orthopaedic surgery patients. *Orthopaedic Nursing, 19*, 55–59.

Smith, S. (1987). Drugs and the gastrointestinal tract. *Nursing Times, 83*(26), 50–52.

Snustad, D., Lee, V., Abraham, I., Alexander, C., Bella, D., and Cumming, C. (1991). Dietary fiber in hospitalized geriatric patients: Too soft a solution for too hard a problem? *Journal of Nutrition for the Elderly, 10*(2), 49–62.

Stewart, E., Innes, J., Mackenzie, J., and Downie, G. (1997). A strategy to reduce laxative use among older people. *Nursing Times, 93*(4), 35–36.

Stewart, R. B., Moore, M. T., Stat, M., Marks, R., and Hale, W. (1992). Correlates of constipation in an ambulatory elderly population. *American Journal of Gastroenterology, 87*, 859–864.

Sunnybrook Health Science Centre (Toronto, Canada). (1992). *Bowel management protocol, extended care.* Unpublished document.

Sunnybrook Health Science Centre (Toronto, Canada). (1994). *Bowel management protocol, acute care.* Unpublished document.

Sunnybrook Health Science Centre Formulary (Toronto, Canada). (1996).

Sykes, N. (1996). A volunteer model for the comparison of laxatives in opioid related constipation. *Journal of Pain and Symptom Management, 11*, 363–369.

Tedesco, F. J., and DiPiro, J. T. (1985). Laxative use in constipation. *American Journal in Gastroenterology, 80*, 303–309.

Tierney, L. M., McPhee, S. J., and Papadakis, M. A.

(1997). *Current medical diagnosis and treatment* (36th ed.). Stamford, CT: Appleton & Lange.

Towers, A. L., Burgion, K. L., Locher, J. L., Merkel, I., Safaeian, M., and Wald, A. (1994). Constipation in the elderly: Influence of dietary, psychological, and physiological factors. *Journal of the American Geriatrics Society, 42,* 701–706.

Turner, J., and Turner, A. (1987). Problems of recognising dehydration in hospital patients. *Nursing Times, 83*(51), 44.

Valle-Jones, J. C. (1985). An open study of oat bran meal biscuits ('Lejfibre') in the treatment of constipation in the elderly. *Current Medical Research and Opinion, 9,* 716–720.

Voderholzer, W. A., Schatke, W., Muhldorfer, B. E., Klauser, A. G., Birkner, B., and Muller-Lissner, S. (1997). Clinical response to dietary fiber treatment of chronic constipation. *American Journal of Gastroenterology, 92,* 95–98.

Wald, A. (1993). Constipation in elderly patients: Pathogenesis and management. *Drugs and Aging, 3,* 220–231.

Wesselius-Descasparis, S., Braadbaart, S., van der Bergh-Bohlken, G., and Mimica, M. (1968). Treatment of chronic constipation with lactulose syrup: Results of a double blind study. *Gut, 9,* 984–986.

Whitehead, W. E., Drinkwater, D., Cheskin, L. J. Heller, B., and Schuster, M. (1989). Constipation in the elderly living at home: Definition, prevalence, and relationship to lifestyle and health status. *Journal of the American Geriatrics Society, 37,* 423–429.

Williams, K., and Rae, B. (1995). Developments in continence care. *Elderly Care, 7*(5), 19–22.

Wright, B. A., and Staats, D. O. (1986). The geriatric implications of fecal impaction. *Nurse Practitioner, 11*(10), 53–66.

Yakabowich, M. (1990). Prescribe with care: The role of laxatives in the treatment of constipation. *Journal of Gerontological Nursing, 17*(7), 4–11.

Ziegenhagen, J., Tewinkel, G., Kruis, W., and Hermann, F. (1991). Adding more fluid to wheat bran has no significant effects on intestinal functions of healthy subjects. *Journal of Clinical Gastroenterology, 13,* 525–530.

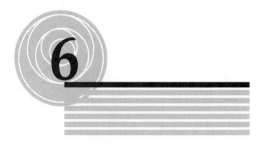

Positioning

Debbie Metzler and Cynthia Finesilver

Positioning, as defined in the *Nursing Interventions Classification (NIC)* (McCloskey & Bulechek, 1996), is moving the patient or patient's body part to provide comfort, reduce the risk of skin breakdown, promote skin integrity, and promote healing. Positioning and turning a patient are an integral part of nursing care and are typically independent nursing actions (Gawlinski, 1993). Nurses are challenged to provide a turning and positioning plan that is based on their particular patient's needs and is cost-effective yet can help prevent the complications of immobility, promote comfort, and facilitate healing. Positioning can be either a dangerous or a beneficial sequence of events depending on the patient's age, pre-existing health problems, and current health status. Assessment of the patient's tolerance of the activities is necessary, as are evaluation and modification of the plan as needed.

This chapter discusses how to implement the current list of NIC positioning activities (Table 6–1), provides research to support use of these activities, makes suggestions on potential additional activities, and discusses how these activities can be applied to specific populations. A case study is included to show how the positioning intervention can be integrated into the nursing process to provide quality patient care.

SPECIFIC USE OF THE CURRENT POSITIONING INTERVENTION

The following information elaborates on some of the positioning activities in NIC (see Table 6–1) and on the underlying research-based rationale for these activities.

Table 6–1 Positioning

DEFINITION: Moving the patient or a body part to provide comfort, to reduce the risk of skin breakdown, promote skin integrity, and/or promote healing.

ACTIVITIES:

Place on an appropriate therapeutic mattress/bed

Provide a firm mattress

Place in the designated therapeutic position

Position in proper body alignment

Immobilize or support the affected body part, as appropriate

Elevate the affected body part, as appropriate

Avoid placing the amputation stump in the flexion posture

Position to alleviate dyspnea (e.g., semi-Fowler position), as appropriate

Provide support to the edematous area (e.g., pillow under arms and scrotal support), as appropriate

Position to facilitate ventilation/perfusion matching ("good lung down"), as appropriate

Encourage active range-of-motion exercises

Provide appropriate support for neck

Apply a footboard to the bed

Turn using the log roll technique

Position to promote urinary drainage, as appropriate

Position to avoid placing tension on the wound, as appropriate

Prop with a backrest, as appropriate

Elevate the affected limb 20 degrees or greater, above the level of the heart, to improve venous return, as appropriate

Instruct the patient to use good posture and good body mechanics while performing any activity

Monitor traction devices for proper setup

Maintain position and integrity of traction

Elevate the head of the bed, as appropriate

Turn as indicated by skin condition

Turn an immobilized patient at least every 2 hr, according to a specific schedule

Use appropriate devices to support limbs (e.g., hand roll and trochanter roll)

Place frequently-used objects within reach

Place bed-positioning switch within easy reach

Place the call light within reach

Source: McCloskey, J. C., and Bulechek, G. M. (Eds.) (1996). *Nursing interventions classification (NIC)* (2nd ed., p. 437). St. Louis: Mosby–Year Book.

Place on appropriate therapeutic mattress/bed

A variety of pressure-reducing mattresses are available, including foam, static air, alternating air, gel, or water. These devices decrease the incidence of pressure ulcers; however, there is no evidence to suggest that one type of mattress is more effective than another in preventing pressure ulcers (Whitney, Fellows, & Larson, 1984). Alterescu (1983) noted that proper selection of mechanical devices can result in a reduction of 5% to 30% in the institutional incidence of pressure sores.

A nurse, however, should not develop a false sense of security when using replacement mattresses that reduce pressure but do not totally relieve it (Whittemore, Bautista, Smith, & Bruttomesso, 1993). Even though these mattresses reduce pressure under the sacrum, the heels may still require additional pressure-relieving measures to prevent cellular ischemia (Whittemore et al., 1993).

Provide a firm mattress

It is generally believed that a firm mattress provides better support than a soft mattress. Research by Seiler, Allen, and Staheli (1986) on healthy subjects, however, indicated that bony prominences became anoxemic when the subject was lying on a typical firm mattress. This was only one study, and it was not done on ill patients; therefore, more research is needed before drawing any conclusions about the use of firm mattresses.

Position in proper body alignment

Positioning the patient in proper body alignment is necessary to prevent development of musculoskeletal deformities, such as contractures and ankylosis. A sufficient number of pillows should be available to maintain body alignment. If an arm is weak or paralyzed, it should be positioned to approximate the joint space in the glenoid cavity. The affected arm should not be pulled. A small pillow or wedge in the axillary region will help prevent adduction of the shoulder. Special resting splints may be ordered to prevent contractures. They should be removed periodically to assess for pressure areas (Hickey, 1996).

Improper positioning can result in peripheral nerve and blood vessel damage, especially if pre-existing conditions such as peripheral vascular disease or diabetes are present. External pressure on, or stretching of, the peripheral blood vessels and nerves is the main cause of damage to these structures (Cantin, 1989). To prevent this from occurring, it is important to have a knowledge of the origins and pathways of the major blood vessels and nerves, in particular those of the extremities. A good rule of thumb for ascertaining nerve pathways is to follow the major blood vessels, because the neurological supply closely parallels the vascular supply (Smith, 1990). Knowing this will help the nurse maintain correct positions that prevent peripheral blood and nerve vessel compromise. In addition to mechanical pressure, vessels can also be occluded by hyperextending or twisting a limb. This action blocks the blood flow by compressing the vessels against the body's skeleton. Therefore, avoid hyperextension of the limbs and pressure on the vessels and nerves.

Brachial plexus damage is a common peripheral nerve injury that can occur when there is hyperextension of the arm (greater than 90 degrees of abduction). This results in motor and sensory loss in the arm and shoulder girdle. Subclavian and axillary arteries may also become compressed with this hyperextension when the patient is unable to move his or her limbs independently (Cantin, 1989). To prevent this injury, do not lift the patient up in bed by grasping under the axillae and shoulders. Instead, use a draw sheet under the patient to lift him or her up in bed.

Wristdrop can be caused by compressing the arm against the side of the bed, causing damage to the radial nerve (Cantin, 1989). A hand deformity may be caused by injury to the median or ulnar nerve. Patients who are emaciated are at even greater risk for nerve damage because there is less soft tissue to protect the nerves. Large vessels may become damaged by the mechanical obstructions associated with tight-fitting elastic stockings or misplaced pillows under the popliteal space. This nerve damage results in numbness on the plantar surface of the foot (Metzler & Harr, 1996).

Elevate the affected body part, as appropriate

Hickey (1996) showed that edema of the extremities, especially the hands, can be controlled by positioning and elevating the hand higher than the elbow.

Position to alleviate dyspnea (e.g., semi-Fowler position), as appropriate

Altering patient position may improve oxygenation status and reduce the need for supplemental oxygen and mechanical ventilation (Yeaw, 1992). When positioning a patient to alleviate dyspnea, the nurse must realize that the presence of pre-existing or current lung disease, the relationship of ventilation and perfusion in the lungs, and the presence of conditions that increase oxygen demand or decrease oxygen supply affect oxygenation status just as the position of the patient does.

It has been demonstrated that when a patient has unilateral lung disease, the "good lung down" position will reduce dyspnea. Patients with bilateral lung disease experience increased dyspnea when turned to the left side (see discussion in "Positioning Activities with Clients Who Have Altered Respiratory Function").

The matching of ventilation and perfusion in the lung is a major factor affecting oxygenation and dyspnea. The force of gravity increases hydrostatic pressure and perfusion in the dependent portions of normal or diseased lungs. However, when pulmonary disease causes decreased ventilation of a lobe or one lung, the increased perfusion results in a ventilation-perfusion mismatch with subsequent tissue hypoxemia and dyspnea (Gawlinski, 1993; Hudak & Gallo, 1992; Swanlund, 1996).

If conditions that increase oxygen demand are present before position change, there may be an increase in dyspnea when the patient is repositioned. Factors that increase oxygen demand include increased body temperature, pain, agitation, increased respiratory rate and effort, and muscle rigidity. A decrease in oxygen delivery due to anemia, decreased cardiac output, airway obstruction, or bleeding may result in dyspnea when a patient is repositioned (Gawlinski, 1993).

If dyspnea occurs during or after a position change, it is generally transient and will improve in 4 to 15 minutes (Shively, 1988; Winslow, Clark, White, & Tyler, 1990). If patients have significant lung disease, bilateral lung disease, or the presence of factors that affect oxygen demand or delivery, they are at greater risk for ongoing dyspnea after position change.

The nurse should monitor oxygenation status before and at frequent intervals after any positioning change (Fontaine & McQuillan, 1989; Gawlinski, 1993). If dyspnea occurs or is increased with a position change, the patient should be placed in the supine position, and oxygenation status and the factors affecting oxygen delivery should be reassessed (Gawlinski, 1993).

Encourage active range-of-motion exercises

The benefits of active and passive range-of-motion exercises include promotion of activity and reduction of pressure on tissue (Colburn, 1987; Dimant & Francis, 1988). If the patient is able, have him or her perform active range-of-motion exercises. This activity can help maintain muscle strength and bone density. Range-of-motion exercises also promote skin integrity secondary to increased blood flow (Vanderber, Gallagher, & Severino, 1995). Be aware of any medical conditions the patient has that affect his or her ability to do range-of-motion exercises, such as arthritis, osteoporosis, muscle weakness or paralysis, decreased mental status, or malnutrition. Movement should never cause or increase pain. Joint movement should never be forced and is more beneficial when the patient is relaxed.

Both active and passive range-of-motion exercises to a joint are contraindicated whenever motion would be disruptive to the healing process, such as with an unhealed fracture or with terminally ill clients who have pathological fractures (McCaffery & Wolff, 1992). When active range-of-motion exercises are done, isometric exercise and the Valsalva maneuver should be avoided because these activities will increase intrathoracic pressure, which may lead to hemodynamic changes as well as increased intracranial pressure (Hickey, 1996).

Apply a footboard to the bed

A footboard may be useful when the patient is in the semi-Fowler position; however, it may increase intracranial pressure, which is contraindicated in patients with altered neurological function (see "Additional Positioning Considerations with Specific Positions" and "Positioning Activities with Clients Who Have Altered Neurological Function") (Hickey, 1996).

Turn using the log roll technique

Log rolling facilitates alignment and avoids angulation of body parts while turning. Special attention must be given to the neck and hips while turning (Kozier, Erb, Blais, & Wilkinson, 1995).

Maintain position and integrity of traction

If the patient has any external devices such as orthotics, slings, braces, casts, traction apparatus, prostheses, or splints, assess for pain, tightness, or changes in sensitivity resulting from pressure and friction of these devices (Wienke, 1987).

Elevate the head of the bed, as appropriate

To reduce shear forces, which increase the risk of sacral tissue necrosis, the head of the bed should be maintained at the lowest degree of elevation consistent with the patient's medical condition (Reichel, 1958).

Turn as indicated by skin condition
Turn an immobilized patient at least every 2 hours, according to a specific schedule

When changing the patient's position, inspect the skin, with increased attention to bony prominences. Ninety percent of pressure ulcers develop over bony prominences of the lower half of the body, with 50% occurring at the sacral and trochanteric areas (Michocki & Lamy, 1976; Rousseau, 1988).

Assessment of the skin should include close observation for redness, which is called hyperemia phenomenon. Hyperemia occurs when an underperfused area regains perfusion with subsequent blood flow into the area and correction of tissue hypoxia (Maklebust, 1987). Recognition of hyperemia is an indication that the patient requires more frequent positioning. When hyperemia persists for more than 15 minutes after pressure has been removed, tissue damage may be present. In dark-skinned patients, a red color change may indicate hyperemia. Tissue hyperemia in very dark-skinned patients may be indicated by an increase in skin temperature, darkening of normal skin color, or lightening of normal skin color (Feustel, 1982). Skin assessments should be documented in addition to the patient's turning schedule.

Use appropriate devices to support limbs (e.g., hand roll and trochanter roll)

Pillows and foam wedges keep bony prominences from direct skin-on-skin contact. If a patient is immobilized, the highest pressure areas are the heels, which require additional interventions. Pillows placed under the lower leg will elevate the heels and relieve pressure (Parish & Witkowski, 1980). The use of donut or ring cushions is controversial because it has been shown that they will cause venous congestion, edema, and possibly pressure ulcers (Crewe, 1987).

Place frequently used objects within reach

Place bed-positioning switch within easy reach

Place the call light within reach

The call light, personal hygiene items, water pitcher, and other items should be placed on the unaffected side of patients with visual problems, unilateral muscle weakness or paralysis, or unilateral neglect (Hickey, 1996).

RESEARCH IS NEEDED ON THE FOLLOWING POSITIONING ACTIVITIES

These activities are also included in the NIC list of activities. Some of the research for these activities is addressed later, related to specific clients. The research for other activities may be covered in a review of other populations not addressed in this chapter.

Place in the designated therapeutic position (Refer to sections of this chapter on positioning activities for specific clients.)

Immobilize or support the affected body part, as appropriate

Avoid placing the amputation stump in the flexion position

Provide support to the edematous areas (e.g., pillow under arms and scrotal support), as appropriate

Position to facilitate ventilation-perfusion matching ("good lung down"), as appropriate (See "Positioning Activities with Clients Who Have Altered Respiratory Function.")

Provide appropriate support for the neck (See "Positioning Activities with Patients Who Have Altered Neurological Function.")

Position to promote urinary drainage, as appropriate

Position to avoid placing tension on the wound, as appropriate

Prop with a backrest, as appropriate

Elevate affected limb 20 degrees or greater above the level of the heart to improve venous return, as appropriate

Instruct the patient to use good posture and good body mechanics while performing any activity

Monitor traction devices for proper setup

ADDITIONAL POSITIONING ACTIVITIES TO CONSIDER

1. Monitor oxygenation status before and after position change. Measurements should include pulse oximetry, respiratory rate and pattern, mental

status, level of comfort, and arterial blood gases, if indicated. Blood for measurement of arterial blood gases should be drawn one-half hour after position change. Record the patient's position along with the blood gas results (Schmitz, 1991).

2. Premedicate patients as indicated before turning. Pain and discomfort experienced during repositioning are major causes of increased energy expenditure during turning (Vanderber et al., 1994). Assess for respiratory depression if analgesic medication is given.

3. Never place the patient in a position that increases pain.

4. Encourage the patient to get involved in positioning changes (Metzler & Harr, 1996).

5. Assess the patient's preferred sleeping position and record it on the care plan. If it is not contraindicated, incorporate this position into the positioning plan (Metzler & Harr, 1996).

6. Explain to the patient that he or she is being repositioned, so that he or she is not frightened or surprised. These activities may cause an increase in oxygen demand (Gawlinski, 1993).

7. Avoid massage over bony prominences because this increases tissue trauma and skin tearing (Ek, Gustavsson, & Lewis, 1985).

8. Minimize friction and shearing forces when positioning and turning the patient to avoid skin injury. Friction injuries to the skin occur when the skin moves across a coarse surface such as bed linens. Many friction injuries can be avoided if, when patients are moved, their skin is never dragged across the linen. Draw sheets should be used to lift the patient. Voluntary and involuntary movements by the patient can also lead to friction. Applying agents such as lubricants, protective films, and padding to elbows and heels can help reduce the potential for injury (Agency for Health Care Policy and Research [AHCPR], 1992). A sheepskin can initially reduce friction, but after several launderings it can actually increase friction (Berecek, 1975). High-top sneakers or snug-fitting socks in bed can also decrease heel friction (Slater, 1985). Shearing injuries occur when the skin remains stationary and the underlying tissue shifts. This shift diminishes blood supply to the skin and soon results in ischemia and tissue damage. Shearing frequently happens when the head of the bed is elevated. This can cause coccygeal pressure ulcers. To help prevent this from occurring, patients in the semi-Fowler or high Fowler's position should have the protection of flexing the knee of the bed or the presence of a footboard to limit downward motion (Slater, 1985).

9. Develop a written schedule for repositioning. Monitor and document activities and patient progress toward outcomes, and modify plan as necessary.

10. Identify patients who are at increased risk for pressure ulcers, because they may need more frequent repositioning. Individuals with an elevated temperature are at increased risk. Skin temperature increases can contribute to pressure ulcer formation. Each degree centigrade rise in temperature can increase tissue metabolism and oxygen demand by 10% (Fisher, Szymke, Apte, & Kosiak, 1978). Plastic-coated mattresses that are used in

institutional settings prevent air circulation. Without air circulation, the body's heat production increases at contact points rather than being conducted away from the skin (Knox, Anderson, & Anderson, 1994). Individuals with inadequate nutrition, especially those with hypoproteinemia and anemia, are also at increased risk for pressure ulcers. Low albumin and hemoglobin levels can lead to poor quality and integrity of the soft tissue, resulting in decreased tolerance to pressure (Braden & Bergstrom, 1987). Additional patient groups at higher risk for pressure ulcers include patients who are unconscious or have compromised circulatory status, such as peripheral vascular disease or diabetes mellitus.

ADDITIONAL POSITIONING CONSIDERATIONS WITH SPECIFIC POSITIONS

When nurses use the traditional positions, there are risks and benefits that must be considered. In addition, the patient's specific health status must be incorporated into the positioning plan.

Supine Position

Placing a patient supine is one of the most frequently selected options when beginning a plan of care (Loeper, 1992). Additionally, the supine position is the most frequently used position in the critical care unit when hemodynamic instability is a concern (Evans, 1994). The supine position, however, may be uncomfortable for patients with back problems and may be contraindicated for clients with respiratory, neurological, or cardiovascular problems (Wilson, Bermingham-Mitchell, Wells, & Zachary, 1996). In the supine position, the abdominal contents are pushed up against the diaphragm, which impedes inspiration (Krayer, Rehder, Vetterman, Didier, & Ritman, 1989). Abdominal muscles also are inactive in the supine position (DeTroyer, 1983). Therefore, it has been suggested that a side-lying or semi-Fowler position promotes better respiratory function (Crosbie & Myles, 1985; Crosbie & Sim, 1986; Hough, 1984). Another study suggests that angina occurs more frequently when patients with stable cardiac disease are positioned in the supine position as compared with the upright position during exercise (Quinn, Smith, Vroman, Kertzer, & Olney, 1995). Other studies indicate that the supine position is a potentiator of myocardial ischemia (Dhainaut, Bons, Bricard, & Monsallier, 1980).

Lateral Position

There are many advantages to the lateral position for patients with and without lung disease. The lateral position increases functional residual capacity (FRC), decreases the risk of airway obstruction and aspiration, enhances secretion removal from the lungs, relieves sacral pressure, and reduces muscle spasticity (Hickey, 1996; Quittenton, 1993; Zejdlik, 1992).

Research has demonstrated increased lung volumes with decreased atelectasis when mechanically ventilated patients with positive end-expiratory pressure are turned to the lateral position (Evans, 1994). Improved skin temperature and transcutaneous oxygen levels of the dependent sides have been demonstrated when adults were placed in the lateral position (Knox et al., 1994; Vanderber et al., 1995).

However, turning an acutely ill patient to the lateral side may cause severe hypoxemia, increased oxygen demand, decreased cardiac output, hypotension, and cardiac dysrhythmias (Evans, 1994; Gawlinski, 1993; Gillespie & Rehder, 1987; Remolina, Khan, Santiago, & Edelman, 1981; Rivara, Artucio, & Hiriart, 1984). Because of the severity of patient illness and the possibility of these complications, studies have demonstrated that nurses turn critically ill clients cautiously. One study of 113 critically ill clients demonstrated that the average rotation was only 24 degrees (Evans, 1994).

Other potential problems with the lateral position include undue curvature of the cervical and thoracic spine, pressure on bony prominences (especially on the trochanter), damage to the nerve plexus in the dependent shoulder, decreased skin perfusion, respiratory muscle fatigue, limited chest expansion, malalignment of the back and extremities, and increased edema of the dependent areas (Zejdlik, 1992).

Patients with severe heart failure may have a dramatic fall in cardiac output with increased shortness of breath when positioned in the left lateral position (Gawlinski, 1993). When the patients were positioned in the right lateral position, the dyspnea improved dramatically (Berensztein, Pineiro, Luis, Iavocoli, & Lerman, 1996; Gawlinski, 1993; Lasater-Erhard, 1995). On the other hand, the hemodynamic changes and decreased arterial oxygenation levels have been shown to be transient with lateral positioning. Even though the benefits of lateral positioning may outweigh the risks, baseline respiratory and hemodynamic status should be determined, with subsequent measurements of parameters after positioning (Aitken, 1995; Banasik & Emerson, 1996).

When turning a patient to the lateral position, a one-quarter, three-quarter, or full turn may be used. Use firm pillows to maintain alignment and relieve pressure on the extremities. A turning clock may be used as a reminder for positioning change. Even though turning clocks are designed to meet the individual needs of the patient, all are designed to facilitate turning the patient at specific time intervals (Helme, 1994; Jacobs, 1994; Lowthian, 1979).

Prone Position

The prone position has been shown to improve ventilation and respiratory status in a variety of clients (Gillespie & Rehder, 1987; Langer, Mascheroni, Marcolin, & Gattinoni, 1988; Pappert, Rossaint, Slama, Gruning, & Falke, 1994; Ryan & Pelosis, 1996; Wolf, 1996). The reasons for the improvement include reexpansion of gravity-induced atelectasis, improved ventilation-perfusion matching, increased tidal volume compared with the supine position, increased contraction of the diaphragm, increased functional residual capacity, redistribution of edema fluid, and improved lymphatic drainage (Douglas, Rehder, Beynen, Sessler, & Marsh, 1977; Evans, 1994; Gawlinski, 1993; Gillespie & Rehder, 1987; Langer et al., 1988; Pappert et al., 1994; Ryan & Pelosis, 1996). The prone position also reduces the risk of hip flexion and reduces pressure on the buttocks from prolonged sitting periods (Zejdlik, 1992).

Traditionally, nurses have been hesitant to turn patients to the prone position because of difficulty maintaining the airway and the parenteral therapy equipment as well as the potential for bruising, facial edema, and nerve damage. Patients fear breathing difficulties or increased discomfort when placed in the prone position (Evans, 1994; Ryan & Pelosis, 1996; Zejdlik, 1992). Although the prone position increases oxygenation in critically ill clients, there are a number of precautions as well as potential problems when using this position. The effect of the prone position on hemodynamic and respiratory status must be carefully monitored (Schmitz, 1991).

Potential problems associated with the prone position include malalignment of the back and extremities; limitation of respiratory function; pressure on iliac crests, genitalia, and breast; hyperextension of the knees; decreased peripheral circulation; nerve damage; and footdrop (Jacobs, 1994; Zejdlik, 1992).

Before using the prone position, determine whether there are any potential problems such as recently performed orthopedic surgery or the inability to extend hips or knees (Jacobs, 1994). Firm pillows should be placed along the chest, thighs, lower legs, and head (Jacobs, 1994). As with other position changes, baseline comfort levels, cardiorespiratory status, and skin perfusion should be established and monitored during and after the position change.

Trendelenburg Position

Since the early days of medicine, the Trendelenburg position has been used to help treat the signs and symptoms of hemorrhage hypovolemia (Zotti, 1994). The theory behind using this position is that by tilting a patient's head down 10 to 30 degrees, the blood in the nonessential areas of the legs and pelvis is shifted by gravity toward the more central circulation of the heart and lungs, thus helping perfuse critical organs (Bivens, 1985).

In studies done on healthy people, the Trendelenburg position causes an increase in preload (the amount of blood in the heart chamber while in the relaxing phase), reduces systemic vascular resistance (the amount of elastic resistance in the arteries against which the heart pumps), and increases cardiac output (the amount of blood pumped with each cardiac contraction) (Sibbald, 1979).

However, when patients with cardiac or hypovolemic shock were placed in the Trendelenburg position, the results were quite different. These patients still had a shift in blood volume from the lower extremities to the upper torso but showed no significant change in preload, systemic vascular resistance, or cardiac output, which would be needed for a positive therapeutic effect (Bivens, 1985).

In the healthy person, the baroreceptors are responsible for regulating the preload, systemic vascular resistance, and cardiac output when increased vascular pressure occurs. However, in a state of physiological shock, the baroreceptors do not function properly secondary to a decreased blood volume and certain cardiorespiratory changes, such as tachycardia and hypotension.

The Trendelenburg position can be of no value to a patient in shock and may be detrimental. Placing the shock patient in the Trendelenburg position can cause a 15% to 20% decrease in pulmonary vital capacity (Bivens, 1985). This occurs secondary to diaphragmatic elevation, including the abdominal compartment's placing pressure on the lung fields. Placing the patient's head in the downward position increases his or her risk for gastric aspiration. Narrowing of the airway is another concern, because the Trendelenburg position allows the tongue and oropharyngeal muscles to fall back, with subsequent airway occlusion (Heinonen, 1969). For patients with neurological problems, the Trendelenburg position can cause increased cerebral edema due to increased cranial venous pressure. The head-down position can increase the intraocular pressure and may be detrimental to patients with glaucoma or eye injuries (Reich, 1989). Because the Trendelenburg position causes increased myocardial workload, increased myocardial oxygen requirements, and a decrease in stroke volume, it should be used cautiously with patients who have myocardial ischemic disease (Biddle & Aker, 1989).

The Trendelenburg position, however, has not been shown to be detrimental in patients with psychogenic shock or syncope in which there is no fluid loss. Several situations where the Trendelenburg position may be appropriate and helpful include positioning for central line insertion via the jugular or the subclavian approach, treatment for suspected air embolism, and pelvic surgery (Bivens, 1985; Roberts & Hedges, 1991; Schwartz, 1992).

POSITIONING ACTIVITIES WITH CLIENTS WHO HAVE ALTERED RESPIRATORY FUNCTION

It is necessary to determine whether the patient has unilateral or bilateral lung disease before positioning him or her in the lateral position. For many years, nurses have followed the "good lung down" practice when caring for patients who have unilateral lung disease or surgery, including pneumothorax, atelectasis, pneumonia, lung cancer, thoracotomy, or lobectomy.

The reason for improved oxygenation status with the "good lung down" is the improved ventilation-perfusion matching in the healthy dependent lung. If the affected lung is in the dependent position, the increased perfusion is not matched by increased ventilation (Wolf, 1996; Yeaw, 1996). There is also shifting of secretions and increased airway obstruction when the affected lung is in the dependent position (Chang, Chang, Shiao, & Perng, 1993).

More recent research has questioned the "good lung down" practice. Two research studies found no difference in the arterial oxygen saturation levels after positioning the patient with the affected and unaffected lungs in the dependent position (Chang et al., 1993; Yeaw, 1996). Several reasons for the conflicting results with previous studies include study of patients with only unilateral disease, larger sample size, and use of multiple measurements over time (Chang et al., 1993; Yeaw, 1996).

The effect of the lateral position on oxygenation status has been evaluated in clients with bilateral lung disease. Patients with bilateral lung disease have a greater decrease in oxygen saturation levels when placed in the right lateral position as compared with the left lateral position. The greater size and vascularity of the right lung along with the weight of the heart and mediastinum compress the left lung with a subsequent decrease in ventilation and perfusion when the client is placed in the left lateral position (Gawlinski, 1993).

POSITIONING ACTIVITIES WITH CLIENTS WHO HAVE ALTERED NEUROLOGICAL FUNCTION

Because of increased venous and cerebrospinal fluid drainage from the cranium, patients who are at risk for increased intracranial pressure have traditionally been positioned with the head of the bed elevated 30 degrees (Arbour, 1993; Hickey, 1996; Mitchell & Mauss, 1978; Williams & Coyne, 1993; Winkelman, 1994).

More recent research studies have questioned the use of the 30-degree elevation and have advocated the flat position for patients who are at risk for increased intracranial pressure. Although elevation of the head may decrease intracranial pressure, variable and transient responses have been noted in clients with alterations in neurological function. Because perfusion of the brain increased and intracranial pressure decreased in some patients while in the flat position, it has been advocated that patients with increased intracranial pressure remain in the flat position unless intracranial pressure rises and cerebral perfusion decreases (Hickey, 1996; Lee, 1989; Winkelman, 1994).

The main consideration for any position change for patients with altered neurological function is to avoid extreme neck flexion or rotation (Arbour, 1993; Lipe & Mitchell, 1980; Mitchell & Mauss, 1978; Williams & Coyne, 1993). Pillows placed behind the neck of a patient in the flat position may reduce venous outflow from the brain with a subsequent increase in intracranial pressure (Hickey, 1996; Jones, 1995; Mitchell & Mauss, 1978; Williams & Coyne, 1993).

Patients should be instructed to exhale and avoid isometric exercise during position changes, which prevents increased intrathoracic and intracranial pressures. Using trapeze bars and pushing against footboards should be avoided because of the resulting increase in intracranial pressure (Hickey, 1996).

No matter what position is used with patients who have altered neurological function, baseline neurological and respiratory status, intracranial and cerebral perfusion pressures, and patient comfort should be established and monitored. Additional factors that increase intracranial pressure need to be reduced or eliminated before position change (Jones, 1995).

POSITIONING CONSIDERATIONS WITH ELDERLY PATIENTS

Because of the normal physiological changes that occur with aging, there are some more specific turning and positioning activities that need to be included in the plan of care of elderly patients. However, it is important to realize that these physiological changes occur at individual rates. Older adults are particularly vulnerable to the development of pressure ulcers as a result of changes in skin and subcutaneous tissues. With aging, the local blood supply to the skin decreases, the epithelial layers flatten and thin, subcutaneous fat decreases, subcutaneous and sweat gland function decreases, and skin sensitivity to pain, touch, and pressure decreases (Kelley & Mobily, 1991).

The traditional regimen of turning every 2 hours may be detrimental to the skin integrity of older adults. It has been estimated that 33% of the elderly population have pressure ulcers (Brown, Boosinger, Black, & Gaspar, 1985), with 7% of these ulcers occurring in hospitalized patients and 20% occurring in those in nursing homes (Rousseau, 1988). In a study done by Knox et al. (1994), it was concluded that an older person may need to be turned every 1 to 1½ hours. It is also recommended that if the individual has redness of the skin (due to hyperemia) when turning is done every 1½ hours, then the turning should be done every hour. If the redness occurs after 1 hour, a pressure-reducing support surface should be used.

Even if the older patient does not have unilateral or bilateral lung disease, some of the same positioning precautions that are taken with those individuals with lung disorders need to be considered when changing the position of an elderly patient. These precautions are indicated because of the normal physiological changes that occur in the respiratory system of elderly patients. With aging, there is a decline in tissue elasticity, a weakening of the respiratory muscles, a decrease in compliance of the spine and rib cage, alveolar thickening, and decreased alveolar numbers. These changes lead to a decrease in lung volumes, impaired gas exchange, and a pooling of secretions that can lead to pneumonia and low arterial oxygen levels when the patient's position is changed (Kelley & Mobily, 1991). The nurse must carefully monitor how these patients are tolerating the position change by assessing their oxygenation status. Additionally, if the patient has lung problems, there may be certain positions that are better tolerated.

Another positioning consideration for aged individuals is keeping the head of the bed elevated at least 30 to 45 degrees for 30 minutes after eating because their cough and gag reflexes are weakened. Perform range-of-motion exercises and position changes slowly and carefully because of bone demineralization and patients' increased risk of fractures, which may occur because their articular cartilage becomes less flexible with less synovial fluid, limiting movement or making movements more painful.

Whether the cardiac system declines as a result of normal aging changes or because of a disease process such as coronary artery disease or heart failure is controversial. Some of these changes include a decrease in cardiac output, venous stasis, and a slower physiological hemodynamic response to physical activity. During position changes of elderly patients, the nurse should assess for orthostatic hypotension, avoid dependent extremity positions, and minimize the crossing of the lower extremities (Miller, 1995).

EDUCATION RELATED TO POSITIONING

Once an individualized positioning plan is developed, the implementation of the plan must be considered a team approach. Each team member must understand the positioning plan and know his or her responsibilities for carrying it out to ensure success. In many health care settings the nursing assistants are primarily responsible for turning and repositioning patients. Educating these caregivers is essential. Therefore, staff inservice training sessions that include simple written guidelines along with demonstrations and illustrations regarding turning and positioning techniques can be useful teaching tools. It is also important to explain to staff the rationale and importance of following the specific plan. Including the caregivers in the evaluation and modification of the plan can increase their involvement in and compliance with the plan.

In spite of educational efforts, frustration and lack of follow-through of the plan can develop. A study done by Helme (1994) showed that there was a deficit in performance of 2-hour turning even though the staff stated that turning should be done every 2 hours. The reasons cited for the deficit in turning were lack of specific turning responsibilities, lack of time, and too few staff.

Nurses need to remember that preventing the adverse effects of immobility is less costly than treating them and that positioning activities are invaluable to this prevention process (Oot-Giromini, 1989).

CASE STUDY

GV, a 78-year-old woman, was admitted to the hospital with right-sided paralysis, decreased peripheral sensation of the right extremities, slurred speech, and difficulty swallowing. She was oriented to time, place, and person and was able to respond to questions appropriately. She was diagnosed with a thrombotic brain attack. Past health problems included arthritis and mild hypertension.

Based on the assessment data, the nursing diagnoses that relate to positioning include

Impaired physical mobility related to necrosis of neurons in the left motor strip, evidenced by inability to voluntarily move right arm and leg

Sensory-perceptual alteration (tactile) related to necrosis of neurons in the left sensory strip, evidenced by inability to detect light or painful touch on right arm and leg

Impaired swallowing related to decreased perfusion of the cranial nerves and damage to laryngeal and pharyngeal muscles, evidenced by choking and coughing when attempting to swallow water

Using the North American Nursing Diagnosis Association (NANDA)–Nursing Outcomes Classification (NOC) linkages in the *Nursing Outcomes Classification (NOC)* (Johnson & Maas, 1997), the following outcomes based on Table 6–2 were identified for GV.

Joint Movement: Active	#1 (No motion: right fingers, thumb, wrist, elbow, shoulder, ankle, knee, hip)
Mobility Level	#1 (Dependent, does not participate)
Self-Care: Activities of Daily Living (ADL)	#2 (Requires assistive person and devices)
Immobility Consequences: Physiological	#2 (Substantial)
Tissue Perfusion: Peripheral	#4 (Mildly compromised)
Safety Status: Physical Injury	#1 (Severe)
Neurological Status	#2 (Substantially compromised)
Self-Care: Eating	#1 (Dependent, does not participate)

Appropriate short-term goals (24 hours) for GV include

Patient will have full range of motion of joints on right side.

Patient will demonstrate no evidence of contractures or footdrop.

Blood pressure will be within normal limits with head-of-bed elevation.

Skin over sacral and trochanter areas will not show hyperemia.

Patient will be free of injury.

Patient will have clear breath sounds and normal body temperature.

Using the NIC intervention of Positioning (see Table 6–1), the following individualized activities were selected for GV:

1. Provide active range-of-motion exercises bilaterally
2. Premedicate with analgesics prior to range-of-motion exercises
3. Do not force joint movement
4. Maintain joints in neutral position with pillow or foam support
5. Avoid pulling the arm or forcing the shoulder through painful range of motion

Table 6–2   NOCs That May Be Affected by the Intervention Positioning

Self-initiated body positioning	Neurological status
Bone healing	Neurological status: central motor control
Cardiac pump effectiveness	Pain control behavior
Caregiver performance: direct care	Pain level
Circulation status	Respiratory status: gas exchange
Comfort level	Respiratory status: ventilation
Dignified dying	Rest
Fluid balance	Safety status: physical injury
Hydration	Self-care: activities of daily living (ADL)
Immobility consequences: physiological	Self-care: eating
Immobility consequences: psychosocial-cognitive	Sleep
Immune hypersensitivity control	Tissue integrity: skin and mucous membrane
Infection status	Tissue perfusion: cardiac
Joint movement: active	Tissue perfusion: cerebral
Joint movement: passive	Tissue perfusion: peripheral
Knowledge: prescribed activity	Tissue perfusion: pulmonary
Knowledge: treatment procedures	Urinary elimination
Loneliness	Vital sign status
Mobility level	Wound healing: primary intention
Muscle function	Wound healing: secondary intention

Source: Johnson, M., and Maas, M. (Eds.) (1997). *Nursing outcomes classification (NOC).* St. Louis: C.V. Mosby.

6. Place small pillow in the right axillary region
7. Elevate the right hand above the elbow
8. Turn every 2 hours, maintaining proper body alignment
9. Assess oxygenation status and comfort before and after position changes
10. Develop written schedule for positioning
11. Monitor and document activities and patient's progress toward outcomes
12. Provide therapeutic mattress
13. Monitor for hyperemia and edema over pressure points every 2 hours
14. Position pillow under lower legs when in supine position
15. Monitor coughing, gagging, and increased salivation during each position change
16. Maintain 30-degree head elevation during meals and for 30 minutes after meals

References

Agency for Health Care Policy and Research (AHCPR), Panel for the Prediction and Prevention of Pressure Ulcers in Adults. (1992). *Pressure ulcers in adults: Prediction and prevention* (Clinical practice guideline, No. 3. AHCPR Publication No. 92-0047). Rockville, MD: Author.

Aitken, L. (1995). Comparison of pulmonary artery pressure measurements in the supine and 60 degree lateral positions. *Australian Critical Care, 8*(4), 22, 24–29.

Alterescu, V. (1983). Prevention and treatment of pressure sores. In D. Cooper, R. Watt, and V. Alterescu (Eds.), *Guide to wound care* (pp. 56–71). Libertyville, IL: Hollister.

Arbour, R. (1993). What you can do to reduce ICP. *Nursing, 23*(11), 41–46.

Banasik, J., and Emerson, R. (1996). Effect of lateral position on arterial and venous blood gases in postoperative cardiac surgery patients. *American Journal of Critical Care, 5*(2), 121–126.

Berecek, K. H. (1975). Treatment of decubitus ulcers. *Nursing Clinics of North America, 10*(1), 171–209.

Berensztein, C. S., Pineiro, D., Luis, J. F., Iavocoli, D., and Lerman, J. (1996). Effect of left and right lateral decubitus positions on doppler mitral flow patterns in patients with severe congestive heart failure. *Journal of the American Society of Echocardiography, 9*(1), 86.

Biddle, C., and Aker, J. (1989). Cardiovascular and ventilatory effects of surgical positioning. *Current Reviews for Post Anesthesia Care Nurses, 11*(4), 25–32.

Bivens, H. (1985). Blood volume distribution in the Trendelenburg position. *Annals of Emergency Medicine, 14*, 642.

Braden, B., and Bergstrom, N. (1987). A conceptual schema for the study of the etiology of pressure sores. *Rehabilitation Nursing, 12*(1), 8–12.

Brown, M. M., Boosinger, J., Black, J., and Gaspar, T. (1985). Nursing innovation for prevention of decubitus ulcers in long term care facilities. *Plastic Surgical Nursing, 5*(57), 62–64.

Cantin, J. E. (1989). Proper positioning eliminates patient injury. *Today's OR Nurse, 11*(4), 18–21.

Chang, S. C., Chang, H. I., Shiao, C. M., and Perng, R. (1993). Effect of body position on gas exchange in patients with unilateral central airway lesions: Down with the good lung? *Chest, 103*(3), 787–791.

Colburn, L. (1987). Pressure ulcer prevention in the hospice patient: Strategies for care to increase comfort. *American Journal of Hospital Care, 4*(2), 22–26.

Crewe, R. A. (1987). Problems of rubber ring nursing cushions and a clinical survey of alternative cushions for ill patients. *Care Science Practice, 5*(2), 9–11.

Crosbie, W. J., and Myles, S. (1985). An investigation into the effect of postural modification on some aspects of normal pulmonary function. *Physiotherapy, 71*, 311–314.

Crosbie, W. J., and Sim, D. T. (1986). The effect of postural modification on some aspects of pulmonary function following surgery of the upper abdomen. *Physiotherapy, 72*, 487–492.

DeTroyer, A. (1983). Mechanical role of the abdominal muscles in relation to posture. *Respiration Physiology, 53*, 341–353.

Dhainaut, J., Bons, J., Bricard, C., and Monsallier, H. (1980). Improved oxygenation in patients with extensive unilateral pneumonia using the lateral decubitus position. *Thorax, 35*, 792–793.

Dimant, J., and Francis, M. E. (1988). Pressure sore prevention and management. *Journal of Gerontological Nursing, 14*(8), 18–25.

Douglas, W. W., Rehder, K., Beynen, F. M., Sessler, A. D., and Marsh, H. M. (1977). Improved oxygenation in patients with acute respiratory failure: The prone position. *American Review of Respiratory Disease, 115*, 559–566.

Ek, A. C., Gustavsson, G., and Lewis, D. H. (1985). The local skin blood flow in areas at risk for pressure sores treated with massage. *Scandinavian Journal of Rehabilitation Medicine, 17*(2), 81–86.

Evans, D. (1994). The use of position during critical illness: Current practice and review of the literature. *Australian Critical Care, 7*(3), 16–21.

Feustel, D. (1982). Pressure sore prevention: Aye, there's the rub. *Nursing, 12*(4), 78–83.

Fisher, S. V., Szymke, T. E., Apte, S. Y., and Kosiak, M. (1978). Wheelchair cushion effect on skin temperature. *Archives of Physical Medicine and Rehabilitation, 59*, 68–72.

Fontaine, D., and McQuillan, K. (1989). Positioning as a nursing therapy in trauma care. *Critical Care Nursing Clinics of North America, 1*(1), 105.

Gawlinski, A. (1993). Effect of positioning on mixed venous oxygen saturation. *Journal of Cardiovascular Nursing, 7*(4), 71–81.

Gillespie, D. J., and Rehder, K. (1987). Body position and ventilation-perfusion relationships in unilateral pulmonary disease. *Chest, 91*(1), 75.

Heinonen, J. (1969). Effect of Trendelenburg tilt and other procedures on the position of endotracheal tubes. *Lancet, 1*, 850.

Helme, T. (1994). Position changes for residents in long-term care. *Advances in Wound Care, 7*(5), 57–58, 60–61.

Hickey, J. A. (1996). Rehabilitation for neuroscience patients. In J. A. Hickey, *The clinical practice of neurological and neurosurgical nursing* (4th ed.). Philadelphia: J.B. Lippincott.

Hough, A. (1984). The effect of posture on lung function. *Physiotherapy, 70*(3), 101–104.

Hudak, C. M., and Gallo, B. M. (Eds.) (1992). *Critical care nursing: A holistic approach* (6th ed., p. 349). Philadelphia: J.B. Lippincott.

Jacobs, B. W. (1994). Working on the right moves: Part 1. *Nursing, 24*(11), 52–54.

Johnson, M., and Maas, M. (Eds.) (1997). *Nursing outcomes classification (NOC).* St. Louis: C.V. Mosby.

Jones, B. (1995). The effects of repositioning on intracranial pressure. *Australian Journal of Advanced Nursing, 12*(2), 32–39.

Kelley, L. S., and Mobily, P. R. (1991). Iatrogenesis in the elderly: Impaired skin integrity. *Journal of Gerontological Nursing, 17,* 24–28.

Knox, D. M., Anderson, T. M., and Anderson, P. S. (1994). Effects of different turn intervals on skin of healthy older adults. *Advances in Wound Care, 7*(1), 48–52, 54–56.

Kozier, B., Erb, G., Blais, K., Wilkinson, J. (1995). *Fundamentals of Nursing: Concepts, process, and practice* (5th ed.). Redwood City, CA: Addison-Wesley.

Krayer, S., Rehder, K., Vetterman, J., Didier, E. P., and Ritman, E. L. (1989). Position and motion of the human diaphragm during anesthetic paralysis. *Anesthesiology, 70,* 891–898.

Langer, M., Mascheroni, D., Marcolin, R., and Gattinoni, L. (1988). The prone position in ARDS patients: A clinical study. *Chest, 94*(1), 103–107.

Lasater-Erhard, M. (1995). The effect of patient position on arterial oxygen saturation. *Critical Care Nurse, 15*(4), 31–36.

Lee, S. T. (1989). Intracranial pressure changes during positioning of patients with severe head injury. *Heart and Lung, 18,* 411–414.

Lipe, H., and Mitchell, P. (1980). Positioning the patient with intracranial hypertension: How turning and head rotation affect the internal jugular vein. *Heart and Lung, 9,* 1031–1037.

Loeper, J. M. (1992). Positioning. In G. M. Bulechek and J. C. McCloskey (Eds.), *Nursing interventions: Essential nursing treatments* (2nd ed., pp. 86–93). Philadelphia: W.B. Saunders.

Lowthian, D. J. (1979). Turning clock system to prevent pressure sores. *Nursing Mirror, 148,* 30–31.

Maklebust, J. A. (1987). Pressure ulcers: Etiology and prevention. *Nursing Clinics of North America, 22,* 359–377.

McCaffery, M., and Wolff, M. (1992). Pain relief using cutaneous modalities, positioning and movement. *Hospital Journal, 8*(1/2), 121–153.

McCloskey, J. C., and Bulechek, G. M. (1996). Positioning. In G. M. Bulechek and J. C. McCloskey (Eds.), *Nursing interventions classification* (2nd ed., p. 437). St. Louis: C.V. Mosby.

Metzler, D., and Harr, J. (1996). Positioning your patient properly. *American Journal of Nursing, 96*(3), 33–37.

Michocki, R. J., and Lamy, P. P. (1976). The problem of pressure sores in a nursing home population: Statistical data. *Journal of the American Geriatrics Society, 24,* 323–328.

Miller, C. A. (Ed.) (1995). *Nursing care of older adults* (2nd ed.). Philadelphia: J.B. Lippincott.

Mitchell, P., and Mauss, N. (1978). The relationship of patient and nurse activity to intracranial pressure variations. *Nursing Research, 27,* 4–10.

Oot-Giromini, B. (1989). Pressure ulcer prevention versus treatment, comparative product cost study. *Decubitus, 23,* 52–53.

Pappert, D., Rossaint, R., Slama, K., Gruning, T., and Falke, K. (1994). Influence of positioning on ventilation-perfusion relationships in severe adult respiratory distress syndrome. *Chest, 106,* 1511.

Parish, L. C., and Witkowski, J. A. (1980). Clinitron therapy and the decubitus ulcer: Preliminary dermatologic studies. *International Journal of Dermatology, 19,* 517–518.

Quinn, T. J., Smith, S. W., Vroman, N. B., Kertzer, R., and Olney, W. B. (1995). Physiologic responses of cardiac patients to supine, recumbent, and upright cycle ergometry. *Archives of Physical Medicine and Rehabilitation, 76,* 257–261.

Quittenton, E. (1993). Altering patient position improves oxygenation and ventilation. *Canadian Journal of Respiratory Therapy, 29*(2), 75.

Reich, D. (1989). Trendelenburg and passive leg raising do not significantly improve cardiopulmonary performance in the anesthetized patient with coronary artery disease. *Critical Care Medicine, 17,* 317.

Reichel, S. M. (1958). Shearing force as a factor in decubitus ulcers in paraplegics. *Journal of the American Medical Association, 166,* 762–763.

Remolina, C., Khan, A. U., Santiago, T. V., and Edelman, N. (1981). Positional hypoxemia in unilateral lung disease. *New England Journal of Medicine, 304,* 523.

Rivara, D., Artucio, H., Arcos, J., and Hiriart, C. (1984). Positional hypoxemia during artificial ventilation. *Critical Care Medicine, 12,* 436.

Roberts, J., and Hedges, J. (1991). *Clinical procedures in emergency medicine.* Philadelphia: W.B. Saunders.

Rousseau, P. (1988). Pressure ulcers in the aged: A preventable problem? *Continuing Care, 17,* 35–42.

Ryan, D. W., and Pelosis, P. (1996). The prone position in acute respiratory distress syndrome: Small studies have shown that it improves oxygenation. *British Medical Journal, 312,* 860–861.

Schmitz, T. (1991). The semi-prone position in ARDS: Five case studies. *Critical Care Nursing Quarterly, 11*(5), 22–23.

Schmitz, T. (1991). Fact or myth? Patients with pulmonary disease should be placed in the semi-Fowler's position. *Focus on Critical Care, 18*(1), 58–64.

Schwartz, G. (1992). *The principles and practices of emergency medicine.* Philadelphia: Lea & Febiger.

Seiler, W. O., Allen, S., and Stahelin, H. B. (1986). Influence of the 30 degrees laterally inclined position and the "super-soft" 3-piece mattress on skin oxygen tension on areas of maximum pressure—implications for pressure sore prevention. *Gerontology, 32*(3), 158–166.

Shively, M. (1988). Effect of position change on mixed venous oxygen saturation in the coronary artery bypass surgery patient. *Heart and Lung, 17*(1), 51–59.

Sibbald, W. (1979). The Trendelenburg position: Hemodynamic effects in hypotensive and normotensive patients. *Critical Care Medicine, 7*(5), 218.

Slater, H. (1985). *Pressure ulcers in the elderly.* Pittsburgh, PA: Synapse Publications.

Smith, K. A. (1990). Positioning principles: an anatomic review. *AORN Journal, 52,* 1196–1208.

Swanlund, S. L. (1996). Body positioning and the elderly with adult respiratory distress syndrome: Implications for nursing care. *Journal of Gerontological Nursing, 22*(2), 46–50.

Vanderber, A., and Gallagher, K. (1994). Effects of bathing, passive range-of-motion exercises, and turning on oxygen consumption in healthy men and women. *American Journal of Critical Care, 3,* 374–381.

Vanderber, A., Gallagher, K., and Severino, R. (1995). The effect of nursing interventions on transcutaneous oxygen and carbon dioxide tensions. *Western Journal of Nursing Research, 17*(1), 76–90.

Whitney, J. D., Fellows, B. J., and Larson, E. (1984). Do mattresses make a difference? *Journal of Gerontological Nursing, 10,* 20–25.

Whittemore, R., Bautista, C., Smith, C., and Bruttomesso, K. (1993). Interface pressure measurements of support surfaces with subjects in the supine and 45-degree Fowler positions. *Journal of ET Nursing, 20*(3), 111–115.

Wienke, V. K. (1987). Pressure sores: Prevention is the challenge. *Orthopaedic Nursing, 6*(4), 26.

Williams, A., and Coyne, S. M. (1993). Effects of neck position on intracranial pressure. *American Journal of Critical Care, 2*(1), 68–71.

Wilson, A., Bermingham-Mitchell, K., Wells, N., and Zachary, K. (1996). Effect of backrest position on hemodynamic and right ventricular measurements in critically ill adults. *American Journal of Critical Care, 5,* 264–270.

Winkelman, C. (1994). Advances in managing increased intracranial pressure: A decade of selected research. *ACCN's Clinical Issues in Critical Care Nursing, 5*(1), 9–13.

Winslow, E., Clark, P., White, K. M., and Tyler, D. O. (1990). Effects of lateral turn on mixed venous oxygen saturation and heart rate in critically ill adults. *Heart and Lung, 19*(5), S557–S561.

Wolf, Z. R. (1996). Positioning your patient for better breathing. *Nursing, 26*(5), 10.

Yeaw, E. (1992). How position affects oxygenation: Good lung down? *American Journal of Nursing, 92*(3), 27–29.

Yeaw, E. (1996). The effect of body positioning upon maximal oxygenation of patients with unilateral lung pathology. *Journal of Advanced Nursing, 23*(1), 55–61.

Zejdlik, C. P. (1992). Maintaining skeletal system integrity. In C. P. Zejdlik, *Management of spinal cord injury* (pp. 422–425). Boston: Jones & Bartlett.

Zotti, R. D. (1994). Trendelenburg: To tilt or not to tilt. *Journal of the Emergency Medical Services, 19*(9), 71–73.

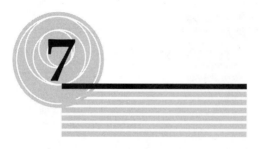

Exercise Promotion

Janet D. Allan and Diane O. Tyler

The need to change the sedentary habits of the adult American population is well recognized. Physical inactivity has been linked to premature cardiovascular disease, obesity, orthopedic problems, and emotional distress. Despite the tremendous public interest in exercise, recent estimates suggest that 25% of U.S. adults are sedentary (defined as no leisure-time activity in the previous month) and that another 54% are somewhat active but do not meet the objective of regular, light to moderate physical activity for at least 30 minutes per day (Pate et al., 1995). Although great strides have been made in getting more Americans to be physically active, the percentage of exercising adults falls far short of the *Healthy People 2000* objectives for physical activity and fitness as revised in 1995 (U.S. Department of Health and Human Services [USDHHS], 1995). Evidence for the role of regular activity in the primary and secondary prevention of cardiovascular disease and numerous other prevalent health problems continues to accumulate (Blair, 1994; USDHHS, 1996). Most health promotion recommendations advocate modification of lifestyles to include regular, moderate-intensity physical activities and resistance training (American College of Sports Medicine [ACSM], 1995). Nurses, as part of their involvement in health promotion and risk reduction, need knowledge of physical activity and exercise training in order to make appropriate assessments and develop interventions for exercise promotion programs with clients.

WHAT IS EXERCISE?

This chapter focuses on helping adults incorporate sufficient exercise into their lives to improve health. Recommendations from *Physical Activity and Health: A*

Report of the Surgeon General (USDHHS, 1996) state that all Americans should accumulate at least 30 minutes of moderate-intensity physical activity on most, and preferably all, days of the week. Moderate physical activity includes activities that can be comfortably sustained for at least 60 minutes, such as walking 3 to 4 miles per hour (mph), raking leaves, lawn mowing with a power push mower, and social dancing. Vigorous activity produces fatigue within 20 minutes (e.g., jogging 5 mph, shoveling snow).

Exercise is technically defined as "physical activity that is planned, structured, repetitive, and results in the improvement or maintenance of one or more facets of physical fitness," whereas physical activity is broader in scope and is defined as "any body movement produced by skeletal muscles that results in caloric expenditure" (Caspersen, Powell, & Christenson, 1985; USDHHS, 1996). Thus, exercise is a subcategory of physical activity, which by definition affects physical fitness. Physical fitness is an aspect of health that relates to body composition, flexibility, aerobic power, endurance, and strength. Based on current health promotion recommendations and research that examines the relationships among various types and amounts of physical activity with a wide spectrum of health indicators and outcomes, the terms *physical activity* and *exercise* are used synonymously in this chapter to represent behaviors that produce numerous health improvements.

OUTCOMES OF EXERCISE

A substantial body of research documents that physical activity and fitness reduce morbidity and mortality for the leading causes of death and disability (Blair et al., 1995; Paffenbarger et al., 1993; USDHHS, 1996). Protective effects of activity on coronary heart disease (Berlin & Coditz, 1990), hypertension (Hagberg, 1990), obesity (DiPietro, 1995), non–insulin-dependent diabetes mellitus (NIDDM) (Helmrich, Ragland, Leung, & Paffenbarger, 1991), and colon cancer (Lee, Paffenbarger, & Hsieh, 1991) are well established. The literature also shows beneficial effects of physical activity in relieving symptoms of depression, anxiety, and osteoarthritis; reducing the risk of falling and preserving ability to maintain independent living status among older adults; and enhancing physical function and psychological well-being in persons compromised by poor health (USDHHS, 1996).

A compelling reason for exercise promotion in the general population is the large body of evidence that moderate-intensity activity performed on a regular basis is associated with lower all-cause mortality (Blair et al., 1989; Paffenbarger, Hyde, & Wing, 1986). Studies also report that changing from a lower to a higher level of physical activity or fitness extends longevity (Blair et al., 1995; Paffenbarger et al., 1993). In a study of 17,321 sedentary male Harvard alumni, Paffenbarger et al. (1993) found that those who began moderately intense sports activity had a 23% lower death rate than those who remained sedentary. Among those who became physically active, added years of life were noted across all age groups. Blair et al. (1995) studied 9,777 men and found a 44% reduction in mortality among those who initially had low levels of cardiovascular fitness and then improved fitness over an average of 5 years.

Multiple physiological mechanisms may contribute to the protective effects of physical activity. Bodily responses to activity produce alterations in the cardiovascular, musculoskeletal, respiratory, endocrine, and immune systems (McArdle, Katch, & Katch, 1994; USDHHS, 1996). The most widely appreciated effects are in the cardiovascular system. Regular exercise appears to reduce the risk of fatal ventricular arrhythmias; decrease myocardial oxygen requirements; improve blood flow and capillary exchange capacities; alter vascular resistance; reduce risk of thrombosis through advantageous effects on blood clotting and fibrinolytic mechanisms; improve lipid profile by influencing key enzymes in lipoprotein metabolism; lower blood pressure, possibly through its effects on the sympathetic nervous system or decrease in cardiac output or peripheral resistance; and promote and maintain weight loss (Blair et al., 1995; USDHHS, 1996).

The relationship between physical activity and coronary heart disease (CHD) has been studied for several decades (Morris, Meady, Raffle, Roberts, & Parks, 1953; Paffenbarger, Laughlin, Gima, & Black, 1970; Paffenbarger, Hale, Brand, & Hyde, 1977; Paffenbarger et al., 1986). Comprehensive reviews and meta-analyses indicate the relative risk of death from CHD is 1.9 for sedentary persons, suggesting that inactive adults are twice as likely to have a coronary event as physically active adults (Berlin & Coditz, 1990; Powell, Thompson, Caspersen, & Kendrick, 1987). In another report of the male Harvard alumni study, Paffenbarger et al. (1986) found that men between the ages of 35 and 74 who walked, climbed stairs, and played sports had fewer incidents of CHD than those who were less active. Supporting these results are the findings from the Framingham study of white men, which found that cardiovascular and coronary heart disease mortality decreased with increasing levels of physical activity at all ages, including in the elderly (Kannel, Belanger, D'Agostino, & Israel, 1986). These classic studies emphasize the beneficial effect of lifetime habitual physical activity, whereas more current research documents the ability to improve health after being sedentary (Blair et al., 1995; Paffenbarger et al., 1993).

A significant cardiovascular beneficial effect of exercise is the reduction of atherosclerosis and improvement in lipid profiles. Studies have found that plasma levels of high-density lipoproteins (HDL) protect against atherosclerosis by transporting cholesterol to the liver for elimination, that elevated HDL levels are associated with a lower risk of CHD (Haskell, 1986; Haskell et al., 1994; Kannel, 1983), that HDL levels increase following moderate and vigorous exercise (Haskell, 1986), and that even a single episode of physical activity can improve blood lipid levels for several days (Durstine & Haskell, 1994; Tsopanakis, Sgouraki, Nadel, Pavlou, & Bussolari, 1989). Although most studies show a dose-response relationship between amount of regular physical activity and plasma HDL levels, moderate-intensity exercise has produced the same or a greater increase in HDL as that seen following vigorous exercise (Duncan, Gordon, & Scott, 1991).

Hypertension increases the risk of CHD twofold. Meta-analyses of the effects of habitual physical activity on blood pressure conclude that aerobic exercise of moderate to vigorous intensity, approximately three to four times per week for 30 to 60 minutes per session, decreases systolic and diastolic blood pressure by approximately 6 to 7 mm Hg (Arroll & Beaglehole, 1992; Kelley & McClellan, 1994). An immediate and temporary effect of a single episode of physical activity is lowered blood pressure through dilating of the peripheral blood vessels; habitual exercise may lower blood pressure by attenuating the sympathetic system (USDHHS, 1996).

Physical activity also affects obesity, which is associated with reduced longevity, increased incidence of cardiovascular disease, diabetes mellitus, osteoarthritis, and certain types of cancer, as well as adverse psychosocial factors such as distorted body image and discrimination (Blair et al., 1995). Several studies show an increased risk for significant weight gain for persons who have lower levels of physical activity than for those with higher levels of activity (Blair, 1993;

DiPietro, 1995; Williamson et al., 1993). Although most research suggests a greater amount of weight loss occurs with caloric restriction only when compared with exercise-only groups, weight loss initiation and maintenance are often found to be more successful when exercise is combined with diet alterations (Blair, 1993; Blair et al., 1995; USDHHS, 1996). Thus, both diet and exercise should be considered when weight loss is a goal.

Exercise also is effective in reducing the risk of NIDDM and the effect is especially pronounced in persons at highest risk for the disease (i.e., those with positive family history, obesity, or hypertension) (Helmrich et al., 1991). One study found that the age-adjusted risk of NIDDM was reduced by 6% for every 500 kcal increase in energy expenditure per week (Helmrich et al., 1991). The benefits of physical activity on preventing and managing NIDDM are attributed to lowering insulin concentrations and increasing insulin sensitivity, glucose transporter-4 concentration, and glucose disposal (Blair et al., 1995).

The elderly are particularly vulnerable to the effects of inactivity, which is associated with osteoporosis, muscle weakness, balance problems, and subsequent hip fractures. By age 90, about one third of women and one sixth of men will have sustained a hip fracture, which has excessively high mortality and permanent disability rates and medical/institutional costs. Physical activity, including muscle-strengthening (resistance) exercises, appears to be protective against falling and fractures among the elderly, probably by increasing muscle strength and balance (USDHHS, 1996).

Habitual exercise also reduces anxiety, improves psychological well-being, and reduces depression. Studies generally indicate that (1) improvements are greatest in those who are the most anxious and depressed; (2) improved cardiovascular fitness is not necessary to achieve psychological effect; (3) moderately intensive activities may improve symptoms better than high-intensity activities; and (4) physical activity has preventive mental health effects (U.S. Preventive Services Task Force, 1996).

Based on the wide spectrum of beneficial effects of physical activity on physical and mental health, many of the outcomes identified in the Nursing-sensitive Outcomes Classification (NOC) (Maas & Johnson, 1997) system may relate to exercise promotion. These include Adherence Behavior; Anxiety Control; Balance; Body Image; Cardiac Pump Effectiveness; Circulation Status; Coping; Endurance; Energy Conservation; Health Beliefs: Perceived Ability to Perform; Health Beliefs: Perceived Control; Health Promoting Behavior; Health Seeking Behavior; Immune Status; Leisure Participation; Mobility Level; Mood Equilibrium; Muscle Function; Nutritional Status; Physical Aging Status; Quality of Life; Safety Behavior: Fall Prevention; Self-Esteem; Sleep; Tissue Perfusion: Cardiac; Tissue Perfusion: Peripheral; and Well-Being.

QUANTIFICATION OF EXERCISE

Current physical activity recommendations emphasize measuring the amount of physical activity, whereas previous recommendations predominantly focused on dose response improvements in performance capacity, primarily the effects of exercise training on maximal oxygen consumption (VO_{2max}) (Pate et al., 1995; USDHHS, 1996). Amount of activity is measured either in the number of minutes activity is performed or in the amount of calories expended. Paffenbarger et al. (1986) calculated activity level and energy expenditure among male Harvard alumni and found that compared with men who were the least active, those who expended 71 to 143 kcal/day had a 22% reduction in overall mortality and those who expended 143 to 214 kcal/day had a 27% reduction. Other studies have reported similar findings (Helmrich et al., 1991; Leon, Connetti, Jacobs, & Rauramad, 1987; Slattery, Jacobs, & Michaman, 1989). Based on an extensive review of the literature, national recommendations for physical activity are to expend an average of 150 kcal/day or 1,000 kcal/wk. This level of activity could be achieved by walking briskly for 30 minutes a day; by performing a more vigorous activity for a shorter duration, such as 15 minutes of running at 10 mph, or by engaging in activity for a longer duration but less frequently, such as 35 minutes of running at 10 mph three times per week (USDHHS, 1996).

Because of the linear relationship between amount of physical activity and health benefit, a key message health care providers must deliver to clients is that some exercise is better than no exercise and that, for those who are active, increasing activity will provide an even greater degree of protection. Furthermore, a pattern of regular physical exercise is essential to attain and maintain maximal lifetime benefit.

ASSESSMENT

Most adults lead sedentary lives and can be considered unconditioned. Most adults also have varying risk factors for cardiovascular disease or other functional impairments. Clear guidelines are needed to identify those clients who require extensive evaluation, including graded exercise testing or physician supervision, and to identify those clients who do not need further evaluation and for whom the nurse can use an Exercise Promotion intervention. These guidelines are useful whether the nurse has primary responsibility for a client's care or is working in collaboration with another health professional.

Assessment of the individual before implementing an Exercise Promotion intervention as specified by the Nursing Interventions Classification (NIC) (McCloskey & Bulechek, 1996) (Table 7–1) should include a focused health history and physical examination and selected laboratory parameters. The purposes of the assessment are (1) to determine the presence of risk factors for or presence of coronary artery disease (CAD), (2) to identify the existence of other health problems or functional difficulties that might modify or preclude exercise prescription, and (3) to collect psychosocial and environmental data that would individualize the exercise plan. Table 7–2 outlines a health history to be used to evaluate an individual before providing the exercise intervention (ACSM, 1995). It incorporates a focused assessment for the presence of risk factors and other health problems that might modify or preclude exercise. For the elderly, major hearing or vision losses are particularly important to evaluate. The psychosocial history provides important data about the individual's current health beliefs, feelings about exercise, lifestyle, and past experiences that will provide clues about motivation for exercising. Another simple screening tool is the Physical Activity Readiness Questionnaire (PAR-Q) (Thomas, Reading, & Shephard, 1992). This seven-item questionnaire can be used with individuals from age 15 to 69 to identify those clients who require further evaluation before exercise prescription.

The physical examination should parallel the history by focusing primarily on the cardiac, respiratory, and musculoskeletal systems. Laboratory studies should include determination of lipid levels, urinalysis, complete blood count (for heavily menstruating women and the elderly), and any other studies indicated by the history and physical examination.

This assessment enables the nurse to identify individuals who can safely use the Exercise Promotion intervention and those who require further evaluation,

Table 7–1   Exercise Promotion

DEFINITION: Facilitation of regular physical exercise to maintain or advance to a higher level of fitness and health.

ACTIVITIES:

Appraise patient's health beliefs about physical exercise

Encourage verbalization of feelings about exercise or need for exercise

Assist in identifying a positive role model for maintaining the exercise program

Include patient's family/caregivers in planning and maintaining the exercise program

Inform patient about health benefits and physiological effects of exercise

Instruct patient about appropriate type of exercise for level of health, in collaboration with physician and/or exercise physiologist

Instruct patient about desired frequency, duration, and intensity of the exercise program

Assist patient to prepare and maintain a progress graph/chart to motivate adherence with the exercise program

Instruct patient about conditions warranting cessation of or alteration in the exercise program

Instruct patient on proper warm-up and cool-down exercises

Instruct the patient in techniques to avoid injury while exercising

Instruct patient in proper breathing techniques to maximize oxygen uptake during physical exercise

Assist patient to develop an appropriate exercise program to meet needs

Assist patient to set short-term and long-term goals for the exercise program

Assist patient to schedule regular periods for the exercise program into weekly routine

Provide reinforcement schedule to enhance patient's motivation (e.g., weekly weigh-in)

Monitor patient's response to exercise program

Provide positive feedback for patient's efforts

Source: McCloskey, J. C., and Bulechek, G. M. (Eds.). (1996). *Nursing interventions classification (NIC)* (2nd ed.). St. Louis: Mosby–Year Book.

perhaps even a professionally supervised exercise program. A two-category system originally developed by Fair, Allan-Rosenaur, and Thurston (1979) has been modified to incorporate the most recent American College of Sports Medicine (ACSM) guidelines (1995) with regard to referral for further evaluation before exercise prescription.

Category I: No Risk Factors or Disease

The nurse and client can use the Exercise Promotion intervention to plan a moderate exercise program for men and women of any age. For men 40 and younger and women 50 and younger, the nurse can plan a vigorous exercise program. Men older than 40 and women older than 50 should be referred for further evaluation, such as exercise stress testing and specialized risk appraisal, before prescribing a vigorous exercise program.

Category II: Risk Factors and/or Disease

The nurse and client can use the Exercise Promotion intervention to plan a moderate exercise program for men and women of any age who have two or more risk factors but are asymptomatic. If individuals have symptoms or known disease, they should be referred for further evaluation before planning a moderate exercise program. All individuals at increased risk or with known disease should be referred for further evaluation before planning a vigorous exercise program.

Table 7–2   Health History for Exercise Promotion Intervention

I. Present Health Status (includes aspects of past health and family history)
  A. Presence of Coronary Artery Disease (actual or suspected)
    1. Do you have angina pectoris (or do you ever get a pressure, pain, or tightness in your chest if excited, exercising, eating, or walking against a cold wind)?
    2. Do you have or have you had palpitations or rapid heartbeats or irregular heartbeats?
    3. Have you ever had a heart attack (myocardial infarction, coronary occlusion, or coronary thrombosis)?
    4. Have you ever had rheumatic fever?
    5. Have you had a cardiogram taken while exercising that was not normal?
    6. Do you take or have you taken any of the following: nitroglycerin (small pill that you put under your tongue for chest pain), digitalis, or quinidine for your heart?
  B. Risk Factors for Coronary Heart Disease
    1. Are you 45 or older (men) or 55 or older (women)?
    2. Did you have a premature menopause (before 50) and not take hormone replacement therapy?
    3. Do you have hypertension or high blood pressure (>140/90)? What is the treatment plan (diet, drugs, exercise, relaxation, herbal remedies)?
    4. Do you have elevated cholesterol (high fat in the blood)? Are you on a special diet or taking medication?
    5. Do you smoke now? How much? Did you ever smoke? When did you quit?
    6. Has anyone in your family had a heart attack or heart trouble or high cholesterol (for father before age 50 and for mother before age 65)?
    7. Do you have diabetes mellitus or high blood sugar? What is the treatment plan (diet, oral agents, insulin)?
  C. Other Potentially Limiting Conditions
    1. Do you have any chronic illnesses?
    2. Ask about asthma; emphysema; hyperthyroidism; anemia; any arthritis, back, joint, visual, or auditory problems (current or past) that limit activity; renal disease; chronic infectious processes (chronic hepatitis); and obesity (greater than 30% of ideal weight).
II. Past Health History
  Ask about any other major hospitalizations and surgeries; medications (prescribed and over-the-counter); major allergies; immunization status; and last skin test for tuberculosis.
III. Personal Social History
  A. Explore individual's health beliefs about health in general and exercise specifically. Include data on the following: general concern about health; priorities and positive health activities; past experience with health care system and providers; perceptions about susceptibility to heart disease and the potential severity of heart disease.
  B. Explore reasons for wishing to start an exercise program and expectations. Include data on the following: past exercise experiences; knowledge about exercise; beliefs in the benefits of exercise; exercise interests; daily schedule (work and home); personal (financial) and community resources and client support systems (family and friends' concerns and knowledge about exercise).

For men younger than 40 and women younger than 50, the nurse should seek consultation to determine whether the risk factors or other health problems are benign enough to allow the exercise prescription or severe enough to warrant referral for exercise stress testing and additional consultation. A 35-year-old man who smokes and has moderate hypertension should be referred for evaluation before prescribing an exercise program. A 43-year-old woman with moderately elevated lipid levels who smokes five cigarettes a day and has chronic mild musculoskeletal low back strain presents a common clinical situation for which the literature offers no clear guidelines. The nurse is left to apply clinical judgment and seek consultation in making decisions about these marginal situations.

Nursing Diagnoses and Exercise Promotion Intervention

Within these broad parameters, the intervention of Exercise Promotion is a treatment option for the resolution of several of the 137 North American Nursing Diagnosis Association (NANDA) nursing diagnoses (NANDA, 1994). The two most general diagnoses for which Exercise Promotion intervention is a treatment option are Health Seeking Behaviors related to effective activity pattern and Altered Health Maintenance due to a sedentary lifestyle (McCloskey & Bulechek, 1996). More specifically, Exercise Promotion, although not the treatment of choice, is an essential intervention in clients with the following diagnoses (McCloskey & Bulechek, 1996): Activity Intolerance, Risk for; Fatigue; Gas Exchange, Impaired; Infection, Risk for; Nutrition, More Than Body Requirements, Altered; Nutrition, Potential for More Than Body Requirements, Altered; and Physical Mobility, Impaired. Exercise Promotion is considered an optional intervention for several diagnoses including Activity Intolerance; Breathing Pattern, Ineffective; Constipation; Diversional Activity Deficit; Hopelessness; Pain; Peripheral Neurovascular Dysfunction, Risk for; Sleep Pattern Disturbance; and Social Isolation.

INTERVENTION ACTIVITIES

Translating an awareness of the need for physical activity into action or behavioral change is crucial to a successful Exercise Promotion intervention. A successful Exercise Promotion intervention includes the designing of an exercise program that has three major goals: (1) increasing the likelihood that an individual will engage in an exercise program, (2) teaching the individual how to achieve physical fitness safely, and (3) assisting the individual in maintaining the exercise program.

Increasing the Likelihood of Engaging in Physical Activity and Exercise

Although there is a vast amount of literature on health behavior, little is known about what motivates individuals to make changes in their lifestyles. The behavioral and environmental determinants of exercise adoption and maintenance are still poorly understood. Dishman and Sallis (1994) concluded that knowledge of and beliefs about health and activity, perceived needs and abilities, expectations, gender, ethnicity, and environmental factors were the most relevant influences in adoption and maintenance of an exercise program. Persons who perceive their health as poor (Broman, 1995; Weitzel & Waller, 1990) and believe that exercise has little value (Marcus, Rakowski, & Rossi, 1992) are less likely to exercise. Environmental factors such as social support of family and friends (Felton & Parsons, 1994; Hovell, Hofstetter, Sallis, Rauh, & Barrington 1992; Hovell et al., 1991) are important influences in initiating and maintaining an exercise program, whereas other environmental factors, such as lack of time (Marcus et al., 1992) and lack of access to an exercise site (Godin et al., 1991) may outweigh personal intention (Dishman & Sallis, 1994; Godin & Shephard, 1990).

Research that has focused on the determinants of health protecting or health promoting behavior provides some direction to the clinician in increasing the likelihood of an individual's participating in physical activity. The best-known health behavior models are the Health Belief Model (HBM) (Kasl & Cobb, 1966), Transtheoretical Model (Armstrong, Sallis, Hovell, & Hofstetter, 1993; Prochaska, DiClemente, & Norcross, 1992), the Theory of Planned Behavior (Fishbein & Ajzen, 1975; Godin & Kok, 1996), and Pender's Health Promotion Model (Ahijevtch & Bernhard, 1994; Pender, 1996).

The revised Health Promotion Model, derived from social learning theory (Bandura, 1986), provides a theoretical approach for predicting the likelihood of an individual's engaging in a health promoting action such as exercise. The model argues that whether an individual will undertake a health action depends on specific individual characteristics, behavior-specific cognitions and affect, and commitment to a plan of action. The relevant cognitive-perceptual factors postulated to determine a health decision include individual perceptions concerning self-efficacy, activity-related affect, benefits and barriers to action, and interpersonal and situational influences. For example, perceived self-efficacy in one's ability to exercise predicts exercise activity (Rudolph & McAuley, 1995). In a survey study of physical activity of 127 Hispanic adults, Hovell et al. (1991) reported that self-efficacy, a friend's support, childhood physical activity, and eating a heart-healthy diet were positively related to vigorous activity. Individual characteristics and experiences that influence decision making include personal factors and prior related behavior. Dishman and Sallis (1994) identified past experiences with fitness programs as a major factor influencing involvement in exercise. Personal factors such as socioeconomic status, perceived health status, or body size indirectly influence behavior-specific cognitions and affect and commitment to action. Ahijevtch & Bernhard (1994), in a study of 187 African-American women, reported that participants who had a medical diagnosis engaged in more health promoting behaviors. They concluded that the illness served as a motivator to improve health. By contrast, Broman (1995), in a telephone survey of 495 African-American adults, reported that individuals with a larger number of health problems were less likely to believe in the efficacy of preventive health behavior than individuals with a smaller number of health problems. Although the Pender Health Promotion Model continues to be tested, the clinician can use the concepts from the model in assessing a client's readiness to engage in an exercise program (see Table 7–2).

In developing an exercise intervention with a client, the nurse must have knowledge of the factors that influence health behavior. The factors outlined in the Pender Model (Pender, 1996) can be integrated into the health history and intervention plan. As research indicates, beliefs change as the individual has positive experiences with the health intervention (Dishman & Sallis, 1994; Godin & Shephard, 1990). The nurse needs to reassess the client's beliefs periodically during the monitoring phase of the intervention.

FURTHERING THE PROCESSES OF BEHAVIOR CHANGE

Pender (1996) advocates using the stages of health behavior change from the Transtheoretical Model (Prochaska et al., 1992) as a guide to structure nursing interventions for behavior change. These stages are (1) precontemplation (not considering change), (2) contemplation (considering change in the next 6 months), (3) planning (considering change within the next month), (4) action (change has been initiated), and (5) maintenance (begins 6 months after the change was made). Research of Prochaska et al. (1992) has suggested that different intervention processes should be emphasized at different stages of change.

When individuals are in the contemplation stage, nursing actions should focus on raising consciousness about being sedentary. Common actions include providing information about health and physical activity and the consequences of inactivity, risk appraisal or self-awareness counseling, and engaging family members in discussions about the client's contemplated behavior change. The power of health assessment and health diagnosis in increasing individual awareness of the risks of a sedentary lifestyle should not be underestimated. Despite the wide distribution of the Put Prevention into Practice (PPIP) program (USDHHS, 1994) into primary care and community settings, there remains insufficient emphasis on health promotion in our health care system. However, the nurse who focuses on health promotion issues often receives a positive response. In that regard, the provision of health information, specifically about physical fitness, cannot be overemphasized. Consistent with PPIP counseling guidelines and the Transtheoretical Model of behavior change (Prochaska et al., 1992), using the "teachable moment" to provide health information, specifically about physical activity, may provide a stimulus to change through consciousness raising.

In preparation for the planning and action stages, several techniques are recommended that include self-reevaluation, cognitive restructuring, reinforcement, modeling, and stimulus control (Pender, 1996; Prochaska et al., 1992). (See Table 7–1 for a listing of several of these techniques.) Self-reevaluation involves working with the client to identify personal beliefs, values, and barriers to being an active person. The individual should list his or her current beliefs about exercise, benefits from change, and barriers to change. The client can do this task orally or keep a written log and bring it to a subsequent visit. Reinforcement management involves the client's selecting behaviors to be changed and rewards for those changes. One technique is to have the client keep an activity/inactivity daily record of behavior, times, and situations to establish a baseline. These data can be used to establish realistic short-term activity goals and rewards for achieving the goals. The reader is referred to Pender (1996) for a more detailed description of these nursing actions. Clients will be at different stages of readiness (Prochaska et al., 1992) for proceeding to the actual Exercise Promotion intervention. Often health professionals move directly from identification of the client as sedentary into a plan for an Exercise Promotion intervention and wonder why the client frequently does not adhere to the program or even return for future visits.

Designing an Exercise Program

The goal of the Exercise Promotion intervention is to design with the client a program that will safely achieve or maintain general health benefits of regular physical activity. An exercise program has eight major aspects: type of activity, intensity, frequency, duration of the exercise, warm-up/cool-down exercises, education about conditions warranting cessation or modification of the program, method for monitoring intensity (ACSM, 1995; Pate et al., 1995; USDHHS, 1996), and an individualized program, which also constitutes the third step of the nursing intervention. Table 7–3 summarizes the Centers for Disease Control and Prevention (CDC)–ACSM (Pate et al., 1995) and ACSM (1995) recommendations for exercise. The 1995 ACSM recommendations are included in the text later. Current consensus is that in Exercise Promotion the focus is on the amount of physical activity performed, which is considered more important than the specific manner (i.e., the mode, frequency, intensity, and duration) in which activity is performed (Pate et al., 1995; USDHHS, 1996). An initial target goal of expending 1,000 kcal/wk (150 kcal/day) is recommended but may require revision depending on individual abilities, needs, and interests (USDHHS, 1996).

TYPE OF ACTIVITY

The most appropriate mode of activity is best determined by individual preferences and what the client decides he or she is willing to do on a regular basis.

Table 7–3 CDC-ACSM Recommendations for Exercise Prescription

Frequency	All or most days of the week
Intensity	Moderate/hard
Duration	>30 min/day in bouts of at least 8–10 min
Mode of activity	Endurance activity that uses large muscles: walking, hiking, running or jogging, cycling-bicycling, dance, rope skipping, stair climbing, swimming
Resistance training	Not specified

Source: Pate et al. (1995). Physical activity and public health: A recommendation from the Centers for Disease Control and Prevention and the American College of Sports Medicine. *JAMA, 273,* 402–407.

For a given week, a combination of endurance types of exercise, especially those that use large muscle groups, is appropriate for most healthy active or sedentary adults. Such activities include walking, stair climbing, rope skipping, cycling (rolling or stationary bicycle), swimming, jogging, or running. Recreational activities such as gardening, dancing, bowling, and martial arts are also recommended. Physically disabled clients may use walking, riding modified stationary bicycles, or wheelchair propulsion (Lampman, 1987; Shephard, 1986). Walking and running are particularly suited to older clients because they avoid the isometric tension in upper body limbs created by cycling (Buchner, 1997), a tension that increases blood pressure. In addition, everyone should be urged to make small lifestyle changes to increase activity, such as parking the car three blocks from work or taking the stairs instead of the elevator.

Resistance and strength training enables all major muscle groups to be exercised. Examples of this type of exercise include weightlifting, pushups, and sit-ups. Weight training is superior for strengthening; however, calisthenics are economical and convenient methods for improving strength. The 1995 ACSM guidelines recommend 8 to 10 exercises of the various large muscle groups with 8 to 12 repetitions per set, 2 days per week.

FREQUENCY, INTENSITY, AND DURATION

The frequency, intensity, and duration of exercise are interrelated, such that the number of episodes of activity per day or week (frequency) depends on the intensity level and duration of activity. For example, activity of higher intensity or longer duration could be performed approximately three times a week, whereas similar benefit is attained with lower-intensity or shorter-duration activities that are performed more often (i.e., 5 to 7 days/wk) (ACSM, 1995).

Intensity and duration of exercise determine the total caloric expenditure during an exercise session. Several methods are used to measure energy expenditure. Exercise and sport scientists advocate obtaining VO_{2max} and maximal heart rate (HR_{max}). Methods commonly used in the community include metabolic equivalents (METs) and ratings of perceived exertion. The Borg Rating of Perceived Exertion (RPE) scale (Borg, 1974; Pollock & Wilmore, 1990) allows individuals to classify intensity along a rank order scale of "very light" exertion to "very heavy" exertion (Table 7–4). The scale has been used extensively in exercise laboratories as well as cardiac rehabilitation programs. METs are calculated energy costs of various physical activities and represent the amount of oxygen used to perform the activity. One MET is the oxygen uptake at rest, which equals 3.5 mL/kg/min. Both methods, METs and RPE, have strong correlations with VO_{2max} and HR_{max} (Pollock & Wilmore, 1990).

Duration refers to the specific length of time the individual should exercise.

Table 7–4 Duration of Various Activities to Expend 150 kcal for an Average 70-kg Adult

Intensity	Activity	RPE*	Metabolic Equivalents (METs)	Approximate Duration in Minutes†
LIGHT	Driving a car, shopping, bowling, fishing, pleasure sailing, golf (with a power cart), slow walk	9–11	1.5–2.5	60
MODERATE	Pleasure cycling, dancing, volleyball (noncompetitive), table tennis, calisthenics, walking 3–4 mph, raking leaves, social dancing, lawn mowing	12–13	3–5	30–45
HARD	Jogging 5 mph, ice skating, competitive tennis, field hockey, swimming	14–16	6–8	15–20
VERY HARD	Running 6 mph, touch football, basketball	17–19	9–10	10–15

*RPE: Borg Rating of Perceived Exertion, 6–20 Scale.

†Formula: $\dfrac{150 \text{ kcal} \times 60 \text{ min/hr}}{\text{METs (kcal/kg/hr)} \times \text{kg}}$ = minutes.

Sources: U.S. Department of Health and Human Services. (1996). *Physical activity and health: A report of the Surgeon General.* Atlanta, GA: U.S. Department of Health and Human Services, Centers for Disease Control and Prevention, National Center for Chronic Disease Prevention and Health Promotion; Pollock, M., and Wilmore, J. H. (1990). *Exercise in health and disease: Evaluation and prescription for prevention and rehabilitation* (2nd ed.). Philadelphia: W.B. Saunders.

For many sedentary adults, a less intense program of longer duration is realistic. Thus, lower-intensity activity needs to be offset by increased duration and frequency. Another approach for clients with reduced performance capacity (i.e., those able to perform only light-intensity activities) is to engage in multiple short daily exercise sessions rather than attempt a lengthy workout a few times a week (ACSM, 1995).

Table 7–4 shows the relationship of activity mode, frequency, intensity, and duration in achieving the caloric goals of the program. A precise method to determine quantity of exercise is as follows: if the goal is set at 1,000 kcal/wk, the individual weighs 70 kg, and moderate-intensity exercise of 5 to 6 METs is selected, the caloric expenditure would be 7.35 kcal/min (METs × 3.5 mL × body weight in kg/200 = kcal/min), which requires 136 minutes of exercise per week. To achieve the 1,000 kcal/wk goal, the individual may choose to exercise 5 days/wk for 27 minutes a day, 4 days/wk for 34 minutes, 3 days/wk for 45 minutes, and so forth (ACSM, 1995).

WARM-UP AND COOL-DOWN PHASES

These periods are integral parts of all exercise programs. The warm-up phase prepares the body for sustained activity by increasing blood flow and stretching postural muscles. It is a period of adaptation that prevents a sudden increase in workload on the heart, the circulatory system, and the muscles and joints. The warm-up sequence should be designed to increase the intensity of exercise gradually, include rhythmic exercises that stretch muscles, and put joints through their full range of motion (Safren, Seaber, & Garret, 1989). For 5 to 10 minutes, as the heart rate slowly reaches its target zone, this sequence should be followed (Pollock & Wilmore, 1990):

1. Initiate rhythmic movements starting with joint range of motion, such as performing a forward and backward crawl (circumduction, extension, and flexion of shoulder girdle); walk with hands clasped behind head while twisting side to side (circulation, rotation of trunk); or do knee bends.

2. Do stretching exercises, such as touching toes (hip, thigh, and back extensors), raising hands over head and bending from side to side (lateral trunk muscles), progressing to alternate knee hugs (back muscles), performing straight leg raises (knee and hip muscles), assuming sprinter's position with heel pointed (hamstrings), and walking rapidly in a circle.

The cool-down period is equally important after the period of endurance exercise to prevent syncope, which can result from a sudden decrease in the supply of blood to large muscle groups. For 5 to 10 minutes, the individual should continue to use large muscle groups (for example, jogging at a slower pace), slow down to a few minutes of walking, and use range of motion, stretching, and static muscle contraction and relaxation activities.

CONDITIONS WARRANTING CESSATION OF OR ALTERATION IN THE EXERCISE PROGRAM

The nurse needs to provide clear instructions to clients to stop exercising and seek health advice if they experience any of the following conditions: pain in chest, arm, neck, or jaw; irregular heart rate; dizziness; persistent shortness of breath after exercise; nausea or vomiting during or after exercise; prolonged fatigue; uncoordinated gait or weakness; or muscle or joint swelling (American Heart Association [AHA], 1991; Pollock & Wilmore, 1990). Investigation of the cause of these symptoms must be made before a client resumes exercising. Every prescription should include a written list of these symptoms, which often occur because individuals do not progress slowly in their training program.

Clients need to consider discontinuation of their training program during episodes of minor illness. Deconditioning occurs very rapidly; studies report an initial loss beginning in 3 days and a 50% loss of the original improvement in 3 months (Froelicher, 1987). The implication of these data is that the intensity of the exercise prescription needs to be decreased when the individual resumes an exercise program.

MONITORING AND INDIVIDUALIZING THE PROGRAM

Program monitoring primarily focuses on evaluating the client's activity performance and satisfaction with the selected program design and on altering aspects of the program as needed. Specific questions should be directed at determining whether the client is having difficulty implementing any of the planned activities, assessing the quantity of activity performed weekly, identifying what the client enjoys and does not enjoy about the program, and asking what he or she would like to change. Follow-up sessions are helpful in tailoring programs to meet the individual's goals.

Most sources (ACSM, 1995; Pollock & Wilmore, 1990; USDHHS, 1996) suggest that sedentary individuals begin with a walking program. Such a program provides an opportunity not only to work out an exercise schedule but also to practice monitoring intensity. Table 7–5 provides examples of a walking program for two different age groups. Walking is a particularly good exercise for the elderly; an individual who is not able to progress to jogging can receive major benefits from a walking program. For some individuals who are unable to be outside, a walking program can be carried out in a gym or recreation center.

Other exercises such as swimming, biking (indoor and outdoor), and rope jumping should be planned in a similar manner. Swimming is an excellent exercise for individuals of all ages. It has the advantage of being useful for clients who have musculoskeletal or neurological disabilities that make walking or jogging too difficult.

Table 7-5 Progressive Walking Program

Week	Frequency/wk	Distance (miles)	Duration (min) <30 yr/>50 yr
1-2	4-5	1.0	15.0/18-20
3	4-5	1.0	13.0/15-17
4	4-5	1.5	21.5/24
5	4-5	1.5	21.0/22.5
6	4-5	1.5	20.5/21.5
7	4-5	2.0	28.0/32
12	3-4	3.0	40.0/44

Sources: Blocker (1976); Cooper (1972); Pollock, M., and Wilmore, J. H. (1990). *Exercise in health and disease: evaluation and prescription for prevention and rehabilitation* (2nd ed.). Philadelphia: W.B. Saunders.

Preventing Common Injuries

Approximately 60% of all aches, pains, and injuries suffered by runners, joggers, and walkers are related to excessive speed work on hills, a lack of shock absorption, and a lack of motion control (Cook, Brinker, & Poche, 1990). Low-impact activities should be emphasized for deconditioned individuals and those susceptible to orthopedic injury, such as postmenopausal women, overweight persons, and the elderly (Jones & Eaton, 1995). Shoes are the most important clothing investment for a runner, jogger, or walker for the prevention of injuries. Running shoes need to provide maximum cushioning to prevent overstretching of muscles and tendons and to provide strong support to control excess motion and guide the foot as it moves (Cook et al., 1990). (Readers desiring more information should seek other sources for specific details about jogging and running injuries, such as Rolf [1995].)

Individualized Program: Maintaining the Exercise Program

Successful maintenance of a change in behavior or lifestyle is vital but notoriously difficult (Neale, Singleton, Dupuis, & Hess, 1990; Pender, 1996). Attrition is a serious problem in most exercise programs, with more than 50% of participants dropping out in the first 6 months (McAuley & Jacobson, 1991). Research on adherence (Dishman, 1990; Hovell et al., 1991; Sallis, Hovell, Hofstetter, & Barrington, 1992; Sallis, Hovell, & Hofstetter, 1992) suggests that self-motivation, personal feedback, and social support are key factors in maintenance of exercise programs. McAuley and Jacobson (1991), in a study of 58 overweight women in an 8-week aerobic exercise class, reported that the factors influencing continued participation included instructor fit, self-efficacy, cognitions about commitment, positive regard for the program, and persistence in exercise. Although this aspect of exercise as a nursing intervention is discussed last, it is probably the most important. The process of individualizing or tailoring a prescription for the individual is the major strategy used not only for initiation of change but also for maintenance (Pender, 1996). This process of tailoring, which underpins the entire exercise intervention, is the cornerstone to successful initiation of and adherence to a particular plan, and it begins when the nurse first encounters the client. A variety of techniques can be used to individualize the intervention: focused nursing assessment, patient self-assessment, client self-monologues, and a specific weekly exercise program. Data related to daily patterns, preferences, past experience, health beliefs, personal resources, and social supports are used

Goal: Establish regular walking program (Week 1):
1. Keep written diary of all activities for 1 week.
2. List pros and cons of exercise.
3. List resources in neighborhood and work.
4. List social support from work colleagues and family.

Contract:
I, Mr. Wiley, will bring diary of list of exercise activities, pros and cons, resources, and social supports from work and home to the next visit. The nurse will evaluate my current activities and help me plan a beginning walking program.

Signed: Ms. Franks, MS, RN, CS, ANP
Signed: Mr. Wiley
Date: 6/3/98
Reward: I will buy a new shirt.

Figure 7–1 Contract for exercise.

not only to increase client readiness but also to tailor the exercise plan (see Table 7–1).

Devising a plan with the client should involve an agreement about objectives or goals of care and mutual expectations. Goals of care are important because they provide clear direction for the nurse and client, guide the selection of specific intervention techniques, and provide a means for evaluation and recognition of change. One technique that is particularly helpful in developing a plan of action is the contract (Neale et al., 1990; Pender, 1996).

Contracting as an intervention is specifically described in Chapter 23. An example of a contract for the intervention of exercise appears in Figure 7–1. Contracting is an ideal strategy for providing clients with an individualized experience in behavioral change and concurrent means of developing positive health beliefs about that change. The use of other patient education techniques, the development of a positive therapeutic relationship, working with the client's support networks, and regular follow-up visits may enhance the client's successful execution of the exercise plan (Jones & Eaton, 1995; Pender, 1996; USDHHS, 1994).

CASE STUDY

CW is a 40-year-old married computer programmer who comes to the clinic concerned about being overweight and having a family history of heart disease. He feels that he is unhealthy and needs to change his lifestyle.

CW, who is 6 feet tall, has weighed 200 pounds since age 30 and has unsuccessfully attempted to lose weight numerous times using self-initiated fad diets. He eats two meals per day, lunch (at work) and dinner (at home), and has a diet consisting of high-cholesterol and high-salt foods—bread or pasta products and few fruits and vegetables. He has never had his blood cholesterol level measured. CW's father, who is living, had a myocardial infarction (MI) at age 45. CW believes that he is at risk for an MI because

he is overweight and sedentary like his father. The rest of the family history is negative for diabetes, heart disease, hypertension, and hypercholesterolemia. CW denies chest pain, high blood pressure, palpitations, or any history of rheumatic fever. He has never had an electrocardiogram (ECG), and he has no history of rheumatic fever or other chronic illness. He has no current concerns. CW does not smoke, drinks 2 ounces of whiskey per day, and does not exercise regularly.

His history reveals no major surgeries or hospitalizations. CW takes no prescribed medication, has no allergies, and was last skin-tested for tuberculosis and immunized in 1992.

CW has been married for 15 years, has two

children, age 12 and 10, and describes his relationship with his wife, who is a high school biology teacher, as very good. His wife, in fact, urged the client to have a checkup and get help for his concerns. CW has worked at the same company for 10 years and generally enjoys his job. He is financially secure. Until recently, CW felt that he was young, had no illnesses, and did not need to be concerned about his health. At a recent college reunion, however, he was shocked both by the early death of a few friends and by the youthfulness of others. As he stated, "I suddenly felt old, ugly, and worried that I'd have an MI like my dad and not be able to fully participate in life's activities." His past experiences with the health care system have been minimal but positive. With regard to exercise, CW wishes to learn how to jog, because it will "improve my heart," but he is afraid it will be too hard to maintain: "I'm lazy." He has not exercised since college and has never run. He would like to exercise at lunch but does not know how to go about this. He thinks that his family will be supportive of his plan.

Physical examination showed an overweight man in no distress (blood pressure, 130/84; pulse, 84; respirations, 18), with the following findings:

Thorax/lungs: No lung abnormalities; equal expansion and diaphragmatic excursion 3 cm bilaterally; resonant to percussion and clear to auscultation.

Cardiovascular: Normal sinus rhythm; $S_1 > S_2$; no murmurs or extra sounds; no bruits; pulses 2 + and equal.

Musculoskeletal: No spinal deformities; full range of motion in all joints; good muscle mass.

Laboratory: ECG and urinalysis results normal; cholesterol level, 240 mg/dL.

Nursing diagnoses for CW are Altered Health Maintenance related to sedentary lifestyle; Altered Nutrition: More Than Body Requirements; and Risk for Activity Intolerance related to sedentary lifestyle.

The exercise program for CW will begin with a progressive walking program (see Table 7–5). Initially, to enhance cognitive structure and motivation and to obtain more specific data, a contract was established with CW. In progressive visits, the nurse will move to assist CW with specific aspects of initiating and maintaining an exercise program, helping him develop a specific exercise plan, and selecting the appropriate time, climate, and clothing. Concurrently, the nurse will work with CW to develop a plan for improving his nutritional intake and weight loss.

SUMMARY

The need to change the sedentary habits of adult Americans is well recognized. With the increasing emphasis on exercise as a significant health promoting behavior, it is important that nurses have knowledge of Exercise Promotion in order to assess and develop management plans with the healthy exercising adult. This chapter provides a review of the fundamental elements of physical activity and the beneficial effects of regular exercise; a model for assessing the adult client; and specific strategies for the development of an Exercise Promotion program with the client. The mechanics of the exercise prescription are straightforward, but the tailoring of an individualized program that provides the guidance and support necessary for the initiation and maintenance of lifestyle change is more difficult.

Although there is a growing body of knowledge that nurses can use in developing Exercise Promotion interventions, more research needs to be done. We know very little about those factors that prompt individuals to make a decision to pursue a new course of action or to maintain this new behavior. Nurses have an important role as researchers and as skilled clinicians in taking leadership in the neglected area of promotion of health in the adult population.

References

Ahijevtch, K., and Bernhard, L. (1994). Health-promoting behaviors of African-American women. *Nursing Research, 43*(2), 86–89.

American Heart Association. (1991). *Exercise standards: A statement for health professionals*. Dallas: Author.

American College of Sports Medicine. (1995). *ACSM's guidelines for exercise testing and prescription* (5th ed.). Baltimore: Williams & Wilkins.

Armstrong, C., Sallis, J., Hovell, M., and Hofstetter, C. (1993). Stages of change, self-efficacy, and the adoption of vigorous exercise: A prospective analysis. *Journal of Sports and Exercise Psychology, 15*, 390–402.

Arroll, B., and Beaglehole, R. (1992). Does physical activity lower blood pressure? A critical review of the clinical trials. *Journal of Clinical Epidemiology, 45*, 439–447.

Bandura, A. (1986). *Social foundations of thought and action: A social-cognitive theory*. Englewood Cliffs, NJ: Prentice-Hall.

Berlin, J. A., and Coditz, G. A. (1990). A meta-analysis of physical activity in the prevention of coronary heart disease. *American Journal of Epidemiology, 132*, 612–628.

Blair, S. N. (1993). Evidence for success of exercise in weight loss and control. *Annals of Internal Medicine, 119*(7 Pt. 2), 702–706.

Blair, S. (1994). McCloy research lecture: Physical activity, physical fitness, and health. *Research Quarterly for Exercise and Sport, 64*, 365–376.

Blair, S. N., Horton, E., Leon, A. S., Lee, I., Drinkwater, B., Dishman, R., and Mackey, R. (1995). Physical activity, nutrition, and chronic disease. *Medicine and Science in Sports and Exercise, 28*, 335–349.

Blair, S. N., Kohl, H. W., III, Barlow, C. E., Paffenbarger, R. S., Gibbons, L., and Macera, C. (1995). Changes in physical fitness and all-cause mortality: A prospective study of healthy and unhealthy men. *JAMA, 273*, 1093–1098.

Blair, S. N., Kohl, H. W., III, Paffenbarger, R. S., Jr., Clark, D., Cooper, K., and Gibbons, L. (1989). Physical fitness and all-cause mortality: A prospective study of healthy men and women. *Journal of the American Medical Association, 262*, 2395–2401.

Blocker, W. (1976). Physical activities. *Postgraduate Medicine, 60*, 56–61.

Borg, G. (1974). Perceived exertion. *Exercise and Sports Science Reviews, 2*, 131.

Broman, C. (1995). Leisure-time physical activity in an African-American population. *Journal of Behavioral Medicine, 18*, 341–353.

Buchner, D. (1997). Physical activity and quality of life in older patients. *JAMA, 277*, 64–66.

Caspersen, C. J., Powell, K. E., and Christenson, G. M. (1985). Physical activity, exercise, and physical fitness: Definitions and distinctions for health-related research. *Public Health Report, 100*, 126–131.

Cook, S. D., Brinker, M. R., and Poche, M. (1990). Running shoes: Their relationship to running injuries. *Sports Medicine, 10*(1), 1–8.

Cooper, K. (1972). *The new aerobics*. New York: Bantam Books.

DiPietro, L. (1995). Physical activity, body weight, and adiposity: An epidemiologic perspective. *Exercise and Sport Sciences Reviews, 23*, 275–303.

Dishman, R. (1990). Determinants of participation in physical activity. In C. Bouchard, R. Shephard, T. Stephens, J. Sutton, and R. McPherson (Eds.), *Exercise, fitness, and health* (pp. 75–101). Champaign, IL: Human Kinetics.

Dishman, R., and Sallis, J. (1994). Determinants and interventions for physical activity. In C. Bouchard, R. Shephard, T. Stephens, J. Sutton, and R. McPherson (Eds), *Exercise, fitness, and health* (pp. 102–140). Champaign, IL: Human Kinetics.

Duncan, J. J., Gordon, N. F., and Scott, C. B. (1991). Women walking for health and fitness: How much is enough? *JAMA, 266*, 3295–3299.

Durstine, J. L., and Haskell, W. L. (1994). Effects of exercise training on plasma lipids and lipoproteins. *Exercise and Sport Sciences Reviews, 22*, 477–521.

Fair, J., Allan-Rosenaur, J., and Thurston, E. (1979). Exercise management. *Nurse Practitioner, 3*, 13–18.

Felton, G., and Parsons, M. (1994). Factors influencing activity in average weight and overweight young women. *Journal of Community Health Nursing, 11*, 109–119.

Fishbein, M., and Ajzen, I. (1975). *Belief, attitude, intention, and behavior: An introduction to theory and research*. Boston: Addison-Wesley.

Froelicher, V. F. (1987). *Exercise and the heart: Clinical concepts* (2nd ed.). Chicago: Year Book Medical Publishers.

Godin, G., Desharnais, R., Valois, P., Lepage, L., Jobin, J., and Bradet, R. (1991). Differences in perceived barriers to exercise between high and low intenders: Observations among different populations. *American Journal of Health Promotion, 8*, 279–285.

Godin, G., and Kok, G. (1996). The theory of planned behavior: A review of its application to health-related behaviors. *American Journal of Health Promotion, 11*(2), 87–98.

Godin, G., and Shephard, R. (1990). Use of attitude-behavior models in exercise promotion. *Sports Medicine, 10*(2), 103–121.

Hagberg, J. M. (1990). Exercise fitness and hypertension. In C. Bouchard, R. J. Shephard, T. Stephens, J. Sutton, and R. McPherson (Eds.), *Exercise, fitness and health* (pp. 455–566). Champaign, IL: Human Kinetics.

Haskell, W. L. (1986). The influence of exercise training on plasma lipids and lipoproteins in health and disease. *Acta Medica Scandinavica* (Suppl. 12), 25–37.

Haskell, W. L., Alderman, E. L., Fair, J. M., Maron, D., Mackey, S., and Superko, H. (1994). Effects of intensive multiple risk factor reduction on coronary atherosclerosis and clinical cardiac events in men and women with coronary artery disease: The Stanford Coronary Risk Intervention Project (SCRIP). *Circulation, 89*, 975–990.

Helmrich, S. P., Ragland, D. R., Leung, R. W., and Paffenbarger, R. S. (1991). Physical activity and reduced occurrence of non-insulin-dependent diabetes mellitus. *New England Journal of Medicine, 325*, 147–152.

Hovell, M., Hofstetter, R., Sallis, J., Rauh, M., and Barrington, E. (1992). Correlates of change in walking for exercise: An exploratory study. *Research Quarterly for Exercise and Sport, 63*, 425–434.

Hovell, M., Sallis, J., Hofstetter, R., Barrington, E., Hackley, M., Elder, J., et al. (1991). Identification of correlates of physical activity among Latino adults. *Journal of Community Health, 16*, 23–36.

Jones, T., and Eaton, C. (1995). Exercise prescription. *American Family Physician, 522*, 543–550.

Kannel, W. B. (1983). High-density lipoproteins: Epidemiologic profile and risks of coronary artery disease. *American Journal of Cardiology, 52*, 98–128.

Kannel, W. B., Belanger, A., D'Agostino, R., and Israel, I. (1986). Physical activity and physical demand on the job and the risk of cardiovascular disease and death: The Framingham study. *American Heart Journal, 112,* 820–825.

Kasl, S. V., and Cobb, S. (1966). Health behavior, illness behavior, and sick role behavior. Part I. *Archives of Environmental Health, 12,* 246–266.

Kelley, G., and McClellan, P. (1994). Antihypertensive effects of aerobic exercise: A brief meta-analytic review of randomized controlled trials. *American Journal of Hypertension, 7,* 115–119.

Lampman, R. (1987). Evaluating and prescribing exercise for elderly patients. *Geriatrics, 8*(42), 63–65, 75.

Lee, I. M., Paffenbarger, R. S., Jr., and Hsieh, C. C. (1991). Physical activity and risk of developing colorectal cancer among college alumni. *Journal of the National Cancer Institute, 83,* 1324–1329.

Leon, A. S., Connett, J., Jacobs, D. R., Jr., and Rauramad, R. (1987). Leisure-time physical activity levels and risk of coronary heart disease and death: The Multiple Risk Factor Intervention Trial. *JAMA, 258,* 2388–2395.

Maas, M., and Johnson, M. (Eds.). (1997). *Nursing outcomes classification (NOC).* St. Louis: Mosby.

Marcus, B., Rakowski, W., and Rossi, J. (1992). Assessing motivational readiness and decision-making for exercise. *Health Psychology, 11,* 257–261.

McArdle, W. D., Katch, F. I., and Katch, V. L. (1994). *Essentials of exercise physiology.* Philadelphia: Lea & Febiger.

McAuley, E., and Jacobson, L. (1991). Self-efficacy and exercise participation in sedentary adult females. *American Journal of Health Promotion, 5,* 185–191.

McCloskey, J. C., and Bulechek, G. M. (Eds.). (1996). *Nursing interventions classification (NIC) (2nd ed.).* St. Louis: Mosby–Year Book.

Morris, J., Heady, J., Raffle, P., Roberts, C., and Parks, J. (1953). Coronary heart disease and physical activity work. *Lancet, 2,* 1053–1057, 1111–1120.

Neale, A., Singleton, S., Dupuis, M., and Hess, J. (1990). The use of behavioral contracting to increase exercise activity. *American Journal of Health Promotion, 4,* 441–447.

North American Nursing Diagnosis Association. (1994). *NANDA nursing diagnoses: Definition and classification 1995–1996.* Philadelphia: Author.

Paffenbarger, R. S., Laughlin, M., Gima, A., and Black, R. (1970). Work activity of longshoremen as related to death from coronary heart disease and stroke. *New England Journal of Medicine, 282,* 1109–1114.

Paffenbarger, R. S., Hale, W., Brand, R., and Hyde, R. (1977). Work-energy level, personal characteristics, and fatal heart attack: A birth cohort affect. *American Journal of Epidemiology, 105,* 200–213.

Paffenbarger, R. S., Jr., Hyde, R. T., and Wing, A. L. (1986). Physical activity level, all-cause mortality, and longevity of college alumni. *New England Journal of Medicine, 314,* 605–613.

Paffenbarger, R. S., Jr., Hyde, R. T., Wing, A. L., Lee, I-M., Jung, D., and Kampert, J. (1993). The association of changes in physical activity level and other lifestyle characteristics with mortality among men. *New England Journal of Medicine, 328,* 538–545.

Pate, R., Pratt, M., Blair, S., Haskell, W. L., Macera, C., Bouchard, C., et al. (1995). Physical activity and public health: A recommendation from the Centers for Disease Control and Prevention and the American College of Sports Medicine. *JAMA, 273,* 402–407.

Pender, N. (1996). *Health promotion in nursing practice* (3rd ed.). Stamford, CT: Appleton-Lange.

Pollock, M., and Wilmore, J. H. (1990). *Exercise in health and disease: Evaluation and prescription for prevention and rehabilitation* (2nd ed.). Philadelphia: W. B. Saunders.

Powell, K. E., Thompson, P. D., Caspersen, C. J., and Kendrick, J. (1987). Physical activity and the incidence of coronary heart disease. *Annual Reviews in Public Health, 8,* 253–287.

Prochaska, J., DiClemente, C., and Norcross, J. (1992). In search of how people change: Applications to addictive behaviors. *American Psychology, 47,* 1102–1114.

Rolf, C. (1995). Overuse injuries of the lower extremity in runners. *Scandinavian Journal of Medicine and Science in Sports, 5,* 181–190.

Rudolph, D., and McAuley, E. (1995). Self-efficacy and salivary cortisol responses to acute exercise in physically active and less active adults. *Journal of Sport and Exercise Physiology, 17,* 206–213.

Safren, M., Seaber, A., and Garret, W. (1989). Warm-up and muscular injuries. *Sports Medicine, 8,* 239–249.

Sallis, J., Hovell, M., and Hofstetter, C. (1992). Predictors of adoption and maintenance of vigorous physical activity in men and women. *Preventive Medicine, 21,* 237–251.

Sallis, J., Hovell, M., Hofstetter, C., and Barrington, E. (1992). Explanation of vigorous physical activity during two years using social learning variables. *Social Sciences and Medicine, 34*(1), 25–32.

Shephard, R. (1986). Physical training for the elderly. *Clinics in Sports Medicine, 5,* 517–530.

Slattery, M. L., Jacobs, D. R., Jr., and Michaman, M. Z. (1989). Leisure-time physical activity and coronary heart disease death: The U.S. Railroad Study. *Circulation, 127,* 571–580.

Thomas, S., Reading, J., and Shephard, R. (1992). Revision of the Physical Activity Readiness Questionnaire (PAR-Q). *Canadian Journal of Sport Sciences, 17,* 338–345.

Tsopanakis, A. O., Sgouraki, E. P., Pavlou, K. N., Nadel, E., and Bussolari, S. (1989). Lipids and lipoprotein profiles in a 4-hour endurance test on a recumbent cycloergometer. *American Journal of Clinical Nutrition, 49,* 980–984.

U.S. Department of Health and Human Services. (1994). *Clinician's handbook of preventive services.* Washington, DC: U.S. Government Printing Office.

U.S. Department of Health and Human Services. (1995). *Healthy People 2000: Mid course review and 1995 revisions.* Washington, DC: U.S. Department of Health and Human Services, Public Health Service.

U.S. Department of Health and Human Services. (1996). *Physical activity and health: A report of the Surgeon General.* Atlanta, GA: U.S. Department of Health and Human Services, Centers for Disease Control and Prevention, National Center for Chronic Disease Prevention and Health Promotion.

U.S. Preventive Services Task Force. (1996). *Guide to clinical preventive services* (2nd ed.). Baltimore: Williams & Wilkins.

Weitzel, M., and Waller, P. (1990). Predictive factors for health-promotive behaviors in white, hispanic and black blue-collar workers. *Family and Community Health, 13*(10), 23–33.

Williamson, D. F., Madans, J., Anda, R. F., Kleinman, J., Kahn, H., and Byers, T. (1993). Recreational physical activity and ten-year weight change in a US national cohort. *International Journal of Obesity, 17,* 279–286.

Pain Management

Keela A. Herr and Paula R. Mobily

Pain is a common symptom and frequent diagnosis that has been addressed extensively in the literature and in clinical practice during the 1990s. Although major advances have been made through the release of federal guidelines on the clinical management of acute and cancer pain, research continues to document inadequate and inappropriate care of persons experiencing pain (Cleeland et al., 1994; Ferrell, McCaffery, & Ropchan, 1992; Jacox, Ferrell, Heidrich, Hester, & Miaskowski, 1992; Miaskowski, Nichols, Brody, & Synold, 1994; Ward & Gordon, 1994).

The experience of pain is a complex and multidimensional phenomenon, mediated by specific sensory processes or nociceptive events, but also influenced by social history, cultural expectations, individual differences concerning the meaning of pain, and effectiveness of personal and social coping resources (Harkins & Price, 1992; Melzack & Wall, 1965; Turk & Rudy, 1988). A concept analysis of pain demonstrates the diversity of definitions attributed to pain, which incorporate physiological components causing the experience; the personal and subjective nature of the experience, often expressed in unpleasant adjectival descriptors; and the consequence of the experience, which includes its tiring and unending nature, its interference with relationships, and its life-giving meaning (Mahon, 1994). The intervention Pain Management is defined in the Nursing Interventions Classification (NIC) as the "alleviation of pain or a reduction in pain to a level of comfort that is acceptable to the patient" (McCloskey & Bulechek, 1996) (Table 8–1). The focus of this intervention is consistent with any of the definitions of pain and can encompass the many components of pain regardless of how they are defined.

Pain Management is a comprehensive intervention intended to address the

Table 8–1   Pain Management

DEFINITION: The alleviation of pain or a reduction in pain to a level of comfort that is acceptable to the patient.

ACTIVITIES

Perform a comprehensive assessment of pain to include location, characteristics, onset/duration, frequency, quality, intensity or severity of pain, and precipitating factors

Observe for nonverbal cues of discomfort, especially in those unable to communicate effectively

Ensure that the patient receives appropriate analgesic care

Use therapeutic communication strategies to acknowledge the pain experience and convey acceptance of the patient's response to pain

Consider cultural influences on pain response

Determine the impact of the pain experience on quality of life (e.g., sleep, appetite, activity, cognition, mood, relationships, performance of job, and role responsibilities)

Evaluate past experiences with pain to include individual or family history of chronic pain or resulting disability, as appropriate

Evaluate, with the patient and the health care team, the effectiveness of past pain control measures that have been used

Assist patient and family to seek and provide support

Use a developmentally-appropriate assessment method that allows for monitoring of change in pain and that will assist in identifying actual and potential precipitating factors, flow sheet, and daily diary

Determine the needed frequency of making an assessment of patient comfort, and implement monitoring plan

Provide information about the pain, such as causes of the pain, how long it will last, and anticipated discomforts from procedures

Control environmental factors that may influence the patient's response to discomfort (e.g., room temperature, lighting, and noise)

Reduce or eliminate factors that precipitate or increase the pain experience (e.g., fear, fatigue, monotony, and lack of knowledge)

Consider the patient's willingness to participate, ability to participate, preference, support of significant others for method, and contraindications when selecting a pain relief strategy

Select and implement a variety of measures (e.g., pharmacological, nonpharmacological, and interpersonal) to facilitate pain relief, as appropriate

Consider type and source of pain when selecting pain relief strategy

Encourage patient to monitor own pain and to intervene appropriately

Teach the use of nonpharmacological techniques (e.g., biofeedback, TENS, hypnosis, relaxation, guided imagery, music therapy, distraction, play therapy, activity therapy, acupressure, heat/cold application, and massage) before, after, and, if possible, during painful activities; before pain occurs or increases; and along with other pain relief measures

Collaborate with the patient, significant other, and other health professionals to select and implement nonpharmacological pain relief measures, as appropriate

Provide the person optimal pain relief with prescribed analgesics

Implement the use of patient-controlled analgesia (PCA), if appropriate

Use pain control measures before pain becomes severe

Medicate before an activity to increase participation, but evaluate the hazard of sedation

Ensure pretreatment analgesia and/or nonpharmacologic strategies before painful procedures

Verify level of discomfort with patient, note changes in the medical record, and inform other health professionals working with the patient

Evaluate the effectiveness of the pain control measures used through ongoing assessment of the pain experience

Institute and modify pain control measures on the basis of the patient's response

Promote adequate rest/sleep to facilitate pain relief

Table 8–1 Pain Management *Continued*

DEFINITION: The alleviation of pain or a reduction in pain to a level of comfort that is acceptable to the patient.

ACTIVITIES *Continued*

Encourage patient to discuss the pain experience, as appropriate

Notify physician if measures are unsuccessful or if current complaint is a significant change from patient's past experience of pain

Inform other health care professionals/family members of nonpharmacologic strategies being used by the patient to encourage preventive approaches to pain management

Use a multidisciplinary approach to pain management, when appropriate

Consider referrals for patient, family, and significant others to support groups and other resources, as appropriate

Provide accurate information to promote family's knowledge of and response to the pain experience

Incorporate the family in the pain relief modality, if possible

Monitor patient satisfaction with pain management at specified intervals

Source: McCloskey, J. C., and Bulechek, G. M. (Eds.). (1996). *Nursing interventions classification (NIC)* (2nd ed., pp. 412–413). St. Louis: Mosby–Year Book.

problem of pain in patients of all ages and settings (see Table 8–1). It incorporates assessment and evaluation guidelines, factors affecting the success of pain management, and strategies for selecting and implementing more specific pain interventions, including NIC interventions using physical techniques (e.g., Acupressure, Analgesic Administration, Cutaneous Stimulation, Environmental Management: Comfort, Heat/Cold Application, Patient-Controlled Analgesia [PCA] Assistance, Progressive Muscle Relaxation, Simple Massage, Therapeutic Touch, and Transcutaneous Electrical Nerve Stimulation [TENS]) and those NIC interventions using psychological techniques (e.g., Anxiety Reduction, Autogenic Training, Biofeedback, Calming Technique, Distraction, Hypnosis, Meditation, Simple Guided Imagery, Simple Relaxation Therapy) (Table 8–2). The user of the Pain Management intervention should be familiar with specific resources that assist with individualization of the activities suggested to promote Pain Management with different populations.

Nurses play a pivotal role in the assessment and management of pain. The Pain Management intervention is one of a group of interventions developed to address the comprehensive nature of pain and to identify activities that address the barriers to successful pain management identified in the literature (Herr & Mobily, 1992). This chapter discusses some of the specific activities of the Pain Management intervention as well as suggestions for use of the intervention in practice, related nursing diagnoses, and patient outcomes associated with Pain Management.

Attempts to improve the assessment and management of pain have led to a number of interdisciplinary efforts to develop clinical practice guidelines for the management of acute and cancer pain (Acute Pain Management Guideline Panel, 1992; Jacox et al., 1994). Additionally, the American Pain Society (APS) has presented revised guidelines for analgesic use and quality improvement guidelines for treating acute and cancer pain (APS, 1992; American Pain Society Quality of Care Committee, 1995). Other organizations (e.g., American Geriatrics Society, Oncology Nursing Society, Association of Pediatric Nurse Practitioners) continue to review accruing research and make recommendations for pain man-

Table 8–2 NIC Interventions Related to Pain

NIC Intervention Label	Definition
Pain Management	Alleviation of pain or a reduction in pain to a level of comfort that is acceptable to the patient
Analgesic Administration	Use of pharmacological agents to reduce or eliminate pain
Environmental Comfort Measures	Environmental measures to promote optimal comfort
Cutaneous Stimulation	Stimulation of the skin and underlying tissues for the purpose of decreasing undesirable signs and symptoms (such as pain, muscle spasm, or inflammation)
Heat/Cold Application	Stimulation of the skin and underlying tissues with heat or cold for the purpose of decreasing pain, muscle spasms, or inflammation
Simple Massage	Stimulation of the skin and underlying tissues with varying degrees of hand pressure to decrease pain, produce relaxation, and/or improve circulation
Transcutaneous Electrical Nerve Stimulation (TENS)	Stimulation of skin and underlying tissues with controlled, low-voltage electrical vibration by electrodes to alter pain sensation
Distraction	Purposeful focusing of attention away from undesirable sensations
Simple Guided Imagery	Purposeful use of imagination to achieve relaxation and/or direct attention away from undesirable sensations
Simple Relaxation Therapy	Techniques to encourage and elicit relaxation for the purpose of decreasing undesirable signs and symptoms (such as pain, muscle tension, or anxiety)

Source: McCloskey, J. C., and Bulechek, G. M. (Eds.). (1996). *Nursing interventions classification (NIC)* (2nd ed., pp. 412–413). St. Louis: Mosby–Year Book.

agement strategies that are most appropriate for given populations and can be used in conjunction with the NIC Pain Management intervention.

ASSESSMENT/EVALUATION ACTIVITIES

Pain assessment has been found to be performed inadequately and inconsistently by nurses in a variety of settings (Clarke et al., 1996; McCaffery & Ferrell, 1991; Paice, Mahon, & Faut-Callahan, 1991; Tittle & McMillan, 1994), a factor that contributes to inadequate pain management. Researchers report inadequacies due to primary reliance on the patient's self-report of pain or incongruencies in nurse-patient judgments of pain intensity (Ferrell, Wisdom, Rhiner, & Alletto, 1991; McCaffery & Ferrell, 1992; Walker, Akinsanya, David, & Marcer, 1990), inability to distinguish acute from chronic pain (Ferrell, Eberts, McCaffery, & Grant, 1991; McCaffery & Ferrell, 1991), lack of ongoing assessment and documentation of medication efficacy and side effects (Choiniere, Melzack, Girard, Rondeau, & Paquin, 1990; Morgan, Lindley, & Berry, 1994; Tittle & McMillan, 1994), and lack of knowledge of cultural differences (Martin & Belcher, 1986). The NIC intervention Pain Management incorporates activities related to assessment that are essential for successful and individualized management of a patient's pain and thus are a key aspect of any Pain Management intervention.

Reflective of the multidimensional and complex phenomenon of pain, careful evaluation of a variety of components is required, including, but not limited to, location, pain characteristics (including intensity, quality, and chronology), response to pain, precipitating and alleviating factors, meaning of pain, typical coping methods, and factors affecting pain (such as fatigue, anxiety, depression, fear, and expectations). Pain often interferes with physical and psychological functioning, resulting in disability and impairment in a number of factors associated with quality of life (e.g., sleep, appetite, daily activities, relationships, role performance) that have been correlated with pain (Haythornthwaite, Seiber, & Kerns, 1991; Herr, Mobily, & Smith, 1993; Mobily, Herr, Clark, & Wallace, 1994). These become critical variables for the evaluation of Pain Management activities, particularly for those with chronic pain conditions. Resources are available to guide the practitioner in identification of the multitude of factors that contribute to pain and need to be considered when evaluating pain (e.g., Allcock, 1996; Kerns, Turk, & Rudy, 1985; McCaffery & Beebe, 1989; Simon, 1996; Simon & McTier, 1996; Watt-Watson & Donovan, 1992).

Communication skills on the part of both patients and health care providers are essential for obtaining accurate information regarding the patient's pain experience and for successful management of pain. The single most reliable indicator of the presence and level of pain is the patient's self-report (Acute Pain Management Guideline Panel, 1992; APS, 1992; Jacox et al., 1994; National Institutes of Health [NIH], 1986). If at all possible, the patient's self-report should take precedence over behavior or vital signs (Beyer, McGrath, & Berde, 1990), and the patient and family should be believed. Patients may not report pain for a variety of reasons such as thinking the pain is not bad enough (Taylor & Curran, 1985), fear of what the pain means (Ahles, Blanchard, & Ruckdeschel, 1983), fear of consequences of acknowledging pain such as the need for hospitalization or diagnostic tests or the loss of independence (Hofland, 1992; Watt-Watson, Evernden, & Lawson, 1990), and the desire to be a "good" patient (Cleeland, 1984; Ward et al., 1993). Establishment of a positive relationship with the patient and his or her significant others and the use of therapeutic communication techniques acknowledge the importance of the pain experience, convey acceptance of the patient's pain situation, and facilitate the sharing of information necessary for effective pain management.

Many factors influence expression of pain, including age, gender, education, religion, socioeconomic class, and acculturation, in addition to ethnicity and cultural differences (Faucett, Gordon, & Levine, 1994). Assessment instruments are culturally influenced and may not provide opportunity for exchange of pain-related information. Starting with standard approaches to data gathering regarding pain is appropriate, but one must avoid drawing stereotypical conclusions (Geissler, 1994). Establishing a nonthreatening, comfortable atmosphere and eliciting information about personal preferences and customs that affect pain expression and interpretation is a key strategy (Pachter, 1994).

In addition to qualitative assessment of pain and its related components, selected measurement instruments can be used to help quantify the pain experience and provide outcome indicators useful in evaluating response to nursing intervention. Assessment strategies must be developmentally appropriate to meet the needs of various patient populations. A variety of established pain assessment instruments are available for the adult population, and pediatric assessment instruments have also become more prevalent. Assessment instruments and strategies for elderly or impaired individuals are less available; however, work is ongoing to provide psychometric support for methods to assess pain in these groups.

Assessment of acute pain usually includes an evaluation of pain intensity or severity, for which a number of scales are available. Three brief, easy-to-use self-report measurement tools for assessing pain intensity and affective distress in adults include the numeric rating scale (NRS), the visual analogue scale (VAS), and the verbal descriptor scale (VDS) (Fig. 8–1). Substantial literature supports the reliability and validity of these instruments with adults (Jensen & Karoly, 1992). The NRS and VDS consist of a series of numbers or words that represent different levels of pain intensity. The VAS is a continuum of pain along a line with extremes at either end offering more options for designating level of pain severity. Variations on these traditional scales have been developed and can be valid and reliable when the endpoints and adjective descriptors are carefully selected (Graceley & Wolskee, 1983; Sriwatanakul, Kelvie, & Lasagna, 1982). A variation commonly used in clinical practice, because of its ease of use, is the verbal numeric rating scale, in which the patient is asked to rate his or her pain from 0 to 10 with 0 representing "no pain" and 10 representing "the worst pain possible" (Murphy, McDonald, Power, Unwin, & MacSullivan, 1988; Paice & Cohen, 1997).

Although some older children are able to use the NRS (McGrath & Unruh, 1987) and the VAS (McGrath, 1990), a number of pain assessment tools have been developed specifically for use with children that address their ability to conceptualize and communicate pain. Generally, children older than 4 years of age can verbalize pain (McGrath, 1990) and should be asked about their pain. Parents can help provide specific words typically used by the child to express pain, valuable information about how the child deals with pain, and preferences for treatment (Hester & Barcus, 1986). A number of assessment tools have research substantiating their psychometric soundness and merit consideration, including, but not limited to, the Poker-Chip Scale (Hester, Foster, & Kristensen,

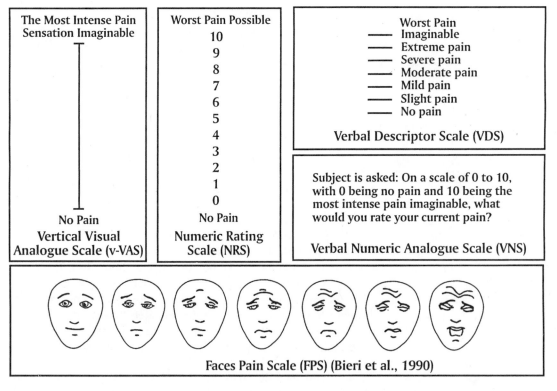

Figure 8–1   Illustration of pain intensity assessment scales. (From Mobily, P., and Herr, K. [in press]. Pain. In M. Maas, K. Buckwalter, M. Hardy, T. Reimer, and M. Titler [Eds.], *Nursing diagnoses and interventions for the elderly* [2nd ed.]. Thousand Oaks, CA: Sage Publications.)

1990), the Oucher Scale (Beyer, Villarruel, & Denyes, 1993), Facial Affective Scale (McGrath, 1990), and the Faces Pain Scale (Bieri, Reeve, Champion, Addicoat, & Aiegler, 1990) (see Fig. 8–1). Other instruments continue to be developed and tested, such as the Coloured Analogue Scale (McGrath et al., 1996) and the CRIES scale for use with neonates (Krechel & Bildner, 1995), in efforts to identify the most clinically useful approach to assessing children's pain.

Instruments currently accepted for use with adults, such as the VDS, NRS, and VAS, can be adapted for use with elderly patients (e.g., larger type, darker lines, selection of simple endpoints); however, empirical evidence of reliability and validity in this population is still scant (Ferrell & Ferrell, 1993; Herr & Mobily, 1991). Facial scales developed for use with children have also been suggested for use with the elderly (Ferrell, Ferrell, & Rivera, 1995; Mobily & Herr, in press). Careful explanation of the use of the instruments is necessary to promote patient understanding and accurate use of the tools, particularly the VAS (Scott & Huskisson, 1976). Although patient preference for a specific tool has not been shown to confound pain measurement (Kremer, Atkinson, & Ignelzi, 1981), elderly patients do differ in their preference for using a particular tool (Herr & Mobily, 1993). Consideration of patient preference should be incorporated into planning with the patient the method of assessing pain to be used, regardless of patient age.

To address the needs of patients unable to communicate their experience and needs, the practitioner will need to select simpler or modified pain scales or alternative assessment strategies. Patients in the immediate postoperative period or in critical care situations, infants and young children, mentally challenged patients, and elderly patients with dementia are all examples of individuals who require special attention when gathering data about their pain. Self-report should be attempted initially and has been shown to be effective in some cognitively impaired persons (Ferrell, Ferrell, & Rivera, 1995; Parmalee, Katz, & Lawton, 1993); however, dependence on behavioral observation may be the strategy of choice for assessment in many of these populations. Developmental factors, as well as situational circumstances, affect behavioral responses and pain expression in infants, toddlers, children, and adolescents (McGrath, 1990), as well as in mentally challenged and cognitively impaired patients. Behaviors (e.g., grimaces, cries, protective posturing) and physiological measures (e.g., heart rate, blood pressure) provide indirect measures from which presence and intensity of pain are inferred; however, additional validation of pain should be solicited. Gathering data from observation of the patient, as well as from significant others, can be valuable in validating the pain problem and the effectiveness of intervention. A parent or spouse can provide invaluable information about past or usual behavior patterns and expressions of discomfort to assist the practitioner in making judgments about the patient's pain. It is important to consider, however, that family members' assessment of pain is significantly related to appropriate knowledge and attitudes and is based on their own perception of the pain experienced by the patient (Elliott, Elliott, Murray, Braun, & Johnson, 1996).

A variety of behavioral scales are available for use with infants and children, such as the Children's Hospital of Eastern Ontario (CHEOPS) scale (McGrath et al., 1985) and the Pain Assessment Inventory for Neonates (Johnson, 1990); however, additional study of validity and reliability is needed. Although development of valid and reliable behavioral scales for the elderly is just beginning, the literature identifies strategies for observing behavior for making judgments regarding pain severity in the elderly (Baker, Bowring, Brignell, & Kafford, 1996; Hurley, Volicer, Hanrahan, Houde, & Volicer, 1992; Marzinksi, 1991). For additional discussion of strategies for assessing pain in the elderly, the reader is referred to Herr and Mobily (1997) or Ferrell (1991).

Nurses often fail to gather data about the effect of pain on quality of life (Dalton, 1989); however, for those with chronic pain conditions, in particular, impact on quality of life can be the most important indicator of pain control. Assessment must be more comprehensive and include evaluation of quality-of-life factors such as mood, relationships, activity, role function, and social engagement. The Multidimensional Pain Inventory (Kerns et al., 1985), the Pain Disability Index (Tait, Chibnall, & Krause, 1990), and the Brief Pain Inventory (Daut, Cleeland, & Flanery, 1983) are instruments for evaluating several domains of quality of life related specifically to pain. Because of the strong association between chronic pain and depression, evaluation of this mood state is also important using a psychometrically sound instrument such as the Beck Depression Inventory (Beck, Ward, Mendelson, Mock, & Erbaugh, 1961), the Center of Epidemiologic Studies Depression Scale (CES-D) (Radloff, 1977), or the Geriatric Depression Scale (Yesavage et al., 1983).

Selection of assessment instruments that are valid and reliable is an important responsibility for the practitioner. Because of the many different tools available, several factors should be considered in determining the best choice for a given patient. Factors to consider include (1) the patient's age; developmental status; physical, emotional, or cognitive condition; and preference; (2) the expertise, time, and effort available from the practitioner; and (3) the institution's requirements for monitoring and documenting for quality assurance purposes (Chapman & Syrjala, 1990). No single scale is ideal for all age groups or situations, and a number of reviews and references are available to guide the clinician in approaching pain assessment and identifying appropriate instrumentation in infants and children (e.g., Barr, 1994; Karoly, 1991; McGrath, 1990; McGrath & Brigham, 1992; Schechter, Berde, & Yaster, 1993) and other special populations (Acute Pain Management Guideline Panel, 1992; Jacox et al., 1994).

Establishment of a score (e.g., 3 on a 10-point scale) that the patient believes is acceptable for the level of pain should be used to determine when intervention is needed, when dose escalation is warranted, and when adjustments in intervention strategies are needed and to evaluate the efficacy of interventions. The patient's preferred tool for pain assessment and the goal for pain management should be recorded and readily available to any health team member assisting with pain control.

Use of a planned monitoring mechanism, such as a pain flow sheet, can be invaluable in assessing, monitoring, managing, and documenting pain and related activities. In addition to evaluating the response to intervention, flow sheets also can provide positive reinforcement of progress toward pain relief and can facilitate communication related to pain problems among health care providers. Readily available information on the patient's pain state and response to intervention can assist in recognizing the need for changes in intervention approach. Figure 8–2 presents an example of a flow sheet developed for use in an acute care setting with patients of all ages and pain problems. Various examples are available in the literature and can be adapted for the setting and population of interest (Jadlos, Kelman, Marra, & Lanoue, 1996; McCaffery & Beebe, 1989). Patients with chronic pain conditions, such as cancer, and their families should be taught to use the assessment instruments in their homes in order to promote continuity of assessment and communication of the pain experience (Jacox et al., 1994).

Although the frequency of assessment is variable depending on a number of

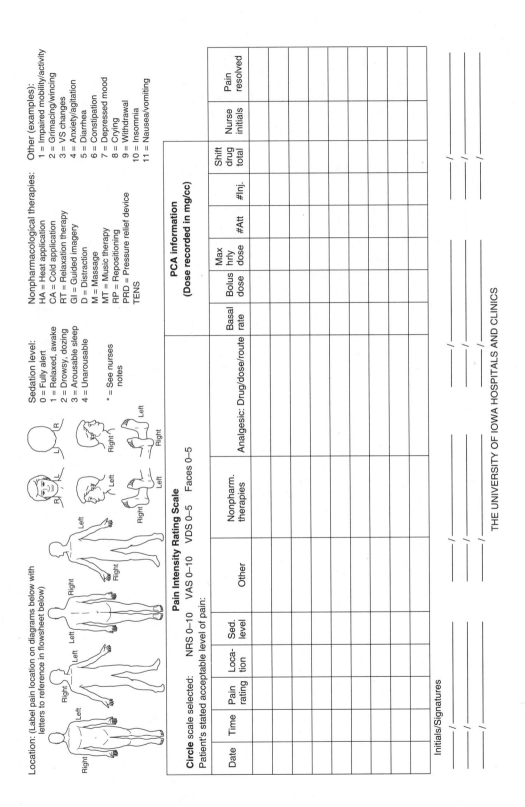

Figure 8–2 Nursing pain assessment and intervention flow sheet. (From Schmidt, K., Alpen, M., and Rakel, B. [1996]. Implementation of the Agency for Health Care Policy and Research pain guidelines. *AACN Clinical Issues, 7*[3], 430.)

157

factors (e.g., chronicity/acuity of the pain problem, success of intervention), data gathering related to pain is not a one-time activity. It must occur on a regular basis to evaluate the progress of pain control. It is recommended that pain be assessed and documented (1) at regular intervals after starting the treatment plan, (2) with each new report of pain, and (3) at a suitable interval after each pharmacological or nonpharmacological intervention, such as 15 to 30 minutes after parenteral drug therapy and 1 hour after oral administration (Jacox et al., 1994).

ACTIVITIES ADDRESSING FACTORS AFFECTING SUCCESS OF PAIN MANAGEMENT

A number of barriers to pain relief have been identified and include inadequate or inappropriate knowledge, beliefs, and attitudes about pain management held by patients (Ferrell, Ferrell, Ahn, & Tran, 1994; Ward et al., 1993), their families (Grossman, Shiedler, Swedeen, Mucenski, & Piantadosi, 1991; Taylor, Ferrell, Grant, & Cheynoy, 1993; Ward, Berry, & Misiewicz, 1996), and nurses (Clark et al., 1996; McCaffery, Ferrell, O'Neil-Page, Lester, & Ferrell, 1990; O'Brien, Dalton, Konsler, & Carlson, 1996; Schmidt, Eland, & Weiler, 1994; Sheidler, McGuire, Grossman, & Gilbert, 1992; Vortherms, Ryan, & Ward, 1992).

Patient and family knowledge and beliefs regarding pain and pain management strategies can have a major impact on the patient's willingness to share information about his or her pain experience, on compliance with a pain protocol, and, ultimately, on the outcome of pain intervention. The idiom *knowledge is power* applies to pain intervention as well.

A number of misbeliefs and concerns have been identified that affect patient/family receptivity to pain intervention strategies. Fears or concerns regarding analgesic use, particularly fear of addiction and respiratory depression, are major concerns for health professionals, as well as their patients (Lander, 1990; McCaffery et al., 1990; Short, Burnett, Egbert, & Parks, 1990). These have been correlated with inadequate use of pain medications (Ward et al., 1993) and interfere with following analgesic guidelines by health professionals and patients in pain.

Determination of the patient's attitude toward the use of opioids or other medications, as well as his or her receptivity to alternative interventional approaches such as relaxation therapy, can be important. Research has demonstrated that patients' attitudes, beliefs, and expectations about their situation, themselves, their coping resources, and the health care system affect their report of pain, activity, disability, and response to treatment (Flor & Turk, 1988; Jensen, Turner, & Romano, 1994; Tota-Faucette, Gil, Williams, & Goli, 1993). Fear of overmedication, resulting in addiction or respiratory depression, concerns about unpleasant side effects, and concerns about becoming tolerant to pain medications can result in noncompliance with analgesic management of pain. Educating patients and families about common fears and misbeliefs related to pain treatment can be an effective pain management strategy (Devine & Westlake, 1995; Ferrell et al., 1994; Rimer et al., 1987). Misconceptions regarding the use of pharmacological or nonpharmacological strategies should be corrected and reinforced by different health team members. Talking with clinicians knowledgeable about pain management and reading the consumer versions of the Agency for Health Care Policy and Research (AHCPR) guidelines (Acute Pain Management Guideline Panel, 1992; Jacox et al., 1994) can help patients and their families overcome fears and concerns regarding pain management strategies.

Unfortunately, many of the misbeliefs are held by health professionals as well, and changes in the educational system and continuing education are needed to remedy these misconceptions (Dalton et al., 1996; Ferrell, Eberts, McCaffery, & Grant, 1991; McCaffery & Ferrell, 1996; Sheidler et al., 1992; Zalon, 1995). Watt-Watson (1992) presents an excellent review of the many misbeliefs regarding the pain experience, pain management, and pain and age and is suggested as a resource for nurses needing to validate or correct their knowledge regarding pain.

Preprocedural and preoperative preparation is quite important in helping patients understand what will occur and how they can play a role in effectively controlling their pain. Preoperative provision of information related to physiological coping and procedural and sensory information has demonstrated decreased pain and less analgesic use (Fortin & Kirouac, 1976; Mogan, Wells, & Robertson, 1986; Reading, 1982). Explanations regarding the cause of the pain, how long it will last, and the anticipated discomforts from procedures can provide the anticipatory guidance that has been shown to decrease level of pain (Routh & Sanfilippo, 1991; Siegel & Peterson, 1981). In general, the following have been shown to lessen pain in children, and most likely also apply to adults: providing accurate, age-appropriate information about pain, particularly the specific sensations that will be experienced; increasing control by offering simple choices; explaining the rationale for what is happening and what can be done to reduce pain; and teaching simple pain-reducing strategies (Beales, 1983; McGrath, 1993; Peterson & Shigetomi, 1981). In adults, pain control can be improved when psycho-educational methods are used to address patient fears, potential side effects, effective communication with health care providers, and use of medications to manage symptoms (Devine & Westlake, 1995; Ferrell et al., 1994; Rimer et al., 1987; Roth-Roemer, Abrams, & Syrjala, 1996).

Collaboration between the health care team and the patient and family is useful for developing a Pain Management plan. Encouraging the patient and significant other to discuss pain and to become involved in the approach to Pain Management can facilitate a successful outcome. Again, cultural sensitivity is essential in developing and implementing a Pain Management plan that meets the patient's and family's needs and addresses the uniqueness of each patient (Juarez, 1997).

Involvement of the family caregiver is essential in the planning and implementation of a pain management plan (Juarez & Ferrell, 1996; Magrum, Bentzen, & Landmark, 1996). Family caregivers are often responsible for the burden of pain management in the home setting and often suffer from demands on time, emotional adjustment, distressing symptoms, work adjustment, sleep adjustment, family/relationship adjustments, and feelings of helplessness and uncertainty (Ferrell & Ferrell, 1991; Ferrell, Taylor, Grant, Fowler, & Corbisiero, 1993). Educational and emotional support for caregivers may be a key factor in pain outcome. Informational needs about symptoms and treatment side effects are important to family members (Hileman, Lackey, & Hassanein, 1992; Juarez & Ferrell, 1996) and include education and repeated reassurances regarding fears related to drug addiction and concerns about dangerous side effects of analgesic use as well as safe and effective drug administration and scheduling. Depending on the patient's support network and family situation, the practitioner may need to assist the patient and family in identifying appropriate resources and support services to meet individual Pain Management needs. Studies have documented the importance of structured support in managing pain (Spiegel & Bloom, 1983; Syrjala, Donaldson, Davis, Kippes, & Carr, 1995). Evaluation of the effect of interventions with the patient and family is essential to problem resolution, as is providing information for strategy selection when, and if, pain recurs.

Factors identified through the assessment phase that precipitate or increase the pain experience (e.g., fear, fatigue, monotony, lack of knowledge) should be addressed. For example, during procedures, environmental factors such as cold or crowded rooms or "beepers" on machines can escalate distress in children (Hester, 1989). Simple comfort measures found in the NIC intervention Environmental Management: Comfort, such as quieting the room, decreasing the lighting, sponging the patient, and providing warm blankets, can assist in decreasing pain.

SELECTION AND IMPLEMENTATION OF SPECIFIC PAIN MANAGEMENT STRATEGIES/TECHNIQUES

Because of the multidimensional nature of pain and the impact of individual experience and preferences, a multimodal approach, incorporating both pharmacological and nonpharmacological intervention strategies, is often most effective in managing pain and can result in more positive patient outcomes including more effective pain control, less reliance on medications, fewer side effects, and less clinical impairment (Ferrell, 1991; Jay & Miller, 1990; Owens & Ehrenreich, 1991; Tait, 1993). The research literature provides support for the use of a variety of pain relief strategies; however, the population and conditions for which each is best used can vary.

As discussed earlier, a number of factors must be taken into consideration when choosing the pain intervention strategy. Consideration of the individual's past experience with pain, particularly the effectiveness of past pain control measures; knowledge of pain management strategies; personal preferences for pain management techniques; and the willingness and ability to participate in a particular strategy, can assist the practitioner in selecting options with the most likelihood for success. Collaboration with the patient, the patient's significant other, and other health professionals in selection of the techniques to be used will facilitate a more positive response and clinical outcome.

The NIC Pain Management intervention identifies many of the factors to be evaluated or considered and presents options for pain relief strategies. The practitioner should select more specific NIC interventions related to pain control, such as Simple Relaxation, Analgesic Administration, or Guided Imagery, to identify specific activities directly related to the technique to be implemented.

Because patient responses to pharmacological and nonpharmacological strategies can vary widely, it is important to individualize the approach and implementation of the strategy as needed. A number of pain relief techniques, particularly nonpharmacological strategies, require the assistance of a significant other; thus, the importance of exploring the support network and availability of someone to assist with the intervention, particularly in the home setting, cannot be overstated. Several interventions have identified contraindications that must be taken into consideration. For example, individuals with pacemakers should not use TENS, those allergic to codeine should avoid some oral opioids, and those with pain in the calf should avoid massage to that area. Consideration of the type and source of pain can also direct the intervention selection. For example, a middle-aged man with muscle spasms in the upper back related to strenuous work might benefit most from Simple Massage Therapy, a young woman with stress-related headaches might achieve relief from learning and regularly practicing Relaxation or Guided Imagery interventions, or an elderly gentleman with episodes of rheumatoid arthritic pain in his hands might respond well to Heat/ Cold Application.

Regardless of the pain relief strategy chosen, education of the patient and family or significant other is key to a successful outcome (Roth-Roemer et al., 1996). Aside from careful instruction on the nature of the intervention and its expected outcome, patients should be taught the best times to use techniques to manage their pain: before, after, and, if possible, during painful activities; before pain occurs, increases, or becomes severe; and concomitant with other pain relief measures (Jacox et al., 1994). Educating the patient and family regarding potential side effects, preventive actions, and safety considerations should be incorporated. For example, when medicating before activity with opioids, it is important to evaluate for the possibility of sedative effects that could endanger the patient (McCaffery & Beebe, 1989).

The use of analgesics, singly or in combination, has been the dominant approach to Pain Management, particularly with acute pain conditions (e.g., postoperative pain) and many severe chronic pain conditions (e.g., cancer pain). It is essential that nurses working with patients experiencing pain be knowledgeable about analgesics, and appropriate resources should be consulted that address population-specific considerations. Three major classes of analgesic drugs are used for management of acute and cancer pain: nonopioid analgesics, opioid analgesics, and analgesic adjuvants (APS, 1992). The World Health Organization Expert Committee (1990) has recommended use of an analgesic ladder to assist with analgesic selection for three different levels of pain intensity and serve the practitioner as a beginning point for titration (Table 8–3). Mild pain may be treated with a non-opioid drug, such as a nonsteroidal anti-inflammatory agent (NSAID), whereas more severe pain requires the addition of a weak opioid to the non-opioid. Pain of severe intensity usually requires a strong opioid added to the non-opioid. Analgesic adjuvants, including tricyclic antidepressants, antihistamines, benzodiazepines, caffeine, dextroamphetamines, steroids, phenothiazines, and anticonvulsants, can enhance the effects of opioids, demonstrate independent analgesic activity in certain situations, or counteract the side effects of analgesics and can be incorporated into the analgesic regimen at any step (APS, 1992).

Although more detailed guidelines regarding analgesic use can be found in the NIC intervention Analgesic Administration, a few specific issues are ad-

Table 8–3   Analgesic Ladder

Ladder Step	Level of Pain Severity	Analgesic Recommended
Step 1	Mild pain	Nonopioid NSAID (e.g., acetylsalicylic acid, acetaminophen, ibuprofen, naproxen) $\pm$ Adjuvant (e.g., anticonvulsant, antidepressant, antihistamine, steroid)
Step 2	Mild to moderate pain	Weak opioid (e.g., codeine, hydrocodone, oxycodone) $+$ Nonopioid $\pm$ Adjuvant
Step 3	Moderate to severe pain	Strong opioid (e.g., morphine, hydromorphone, fentanyl, methadone) $\pm$ Nonopioid $\pm$ Adjuvant

Source: Data from World Health Organization. (1990, 1996). *Cancer pain relief and palliative care.* Geneva, Switzerland: Author.

dressed here. General approaches to the use of analgesics include (1) selecting the simplest dosage schedule and the least invasive modality first, (2) basing drug selection on the analgesic ladder, and (3) monitoring for side effects and treating prophylactically (Jacox et al., 1994). Principles of opioid use can guide the practitioner in providing maximum analgesic intervention that meets individual patient needs and includes the following: individualization of the route, dosage, and schedule; administering analgesics regularly (not as needed) if pain is present most of the day; familiarization with the dose and time-course of several strong opioids; administering adequate doses of opioids to infants and children; following up patients closely, particularly when beginning or changing analgesic regimens; use of equianalgesic dosing when changing drugs; recognizing and treating side effects; being aware of the potential hazards of meperidine and mixed agonist-antagonists; avoiding use of placebos to assess the nature of pain; watching for the development of tolerance and treating appropriately; being aware of the development of physical dependence and preventing withdrawal; not labeling patients "addicted" when they are physically dependent on or tolerant to opioids; and being alert to the psychological state of the patient (Acute Pain Management Guideline Panel, 1992; APS, 1992; Foley, 1985; Jacox et al., 1994; Twycross & Lack, 1983).

Patient-controlled analgesia (PCA) is a technique by which the patient administers small doses of drug on demand by one of several routes using a microprocessor-controlled infusion pump. Research has demonstrated that, in adults, PCA produces an overall improvement in analgesia (White, 1989) without an increase in sedation (Ferrante, Orav, Rocco, & Gallo, 1988). PCA also has demonstrated effectiveness with adolescents and older children (Berde, Lehn, Yee, Sethna, & Russo, 1991) as well as with older adults (Duggleby & Lander, 1992) and is an option for promoting a positive pain outcome in selected situations. Cognitive awareness and ability to follow directions and make judgments regarding pain are necessary to use PCA effectively. Careful evaluation of patient understanding and monitoring of usage is still important.

The practitioner should anticipate the development of pain and intervene to ensure patients receive pretreatment analgesia and/or nonpharmacological strategies before painful procedures to avoid severe pain. When pain is established or severe, it is more difficult to control (Wall, 1988). Patients and families should be taught the procedures and techniques involved in nonpharmacological modalities or interventions before an episode of acute pain, if possible, when learning is more likely. Opportunity to practice the procedures before the immediate need occurs also enhances the patient's ability to effectively implement the techniques.

Nonpharmacological techniques can be classified as either (1) physical or cutaneous stimulation interventions involving stimulating the skin and the underlying tissues to moderate or relieve pain, or (2) cognitive-behavioral interventions focusing on helping the individual cope with the pain being experienced by altering the interpretation of the sensation of pain and enhancing self-control (Mobily & Herr, in press). Cutaneous stimulation interventions, such as TENS, Heat/Cold Application, and Simple Massage, provide relief by increasing blood flow to the skin and superficial organs, reducing inflammation and edema to injured areas, and relaxing tightened musculature (Mobily, 1994). Cognitive-behavioral interventions, such as Distraction, Simple Guided Imagery, Humor, Music Therapy, Play Therapy, Preparatory Sensory Information, and Simple Relaxation Therapy, help patients develop the expectation that they can learn to manage their pain effectively and provide them with the skills to respond to their pain (Bradley, 1996).

The NIC provides interventions and activities for implementing nonpharmacological strategies (McCloskey & Bulechek, 1996). Most of these interventions can be implemented with basic education and practice (e.g., Heat/Cold Application, Simple Massage, Simple Relaxation Therapy, Simple Guided Imagery, Music Therapy); however, others require specialized education and training (e.g., Biofeedback Therapy, Hypnosis, TENS). Reported limitations in exposure to these techniques in basic nursing education curriculums suggest the importance of incorporating additional education and skill development into nonpharmacological techniques to promote use of these approaches in pain management (Zalon, 1995).

Nonpharmacological strategies, such as progressive muscle relaxation, guided imagery, music therapy, massage, and hypnosis, have been shown to work independently to achieve pain control and, when used concomitantly, to enhance the effects of analgesia and reduce the amount of analgesia required (Sloman, 1995; Speigel & Bloom, 1983; Syrjala, Cummings, & Donaldson, 1992; Syrjala et al., 1995; Zimmerman, Nieveen, Barnason, & Schmaderer, 1996). When used in chronic pain conditions, nonpharmacological interventions have resulted in reductions in patients' self-report of pain, observable pain behaviors, and disease activity (Edgar & Smith-Hanrahan, 1992; Keefe et al., 1990; Mobily, 1994). The type of pain and nature of pain contribute to the usefulness of specific nonpharmacological strategies for a given patient.

Nonpharmacological interventions might be useful for patients experiencing any of the following: (1) interest or desire to try the intervention, (2) anxiety or fear that is not incapacitating or related to a psychiatric or medical condition, (3) benefit from avoiding or reducing drug therapy, (4) pain likely to last for a prolonged period, or (5) incomplete pain relief following appropriate pharmacological intervention (Acute Pain Management Guideline Panel, 1992). Research provides support for the use of all the nonpharmacological interventions with selected pain populations; however, the nurse must be familiar with the literature that addresses specific uses and adaptations appropriate for a specific population or pain condition. For example, for a young child, puppet play might be used as a distraction technique, whereas for an elderly patient, reading, prayer, or socialization might be more appropriate distraction techniques.

Many of the strategies require limited time to teach the patient, but periodic reinforcement through encouragement, coaching, and family support is necessary to sustain the skills and motivate use. Positive relationships found between patients' adherence to their medical regimen and their social support systems (Sackett & Haynes, 1976) suggest that the family caregiver can play a key role in ensuring that both analgesic and nonpharmacological interventions are used. Several nonpharmacological strategies can be implemented with the use of audiotapes, which decreases the amount of time required of the practitioner to implement the therapy (Sloman, 1995), particularly for patients needing repeated coaching and reinforcement.

Because of the complexity of the pain experience and the knowledge and expertise required in many different areas to wholly address the pain problem, a multidisciplinary approach to pain management is desirous to achieve the best possible outcome (Ashburn, 1994; Miller, Bruno, & Kinzbrunner, 1996), and nurses are pivotal in fostering multidisciplinary efforts to improve pain management (Benoliel, 1995). Working together to plan and implement a pain management plan, health team members should keep each other informed of the treatment strategies being implemented, as well as their effectiveness for the individual patient, to ensure consistency and reinforce the positive aspects of the strategies chosen. Involvement of the family in the implementation of the selected pain relief modality is especially helpful with young or elderly patients and those in the community setting. Because of the positive effects of support groups noted in the literature (Fawzy, Fawzy, Arndt, & Pasnau, 1995; Syrjala et al., 1995), the practitioner should develop awareness of the availability of local support groups and make referrals when appropriate. Also, other resources in the community should be identified, such as medical supply companies, activities of daily living (ADL) supports, and home health care options, to assist the patient and family in coping with the pain problem and in the delivery of pain strategies.

ASSOCIATED NURSING DIAGNOSES AND APPROPRIATE CLIENT GROUPS

Linkages have been developed between North American Nursing Diagnosis Association (NANDA) nursing diagnoses and NIC interventions (McCloskey & Bulechek, 1996) to provide beginning help to nurses selecting individual interventions for patients. Pain Management has been identified as the primary intervention for two NANDA nursing diagnoses (Pain, Chronic Pain). These two diagnoses address the basic differences in duration, defining characteristics, and related factors of pain for pain problems that can require very different intervention approaches. It is important that nurses not only be able to diagnose pain, but also be able to distinguish between acute and chronic pain (Simon, Nolan, & Baumann, 1995). Typically, acute and chronic pain are differentiated according to onset, duration, and cause of pain. Acute pain is associated with recent, sudden onset, usually a result of disease, treatment or operative procedures, or trauma, and is limited in duration, typically subsiding as healing occurs. Conversely, chronic pain is caused by chronic pathological processes, may be caused by psychological or environmental factors, and is less easily differentiated, with less obvious defining characteristics. The intensity of chronic pain is more difficult to evaluate, suffering usually increases over time, pain duration continues for 3 months or longer, and the likelihood of complete relief is diminished (Bonica, 1990; McFarland & McFarlane, 1997).

The diagnoses associated with the phenomenon of pain are interrelated with many other diagnoses and often contribute to or are a result of other problems. Thus, the Pain Management intervention may be useful for alleviation of other diagnosed problems. The linkage work completed at the University of Iowa (McCloskey & Bulechek, 1996) identified Pain Management as a suggested intervention for eight NANDA nursing diagnoses (Body Image Disturbance; Acute Confusion; Energy Field Disturbance; Disorganized Infant Behavior; Potential for Enhanced Organized Infant Behavior; Risk for Disorganized Infant Behavior; Rape-Trauma Syndrome: Compound Reaction; Rape-Trauma Syndrome: Silent Reaction) and as an optional intervention for 25 NANDA nursing diagnoses (Activity Intolerance, Risk for Activity Intolerance, Ineffective Breathing Pattern, Decreased Cardiac Output, Constipation, Colonic Constipation, Risk for Disuse Syndrome, Diversional Activity Deficit, Impaired Gas Exchange, Knowledge Deficit, Altered Oral Mucous Membrane, Risk for Peripheral Neurovascular Dysfunction, Impaired Physical Mobility, Rape-Trauma Syndrome, Self Care Deficit: Dressing/Grooming, Self Care Deficit: Feeding, Self Care Deficit: Toileting, Sexual Dysfunction, Sleep Pattern Disturbance, Altered Thought Processes, Altered Tissue Perfusion: Cardiopulmonary, Altered Tissue Perfusion: Cerebral, Altered Tissue Perfusion: Peripheral, Altered Tissue Perfusion: Renal, Altered Urinary Elimination). This linkage work demonstrates the Pain Management intervention's ability to contribute to a large variety of nursing diagnoses yet should not exclude the possibility of Pain Management as an intervention option for other NANDA diagnoses not identified. The Pain Management intervention is written in a general manner and can be useful in identifying activities that can be suitable for any patient, with appropriate developmental alterations. The user of the NIC Pain Management intervention must use resources that provide specific content and guidance for implementation of many of the population-specific activities.

PATIENT OUTCOMES AFFECTED BY PAIN MANAGEMENT

A variety of patient outcomes could be identified to serve as measures of the effectiveness of the Pain Management intervention. The approach selected should serve as a mechanism for gathering initial baseline data, monitoring ongoing progress toward outcome attainment, and evaluating the effectiveness of the Pain Management intervention. The patient is an integral partner in the evaluation process and should be involved in establishing goals for pain relief early in the care relationship.

Documentation of changes in subjective and objective data gathered from repeat assessment should include parameters such as decrease in pain complaints, qualitative change in description of pain intensity, relaxation of skeletal muscles, elimination of pain posturing, decrease in verbalization (moaning, crying), widening of focus, increased participation in activities, and increased ability to rest, relax, or sleep. Standardized measures of pain, such as intensity measures (Dalton, 1995) and the impact of pain reflected in quality-of-life measures (Ferrell, Wisdom, & Wenzl, 1989), also provide evidence of treatment effectiveness. Patient satisfaction also has been used to measure outcomes of Pain Management; however, patients tend to report satisfaction even with high levels of pain (Miaskowski et al., 1994; Ward & Gordon, 1994). Outcome questionnaires have been developed that attempt to sort through the complicating factors (e.g., satisfaction with nursing care, satisfaction with caring attitudes of staff, interference in activities caused by pain) to determine actual response to pain management programs (American Pain Society Quality of Care Committee, 1995; Ferrell, Whedon, & Rollins, 1995).

In an effort to standardize the language used in documenting patient outcomes, nursing-sensitive patient outcomes have been developed as the Nursing Outcomes Classification (NOC) (Maas & Johnson, 1997). Four outcomes clearly reflect the variables in the patient situation that the intervention of Pain Management addresses; they are Pain Level, Pain Control Behavior, Pain: Disruptive Effects, and Comfort Level. These outcomes incorporate many of the defining characteristics used to identify pain as a problem in the NANDA diagnoses of Pain and Chronic Pain, as well as other indicators noted in clinical practice related to pain.

The outcome Pain Level is especially useful to evaluate the effect of interventions for acute pain. Most of the defining characteristics identified by NANDA are incorporated into the indicators of the outcome, and additional defining characteristics such as percentage of body affected, frequency of pain, and length of pain episodes provide data to support a change in the pain state.

The outcomes Pain Control Behavior and Pain: Disruptive Effects are particularly important in evaluating intervention effectiveness for those with chronic pain. Because of the long-term management required for chronic pain, factors related to compliance and interruption of life activities need to be addressed. These two outcomes identify indicators that promote a more comprehensive evaluation of the effect of intervention for chronic pain problems to add to the Pain Level outcome.

Additionally, overall feelings of psychological and physical comfort that are often affected by pain are addressed in the outcome Comfort Level. These four outcome measures provide a consistent approach for documenting response to the Pain Management intervention. However, empirical testing of these NOC scales is needed to support their reliability and validity as measures of patient outcome in clinical practice with different patient populations.

The timing and use of several evaluative criteria to judge the success or failure of interventions for pain is important. For acute pain, the evaluation may occur very quickly (e.g., in 10 to 30 minutes). For chronic pain problems, outcome measurement at admission, discharge, and 1 month, 3 months, and 6 months post discharge is common practice.

CASE STUDY

Mrs. T is an 82-year-old woman living at home who was visited by the home health nurse following a request by Mrs. T's daughter. Mrs. T was diagnosed with degenerative joint disease 20 years ago and underwent a right knee replacement 5 years ago. On arrival, Mrs. T was observed lying in her bed quietly, her brow wrinkled and her eyes clenched tightly. The nurse sat by Mrs. T, gently touched her arm, and asked her to describe what was the matter. Mrs. T indicated she had pain in her left knee so bad that she couldn't walk. She described a nagging, aching discomfort that got worse when she was up and walking and didn't let up until she was resting for several hours. When asked to rate the pain severity on a scale from 0 to 10, with 0 being no pain and 10 being the most severe pain imaginable, Mrs. T rated her current pain an 8 and stated that it was usually a 6. She stated she had given up her twice-weekly bridge game and her weekly church social event and no longer went to the store down the street for her groceries. She stated she missed seeing her friends and didn't have much enjoyment in her life anymore. She has difficulty falling asleep at night because of the pain. The nurse asked Mrs. T what she had done in the past to help relieve the pain. Mrs. T indicated she had a prescription for Nalfon, a nonsteroidal anti-inflammatory drug (NSAID), but that she didn't take it because she had heard it could cause kidney failure. The nurse talked with Mrs. T and her daughter about keeping a pain diary

for a week to help identify activities or events that seemed to make the pain better or worse and to record how severe the pain was at different times throughout the week. In the meantime, the nurse encouraged Mrs. T to begin taking the prescribed analgesic around the clock and explained the purpose of the medication and what could be expected as far as side effects and pain relief. They planned an appointment in 1 month to evaluate laboratory work related to gastrointestinal bleeding and renal function. In addition, Mrs. T agreed to try using alternating hot- and cold-pack application to the left knee during painful episodes. Instructions regarding safety and convenience of application were provided. Mrs. T also agreed to try music therapy. She selected an audiotape of classical tunes and was given instructions on how and when to use the tape. The nurse contacted Mrs. T's primary care physician and the physical therapist who had been working with Mrs. T after her joint replacement to discuss her assessment and plan of action. They concurred with the intervention plan and also suggested referral to an arthritis support group in her locale. The nurse discussed with Mrs. T and her daughter the importance of monitoring her discomfort level and noting response to the different intervention strategies.

The nurse called Mrs. T the following day to evaluate the effectiveness of the plan of care. Mrs. T indicated she was taking the medication and had listened to the audiotape at bedtime but stated that the cold packs were uncomfortable so she didn't use them. She said she was able to fall asleep earlier than usual and felt a bit more rested. She rated her current pain a 4. The nurse encouraged Mrs. T to continue with the analgesic and music therapy and to use a warm blanket around the rest of her body while the cold packs were on. She explained in more detail the reason for using both hot and cold and their ability to reduce inflammation and muscle spasm. The nurse also encouraged Mrs. T to use the hot- and cold-pack applications 20 minutes before and immediately after increased activity periods. One week later, Mrs. T reported much improvement in her knee pain. She stated she was able to attend bridge club and was planning to go to next week's church social. She indicated that her pain was now a 3 on the average and was no longer interfering with her ability to engage in activities that required mobilization. She planned to continue with the interventions and report to her physician in 1 month for follow-up blood tests related to her NSAID therapy.

SUMMARY

Pain Management is a comprehensive intervention developed to address the primary NANDA diagnoses of Pain and Chronic Pain, but it can also serve to alleviate many other patient diagnoses. The intervention identifies activities to address key issues for successful pain relief. Assessment concerns and factors that contribute to the effectiveness of overall pain management, as well as specific activities that address selection and implementation protocols for pain management, are incorporated. The user of the Pain Management intervention must have a sound knowledge base in pain management, particularly as it relates to adaptations in assessment and intervention techniques appropriate for different age groups, as well as referral to other, more specific NIC interventions related to pain for the most effective outcomes. Ultimately, use of Pain Management will contribute to effective pain relief and enhanced quality of life for patients of all ages and settings.

References

Acute Pain Management Guideline Panel. (1992). *Acute pain management: Operative or medical procedures and trauma. Clinical practice guideline* (AHCPR Publication No. 92-0032). Rockville, MD: Agency for Health Care Policy and Research, Public Health Services, U.S. Department of Health and Human Services.

Ahles, T. A., Blanchard, E. B., and Ruckdeschel, J. C. (1983). The multidimensional nature of cancer-related pain. *Pain, 17,* 277–288.

Allcock, N. (1996). Factors affecting the assessment of postoperative pain—A literature review. *Journal of Advanced Nursing, 24,* 1144–1151.

American Pain Society. (1992). *Principles of analgesic use in the treatment of acute pain and cancer pain* (3rd ed.). Skokie, IL: Author.

American Pain Society Quality of Care Committee. (1995). Quality improvement guidelines for the treatment of acute pain and cancer pain. *JAMA, 274,* 1874–1880.

Ashburn, M. A. (1994). Interdisciplinary chronic pain management programs. *Journal of Pharmaceutical Care in Pain and Symptom Control, 2*(3), 7–24.

Baker, A., Bowring, L., Brignell, A., and Kafford, D. (1996). Chronic pain management in cognitively impaired patients: A preliminary research report. *Perspectives, 20*(2), 4–8.

Barr, R. G. (1994). Pain experience in children: Developmental and clinical characteristics. In P. D. Wall and R. Melzack (Eds.), *Textbook of pain* (3rd ed., pp. 739–765). Edinburgh: Churchill Livingstone.

Beales, J. G. (1983). Factors influencing the expectation of pain among patients in a children's burn unit. *Burns, 9,* 187–192.

Beck, A. T., Ward, C., Mendelson, M., Mock, J., and Erbaugh, J. (1961). An inventory for measuring depression. *Archives of General Psychiatry, 4,* 561–571.

Benoliel, J. (1995). Multiple meanings of pain and complexities of pain management. *Nursing Clinics of North America, 30,* 583–596.

Berde, C. B., Lehn, B. M., Yee, J. D., Sethna, N. F., and Russo, D. (1991). Patient-controlled analgesia in children and adolescents: A randomized, prospective comparison with intramuscular administration of morphine for postoperative analgesia. *Journal of Pediatrics, 118,* 460–466.

Beyer, J. E., McGrath, P. J., and Berde, C. B. (1990). Discordance between self-report and behavioral pain measures in children aged 3-7 years after surgery. *Journal of Pain and Symptom Management, 5,* 350–356.

Beyer, J. E., Villarruel, A. M., and Denyes, M. (1993). *The Ouchers: The new user's manual and technical report.* Denver: University of Colorado Health Sciences Center.

Bieri, D., Reeve, R. A., Champion, G. D., Addicoat, L., and Aiegler, J. B. (1990). The Faces Pain Scale for the self-assessment of the severity of pain experienced by children: Initial validation, and preliminary investigation for ratio scale properties. *Pain, 41,* 139–150.

Bonica, J. J. (1990). General considerations of chronic pain. In J. J. Bonica (Ed.), *The management of pain* (2nd ed., pp. 180–196). Philadelphia: Lea & Febiger.

Bradley, L. A. (1996). Cognitive-behavioral therapy for chronic pain. In R. J. Gatchel and D. C. Turk (Eds.), *Psychological approaches to pain management—A practitioner's handbook* (pp. 131–147). New York: The Guilford Press.

Chapman, C. R., and Syrjala, K. L. (1990). Measurement of pain. In J. J. Bonica (Ed.), *The management of pain* (2nd ed., pp. 580–594). Philadelphia: Lea & Febiger.

Choiniere, M., Melzack, R., Girard, N., Rondeau, J., and Paquin, M. J. (1990). Comparisons between patients' and nurses' assessment of pain and medication efficacy in severe burn injuries. *Pain, 40,* 143–152.

Clarke, E., French, B., Bilodeau, M., Capasso, V., Edwards, A., and Empliti, J. (1996). Pain management knowledge, attitudes and clinical practice: The impact of nurses' characteristics and education. *Journal of Pain and Symptom Management, 11*(1), 18–31.

Cleeland, C. (1984). The impact of pain on the patient with cancer. *Cancer, 54,* 2635–2641.

Cleeland, C. S., Gonin, R., Hatfield, A. K., Edmonson, J. H., Blum, R. H., Stewart, J. A., and Pandya, K. J. (1994). Pain and pain treatment in outpatients with metastatic cancer: The Eastern Cooperative Oncology Group's outpatient pain study. *New England Journal of Medicine, 330,* 592–596.

Dalton, J. (1989). Nurses' perceptions of their pain assessment skills, pain management practices, and attitudes toward pain. *Oncology Nursing Forum, 16,* 225–231.

Dalton, J. (1995). Outcomes that provide evidence of change in cancer pain management. *Nursing Clinics of North America, 30,* 683–695.

Dalton, J., Blau, W., Carlson, J., Mann, J., Bernard, S., Toomey, T., Pierce, S., and Germino, B. (1996). Changing the relationship among nurses' knowledge, self-reported behavior, and documented behavior in pain management: Does education make a difference? *Journal of Pain and Symptom Management, 12,* 308–319.

Daut, D. L., Cleeland, C. S., and Flanery, R. C. (1983). The development of the Wisconsin Brief Pain Questionnaire to assess pain in cancer and other diseases. *Pain, 17,* 197–210.

Devine, E. C., and Westlake, S. K. (1995). The effects of psychoeducational care provided to adults with cancer: Meta-analysis of 116 studies. *Oncology Nursing Forum, 22,* 1369–1379.

Duggleby, W., and Lander, J. (1992). Patient-controlled analgesia for older adults. *Clinical Nursing Research, 1*(1), 107–113.

Edgar, L., and Smith-Hanrahan, C. (1992). Nonpharmacologic pain management. In J. H. Watt-Watson and M. I. Donovan (Eds.), *Pain management: Nursing perspective* (pp. 162–202). St. Louis: Mosby-Year Book.

Elliott, B., Elliott, T., Murray, D., Braun, B., and Johnson, K. (1996). Patients and family members: The role of knowledge and attitudes in cancer pain. *Journal of Pain and Symptom Management, 12,* 209–220.

Faucett, J., Gordon, N., and Levine, J. (1994). Differences in post-operative pain severity among four ethnic groups. *Journal of Pain and Symptom Management, 9,* 383–389.

Fawzy, F. J., Fawzy, N. W., Arndt, L. A., and Pasnau, R. O. (1995). Critical review of psychosocial interventions in cancer care. *Archives of General Psychiatry, 52,* 100–113.

Ferrante, F. M., Orav, E. J., Rocco, A., and Gallo, J. (1988). A statistical model for pain in patient-controlled analgesia and conventional intramuscular opioid regimens. *Anesthesiology and Anesthesia, 67,* 457–461.

Ferrell, B., Whedon, M., and Rollins, B. (1995). Pain and quality assessment/improvement. *Journal of Nursing Care Quality, 9*(3), 69–85.

Ferrell, B. A. (1991). Principles of pain management in older people. *Comprehensive Therapy, 17,* 53.

Ferrell, B. A., and Ferrell, B. A. (1991). Pain management at home. *Clinics of Geriatric Medicine, 7,* 765–776.

Ferrell, B. A., and Ferrell, B. R. (1993). Pain assessment among cognitively impaired nursing home residents. *Journal of the American Geriatrics Society, 41,* 24–27.

Ferrell, B. A., Ferrell, B. R., and Rivera, L. (1995). Pain in cognitively impaired nursing home patients. *Journal of Pain and Symptom Management, 10,* 591–598.

Ferrell, B. R., Eberts, M., McCaffery, M., and Grant, M. (1991). Clinical decision-making and pain. *Cancer Nursing, 14,* 289–297.

Ferrell, B. R., Ferrell, B. A., Ahn, C., and Tran, K. (1994). Pain management for elderly patients with cancer at home. *Cancer, 74,* 2139–2146.

Ferrell, B. R., McCaffery, M., and Ropchan, R. (1992). Pain management as a clinical challenge for nursing administration. *Nursing Outlook, 40,* 263–268.

Ferrell, B. R., Taylor, E. J., Grant, M., Fowler, M., and Corbisiero, R. (1993). Pain management at home: Struggle, comfort and mission. *Cancer Nursing, 16,* 169–178.

Ferrell, B. R., Wisdom, C., Rhiner, M., and Alletto, J. (1991). Pain management as a quality of care outcome. *Journal of Nursing Quality Assurance, 5*(2), 50–58.

Ferrell, B. R., Wisdom, C., and Wenzl, C. (1989). Quality of life as an outcome variable in the management of cancer pain. *Cancer, 63,* 2321–2327.

Flor, H., and Turk, D. C. (1988). Chronic back pain and rheumatoid arthritis: Predicting pain and disability from cognitive variables. *Journal of Behavioral Medicine, 11,* 251–265.

Foley, K. (1985). Treatment of cancer pain. *New England Journal of Medicine, 113,* 84–95.

Fortin, F., and Kirouac, S. (1976). A randomized controlled trial of preoperative patient education. *International Journal of Nursing Studies, 13,* 11–24.

Geissler, E. (1994). *Pocket guide to cultural assessment* (pp. xiii–xv). St. Louis: Mosby.

Graceley, R. H., and Wolskee, P. J. (1983). Semantic functional measurement of pain: Integrating perception and language. *Pain, 15,* 389–398.

Grossman, S. A., Shiedler, V. R., Swedeen, K., Mucenski, J., and Piantadosi, S. (1991). Correlation of patient and caregiver ratings of cancer pain. *Journal of Pain and Symptom Management, 6,* 53–57.

Harkins, S. W., and Price, D. D. (1992). Assessment of pain in the elderly. In D. Turk & R. Melzack (Eds.), *Handbook of pain assessment* (pp. 315–331). New York: The Guilford Press.

Haythornthwaite, J., Seiber, W., and Kerns, R. (1991). Depression and the chronic pain experience. *Pain, 46,* 177–184.

Herr, K., and Mobily, P. (1991). Complexities of pain assessment in the elderly: Practical considerations. *Journal of Gerontological Nursing, 17*(4), 12–19.

Herr, K., and Mobily, P. (1992). Interventions related to pain. In G. M. Bulechek and J. C. McCloskey (Eds.), *Symposium on nursing interventions. Nursing Clinics of North America, 27,* 347–370.

Herr, K., and Mobily, P. (1993). Comparison of selected pain assessment tools for use with the elderly. *Applied Nursing Research, 6,* 39–46.

Herr, K., and Mobily, P. (1997). Chronic pain in the elderly. In E. A. Swanson and T. T. Reimer (Eds.), *Advances in gerontological nursing: Vol. 2. Chronic illness in the older adult* (pp. 82–111). New York: Springer Publishing.

Herr, K., Mobily, P., and Smith, C. (1993). Depression and the experience of chronic back pain: A study of related variables and age differences. *Clinical Journal of Pain, 9,* 104–114.

Hester, N. O. (1989). Comforting the child in pain. In S. G. Funk, E. M. Tornquist, M. T. Champagne, L. A. Copp, and L. A. Weise (Eds.), *Key aspects of comfort: Management of pain, fatigue, and nausea* (pp. 290–298). New York: Springer Publishing.

Hester, N. O., and Barcus, C. S. (1986). Assessment and management of pain in children. *Pediatrics: Nursing Update, 1,* 1–8.

Hester, N. O., Foster, R., and Kristensen, K. (1990). Measurement of pain in children: Generalizability and validity of the Pain Ladder and the Poker Chip Tool. In D. C. Tyler and E. J. Drane (Eds.), *Pediatric pain: Vol. 15. Advances in pain research and therapy* (pp. 79–84). New York: Raven Press.

Hileman, J. W., Lackey, N. R., and Hassanein, R. S. (1992). Identifying the needs of home caregivers of patients with cancer. *Oncology Nursing Forum, 1,* 8–17.

Hofland, S. L. (1992). Elder beliefs: Blocks to pain management. *Journal of Gerontological Nursing, 18*(6), 19–24, 39–40.

Hurley, A. C., Volicer, B. J., Hanrahan, P. A., Houde, S., and Volicer, L. (1992). Assessment of discomfort in advanced Alzheimer's patients. *Research in Nursing and Health Care, 15,* 369–377.

Jacox, A., Carr, D. B., Payne, R., et al. (1994). *Management of cancer pain. Clinical practice guideline no. 9* (AHCPR Publication No. 94-0592). Rockville, MD: Agency for Health Care Policy and Research, U.S. Department of Health and Human Services, Public Health Services.

Jacox, A., Ferrell, B., Heidrich, G., Hester, N., and Miaskowski, C. (1992). A guideline for the nation: Managing acute pain. *American Journal of Nursing, 92*(5), 49–55.

Jadlos, M. A., Kelman, G. B., Marra, K., and Lanoue, A. (1996). Documentation. A pain management documentation tool. *Oncology Nursing Forum, 23,* 1451–1454.

Jay, L., and Miller, T. (1990). Chronic pain and the geriatric patient. In T. Miller (Ed.), *Chronic pain* (Vol. 2, pp. 821–838). Madison, WI: International Universities Press.

Jensen, M., and Karoly, P. (1992). Self-report scales and procedures for assessing pain in adults. In D. Turk and R. Melzack (Eds.), *Handbook of pain assessment* (pp. 295–314). New York: Guilford Press.

Jensen, M. P., Turner, J. A., and Romano, J. M. (1994). Correlates of improvement in multidisciplinary treatment of chronic pain. *Journal of Consulting and Clinical Psychology, 62,* 172–179.

Johnson, M. R. (1990). Pain response in preterm infants. *Infant Behavioral Development, 67,* A440.

Juarez, G., and Ferrell, B. R. (1996). Family and caregiver involvement in pain management. *Clinics in Geriatric Medicine, 12,* 531–547.

Juarez, G. (1997). Culture and pain. *Quality of Life—A Nursing Challenge, 4*(4), 86–90.

Karoly, P. (1991). Assessment of pediatric pain. In J. P. Bush and S. W. Harkins (Eds.), *Children in pain: Clinical and research issues from a developmental perspective* (pp. 59–82). New York: Springer-Verlag.

Keefe, F. J., Caldwell, D. S., Williams, D. A., Gil, K. M., Mitchell, D., Robertson, C., Martinez, S., Nunley, J., Beckham, J., Crisson, J. E., and Helms, M. (1990). Pain coping skills training in the management of osteoarthritic knee pain: A comparative study. *Behavior Therapy, 21,* 49–62.

Kerns, R., Turk, D., and Rudy, T. (1985). The West Haven-Yale Multidimensional Pain Inventory (WHYMPI). *Pain, 23,* 345–356.

Krechel, S. W., and Bildner, J. (1995). CRIES: A new neonatal post-operative pain measurement score. Initial testing of validity and reliability. *Pediatric Anesthesia, 5,* 53–61.

Kremer, E., Atkinson, J. H., and Ignelzi, R. J. (1981). Measurement of pain: Patient preference does not confound pain measurement. *Pain, 10,* 241–248.

Lander, J. (1990). Clinical judgments in pain management. *Pain, 42,* 15–22.

Maas, M., and Johnson, M. (Eds.) (1997). *Nursing outcomes classification (NOC).* St. Louis: Mosby-Year Book.

Magrum, L. C., Bentzen, C., and Landmark, S. (1996). Pain management in home care. *Seminars in Oncology Nursing, 12*(3), 202–218.

Mahon, S. (1994). Concept analysis of pain: Implications related to nursing diagnoses. *Nursing Diagnosis, 5*(1), 14–25.

Martin, B. A., and Belcher, J. V. (1986). Influence of cultural background on nurses' attitudes and care of the oncology patient. *Cancer Nursing, 9*(5), 230–237.

Marzinski, L. R. (1991). The tragedy of dementia: Clinically assessing pain in the confused, nonverbal elderly. *Journal of Gerontological Nursing, 17*(6), 25–28.

McCaffery, M., and Beebe, A. (1989). *Pain: Clinical manual for nursing practice.* St. Louis: C. V. Mosby.

McCaffery, M., and Ferrell, B. (1992). Opioid analgesics: Nurses' knowledge of doses and psychological dependence. *Journal of Nursing Staff Development, 8*(2), 77–84.

McCaffery, M., and Ferrell, B. R. (1991). Assessment of pain intensity and choice of analgesic dose. *Nursing, 21,* 24–27.

McCaffery, M., and Ferrell, B. R. (1996). Correcting misconceptions about pain management and use of opioid analgesics: Educational strategies aimed at public concerns. *Nursing Outlook, 44*(4), 184–190.

McCaffery, M., Ferrell, B., O'Neil-Page, E., Lester, M., and Ferrell, B. (1990). Nurses' knowledge of opioid analgesic drugs and psychological dependence. *Cancer Nursing, 13,* 21–27.

McCloskey, J. C., and Bulecheck, G. M. (Eds.). (1996). *Nursing interventions classification (NIC)* (2nd ed.). St. Louis: Mosby-Year Book.

McFarland, G. K., and McFarlane, E. A. (1997). *Nursing diagnosis and intervention* (3rd ed.). St. Louis: Mosby-Year Book.

McGrath, P. (1990). *Pain in children. Nature, assessment and treatment.* New York: Guilford Press.

McGrath, P., and Brigham, M. (1992). The assessment of pain in children and adolescents. In D. Turk and R. Melzack (Eds.), *Handbook of pain assessment* (pp. 295–314). New York: Guilford Press.

McGrath, P., Seifert, C., Speechley, K., Booth, J., Stitt, L., and Gibson, M. (1996). A new analogue scale for assessing children's pain: An initial validation study. *Pain, 64,* 435–443.

McGrath, P., and Unruh, A. M. (1987). *Pain in children and adolescents.* New York: Elsevier Science Publishers.

McGrath, P. A. (1993). Psychological aspects of pain perception. In N. L. Schecter, C. B. Berde, and M. Yaster (Eds.), *Pain in infants, children, and adolescents* (pp. 39–63). Baltimore: Williams & Wilkins.

McGrath, P. J., Johnson, G., Goodman, J. T., Schillinger, J., Dunn, J., and Chapman, J. (1985). The CHEOPS: A behavioral scale to measure post-operative pain in children. In H. L. Fields, R. Dubner, and F. Cervero (Eds.), *Advances in pain research and therapy* (pp. 395–402). New York: Raven Press.

Melzack, R., and Wall, P. D. (1965). Pain mechanisms: A new theory. *Science, 150,* 971–979.

Miaskowski, C., Nichols, R., Brody, R., and Synold, T. (1994). Assessment of patient satisfaction utilizing the American Pain Society's quality assurance standards on acute and cancer-related pain. *Journal of Pain and Symptom Management, 9,* 5–11.

Miller, B., Bruno, S., and Kinzbrunner, B. (1996). Team approach to pain management. In E. Salerno and J. Willens (Eds.), *Pain management handbook—An interdisciplinary approach* (pp. 179–200). St. Louis: Mosby-Year Book.

Mobily, P. (1994). Nonpharmacologic interventions for the management of chronic pain in older women. *Journal of Women and Aging, 6*(4), 89–109.

Mobily, P., and Herr, K. (in press). Pain. In Maas, M., Buckwalter, K., Hardy, M., Tripp-Reimer, T., and Titler, M. *Nursing diagnoses and interventions for the elderly.* Thousand Oaks, CA: Sage Publications.

Mobily, P., Herr, K., Clark, M. K., and Wallace, R. (1994). An epidemiologic analysis of pain in the elderly. *Journal of Aging and Health, 6*(2), 139–154.

Mogan, J., Wells, N., and Robertson, E. (1986). Effects of pre-operative teaching on post-operative pain: A replication and expansion. *Pain, 26*(1), 124.

Morgan, A. E., Lindley, C. M., and Berry, J. I. (1994). Assessment of pain and patterns of analgesic use in hospice patients. *American Journal of Hospice and Palliative Care, 11*(1), 13–19.

Murphy, D., McDonald, A., Power, A., Unwin, A., and MacSullivan, R. (1988). Measurement of pain: A comparison of the visual analogue with a nonvisual analogue scale. *Clinical Journal of Pain, 3,* 197–219.

National Institutes of Health. (1986). The integrated approach to the management of pain. *National Institutes of Health Consensus Development Conference Statement, 6*(3).

O'Brien, S., Dalton, J., Konsler, G., and Carlson, J. (1996). The knowledge and attitudes of experienced oncology nurses regarding the management of cancer-related pain. *Oncology Nursing Forum, 23,* 515–520.

Owens, M. K., and Ehrenreich, D. (1991). Literature review of nonpharmacologic methods for the treatment of chronic pain. *Holistic Nursing Practice, 6*(1), 24–31.

Pachter, L. M. (1994). Culture and clinical care—Folk illness beliefs and behaviors and their implications for health care delivery. *Journal of the American Medical Association, 271,* 690–694.

Paice, J., Mahon, S., and Faut-Callahan, M. (1991). Factors associated with adequate pain control in hospitalized postsurgical patients diagnosed with cancer. *Cancer Nursing, 14,* 298–305.

Paice, J. A., and Cohen, F. L. (1997). Validity of a verbally administered numeric rating scale to measure cancer pain intensity. *Cancer Nursing, 20*(2), 88–93.

Parmalee, P. A., Katz, I. R., and Lawton, M. P. (1993). Pain complaints and cognitive status among elderly institution residents. *Journal of the American Geriatrics Society, 41,* 395–465.

Peterson, L., and Shigetomi, C. (1981). The use of coping techniques to minimize anxiety in hospitalized children. *Behavior Therapy, 12,* 1–14.

Radloff, L. (1977). The CES-D Scale: A self-report depression scale for research in the general population. *Applied Psychological Measurement, 1,* 385–401.

Reading, A. E. (1982). The effects of psychological preparation on pain and recovery after minor gynecological surgery: A preliminary report. *Journal of Clinical Psychology, 38,* 504–512.

Rimer, B., Levy, M. H., Keintz, M. K., Fox, L., Engstrom, P., and MacElwee, N. (1987). Enhancing cancer pain control regimens through patient education. *Patient Educational Counseling, 10,* 267–277.

Roth-Roemer, S., Abrams, J., and Syrjala, K. (1996). Nonpharmacologic approaches to adult cancer pain management. *APS Bulletin, 6*(5), 1–4, 9.

Routh, D. K., and Sanfilippo, M. D. (1991). Helping children cope with painful medical procedures. In J. P. Bush and S. W. Harkins (Eds.), *Children in pain: Clinical and research issues from a developmental perspective* (pp. 397–424). New York: Springer-Verlag.

Sackett, D. L., and Haynes, R. B. (1976). *Compliance with therapeutic regimens.* Baltimore: Johns Hopkins University Press.

Schechter, N. L., Berde, C. B., and Yaster, M. (Eds.). (1993). *Pain in infants, children, and adolescents.* Baltimore: Williams & Wilkins.

Schmidt, K., Eland, J., and Weiler, K. (1994). Pediatric cancer pain management: A survey of nurses' knowledge. *Journal of Pediatric Oncology Nursing, 11,* 4–12.

Scott, J., and Huskisson, E. C. (1976). Graphic representation of pain. *Pain, 2,* 175–184.

Sheidler, V. R., McGuire, D. B., Grossman, S. A., and Gilbert, M. R. (1992). Analgesic decision-making skills of nurses. *Oncology Nursing Forum, 19,* 1531–1534.

Short, L. M., Burnett, M. S., Egbert, A. M., and Parks, L. H. (1990). Medicating the postoperative elderly: How do nurses make their decisions? *Journal of Gerontological Nursing, 16*(7), 12–17.

Siegel, L. J., and Peterson, L. (1981). Maintenance effects of coping skills and sensory information on young children's response to repeated dental procedures. *Behavior Therapy, 12,* 530–535.

Simon, J. (1996). Chronic pain syndrome: Nursing assessment and intervention. *Rehabilitation Nursing, 21*(1), 13–19.

Simon, J., and McTier, C. L. (1996). Development of a chronic pain assessment tool. *Rehabilitation Nursing, 21*(1), 20–24.

Simon, J. M., Nolan, L., and Baumann, M. A. (1995). Validation of the nursing diagnoses acute pain and chronic pain. *Nursing Diagnosis, 6*(2), 199–203.

Sloman, R. (1995). Relaxation and the relief of cancer pain. *Nursing Clinics of North America, 30,* 697–709.

Speigel, D., and Bloom, J. R. (1983). Group therapy and hypnosis reduce metastatic breast carcinoma pain. *Psychosomatic Medicine, 45,* 333–339.

Sriwatanakul, K., Kelvie, W., and Lasagna, L. (1982). The quantification of pain: An analysis of words used to describe pain and analgesia in clinical trials. *Clinical Pharmacology and Therapeutics, 32*(2), 143–148.

Syrjala, K. L., Cummings, C., and Donaldson, G. (1992). Hypnosis or cognitive-behavioral training for the reduction of pain and nausea during cancer treatment: A controlled clinical trial. *Pain, 48,* 137–146.

Syrjala, K. L., Donaldson, G. W., Davis, M. W., Kippes, M. E., and Carr, J. E. (1995). Relaxation and imagery and cognitive-behavioral training reduce pain during cancer treatment: A controlled clinical trial. *Pain, 63,* 189–198.

Tait, R. C. (1993). Management of pain in the elderly. In P. A. Szwabo and G. T. Grossberg (Eds.), *Problem behaviors in long-term care: Recognition, diagnosis, & treatment.* New York: Springer Publishing.

Tait, R. C., Chibnall, J., and Krause, S. (1990). The Pain Disability Index: Psychometric properties. *Pain, 40,* 171–182.

Taylor, E. J., Ferrell, B. R., Grant, M., and Cheynoy, L. (1993). Managing cancer pain at home: The decisions and ethical conflicts of patients, family caregivers and homecare nurses. *Oncology Nursing Forum, 20,* 919–927.

Taylor, H., and Curran, N. M. (1985). *The Nuprin pain report* (No. 851017). New York: Louis Harris and Associates.

Tittle, M., and McMillan, S. (1994). Pain and pain-related side effects in an ICU and on a surgical unit: Nurses' management. *American Journal of Critical Care, 3,* 25–30.

Tota-Faucette, M. E., Gil, K. M., Williams, F. J., and Goli, V. (1993). Predictors of response to pain management treatment: The role of family environment and changes in cognitive processes. *Clinical Journal of Pain, 9,* 115–123.

Turk, D. C., and Rudy, T. E. (1988). Toward an empirically derived taxonomy of chronic pain patients: Integration of psychological assessment data. *Journal of Clinical and Consulting Psychology, 56,* 233–238.

Twycross, R. G., and Lack, S. A. (1983). *Symptom control in far advanced cancer: Pain relief.* London: D Pittman.

Vortherms, R., Ryan, P., and Ward, S. (1992). Knowledge of, attitudes toward, and barriers to pharmacologic management of cancer pain in a statewide random sample of nurses. *Research in Nursing and Health, 15,* 459–466.

Walker, J. M., Akinsanya, J. A., David, B. D., and Marcer, D. M. (1990). The management of elderly patients with pain in the community: Study and recommendations. *Journal of Advanced Nursing, 15,* 1154–1161.

Wall, P. D. (1988). The prevention of postoperative pain. *Pain, 33,* 289–290.

Ward, S., Goldberg, N., Miller-McCauley, V., Mueller, C., Nolan, A., Pawlik-Plank, D., Robbins, A., Stormoen, D., and Weissman, D. E. (1993). Patient-related barriers to management of cancer pain. *Pain, 52,* 319–324.

Ward, S., and Gordon, D. (1994). Application of the American Pain Society quality assurance standards. *Pain, 56,* 299–306.

Ward, S. E., Berry, P. E., and Misiewicz, H. (1996). Concerns about analgesics among patients and family caregivers in a hospice setting. *Research in Nursing and Health, 19*(3), 205–211.

Watt-Watson, J. (1992). Misbeliefs about pain. In J. Watt-Watson and M. Donovan (Eds.), *Pain management—Nursing perspective* (pp. 36–58). St. Louis: Mosby-Year Book.

Watt-Watson, J., and Donovan, M. (Eds.). (1992). *Pain management—Nursing perspective.* St. Louis: Mosby-Year Book.

Watt-Watson, J. H., Evernden, C., and Lawson, C. (1990). Parents' perceptions of their child's acute pain experience. *Journal of Pediatric Nursing, 5,* 344–349.

White, P. F. (1989). Patient-controlled analgesia: An update on its use in the treatment of postoperative pain. *Anesthesiology Clinics of North America, 7,* 63–78.

World Health Organization Expert Committee. (1990). *Cancer pain relief and palliative care.* Geneva, Switzerland: World Health Organization.

Yesavage, J., Brink, T., Rose, T., Lum, O., Huang, V., Adey, M., and Leirer, V. (1983). Development and validation of a geriatric screening scale: A preliminary report. *Journal of Psychiatric Research, 17,* 37–49.

Zalon, M. (1995). Pain management instruction in nursing curricula. *Journal of Nursing Education, 34*(6), 262–267.

Zimmerman, L., Nieveen, J., Barnason, S., and Schmaderer, M. (1996). The effects of music interventions on postoperative pain and sleep in coronary artery bypass graft (CABG) patients. *Scholarly Inquiry for Nursing Practice, 10*(2), 153–174.

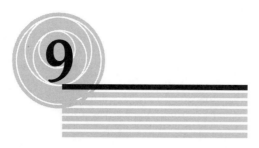

Therapeutic Touch

Therese Connell Meehan

Some of the earliest symbolism in nursing history reflects the importance of nurses' use of their hands as a mediating focus for their therapeutic intent (Connell, 1983). In 1956, Mead observed that nurses' compassionate use of their hands is one of the unique functions of nursing in modern society. The development and use of Therapeutic Touch as a nursing intervention is one way in which nurses have sought to become more consciously aware of how they use their hands to facilitate patient comfort and healing.

Therapeutic Touch was developed by Kunz and Krieger in the early 1970s following Kunz's systematic observation of the practice of laying-on of hands. Kunz was impressed with practitioners' gentleness, their focused intent to help, the specially developed sensitivity of their hands, and the fact that ill patients were frequently helped to feel more relaxed, comfortable, and energetic. Although she recognized that the laying-on of hands was done within a religious context, she proposed that it would be possible to develop a similar practice within the context of a broad philosophical framework that would be understandable and acceptable to a wide range of people and health care organizations. She also proposed that the ability to facilitate healing in another person was a natural human potential and could be learned by those who were sincerely interested, healthy, compassionate, and dedicated to helping others. With the assistance of Krieger, she developed the new practice, which Krieger named Therapeutic Touch.

Kunz chose to teach the new practice primarily to nurses because she believed that they had the professional dedication necessary to learn to use it most effectively and spent the most time with ill people. Krieger observed that nurses' use of Therapeutic Touch appeared to be effective in helping ill patients and introduced it to the profession at large as a nursing intervention in 1975. Since that time, many nurses have learned Therapeutic Touch and used it to help promote relaxation, comfort, and healing in their patients. It received formal recognition as a nursing intervention from the Iowa Intervention Project in the Nursing Interventions Classification (NIC) (McCloskey & Bulechek, 1996). A considerable body of Therapeutic Touch literature is now available and includes discussion of its theoretical rationale, practice reports, research findings, critical commentary, and its definition as a nursing intervention.

RELATED LITERATURE

Theoretical Rationale

Two similar frameworks are used to describe and explain Therapeutic Touch. A general energy field framework proposed by Weber (1981, 1990) is rooted in philosophical propositions common in many cultures. It posits that aside from the physical matter, separateness, and multiplicity of causal and local events so predominantly evident in ordinary experience, there exists a fundamental, unitary, universal flow of energy within which all matter, consciousness, and events are grounded and interconnected. Over the past 50 years, the concept of a fundamental, universal energy has become linked to and developed within field theory. Support for the view that energy fields are the basic organizing forces of the universe and that quanta, the solidlike particles of matter, are momentary manifestations of interacting fields is provided by the relativistic quantum field theories of modern physics (Bohm, 1973, 1986; Cushing & McMullin, 1989; Josephson & Pallikari-Viras, 1991; Stapp, 1993). Studies of plants, animals, and humans have suggested that energy fields are of fundamental significance in establishing and maintaining pattern and organization in living systems (Burr, 1972).

It is proposed that from within this universal energy flows a life-giving, healing energy that is present in all living systems and is composed of intelligence, order, and compassion (Weber, 1981, 1990). In a state of health, the healing energy flows with freedom and abundance, whereas in a state of illness, the flow has become blocked and depleted. Conscious awareness of this healing energy and the ability to facilitate its flow within oneself arises through the spiritual dimension of human experience and is considered a natural human potential. Human beings also have the potential to facilitate this flow of healing energy in others, given a relative state of health, the ability to center themselves, and a nonattached intent to help and facilitate healing in others (Kunz, 1985).

A nursing theoretical framework, the Science of Unitary Human Beings (Rogers, 1970, 1990), also provides a theoretical rationale for Therapeutic Touch (Biley, 1996; Malinski, 1993; Meehan, 1990a; Miller, 1979; Samarel, 1997). It posits that energy fields are the basic organizing forces of the human being and environment. Thus, human beings and the environment are viewed as unitary phenomena integral with one another in a continuous process of energy field patterning and innovative change. The nurse providing an intervention for a patient is viewed as an energy field pattern integral with the patient's environmental field patterning, and the patient is viewed as an energy field pattern integral with the nurse's environmental field patterning. In Rogers's view, Therapeutic Touch is one example by which "professional practice in nursing seeks to strengthen the coherence and integrity of human and environmental fields and to knowingly participate in the patterning of human and environmental fields for the realization of optimum well-being" (M. E. Rogers, personal communication, June 1988).

Practice Literature

Since the late 1970s, nurses' use of Therapeutic Touch has been documented in a growing body of literature. Books by Krieger (1979), Macrae (1988), and Sayre-Adams (1995) describe the intervention in detail. The integration of Therapeutic Touch into nursing practice has been described by Boguslawski (1979), Egan (1992), Fanslow (1983), Feltham (1991), the Hospital Satellite Network (1986), Jurgens, Meehan, and Wilson (1987), Keller (1984), Lionberger (1986), Mackey (1995), Meehan (1990b), Mulloney & Wells-Federman (1996), the National League for Nursing (1992), and Wyatt (1989). The most frequently reported effect of Therapeutic Touch is a generalized relaxation response, which has led to the belief that it can be effective in helping to relieve a wide variety of symptoms (Borelli & Heidt, 1981; Krieger, 1979). Its use to reduce pain has been described by Biley (1996), Boguslawski (1980), Meehan (1990b), Peric-Knowlton (1984), and Wright (1987). In addition, it has been reported to be effective in relieving anxiety (Olson & Sneed, 1995); promoting rest (Heidt, 1991) and sleep (Braun, Layton, & Braun, 1986; Dall, 1993); calming hospitalized infants (Leduc, 1987), patients undergoing anesthesia and surgery (Jonasen, 1981, 1994; Ledwith, 1995), clinic patients (Wytias, 1994), the elderly (Fanslow, 1990; Simington, 1993), and women in childbirth (Lothian, 1988, 1993; Wolfson, 1990); providing support and comfort for hospitalized children (Finnerin, 1981; Macrae, 1979; Thayer, 1990), patients receiving psychotherapy (Hill & Oliver, 1993), patients with acquired immunodeficiency syndrome (AIDS) (Newshan, 1989), and patients who are dying (Fanslow, 1983; Jackson, 1981); and facilitating physical rehabilitation (Payne, 1989) and drug rehabilitation (Macrae, 1989).

Nurses also report integrating the concepts of centering and focused intent, which underlie their practice of Therapeutic Touch, into a wide range of other nursing activities. Centering refers to a simple form of meditation in which the nurse shifts his or her awareness from a direct focus on the physical environment to an inner focus on what he or she perceives as the center of life within himself or herself—a center of peace and order through which the nurse perceives himself or herself and the patient as unitary wholes. From this centered perspective, the nurse's attitude becomes one of clear, gentle, and compassionate attention to the patient and, ideally, is detached from personal feelings or emotions. The nurse's intent, or intentionality, to help and facilitate healing in the patient is focused from this centered perspective of nonattached compassion. From this perspective, nursing activities such as giving a back rub or doing a patient assessment are conducted in a calm and receptive manner that allows the nurse to observe the patient's condition intuitively as well as objectively. The introduction of these concepts into nurses' practice at a major medical center, through an inservice education program, has been shown to contribute to a significant decrease in work-related stress and emotional exhaustion and an increase in personality hardiness and self-actualization (Meehan, Mahoney, et al., 1990).

Many nurses who have integrated Therapeutic Touch into their practice report that it has changed their professional lives (Kunz & Krieger, 1975–1997; Quinn, 1979; Simeone, 1985; Woods-Smith, 1988). Generally, they report that they feel more enthusiastic, confident, and satisfied in their work; that their work has become more meaningful to them; and that aside from the frequent stresses of day-to-day practice, they have a greater sense of well-being. Simeone (1985) writes that "the little tasks of nursing seem less tedious and I feel strongly that my relationships with patients have grown more beneficial to both them and me. . . . I still get flustered and frustrated by things that happen on our floor, but I now have a tool to help me revitalize and see things more clearly" (p. 618). These changes are probably brought about through learning the centering meditation, which is basic to the practice of Therapeutic Touch. Learning this relatively simple form of meditation appears to promote a process of self-healing in the nurse. During the practice of Therapeutic Touch, this meditative perspective brings about an attitude of nonattached compassion and enables the nurse to perceive the inherent beauty of the patient as a unitary whole, aside from whatever the ordinary circumstances of the interaction might be. Such experiences and the development of an underlying meditative perspective alter the nurse's view of nursing practice and the role it plays in his or her life.

Research Findings

Research on Therapeutic Touch was initiated by Krieger and has continued to develop, despite a wide range of methodological problems confronted by investigators. Qualitative designs have been used to try to clarify the nature of the intervention and how it is experienced by patients and nurses. Quantitative designs have been used to test its effectiveness in facilitating health-related outcomes, but difficulties have arisen in attempting to differentiate between the effects of Therapeutic Touch and the placebo effect. Most studies reported after 1983 included a control group that received a mimic Therapeutic Touch intervention, developed and validated by Quinn (1982), as a single-blind placebo control. Full control for the placebo effect through a double-blind design is not possible because the placebo effect that arises from implicit and explicit expectation and suggestion by the nurse administering the intervention cannot be eliminated. Some studies include a control group that received another touch intervention or a standard intervention of known effectiveness, and some also include a nonintervention group.

Originally, Krieger (1975) derived a theory from Eastern philosophy that led her to investigate the effect of Therapeutic Touch on hemoglobin values in ill patients. Although the study findings appeared to suggest that Therapeutic Touch could have the potential to increase hemoglobin values, methodological problems precluded scientific support for this outcome. In subsequent studies, no significant relationship has been found between Therapeutic Touch and increased hemoglobin values (Meehan, Mersmann, Wiseman, Wolff, & Malgady, 1991) or transcutaneous oxygen blood gas pressure (Fedoruk, 1984).

Observations by Krieger, Peper, and Ancoli (1979) suggested that Therapeutic Touch could have the potential to promote a relaxation response. Heidt (1981) and Quinn (1984) found that hospitalized cardiovascular patients who received Therapeutic Touch had a significant decrease in anxiety immediately following the intervention. Turner, Clark, Gauthier, and Williams (1998) found that patients hospitalized for burn injuries who received Therapeutic Touch over a 5-day period experienced significantly less anxiety on the sixth hospital day. Simington and Laing (1993) found that elderly institutionalized patients who received Therapeutic Touch incorporated into a back rub procedure also experienced a significant decrease in anxiety. Gagne and Toye (1994) found that hospitalized psychiatric patients who received Therapeutic Touch experienced a very significant decrease in anxiety. However, in other studies using hospitalized patients as subjects (Hale, 1986; Quinn, 1989; Parkes, 1985), no decrease in anxiety was found. In a study of preoperative patients, Meehan et al. (1991) found approximately the same mean decrease in anxiety in the Therapeutic Touch group as was found in the Heidt (1981) and Quinn (1984) studies, but this decrease was not significantly greater than that in the mimic control group. In the same study, patients who received Therapeutic Touch morning and evening over a 3-day postoperative period had no significant decrease in anxiety or fatigue and no significant increase in vigor over the intervention period.

Findings of exploratory studies suggest that Therapeutic Touch may have the potential to reduce stress (Olson, Sneed, Bonadonna, Ratliff, & Dias, 1992) and adverse immunological effects of stress (Olson et al., 1997) and facilitate health-related changes in the immune system (Quinn & Strelkauskas, 1989). Fedoruk (1984) found that treatment by Therapeutic Touch was significantly associated with reduction in a behavioral indicator of stress in hospitalized premature infants. Kramer (1990) reported that Therapeutic Touch significantly reduced stress in hospitalized children. However, Randolph (1984) found that healthy females who received Therapeutic Touch while being subjected to artificially induced stress had no significant decrease in physiological indicators of stress. Snyder, Egan, and Burns (1995) tested the effects of Therapeutic Touch on relaxation and stress-related agitation behaviors in patients suffering from Alzheimer's disease. Therapeutic Touch was found to be as effective as hand massage in increasing relaxation, but no decrease was found in agitation behavior. Mersmann (1993) linked the potential of Therapeutic Touch to increase relaxation and decrease stress to milk letdown in nonnursing mothers of premature infants. Mothers experienced significantly more leaking of milk while receiving Therapeutic Touch and expressed significantly more milk following the intervention.

These findings are confounded by some methodological limitations. For example, the Kramer (1990) study contained serious methodological flaws. Parkes's (1985) elderly subjects had difficulty completing the anxiety questionnaire; the Hale (1986), Olson et al. (1992, 1997), and Quinn and Strelkauskas (1989) sample sizes were small; the Quinn (1984) and Turner et al. (1998) studies did not include a standard control group to control for the ordinary presence of a nurse; Quinn's (1989) findings were confounded by effects of tranquillizing medications; Fedoruk (1984) reported variability in lengths of intervention times; Randolph (1984) and Snyder et al. (1995) used a significantly modified Therapeutic Touch procedure; and in the Heidt (1981), Hale (1986), Quinn (1989), and Snyder et al. (1995) studies, the investigators administered the interventions. In the Meehan et al. (1991) study, postoperative measurements were taken several hours after the intervention in an attempt to detect generalized effects. Constructive replication and extension of these studies is needed. To date, scientific support for the view that Therapeutic Touch decreases anxiety beyond a placebo effect and decreases stress is somewhat equivocal.

The proposition that Therapeutic Touch can decrease pain has also been tested. Keller and Bzdek (1986) found that Therapeutic Touch significantly reduced tension headache pain in otherwise healthy subjects immediately after the intervention and 4 hours later. Meehan (1993) found that Therapeutic Touch did not significantly reduce postoperative pain but that patients waited significantly longer before requesting more analgesic medication. Meehan, Mersmann, Wiseman, Wolff, and Malgady (1990) found that postoperative patients who received Therapeutic Touch in conjunction with a narcotic analgesic as needed (prn) had no significant decrease in pain over the first 3 hours after the intervention but that, again, patients waited significantly longer before requesting further analgesic medication. Turner et al. (1998) found that patients hospitalized for burn injuries who received Therapeutic Touch over a 5-day period reported significantly less pain according to the sensory and affective subscales of the McGill Pain Questionnaire but not the evaluative subscale. Mueller Hinze (1988) found that Therapeutic Touch had no significant effect on experimentally induced pain. Peck (1997) found that Therapeutic Touch treatments given weekly over a 6-week period significantly reduced pain and distress in elderly patients with degenerative arthritis, compared with routine treatment. Compared with a progressive muscle relaxation intervention, Therapeutic Touch was as effective in reducing pain but significantly less effective in reducing distress.

Again, methodological limitations confound interpretation of some findings. Measurement of effects in the Meehan (1993) study was complicated by the fact that some patients required analgesic medication before the 1-hour postintervention time was completed. Turner et al. (1998) did not include a standard control group to allow for the ordinary presence of a nurse. The sample size was very small in the Mueller Hinze (1988) study, and the study interventions were administered by the principal investigator in the Keller and Bzdek (1986) study. In the Peck (1997) study, the role of the placebo effect in the progressive muscle relaxation intervention is not clear. Thus, it is difficult to determine whether control for the placebo was, in fact, included in the study design. Constructive replication of these studies and extension to include patients with different types of mild to moderate pain and repeated treatments and measures, as well as consistent control for the placebo effect, are needed. So far, study findings suggest that Therapeutic Touch may have the potential, beyond a placebo effect, to reduce headache pain and decrease the need for prn analgesic medication.

Four qualitative studies and one descriptive study of Therapeutic Touch have been reported. Lionberger (1985) interviewed 51 nurses, who had practiced Therapeutic Touch for at least 6 months, and 20 patients. She found that many nurses modified the standardized assessment and treatment phases of the procedure because of difficulty explaining the intervention in environments dominated by the medical model. Lionberger (1986) suggested that Therapeutic Touch be developed as a caring strategy rather than as a healing modality. Wyatt (1988) examined conceptual change in 11 nurses who had completed a 2-day advanced continuing education seminar on Therapeutic Touch. Data from surveys and interviews over a 2-month period indicated that although knowledge and application were high 1 week after the seminar, they were not maintained over time because of perceived barriers to implementation in the workplace. Heidt (1990) interviewed and observed seven nurses, who had practiced Therapeutic Touch for at least 3 years, and seven patients. She found that all nurses conformed to the standardized practice procedure, that the primary experience of Therapeutic Touch was that of opening to the flow of the universal life energy, and that during the intervention the patient's experience of Therapeutic Touch frequently paralleled that of the nurse. Samarel (1992) described the experience of receiving Therapeutic Touch in 20 patients with a range of chronic illnesses. Patients' experience encompassed increased personal awareness and change and a sense of fulfillment and well-being. Using a simple descriptive approach, Sneed, Olson, and Bonadonna (1997) explored 11 graduate students' experiences of receiving Therapeutic Touch for the first time as participants in a randomized experimental study. All reported feelings of relaxation and a range of physical sensations, and most reported positive mental or emotional responses. In the future, comparison of such experiences with the experiences of control group participants could help identify experiences particular to receiving Therapeutic Touch. More qualitative and descriptive studies are needed to clarify and verify themes already identified and contribute to theory building.

Critical Commentary

The development of Therapeutic Touch as a nursing intervention has engendered considerable criticism. This is to be expected because of its unusual nature and welcomed considering its development within the context of nursing as a professional discipline. Critical commentary has focused on the theoretical frameworks, the spiritual dimension of the intervention, and the meaning of research findings.

The concepts and propositions of both theoretical frameworks are complex and highly speculative. However, very little specific explication, logical analysis, or critical evaluation of either framework as an explanation for Therapeutic Touch appears in the nursing literature. For example, in neither framework is the concept of an energy field precisely defined, apparent inconsistencies between the frameworks are not addressed, and possible alternative explanations for Therapeutic Touch, such as the psychological-humanistic framework identified by Weber (1990), are not explored. Since its introduction, descriptions of Therapeutic Touch have been criticized for being enigmatic and lacking in clear definitions of concepts (Walike et al., 1975). Continued absence of scholarly response to criticism has led to charges of blatant "nurse quackery" (Levine, 1979), unprofessional association with the occult and mystical (Curtin, 1980), engaging in pseudoscience (Bullough & Bullough, 1993) and fuzzy metaphysics (Stahlman, 1995), misrepresentation and fraud (Oberst, 1995a), and being a source of embarrassment to the profession (Bullough & Bullough, 1995). It is urgent that nurses address these issues through scholarly analysis and argumentation. The work of Weber (1981, 1990), a philosopher, requires critical analysis and development in the nursing literature. More precise analysis of the Science of Unitary Human Beings model concepts and comparison with Therapeutic Touch concepts, as well as explication of links between these concepts and related concepts from philosophy and physics, are needed.

It seems clear that there is a central spiritual dimension to Therapeutic Touch that is linked to facilitating the healing process. However, this is not clearly explicated, and references made to the source of the healing impetus are inconsistent. In developing Therapeutic Touch, Kunz and Krieger were guided by the general energy field framework described by Weber. In this framework, the nurse practicing Therapeutic Touch seeks to become conscious of and act as an instrument for a universal healing energy that arises from the spiritual dimension of human experience and permeates all living systems. Although some sources suggest the very different view that the nurse is drawing upon and using personal excess energy, Kunz (personal communication, July 1998) and most nurses maintain that the nurse's role in seeking to act as an instrument for a universal healing energy is a central and essential aspect of the practice of Therapeutic Touch.

A related inconsistency concerns the relationship between Therapeutic Touch and religion. It is frequently claimed that Therapeutic Touch is not practiced within a religious context, but Kunz has pointed out that it can be practiced within a religious context (D. Kunz, personal communication, August 1995). The important point is that a particular religious context is not necessary. The broad philosophical framework outlined by Weber (1981, 1990) may serve as a foundation for any practitioner, and, at the same time, this framework may also be linked to most religious systems of thought. Thus, particular religious backgrounds can be drawn upon naturally to help nurses facilitate their ability to practice Therapeutic Touch effectively. Lack of clarity on such issues is likely to be of concern to some nurses (Wuthnow & Miller, 1987) and lead to misunderstanding and misinterpretation of the intervention.

Most critical commentary concerns interpretation of research findings related to proposed effects of Therapeutic Touch. Nurses who use the intervention are convinced that it is effective in relieving a wide range of stress-related conditions. However, it appears that many do not critically evaluate research reports and possibly allow "the enthusiasm of discovery" (Johnson, 1994) to cloud their scientific judgment. Even reviews of Therapeutic Touch research (Krieger, 1990; McKinney, 1995; Quinn, 1988) tend to lack critical analysis. Critics have pointed out that Therapeutic Touch research is often flawed and that there is little or no evidence that it is more effective than a placebo (Clark & Clark, 1984; Curtin, 1980; Levine, 1979; Meehan, 1995b; Oberst, 1995a; Stahlman, 1995). Debate about differing views of the meaning of research findings is well illustrated in an editorial (Oberst, 1995a), a series of letters to the editor (Barrett, 1995; Baun, 1995; Bright, 1995; Bullough & Bullough, 1995; Heidt, 1995; Keller, Lauver, McCarthy, & Ward, 1995; Malinski, 1995; Meehan, 1995a; Straneva, 1995; Wells-Federman, 1995), and a further editorial (Oberst, 1995b), which appeared in a prominent nursing research journal. Some comments about research standards and findings on both sides of the debate could be considered extreme. With regard to a similar debate, Joel (1995) reminded the profession that "an open mind is the first and foremost quality of a scholar" (p. 7). Scholarly debate is of critical importance in the development of Therapeutic Touch as a nursing intervention. More logical analysis and scientific evidence is needed in order to clarify the nature of the intervention and determine whether its proposed effects can be considered either refuted or verified.

THE INTERVENTION

Intervention Tools

The Subjective Experience of Therapeutic Touch Survey (SETTS), a 68-item, self-report tool, was developed by Krieger and Wilcox (Winstead-Fry, 1983) to measure how well individuals perform Therapeutic Touch. Their analysis indicated that the tool could reliably distinguish between experienced and nonexperienced practitioners. Extension of this work by Ferguson (1986) indicated that the SETTS could reliably differentiate among experienced practitioners, inexperienced practitioners, and nurses who did not practice Therapeutic Touch and that experienced practitioners were significantly more effective in reducing anxiety in patients compared with inexperienced practitioners. Despite some limitations, the SETTS may be useful in selecting nurses who are experienced and effective in the practice of Therapeutic Touch.

The Energy Field Assessment was developed to record specific qualities of the Therapeutic Touch energy field assessment (Wright, 1991). This one-page, three-part tool is designed to translate the subjective experience of energy field assessment into measurable terms. Wright (1991) demonstrated beginning content and construct validity for the tool. She found significant relationships between location of field disturbance and physical location of pain and between decreased background strength of the field and fatigue, but no significant relationship between field disturbance and pain intensity. Although the tool requires further testing, it could serve as a useful guide for nurses learning Therapeutic Touch.

Intervention Process

A standardized definition of Therapeutic Touch has been developed by Kunz and Krieger (1975–1997) and is used in most intervention research. The operational definition includes the following steps: the nurse (1) assumes a centered (meditative) state of consciousness; (2) makes the conscious intent to therapeutically assist the patient; (3) moves his or her hands, at a distance of approximately 2 inches, over the patient's body from head to feet, attuning to the condition of the patient and becoming aware of differences in sensory cues in his or her hands; (4) redirects areas of accumulated tension in the patient by movement of the hands; (5) focuses intent on the specific direction of energy using his or her hands as focal points; and (6) places the hands over the area of the solar plexus (just below the sternum) and directs energy to the patient. Therapeutic Touch may include physical contact but usually does not. Minor variations in the definition are acceptable, and the intervention may be incorporated naturally into other nursing interventions. However, it is evident that some interventions or procedures are being called Therapeutic Touch when, in fact, they are not. For example, "healing touch," "touch for health," and "magnetic unruffling" are not Therapeutic Touch, and they are not variations of Therapeutic Touch. Wirth and Cram (1993) and Wirth, Richardson, Eidelman, and O'Malley (1993) claim to test the effects of Therapeutic Touch; however, the operational definitions of the procedures used in these studies indicate clearly that it is not Therapeutic Touch that is being tested. In a research review, Easter (1997) examined the findings of 23 studies she purports to be of Therapeutic Touch; however, only seven of the reports actually concern Therapeutic Touch research.

The intervention of Therapeutic Touch as it appears in the *Nursing Interventions Classification (NIC)* (McCloskey & Bulecheck, 1996) is shown in Table 9–1. The following comments on the definition and each activity of the NIC intervention are summarized from reviews of the definition by five nurses who have been closely involved with the practice and research of Therapeutic Touch for several years. Following the comments, revisions are suggested to attain congruence with the standardized definition developed by Kunz and Krieger, the research findings, and current use in practice.

NIC Conceptual Definition: "Directing one's own interpersonal energy to flow through the hands to help or heal another." Although in early writings Krieger (1979) and Krieger et al. (1979) state that the nurse's personal energy is used, most of the literature indicates, and all of the reviewers stress emphatically, that during the practice of Therapeutic Touch the nurse attunes to the universal healing energy and acts as an instrument for its healing influence. Kunz stresses the importance of this principle (D. Kunz, personal communication, May 1997). *Suggested revision: Facilitating the flow of a universal healing energy through centering, intentionality, and the use of the hands to help or promote healing in another.*

NIC Activity 1: "Center oneself physically and psychologically to purposefully relax tensions." Centering is not a particulate physical and psychological activity; it is a simple form of meditation and a unitary process. *Suggested revision: Focus*

Table 9–1   Therapeutic Touch

DEFINITION: Directing one's own interpersonal energy to flow through the hands to help or heal another.

ACTIVITIES:
Center oneself physically and psychologically to purposefully relax tensions
Sit in a relaxed position with body in alignment and hands in lap
Close eyes and breathe evenly and slowly
Attain a sense of inner equilibrium in preparation for directing physical and psychodynamic energies
Place the hands 2 to 3 inches from the patient's skin
Move hands slowly and steadily over patient
Complete total body assessment, typically working from head to toe, front to back
Note any sign of temperature change, tingling, pressure, electric shock, or pulsation in your hands
"Unruffle the field" around pressure areas by placing the hands with palms away from the body and moving hands away in a sweeping gesture
Directs energies to patient's areas of imbalances
Stop when there are no longer bilateral differences in the patient's field
Note objective signs of patient's experience: relaxation, slow respirations, peripheral flush, relief of pain, relief of nausea, and increased peristalsis

Source: McCloskey, J. C., and Bulechek, G. M. (Eds.). (1996). *Nursing interventions classification (NIC)* (2nd ed., p. 564). St. Louis: Mosby–Year Book.

awareness through the inner self and experience its peace and order; perceive the patient to be always striving toward wholeness.

NIC Activities 2 and 3:   "Sit in relaxed position with body in alignment and hands in lap," and "Close eyes and breathe evenly and slowly." These steps are unnecessary to the success of the intervention but may sometimes be done to create a sense of calmness in the patient's environment.

NIC Activity 4:   "Attain a sense of inner equilibrium in preparation for directing physical and psychodynamic energies." The term *inner equilibrium* does not convey the awareness of the inner self of the human person and its peace and order, which is the essential ingredient of centering. The term *physical and psychodynamic energies* is particulate rather than holistic. This step is part of centering and thus unnecessary, but it could be included. *Suggested revision: Attain a sense of the peace and order of the inner self.*

NIC Activity 5:   "Place the hands 2 to 3 inches from the patient's skin." The distance of 2 to 3 or 4 inches is frequently referred to in the nursing literature; however, Kunz states that the hands should be "just an inch, not 3 inches" from the patient's body (D. Kunz, personal communication, May 1997). *Suggested revision: Place the hands 1 to 2 inches from the patient's body.*

NIC Activity 6:   "Move hands slowly and steadily over patient." This statement needs to be extended to indicate what is occurring. *Suggested revision: Begin the energy field assessment by moving the hands slowly and steadily over the patient.*

NIC Activity 7:   "Complete total body assessment, typically working from head to toe, front to back." This statement needs to be clarified to mean an energy field assessment, not a body assessment. *Suggested revision: Carry out the energy field assessment, typically moving the hands over the whole person from head to toe, front to back.*

NIC Activity 8: "Note any sign of temperature change, tingling, pressure, electric shock, or pulsation in your hands." The changes perceived by the hands are extremely subtle and are usually referred to as cues. The most commonly perceived cues are warmth and tingling. Although there may be some perception of movement, pulsation is not an accurate choice of words. The term *electric shock* is definitely not appropriate. *Suggested revision: Note the overall pattern of the energy flow and especially any areas of disturbance, such as congestion or unevenness, which may be perceived through very subtle cues in the hands—for example, temperature change, tingling, or other subtle feelings of movement.*

NIC Activity 9: " 'Unruffle the field' around pressure areas by placing the hands with palms away from the body and moving hands away in a sweeping gesture." Although the term *unruffle* has crept into some of the nursing literature, it is not useful because it does not convey what is occurring. The phrase *palms away from the body* and the term *pressure areas* are confusing. The term *sweeping gesture* is inappropriate because it does not convey the most important aspect of this step, which is gentleness. *Suggested revision: Focus intention on facilitating the flow and symmetry of the patient's energy field. Begin by moving the hands in very gentle downward movements through the patient's energy field, thinking of the patient as a unitary whole.*

NIC Activity 10: "Directs energies to patient's areas of imbalances." It is not clear what this means. In continuing the treatment, the nurse focuses on particular areas of disturbance in the patient's energy field and on facilitating symmetry and healing in disturbed areas. In completing the treatment, the hands may be placed for 1 or 2 minutes over the area of the solar plexus (just below the sternum) while intention is focused on facilitating the flow of healing energy in the patient. *Suggested revision: Continue the treatment by very gently facilitating the flow of healing energy into areas of disturbance. Complete the treatment by placing the hands over the area of the patient's solar plexus for 1 or 2 minutes and facilitating the flow of healing energy in the patient.*

NIC Activity 11: "Stop when there are no longer bilateral differences in the patient's field." Only a certain amount of change can occur in any one treatment. In many cases, especially when the patient is acutely or chronically ill, there may still be areas of disturbance and asymmetry, even though the energy field will flow more openly and symmetrically than before the treatment. The decision to finish the treatment is based on the nurse's sense of the amount of change that has taken place in relation to what is possible for the particular patient at the time of the treatment. The phrase *there are no longer bilateral differences* does not have the same meaning as symmetry. The length of treatment time varies according to the age and needs of the patient. It is generally suggested that for premature or small infants it can range from 1 to 2 minutes and that for adults it can range from 5 to 10 minutes. Kunz has recommended that generally, for an adult, no more than a 5- to 7-minute treatment time is needed (D. Kunz, personal communication, August 1995). *Suggested revision: Finish when you judge that the appropriate amount of change has taken place (guidelines: an infant, 1 to 2 minutes; an adult, 5 to 7 minutes), keeping in mind the importance of gentleness.*

NIC Activity 12: "Note objective signs of patient's experience: relaxation, slow respirations, peripheral flush, relief of pain, relief of nausea, and increased peristalsis." The most important response to observe for related to the effectiveness of the intervention is relaxation. Any additional responses follow from this. Based on research findings, relief from pain may or may not occur. There is no scientific evidence to support any expectation of a peripheral flush, relief from nausea, or increased peristalsis. *Suggested revision: Note whether the patient has experienced a relaxation response, relief from pain, or a general sense of comfort and well-being.*

It is recommended that before using Therapeutic Touch in their care of patients, nurses complete at least 6 months' experience in professional practice. It is also strongly recommended that they receive appropriate educational preparation within a recognized professional basic or continuing educational program that, at a minimum, includes the following: (1) teaching by nurses who have had at least 2 years' experience using Therapeutic Touch, preferably have a master's degree in nursing, and conform to the practice guidelines developed by Kunz and Krieger (1975–1997); (2) 30 hours of instruction in the theory and practice of Therapeutic Touch and 30 hours of supervised practice with relatively healthy individuals; (3) evaluation methods that ensure a basic understanding of the theoretical frameworks used to describe and explain Therapeutic Touch, the ability to discuss the peer-reviewed literature and critically evaluate research reports, and the ability to discuss the intervention in terms that can be understood by health professionals and patients who are not familiar with it.

NURSING DIAGNOSES AND APPROPRIATE PATIENT GROUPS

Because Therapeutic Touch generally promotes relaxation and thereby appears to facilitate the natural healing process in the patient, it can be used with a wide variety of patient groups. The research literature suggests that Therapeutic Touch may be useful for the North American Nursing Diagnosis Association (NANDA) diagnoses of Anxiety and Pain. The practice literature suggests that Therapeutic Touch may be useful for the NANDA diagnoses of Ineffective Individual Coping, Fear, Anticipatory Grieving, Impaired Physical Mobility, Powerlessness, and Sleep Pattern Disturbance.

There is essentially no risk in using Therapeutic Touch, but there are some patient groups with which caution is suggested. For many patients, Therapeutic Touch appears to be a new and very different kind of intervention. Therefore, it is generally not wise to use it to treat patients with critical, labile conditions, such as a bleeding intracranial aneurysm awaiting surgery, where absolute quiet is required and it is better not to introduce different and nonessential circumstances. For patients with psychiatric illnesses for whom the NANDA diagnosis Alteration in Thought Processes applies, Therapeutic Touch should be used only by nurses who have had several years' experience with Therapeutic Touch and with caring for such patients and who have excellent clinical judgment. Such patients are often extremely sensitive to close human interaction and to its meaning for them.

NURSING-SENSITIVE PATIENT OUTCOMES

Although the practice literature suggests that there is a wide range of nursing-sensitive patient outcomes related to Therapeutic Touch, it must be borne in mind that most of these would be due to the probable role of Therapeutic Touch in enhancing the placebo effect. From this perspective, any nursing-sensitive outcome that could be expected to follow from a relaxation response could possibly be expected following Therapeutic Touch. Based on the research literature, the outcomes identified in the Nursing Outcomes Classification (NOC) (Johnson & Maas, 1997) that could be linked to Therapeutic Touch are Anxiety Control, Comfort Level, and Pain Level.

CASE STUDY

Mrs. M was hospitalized for a total abdominal hysterectomy because of fibroids. She was 55 years old, otherwise healthy, and of medium build and weight with a groomed appearance. She was a widow of 2 years, was financially secure, had two grown sons who lived some distance away, and gave the impression of being self-sufficient. She lived an intensely active professional life as a stock analyst for a prominent financial organization and took little time to pursue her more light-hearted interests.

Her surgery was straightforward, and her postoperative condition was stable. By her third postoperative day, her urinary catheter had been removed, and she was voiding without difficulty. She had progressed to a soft diet and was able to get out of bed and walk by herself. She reported a moderate amount of incisional pain, for which she received two tablets of Percocet every 4 to 6 hours. She experienced difficulty sleeping and was prescribed Nembutal 100 mg to settle at night and a repeat dose in 4 hours as needed, which she took. But this had not helped her, and a switch to chloral hydrate had been made.

Although she was making good physical progress and said that she was "just fine," she was becoming increasingly tense and irritable. Mrs. M's primary nurse took extra time to attend to Mrs. M, using the NIC interventions Presence and Active Listening. During this interaction, some of Mrs. M's self-sufficient manner began to dissipate. It

emerged that she was not sleeping despite the hypnotic medication and was beginning to feel "spaced out." She felt anxious about not being able to cope by herself and profoundly sad about the loss of "part of myself." In addition, although she thought that she had adjusted well to her husband's death, she really missed him now. In her words, "Everything seems just pent up inside of me, and I do wish he was here."

Her primary nursing diagnoses were Anxiety, Pain, and Sleep Pattern Disturbance. The nurse's use of Presence and Active Listening comforted Mrs. M and helped her relax. The nurse explained Therapeutic Touch to her, and Mrs. M said that she would like to try it with her pain medication and instead of her sleeping medication. The first night, Mrs. M received Therapeutic Touch when she settled to sleep and again when she awoke at 3 AM. She felt more rested in the morning. On subsequent nights she received Therapeutic Touch when she settled to sleep and then slept through the night. She felt that receiving Therapeutic Touch with her analgesic (which had been decreased to Tylenol) facilitated her naturally decreasing need for analgesia. Overall, she began to feel more energetic and also relieved that she could take care of herself again.

For about 2 months after discharge, she continued to receive a Therapeutic Touch treatment once a week at a Saturday-morning nursing clinic. She felt that it helped her "get settled into my life again."

CONCLUSION

For many nurses, the use of Therapeutic Touch seems close to the heart of nursing practice. They feel that, to borrow a phrase from Nightingale (1859/ 1969, p. 110), it is one way by which they can truly "put the patient in the best condition for nature to act upon him." Others nurses have questioned its appropriateness and effectiveness as a nursing intervention. Further investigation of its nature and effects is clearly necessary and should include a wide range of carefully designed quantitative and qualitative studies. In the meantime,

Therapeutic Touch will continue to play a significant role in helping patients, in strengthening nurses' commitment to nursing, and in contributing moments of nurturance and peacefulness in the often stressful and troubled world.

References

Barrett, E. A. M. (1995). More on therapeutic touch [Letter to the editor]. *Research in Nursing and Health, 18*, 378.

Baun, M. M. (1995). Therapeutic touch [Letter to the editor]. *Research in Nursing and Health, 18*, 287.

Biley, F. (1996). Rogerian science, phantoms, and therapeutic touch: Exploring potentials. *Nursing Science Quarterly, 9*, 165.

Boguslawski, M. (1979). The use of therapeutic touch in nursing. *Journal of Continuing Education in Nursing, 10*(4), 9.

Boguslawski, M. (1980). Therapeutic touch: A facilitator of pain relief. *Topics in Clinical Nursing, 2*(1), 27.

Bohm, D. (1973). Quantum theory as an indication of a new order in physical law. *Found Physics, 3*(2), 144.

Bohm, D. (1986). The implicate order and the superimplicate order. In R. Weber (Ed.), *Dialogues with scientists and sages: The search for unity* (pp. 23–52). New York: Routledge & Kegan Paul.

Borelli, M. D., and Heidt, P. (Eds.). (1981). *Therapeutic touch.* New York: Springer Publishing.

Braun, C., Layton, J., and Braun, J. (1986). Therapeutic touch improves residents' sleep. *American Health Care Association Journal, 12*(1), 48.

Bright, M. A. (1995). Therapeutic touch [Letter to the editor]. *Research in Nursing and Health, 18*, 285.

Bullough, V. L., and Bullough, B. (1993). Therapeutic touch. Why do nurses believe? *Skeptical Inquirer, 17*, 169.

Bullough, V. L., and Bullough, B. (1995). More on therapeutic touch [Letter to the editor]. *Research in Nursing and Health, 18*, 377.

Burr, H. S. (1972). *Blueprint for immortality: The electric patterns of life.* London: Neville Spearman.

Clark, P. E., and Clark, M. J. (1984). Therapeutic touch: Is there a scientific basis for practice? *Nursing Research, 33*(1), 37.

Connell, M. T. (1983). Feminine consciousness and the nature of nursing practice: A historical perspective. *Topics in Clinical Nursing, 5*(3), 1.

Curtin, L. (1980). Nurse quackery [Editorial]. *Supervisor Nurse, 11*(3), 9.

Cushing, J., and McMullin, E. (Eds.). (1989). *Philosophical consequences of quantum theory.* Notre Dame, IN: University of Notre Dame Press.

Dall, J. V. (1993). Promoting sleep with therapeutic touch. *Addictions Nursing Network, 5*(1), 23.

Easter, A. (1997). The state of research on the effects of therapeutic touch. *Journal of Holistic Nursing, 15*(2), 158.

Egan, E. C. (1992). Therapeutic touch. In M. Snyder M. (Ed.), *Independent nursing interventions* (p. 173). Albany, NY: Nyelmar Publishers.

Fanslow, C. A. (1983). Therapeutic touch: A healing modality throughout life. *Topics in Clinical Nursing, 5*(2), 72.

Fanslow, C. A. (1990). Touch and the elderly. In K. E. Barnard and T. B. Brazelton (Eds.), *Touch: The foundation of experience* (p. 541). Madison, WI: International Universities Press.

Fedoruk, R. B. (1984). *Transfer of the relaxation response: Therapeutic touch B as a method for reduction of stress in premature neonates.* Doctoral dissertation, University of Maryland (UMI No. 8509162).

Feltham, E. (1991). Therapeutic touch and massage. *Nursing Studies, 31*(5), 26.

Ferguson, C. (1986). *Subjective experience of therapeutic touch survey (SETTS): Psychometric examination of an instrument.* Doctoral dissertation, University of Texas, Austin (UMI No. 8618464).

Finnerin, D. (1981). Therapeutic touch for children and their families. In M. D. Borelli and P. Heidt (Eds.), *Therapeutic touch* (p. 64). New York: Springer Publishing.

Gagne, D., and Toye, R. C. (1994). The effects of therapeutic touch and relaxation therapy in reducing anxiety. *Archives of Psychiatric Nursing, 7*(3), 184.

Hale, E. H. (1986). *A study of the relationship between therapeutic touch and the anxiety levels of hospitalized adults.* Doctoral dissertation, Texas Women's University (UMI No. 8618897).

Heidt, P. R. (1981). Effect of therapeutic touch on anxiety level of hospitalized patients. *Nursing Research, 30*, 33.

Heidt, P. R. (1990). Openness: A qualitative analysis of nurses' and patients' experiences of therapeutic touch. *Image, 22*(3), 180.

Heidt, P. R. (1991). Helping patients rest: Clinical studies in therapeutic touch. *Holistic Nursing Practice, 5*(4), 57.

Heidt, P. R. (1995). More on therapeutic touch [Letter to the editor]. *Research in Nursing and Health, 18*, 377.

Hill, L., and Oliver, N. (1993). Therapeutic touch and theory-based mental health nursing. *Journal of Psychosocial Nursing, 31*(2), 19.

Hospital Satellite Network (Producer), and American Journal of Nursing Company (Distributor). (1986). *Therapeutic touch: A new skill from an ancient practice* (Videocassette No. 7538). New York: American Journal of Nursing Company.

Jackson, M. E. (1981). The use of therapeutic touch in the nursing care of the terminally ill person. In M. D. Borelli and P. Heidt (Eds.), *Therapeutic touch* (p. 72). New York: Springer Publishing.

Joel, L. A. (1995). Alternative solutions to health problems. *American Journal of Nursing, 95*(7), 7.

Johnson, M., and Maas, M. (Eds.). (1997). *Nursing outcomes classification (NOC).* St. Louis: Mosby-Year Book.

Johnson, P. (1994 September). Why all of us should observe the eleventh commandment of Karl Popper. *The Spectator, 24.*

Jonasen, A. M. (1981). Therapeutic touch in the operating room: Best of both worlds. In M. D. Borelli and P. Heidt (Eds.), *Therapeutic touch* (p. 80). New York: Springer Publishing.

Jonasen, A. M. (1994). Therapeutic touch: A holistic approach to perioperative nursing. *Today's OR Nurse, 16*(1), 7.

Josephson, B. D., and Pallikari-Viras, F. (1991). Biological utilization of quantum nonlocality. *Found Physics, 21*(2), 197.

Jurgens, A., Meehan, T. C., and Wilson, H. L. (1987). Therapeutic touch as a nursing intervention. *Holistic Nursing Practice, 2*(1), 1.

Keller, E. K. (1984). Therapeutic touch: A review of the literature and implications of a holistic nursing modality. *Journal of Holistic Nursing, 2*(1), 24.

Keller, E., and Bzdek, V. M. (1986). Effects of therapeutic touch on tension headache pain. *Nursing Research, 35*(2), 101.

Keller, M., Lauver, D., McCarthy, D., and Ward, S. (1995). Therapeutic touch [Letter to the editor]. *Research in Nursing and Health, 18*, 286.

Kramer, N. A. (1990). Comparison of therapeutic touch and casual touch in stress reduction of hospitalized children. *Pediatric Nursing, 16*, 483.

Krieger, D. (1975). Therapeutic touch: The imprimatur of nursing. *American Journal of Nursing, 75*, 784.

Krieger, D. (1979). *The therapeutic touch: How to use your hands to help or to heal.* Englewood Cliffs, NJ: Prentice-Hall.

Krieger, D. (1990). Therapeutic touch: Two decades of research, teaching and clinical practice. *Imprint, 37*(3), 83.

Krieger, D., Peper, E., and Ancoli, S. (1979). Therapeutic touch: Searching for evidence of physiological change. *American Journal of Nursing, 79*, 660.

Kunz, D. (1985). Compassion, rootedness and detachment: Their role in healing. In D. Kunz (Ed.), *Spiritual aspects of the healing arts* (p. 289). Wheaton, IL: Theosophical Publishing House.

Kunz, D., and Krieger, D. (1975–1997). *Annual invitational workshops on therapeutic touch.* Craryville, NY: Pumpkin Hollow Foundation.

Leduc, E. (1987). Therapeutic touch [Letter to the editor]. *Neonatal Network, 5*(6), 46.

Ledwith, S. P. (1995). Therapeutic touch and mastectomy: A case study. *RN, 58*(7), 51.

Levine, M. E. (1979). "The science is spurious . . ." [Letter to the editor]. *American Journal of Nursing, 79*, 1379.

Lionberger, H. (1985). *An interpretative study of nurses' practice of therapeutic touch.* Doctoral dissertation, University of California, San Francisco (UMI No. 8524008).

Lionberger, H. J. (1986). Therapeutic touch: A healing modality or a caring strategy. In P. L. Chin (Ed.), *Methodological issues in nursing.* Gaithersburg, MD: Aspen.

Lothian, J. A. (1988). Therapeutic touch. In F. Nichols and S. Humenick (Eds.), *Childbirth education, practice, research, and theory.* Philadelphia: W. B. Saunders.

Lothian, J. A. (1993). Therapeutic touch. *Childbirth Instructor,* Sp, 32.

Mackey, R. B. (1995). Discover the healing power of therapeutic touch. *American Journal of Nursing, 95*(4), 27.

Macrae, J. (1979). Therapeutic touch in practice. *American Journal of Nursing, 79*, 664.

Macrae, J. (1988). *Therapeutic touch: A practical guide.* New York: Knopf.

Macrae, J. (1989). Principles of therapeutic touch applied to the treatment of addiction. *Addictions Nursing Network, 1*(2), 4.

Malinski, V. (1993). Therapeutic touch: The view from Rogerian nursing science. *Visions, 1*, 45.

Malinski, V. (1995). Therapeutic touch [Letter to the editor]. *Research in Nursing and Health, 18*, 286.

McCloskey, J. C., and Bulecheck, G. M. (Eds.). (1996). *Nursing interventions classification (NIC)* (2nd ed., p. 564). St. Louis: Mosby–Year Book.

McKinney, J. B. (1995). Therapeutic touch in nursing practice: Building the knowledge. *Online Journal of Knowledge Synthesis in Nursing, 2*(11 #23), 1.

Mead, M. (1956). Nursing—primitive and civilized. *American Journal of Nursing, 56*(8), 101.

Meehan, T. C. (1990a). The science of unitary human beings and theory-based practice: Therapeutic touch. In E. A. M. Barrett (Ed.), *Visions of Rogers' science-based nursing* (p. 67). New York: National League for Nursing.

Meehan, T. C. (1990b). Theory development. In E. A. M. Barrett (Ed.), *Visions of Rogers' science-based nursing* (p. 197). New York: National League for Nursing.

Meehan, T. C. (1993). Therapeutic touch and postoperative pain: A Rogerian research study. *Nursing Science Quarterly, 6*(2), 62.

Meehan, T. C. (1995a). And still more on TT [Letter to the editor]. *Research in Nursing and Health, 18*, 471.

Meehan, T. C. (1995b). Quackery and pseudo-science [Letter to the editor]. *American Journal of Nursing, 95*(7), 17.

Meehan, T. C., Mahoney, K., Ake, J., Iervolino, L., Glassman, K., Tedesco, P., and Mariano, C. (1990). *A professional self-development program for nurses: Final project report to the United Hospital Fund.* New York: Department of Nursing, New York University Medical Center.

Meehan, T. C., Mersmann, C. A., Wiseman, M., Wolff, and Malgady (1990). The effects of therapeutic touch on postoperative pain [Abstract]. *Pain* (Suppl. 5), 149.

Meehan, T. C., Mersmann, C. A., Wiseman, M., Wolff, and Malgady. (1991). *Therapeutic touch and surgical patients' stress reactions: Final project report to National Center for Nursing Research, NIH.* New York: Department of Nursing, New York University Medical Center.

Mersmann, C. A. (1993). *Therapeutic touch and milk letdown in mothers of non-nursing preterm infants.* Doctoral dissertation, New York University (UMI No. 9333919).

Miller, L. (1979). An explanation of therapeutic touch using the science of unitary man. *Nursing Forum, 18*, 278.

Mueller Hinze, M. L. (1988). *The effects of therapeutic touch and acupressure on experimentally-induced pain.* Doctoral dissertation, University of Texas, Austin (UMI No. 8901377).

Mulloney, S. S., Wells-Federman, C. (1996). Therapeutic touch: A healing modality. *Journal of Cardiovascular Nursing, 10*(3), 27.

National League for Nursing. (1992). *Therapeutic touch: Healing through human energy fields* (Videotape Series Publication no. 42-2485, 42-2486, 422487). New York: National League for Nursing.

Newshan, G. (1989). Therapeutic touch for symptom control in persons with AIDS. *Holistic Nursing Practice, 3*(4), 45.

Nightingale, F. (1859/1969). *Notes on nursing: What it is and what it is not.* New York: Dover.

Oberst, M. (1995a). Our naked emperor [Editorial]. *Research in Nursing and Health, 18*, 1.

Oberst, M. (1995b). The naked emperor revisited [Editorial]. *Research in Nursing and Health, 18*, 383.

Olson, M., and Sneed, N. (1995). Anxiety and therapeutic touch. *Issues in Mental Health Nursing, 16*, 97.

Olson, M., Sneed, N., Bonadonna, R., Ratliff, J., and Dias, J. (1992). Therapeutic touch and post–hurricane Hugo stress. *Journal of Holistic Nursing, 10*, 120.

Olson, M., Sneed, N., LaVia, M., Virella, G., Bonadonna,

R., and Michel, Y. (1997). Stress-induced immuno-suppression and therapeutic touch. *Alternative Therapies in Health and Medicine, 3*(2), 68–74.

Parkes, B. S. (1985). Therapeutic touch as an intervention to decrease anxiety in elderly hospitalized patients. Doctoral dissertation, University of Texas, Austin (UMI No. 8609563).

Payne, M. B. (1989). The use of therapeutic touch with rehabilitation clients. *Rehabilitation Nursing, 15*(2), 69.

Peck, S. D. E. (1997). The effectiveness of therapeutic touch for decreasing pain in elders with degenerative arthritis. *Journal of Holistic Nursing, 15*(2), 176.

Peric-Knowlton, W. (1984). The understanding and management of acute pain in adults: The nursing contribution. *International Journal of Nursing Studies, 21*, 141.

Quinn, J. F. (1979). One nurse's evolution as a healer. *American Journal of Nursing, 79*, 662.

Quinn, J. F. (1982). *An investigation of the effects of therapeutic touch done without physical contact on state anxiety of hospitalized cardiovascular patients.* Doctoral dissertation, New York University (UMI No. 8226788).

Quinn, J. F. (1984). Therapeutic touch as energy exchange: Testing the theory. *Advances in Nursing Science, 6*(2), 42.

Quinn, J. F. (1988). Building a body of knowledge: Research on therapeutic touch 1974–1986. *Journal of Holistic Nursing, 6*(1), 37.

Quinn, J. F. (1989). Therapeutic touch as energy exchange: Replication and extension. *Nursing Science Quarterly, 2*(2), 79.

Quinn, J. F., and Strelkauskas, A. J. (1989). Psychoimmunologic effects of therapeutic touch on practitioners and recently bereaved recipients: A pilot study. *Advances in Nursing Science, 15*(4), 13.

Randolph, G. L. (1984). Therapeutic and physical touch: Physiological response to stressful stimuli. *Nursing Research, 33*, 33.

Rogers, M. E. (1970). *An introduction to the theoretical basis of nursing.* Philadelphia: F. A. Davis.

Rogers, M. E. (1990). Nursing: Science of unitary, irreducible human beings: Update 1990. In E. A. M. Barrett (Ed.), *Visions of Rogers' science-based nursing* (p. 5). New York: National League for Nursing.

Samarel, N. (1992). The experience of receiving therapeutic touch. *Journal of Advanced Nursing, 17*, 651.

Samarel, N. (1997). Therapeutic touch, dialogue, and women's experiences in breast cancer surgery. *Holistic Nursing Practice, 12*(1), 62.

Sayre-Adams, J. (1995). *The theory and practice of therapeutic touch.* London: Churchill Livingstone.

Simeone, C. (1985). Changing practice through therapeutic touch. *California Nursing, 80*, 618.

Simington, J. A. (1993). The elderly require a "special touch." *Nursing Homes, 4*, 30.

Simington, J. A., and Laing, G. P. (1993). Effects of therapeutic touch on anxiety in the institutionalized elderly. *Clinical Nursing Research, 2*, 438.

Sneed, N. V., Olson, M., and Bonadonna, R. (1997). The experience of therapeutic touch for novice recipients. *Journal of Holistic Nursing, 15*, 243.

Snyder, M., Egan, E. C., and Burns, K. R. (1995). Interventions for decreasing agitation behaviors in persons with dementia. *Journal of Gerontological Nursing, 21*(4), 34.

Stahlman, J. (1995). Therapeutic touch: Fuzzy metaphysics [Letter to the editor]. *American Journal of Nursing, 95*(7), 17.

Stapp, H. P. (1993). *Mind, matter, and quantum mechanics.* Berlin: Springer-Verlag.

Straneva, J. (1995). More on TT [Letter to the editor]. *Research in Nursing and Health, 18*, 379.

Thayer, M. B. (1990). Touching with intent: Using therapeutic touch. *Pediatric Nursing, 16*, 70.

Turner, J., Clark, A., Gauthier, D., and Williams, M. (1998). The effect of therapeutic touch on pain and anxiety in burn patients. *Journal of Advanced Nursing, 28*, 10–20.

Walike, B., Bruno, P., Donaldson, S., Erickson B., Giblin, E., Hanson, R., Mitchel, P., Sharp, B., Mahomet, A., Bolin, R., Craven, R., and Enloe, C. (1975). Attempts to embellish a totally unscientific process with an aura of science [Letter to the editor]. *American Journal of Nursing, 75*, 1275.

Weber, R. (1981). Philosophical foundations and frameworks for healing. In M. A. Borelli and P. Heidt (Eds.), *Therapeutic touch: A book of readings* (p. 13). New York: Springer Publishing.

Weber, R. (1990). A philosophical perspective on touch. In K. E. Barnard and T. B. Brazelton (Eds.), *Touch: The foundation of experience* (p. 11). Madison, WI: International Universities Press.

Wells-Federman, C. L. (1995). And still more on TT [Letter to the editor]. *Research in Nursing and Health, 18*, 472.

Winstead-Fry, P. (1983). *A report to the profession: Nursing research emphasis grant: Families and parenting.* New York: Division of Nursing, New York University.

Wirth, D. P., and Cram, J. R. (1993). Multi-site electromyographic analysis of non-contact therapeutic touch. *International Journal of Psychosomatics, 40*(1), 47.

Wirth, D. P., Richardson, J. T., Eidelman, W. S., and O'Malley, A. (1993). Full thickness dermal wounds treated with non-contact therapeutic touch: Replication and extension. *Complementary Therapies in Medicine,* 127.

Wolfson, I. S. (1990). Therapeutic touch and midwifery. In K. E. Barnard and T. B. Brazelton (Eds.), *Touch: The foundation of experience* (p. 383). Madison, WI: International Universities Press.

Woods-Smith, D. (1988). Therapeutic touch: A healing experience. *Maine Nursing, 74*(2), 3, 7.

Wright, S. M. (1987). The use of therapeutic touch in the management of pain. *Nursing Clinics of North America, 22*, 704.

Wright, S. M. (1991). Validity of the human energy field assessment form. *Western Journal of Nursing Research, 13*, 635.

Wuthnow, S. W., and Miller, A. (1987). Should Christian nurses practice therapeutic touch? *Journal of Christian Nursing, 4*(4), 15.

Wyatt, G. (1988). *Therapeutic touch: promoting and assessing conceptual change among health care professionals.* Doctoral dissertation, Michigan State University (UMI No. 8900128).

Wyatt, G. (1989). Keeping the caring touch in the high-tech maze. *Michigan Hospital, 25*(5), 6.

Wytias, C. A. (1994). Therapeutic touch in primary care. *Nurse Practitioner Forum, 5*(2), 91.

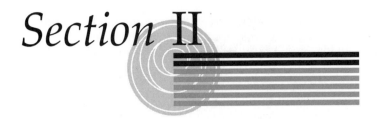

Section II

Physiological: Complex Interventions

Overview: Care That Supports Homeostatic Regulation

Gloria M. Bulechek

Joanne C. McCloskey

The interventions in this section require an in-depth understanding of normal body function, compensatory mechanisms for alterations in function, and the use of technology and drugs to treat dysfunction. These interventions are now used in settings other than hospitals and critical care units and are often done in long-term care settings, schools, and the home. The 12 interventions in this section illustrate the complex nature of clinical judgment required of the nurse and the comprehensive responsibility that is assumed.

Pressure Ulcer Prevention involves a constellation of activities designed to alleviate risk factors for pressure sore development. In Chapter 10, Barbara J. Braden and Nancy Bergstrom review the many factors that lead to pressure sore development and provide a conceptual model of these factors. The chapter also features the Braden Scale for assessing pressure sore risk. The research base and the appropriate use of various intervention activities are discussed. Activities include frequent repositioning, use of pillows or wedges, use of protective devices for bony prominences, monitoring the elevation of the head of the bed, use of lifting devices, and use of special mattresses and beds. The choice of activities depends on the goal of the intervention and the level of risk. Two case studies demonstrate the use of the Braden Scale to determine the level of risk and the choice of intervention activities.

In Chapter 11, **Pressure Ulcer Care,** Rita A. Frantz and Sue Gardner review the phases of pressure ulcer healing to provide a framework for clinical decision making in application of the intervention's activities. The inflammatory phase begins with tissue injury and tissue death and concludes with complete removal of necrotic tissue from the wound. The second phase of pressure ulcer healing is the proliferative phase. Cells regenerate and granulation tissue fills the wound, with re-epithelialization of the wound surface. The final phase of maturation takes place over a period of years as new collagen fibers add strength to the wound. Nursing action during the inflammatory phase focuses on provision of a moist wound environment, control of bacteria, provision of essential substrates, and prevention of further injury. Frantz was a member of the Agency for Health Care Policy and Research (AHCPR) guideline panel that developed *Treatment of Pressure Ulcers,* and the authors illustrate the congruence between the activities in the intervention Pressure Ulcer Care and the activities in the AHCPR guideline. The authors recommend that the diagnosis Pressure Ulcer be added to the North American Nursing Diagnosis Association (NANDA) taxonomy. The Nursing Outcomes Classification (NOC) outcome Wound Healing: Secondary Intention articulates with the Nursing Interventions Classification (NIC) intervention of Pressure Ulcer Care, but the authors speculate that intermediate measures of progress will be needed to capture the sequential nature and prolonged time for wound closure. The case study illustrates this point very clearly.

Teaching: Preoperative is an intervention that is widely used. It consists of structured information tailored to levels of anxiety. The nurse prepares patients for what to expect postoperatively and to cope with the threat behind the anxiety about surgery. In Chapter 12, Lori Butcher first reviews the research base that supports the design of the intervention and then summarizes the research base in a model for research-based preoperative teaching. The intervention, which is both structured and flexible, promotes a sense of control over the situation. Butcher offers creative ways to deliver the known, effective components of this intervention in the current health care environment of same-day surgery and early discharge. Butcher identifies several patient outcomes that can be influenced by this intervention. The chapter concludes with a case study.

Medication Management is defined as the facilitation of safe and effective use of prescription and over-the-counter drugs. In Chapter 13, Madeline A. Naegle reviews the broad base of nursing knowledge required to implement this intervention. This includes knowledge about the medication, a complete assessment of the client and family, and understanding of the nurse's scope of practice. Agency policies and procedures, as well as practice protocols, provide guidance in implementation of this intervention. Collaboration with other health professionals is essential. The chapter contains two case studies, one of a chronic drug abuser and another of a patient with a newly diagnosed condition, that illustrate the implementation of the intervention. Associated NANDA diagnoses and NOC outcomes are listed in tables.

Another important intervention in the Physiological: Complex Interventions domain is **Fluid Management.** In Chapter 14, Alice S. Poyss reviews the extensive knowledge base needed to implement this intervention. This includes an excellent review of normal fluid balance, thirst, output, and fluid volume imbalances. The cornerstone of achieving fluid balance is the daily intake and output record. Close monitoring can detect fluid imbalance while it can still be corrected with oral fluids. Although the prescription of the specific intravenous fluid is the usual role of the physician, this author has demonstrated that the nursing role in Fluid Management is important for early detection and prevention of complications. The associated nursing diagnoses are specified, and two new diagnoses are suggested. The associated nurse-sensitive outcomes are identified, and a case study of an elderly woman shows how the intervention can be applied.

In Chapter 15, Marita G. Titler and Michele A. Alpen present the intervention of **Airway Management.** The authors synthesize the large literature base surrounding this intervention into four parts: monitoring, positioning, artificial airway insertion, and secretion removal. Considerable research has been done that is giving direction to practice, and the authors identify additional areas where study is needed. Airway Management is a global intervention that can be used with diverse patient populations. The authors identify several other NIC interventions that could be an adjunct to Airway Management. Associated NANDA diagnoses and NOC outcomes are also identified. A table lists associated diagnoses, interventions, and outcomes, showing the various appropriate linkages, and a case study illustrates application of the intervention with a trauma patient. The chapter also includes an extensive reference list.

The administration of chemotherapy, like many other complex medical therapies, is moving to the outpatient and home setting. In Chapter 16, Mary H. Wegenka describes the intervention of **Chemotherapy Management,** which includes nursing activities that prepare the patient and family to manage the self-care activities needed to respond to the side effects and toxicities of chemotherapy. Common side effects such as myelosuppression, nausea and vomiting, alopecia, stomatitis, anorexia, altered elimination, and fatigue are reviewed. Nationally accepted guidelines for administration of chemotherapy are identified, as are tools for teaching to help the reader find the specific information needed to work with this population. The associated list of nursing diagnoses and nurse-sensitive outcomes is lengthy for this important nursing intervention. The chapter concludes with a case study of a 38-year-old woman receiving chemotherapy for breast cancer.

Conscious Sedation is an intervention that has become more widely used as invasive medical treatments and procedures have moved to the outpatient setting. Nurses who are involved with implementing this intervention need specialized knowledge and skill in required administration and monitoring activities. In Chapter 17, Steven J. Somerson, Susan W. Somerson, and Michael R. Sicilia review the commonly used drugs and summarize the drug action in a table. They present an overview of the levels of sedation as well as the symptoms that should be monitored. The authors stress that the nurse must be able to quickly recognize signs of respiratory or cardiovascular complications and be prepared to resuscitate the patient if necessary. The patient must be positioned and protected to prevent injury while in an altered state of consciousness. Standards and guidelines are available from national bodies to help agencies develop a safe protocol and adequately train staff to conduct this intervention. The chapter concludes with a case study.

In Chapter 18, Meg Gulanick and Carol Ruback review the various types of shock and outline the nursing diagnoses and nursing outcomes associated with this life-threatening event. They overview **Shock Management** as an intervention with four components: prioritizing surveillance, maintaining tissue perfusion, maintaining vital organ function, and providing emotional support. The numerous nursing activities required to carry out the components of the intervention are described and displayed in a table. A case study illustrates that nursing judgment and action to implement the intervention are the key factors in patient survival.

The intervention of **Hypoglycemia Management** is a treatment that every nurse needs to be able to implement. According to the American Diabetes Association (ADA), 1,700 people are diagnosed with diabetes every day. Current recommendations established by the ADA are based on evidence that strict control of blood glucose levels in persons with type 1 and type 2 diabetes reduces the risk of long-term complications. Intensified regimens to normalize blood glucose levels are increasing the frequency and severity of hypoglycemic episodes. In Chapter 19, Vicki L. Kraus describes the symptoms and incidence of hypoglycemia and stresses the individualized nature of the event. All patients, and those around them, must learn to recognize early symptoms and be prepared to take immediate action. The chapter gives recommendations on 15 g sources of carbohydrate, with guidelines on frequency of administration to keep blood glucose at a safe level and a case study illustrating application of the guidelines.

In Chapter 20, Mary Kay Bader and Linda Littlejohns describe implementation of **Intracranial Pressure Monitoring.** They identify six categories of activities: (1) preparation and monitoring, (2) airway management, (3) cerebral perfusion management, (4) positioning, (5) stimulation and regulation of the environment, and (6) thermoregulation. Types of intracranial pressure devices and their correct placement are described. Normal and abnormal waveform patterns are illustrated. The authors stress that intracranial pressure is just one variable to consider in the total clinical picture. The nurse must be knowledgeable about neurological assessment and the pathophysiological changes of the clinical state to successfully perform this intervention. The authors identify clinical guidelines to direct nursing action. The chapter concludes with a case study.

Barbara J. Holtzclaw begins Chapter 21 with a review of fever, and the febrile episode is illustrated in a figure. Mildly elevated fever is viewed as a benefit that can create a hostile environment for several microorganisms. Current work on the substances that evoke fever is producing emerging information about approaches to clinical management of fever. Holtzclaw discusses implementation of **Fever Treatment** in three areas. First, she discusses the instruments and techniques for detecting temperature elevation. It cannot be assumed that skin, oral, rectal, or tympanic membrane temperatures vary consistently. Second, she discusses the activities used to stabilize the thermoregulatory set point. Medications to treat an infection or allergic response are often needed. Antipyretic drugs are used more for comfort than for reducing mild temperature elevations. Supportive care to maintain fluid balance is crucial. The third set of activities to suppress febrile shivering includes supportive care and, possibly, medications. The author describes the best practice for use of a cooling blanket for dangerously high temperatures. Relevant diagnoses and outcomes are identified, and the chapter concludes with a case study.

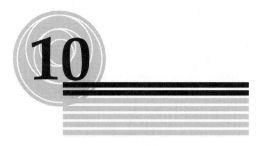

Pressure Ulcer Prevention

Barbara J. Braden and Nancy Bergstrom

DEFINITION AND DESCRIPTION OF THE INTERVENTION

Pressure Ulcer Prevention involves a constellation of activities designed to alleviate or eliminate risk factors for pressure sore development. These risk factors may be classified as contributing either to the intensity and duration of pressure or to diminished tissue tolerance for pressure (Braden & Bergstrom, 1987) (Fig. 10–1). Intensity and duration of pressure are, by definition, the most important factors in pressure ulcer development. Tissue tolerance, however, refers to the ability of the skin and supporting structures to resist or succumb to the adverse effects of pressure.

The primary clinical determinants of exposure to intense and prolonged pressure are activity, mobility, and sensory perception. The clinical determinants of tissue tolerance for pressure can be classified as either intrinsic or extrinsic. Extrinsic factors are physical factors that weaken the outer layers of the skin, making it more susceptible to the effects of pressure. Examples of these factors are moisture, friction, and shear. Intrinsic factors are those influencing either the supporting structures of the skin or the physiological processes in such a way that tissue injury occurs at lower external pressures. These factors include such conditions as low arteriolar pressure, aging skin, and malnutrition.

Prevention of pressure ulcers involves intervening to eliminate or ameliorate these risk factors in the hope of mitigating the potentially negative effect. Because a pressure ulcer does not occur without exposure to pressure, the most crucial intervention is pressure reduction. Pressure reduction refers to an abatement of the mechanical load exerted over parts of the body that interface with another surface. This external mechanical load may be experienced as

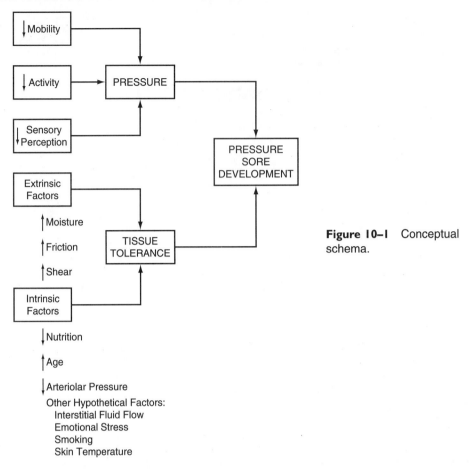

Figure 10–1 Conceptual schema.

either normal (direct) pressure or tangential loading (shear) (Bennett, Kavner, Lee, Trainor, & Lewis, 1984). The primary objective of pressure reduction as a nursing intervention is to maintain capillary blood flow to prevent ischemic injury to the tissues. Provision of comfort may be either a primary or a secondary objective of pressure reduction. Even in cases where tissue tolerance for pressure is a serious problem (e.g., the person is severely hypotensive or malnourished), pressure reduction is paramount.

Pressure reduction is an intervention that may be achieved by using a variety of strategies. Those strategies can be generally characterized as involving either (1) repositioning to achieve temporary pressure reduction and relief over some bony prominence or (2) altering the physical properties of the support surface. Reduction of pressure at the interface of a support surface is usually achieved by providing a surface for sitting or lying positions that disperses pressure over a larger surface area of the body, thereby reducing pressure over bony prominence. Complete pressure relief at a support surface–bony prominence interface is difficult, if not impossible, to achieve. Pressure relief over a given bony prominence, however, may be achieved for a period of time by frequent repositioning.

LITERATURE RELATED TO THE INTERVENTION

The relationship of pressure to tissue necrosis has been studied extensively, and several features of this phenomenon are well documented. Important features of

the pressure-tissue necrosis phenomenon are that low external loads of prolonged duration are at least as likely to damage tissues as is high pressure of
shorter duration (Daniel, Priest, & Wheatley, 1981; Dinsdale, 1974; Husain, 1953)
and that muscle is much more susceptible to the destructive effects of pressure
than is normothermic skin (Daniel et al., 1981).

A great deal of variability has been found in the intensity and duration of
pressure required to produce necrosis. It appears that the amount and duration
of pressure required to damage the skin can be mediated by intrinsic and
extrinsic factors that alter the ability of the tissues to tolerate pressure.

Friction is a classic example of a factor that alters tissue tolerance for pressure.
Dinsdale (1974) found that the skin of normal swine, when pretreated with
friction, sustained ischemic injury after being subjected to only 45 mm Hg of
pressure, whereas in the absence of friction a pressure of 290 mm Hg was
required to produce ischemic injury.

Other examples of factors that alter tissue tolerance abound. Maceration of
the skin from excess exposure to moisture can decrease tissue tolerance by
decreasing tensile strength of the skin (Flam, 1987), and certain sources of
moisture, such as loose stools, are particularly harmful. Normal changes in the
mechanical properties of collagen and elastin that occur with aging can increase
the compressibility of the tissues (Kenney, 1982; Krouskop, 1983) and make the
tissues more susceptible to both direct pressure and shearing forces (Bennett et
al., 1984). Likewise, persons who are undernourished and underweight have
tissues that deform more easily and therefore tend to develop higher interface
pressures than do persons who are overweight (Ferguson-Pell, 1990). Bergstrom
and Braden (1992) found that current dietary intake of protein was a particularly
strong predictor of which subjects would develop pressure ulcers. Finally, blood
pressure has been found to affect capillary dynamics to the extent that subjects
who were hypertensive were able to withstand higher external loads before
vascular occlusion occurred than those subjects who were normotensive (Larsen,
Holstein, & Lassen, 1979), whereas subjects who were hypotensive were more
likely to develop pressure ulcers than those who were normotensive (Bergstrom & Braden, 1992). These and many other individual differences can contribute to diminished tissue tolerance and therefore to differences in the intensity
and duration of pressure required to produce necrosis.

Because there is no single answer to questions regarding the intensity and
duration of pressure required to produce tissue necrosis at various sites on
the human body, certain generalities apply to preventive protocols. Frequent
repositioning as a means of temporary pressure relief and reduction has long
been the backbone of preventive protocols. Frequent pressure relief is essential,
not only to prevent direct tissue injury, but also to allow occult tissue injury to
heal before repetitive subclinical pressure insults lead to perceptible skin breakdown. Norton, McLaren, and Exton-Smith (1962) found that a program of
repositioning high-risk patients every 2 to 3 hours was successful in decreasing
the number and severity of pressure ulcers as compared with a program in
which similar groups received local skin care (creams and cleansers) only. Still,
nine of these patients developed pressure ulcers that might have been prevented
by more frequent turning or a pressure-reducing support surface.

There is some evidence that small shifts in body weight might be important
in preventing pressure ulcers. Exton-Smith and Sherwin (1961) studied the
relationship between pressure ulcer development and the mean number of
spontaneous body movements that elderly patients newly admitted to a geriatric
unit made from 11 PM to 6 AM. Of the 50 subjects studied, 10 subjects had, on

the average, fewer than 20 spontaneous body movements per night, and 9 of these subjects developed a pressure ulcer. Only one other subject developed a pressure ulcer, and while her mean movement score was 23, erythema developed on a night the score fell to 15, and a frank sacral sore was seen two nights later when the score for that night had fallen to 7. Twenty-eight of the 50 subjects had mean nightly movement scores greater than 50, and, of these, 9 had mean scores greater than 110. Because of instrumentation artifacts that occurred with major movements, the movements recorded in the lower ranges have been assumed to represent small shifts in body weight.

Several investigators have attempted to demonstrate that protocols incorporating small shifts in body weight (whether provided by the nurse or by the patient) are effective in preventing pressure ulcers. Brown, Boosinger, Black, and Gaspar (1985) studied 15 at-risk subjects: 7 receiving usual care and 8 receiving usual care and small shifts in body weight. None of the subjects receiving small shifts in body weight developed pressure ulcers, whereas one of the seven subjects receiving usual care developed two pressure ulcers. In a subsequent study, researchers examined the effects of small shifts on interface pressure by measuring interface pressure at 5-minute intervals over a 15-minute period of time before and after a small shift. They found that small shifts significantly decreased interface pressure, although they were unable to conclude whether this difference would be great enough to prevent pressure ulcers (Oertwich, Kindschuh, & Bergstrom, 1995).

Other investigators, using instrumented wheelchair seating, attempted to demonstrate that pressure ulcer development in a spinal-cord-injured patient would be related to the frequency of small shifts in body weight performed by the patient (Merbitz, King, Bleiberg, & Grip, 1985; Patterson & Fisher, 1986). They found, instead, that no pressure ulcers developed despite widely varying and sometimes multihour periods of exposure to sitting pressures exceeding the usual acceptable intensity level. None of these studies, however, had a large enough sample to warrant acceptance or rejection of small shifts in body weight as a preventive strategy.

Other investigators have examined the effect of various body positions on interface pressure. Garber, Campion, and Krouskop (1982) found that the traditional side-lying position in which the superior leg is flexed (55- to 65-degree hip flexion, 80-degree knee flexion), positioned ahead of the midline of the body, and supported by a pillow produced very high trochanteric pressures in normal and spinal-cord–injured subjects. Significant reduction in trochanteric pressure ($p<.001$) was achieved in spinal-cord–injured subjects when the superior leg was extended (30-degree hip flexion, 35-degree knee flexion) and positioned behind the midline of the body. Seiler, Allen, and Stahelin (1986), in a related study, examined differences in transcutaneous partial pressure of oxygen (tc PO_2) at the site of the trochanter when subjects were positioned in a 90-degree lateral position and a 30-degree lateral position on a normal hospital mattress and on a "super-soft" mattress. They found that, regardless of mattress, trochanteric tc PO_2 decreased significantly from baseline when the subject was positioned in the 90-degree lateral position but did not decrease significantly when the subject was positioned in the 30-degree lateral position. Consequently, these researchers recommend the 30-degree lateral position, with the patient's leg position determined by comfort alone.

Although good positioning and frequent repositioning can do much to prevent pressure ulcers, it may also be necessary to provide a support surface that reduces interface pressure over bony prominence. In the literature, these surfaces are generally categorized as mattress (or wheelchair) overlays, mattress replacements, or specialty beds. Mattress overlays and mattress replacements are considered to be either static (e.g., foam, gels) or dynamic (e.g., alternating pressure surfaces). Specialty beds are described as either low air loss or air fluidized. Investigators, then, evaluate these surfaces in either clinical trials or laboratory studies using such measures as interface pressures, skin oxygen tension, and blood flow. Both types of studies are important, but the strongest evidence would come from large randomized clinical trials.

There is a common and persistent perception that a support surface that consistently produces interface pressures of less than 32 mm Hg when tested with a variety of patients will prevent closure of the capillary bed and reduce the opportunity for ischemic injury. This figure represents the mean blood pressure obtained by Landis (1930) through cannulation of the arteriolar limb of capillaries in the fingernail beds. Interface pressures of 32 mm Hg obtained at other body sites cannot be assumed to protect against closure of the capillary beds at that site. Transmission of load through tissue and muscle mass may decrease or increase, depending on the body site and characteristics of the tissue at that site for any specific person (Ferguson-Pell, 1990; Le et al., 1984). For this reason and others, an interface pressure of 32 mm Hg should not be viewed as an absolute standard for evaluation of support surfaces. Interface pressure values may, however, be used as an index to compare pressure-reduction capabilities of support surfaces in circumstances where similar subjects and identical instruments and protocols are ensured.

Mattress overlays, mattress replacements, and specialty beds are commonly used to achieve pressure reduction. Research into the effectiveness of these devices is difficult to evaluate because differences in surfaces, subjects, instrumentation, and protocol invalidate many comparisons. There are a few areas, however, on which findings converge: (1) almost any surface tested reduced pressure below that of a standard hospital mattress (Bliss, McLaren, & Exton-Smith, 1967; Goldstone, Norris, O'Reilly, & White, 1982; Jacobs, 1989); (2) foam overlays that were 2 to 3 inches thick did not compare favorably with other pressure-reduction surfaces, including thicker foam overlays and mattress replacements (Krouskop, 1986; Stapleton, 1986); (3) high-density foam replacement mattresses are more effective in reducing pressure and preventing pressure ulcers than are foam overlays (Vyhlidal, Moxness, Bosak, Van Meter, & Bergstrom, 1997); (4) gel-filled overlays and mattresses reduce pressure better than most foam overlays (Berjian, Douglass, Holyoke, Goodwin, & Priore, 1983; Krouskop, 1986); (5) modular air mattresses and water mattresses reduce pressure better than foam mattress replacements; and (6) the air-fluidized bed results in substantial pressure reduction and appears to be beneficial in healing pressure ulcers, although results are not always dramatic (Allman et al., 1987; Bennett, Bellantoni, & Ouslander, 1989; Jackson, Chagares, Nee, & Freeman, 1988). Whatever support surface is used, it is important that the patient at risk for pressure ulcers be placed on the surface immediately, because Vyhlidal et al. (1997) found that several subjects developed ulcers between the time the foam was ordered and the time it was received and placed on the bed.

Foam is one of the products most frequently used in achieving pressure reduction. Kemp and Krouskop (1994) state that the nurse must be concerned with the thickness, stiffness, and density of the foam. Stiffness is measured by pressing a circular object (planten) 8 inches in diameter a certain percentage (usually 25%) into a 16 × 16 inch slab of foam and determining the force (in pounds) required to accomplish the compression. This measure is referred to as indentation load deflection (ILD). Density is a measure of the amount of material in foam, and the unit of measure is pounds per cubic foot. Kemp and Krouskop (1994) make recommendations for wheelchair seating and foam mattresses or overlays based on these measures. When the patient weighs between 50 and 300 pounds, foam wheelchair cushions should be 3 to 4 inches thick and have a 25% ILD between 40 and 70 pounds and a density between 1.3 and 2.8 pounds per cubic foot. The mattress overlay for the same patient should also be 3 to 4 inches thick and exhibit a 25% ILD of 30 pounds and a density of 1.3 to 2.5 pounds per cubic foot.

Other characteristics must be considered in a surface intended to reduce pressure and prevent pressure ulcers. According to Ferguson-Pell (1990), factors to appraise are (1) moisture accumulation and moisture resistance, (2) heat accumulation or loss, (3) sufficient stability to allow for ease of turning, (4) shifting and transferring, (5) frictional properties of the surface and cover, (6) cost, (7) durability and maintenance requirements, (8) flammability, and (9) safety. Because different products have differing abilities to reduce pressure, these additional factors may be used to evaluate the advantages and disadvantages of certain surfaces under individualized circumstances. For example, although there is some evidence that gel pads are somewhat more effective than thick foam in reducing pressure, it should be considered that gel pads or mattresses are heavy and difficult to handle and contribute to heat loss. This last factor would be a distinct disadvantage for a thin, elderly person who might become very cold if placed on gel, whereas it would be a distinct advantage for a person who is overweight and prone to heat accumulation.

In addition to these characteristics, nurses will be interested in whether special linens or bedmaking procedures are necessary and whether the surface is easy to clean, disinfect, and deodorize. Safety issues to consider include whether the surface increases the risk of falls because it raises the level of the support surface above or even with the siderail or is so slick that linens become a "sliding board" when patients are leaving the bed or chair.

Cost, durability, and maintenance requirements are of paramount importance in today's health care market. Although foam mattress replacements are relatively inexpensive and require little maintenance, these products may not retain their pressure-reducing properties for more than 2 to 3 years (Krouskop et al., 1994). In addition to replacement costs every 2 to 3 years, one must also consider the cost of foam disposal.

IDENTIFICATION OF INTERVENTION TOOLS

Instruments are available to measure the level of interface pressure and the effects of that pressure. These instruments include single-cell and multicell electropneumatic pressure sensors, laser Doppler flowmetry, and tc PO$_2$. Although these instruments are primarily research tools, it is becoming common for clinicians to use pressure sensors to assess the pressure-reduction qualities of support surfaces to justify decisions related to buying new surfaces or replacing those that have lost their pressure-reduction effectiveness. Clinicians who use this instrumentation should realize that the consistency of the pressure readings obtained depends greatly on positioning of the sensor and deformability of the tissues at the site (Allen, Ryan, & Murray, 1993).

Screening tools to determine presence and level of risk are, however, the primary clinical tools used to guide nursing activities aimed at Pressure Ulcer Prevention. Rating scales are the most common screening tools used by nurses to identify patients at risk for pressure ulcer development and have the advantage of being lower in cost, less invasive, and more accurate at predicting pressure ulcer development than other screening tools (e.g., serum albumin, hemoglobin). Although there are several rating scales in existence, only the Norton Scale and the Braden Scale for Predicting Pressure Sore Risk are recommended in the guidelines published by the Agency for Health Care Policy and Research (AHCPR) (U.S. Department of Health and Human Services [USDHHS], 1992). The Braden Scale tends to be more commonly used in the United States and has a higher degree of reliability and validity than other rating scales (Smith, Winsemius, & Besdine, 1991; Taylor, 1988).

The Braden Scale is composed of six subscales reflecting sensory perception, skin moisture, activity, mobility, nutritional intake, and friction and shear. All subscales are rated from 1 to 4, with the exception of the friction and shear subscale, which is rated from 1 to 3. Each rating is accompanied by a description of criteria for rating. Potential scores range from 6 to 23. The Braden Scale has been extensively tested (Bergstrom, Braden, Laguzza, & Holman, 1987; Bergstrom, Demuth, & Braden, 1987; Braden & Bergstrom, 1989). Interrater reliability for 86 pairs of observations by a graduate student and a registered nurse primary caregiver was reported to be r = 0.99 (p<.001). In two studies of predictive validity in hospitalized patients (N = 99, N = 100), sensitivity was 100%, and specificity ranged from 90% to 64% at a cut score of 16. Subsequent studies, however, indicate that a cut score of 18 may be more appropriate (Bergstrom, Braden, Champagne, Kemp, & Rudy, 1998; Ramundo, 1995).

SUGGESTED PROTOCOL

As nursing science develops, it is important that nursing interventions be evidenced based. The evaluation of the state of the science of interventions that involve multiple activities is arduous but important. The Clinical Guideline Panels convened by the AHCPR have conducted this evaluation. These guidelines should be incorporated into intervention protocols, provided clinicians continue to review and take into consideration more recent evidence. The following protocol is congruent with the related AHCPR Clinical Practice Guideline (USDHHS, 1992) and with the nursing activities associated with Pressure Ulcer Prevention as developed by the Iowa Intervention Project (McCloskey & Bulechek, 1996) (Table 10–1).

Risk Assessment

Pressure Ulcer Prevention involves multiple activities that may vary in degree of intensity. The intensity of a nursing intervention is strongly related to the specific risk factors being exhibited by the patient and the degree to which these risk factors are problematic. For this reason, nursing activities should be prescribed according to the total risk score as well as to scores on individual subscales of the risk assessment scale. Patients at risk for pressure ulcers should be identified on admission to health care agencies. All individuals at risk for developing pressure ulcers by virtue of their bedfast or chairfast status should be further assessed using an assessment tool to determine the level of risk and other associated risk factors. This assessment should take place on admission and 48 hours later. Reassessment should take place at periodic intervals, depending on the rapidity with which the condition changes, and whenever a major change occurs in the condition.

Risk assessment should be performed using an adequately tested risk assessment tool like the Braden Scale or the Norton Scale. The Braden Scale for

Table 10–1 Pressure Ulcer Prevention

DEFINITION: Prevention of pressure ulcers for a patient at high risk for developing them.

ACTIVITIES:
Use an established risk assessment tool to monitor patient's risk factors (e.g., Braden Scale)
Document skin status on admission and daily
Remove excessive moisture on the skin resulting from perspiration, wound drainage, and fecal or urinary incontinence
Apply protective barriers, such as creams or moisture-absorbing pads, to remove excess moisture, as appropriate
Apply transparent film occlusive dressing to areas at risk to protect skin from wetness
Turn every 1 to 2 hr continuously, as appropriate
Position prone, as appropriate
Turn with care to prevent injury to fragile skin
Post turning schedule at the bedside
Inspect skin over bony prominences and other pressure points when repositioning at least daily
Position with pillows to elevate pressure points off the bed
Keep bed linens clean, dry, and wrinkle free
Make bed with toe pleats
Avoid massaging pressure points
Moisturize dry, unbroken skin
Monitor any reddened areas closely
Apply elbow and heel protectors, as appropriate
Facilitate small shifts of body weight frequently
Provide trapeze to assist patient in shifting weight frequently
Ensure adequate nutrition, especially protein, vitamins B and C, iron, and calories, using supplements as appropriate

Source: McCloskey, J. C., and Bulechek, G. M. (1996). *Nursing interventions classification (NIC)* (p. 286). St. Louis: Mosby–Year Book.

Predicting Pressure Sore Risk (Bergstrom, Braden, et al., 1987) has demonstrated reliability and validity, has been tested in numerous clinical settings with easily achieved interrater reliability, and requires little time to administer (less than a minute when administered by the primary caregiver) (Fig. 10–2). The Norton Scale does not have operationalized levels for each of the subscales, and reliability has not been demonstrated through clinical studies. For this reason, the Braden Scale is recommended as the basis for risk assessment and clinical decision making.

Pressure ulcer risk increases as scores on the Braden Scale decrease. Scores of 15 to 18 indicate mild risk; scores of 12 to 14 indicate moderate risk; and scores below 12 indicate serious risk. The most important initial intervention for any level of risk is pressure reduction. The manner in which pressure reduction is achieved depends on the level of risk as indicated by the mobility and activity subscales of the Braden Scale. This can be further refined by an understanding of the sensory perception and friction and shear subscales. Individuals who are at mild to moderate risk based on scores of 2 or 3 on the activity or mobility subscales and who have other risk factors (e.g., incontinence, malnutrition) may need more protection from pressure than individuals without the additional risk factors.

Pressure-Reduction Strategies

Pressure reduction may be achieved through a variety of nursing activities and assistive devices. To reiterate briefly, these activities include frequent repositioning (q 2 hr in bed, q 1 hr in wheelchair), the use of pillows or wedges to keep bony prominence from direct contact, heel and other specific contact point protective devices, monitoring the elevation of the head of the bed, and using mattresses, overlays or replacements, seat cushions, specialty beds, and trapezes and other lifting devices. Nurses who are involved in making facilitywide or agencywide decisions concerning specific support surfaces should seek published data. The most useful data are provided by clinical trials that show that subjects using the device of interest develop fewer pressure ulcers than a group of subjects receiving basic nursing care. When this type of information is not available, comparisons of mean interface pressures for various surfaces may be used to estimate effectiveness of these products in producing pressure reduction. In addition to mean interface pressures, the nurse should examine the standard deviations surrounding mean interface pressures to determine the consistency with which the surface reduces pressure (Kemp & Krouskop, 1994).

Mild Risk

Mild risk is present when Braden Scale scores are 15 to 18 or activity and mobility subscale scores are 2 to 3. If other major risk factors not measured by the Braden Scale (low blood pressure, elevated temperature, fecal incontinence, advanced age, severe emaciation) are present, the nurse should advance to strategies appropriate for the next level of risk. Repositioning-related strategies may include using a turning or positioning schedule that is individualized to the patient's needs and planned around meals, bathing, and therapies. It is helpful to have the schedule at the bedside or to ensure in some other way that all staff caring for the patient are aware of the turning schedule. If the patient is thin and has poor muscle tone, only 30-degree lateral turns should be used. More assistance may be needed with positioning during the night or any time sedatives or narcotics are being used. If the turning schedule is faithfully followed, or the patient's mobility is expected to improve rapidly (e.g., postsurgical patient without complications), a pressure-reduction support surface may not be necessary. Individuals having difficulty with bed mobility may benefit from heel or elbow pads or a trapeze to reduce friction when being repositioned in bed. Comfort and pressure reduction may be enhanced through the use of pillows or other padding in lean individuals.

Moderate Risk

Moderate risk is present when Braden Scale scores are between 12 and 14 points or activity or mobility subscale scores are no higher than 2. Repositioning should be done with assistance and with attention to good body mechanics, using pillows and pads to protect bony prominence and heel and elbow protectors as needed for comfort. Lateral positioning should not exceed 30 degrees. Legs should be supported on pillows with the heels off the mattress when lying in the recumbent position. A pressure-reduction support surface (mattress overlays or mattress replacements) should be used. The pressure-reduction support surface does not reduce the importance of a documented repositioning schedule or the use of other protective devices. Trapezes and foam or stockinette heel and elbow pads may be useful in reducing friction.

High Risk

High risk is present when Braden Scale scores are below 12 points or activity or mobility subscale scores are below 2. This level of risk is even greater when

Braden Scale
FOR PREDICTING PRESSURE SORE RISK

Patient's Name _____ Evaluator's Name _____

	1.	2.	3.	4.	Date of Assessment	CASE 1	CASE 2
SENSORY PERCEPTION ability to respond meaningfully to pressure-related discomfort	1. Completely Limited: Unresponsive (does not moan, flinch, or grasp) to painful stimuli, due to diminished level of consciousness or sedation. OR Limited ability to feel pain over most of body surface.	2. Very Limited: Responds only to painful stimuli. Cannot communicate discomfort except by moaning or restlessness. OR Has a sensory impairment which limits the ability to feel pain or discomfort over ½ of body.	3. Slightly Limited: Responds to verbal commands, but cannot always communicate discomfort or need to be turned. OR Has some sensory impairment which limits ability to feel pain or discomfort in 1 or 2 extremities.	4. No Impairment: Responds to verbal commands. Has no sensory deficit which would limit ability to feel or voice pain or discomfort.		4	2
MOISTURE degree to which skin is exposed to moisture	1. Constantly Moist: Skin is kept moist almost constantly by perspiration, urine, etc. Dampness is detected every time patient is moved or turned.	2. Very Moist: Skin is often, but not always moist. Linen must be changed at least once a shift.	3. Occasionally Moist: Skin is occasionally moist, requiring an extra linen change approximately once a day.	4. Rarely Moist: Skin is usually dry, linen only requires changing at routine intervals.		2	1
ACTIVITY degree of physical activity	1. Bedfast: Confined to bed	2. Chairfast: Ability to walk severely limited or non-existent. Cannot bear own weight and/or must be assisted into chair or wheel-chair.	3. Walks Occasionally: Walks occasionally during day, but for very short distances, with or without assistance. Spends majority of each shift in bed or chair.	4. Walks Frequently: Walks outside the room at least twice a day and inside room at least once every 2 hours during waking hours.		2	1
MOBILITY ability to change and control body position	1. Completely Immobile: Does not make even slight changes in body or extremity position without assistance.	2. Very Limited: Makes occasional slight changes in body or extremity position but unable to make frequent or significant changes independently.	3. Slightly Limited: Makes frequent though slight changes in body or extremity position independently.	4. No Limitations: Makes major and frequent changes in position without assistance.		3	2

	1. Very Poor:	2. Probably Inadequate:	3. Adequate:	4. Excellent:		
NUTRITION *usual* food intake pattern	Never eats a complete meal. Rarely eats more than ⅓ of any food offered. Eats 2 servings or less of protein (meat or dairy products) per day. Takes fluids poorly. Does not take a liquid dietary supplement. OR Is NPO and/or maintained on clear liquids or IV's for more than 5 days.	Rarely eats a complete meal and generally eats only about ½ of any food offered. Protein intake includes only 3 servings of meat or dairy products per day. Occasionally will take a dietary supplement. OR Receives less than optimum amount of liquid diet or tube feeding.	Eats over half of most meals. Eats a total of 4 servings of protein (meat, dairy products) each day. Occasionally will refuse a meal, but will usually take a supplement if offered. OR Is on a tube feeding or TPN regimen which probably meets most of nutritional needs.	Eats most of every meal. Never refuses a meal. Usually eats a total of 4 or more servings of meat and dairy products. Occasionally eats between meals. Does not require supplementation.	3	3
	1. Problem:	2. Potential Problem:	3. No Apparent Problem:			
FRICTION AND SHEAR	Requires moderate to maximum assistance in moving. Complete lifting without sliding against sheets is impossible. Frequently slides down in bed or chair, requiring frequent repositioning with maximum assistance. Spasticity, contractures or agitation leads to almost constant friction.	Moves feebly or requires minimum assistance. During a move skin probably slides to some extent against sheets, chair, restraints, or other devices. Maintains relatively good position in chair or bed most of the time but occasionally slides down.	Moves in bed and in chair independently and has sufficient muscle strength to lift up completely during move. Maintains good position in bed or chair at all times.		2	1
			Total Score		16	10

Figure 10–2   Braden Scale for predicting pressure sore risk. (Copyright 1988, Barbara Braden and Nancy Bergstrom.)

other risk factors are present (e.g., hypotension, hyperpyrexia). Turning schedules should include either increased frequency of turns or assisted frequent, small shifts in body weight, and lateral turns should not exceed 30 degrees. High-quality foam wedges and pads should be used in positioning. When patients can tolerate the prone position, it should be added to the turning schedule, because it allows the most common sites of pressure ulcer formation (sacrum, trochanters, heels) to be totally relieved of pressure while also preventing flexion contractures of the hips. Impeccable padding and positioning are required if the prone position is to be used. A good pressure-reduction support surface is absolutely essential. Continued attention should be given to suspending the heels off the surface of the bed. Specialty beds are not generally required to prevent pressure ulcers in high-risk patients when adequate nursing care is available, unless these specialty beds are useful for prevention of additional problems.

It is also essential to remember that, in a program of Pressure Ulcer Prevention or treatment, pressure-reduction protocols address only one aspect of the problem, albeit the most crucial aspect. Risk factors that affect tissue tolerance (poor nutrition, exposure of the skin to moisture, friction and shear) must be controlled or ameliorated when possible.

Moisture

Activities to decrease exposure of the skin to moisture are indicated in patients who are experiencing urinary incontinence, fecal incontinence, or excessive perspiration. Urinary incontinence can be eliminated or ameliorated through a variety of short-term and long-term nursing interventions and activities (e.g., bladder training, prompted voiding, intermittent catheterization, pelvic floor exercises). Detailed protocols for assessing and intervening in urinary incontinence can be found in the AHCPR guidelines (USDHHS, 1996), and a full discussion of Intermittent Catheterization and Pelvic Floor Exercise can be found in Chapters 3 and 4. When incontinence cannot be or has not been avoided, the nurse should use a very mild soap to gently but thoroughly cleanse the skin, pat the skin dry, and apply a commercial moisture barrier. Absorbent underpads or briefs should be used, checked frequently, and changed as needed.

Fecal incontinence also increases risk for skin injury, but diarrheal stools are especially caustic to the skin and can lead quickly to skin breakdown. An attempt should be made to determine the cause of the diarrhea and eliminate that cause. If this does not bring quick results, a fecal incontinence bag should be used while further attempts are made to control the diarrhea.

Perspiration can also be problematic, especially when experienced in the magnitude seen in patients with neurological injuries accompanied by autonomic instability. Absorbent materials should be used beneath the patient and next to the patient's skin. Absorbent powders are generally not advisable, as the particles may collect in skin folds and actually become a source of skin injury. If perspiration is the result of a nonbreathing support surface, an alternative surface should be sought.

Friction and Shear

In patients whose skin is being exposed to friction and shear, there are several nursing activities that may be appropriate, depending on the areas of the body being exposed and the functional abilities of the patient. When movement in bed is causing friction and shear over the sacrum or trochanter, a trapeze or turning sheet can be very effective in preventing skin exposure. Because shearing and excessive sacral pressure begin to develop when the head of the bed is elevated more than 30 degrees, higher levels of elevation should be avoided when possible. When ankles and heels are exposed to friction and shear, socks or stockinette protectors may provide some protection. Transparent film or hydrocolloid dressings may also be used over exposed bony prominences to protect the underlying skin.

Nutritional Repletion

Patients who have long-term problems with nutrition are more prone to pressure sore development; however, it appears that immediate nutritional repletion, particularly for protein intake, can provide some protection (Bergstrom & Braden, 1992). It may be helpful to raise the protein intake beyond 100% of the recommended daily allowance (RDA), provided the patients have good liver and renal function. It is also helpful to enhance intake of sufficient calories from carbohydrates to spare the proteins. Although there is no direct evidence that any vitamin deficiency increases the risk for developing pressure ulcers, it is known that certain vitamins and minerals are important in building new tissue and healing injured tissue. It is possible, therefore, that a vitamin supplement containing vitamin C, vitamin A, and zinc may be helpful.

A consultation with a registered dietitian should be considered, particularly for patients being fed enterally. Many patients being fed enterally develop diarrhea, and this problem demands immediate attention. The composition of the feeding may require a change to a feeding with a lower osmolality, higher fiber content, or lack of artificial coloring. The potential for bacterial contamination from the feeding equipment should be addressed. Occasionally, antidiarrheal medication may be necessary.

General Care

All individuals found to be at risk for pressure ulcers should have routine, systematic (head-to-toe) examination of the skin. The frequency of this examination will vary with the level of risk and the independence of the individual. As a rule, daily examination of the skin may be adequate in inpatient settings, especially when this is coupled with evaluation of specific sites that become accessible during repositioning. The condition of the skin should be documented daily in acute care settings and weekly in long-term care settings. Tools to guide evaluation and documentation of skin condition are abundant, and one that is similar to those used in most clinical settings and has been tested and documented to be reliable and valid can be seen in Figure 10–3 (Bergstrom, 1990). It is extremely important to document the skin condition, because this documentation is necessary to demonstrate the effectiveness of nursing actions in meeting the goals of pressure reduction.

Good general skin hygiene is important, but it is essential to avoid drying the skin through excessive bathing with any but the mildest soaps. In an effort to keep skin supple and healthy, very mild, nondrying soaps should be used in bathing; skin moisturizers should be applied; adequate humidification of ambient air should be addressed; and good hydration should be maintained. Linens should be clean, dry, and wrinkle free, but it is important that sheets not be pulled taut over a pressure-reduction support surface, because this diminishes

Pressure Sore Data Collection Questionnaire
Skin Assessment Tool (Nurse II)

Name _____   ID Number _____

DATE OF OBSERVATION: _____   _____
                        Month   Day   Year

ASSESSMENT SITE*   SKIN CONDITION

	Size	Depth	Stage
1) Back of head	_____	_____	_____
2) Right ear	_____	_____	_____
3) Left ear	_____	_____	_____
4) Right scapula	_____	_____	_____
5) Left scapula	_____	_____	_____
6) Right elbow	_____	_____	_____
7) Left elbow	_____	_____	_____
8) Vertebrae (upper-mid)	_____	_____	_____
9) Sacrum	_____	_____	_____
10) Coccyx	_____	_____	_____
11) Right iliac crest	_____	_____	_____
12) Left iliac crest	_____	_____	_____
13) Right trochanter (hip)	_____	_____	_____
14) Left trochanter (hip)	_____	_____	_____
15) Right ischial tuberosity	_____	_____	_____
16) Left ischial tuberosity	_____	_____	_____
17) Right thigh	_____	_____	_____
18) Left thigh	_____	_____	_____
19) Right knee	_____	_____	_____
20) Left knee	_____	_____	_____
21) Right lower leg	_____	_____	_____
22) Left lower leg	_____	_____	_____
23) Right ankle (inner/outer)	_____	_____	_____
24) Left ankle (inner/outer)	_____	_____	_____
25) Right heel	_____	_____	_____
26) Left heel	_____	_____	_____
27) Right toe(s)	_____	_____	_____
28) Left toe(s)	_____	_____	_____
29) Other (specify)	_____	_____	_____

*Assess and record each site each observation time. Mark site(s) on figure below.

Stage key
Stage 0 No redness or breakdown
Stage 1 Erythema only: redness does not disappear for 24 hours after pressure is relieved
Stage 2 Break in skin such as blisters or abrasions
Stage 3 Break in skin exposing subcutaneous tissue
Stage 4 Break in skin extending through tissue and subcutaneous layers, exposing muscle or bone
Stage 9 Dark necrotic tissue. (Use this rating until tissue sloughs, then continue staging.)

Figure 10–3 Skin assessment sheet. (Copyright 1989, Nancy Bergstrom.)

its pressure-reducing characteristics. Toe pleats in the top linens should be used to avoid pressure on toes or feet.

Certain nursing activities that were once quite routine are now believed to be harmful and should be avoided. There is a possibility that massage of reddened bony prominences causes decreased perfusion and liquefaction of the underlying tissues, so this practice should be abandoned. This does not mean that massage should be abandoned as a comfort measure, but rather that it should be restricted to areas where skin is unbroken and uninjured, as evidenced by the absence of reactive hyperemia. Likewise, donuts and heat lamps have been found to increase the risk for skin injury rather than prevent it. Therefore, these items should not be used in patient care.

In addition, the overall goals for the patient must be considered when selecting the methods to be used to prevent or manage the treatment of pressure ulcers. Patients who are recovering from acute illness, are chronically ill, or are receiving rehabilitative care should have access to the best preventive and treatment strategies necessary. When patients are terminally ill and pressure ulcers may be a sign of general physical decline, the goal of care should be kept in mind. Terminally ill patients may have comfort as a goal. To meet this goal, less disruption and movement may be desired, and pressure reduction may involve more attention to support surfaces and less attention to turning schedules. The key point is that the goal of care should be known and a rational plan developed. Neglect is not to be condoned.

Finally, because some patients and their families will have to contend with ongoing risk for pressure ulcer development, it is important that a teaching plan be developed and delivered so this complex intervention may be carried out in the absence of a professional nurse. This teaching plan must be based on a thorough assessment of the patient's home environment and support system and recognize the abilities and disabilities of both the patient and the caregiver. It is especially important that patients be as involved as possible in their own repositioning. Patients should be encouraged to shift their weight frequently, make complete turns in bed when possible, and lift their buttocks off their chair seating every 15 minutes if possible. Assistance with patient teaching is available from the AHCPR in the form of consumer guidelines (USDHHS, 1992).

IDENTIFICATION OF ASSOCIATED NURSING DIAGNOSES AND APPROPRIATE CLIENT GROUPS

The primary North American Nursing Diagnosis Association (NANDA) diagnosis that always indicates the necessity for implementing the Pressure Ulcer Prevention intervention is Skin Integrity, Risk for Impaired. It should be noted that the activities included in this intervention are also appropriate for persons who have an existing pressure ulcer or are experiencing pressure-related discomfort or pain with movement. Nursing diagnoses directly associated with these client groups are Skin Integrity, Risk for Impaired; Pain; and Pain, Chronic. Other NANDA diagnoses commonly associated with the diagnosis Skin Integrity, Risk for Impaired are Activity Intolerance; Physical Mobility, Impaired; Nutrition: Less Than Body Requirements, Altered; and Tissue Perfusion, Altered: Peripheral.

PATIENT OUTCOMES SENSITIVE TO THE INTERVENTION

The primary Nursing Outcomes Classification (NOC) outcome affected by this intervention is Tissue Integrity: Skin & Mucous Membranes. In other words, one should expect a decrease in the incidence of pressure ulcers as well as a decrease in the severity of the pressure ulcers that sometimes develop despite use of the intervention. Because the nursing activities undertaken to prevent pressure ulcers are also part of promoting wound healing, it is appropriate to expect that this intervention will have an impact on Wound Healing: Secondary Intention. Additional outcomes that are influenced by this intervention are Pain Level, Immobility Consequences: Physiological, Nutritional Status, and, in some cases, Mobility Level. For patients who have the cognitive ability to learn, the outcomes of the educational activities that are part of the intervention are Knowledge: Treatment Regimen and Risk Control. If the patient with the cognitive ability to learn also has some upper- or low-body muscle function, the intervention should affect the outcome Body Positioning: Self-Initiated. When the patient does not have the functional ability to be independent in self-care, the outcomes affected are Caregiver Home Care Readiness and Caregiver Performance: Indirect Care.

CASE STUDIES

Case Study 1

Mrs. L is a 75-year-old woman who suffered a fractured hip in a fall at the grocery store and was admitted to an extended care facility 5 days after hip pinning surgery. She had a Braden Scale score of 16 when risk was assessed the day following admission, with a score of 2 on the activity, mobility, and friction and shear subscales. These scores were awarded because she was chairfast and too weak to make or maintain major changes in position or to lift up when moved. She had no deficits in sensory perception but was incontinent at night. She had been eating more than half of all meals served, but did not have much appetite and was underweight for her height. Because she was so light, she had a tendency to slide down in bed. Her temperature had been within normal range since admission, but her blood pressure had been only 106/74 mm Hg.

The plan for pressure reduction included a scheduled turning program that included q 2 hr turning from 8 PM to 10 AM, with lateral turns not to exceed 30 degrees and head-of-bed elevation not to exceed 30 degrees. Following morning care, when Mrs. L was up in a chair, the repositioning schedule increased to hourly. Mrs. L was not sufficiently strong to change her position in the chair but was encouraged to shift her weight as often as possible (leaning forward, leaning sideways). Ordinarily, at this level of risk, a meticulous turning schedule would have been sufficient, but because Mrs. L had several additional significant risks (low body weight, low blood pressure), the nurses decided to use a 4-inch foam mattress overlay and a 4-inch foam chair pad as well. Elbow and heel protectors were ordered to prevent friction injuries from occurring, but Mrs. L was deemed to have too little upper-arm strength to benefit from a trapeze. A turning sheet was used to reposition Mrs. L in bed. Nutritional supplementation, scheduled nighttime toileting, and a program of remobilization were also instituted.

As nutritional status improved and the program of remobilization began to improve Mrs. L's ability to initiate changes in body position and mobility level, she was able to transfer to a commode without assistance and was no longer incontinent at night. Her skin was inspected daily, and no problems with tissue integrity developed. The Braden Scale score rose to 18. As plans for discharge began to accelerate, she and her husband were instructed in risk control and the treatment regimen. Arrangements were made for a home care agency to provide continuing physical therapy and for a home health aide to assist Mrs. L with ambulation and continued recovery of self-care activities. At the time of discharge from the nursing home, Mrs. L was able to discuss most aspects of risk control and her treatment regimen. Her husband was able to fill in the aspects that Mrs. L sometimes forgot and was judged to be ready to deliver many aspects of her care, monitor her adherence to the treatment regimen, and provide oversight of care delivered by the home health aide.

Case Study 2

Miss W suffered a severe head injury in a car accident and was admitted to a skilled nursing facility in a chronic vegetative state following several weeks of stabilization in an acute care hospital. She was incapable of voluntary movement but moaned and winced occasionally and had some spastic movements in her lower extremities. The gastrostomy feedings she was receiving resulted in occasional liquid stools but eliminated earlier problems of regurgitation that had occurred with a nasogastric tube. Her skin was frequently moist because of bouts of profuse perspiration, and her total Braden Scale score was 10.

A scheduled turning program was implemented that included lateral turns not to exceed 30 degrees and head-of-bed elevation not to exceed 30 degrees. Because there was no possibility of eventual mobilization, the schedule also included positioning in the prone position for 1 to 2 hours every shift as a means to prevent hip flexion contractures and to provide multihour pressure relief on other bony prominences. Foam wedges were ordered to facilitate positioning, and foam-padded boots were obtained to prevent footdrop and decrease heel pressure. A thick foam mattress replacement was placed on the bed, and a schedule for periodic replacement was written in the nursing care plan. The osmolality of the gastrostomy feedings was adjusted to prevent the liquid stools, and bowel elimination was then facilitated with glycerin suppositories on Monday, Wednesday, and Friday.

SUMMARY

Nurses have struggled for many years with prevention and treatment of pressure ulcers, and pressure reduction has been the cornerstone of these efforts. Frequent repositioning is the nursing strategy traditionally used as a means to achieve pressure reduction. An assortment of high-technology approaches to pressure reduction have also become available, consisting primarily of specialty beds, but these are quite costly. Developing a rational plan of nursing actions that is effective in reducing pressure and appropriate to the individual's level of risk can be cost-efficient but requires knowledge of the current scientific base for this intervention. This knowledge, in conjunction with good nursing judgment concerning its appropriate application, will bring nursing closer to the goal of eliminating pressure ulcers from all health care settings.

References

Allen, V., Ryan, D. W., and Murray, A. (1993). Repeatability of subject/bed interface pressure measurements. *Journal of Biomedical Engineering, 15*, 329–332.

Allman, R. M., Walker, J. M., Hart, M., Laprade, C. A., Noel, L. B., and Smith, C. R. (1987). Air-fluidized beds or conventional therapy for pressure sores. *Annals of Internal Medicine, 107*, 641–648.

Bennett, L., Kavner, D., Lee, B. Y., Trainor, F. S., and Lewis, J. M. (1984). Skin stress and blood flow in sitting paraplegic patients. *Archives of Physical Medicine and Rehabilitation, 65*, 186–190.

Bennett, R. G., Bellantoni, M. F., and Ouslander, J. G. (1989). Air-fluidized bed treatment of nursing home patients with pressure sores. *Journal of the American Geriatrics Society, 37*, 235–242.

Bergstrom, N. (1990). *Nursing assessment of pressure sore risk* [Research proposal]. National Institutes of Health, National Center for Nursing Research.

Bergstrom, N., and Braden, B. (1992). A prospective study of pressure sore risk among institutionalized elderly. *Journal of the American Geriatrics Society, 40*, 747–758.

Bergstrom, N., Braden, B., Kemp, M., and Champagne, M. (1998). Reliability and validity of the Braden Scale: A multi-site study. *Nursing Research, 47*, 261–269.

Bergstrom, N., Braden, B., Laguzza, A., and Holman, A. (1987). The Braden Scale for predicting pressure sore risk. *Nursing Research, 36*, 205–210.

Bergstrom, N., Demuth, P. J., and Braden, B. J. (1987). A clinical trial of the Braden Scale for predicting pressure sore risk. *Nursing Clinics of North America, 22*, 417–428.

Berjian, R. A., Douglass, H. O., Jr., Holyoke, E. D., Goodwin, P. M., and Priore, R. L. (1983). Skin pressure measurements on various mattress surfaces in cancer patients. *American Journal of Physical Medicine, 62*, 217–226.

Bliss, M. R., McLaren, R., and Exton-Smith, A. N. (1967). Preventing pressure sores in hospital: Controlled trial of a large-celled ripple mattress. *British Medical Journal, 1*, 394–397.

Braden, B., and Bergstrom, N. (1987). A conceptual schema for the study of the etiology of pressure sores. *Rehabilitation Nursing, 12*(1), 8–12, 16.

Braden, B. J., and Bergstrom, N. (1989). Clinical utility of the Braden Scale for predicting pressure sore risk. *Decubitis, 2*(3), 44–51.

Brown, M. M., Boosinger, J., Black, J., and Gaspar, T. (1985). Nursing innovation for prevention of decubitus ulcers in long term care facilities. *Plastic Surgical Nursing, 5*(2), 57–64.

Daniel, R. K., Priest, D. L., and Wheatley, D. C. (1981). Etiologic factors in pressure sores: An experimental model. *Archives of Physical Medicine and Rehabilitation, 62,* 492–498.

Dinsdale, S. M. (1974). Decubitus ulcers: Role of pressure and friction in causation. *Archives of Physical Medicine and Rehabilitation, 55,* 147–152.

Exton-Smith, A. N., and Sherwin, R. W. (1961). The prevention of pressure sores: Significance of spontaneous bodily movements. *Lancet, 47,* 1124–1126.

Ferguson-Pell, M. W. (1990). Seat cushion selection: Technical considerations. *Journal of Rehabilitation Research and Development,* (Clinical Suppl. 2), 49–73.

Flam, E. (1987). Optimum skin aeration in pressure sore management [Abstract]. *Proceedings of the Annual Conference on Engineering in Medicine and Biology, 29,* 84.

Garber, S. L., Campion, L. J., and Krouskop, T. A. (1982). Trochanteric pressure in spinal cord injury. *Archives of Physical Medicine and Rehabilitation, 63,* 549–552.

Goldstone, L. A., Norris, M., O'Reilly, M., and White, J. (1982). A clinical trial of a bead bed system for the prevention of pressure sores in elderly orthopaedic patients. *Journal of Advanced Nursing, 7,* 545–548.

Husain, T. (1953). An experimental study of some pressure effects on tissues, with reference to the bedsore problem. *Journal of Pathology and Bacteriology, 66,* 347–358.

Jackson, B. S., Chagares, R., Nee, N., and Freeman, K. (1988). The effects of a therapeutic bed on pressure ulcers: An experimental study. *Journal of Enterostomal Therapy, 15,* 220–226.

Jacobs, M. A. (1989). Comparison of capillary blood flow using a regular hospital bed mattress, ROHO mattress, and Mediscus bed. *Rehabilitation Nursing, 14,* 270–272.

Kemp, M. G., and Krouskop, T. A. (1994). Pressure ulcers: Reducing incidence and severity by managing pressure. *Journal of Gerontological Nursing, 20*(9), 27–34, 46–47.

Kenney, R. A. (1982). *Physiology of aging: A synopsis.* Chicago: Year Book Medical Publishers.

Krouskop, T. A. (1983). A synthesis of the factors that contribute to pressure sore formation. *Medical Hypotheses, 11,* 255–267.

Krouskop, T. A. (1986). *The effect of surface geometry on interface pressures generated by polyurethane foam mattress overlays* [Compilation of reports]. Houston, TX: The Rehabilitation Engineering Center, Institute for Rehabilitation and Research.

Krouskop, T. A., Randall, C., Davis, J., Garber, S., Williams, S., and Callaghan, R. (1994). Evaluating the long-term performance of a foam-core hospital replacement mattress. *Journal of WOCN, 21,* 241–246.

Landis, E. (1930). Studies of capillary blood pressure in human skin. *Heart, 15,* 209–228.

Larsen, B., Holstein, P., and Lassen, N. A. (1979). On the pathogenesis of bedsores. *Scandinavian Journal of Plastic and Reconstructive Surgery, 13,* 347–350.

Le, K. M., Madsen, B. L., Barth, P. W., Ksander, G. A., Angell, J. B., and Vistnes, L. M. (1984). An in-depth look at pressure sores using monolithic silicon pressure sensors. *Plastic and Reconstructive Surgery, 74,* 745–754.

McCloskey, J. C., and Bulechek, G. M. (Eds.). (1996). *Nursing interventions classification (NIC)* (2nd ed.). St. Louis: Mosby-Year Book.

Merbitz, C. T., King, R. B., Bleiberg, J., and Grip, J. C. (1985). Wheelchair push-ups: Measuring pressure relief frequency. *Archives of Physical Medicine and Rehabilitation, 66,* 433–438.

Norton, D., McLaren, R., and Exton-Smith, A. N. (1962). *An investigation of geriatric nursing problems in hospitals.* London: National Corporation for the Care of Old People.

Oertwich, P. A., Kindschuh, A. M., and Bergstrom, N. (1995). The effects of small shifts in body weight on blood flow and interface pressure. *Research in Nursing and Health, 18,* 481–488.

Patterson, R. P., and Fisher, S. V. (1986). Sitting pressure-time patterns in patients with quadriplegia. *Archives of Physical Medicine and Rehabilitation, 67,* 812–814.

Ramundo, J. M. (1995). Reliability and validity of the Braden Scale in the home care setting. *Journal of WOCN, 22,* 128–134.

Seiler, W. O., Allen, S., and Stahelin, H. B. (1986). Influence of the 30 degrees laterally inclined position and the "super-soft" 3-piece mattress on skin oxygen tension on areas of maximum pressure—Implications for pressure sore prevention. *Gerontology, 32*(3), 158–166.

Smith, D. M., Winsemius, D. K., and Besdine, R. W. (1991). Pressure sores in the elderly: Can this outcome be improved? *Journal of General Internal Medicine, 6*(1), 81–93.

Stapleton, M. (1986). Preventing pressure sores—An evaluation of three products. *Geriatric Nursing, 6*(2), 23–25.

Taylor, K. J. (1988). Identification of patients at risk for pressure sores. *Journal of Enterostomal Therapy, 15,* 201–205.

U.S. Department of Health and Human Services, Panel for Prediction and Prevention of Pressure Ulcers. (1992). *Preventing pressure ulcers: A patient's guideline* (AHCPR Publication No. 92-0048). Rockville, MD: Author.

U.S. Department of Health and Human Services, Panel for Urinary Incontinence. (1996). *Urinary incontinence in adults: Acute and chronic management* (AHCPR Publication No. 96-0682). Rockville, MD: Author.

Vyhlidal, S. K., Moxness, D., Bosak, K. S., Van Meter, F. G., and Bergstrom, N. (1997). Mattress replacement or overlay: A prospective study on the incidence of pressure ulcers. *Applied Nursing Research. 10,* 111–120.

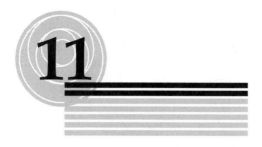

Pressure Ulcer Care

Rita A. Frantz and Sue Gardner

Pressure ulcers commonly occur among aged and functionally impaired patients. A pressure ulcer is a localized area of soft tissue necrosis over a bony prominence resulting from prolonged pressure over the area. Prolonged pressure causes tissue ischemia and necrosis. Pressure ulcers heal slowly, and the management of pressure ulcers must be directed at supporting the normal biological sequences of wound healing.

The integral role of nursing in managing pressure ulcers is delineated in the Nursing Interventions Classification (NIC) intervention Pressure Ulcer Care (McCloskey & Bulechek, 1996), which appears in Table 11–1. The Pressure Ulcer Care intervention is composed of 17 specific activities used by nurses to facilitate pressure ulcer healing. The activities include the assessment and care of the pressure ulcer wound as well as the assessment and support of systemic factors that promote the wound-healing process.

PRESSURE ULCER HEALING

Optimal pressure ulcer management is dependent on a clear understanding of the biological events that lead to pressure ulcer healing. Pressure ulcers are wounds caused by localized ischemic tissue death due to prolonged pressure (Kosiak, 1961). Pressure ulcer healing is a complex biological process of necrotic tissue removal, tissue synthesis, and scar formation. These processes require adequate substrates, including oxygen, vitamins, minerals, amino acids, and energy (Hunt & VanWinkle, 1979). When these substrates are available in adequate amounts, the repair process occurs in a predictable manner, with identifi-

Table 11–1   Pressure Ulcer Care

DEFINITION: Facilitation of healing in pressure ulcers.

ACTIVITIES:

Measure and describe characteristics of the ulcer at regular intervals

Determine level of ulcer formation: stage I to IV

Keep the ulcer moist to aid in healing

Cleanse the skin around the ulcer with mild soap and water

Protect surrounding skin from moisture by using petroleum jelly, if using wet dressings

Cleanse the ulcer with the appropriate nontoxic solution, working in a circular motion from the center

Use a 19-gauge needle and 35-cc syringe to clean deep ulcers

Note characteristics of any drainage

Debride ulcer, as needed

Apply a permeable membrane to the ulcer, as appropriate

Apply saline soaks, as appropriate

Apply ointments, as appropriate

Apply dressings, as appropriate

Position to avoid prolonged pressure on other sites

Monitor for signs and symptoms of infection in the wound

Increase protein intake to help rebuild epidermal tissue, as appropriate

Monitor calorie intake to ensure adequate intake

Source: McCloskey, J. C., and Bulechek, G. M. (1996). *Nursing interventions classification (NIC).* St. Louis: Mosby–Year Book.

able phases that overlap one another. These are the inflammatory, the proliferative, and the maturation phases (Hunt, 1979).

The inflammatory phase begins with tissue injury and tissue death. During the inflammatory phase, neutrophils and monocytes are attracted to the wound site. In the wound, these white blood cells control microorganisms, autolyse and denature the proteins of dead tissue (Majno & Joris, 1995), and stimulate fibroblast production of collagen and angiogenesis (Hunt & VanWinkle, 1979). Of the two white blood cell types, monocytes are believed to play the major role.

Inflammatory processes, including the proteinolytic activity of neutrophils and monocytes, change the cellular characteristics of dead tissue to clinically observable necrotic tissue (Majno & Joris, 1995). Based on experimentally induced ischemic animal wounds (Sakharov, Glyanzev, Litvin, & Savvina, 1993), clinically observable changes are not expressed until 3 to 6 days after tissue death. Because stage 3 and 4 pressure ulcers are the result of ischemic tissue death (Kosiak, 1959), these pressure ulcers contain necrotic tissue in the initial stage of their natural history.

The actions of neutrophils and monocytes (i.e., protein autolysis and denaturation) eventually result in the complete removal of necrotic tissue from the wound bed. However, the time required for complete removal of necrotic tissue and completion of the inflammatory phase of healing is generally more prolonged with a pressure ulcer than with an acute wound (i.e., 3 to 5 days) (McPherson & Piez, 1988). The prolonged inflammatory phase can be attributed to the greater amount of necrotic tissue in pressure ulcers, which results in a large-volume tissue defect (i.e., loss of tissue) as the necrotic tissue is removed. Complete removal of necrotic tissue from the wound is widely regarded as an essential first step in wound healing (Agren & Stromberg, 1985; Bale & Harding, 1990; Bergstrom et al., 1994; Lee & Ambrus, 1975).

The second phase of wound healing is the proliferative phase. The proliferative phase is characterized by fibroblast proliferation, collagen synthesis, and angiogenesis (Hunt & VanWinkle, 1979). The result of collagen deposition and angiogenesis is clinically described as granulation tissue. Granulation tissue fills the tissue defect of the wound and eventually becomes scar tissue. In addition, contraction of the wound during this phase reduces the wound's surface area and volume and is independent of granulation tissue formation (Pai & Hunt, 1972). After the formation of viable granulation tissue, epithelial cells migrate over the wound bed and close the wound. As compared with other processes in the proliferative phase, the rate of re-epithelialization is relatively fast (Rodeheaver et al., 1994). The end of the proliferative phase (i.e., complete re-epithelialization of the wound surface) is generally considered in clinical practice to be the completion of healing, because the final phase of healing is lengthy and difficult to clinically discern.

The maturation, or remodeling, phase of wound healing is the final biological process of tissue repair. This phase is characterized by the turnover of collagen (i.e., synthesis and lysis) and is thought to last at least 2 years (McPherson & Piez, 1988). Re-orientation and restructure of collagen fibers increase the tensile strength of the wound, because new collagen fibers add strength and are re-aligned toward the areas of greatest tension on the wound (Messer, 1989).

LITERATURE AND RESEARCH BASE

The literature and research base of Pressure Ulcer Care addresses assessment and care activities that support the healing process.

Pressure Ulcer Assessment

The initial element in management of an individual with a pressure ulcer involves a comprehensive assessment, with specific attention to assessing the ulcer itself and to the physical and psychological characteristics of the individual relevant to healing. Specific characteristics of the wound to be assessed include the ulcer site, stage, and size (length, width, and depth); the presence of sinus tracts, tunneling, undermining, necrotic tissue, granulation tissue, epithelial tissue, exudate, and pain; and the characteristics of the skin surrounding the ulcer (Bergstrom et al., 1994). This assessment provides information as to which phase of healing the pressure ulcer depicts. For example, a wound bed covered with necrotic tissue exemplifies a pressure ulcer in the inflammatory phase, whereas a wound filled with granulation tissue is characteristic of a pressure ulcer in the proliferative phase.

A nutritional assessment of the person with a pressure ulcer is also required. Factors to be assessed include indicators of both the somatic and the visceral protein compartments, hydration status, and actual protein and calorie intake as well as estimated requirements (Bergstrom et al., 1994). This assessment provides information regarding availability of substrates for the proliferative phase of wound healing, as well as information regarding the ability of the host to resist wound infection.

Pressure Ulcer Care Activities

The literature and research base of substantive pressure ulcer care activities can be linked to the inflammatory and proliferative phases of pressure ulcer healing.

INFLAMMATORY PHASE ACTIVITIES

Debridement During the initial phase of the wound-healing process, necrotic tissue and debris must be removed from the wound bed, because these substances provide a culture medium for bacterial growth (Dhingra, Schauerhamer, & Wangensteen, 1976). The presence of necrotic tissue is associated with large numbers of aerobic and anaerobic bacteria (Sapico et al., 1986). High bacterial levels have been found to be associated with delayed healing of pressure ulcers (Robson & Heggers, 1969).

Removal of adherent necrotic tissue can be accomplished by one of four debridement methods—sharp, mechanical, chemical, and autolytic. Conservative sharp debridement includes the use of scissors or scalpel to remove macroscopically visible necrotic tissue and is the most rapid and efficient debridement method. Although the surgical excision of necrotic tissue from viable tissue is beyond the scope of nursing practice, numerous state nurse practice laws define conservative sharp debridement to be within the scope of nursing practice consequent to appropriate credentials (Fowler, 1992). Mechanical debridement involves the use of wet-to-dry gauze dressings that adhere to necrotic tissue and physically remove it during dressing changes. Chemical debridement involves the use of enzyme agents selected to specifically target the protein that composes the necrotic tissue, such as fibrin, elastin, and collagen. Enzymes are classified into one of three groups—proteinolytics, fibrinolytics, and collagenases (Feedar, 1994). Enzymes are capable of more selective debridement than mechanical debridement. However, enzymes are more expensive and relatively slow in action. Autolytic debridement involves the use of occlusive dressings that concentrate the body's own endogenous enzymes in the wound bed. The naturally occurring neutrophils and macrophages in the wound fluid digest and lyse necrotic tissue. Autolytic debridement is highly selective, but it is also relatively slow.

Although the debridement of necrotic tissue is considered essential during the inflammatory phase of wound healing, research comparing the effectiveness of various debridement methods is scarce. Chemical debridement is the only debridement method that has been subjected to randomized clinical trials. These studies support the superior efficacy of collagenase over a placebo and have demonstrated that collagenase can dissolve undenatured collagen (Boxer, Gottesman, Bernstein, & Mandl, 1969; Lee & Ambrus, 1975; Rao, Sane, & Georgiev, 1975; Varma, Bugatch, & German, 1973). Nonetheless, additional research is needed in order to determine which debridement method is most effective under various wound and patient conditions.

Cleansing Nonadherent foreign material and wound exudate can impede healing. Activities to cleanse the wound of these inflammation-producing materials will promote progression to the proliferative phase of the wound-healing process. Wound cleansing involves the selection of a cleansing solution and a method to deliver the solution to the wound bed. Many wound cleansers are available; however, the most common and inexpensive wound-cleansing solution is isotonic saline (Bergstrom et al., 1994). Research has demonstrated that many wound cleansers are cytotoxic to white blood cells (Foresman, Payne, Becker, Lewis, & Rodeheaver, 1993) and proliferative fibroblast cells (Lineweaver et al., 1985). The method used to deliver the solution to the wound bed must be capable of removing debris without harming underlying viable tissue. Although gentle swabbing of a superficial pressure ulcer with a solution-soaked gauze can effect removal of foreign material and exudate without causing trauma to underlying tissues, deep ulcers require wound irrigation to effectively cleanse the wound bed of exudate. However, irrigation pressures in excess of 15 pounds per square inch (psi) have been shown to damage viable wound tissue and drive bacteria into tissues (Bhaskar, Cutright, Hunsuck, & Gross, 1971; Wheeler, Rodeheaver, Thacker, Edgerton, & Edlich, 1976). Effective removal of debris without harm to underlying tissues can be accomplished with irrigation pressures between 4 and 15 psi (Rodeheaver, Pettry, Thacker, Edgerton, & Edlich, 1975; Stevenson, Thacker, Rodeheaver, Bacchetta, & Edgerton, 1976). Irrigation pressures within this range can be achieved through the use of a 35-mL syringe and a 19-gauge needle (Rodeheaver et al., 1975).

PROLIFERATIVE PHASE ACTIVITIES

Provision of a Moist Wound Environment   Epithelialization of wounds was found to be enhanced by a moist environment (Winter & Scales, 1963). Exposing the wound to air for prolonged periods of time dries out the wound and forces epithelial cells to migrate under the dried crusts or scabs. Covering the wound also decreases contamination with microorganisms.

Hundreds of dressing materials have been developed to provide a moist environment conducive to wound healing, such as gauze dressings soaked in solutions, hydrophilic beads (dextran polymers or dextranomer), copolymer absorption dressings, polyurethane dressings, and hydrocolloid dressings. These dressings are designed to perform other functions in addition to moisture retention, including debridement, absorption of drainage, obliteration of dead space, and protection from trauma and infection. The selection of a dressing material is based on the characteristics of individual wounds, because no single product or dressing is optimal for all wounds. As the wound progresses through the phases of healing, the dressing may need to be modified to match changing wound characteristics. Research has demonstrated that pressure ulcer healing does not differ among the various moist wound dressings available (Alm et al., 1989; Colwell, Foreman, & Trotter, 1992; Neill, Conforti, Kedas, & Burris, 1989; Oleske, Smith, White, Pottage, & Donavan, 1986; Xakellis & Chrischilles, 1992).

Control of Bacteria   High levels of bacteria in pressure ulcers have been associated with impaired healing of pressure ulcers (Bendy et al., 1964). Wound infection occurs when invading organisms overwhelm the immunological response of the host. The type and number of organisms, as well as defects in the immune system, may predispose the wound to infection (Mertz & Ovington, 1993). Wound infection impairs healing because toxic bacterial products and excessive inflammatory host responses cause tissue injury (Robson, Stenberg, & Heggers, 1990). In addition, leukocytes summoned to the area consume large amounts of oxygen needed for the healing process (Pai & Hunt, 1972).

Impaired healing of pressure ulcers has been found to occur when bacterial quantities exceed 10^5 organisms per gram of tissue using tissue biopsies of wound tissue (Robson & Heggers, 1969). Using quantitative swab cultures, impaired healing occurred at quantities exceeding 10^6 organisms per milliliter (Bendy et al., 1964).

In addition to tissue biopsies and quantitative swab cultures, other techniques are available to monitor bacteria levels in wounds (Stotts, 1995). Controversy exists over the appropriate technique for monitoring bacteria levels in pressure ulcers. However, swab cultures of the wound surface are of no value in monitoring quantity of bacteria, because they cannot differentiate between high levels of bacteria in wound tissue and simple wound surface contamination (Bergstrom et al., 1994). The Centers for Disease Control and Prevention (CDC) defines wound infection as the presence of two of the following clinical findings: redness, tenderness, or swelling of wound edges *and* organisms isolated from a needle aspirate, tissue biopsy, or blood culture (Garner, Jarvis, Emori, Horan, & Hughes, 1988).

Although the cornerstone of controlling bacterial levels in pressure ulcers is the effective use of debridement and cleansing procedures, wound infection does occur in "clean" appearing pressure ulcers. Topical antibiotics are indicated for wounds with high bacterial levels despite adequate debridement and cleansing (Bendy et al., 1964; Kucan, Robson, Heggers, & Ko, 1981). Systemic antibiotics are appropriate only in the presence of bacteremia, sepsis, advancing cellulitis, and osteomyelitis and not for locally contained wound infections (Chow, Galpin, & Guze, 1977; Lewis et al., 1988). The use of antiseptics to control bacterial levels has been shown to be detrimental to the wound-healing process. These solutions contain reactive chemicals that are toxic to a number of cells responsible for maintaining the healing trajectory (Lineweaver et al., 1985).

Provision of Essential Substrates   Substrates required for wound healing are proteins, calories, vitamins, and minerals. Deficits or imbalances of dietary protein and amino acids, such as methionine, cysteine, and lysine, impair angiogenesis, fibroblast proliferation, collagen synthesis, and scar remodeling (Irvin, 1978). Adequate amounts of carbohydrates and fats are needed in order to prevent amino acids from being oxidized for caloric needs. Glucose is needed to meet the energy requirements of the cells involved in wound healing, such as fibroblasts and leukocytes. In addition to providing calories for energy, fats provide essential fatty acids, such as arachidonic, linoleic, and linolenic. Vitamins A, B complex, and C are essential for collagen synthesis, re-epithelialization, resistance to infection, and maintenance of newly formed scar tissue. Zinc is a mineral component of many enzymes, including DNA and RNA polymerases (Pollack, 1979). Injury increases the need for zinc and causes zinc levels to drop. The serum level at which zinc deficiency is reported to interfere with wound healing is 100 μg/100 mL. At this level or below, studies have found that wound healing is restored to normal with zinc supplementation (Levenson, Seifter, & Van Winkle, 1979).

Although the amounts of specific substrates required to promote healing remain unclear, nutritional support of patients with pressure ulcers requires placing the patient in a positive nitrogen balance (i.e., approximately 30 to 35 calories/kg/day and 1.25 to 1.50 g of protein/kg/day) (Chernoff, Milton, & Lipschitz, 1991; Kaminski, 1976). When vitamin and mineral deficiencies are suspected, a multivitamin with mineral supplement should be prescribed (Bergstrom & Braden, 1992; Pinchofsky-Devin & Kaminski, 1986).

Prevention of Further Injury   In order for healing to progress, the damaging forces of prolonged pressure must be avoided over the wound area. The patient with a pressure ulcer should be positioned in a manner that avoids external force on the pressure ulcer, if possible. Patients with sacral ulcers should avoid the sitting position until the wound is healed. There are numerous devices (e.g., support mattresses and cushions, specialty beds) available to reduce the force of pressure on overlying tissues. Although these devices reduce interface pressures between support surface and soft tissue, there is little evidence from which to recommend one type of support surface over another (Allman et al., 1987; Conine, Daechsel, & Lau, 1990; Ferrell, Osterwell, & Christenson, 1993; Jackson,

Chagares, Nee, & Freeman, 1988; Munro, Brown, & Heitman, 1989; Strauss, Gong, Gary, Kalsbeek, & Spear, 1991; Warner, 1992). However, Vyhlidal, Moxness, Bosak, Van Meter, and Bergstrom (1997) found that the Maxifloat replacement mattress was more effective in reducing the incidence of pressure ulcers than foam overlays. Nonetheless, the selection of a support surface must be determined by the clinical condition of the patient, the characteristics of the clinical setting, and the characteristics of the support surface.

PRESSURE ULCER CARE GUIDELINE

The Agency for Health Care Policy and Research (AHCPR) Clinical Practice Guideline *Treatment of Pressure Ulcers* (Bergstrom et al., 1994) provides a comprehensive framework for the management of pressure ulcers and represents the best research-based protocol for managing pressure ulcers in clinical practice. This guideline underwent peer review as well as preliminary pilot testing before being published. Implementation of this guideline has been shown to enhance standardization of Pressure Ulcer Care and to reduce treatment costs (Frantz, Bergquist, & Specht, 1995).

Compiled by a 15-member multidisciplinary panel of experts on pressure ulcers and wound healing, the guideline is based on an extensive analysis of the research literature, supplemented, as needed, by expert opinion. Six elements form the framework for the AHCPR guideline on treating pressure ulcers: assessment, managing tissue loads, ulcer care, managing bacterial colonization and infection, operative repair, and education and quality improvement. Within each element are recommendations for activities to promote healing and prevent further trauma to the tissue. In addition to specific recommendations regarding various activities to support repair and prevent further injury to soft tissue, the guideline contains preferred pathways or algorithms to assist clinicians in selecting appropriate strategies for treatment (Bergstrom et al., 1994).

All but one of the 17 specific activities listed in the NIC intervention Pressure Ulcer Care are represented in the elements and algorithms of the AHCPR Clinical Practice Guideline. However, the NIC activities are, in general, less specific and comprehensive than the guideline activities. For example, several activities related to assessment of an ulcer are delineated in the NIC intervention Pressure Ulcer Care. These include measuring and describing the characteristics of the ulcer, determining the level of ulcer formation, noting characteristics of drainage, and monitoring for signs and symptoms of infection. Unlike the AHCPR guideline, there are no assessment activities included in the NIC intervention related to evaluating the periwound area, with the exception of those assessment parameters that would be included in monitoring for infection of the wound. In addition, nursing assessments related to pain management and psychosocial adjustment to the pressure ulcer are also absent from the NIC intervention, although there are other NIC interventions that address these activities. Therefore, in using the AHCPR guideline and algorithms, the nurse may use more activities than identified in the Pressure Ulcer Care intervention, but these activities may be included in other NIC interventions.

Table 11–2 lists the Pressure Ulcer Care intervention activities and the chapter or algorithm of the AHCPR guideline that contains that activity. The 17 activities have been organized according to whether they are related to assessment, are directed toward the inflammatory phase of wound healing, or are directed toward the proliferative phase of wound healing. This organization provides a framework to assist in the appropriate selection of specific care activities. It is

Table 11–2 NIC Pressure Ulcer Care Activities and Their Corresponding Section of the AHCPR Clinical Practice Guideline, *Treatment of Pressure Ulcers*

NIC Pressure Ulcer Care Activity	Corresponding Section of the AHCPR Guideline
ASSESSMENT	
Measure and describe characteristics of the ulcer at regular intervals.	Chapter 2: Assessment at least weekly
Determine level of ulcer formation.	Chapter 2: Assessment
Note characteristics of drainage.	Chapter 2: Assessment
Monitor for signs and symptoms of infection.	Chapter 2: Assessment
Monitor calorie intake to ensure adequate intake.	Algorithm: Nutritional support and assessment
Cleanse the skin around the ulcer with mild soap and water.	Not in AHCPR guideline
DIRECTED TOWARD THE INFLAMMATORY PHASE OF WOUND HEALING	
Debride ulcer, as needed.	Chapter 4: Ulcer Care
Cleanse the ulcer with the appropriate nontoxic solution, working in a circular motion from the center.	Chapter 4: Ulcer Care
Use a 19-gauge needle and 35 mL syringe to clean deep ulcers.	Chapter 4: Ulcer Care
DIRECTED TOWARD THE PROLIFERATIVE PHASE OF WOUND HEALING	
Keep the ulcer moist to aid in healing.	Chapter 4: Ulcer Care
Apply a permeable adhesive membrane to the ulcer, as appropriate.	Chapter 4: Ulcer Care
Protect surrounding skin from moisture by using petroleum jelly, if using wet dressings.	Chapter 4: Ulcer Care
Apply dressings, as appropriate.	Chapter 4: Ulcer Care
Apply saline soaks, as appropriate.	Chapter 4: Ulcer Care
Apply ointments, as approriate.	Chapter 4: Ulcer Care
Position to avoid prolonged pressure on other sites.	Chapter 3: Managing Tissue Loads Algorithm: Management of tissue loads
Increase protein intake to help rebuild epidermal tissue, as appropriate.	Chapter 2: Assessment

important to realize that many of the activities directed toward the proliferative phase can, and should, be instituted during the inflammatory phase of wound healing.

NURSING DIAGNOSES

Linking the NIC intervention Pressure Ulcer Care to associated diagnoses is complicated by the ambiguity of the diagnostic labels applied to this condition. Historically, the terms *decubitus ulcer* or *bedsore* were widely used to describe the pressure-induced injury, because they were observed to occur most frequently in individuals who were confined to bed. Arising from the Latin word *decumbere,* which means "to lie down," the term *decubitus ulcer* implies that the lesion is caused solely by prolonged recumbence. More recent clinical observations have confirmed that the ulcer can occur in any position exposed to excessive, unrelieved pressure. The term *pressure ulcer* or *pressure sore* evolved to reflect more accurately the etiology of the ulceration rather than a specific body position. In an effort to establish consistent terminology, the National Pressure Ulcer Advisory Panel (NPUAP) Consensus Development Conference (1989) determined that the term *pressure ulcer* should be used universally. This label was reaffirmed by the AHCPR Guideline Panel (Clinical Practice Guideline Panel, 1992) in its clinical practice guideline on prediction and prevention of pressure ulcers.

The North American Nursing Diagnosis Association's (NANDA) taxonomy of nursing diagnoses contains two diagnoses that relate to the phenomenon of pressure ulcers: Impaired Skin Integrity and Impaired Tissue Integrity (Carroll-Johnson, 1989). Examination of the definitions for the NANDA diagnoses reveals a lack of specificity for delineating the phenomenon of pressure ulcers. Both Impaired Skin Integrity and Impaired Tissue Integrity are defined as disruptions in the skin or integument. The defining characteristics are identified broadly as disruptions or destruction of skin tissue. Specific, measurable signs and symptoms have not been delineated, although preliminary work has attempted to operationalize the diagnosis of Impaired Skin Intergrity (Cattaneo & Lackey, 1987). Given the lack of a narrowly focused diagnosis, the NIC intervention Pressure Ulcer Care may or may not be appropriate, depending on the nature of the impaired skin integrity or impaired tissue integrity.

In the view of the authors, the diagnostic concept herein described as a pressure ulcer would more accurately be identified by that label. It is conceptually congruent with the well-established etiology of pressure over a bony prominence in excess of a critical pressure-time threshold. This label is consistent with the terminology recommended by other expert panels in skin and wound care. Furthermore, the documented pathological events that occur in the presence of this etiology give rise to a cluster of observable, measurable changes in the skin and underlying tissue. The pattern of these changes would define the signs and symptoms of the diagnosis. The NIC intervention Pressure Ulcer Care would link directly with this diagnostic label.

PATIENT OUTCOMES

The Nursing Outcomes Classification (NOC), developed by the Iowa Outcomes Project (Johnson & Maas, 1997), describes only one outcome pertinent to pressure ulcers, Wound Healing: Secondary Intention. Defined as the extent to which cells and tissues in an open wound have regenerated, it clearly articulates with the NIC intervention Pressure Ulcer Care, which is described as facilitation of healing.

This outcome lists 18 indicators of healing, along with size based on wound area and depth. Each indicator is quantified from *none* to *complete* using a five-point scale. In its current form, NOC provides a starting point for delineating the outcomes relevant to nursing interventions that are implemented to treat pressure ulcers. The indicators specified by NOC are directly linked to the physiological events that characterize secondary wound healing. Some indicators capture changes in drainage from purulent to serous or serosanguineous as the wound moves from the inflammatory phase of healing through proliferation. Other indicators capture the dissipation of necrotic tissue and slough as a result of the autolytic activity that occurs during inflammation. Still others capture the generation of granulation tissue, which becomes observable as new capillary buds proliferate in the wound bed and areas of tunneling and undermining are resolved. The movement of epithelial cells over the granulating wound bed as the proliferative phase of healing continues ultimately produces the NOC indicator of wound size resolution.

It is these authors' view that, given the sequential nature of wound healing and the prolonged time that may elapse before the ultimate endpoint of wound closure is achieved, intermediate measures of progress are essential. This is especially true in settings populated by elderly persons, whose healing is often delayed (Eaglstein, 1986; Grove, 1982). The quarterly assessments mandated by federal regulations of long-term care further reinforce the need for intermediate outcomes that can be used as benchmarks of progress leading to the primary outcome of wound closure. The five-point scale used to quantify each indicator in this NOC label offers the potential to identify quantifiable measures of progress toward wound closure. However, empirical testing of the NOC outcome is needed to determine the correlational and predictive validity of these collective indicators, as well as their sensitivity to change over the natural history of the wound.

CASE STUDY

MS is a 73-year-old man who experienced a right-sided cerebrovascular accident (CVA) resulting in left-sided hemiplegia. The CVA left him physically immobilized and unresponsive to verbal and painful stimuli. During the acute phase of his CVA, he developed two stage IV pressure ulcers, one on each trochanter. At the time of transfer to a long-term care facility, MS had an open ulcer over the right trochanter that extended through the dermis and subcutaneous tissue, exposing deep fascia and bone. Adherent necrotic tissue covered 90% of the floor of the wound. Undermining of 2 to 4 cm extended over 75% of the wound margins. The wound edges were distinct and not attached to the wound bed. Large amounts of purulent exudate were draining from the wound. The periwound skin was intact and pale gray in color. Digitized tracing of the wound revealed a surface area equalling 62 cm².

The left trochanteric ulcer also extended through the soft tissue to the fascial plate. However, no bone was exposed. Adherent necrotic tissue covered 75% of the wound floor, and there were large amounts of purulent exudate draining from the wound. Undermining of up to 2 cm extended over 25% of the wound margins. The wound edges were distinct and not attached to the wound bed. The periwound skin was pale gray and intact. Digitized tracing of the wound perimeter revealed a surface area of 38 cm².

The diagnosis Impaired Tissue Integrity (i.e., pressure ulcer) was inferred from the clinical data. Following consultation with the patient's family to

determine their preferences for MS's care, nursing interventions were planned. Nursing interventions to treat the pressure ulcer were implemented according to the recommendations outlined in the AHCPR guideline *Treatment of Pressure Ulcers,* which contains most of the activities associated with the NIC intervention Pressure Ulcer Care and some of the activities associated with the NIC intervention Pressure Ulcer Prevention.

A comprehensive assessment was completed, including a thorough nutritional evaluation. MS was found to be significantly malnourished. His albumin level was 2.5 mg dL, and his total lymphocyte count was 1,500. He had experienced a 5 kg weight loss during hospitalization. His admission weight was 62 kg, and he was 180 cm tall. He was unable to take food orally and had been receiving only intravenous fluids during his hospitalization. A feeding tube had been placed 2 days before discharge from the hospital.

Other nursing activities focused on nutritional support, management of mechanical load, reduction of bacterial burden, and ulcer care, including cleansing, debridement, and dressings. Nutritional support was provided with around-the-clock half-strength Ensure by feeding tube to ensure 3,000 calories and 100 g of protein per day. Multivitamins and minerals were added to the formula to ensure complete nutritional supplementation. Because of the presence of large amounts of devitalized tissue in the ulcers, sharp debridement of the necrotic tissue was performed weekly.

The wounds were covered with normal-saline-moistened gauze dressings that were changed every 8 hours in an effort to facilitate removal of the adherent necrotic tissue. Cleansing was performed with each dressing change using normal saline and a 35 mL syringe and 19-gauge angiocatheter. MS was placed on a static air mattress and repositioned every 2 hours. Side-lying positions were limited to a 30-degree angle to avoid any pressure directly on the ulcer. Intravenous antibiotics and surgical interventions were not pursued, congruent with the wishes of the patient's family.

MS's pressure ulcers progressed toward healing until his death due to pneumonia 3 months following admission to the long-term care facility. The necrotic tissue slowly decreased in coverage of the wound bed, and granulation tissue began to appear at the edges of each ulcer. The exudate changed from a thick purulent to a thin purulent consistency and decreased from a large to a moderate amount. The ulcers did not change in surface area size because epithelial cell migration had not yet begun. Although ulcer closure was far from complete at the time of MS's death, intermediate outcomes suggested that the selected activities were facilitating pressure ulcer healing.

References

Agren, M. S., and Stromberg, H. (1985). Topical treatment of pressure ulcers: A randomized comparative trial of Varidase® and zinc oxide. *Scandinavian Journal of Plastic and Reconstructive Surgery, 19*, 97–100.

Allman, R. M., Walker, J. M., Hart, M. K., Laprade, C. A., Noel, L. B., and Smith, C. R. (1987). Air fluidized beds or conventional therapy for pressure sores: A randomized trial. *Annals of Internal Medicine, 107*, 641–648.

Alm, A., Hornmark, A. M., Fall, P. A., Linder, L., Bergstrand, B., Ehrnebo, M., Madsen, S. M., and Setterberg, G. (1989). Care of pressure sores: A controlled study of the use of a hydrocolloid dressing compared with wet saline gauze compresses. *Acta Dermato-Venereologica (Stockholm), 149*(Suppl), 1–10.

Bale, S., and Harding, K. G. (1990). Using modern dressings to effect debridement. *The Professional Nurse, 5*, 244–245.

Bendy, R. H., Jr., Nuccio, P. A., Wolfe, E., Collins, B., Tamburro, D., Glass, W., and Martin, C. M. (1964). Relationship of quantitative wound bacterial counts to healing of decubiti: Effect of topical gentamicin. *Antimicrobial Agents and Chemotherapy, 4*, 147–155.

Bergstrom, N., Allman, R. M., Alvarez, O. M., Bennett, M. A., Carlson, C. E., Frantz, R. A., Garber, S. L., Jackson, B. S., Kaminski, M. V., Jr., Kemp, M. G., Kroskop, T. A., Lewis, V. L., Jr., Maklebust, J., Margolis, D. J., Marvel, E. M., Reger, S. I., Rodeheaver, G. T., Salcido, R., Xakellis, G. C., Yarkony, G. M. (1994, December). *Treatment of pressure ulcers* (Clinical Practice Guideline No. 15. AHCPR Publication No. 95-0652). Rockville, MD: Agency for Health Care Policy and Research, Public Health Service, U.S. Department of Health and Human Services.

Bergstrom, N., and Braden, B. (1992). A prospective study of pressure sore risk among institutionalized elderly. *Journal of the American Geriatrics Society, 40*, 747–758.

Bhaskar, S. N., Cutright, D. E., Hunsuck, E. E., and Gross, A. L. (1971). Pulsatile water jet devices in debridement of combat wounds. *Military Medicine, 136*(3), 264–266.

Boxer, A. M., Gottesman, N., Bernstein, H., and Mandl, I. (1969). Debridement of dermal ulcers and decubiti with collagenase. *Geriatrics, 24*(7), 75–86.

Carroll-Johnson, R. (Ed.) (1989). *Classification of nursing diagnoses: Proceedings of the eighth conference.* Philadelphia: J. B. Lippincott.

Cattaneo, C. J., and Lackey, N. R. (1987). Impaired skin intergrity. In A. M. McLane (Ed.), *Classification of nursing diagnoses: Proceedings of the seventh conference* (pp. 129–135). St. Louis: Mosby.

Chernoff, R., Milton, K., and Lipschitz, D. (1991). The effect of a very high-protein liquid formula (Replete®) on decubitus ulcer healing in long-term tube-fed institutionalized patients [Abstract]. *Journal of the American Dietetic Association, 90*(9), A-130.

Chow, A. W., Galpin, J. E., and Guze, L. B. (1977). Clindamycin for treatment of sepsis caused by decubitus ulcers. *Journal of Infectious Disease, 135*(Suppl), S65–68.

Clinical Practice Guideline Panel. (1992). *Clinical practice guideline: Pressure ulcers in adults: Prediction and prevention* (AHCPR Pub. No. 92-0047). Rockville, MD: Agency for Health Care Policy and Research, Public Health Service, U.S. Department of Health and Human Services.

Colwell, J. C., Foreman, M. D., and Trotter, J. P. (1992). A comparison of the efficacy and cost-effectiveness of two methods of managing prssure ulcers. *Decubitus, 6*(4), 28–36.

Conine, T. A., Daechsel, D., and Lau, M. S. (1990). The role of alternating air and Silicore overlays in preventing decubitus ulcers. *Journal of Rehabilitation Research, 13*(1), 57–65.

Dhingra, U., Schauerhamer, R. R., and Wangensteen, O. H. (1976). Peripheral dissemination of bacteria in contaminated wounds; role of devitalized tissue: Evaluation of therapeutic measures. *Surgery, 80*(5), 535–543.

Eaglstein, W. H. (1986). Wound healing and aging. *Dermatologic Clinics, 4*, 481–484.

Feedar, J. A. (1994). Products that facilitate wound healing. *Topics in Geriatric Rehabilitation, 9*(4), 58–81.

Ferrell, B. A., Osterweil, D., and Christenson, P. (1993). A randomized trial of low-air-loss beds for treatment of pressure ulcers. *Journal of the American Medical Association, 269*, 494–497.

Foresman, P. A., Payne, D. S., Becker, D., Lewis, D., and Rodeheaver, G. T. (1993). A relative toxicity index for wound cleansers. *Wounds, 5*, 226–231.

Fowler, E. (1992). Instrument / sharp debridement of

nonviable tissue in wounds. *Ostomy/Wound Management, 38*(8), 26–33.

Frantz, R. A., Bergquist, S., and Specht, J. (1995). The cost of treating pressure ulcers following implementation of a research-based skin care protocol in a long term care facility. *Advances in Wound Care: The Journal for Prevention and Healing, 8*(1), 36–45.

Garner, J. S., Jarvis, W. R., Emori, T. G., Horan, T. C., and Hughes, J. M. (1988). CDC definitions for nosocomial infections. *American Journal of Infection Control, 16*(3), 128–140.

Grove, G. L. (1982). Age related differences in healing superficial skin wounds in humans. *Archives of Dermatological Research, 272,* 381–385.

Hunt, T. K. (1979). Disorders of repair and their management. In T. K. Hunt and J. E. Dunphy (Eds.), *Fundamentals of wound management* (pp. 68–168). New York: Appleton-Century-Crofts.

Hunt, T. K., and VanWinkle, W., Jr. (1979). Normal repair. In T. K. Hunt and J. E. Dunphy (Eds.), *Fundamentals of wound management* (pp. 2–67). New York: Appleton-Century-Crofts.

Irvin, T. T. (1978). Effects of malnutrition on wound healing. *Surgical Gynecology and Obstetrics, 146,* 33–37.

Jackson, B. S., Chagares, R., Nee, N., and Freeman, K. (1988). The effects of a therapeutic bed on pressure ulcers: An experimental study. *Journal of Enterostomal Therapy, 15*(6), 220–226.

Johnson, M., and Maas, M. (1997). *Nursing outcomes classification (NOC).* St. Louis: Mosby–Year Book.

Kaminski, J. V., Jr. (1976). Enteral hyperalimentation. *Surgical Gynecology and Obstetrics, 143*(1), 12–16.

Kosiak, M. (1959). Etiology and pathology of ischemic ulcers. *Archives of Physical Medicine and Rehabilitation, 40*(2), 62–69.

Kosiak, M. (1961). Etiology of decubitus ulcers. *Archives of Physical Medicine and Rehabilitation, 42*(1), 19–29.

Kucan, J. O., Robson, M. C., Heggers, J. P., and Ko, F. (1981). Comparison of silver sulfadiazine, povidone-iodine and physiologic saline in the treatment of chronic pressure ulcers. *Journal of the American Geriatrics Society, 29*(5), 232–235.

Lee, L. K., and Ambrus, J. L. (1975). Collagenase therapy for decubitus ulcers. *Geriatrics, 30*(5), 91–93, 97–98.

Levenson, S., Seifter, E., and VanWinkle, W., Jr. (1979). Nutrition. In T. K. Hunt and J. E. Dunphy (Eds.), *Fundamentals of wound management* (pp. 286–363). New York: Appleton-Century-Crofts.

Lewis, V. L., Jr., Bailey, M. H., Pulawski, G., Kind, G., Bashioum, R. W., and Hendrix, R. W. (1988). The diagnosis of osteomyelitis in patients with pressure sores. *Plastic and Reconstructive Surgery, 81*(2), 229–232.

Lineweaver, W., Howard, R., Soucy, D., McMorris, S., Freeman, J., Crain, C., Robertson, J., and Romley, T. (1985). Topical antimicrobial toxicity. *Archives of Surgery, 120,* 267–270.

Majno, G., and Joris, I. (1995). Apoptosis, oncosis, necrosis: An overview of cell death. *American Journal of Pathology, 146,* 3–15.

McCloskey, J. C., and Bulechek, G. M. (1996). *Nursing interventions classification (NIC).* (2nd ed.). St. Louis: Mosby–Year Book.

McPherson J., and Piez, K. (1988). Collagen in dermal wound repair. In R. Clark and P. Henson (Eds.), *The molecular and cellular biology of wound repair.* New York: Plenum Press.

Mertz, P. M., and Ovington, L. G. (1993). Wound healing microbiology. *Dermatology Clinics, 11,* 739–747.

Messer, M. S. (1989). Wound care. *Critical Care Nursing Quarterly, 11*(4), 17–27.

Munro, B. H., Brown, L., and Heitman, B. B. (1989). Pressure ulcers: One bed or another? *Geriatric Nursing (New York), 10*(4), 190–192.

National Pressure Ulcer Advisory Panel. (1989). *Pressure ulcers: Incidence, economics, risk assessment. Consensus development conference statement,* West Dundee, IL: S-N Publications.

Neill, K. M., Conforti, D., Kedas, A., and Burris, J. F. (1989). Presure sore response to a new hydrocolloid dressing. *Wounds, 1*(3), 173–185.

Oleske, D. M., Smith, X. P., White, P., Pottage, J., and Donavan, M. J. (1986). A randomized clinical trial of two dressing methods for the treatment of low-grade pressure ulcers. *Journal of Enterostomal Therapy, 13*(3), 90–98.

Pai, M. P., and Hunt, T. K. (1972). Effect of varying oxygen tensions on healing of open wounds. *Surgery, Gynecology and Obstetrics, 135,* 756–758.

Pinchcofsky-Devin, G. D., and Kaminski, M. V., Jr. (1986). Correlation of pressure sores and nutritional status. *Journal of the American Geriatrics Society, 34,* 435–440.

Pollack, S. V. (1979). Wound healing: A review 3: Nutritional factors affecting wound healing. *Journal of Dermatology, Surgery, and Oncology, 5,* 615–619.

Rao, D. B., Sane, P. G., and Georgiev, E. L. (1975). Collagenase in the treatment of dermal and decubitus ulcers. *Journal of the American Geriatrics Society, 23*(1), 22–30.

Robson, M. C., and Heggers, J. P. (1969). Bacterial quantification of open wounds. *Military Medicine, 134*(1), 19–24.

Robson, M. C., Stenberg, B. D., and Heggers, J. P. (1990). Wound healing alterations caused by infection. *Clinics in Plastic Surgery, 17*(3), 485–492.

Rodeheaver, G., Baharestani, M. M., Brabee, M. E., Byrd, H. J., Salzberg, C. A., Scherer, P., and Vogelpohl, T. S. (1994). Wound healing and wound management: Focus on debridement. *Advances in Wound Care: The Journal of Prevention and Healing, 17*(1), 22–36.

Rodeheaver, G. T., Pettry, D., Thacker, J. G., Edgerton, M. T., and Edlich, R. F. (1975). Wound cleansing by high pressure irrigation. *Surgical Gynecology and Obstetrics, 141*(3), 357–362.

Sakharov, I. Y., Glyanzev, S. P., Litvin, F. E., and Savvina, T. V. (1993). Potent debriding ability of collagenolytic protease isolated from the hepatopancreas of the king crab Paralithodes camtschatica. *Archives of Dermatological Research, 285,* 32–35.

Sapico, F. L., Ginunas, V. J., Thornhill-Joynes, M., Canawati, H. N., Capen, D. A., Klein, N. E., Khawam, S., and Montgomerie, J. Z. (1986). Quantitative microbiology of pressure sores in different stages of healing. *Diagnostic Microbiology and Infectious Disease, 5,* 31–38.

Stevenson, T. R., Thacker, J. G., Rodeheaver, G. T., Bacchetta, C., and Edgerton, M. T. (1976). Cleansing the traumatic wound by high pressure syringe irrigation. *Journal of the American College of Emergency Physicians, 5*(1), 17–21.

Stotts, N. A. (1995). Determination of bacterial burden in wounds. *Advances in Wound Care: The Journal for Prevention & Healing, 8*(4), 28/46–28/52.

Strauss, M. J., Gong, J., Gary, B. D., Kalsbeek, W. D., and Spear, S. (1991). The cost of home air-fluidized therapy for pressure sores: A randomized controlled trial. *Journal of Family Practice, 33*(1), 52–59.

Varma, A. O., Bugatch, E., and German, F. M. (1973).

Debridement of dermal ulcers with collagenase. *Surgical Gynecology and Obstetrics, 136*(2), 281–282.

Vyhlidal, S. K., Moxness, D., Bosak, K. S., Van Meter, F. G., and Bergstrom, N. (1997). Mattress replacement or foam overlay? A prospective study on the incidence of pressure ulcers. *Applied Nursing Research, 10*(3), 111–120.

Warner, D. J. (1992). A clinical comparison of two pressure-reducing surfaces in the management of pressure ulcers. *Decubitus, 5*(3), 52–55, 58–60, 62–64.

Wheeler, C. B., Rodeheaver, G. T., Thacker, J. G., Edgerton, M. T., and Edlich, R. F. (1976). Side-effects of high pressure irrigation. *Surgical Gynecology and Obstetrics, 143,* 775–778.

Winter, G. D., and Scales, J. T. (1963). Effect of air drying and dressings on the surface of a wound. *Nature, 197,* 91–92.

Xakellis, G. C., and Chrischilles, E. A. (1992). Hydrocolloid versus saline gauze dressings in treating pressure ulcers: A cost-effectiveness analysis. *Archives of Physical Medicine and Rehabilitation, 73,* 463–469.

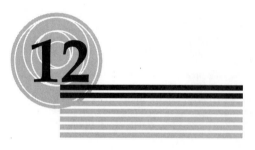

Teaching: Preoperative

Lori Butcher

Preoperative teaching is an essential nursing intervention, and its significant impact on patient outcomes is well documented in nursing research since the late 1970s. Preoperative teaching is conceptually defined by the Nursing Interventions Classification (NIC) as "assisting a patient to understand and mentally prepare for surgery and the postoperative recovery period" (Table 12–1). NIC has identified 31 defining nursing activities associated with preoperative teaching. There is no argument as to whether preoperative teaching should or should not be done, but a quandary arises as to what kind of and how much information should be given to patients, as well as in what form, by whom, and when the information should be given.

The forces of the present health care climate only accentuate nurses' responsibility to provide high-quality preoperative teaching. The strongest forces include cost containment and the pressure to reduce costs and hospitalization days. Another trend is the increase in ambulatory surgery with recovery at home. Patients and family members assume the responsibility for recovery and self-care previously provided by nurses in the hospital setting. These current trends result in a critical need for preoperative patient education. Nurses are thus faced with a challenge because of the increase in outpatient surgery and early-morning admissions, as well as increases in nurse-patient ratios, resulting in decrease in time allotted to nursing staff for education. Nurses must use innovative strategies to provide the necessary nursing activities associated with preoperative teaching. These strategies must be based on research findings to achieve desired patient outcomes.

Table 12–1 Teaching: Preoperative

DEFINITION: Assisting a patient to understand and mentally prepare for surgery and the post-operative recovery period.

ACTIVITIES:

Inform the patient and significant other(s) of the scheduled date, time, and location of surgery

Inform the patient/significant other(s) how long the surgery is expected to last

Determine the patient's previous surgical experiences and level of knowledge related to surgery

Appraise the patient's/significant other's anxiety relating to surgery

Provide time for the patient to ask questions and discuss concerns

Describe the preoperative routines (e.g., anesthesia, diet, bowel preparation, tests/labs, voiding, skin preparation, IV therapy, clothing, family waiting area, and transportation to operating room), as appropriate

Describe any preoperative medications, the effects these will have on the patient, and the rationale for using them

Inform the significant other(s) of the location to wait for the results of the surgery, as appropriate

Conduct a tour of the postsurgical unit(s) and waiting area(s), as appropriate

Introduce the patient to the staff who will be involved in the surgery/postoperative care, as appropriate

Reinforce the patient's confidence in the staff involved, as appropriate

Provide information on what will be heard, smelled, seen, tasted, or felt during the event

Discuss possible pain control measures

Explain the purpose of frequent postoperative assessments

Describe the postoperative routines/equipment (e.g., medications, respiratory treatments, tubes, machines, support hose, surgical dressings, ambulation, diet, and family visitation), and explain their purpose

Instruct the patient on the technique of getting out of bed, as appropriate

Evaluate the patient's ability to return demonstrate getting out of bed, as appropriate

Instruct the patient on the technique of splinting incision, coughing, and deep breathing

Evaluate the patient's ability to return demonstrate splinting incision, coughing, and deep breathing

Instruct patient on how to use the incentive spirometer

Evaluate the patient's use of the incentive spirometer

Instruct the patient on the technique of leg exercises

Evaluate the patient's ability to return demonstrate leg exercises

Stress the importance of early ambulation and pulmonary care

Inform patients about how they can aid in recuperation

Reinforce information provided by other health care team members, as appropriate

Determine the patient's expectations of the surgery

Correct unrealistic expectations of the surgery, as appropriate

Provide time for the patient to rehearse events that will happen, as appropriate

Instruct the patient to use coping techniques directed at controlling specific aspects of the experience (e.g., relaxation and imagery), as appropriate

Include the family/significant others, as appropriate

Source: McCloskey, J. C., and Bulechek, G. M. (Eds.) (1996). *Nursing interventions classification (NIC).* (2nd ed.). St. Louis: Mosby–Year Book.

LITERATURE REVIEW

A number of research studies have been conducted that examine the effectiveness of preoperative teaching. This research can be summarized in two areas: (1) content of information and (2) instructional methods.

Content of Information

A combination of three main content areas—procedural, sensory, and psychological—has been found to be the most effective preoperative instruction program (Devine & Cook, 1983, 1986; Hathaway, 1986; Johnson, 1984; Mumford, Schlesinger, & Glass, 1982; Rothrock, 1989; Theis & Johnson, 1995). Procedural information is concrete and factual, explaining what will occur during a series of events or activities. Sensory information focuses on information describing sensations patients may experience during the procedure. Psychological instruction explores the patient's attitudes and feelings toward the surgical experience. In two studies by Devine and Cook (1983, 1986), multidimensional psychoeducational interventions were found to reduce length of hospital stay, decrease postoperative pain, and increase patient satisfaction. When a combination of types of content was presented during instruction, Hill (1982) found that patients were able to leave their homes sooner following surgery. Hathaway (1986), in a meta-analysis of preoperative teaching research, concluded that the focus of the content of information should be based on the individual patient's level of fear and anxiety. When the level of fear and anxiety is high, outcomes are improved if psychological content is the focus. When the level of fear and anxiety is low, procedural content should be the focus of the instruction.

The inclusion of sensory information in the combination of content improved effectiveness of instructional interventions on patient outcomes and is well documented in the literature (Johnson, Rice, Fuller, & Endress, 1978a, 1978b; Klos, Cummings, Joyce, Graichen, & Quigley, 1980; Levesque, Grenier, Kérouac, & Reidy, 1984; McHugh, Christman, & Johnson, 1982; Morgan, Wells, & Robertson, 1985). Providing information on sensory experiences is especially important for patients who are frightened or experiencing a procedure for the first time. Both subjective and objective content should be included. Subjective information deals with physical sensations that are verified by the person experiencing the event. Spatial and temporal characteristics of the event are considered objective information (McHugh et al., 1982).

Research studies examining perceptions of patients about information needed before surgery revealed that nurses do not always teach what patients perceive as important. Historically, nurses teach what they feel the patient needs to know. In this time of patient-centered care and a move to more self-care activity, we must examine what patients feel is important to their recovery. Yount and Schoessler (1991) compared patient and nurse perceptions of five dimensions of preoperative teaching: (1) situational information, (2) patient role, (3) sensation-discomfort, (4) skills training, and (5) psychosocial support. A discrepancy was noted between nurse and patient rank orderings. Nurses ranked psychosocial support and skills training higher than did patients, whereas patients ranked sensation-discomfort more important than did nurses. Another study found similar findings when comparing rankings of teaching content of 30 ambulatory surgical patients and 29 perioperative nurses. Nurses ranked psychosocial support as most important, and patients ranked situational information such as explaining activities and events as most important (Brumfield, Kee, & Johnson, 1996).

When studying the cardiac surgical patient's needs for preoperative teaching, it was found that patients reported not having the areas of teaching they needed addressed, reinforced, or repeated by the nursing staff, as well as not being adequately prepared for the amount of pain and discomfort resulting from the procedure (Miller & Shada, 1978). In a survey by Lisko (1995), conflicting perceptions of patients' priorities and nurses' assumptions in regard to the appropriateness of information were reported.

Instructional Methods

Another area of study about the value of preoperative teaching involves determining the most effective format and methods of instruction. A landmark study done in 1971 (Lindeman & van Aernam) examined the effects of a structured preoperative teaching program on patient outcomes. A pre-established lesson plan—the structured format—was compared with a vague and inconsistent unstructured approach where each nurse determined what was actually taught. Shorter length of stay, improved ventilatory function, and increased nurse satisfaction were outcomes of the structured approach. King and Tarsitano (1982) replicated the study and found that when a planned, structured teaching protocol was consistently implemented by nursing staff, patient outcomes improved.

The effects of three approaches to preoperative teaching on postoperative complications, psychological well-being, and ventilatory function were studied by Felton, Huss, Payne, and Srsic (1981). Routine preoperative care was compared with a structured format and a therapeutic communications format. Patients who received the structured format reported higher scores of well-being as well as lower levels of anxiety than the other two groups. In a meta-analysis of 73 research studies examining teaching strategies used in patient education, 66% of the subjects who receive planned patient teaching had better outcomes than did subjects receiving routine care (Theis & Johnson, 1995).

A strong research base exists for a structured approach to preoperative teaching, but a challenge arises when nurses try to find the time and the best method to deliver this structured information. Patients no longer are admitted the evening before surgery; instead, they are admitted the morning of surgery. Arrival the morning of surgery does not allow adequate time for preoperative teaching, presenting a dilemma. Research findings have shown that teaching is important, but how do nurses find the time, and what is the best time, to do the teaching that results in positive outcomes for the clients?

In 1976, Fortin and Kirouac examined a pre-admission educational program for surgical patients. Patients who received pre-admission instructions reported higher levels of physical comfort and improved physical function and required less pain medication postoperatively; Johnson (1989) reported that the average time required for adequate preoperative teaching is 30 to 60 minutes. The two most common factors preventing nurses from completing preoperative teaching were time constraints and the unavailability of the patient. Rice and Johnson (1984) studied the effects of a self-instructional booklet sent to patients before admission on teaching time and patient level of performance. More behaviors were learned by those patients who received a specific exercise instruction booklet than by those who were sent nonspecific instructions. The teaching time necessary after admission was significantly reduced also. Wong and Wong (1985) examined the use of written materials before admission and reported increased patient compliance and satisfaction when using the pre-admission materials. In addition, active participation by the patient and family was encouraged with this method. Mikulaninec (1987), when studying effects of preoperative instructions by mail, reported similar findings. Patients were found to be motivated to learn postoperative exercises when receiving preoperative instructions by mail, with an increase in family involvement and promotion of learning noted.

Lepczyk, Raleigh, and Rowley (1990) found that the timing of preoperative teaching did not significantly affect the knowledge and anxiety levels of surgical patients. Little variance was found in test scores, whether patients received teaching up to a week before or only 1 day before surgery. Caldwell (1991) believes that because most patients use emotion-focused coping at the time of surgery, preoperative teaching is beneficial when done well before admission. In a study by Brumfield, Kee, and Johnson (1996), patients preferred to receive teaching before admission for ambulatory surgery. Pre-admission teaching is a cost-effective and time-effective approach to patient education (Theis & Johnson, 1995).

When discussing teaching methods, video instruction and written instruction must be addressed. It is important to note that the written materials sent to patients were generally used in combination with other teaching strategies, such as videotaped instruction or reinforcement by nurses on admission. This combination of strategies was found to improve patient compliance with preoperative activities, improve patient satisfaction, decrease anxiety, improve coping behaviors, increase patient knowledge, and decrease nursing time. Patients are becoming more aware of and involved with self-care activities, are generally healthy participants in their own care, and are able to process information and make informed decisions.

After reviewing studies on video instruction, Gagliano (1988) identified video instruction as an effective method of patient education. It is a cost-effective method that provides standardized education. Videotaped instruction for home viewing is a method of patient education examined by Yale (1993). Yale concluded that it was an economical, self-paced, and convenient method of instruction and that it may lead to increase in motivation to learn. Advantages cited for home viewing of videotapes were ensuring complete information, opportunity for review, comfortable learning environment, decreased interruptions, increased family support, and cost-effectiveness. Disadvantages noted were patients' access to a videocassette recorder, lack of motivation by some patients, and lack of media resource departments for videotape production. In a pilot study by Lisko (1995), there was no significant difference in knowledge scores when using the home viewing videotaped instruction method, but patients reported favorable comments.

Theis and Johnson (1995) found that 65% of subjects receiving alternative methods such as audiovisual or written information reported having better outcomes. Reinforcement of information also had a positive effect on patient outcomes. When using videotape to describe the surgery, pain control, and other necessary information, the nurse can then use her or his limited time to reinforce information; observe return demonstrations of leg exercises, coughing, and deep breathing; and answer questions.

In summary, literature exists to support the nursing intervention of preoperative teaching. This teaching is best if a structured approach is used with a combination of procedural, sensory, and psychological content. Additionally, preoperative teaching before admission using written materials or videotape, with reinforcement and review by nurses on admission, is an effective strategy for nurses to use in addressing the dilemma of preoperative teaching in today's health care environment.

INTERVENTION TOOLS

An excellent tool to guide nurses in the development of a preoperative teaching protocol is the work by the Iowa Intervention Project (McCloskey & Bulechek, 1996). Thirty-one separate nursing activities have been identified (see Table 12–1). The research base discussed earlier supports each nursing activity listed. This basic list can be used as the groundwork in organizing the preoperative teaching necessary for every surgical patient. These activities can be categorized according to the three main content areas (procedural, sensory, and psychological) proven to be most effective as documented in the research. Several of the nursing activities promote self-care and family involvement, which is of utmost importance today with recovery at home.

With the list of nursing activities as a reference, the format of the preoperative teaching intervention must be decided. The format and teaching strategies will be unique to each institution as long as the basic research-based knowledge is presented in a manner that research has shown to be most effective (i.e., structured, combination of content information, and combination of teaching methods). Some institutions may select pre-admission brochures, while others may choose videotaped instruction. Whatever the format, it is important to keep in mind that videotapes and written instructions do not take the place of interventions best suited for nurse-patient interaction.

It might appear overwhelming to nurses to include all 31 activities for each surgical patient, especially with the time constraints nurses are currently experiencing. Nurses must look to research for guidance in prioritizing information based on what patients consider most important. Nurses must become consumer driven and give patients the information they want. Patient access to information will explode with all the health information available to the public through media, especially the Internet. It is imperative that nurses use their assessment skills to evaluate each individual, because each patient is unique and may need a slightly different approach, focusing on different content areas, to have optimal patient outcomes.

A practice level model such as the Butcher Model for Research-Based Preoperative Teaching (Fig. 12–1) is an example of a guide for nurses during the preoperative teaching process. Research findings show that patients with different anxiety levels do better if the focus of content is shifted according to their individual needs. Therefore, the teaching process begins with an assessment of anxiety and fear. This initial nursing activity was identified by NIC as appraising the patient's or significant other's anxiety relating to surgery. This nursing activity then drives the remainder of the teaching intervention. One of three paths is chosen, with each path a systematic, uniform teaching protocol. These protocols contain nursing activities. Examples of NIC nursing activities that could be categorized in the psychological component are as follows:

1. Provide time for the patient to ask questions and discuss concerns.
2. Determine the patient's expectations of the surgery.
3. Correct unrealistic expectations of the surgery, as appropriate.
4. Instruct the patient to use coping techniques directed at controlling specific aspects of the experience, as appropriate.

The nursing activity addressing sensory components includes providing information on what will be heard, smelled, seen, tasted, or felt during the events. The procedural component activities include the following:

1. Describe the postoperative routines and equipment.
2. Discuss possible pain control measures.
3. Instruct the patient on the techniques of getting out of bed.
4. Inform the patient and significant other(s) of the scheduled date, time, and location of the procedure.
5. Conduct a tour of the postsurgical unit(s) and waiting area(s), as appropriate.

Using this model, the structured teaching plan can be adapted to the individual needs of patients by focusing on specific components. The low-anxiety route

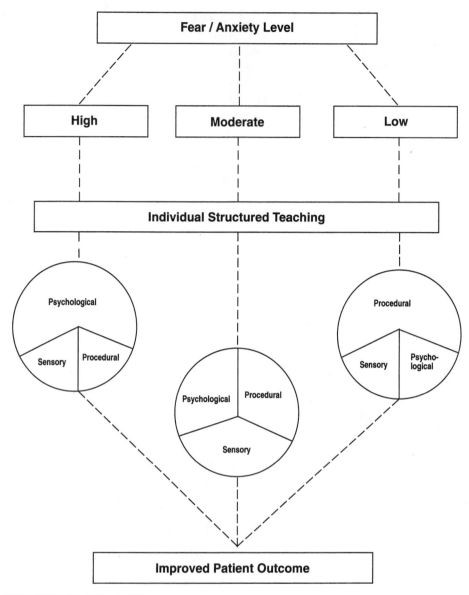

Figure 12-1 Butcher Model for Research-Based Preoperative Teaching. (Courtesy of Horn Video Productions, Ida Grove, IA.)

focuses on procedural information, the middle level has equal emphasis on all three components, and the high-anxiety path focuses on psychological components. The patient's anxiety level may vary from the time when teaching is done to the time of admission before the procedure; therefore, preoperative teaching is an ongoing process. It may be necessary to use a different path during the reinforcement phase of teaching.

NURSING DIAGNOSES

The diagnoses of the North American Nursing Diagnosis Association (NANDA) that have been linked with the NIC intervention of Teaching: Preoperative are

Knowledge Deficit, Fear, and Anxiety. The Teaching: Preoperative intervention is considered a suggested nursing intervention for problem resolution of the diagnosis Knowledge Deficit. It is considered an appropriate intervention when linked to the diagnoses of Fear and Anxiety.

PATIENT OUTCOMES

Patient outcomes are patient states and behaviors that include the state of the patient following an intervention. These outcomes can be measured and compared over time (Maas, Johnson, & Moorhead, 1996). The direct and indirect impacts of preoperative teaching on patient outcomes have been documented in the literature. Any positive effect on patient outcomes, even one of very small significance, provides implications for nursing interventions. The most commonly researched outcomes are fear and anxiety, length of stay, satisfaction with care, physiological variables, family inclusion in teaching, outcome in same-day and ambulatory surgery, and study of specific patient populations (Rothrock, 1989). The Nursing Outcomes Classification (NOC) identifies outcomes that are sensitive to nursing interventions (Maas et al., 1996). Associated patient outcomes that the NIC intervention Teaching: Preoperative would be expected to affect are listed in Table 12–2. The most obvious outcomes would be Anxiety Control, Compliance Behavior, Fear Control, and Knowledge: Treatment Procedure(s).

Table 12–2 Nursing-Sensitive Outcomes Associated with Teaching: Preoperative

Nursing Outcome	Definition
Anxiety Control	Ability to eliminate or reduce feelings of apprehension and tension from unidentifiable source
Circulation Status	Extent to which blood flows unobstructed, unidirectionally, and at an appropriate pressure through large vessels of the systemic and pulmonary circuits
Comfort Level	Feelings of physical and psychological ease
Compliance Behavior	Actions taken on the basis of professional advice to promote wellness, recovery, and rehabilitation
Coping	Actions to manage stressors that tax an individual's resources
Fear Control	Ability to eliminate or reduce disabling feelings of alarm aroused by an identifiable source
Immobility Consequences: Physiological	Compromise in physiological functioning due to impaired physical mobility
Information Processing	Ability to acquire, organize, and use information
Knowledge: Prescribed Activity	Extent of understanding conveyed about prescribed activity and exercise
Knowledge: Treatment Procedure(s)	Extent of understanding and skills conveyed about procedure(s) required as part of a treatment regimen
Pain Control Behavior	Personal actions to control pain
Pain: Disruptive Effects	Observed or reported disruptive effects of pain on emotions and behavior
Pain Level	Amount of reported or demonstrated pain
Respiratory Status: Ventilation	Movement of air in and out of the lungs

Source: Johnson, M., and Maas, M. L. (1997). *Nursing outcomes classification (NOC)*. St. Louis: Mosby–Year Book.

CASE STUDY

Ms. B is a 44-year-old woman who is scheduled to undergo an abdominal hysterectomy at a small rural hospital. Three days before surgery, she goes to the outpatient department of the hospital for laboratory tests. At this time, the operating nurse manager begins the preoperative teaching interventions. Ms. B's anxiety level is assessed using a visual analog scale before any teaching begins. Based on this information, the nurse proceeds with the teaching protocol that includes psychological, sensory, and procedural information. Ms. B's anxiety level is rated in the middle range, so equal emphasis is placed on each content area. A structured format for teaching is used that is a combination of verbal instructions, demonstrations, videotapes, and written instructions.

Verbal instructions are given that include descriptions of the preoperative and postoperative routines, pain control measures, and information about arrival time and scheduled time of surgery. Next, the nurse explains the proper way to get out of bed, cough, deep breathe, and perform leg exercises. These activities are also demonstrated to Ms. B, with her returning the demonstration so the proper technique can be practiced at home. Sensory information is also given to Ms. B. After receiving verbal instructions and demonstration of postoperative activities, Ms. B and her husband watch videotapes on pain management and life after hysterectomy. Before leaving, time is spent on any questions or concerns Ms. B and her husband have about the procedure and what expectations they may have. A booklet that is a condensed version of the information and instruction is given to Ms. B for review at home.

Ms. B arrives 1 hour before surgery. On admission, the nurse reassesses her level of anxiety, determines her knowledge base, and evaluates her coughing, deep breathing, and leg-exercise techniques. Ms. B's anxiety level has decreased, and she has a few questions. She has practiced the postoperative exercises and demonstrated proper technique.

Following surgery, Ms. B uses the proper technique for getting out of bed. She coughs and deep breathes on her own with minimal encouragement necessary from nursing personnel. Her husband actively assists in recovery. Ms. B is kept comfortable with pain management protocols. At dismissal she experiences no signs of infection or respiratory or circulatory problems and is very active in the recovery process. Her fear and anxiety level is low. She and her family are satisfied with the care received.

This case study is an example of positive patient outcomes when the nursing intervention Teaching: Preoperative is implemented. Because today's health care environment is in continual flux, nurses need to continue to examine this intervention, not to substantiate its importance but to find exciting new ways to educate patients, especially presurgical clients. As innovative teaching strategies evolve in this computer age, nursing must be visionary and address the needs of clients by providing information in the most time-effective and cost-effective manner with the most positive outcomes for patients.

References

Brumfield, V. C., Kee, C. C., and Johnson, J. Y. (1996). Preoperative patient teaching in ambulatory surgery settings. *AORN Journal, 64*, 941–946.

Caldwell, L. M. (1991). The influence of preference for information on preoperative stress and coping in surgical outpatients. *Applied Nursing Research, 4*, 177–183.

Devine E. C., and Cook, T. D. (1983). A meta-analytic analysis of effects of psychoeducational interventions on length of postsurgical hospital stay. *Nursing Research, 32*, 267–274.

Devine, E. C., and Cook, T. D. (1986). Clinical and cost-saving effects of psychoeducational interventions with surgical patients: A meta-analysis. *Nursing Research, 9*, 89–105.

Felton, G., Huss, K., Payne, E. A., and Srsic, K. (1981). Preoperative nursing intervention with the patient for surgery: Outcomes of three alternative approaches. In J. Horsley, J. Crane, M. Crabtree, and J. Wood, *Structured preoperative teaching: CURN project* (pp. 43–62). New York: Grune & Stratton. (Reprinted from *International Journal of Nursing Studies, 13*, 83–96.)

Fortin, F., and Kirouac, S. (1976). A randomized controlled trial of preoperative patient education. *International Journal of Nursing Studies, 13*, 11–24.

Gagliano, S. A. (1988). A literature review of the efficacy of video in patient education. *Journal of Medical Education, 63*, 785–792.

Goode, C., Butcher, L., Cipperley, J., Claussen, B., Ekstrom, J., Hayes, J., Lovett, M., and Wellendorf, S. (1986). In *Research utilization: A study guide* (2nd ed.). Ida Grove, IA: Horn Video Productions.

Hathaway, D. (1986). Effect of preoperative instruction on postoperative outcomes: A meta-analysis. *Nursing Research, 35,* 269–275.

Hill, B. J. (1982). Sensory information, behavioral instructions, and coping with sensory alteration surgery. *Nursing Research, 31,* 17–21.

Johnson, J. (1984). Coping with elective surgery. *Annual Review of Nursing Research, 2,* 107–132.

Johnson, J., Rice, V., Fuller, S., and Endress, M. (1978a). Sensory information, instruction in a coping strategy, and recovery from surgery. *Research in Nursing and Health, 1,* 4–17.

Johnson, J. E., Rice, V., Fuller, S., and Endress, M. (1978b). Altering patient's responses to surgery: An extension and replication. *Research in Nursing and Health, 1,* 111–117.

Johnson, S. (1989). Preoperative teaching: A need for change. *Nursing Management, 20*(2), 80B–80H.

King, I., and Tarsitano, B. (1982). The effect of structured and unstructured pre-operative teaching: A replication. *Nursing Research, 31,* 324–329.

Klos, D., Cummings. M., Joyce, J., Graichen, J., and Quigley, A. (1980). A comparison of two methods of delivering presurgical instructions. *Patient Counseling and Health Education, 2*(1), 6–13.

Lepczyk, M., Raleigh, E. H., and Rowley, C. (1990). Timing of preoperative teaching. *Journal of Advanced Nursing, 15,* 300–306.

Levesque, I., Grenier, R., Kérouac, S., and Reidy, M. (1984). Evaluation of a presurgical group program given at two different times. *Research in Nursing and Health, 7,* 227–236.

Lindeman, C. A., and van Aernam, B. V. (1971). Nursing intervention with the presurgical patient—the effects of structured and unstructured preoperative teaching. *Nursing Research, 20,* 319–332.

Lisko, S. A. (1995). Development of use of videotaped instruction for preoperative education of the ambulatory gynecological patient. *Journal of Post Anesthesia Nursing, 10,* 324–328.

Maas, M. L., Johnson, M., and Moorhead, S. (1996). Classifying nursing-sensitive patient outcomes. *Image, 28,* 295–308.

McCloskey, J. C., and Bulechek, G. M. (1996). NIC interventions linked to NANDA diagnoses. In J. C. McCloskey and G. M. Bulechek (Eds.), *Nursing interventions classification (NIC)* (2nd ed., pp. 603–684). St. Louis: Mosby–Year Book.

McHugh, M. G., Christman, N. I., and Johnson, J. E. (1982). Preparatory information: What helps and why. *American Journal of Nursing, 82,* 780–782.

Mikulaninec, C. E. (1987). Effects of mailed preoperative instructions on learning and anxiety. *Patient Education and Counseling, 10,* 253–265.

Miller, P., and Shada, E. A. (1978). Preoperative information and recovery of open-heart surgery patients. *Heart and Lung, 7,* 486–493.

Morgan, J., Wells, N., and Robertson, E. (1985). Effects of preoperative teaching on postoperative pain: A replication and expansion. *International Journal of Nursing Studies, 22,* 267–280.

Mumford, E., Schlesinger, H., and Glass, G. (1982). The effects of psychological intervention on recovery from surgery and heart attacks: An analysis of literature. *American Journal of Public Health, 72*(2), 141–151.

Rice, V., and Johnson, J. E. (1984). Preadmission self-instruction booklets, postadmission exercise performance and teaching time. *Nursing Research, 33,* 147–151.

Rothrock, J. C. (1989). Perioperative nursing research, part 1: Preoperative psycho-educational interventions. *AORN Journal, 49,* 597–619.

Theis, S. L., and Johnson, J. H. (1995). Strategies for teaching patients: A meta-analysis. *Clinical Nurse Specialist, 9,* 100–105.

Wong, J., and Wong S. (1985). A randomized control trial of a new approach to preoperative teaching and patient compliance. *International Journal of Nursing Studies, 22,* 105–115.

Yale, E. (1993). Preoperative teaching strategy: Videotapes for home viewing. *AORN Journal, 57,* 901–908.

Yount, S., and Schoessler, M. (1991). A description of patient and nurse perceptions of preoperative teaching. *Journal of Post Anesthesia Nursing, 6*(1), 17–25.

Medication Management

Madeline A. Naegle

Medication Management is a comprehensive intervention that encompasses the nurse's knowledge and the activities that are undertaken to potentiate the patient's maximum benefit from pharmacotherapeutic agents. The nurse-environment interaction considers characteristics of the individual, the setting, the influence of significant others, and the nature and actions of a variety of potentially therapeutic agents. Recent social changes suggest that trends influence the scope and nature of activities undertaken on behalf of, and with, the client in relation to medication. An informed public now self-medicates with multiple over-the-counter drugs, feels empowered to make decisions about the types and amounts of medication prescribed, chooses alternative therapeutic agents, and uses illicit agents to achieve self-defined positive outcomes not achieved with prescribed products. Interventions require that nursing action derives from a knowledge base. The depth of the required knowledge base is determined by the scope of nursing practice associated with levels of education and regulatory licensure. For example, the generalist practitioner of nursing does not require the depth of knowledge that is required for the advanced practice nurse who has prescribing privileges. Minimum knowledge required by the nurse includes "knowing the patient." This is defined by Radwin (1995) as purposeful action whereby the nurse uses understanding of the patient's experiences, behaviors, and feelings and other perceptions to individualize interventions. In addition, the nurse needs knowledge of the patient's current health status and comprehensive knowledge of the actions of the medication. This includes the chemical structure and expected actions of the drug; probable side effects; drug interaction with foods, other substances, and medications; and considerations related to the route of administration of the drug (Naegle, 1994).

REVIEW OF THE LITERATURE
■

Independent and Collaborative Activities

Depending on which state within the United States the nurse practices, two levels of nursing activity related to Medication Management are now legally recognized: the administration and monitoring of medication and drug use, and the prescription of medication. In all states, registered nurse (RN) licensure grants the privilege to implement physician's orders for medication. While this is a legally dependent function, the nurse is independently responsible and legally accountable for knowing the drug, the appropriate dosage, the anticipated and untoward effects, and the specific drug-related considerations including route of administration. Licensure and certification for advanced practice nurses and nurse midwives specify a range of collaborative and autonomous privileges. Laws vary by state, so that in some states the nurse may be legally able to prescribe according to protocols, in collaboration with the physician, or independently for prescription medications and controlled substances. The nurse must be knowledgeable about state statutes that designate the scope of nursing practice, from which the guidelines for Medication Management derive. Factors contributing to nursing errors in Medication Management include workplace conditions, workload, employer policies and procedures, and levels of nurses' educational preparation and experience. Drug diversion by impaired nurses can result in medication errors and differences in error levels. Some research suggests that seasonal affective disorder (SAD) may play a role in medication errors (Roseman & Booker, 1995; Thompson & Isaacs, 1988). The most common errors occur when nurses administer medications in the wrong doses or by routes other than those ordered (Guido, 1997).

In a New York study of nurses disciplined for medication errors, 57.1% of the nurses were employed in hospitals, with the second most frequent site being long-term care facilities. The disciplined nurses generally had less education and less experience than most New York RNs. More than 50% of them held associate degrees, and 21.5% had been practicing for less than 5 years. Evidence of correlations between working conditions and medication errors included the findings that 53.3% of the disciplined nurses (versus 49.7% of the general nurse population) worked in downsized institutions and that 71.4% of them worked overtime because of unfilled RN positions or decreased RN staff (New York State Nurses Association, 1997). Errors were also found to correlate positively with greater numbers of shifts worked by temporary nursing staff (Roseman & Booker, 1995). In addition to resolving negative workplace factors, there is some evidence that individual medication-related job performance can be improved by medication administration training, credentialing, and attendance at a behavior-oriented safety program (Fuqua & Stevens, 1988).

Peer review is a form of collaboration that can increase the effectiveness of Medication Management. Advanced practice nurses working in collaboration with physicians can successfully form peer-review groups for overall patient case management review. Whether implemented by region or in institutional settings, satisfaction with peer review as a form of quality assurance was reported by participants who were consultation-liaison nurses. In addition to facilitating learning and mastery, the peer-review group process was believed to have effectively served to assure the consumer of the competence of the psychiatric consultation-liaison nurse and the quality of his or her practice (Titlebaum, Hart, & Roman-Egan, 1992).

Peer assistance enhances Medication Management when it provides support to nurses who are in recovery from addiction, burnout, or psychiatric illness. In the case of addiction, peers are often asked to administer narcotics until the recovering nurse is well advanced in his or her sobriety and can resume those role responsibilities. In situations of stress and job overload, peer support can reduce subjective strain and provide affirmation of professional competence.

The use of technology in both the administration of medication and the documentation of Medication Management is central to job performance and quality assurance. The presence of an up-to-date, readily accessed record means that nurses and colleagues can use information to prevent errors and anticipate possible negative outcomes of drug interactions. Many hospitals now use centrally located computer terminals to record medication administration. Bedside computers have also been used in efforts to increase the accuracy and timeliness of medication administration. Research on this innovation, however, has not validated the benefits of bedside terminal use in any consistent way (Marr et al., 1993), and only limited conclusions have been drawn about improvement in the quality of patient care (Simpson, 1997). An innovative point-of-information system used at the bedside, although difficult to implement, has been observed to improve timing, decrease error rate, and increase the accuracy of recording (Puckett, 1995).

Collaboration and Consultation

Collaboration with others is always required in Medication Management. It takes the forms of communication and validation with the physician and pharmacist, communication with other nurses also responsible for Medication Management, and communication and supervision of individuals such as students or licensed practical nurses (LPNs). Consultation responsibilities change as a function of the setting in which the nurse practices and are different in generalist and advanced practice roles. When the nurse functions as a generalist and in collaboration with other team members, responsibilities listed under medication knowledge apply as minimum expectations. Supervision of others in medication administration increases the nurse's responsibilities. Delegation of medication administration responsibilities does not relieve the nurse of the responsibilities outlined under medication knowledge. Management practices should include sufficient knowledge on the part of the delegating nurse to assign medication administration to appropriately educated and licensed personnel. Supervision of personnel not licensed to dispense medication, for example, places the nurse at risk for licensure discipline. When the nurse has prescribing privileges, consultation with physicians and peers should be sought. In some states this is mandated in laws that provide for *complementary authority* in medication prescription. Where nurse practitioners have *substitutive authority* and autonomous prescription-writing authority, consultation with physicians and peers is desirable (Talley & Brooke, 1992).

Collaboration with the patient and family members can increase the accuracy and consistency with which the patient self-administers prescribed medications or receives them from family members or designated caretakers. Medication can be effectively administered by these individuals when the nurse implements strategies related to collaboration in Medication Management. For example, errors in administration of medication by patients and family have actually been observed to occur less frequently than nursing staff errors, errors attributed to equipment defects, or pharmacist errors in a cooperative care unit where nurses educate participants (Phelan, Kramer, Grieco, & Glassman, 1996.) Other research, however, indicates that self-medication rates vary considerably by population and age group. In groups of elders, for example, medication errors persisted despite special education and monitoring (Pereles et al., 1996).

In collaboration with patient and family, the nurse assesses the patient and family for readiness to undertake and comply with a medication regimen. The nurse then educates the patient and family about the properties, side effects, and potential benefits of the medication and the schedule for, and manner of, medication administration.

Knowledge of Lifestyle

Lifestyles emerge as functions of choices by individuals and are based on belief systems, attitudes, and preferences. Assessment provides a database that includes information about the individual's or family's habits, traditions, culture, living environment, and health behaviors, all of which can influence effective nursing interventions. Cultural traditions and beliefs support attitudes about the use of medications and the types of medications considered acceptable to the user (Spector, 1996). Cultural beliefs also support a client's choice to use substances not regulated by the federal government such as herb and vitamin preparations and home remedies. Increasingly, consumers are choosing "natural" products and alternative treatments over prescription drugs as a result of cultural traditions or belief systems. In addition, people are including natural products, vitamin regimens, and home remedies in health seeking behaviors. Nonmedical drugs and alternative methodologies outside the realm of research evaluation may pose risks to health and result in conflict between clients and health care providers over the most beneficial approaches to pharmacological treatment.

Lifestyle includes decisions to use drugs and decisions on which drugs to use. Prescribed, over-the-counter, and legal and illicit drugs all have the potential to be harmful to health. Medication Management as an effective intervention derives from the nurse's knowledge of what drugs are considered by the patient to be part of his or her lifestyle as well as of the way the drugs are used. The legal drugs alcohol and nicotine are the most harmful to health, are frequently used together, and are also the drugs most often used to excess. *Misuse* is the use of a drug for purposes other than that for which it was intended. Misuse applies to the use of illicit drugs to self-medicate moods or uncomfortable states as well as to the use of over-the-counter and prescription drugs; knowledge of misuse is important for effective Medication Management. For example, over-the-counter sleep aids are used in greater proportion than benzodiazepines for the treatment of sleep problems, and their use is consumer initiated (Pilliteri, Kozlowski, Person, & Spear, 1994). In studies of community-dwelling elders, findings not considered to be unusual noted that residents were taking an average of 2.1 prescription and 2.3 over-the-counter medications. At the same time, 16.3% of that population reported sometimes drinking alcohol, and 11.3% reported drinking alcohol regularly (Pollow, Stoller, Forster, & Duniho, 1994). The most common problems result from the use of alcohol in combination with prescribed drugs and illicitly obtained prescription drugs. When psychoactive drugs are taken in combination with prescription stimulants, analgesics, and antianxiety agents, morbidity and mortality are significant (Wilford, Finch, Czechowicz, & Warren, 1994). Prescription drug misuse is a common problem among community-dwelling elderly (Schneitman-McIntire, Farne, Gordon, Chan, & Toy, 1996) and in nursing homes where residents also misuse alcohol, nicotine, and illicit drugs (Joseph, 1995) while commonly taking antihypertensives, cardiac medications, and minor tranquilizers.

Medication Management poses particular challenges when the patient is an actively using or recovering addict. The nurse must know the interaction potential of prescribed drugs in combination with alcohol and illicit drugs, the addictive potential of analgesics and psychotropic drugs, and the safety margins for drugs used in treating addiction, such as methadone and naltrexone. Complex clinical problems are not uncommon with recovering addicts who may be seropositive for human immunodeficiency virus (HIV) secondary to intravenous drug abuse. Medication Management can involve numerous drugs with potentially negative interactions. Education about the potential outcomes of relapses to illicit drug or alcohol use is central to patient teaching. The use of illicit drugs is an important consideration in knowing the patient, because some illicit drugs are more commonly used at various phases in the life cycle. Illicit use of growth-promoting steroids, for example, occurs most often among adolescents and young adults who are enabled by fellow athletes or adults in sports programs. Similarly, over-the-counter and prescription appetite suppressants are misused by men and women concerned with weight. It is conceivable that a client can be taking a prescription drug, using an illicit psychotropic agent like marijuana, and using an over-the-counter stimulant medication like NōDōz or a hypnotic. Without knowledge of this drug-taking lifestyle, nursing action related to Medication Management cannot be expected to result in anticipated outcomes.

In summary, in both institutional and community settings and in the role of direct care provider, administrator, or case manager, the nurse is responsible for complying with established protocols ranging from medication administration to updating medication records as prescriptions are written and changed, in accord with information obtained from the patient about drug use. The nurse should educate the patient about the need to inform health care providers that drug use patterns have changed and about the risks involved when using alcohol or illicit drugs while taking prescription medication. Patient education and patient safety are central components of nursing intervention in Medication Management, but with increasing numbers of states granting prescribing privileges to nurses, responsibilities are changing. The nursing activities for Medication Management incorporate these actions as shown in Table 13–1.

ASSOCIATED NURSING DIAGNOSES

Because Medication Management must consider prescribed, over-the-counter, and social or illicit drugs, several North American Nursing Diagnosis Association (NANDA) diagnoses are applicable to conditions resulting from, or associated with, medication and drug use. Nursing diagnoses may apply to conditions whereby self-medication is practiced, conditions induced by incorrect use of drugs, conditions that reflect self-care deficits, and conditions resulting from the properties of drugs, whether administered by self or others. Table 13–2 lists nursing diagnoses commonly associated with Medication Management.

NURSING OUTCOMES OF MEDICATION MANAGEMENT

Outcomes, such as those defined in the Nursing Outcomes Classification (NOC), describe behaviors, responses, and feelings of the patient in response to, or as a result of, nursing actions (Bulechek & McCloskey, 1992). Outcomes for Medication Management should be established before action is taken and should reflect

Table 13–1   Medication Management

DEFINITION: Facilitation of safe and effective use of prescription and over-the-counter drugs.

ACTIVITIES:

Determine what drugs are needed, and administer according to prescriptive authority and/or protocol

Determine patient's ability to self-medicate, as appropriate

Monitor effectiveness of the medication administration modality

Monitor patient for the therapeutic effect of the medication

Monitor for signs and symptoms of drug toxicity

Monitor for adverse effects of the drug

Monitor for nontherapeutic drug interactions

Review periodically with the patient and/or family types and amounts of medications taken

Facilitate changes in medication with physician, as appropriate

Determine factors which may preclude the patient from taking drugs as prescribed

Develop strategies with the patient to enhance compliance with prescribed medication regimen

Consult with other health care professionals to minimize the number and frequency of drugs needed for a therapeutic effect

Teach patient and/or family members the method of drug administration, as appropriate

Teach patient and/or family members the expected action and side effects of the medication

Provide patient and family members with written and visual information to enhance self-administration of medications, as appropriate

Obtain physician order for patient self-medication, as appropriate

Establish a protocol for the storage, restocking, and monitoring of medications left at the bedside for self-medication purposes

Investigate possible financial resources for acquisition of prescribed drugs, as appropriate

Determine impact of medication use on patient's life-style

Provide alternatives for timing and modality of self-administered medications to minimize life-style effects

Assist the patient and family members in making necessary life-style adjustments associated with certain medications, as appropriate

Instruct patient when to seek medical attention

Identify types and amounts of over-the-counter drugs used

Provide information about the use of over-the-counter drugs and how they may influence the existing condition

Determine whether the patient is using culturally-based home health remedies and the possible effects on use of over-the-counter and prescribed medications

Provide patient with a list of resources to contact for further information about the medication regimen

Contact patient and family postdischarge, as appropriate, to answer questions and discuss concerns associated with the medication regimen

---

Source: McCloskey, J. C., and Bulechek, G. M. (1995). *Nursing interventions classification (NIC).* St. Louis: Mosby–Year Book.

the influence of the relevant variables of behavioral and constitutional patient characteristics, family and environmental factors, the pharmacotherapeutic agent, and the nursing diagnosis. Medication Management is directed toward achieving the most desirable outcome for the patient, whether or not the nurse actually administers or prescribes the medication. In the misuse of over-the-counter medications, for example, the intervention may be directed toward the elimination of medications inappropriately self-administered by the client. Outcomes of Medication Management issue from an interactional process involv-

Table 13–2 NANDA Diagnoses Linked to Medication Management

Acute Confusion
Altered Health Maintenance
Chronic Pain
Diarrhea
Health Seeking Behaviors
Hyperthermia
Ineffective Individual Coping
Knowledge Deficit: health implications of drug, tobacco, alcohol use
Noncompliance: self-medicating
Pain
Risk for Poisoning: drug and alcohol toxicity
Self-Care Deficit: medications
Sexual Dysfunction
Sleep Pattern Disturbance

ing a number of variables that the nurse may influence but over which the nurse has limited control. For example, the nurse practitioner may prescribe a particular medication, but the process by which the prescription is filled involves choice of pharmacy and the actions of the responding pharmacist. Health teaching is a nursing action that is essential to the determination of outcomes for the client. In identifying an outcome, therefore, it is important that the nurse consider all relevant intervening variables and decide which nursing actions are appropriate to influence or change those variables. Table 13–3 delineates some identified potential outcomes of Medication Management.

CASE STUDIES

Case Study 1

Mr. W, a 52-year-old Vietnam veteran, is admitted to an acute care unit with a fever of 102°F, shortness of breath, tachypnea, and diminished appetite. In the last year, he completed a drug and alcohol rehabilitation program, and he reports no use of nonprescription drugs, including alcohol, for 6 months. On assessment, it is noted that he is anxious and tremulous, has difficulty concentrating, and is mildly diaphoretic. He has had a history of substance abuse since high school and

was recently diagnosed as being HIV positive. He started a new regimen of two nucleosides and a protease inhibitor 4 weeks ago. At that time he was also placed on Bactrim as prophylaxis for *Pneumocystis carinii* pneumonia. During the admission interview his wife says, and he concurs, that he has been very upset and anxious since learning of his HIV-positive status and is attempting to comply with his new treatment.

The nurse considers the role that Medication Management may play in his current symptom

Table 13–3 NOC Outcomes Linked to Medication Management

Comfort Level	Pain Control Behavior
Compliance Behavior	Pain Level
Coping	Risk Control: Alcohol Use
Health Beliefs: Perceived Ability to Perform	Risk Control: Drug Use
Health Beliefs: Perceived Threat	Risk Control: Tobacco Use
Health Promoting Behavior	Self-Care: Non-Parenteral Medication
Knowledge: Health Behaviors	Self-Care: Parenteral Medication
Knowledge: Medication	Symptom Severity
Knowledge: Substance Use Control	Well-Being
Knowledge: Treatment Regimen	

profile. The nurse obtains a detailed history of all prescribed medications, considering that Noncompliance: failure to follow prescribed regimen may be an applicable nursing diagnosis. The nurse notes that the diagnosis Ineffective Individual Coping is supported by his anxiety and reported "upset" and disturbed concentration related to his recent HIV diagnosis. Given Mr. W's history of drug and alcohol use, the nurse considers that Noncompliance: self-medicating may be applicable and that Mr. W may have been using alcohol or an illicit drug in an effort to cope with anxiety. The nurse considers that Mr. W could be experiencing withdrawal from heavy alcohol consumption or another drug. Knowledge of the actions and side effects of protease inhibitors and other antiretroviral agents forms the database from which to evaluate the meaning of observed symptoms.

The nurse expands upon the history gathered by talking with Mr. W and his wife in more detail about his declared abstinence from illicit drugs and alcohol, seeking collateral information that might suggest that he has lapsed from his intentions to abstain. They review the protocols for use of all prescribed drugs, and the nurse verifies with the attending physician information about the initiation of a new drug regimen and Mr. W's patterns of use and responses to medication. Once Mr. W is feeling more comfortable, the nurse reviews with him the signs and symptoms that might derive from ineffective medication management. The nurse inquires about Mr. W's knowledge of medication and drug effects and assesses his state of readiness for patient education. Depending on the patient's state of readiness, the nurse reviews information about actions of all the drugs that Mr. W may have used or self-administered, the effects of alcohol on the T cell count, and the interaction of alcohol and other drugs with prescribed medication. The nurse plans a review of the information with Mr. W and his wife before discharge, discusses their concerns about the complex and somewhat burdensome new medication regimen, and assists them in formulating a schedule that can be realistically implemented given their lifestyle.

Case Study 2

A 42-year-old woman, Ms. S, is seen in the outpatient clinic, having been diagnosed with early symptoms of multiple sclerosis. The physician has prescribed diazepam (Valium), 10 mg prn for spasm, and amantadine (Symmetrel), 75 mg a day, to offset fatigue. The nurse is asked to implement health teaching. The nurse considers the nursing diagnoses Altered Health Maintenance, Knowledge Deficit, Risk for Poisoning, and Spiritual Distress secondary to adjustment to diagnosis of a chronic and progressive illness. The nurse interviews Ms. S and develops a knowledge base that includes the patient's knowledge level of the disease, medication regimen, and lifestyle, including the patient's social support systems.

The nurse considers aspects of Ms. S's lifestyle that could influence the effectiveness of the prescribed medications, including her pattern of drinking one to two glasses of wine 3 days a week and smoking half a pack of cigarettes daily, because nicotine can stimulate the sympathetic nervous system and block the parasympathetic nervous system, or vice versa. After exposure to nicotine, the individual may also experience depressive symptoms, aggravating any negative emotional states associated with lifestyle adjustment to the disease.

In implementing Medication Management, the nurse uses printed patient education materials to teach about the actions of the prescribed drugs and their potential side effects. The nurse assists the client in identifying experiences that indicate the need for taking the Valium and works with her to plan a schedule in accord with her work patterns so as to maximize the effects of the Symmetrel. A potential outcome might be Knowledge: treatment regimen, because the teaching involves development of skills about assessing one's emotional state as well as receiving information about the medication. The nurse educates Ms. S about the importance of decreasing or eliminating alcohol use because of its role in increasing depression and producing drowsiness and the potential for poisoning when alcohol is taken while using Valium. Ms. S is cautioned about driving or using machinery because of the psychomotor impairment secondary to Valium use. The nurse informs Ms. S about safe levels for use of Valium in the relief of muscle spasm and discusses the risk for developing benzodiazepine dependence when the dosage is indiscriminately or progressively increased. The nurse instructs Ms. S in alternative modalities like relaxation exercises to induce the relaxation she seeks with alcohol use and to decrease the discomfort of muscle spasms. A potential outcome would be Knowledge: Health Behaviors, because the intervention considers health teaching about the interaction of two self-medicating behaviors that relate to each other. The nurse counsels Ms. S about possible lifestyle changes that could decrease the

stress and fatigue associated with her disease and facilitate her adjustment with minimal spiritual and emotional distress. After information about how to contact the nurse with concerns or questions is provided, arrangements are made to review outcomes of the teaching session with the client when she next visits the clinic.

SUMMARY

■

Medication Management requires a broad base of nursing knowledge about medication, the client and family, and the scope of practice for which the nurse is prepared. The use of quality assurance mechanisms, institutional and agency procedures, and physician or advanced practice nurse protocols provides guidelines for the safe and effective implementation of nursing activities related to Medication Management. The nurse engages in professional role functions, including collaboration with other health care providers and family members, advocacy for obtaining and using safe and cost-effective pharmacotherapeutic agents, and referral when responses to medication regimens or the use of other drugs, including alcohol and nicotine, produce alterations in health maintenance.

References

Bulechek, G. M., and McCloskey, J. C. (1992). *Nursing interventions: essential nursing treatments* (2nd ed.). Philadelphia: W.B. Saunders.

Fuqua, R., and Stevens, K. (1988). What we know about medication errors: A literature review. *Journal of Nursing Quality Assurance, 3*(1), 1–17.

Guido, G. W. (1997). *Legal issues in nursing* (2nd ed.). Stamford, CT: Appleton & Lange.

Joseph, C. L. (1995). Alcohol and drug misuse in the nursing home. *International Journal of Addiction, 30,* 1953–1984.

Marr, P. B., Duthie, E., Glassman, K., Janovas, D. M., Kelly, J. B., Graham, E., Kovner, C., Rienzi, A., Roberts, N. K., and Schick, D. (1993). Bedside terminals and quality of nursing administration. *Computers in Nursing, 11*(4), 176–182.

Naegle, M. A. (1994). Prescription drugs and nursing education: Knowledge gaps and implications for role performance. *Journal of Law, Medicine and Ethics, 22*(3), 257–261.

New York State Nurses Association. (1997 July-August). Understaffing = medication errors. *Report: The Official Newsletter of the New York State Nurses Association,* 3.

Pereles, L., Romonko, L., Muryzn, T., Hogan, D., Silvius, J., Long, S., and Fung, T. (1996). Evaluation of a self-medication program. *Journal of the American Geriatrics Society, 44*(2), 161–165.

Phelan, G., Kramer, E. J., Grieco, A. J., and Glassman, K. S. (1996). Self-administration of medication by patients and family members during hospitalization. *Patient Education and Counseling, 27*(1), 103–112.

Pilliteri, J. L., Kozlowski, L. T., Person, D. C., and Spear, M. E. (1994). Over-the-counter sleep aids: Widely used but rarely studied. *Journal of Substance Abuse, 6*(3), 315–323.

Pollow, R. L., Stoller, E. P., Forster, L. E., and Duniho, T.

S. (1994). Drug combinations and potential for risk of adverse drug reaction among community-dwelling elderly. *Nursing Research, 43*(1), 44–49.

Puckett, F. (1995). Medication management component of a point-of-care information system. *American Journal of Health-System Pharmacy, 52,* 1305–1309.

Radwin, L. E. (1995). Knowing the patient: A process model for individualized interventions. *Nursing Research, 44*(6), 364–370.

Roseman, C., and Booker, J. (1995). Workload and environmental factors in hospital medication errors. *Nursing Research, 44*(4), 226–230.

Schneitman-McIntire, O., Farne, T. A., Gordon, N., Chan, J., and Toy, W. A. (1996). Medication misadventures resulting in emergency department visits at an HMO medical center. *American Journal of Health-System Pharmacy, 53,* 1416–1422.

Simpson, R. L. (1997). Point of care technology: A new perspective. *Nursing Management, 28*(8), 16.

Spector, R. (1996). *Cultural diversity in health and illness.* Stamford, CT: Appleton & Lange.

Talley, S., and Brooke, P. S. (1992). Prescriptive authority for psychiatric clinical specialists: Facing the issues. *Archives of Psychiatric Nursing, 6*(2), 71–82.

Thompson, C., and Isaacs, G. (1988). Seasonal affective disorder: Symptomatology in relation to mode of referral and diagnostic subtype. *Journal of Affective Disorder, 14,* 1–11.

Titlebaum, H., Hart, C. A., and Roman-Egan, J. (1992). Interagency psychiatric consultation-liaison nursing peer review and peer board: Quality assurance and empowerment. *Archives of Psychiatric Nursing, 6*(2), 125–131.

Wilford, B., Finch, J., Czechowicz, D. J., and Warren, D. (1994). An overview of prescription drug misuse and abuse: Defining the problem and seeking the solutions. *Journal of Law, Medicine and Ethics, 22*(3), 197–203.

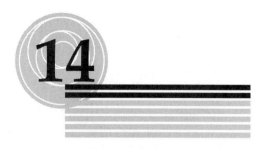

Fluid Management

Alice Poyss

Abnormalities of body fluid and electrolyte metabolism present certain therapeutic problems. When the mechanisms normally regulating fluid volume, electrolyte composition, and osmolality are impaired, therapy becomes complicated. The activities performed by nurses for managing fluids are intended to prevent abnormal or undesired fluid levels. The nurse has the responsibility of recognizing the importance of adverse effects of fluid and electrolyte metabolism. The nurse gathers information through continued physical assessment, weight monitoring, and monitoring of hemodynamics and hydration state. Nurses cannot focus on the effects of fluid balance and electrolyte disturbances because each problem is characterized by myriad symptoms that cut across all systems. The knowledge the nurse uses in recognizing adverse effects contributes to safe, successful Fluid Management in critically ill patients (Jacobs, 1994).

Research demonstrates that there is an inhibitory influence of central volume receptors and an increased fractional sodium excretion in older clients. Age changes the plasma volume baroreceptors, and terminal illness changes osmolality (Stachenfeld, DiPietro, Nadel, & Mack, 1997). An understanding of these metabolic processes enables the nurse to make clinical judgments concerning the outcomes of Fluid Management.

RELATED LITERATURE

The physiological mechanisms of Fluid Management include a basic comprehension of the mechanisms of fluid compartments and fluid movement. The extracellular and intracellular compartments and their electrolytes assist in the basic maintenance of fluid balance. Every body system and body organ is used to maintain the internal environment. The lungs, kidneys, heart, adrenal glands, pituitary gland, and parathyroid glands are involved in regulatory mechanisms.

Water is the sole solvent and the most abundant compound in the human body, constituting 40% to 80% of body weight. The body is essentially an aqueous solution in which a vast complex of solutes is distributed in compartments that vary in size and are bounded by lipid membranes. Water is the environment in which the reactions of life occur. The total body water of an individual varies with body fat. Body fat is essentially water free; the greater the fat content, the less the water content (Narins, 1994).

Fluid housed in the body can be divided into two main compartments: intracellular and extracellular. Intracellular fluid accounts for approximately three fourths of the body's total body fluid. Intracellular fluid compartments provide the cells with the internal aqueous medium necessary for chemical functions. Extracellular fluid accounts for the rest of the body fluid. The extracellular fluid compartments help maintain the internal environment, offering nutrients and other substances to the cells, as well as removal of waste. This is a constant movement throughout the body, assisting the internal cells in maintenance and balance.

Extracellular fluid includes all body water that is external to the cells, including erythrocytes. Thus, extracellular water includes water inside and outside blood vessels, as well as water that is in the interstitium between cells and water that has crossed epithelial cells (for example, gastrointestinal fluids). Other extracellular water compartments include those that contain plasma, interstitial fluid, lymph, inaccessible bone water, and transcellular water (Narins, 1994). The transcellular compartment is the product of cellular metabolism and consists of secretions that assist in tracing lost electrolytes and prescribing proper fluid and electrolyte replacement. Excessive fluid and electrolyte loss in this compartment will affect the balance of the two main fluid compartments (Halperin & Goldstein, 1994). Interstitial fluid accounts for the fluid component of blood and constitutes the remaining 20% of the extracellular fluid (Narins, 1994).

Water distribution into the various body compartments is dependent on the permeability of the barrier between compartments and the solute in each compartment. Almost all compartmental barriers in humans are highly permeable to water. Normal intracellular water varies inversely with extracellular fluid and a decrease in extracellular volume (Halperin & Goldstein, 1994).

The amount of body water loss is easily computed by weighing a patient and noting weight loss; 1 L of body water is equivalent to 1 kg (2.2 lb) of body weight. Weight changes are valuable tools to indicate fluid imbalances (Methany, 1996).

Electrolyte concentration plays a significant role in cellular function and in the distribution of water in the various fluid spaces. The concentration of ions moves from the area of higher concentration to the area of lower concentration until the concentrations are equal. This constant interchange of ions and water between the fluid compartments is dependent on the unique structure of the cell membrane—a structure designed to regulate this exchange between the cell and its surrounding environment. Terms related to movement include osmosis, osmolality, active transport, and oncotic pressure (Lancaster, 1987).

Osmosis is a special type of diffusion in which water is the chief substance to pass through a selectively permeable membrane (Narins, 1994). Water moves freely from a weak solution into a more concentrated one. Osmosis stops when both fluids have the same osmolality.

The number of dissolved particles in a unit of water determines the solution's concentration and can be expressed as either osmolality or osmolarity. Osmolality refers to the number of osmoles per kilogram of water; thus, the total volume will be 1 kg of water plus the relatively small volume occupied by the solute. On the other hand, osmolarity refers to the number of osmoles per liter of solution. In this instance, the volume of water is less than 1 L by amount equal to the solute volume. Because of the very low solute concentration in body fluids, the difference between osmolality and osmolarity is negligible. Nonetheless, *osmolality* is the correct term to use when referring to body fluids, because osmotic activity in the body depends on the concentration of active particles per kilogram of water (Narins, 1994). The term *tonicity* is sometimes used instead of osmolality. Solutions may be termed isotonic, hypotonic, or hypertonic. Isotonic solutions have the same effective osmolality as body fluids (close to 285 milliosmol [mOsm]). An example of an isotonic fluid is 0.9% sodium chloride. In contrast, a hypotonic solution has a lower osmolality than body fluids; an example of a hypotonic fluid is 0.45% sodium chloride. Finally, a hypertonic solution has an effective osmolality greater than that of body fluids; an example of a hypertonic fluid is 3% sodium chloride.

There are a number of terms important to fluid management. *Active transport* is the movement of solutes across a cell membrane in the absence of a favorable electrochemical or concentration gradient; it requires energy. *Oncotic pressure* is the osmotic pressure exerted by protein within the membranes. *Diffusion* is the continual movement of molecules among each other in liquids or in gases (Methany, 1996). *Filtration* is the transfer of water and dissolved substances from a region of high pressure to a region of low pressure. The force behind filtration is hydrostatic pressure. An example of filtration is the passage of water and electrolytes from the arterial capillary bed to the interstitial fluid; in this instance, the hydrostatic pressure is furnished by the pumping action of the heart.

Thirst and Output

Whether primary or secondary to other conditions, all body fluid disturbances are caused by abnormal differences between gains and losses of water and electrolytes. One mechanism for gaining fluid in a healthy adult is stimulating the thirst center (Narins, 1994). The body gains water and electrolytes in various ways; water alone is gained by drinking water and by oxidation of foodstuffs and body tissues. Renal regulation of water assists the body in maintaining fluid loss.

The thirst center functions in a manner similar to that of an osmoreceptor. When the thirst center is stimulated, particularly by a high extracellular osmolality, water leaves the cells by osmosis, causing them to shrink. The shrinking stimulates signals to the cortex indicating the desire to drink (Halperin & Goldstein, 1994). Although the primary stimulus is that of high osmolality, other patient conditions that suggest other causes of thirst include the following.

- Excessive loss of potassium ions (causes cells to shrink)
- Decreased blood volume
- Mucous membrane dehydration
- Psychological illness (e.g., schizophrenia) (Rinard, 1989)

Angiotensin II stimulates the thirst center as well as the secretion of antidiuretic hormone (ADH) and an increase in gastrointestinal water absorption. Angiotensin II is formed in the blood when the kidneys release renin in response to a low blood volume (extracellular volume contracts). Angiotensin II causes aldosterone to be released, more sodium bicarbonate ($NaHCO_3$) to be reabsorbed by the proximal tubule, and thirst to be stimulated. The perception of thirst requires an alert level of consciousness. In an alert person, the thirst mechanism can compensate when antidiuretic hormone mechanisms fail by causing an awareness of the increased need for fluid to replace that being lost in the urine. Infants, persons with impaired levels of consciousness, or those with psychological disturbances may not respond to the stimulants sent out by the thirst center (Rinard, 1989).

Thirst is not always a reliable indicator of need for fluids. Critically ill patients often do not recognize thirst, and even if they do, they may be unable to reach for water (Cogan, 1991; Gaspar, 1988). Patients with fluid volume excesses caused by cardiac or renal damage are sometimes quite thirsty. Patients with burns experience great thirst, but their needs are met with electrolyte solutions. Burn patients' quantity and osmolality of intravenous fluids are carefully monitored. Volume-depleted patients, whether they have malabsorptive gastrointestinal (GI) syndromes or not, and cardiovascular patients should be high priority for careful evaluation of fluid replacement, because the thirst mechanism is altered (Narins, 1994).

When water is ingested without solutes, for balance, water without solutes must be excreted in the urine. There are several nephron sites where sodium (Na^+) and chloride (Cl^-) are reabsorbed but water is not. Of the 180 L/day of water filtered through the glomerulus, about 95% to 99% is reabsorbed throughout the renal tubule. The kidney can produce concentrated urine or a dilute urine, depending on the needs of the body (Halperin & Goldstein, 1994). The most important of these sites is the thick ascending limb of the loop of Henle. Other segments are the early distal convoluted tubule (not sensitive to ADH), the late distal convoluted tubule, and the collecting duct (which requires absence of ADH to maintain impermeability to water). To excrete dilute urine, the following three processes must occur:

- Delivery of saline to the thick ascending limb of the loop of Henle. One third of the glomerular filtration rate (GFR) (60 L/day) is delivered to diluting sites of the nephron. Only a major reduction in the GFR can reduce delivery sufficiently to be the sole cause of a limited excretion of electrolyte-free water.
- Separation of salt and water (reabsorption of sodium chloride without water). In the thick ascending limb of the loop of Henle, there is a net reabsorption of Na^+ and Cl^- without water. In the collecting duct, the urine can be diluted further when sodium chloride is reabsorbed to a greater degree than water. ADH must be absent for this dilution to occur.
- Maintenance of separation. The loop of Henle must remain impermeable to water when ADH is absent. ADH can be released for a variety of reasons unrelated to tonicity. One example is hyperosmolar urine, which can be excreted during a hypo-osmolar state.

Water Reabsorption and Tonicity

Maintenance of tonicity and water reabsorption take place after release of ADH. The cascade of events required for the processes of water reabsorption occur in the distal nephron. The action of ADH stimulates activation of adenylate cyclase and cAMP inside the cell structure. Channels with water receptors (pores) are formed through the initiation of cAMP-dependent protein kinase and phosphorylate elements from intracellular compartments. The membrane of the nephron is transformed as open circles that favor the reabsorption of water through these created water pores. In the medullary collecting duct, ADH also leads to the insertion of a pore that permits urea to diffuse across the luminal membrane (Halperin & Goldstein, 1994; Papadakis, 1996).

The hypothalamus balances fluid and electrolytes by secreting ADH to make the body retain water. Too much ADH means too much retention and a drop in serum sodium levels (Narins, 1994).

ADH secretion may be stimulated or its activity potentiated by factors such as trauma, pain, stress, anxiety, and medications such as morphine, meperidine, and thiazide diuretics. ADH suppression occurs when volume receptors in the heart (atria) sense intravascular volume or when the baroreceptors sense increased blood pressure.

FLUID VOLUME IMBALANCES

Fluid Volume Excess

Edema is a detectable accumulation of excess interstitial fluid. It may be confined to a sharply circumscribed area, as occurs in local inflammation or angioedema, or it may be generalized so that interstitial fluid accumulates in virtually every tissue in the body (Methany, 1996).

The extracellular fluid consists of plasma fluid (4% body weight) and interstitial fluid (i.e., water in tissues between the cells, 16% body weight). Water in the abdominal cavity (ascites) or thoracic cavity (pleural effusion) is a component of the interstitial space. In certain disease states, fluid accumulates in the interstitial space of the extracellular fluid to an appreciable degree and is called edema, ascites, or pleural effusion (Halperin & Goldstein, 1994).

The existence of edema indicates a disturbance in the normal regulation of extracellular volume. Each of the major disorders associated with generalized edema is characterized by a defect in at least one of the Starling capillary forces and by renal retention of Na^+ and water (Narins, 1994). Starling forces include mechanisms that govern the distribution of fluid across capillaries: hydrostatic pressure, decreased colloid osmotic pressure, and increased capillary permeability.

In idiopathic edema, there is an isotonic expansion of the extracellular volume. The extracellular compartments expand in proportion to the fluid infused. The increase in volume of fluid dilutes the concentration of hemoglobin and lowers the hematocrit and total protein levels, but the serum sodium level remains the same (Methany, 1996). Populations at risk for idiopathic edema are elderly persons and early postsurgical or posttrauma patients. Elderly patients have a low tolerance for altered fluid states. Those receiving isotonic saline solutions must be carefully monitored for complications (Halperin & Goldstein, 1994).

In patients with ascites, 10 L or more of fluid can collect in the bowel, resulting in severe extracellular volume loss. Plasma concentration of electrolytes is initially preserved; however, the patient becomes thirsty and drinks water, leading to hyponatremia (Adinaro, 1987). The volume of fluid trapped in the intestines can only be estimated. Weight measurements are valueless in detecting the amount of fluid trapped in the bowel. Careful observation of vital signs, the patient's appearance, urinary volume, and specific gravity are significant. Mild tachycardia may suggest an acute fluid loss of 5% of body weight; an acute fluid loss greater than 10% of body weight can cause hypovolemic shock (Adinaro, 1987).

In severe liver disease, ascites is caused by a decreased plasma albumin, combined with an increased capillary pressure produced by portal hypertension. The combination of both defects allows the albumin-filled fluid to shift out into the peritoneal cavity (Adinaro, 1987). In cirrhosis, specifically, edema is caused by pressure on the vena cava, which impairs the venous drainage from the lower extremities. Low plasma oncotic pressure secondary to hypoalbuminemia may occur when no ascites is present (Box 14–1).

Fluid Volume Deficit

Fluid volume deficit is a result of water and electrolyte loss in an isotonic fashion. Serum electrolyte levels remain unchanged unless other imbalances are also present. Fluid volume deficit is most often the result of body fluid loss or fluid collection in the third space. It is also called hypovolemia. The condition is exacerbated by decreased fluid intake. As a result, the extracellular compartment shrinks. This type of deficit is most commonly caused by fluids lost through the gastrointestinal tract and by conditions that cause polyuria and increase in sensible perspiration, respiratory rate and depth, and body temperature. Hypovolemic shock may result from severe loss of extracellular volume. Prolonged fluid volume deficit may result in renal failure (Methany, 1996).

In the absence of water intake, the tonicity of body fluids rises because there is ongoing water loss. This rise in tonicity leads to cell shrinkage and thereby stimulates the release of ADH from the posterior pituitary gland. Binding of ADH to its receptors on the basolateral membrane of late distal convoluted tubular cells, as well as on cells of the cortical and medullary collecting duct, results in the formation of cAMP, which increases the permeability of the collecting duct to water. Therefore, water is reabsorbed passively down an osmotic difference from the collecting duct lumen to the hyperosmolar renal medullary interstitium; as a result, a hyperosmolar urine is excreted and free water is conserved. To analyze the impact of a given urine excretion on body tonicity, ignore the urine osmolality and consider only the osmoles critical for water distribution across cell membranes: Na^+ and possibly potassium (K^+), with accompanying ions, and the water itself (Halperin & Goldstein, 1994).

In fluid volume deficit, there can be two forms of extracellular defects: isotonic dehydration and hypotonic dehydration. In isotonic dehydration, there is loss of salt and water in proportionate amounts—as occurs, for example, with acute hemorrhage. The intracellular compartment remains unchanged. In hypotonic dehydration, there is hypotonicity of extracellular fluid caused by an osmotic shift of water into the cells. The intracellular volume is actually expanded in patients with hypotonic dehydration and a deficit of total body water (Narins, 1994; Solomon, 1990).

Any disorder or treatment that causes increased urine excretion can lead to

---

Box 14–1   Assessment Parameters for Fluid Volume Excess

• Weight gain over 2 lb in short period of time	• Decreased BUN
• Full pulse, bounding in some adults	• Decreased hematocrit
• Distended neck veins in supine position	• Polyuria
• Peripheral edema	• Distended, slow emptying peripheral veins
• Moist rales in lungs	• Presence of ascites or pulmonary edema

extracellular fluid loss. Examples include diuretic use without careful assessment of renal status, conditions such as salt-losing nephritis and hyperglycemia, and hyperosmolar parenteral-enteral products. All these conditions cause polyuria because of the high load of solutes (dissolved substances) causing extracellular fluid to be removed from the plasma, tissue spaces, and cells in order for the excess solutes to be excreted in the urine (Box 14–2).

Sodium Imbalances

Na^+ is the major cation in the extracellular fluid compartment. Na^+ concentration within the extracellular compartment ranges from 135 mEq/L to 145 mEq/L. Because of its high concentration and inability to cross the cell membrane easily, Na^+ is the primary determinant of extracellular fluid concentration and the primary regulator of extracellular volume (Narins, 1994). Na^+ is reflective of the body's water balance. Na^+ imbalances occur because of a change of Na^+ content in the extracellular fluid as a result of conditions such as excessive vomiting or because of a failure of the body to excrete Na^+.

An excess in Na^+ in extracellular fluid is called hypernatremia, also referred to as an intracellular deficit (Methany, 1996). Initial signs and symptoms of uncompensated hypernatremia are the same as those of dehydration, hyperosmolality, and hypernatremia. On physical examination, the patient reports thirst, and, objectively, a red, dry, swollen tongue, elevated temperature, and neurological manifestations are found. Neurological abnormalities such as disorientation, lethargy, irritability, focal or grand mal seizures, and hallucinations are caused by cellular dehydration (Gasparis, Murray, & Ursomanno, 1989). In severe cases, permanent brain damage can occur because of subarachnoid hemorrhages as a result of brain tissue concentration.

Causes of hypernatremia include lack of fluid intake, largely because of inability to respond to thirst (Gaspar, 1988). Other causes of hypernatremia include diarrhea, ingestion of salt in abnormal amounts, profuse perspiration (as in athletic competition), diabetes insipidus, hyperalimentation without fluid correction, increase in loss of water vapor by the respiratory tract, excessive intravenous therapy using sodium-containing fluids, heart disease progressing to congestive heart failure, and chronic renal failure.

Offering fluids at regular intervals or through alternative routes such as tube feedings or parenteral therapy prevents hypernatremia. Check for excessive thirst and for an increase in body temperature. Check the mouth, tongue, and mucous membranes and provide frequent mouth care. Monitor and report

---

Box 14–2   Assessment Parameters for Fluid Volume Deficit

- Dry mucous membranes—especially dry mouth in adults
- Pinched facial expression
- Decreased intraocular pressure, making eyes appear sunken and feel soft to touch
- Thirst, in a neurologically intact individual
- Flat skin with slow turgor (known as tenting)
- Additional tongue furrows—useful in all age groups, because in normal fluid states the tongue has only one furrow
- Pale, cool skin
- Flat neck veins in supine adults
- Neuromuscular irritability, particularly in the presence of other electrolyte imbalances (e.g., calcium, magnesium, sodium)
- Changes in behavior or sensation and easy fatigability, especially in older patients

Box 14–3   Symptoms of Hypernatremia

Excessive thirst	Disorientation
Red, swollen tongue	Hallucination
Restlessness	Lethargy
Increased irritability	Stupor or coma

changes in sensorium, such as restlessness, increased irritability, disorientation, hallucinations, lethargy, stupor, or coma. (See Box 14–3 for a summary of symptoms of hypernatremia.)

Hyponatremia is a condition in which the serum sodium level is below normal. It may be caused by an excessive loss of Na^+ or by excessive fluid volume. It is generally synonymous with a hypo-osmolar state with a relatively greater concentration of water than Na^+. It can be thought of as a condition of water excess resulting in diluted serum. Hyponatremia may also be associated with abnormal extracellular volume because of excessive antidiuretic hormone activity. Hyponatremia may occur in heart failure, nephrotic syndrome, and cirrhosis of the liver. (See Box 14–4 for a summary of symptoms of hyponatremia.)

Na^+ losses in disease states are related to gastrointestinal, renal, and third-space fluid losses. Skin losses occur because of profuse perspiration and drainage from lesions. Other causes include profuse perspiration with increased fluid intake (as in athletes), low salt intake, use of diuretics, and aldosterone deficiency caused by adrenal insufficiency (Halperin & Goldstein, 1994). In excessive parenteral administration of dextrose and water, there is a gain of free body water. This is due to the breakdown of dextrose leaving the hypotonic water solution. This solution pulls K^+ and intracellular fluid out of the cell into the extracellular fluid, diluting the serum sodium and increasing total body volume (Halperin & Goldstein, 1994). Later signs include symptoms of increased intracranial pressure, such as lethargy, weakness, confusion, focal weakness, ataxia, hemiparesis, Babinski reflex, convulsions, papilledema, and coma (Methany, 1996).

DESCRIPTION OF THE INTERVENTION

Implementation of Fluid Management requires the integration of knowledge of common causes and manifestations of fluid imbalances, as well as recognition of daily fluid requirements in critically ill patients. The definion and related activities appear in Table 14–1. Organizing nursing assessment and using a fluid management tool will facilitate the collection of data. Actions appropriate to evaluating fluid therapy and identifying sources of imbalances will lead to accurate outcome identification and goal-directed nursing care.

Intake and Output

All intake and output should be carefully measured and recorded. Hourly urine measurements may be in order if the medical treatment order is to maintain

Box 14–4   Symptoms of Hyponatremia

Anorexia, nausea, and vomiting	Postural blood pressure changes
Body water gain	Full neck veins
Muscle cramps and fatigue	Flushed skin
Dyspnea on exertion	Poor skin turgor

Table 14–1 Fluid Management

DEFINITION: Promotion of fluid balance and prevention of complications resulting from abnormal or undesired fluid levels.

ACTIVITIES:

Weigh daily and monitor trends

Count or weigh diapers, as appropriate

Maintain accurate intake and output record

Insert urinary catheter, if appropriate

Monitor hydration status (e.g., moist mucous membranes, adequacy of pulses, and orthostatic blood pressure), as appropriate

Monitor laboratory results relevant to fluid retention (e.g., increased specific gravity, increased BUN, decreased hematocrit, and increased urine osmolality levels)

Monitor hemodynamic status, including CVP, MAP, PAP, and PCWP, if available

Monitor vital signs, as appropriate

Monitor for indications of fluid overload/retention (e.g., crackles, elevated CVP or pulmonary capillary wedge pressure, edema, neck vein distention, and ascites), as appropriate

Monitor patient's weight change before and after dialysis, if appropriate

Assess location and extent of edema, if present

Monitor food/fluid ingested and calculate daily caloric intake, as appropriate

Administer IV therapy, as prescribed

Monitor nutrition status

Give fluids, as appropriate

Administer prescribed diuretics, as appropriate

Administer IV fluids at room temperature

Promote oral intake (e.g., provide a drinking straw, offer fluids between meals, and change ice water routinely), as appropriate

Instruct patient on nothing by mouth (NPO) status, as appropriate

Administer prescribed nasogastric replacement based on output, as appropriate

Distribute the fluid intake over 24 hr, as appropriate

Encourage significant other to assist patient with feedings, as appropriate

Offer snacks (e.g., frequent drinks and fresh fruits/fruit juice), as appropriate

Restrict free water intake in the presence of dilutional hyponatremia with serum Na level below 130 mEq per liter

Monitor patient's response to prescribed electrolyte therapy

Consult physician, if signs and symptoms of fluid volume excess persist or worsen

Arrange availability of blood products for transfusion, if necessary

Prepare for administration of blood products (e.g., check blood with patient identification and prepare infusion setup), as appropriate

Administer blood products (e.g., platelets and fresh frozen plasma), as appropriate

Source: McCloskey, J. C., and Bulechek, G. M. (1996). *Nursing interventions classification (NIC)* (p. 292). St. Louis: Mosby–Year Book.

urine output between 30 mL/hr and 50 mL/hr. All body fluids must be measured and recorded on the record. Body fluids should not be estimated, and ice offered must be calculated as measurable intake. In cases of diarrhea, volume and consistency must be documented. If incontinence is a problem, absorbent pads must be weighed. With careful nursing management, fluids lost through incontinence and perspiration can be weighed. Wound drainage, including its pH, should be documented. Decreased urinary output can be caused by a deficit of extracellular volume filtering through the kidney. In severe cases of fluid volume deficit, oliguria occurs and may lead to damage to the renal tubules (Halperin & Goldstein, 1994).

Offer oral rehydration solutions, if appropriate. The World Health Organization (WHO) has a formula useful for adults who cannot maintain adequate oral intake to compensate for large-volume diarrhea (e.g., adults with acquired immunodeficiency syndrome [AIDS], diabetic diarrhea, or vancomycin resistant enterococcus [VRE]; elderly patients with *Clostridium* diarrhea). The formula is easy to prepare and can be offered in place of plain water (Box 14–5). Research has demonstrated its effectiveness, although lower-osmolarity (245 mOsm/L) oral solutions such as those made with rice do decrease stool volume and prevent complications of severe fluid volume deficit (Islam, Molla, Ahmed, et al. 1994; Santosham et al., 1996).

Water lost via the skin and respiratory tract is a hypotonic solution with an even lower Na^+ level than that when fluid volume is high. On average, just over 1 L is lost each day. Losses in perspiration can increase dramatically in hot environments and with exercise. Similarly, water losses in patients who are febrile and hyperventilating are higher. Patients with space-occupying lesions, infection, sarcoid, hypoxic states, and trauma are at risk for developing diabetes insipidus (DI). The mechanism begins with hypernatremia and an intact renal system that excretes large volumes of hypo-osmolar urine (Halperin & Goldstein, 1994). This disorder is termed *central DI* and can be treated by raising the urine osmolality and administering ADH. The urine Na^+ and K^+ levels are useful in detecting the kidney's influence on the tonicity of the body (Halperin & Goldstein, 1994).

A sudden gain or loss in weight is a significant sign of a change in the fluid volume. A change in the volume of body fluid can be calculated by weighing the patient daily at the same time of day, on the same scales, with the same amount of clothing. A sudden weight loss or gain of 2 pounds or more in a short time is significant for a change in the patient's fluid status.

Additional water is particularly important for patients receiving enteral nutrition. The wide range of different formulas assists providers in matching appropriate formulas to the patient's disease and nutrition state, but sufficient water must be provided. Ross Product Division (1989) published a fluid calculation estimation that assists practitioners in estimating appropriate fluid therapy with the patient's tube feeding. Estimate approximately 1 mL of water for every calorie of formula delivered.

Intravenous Therapy

Fluid replacement by the parenteral route is used to correct any pre-existing deficit of fluids and electrolytes, maintain fluid and electrolyte balance, or replace losses of electrolytes and fluids in such conditions as burns, draining fistulas, vomiting, and diarrhea. Patients whose fluid volume is normal at the time therapy is initiated will require a solution to maintain fluid equilibrium. For the

---

Box 14–5   CDC/WHO Recipe for Volume Replacement

• 3/4 teaspoon table salt	• 4 tablespoons sugar	• 1 L clean water (not distilled)
• 1 teaspoon baking powder	• 1 cup orange juice	

replacement of an abnormal loss of fluid or electrolytes, replacement fluids are selected with a composition resembling the body fluid lost.

The goal in fluid replacement is to restore volume without altering the electrolyte balance. Until the 1960s, intravenous therapy was the sole responsibility of the physician. Today, hospital policies identify essential guidelines for hospital personnel to follow in inserting and maintaining intravenous lines and peripherally inserted central catheter (PICC) lines, as well as preparing and administering admixtures to patients. Parenteral fluids are classified according to the tonicity of the fluid in relation to the normal blood plasma. The osmolarity of blood plasma is between 280 mOsm/L and 300 mOsm/L. Fluid that approximates 290 mOsm/L is considered isotonic. Intravenous fluids with an osmolarity significantly higher than 290 mOsm/L (by 50 mOsm/L or more) are considered hypertonic; those with an osmolarity significantly lower than 290 mOsm/L are hypotonic (Halperin & Goldstein, 1994). In a healthy body, the number of cations equals the number of anions. When added together, cations and anions equal 290 mEq/L in extracellular fluid. Intravenous solutions may be equal to (isotonic), less than (hypotonic), or more than (hypertonic) 310 mEq/L (Gasparis et al., 1989; Methany, 1996).

The tonicity of the fluid when infused into the circulation has a direct effect on the patient. Hypertonic fluids increase the osmotic pressure of the blood plasma, drawing fluid from the cells; excessive infusions of such fluids can cause cellular dehydration. Hypotonic fluids lower the osmotic pressure, causing fluid to invade cells; when fluid is infused beyond the patient's tolerance for water, water intoxication results. Isotonic fluids cause increased extracellular fluid volume, which can result in circulatory overload (Methany, 1996). Because of the direct and effective role osmolarity plays in intravenous therapy, it is helpful for the nurse involved in the administration of intravenous fluids to be able to identify the patient's osmolarity. The serum osmolarity is calculated by identifying the patient's sodium level, blood urea nitrogen (BUN) level, and glucose level using the following formula:

$$2(Na) + \frac{BUN}{5} + \frac{Glucose}{20} = 280\text{--}300 \, mOsm/L$$

Crystalloids are electrolyte solutions named for their potential to form crystals. After being infused into the bloodstream, they act much like extracellular fluid, diffusing through the capillary endothelium to the interstitium as necessary to maintain fluid balance (Horne, Heitz, & Swearingen, 1991).

Colloidal solutions are used as plasma expanders and are obtained from sources other than blood. These solutions exert a colloidal pressure similar to that of plasma proteins. By increasing the colloidal pressure in the vascular bed, fluid is pulled from the extracellular compartments, and increasing the colloidal pressure in the vascular bed increases the total blood volume. Types of colloidal fluids include normal saline and lactated Ringer's solution; each of these solutions has a sodium concentration similar to that of extracellular fluids. Isotonic fluids have the same osmolarity as intracellular fluids. The fluids fill the extracellular fluid compartment without changing the osmolarity.

Hypertonic fluids pull fluid from the intracellular compartment into the extracellular volume. Hypertonic solutions have a lower concentration of free water but a higher osmotic weight (greater than 375 mOsm/L). Types of fluids include 10% to 50% dextrose in water and 5% dextrose in Ringer's solution.

Hypertonic fluids increase intravascular osmolarity, which results in intracellular and interstitial dehydration. Hypertonic solutions can be used carefully in

Box 14–6 Maintaining Balance

Visible Fluids = 1,200 mL
+
Three Meals = 100 mL
+
Oxidation = 300 mL
Fluids should exceed urine output by 500 mL.

peripheral lines but are effectively monitored and assessed through central lines and PICC lines.

Hypotonic fluids are used strictly for rehydration states. These solutions give water to dehydrated cells. Hypotonic solutions are given slowly because of shifting of fluid into the cells. Types of fluids include one-half Ringer's solution, 2.5% dextrose in water, and 0.45% physiological saline solution. Hypotonic solutions decrease intravascular osmolarity (Horne, Heitz, & Swearingen, 1991).

Colloids are used when the goal is to replace intravascular volume only. Colloids are fluids containing proteins or starch molecules that remain uniformly distributed in fluid and do not form a true solution. Examples of colloids are albumin, plasma protein fraction, dextran, and hetastarch. Colloids draw fluid in from other compartments to increase the vascular volume by increasing the osmotic pressure within the bloodstream.

Crystalloids are used to replace concurrent losses of water, carbohydrates, and electrolytes. Most of those who require water and electrolytes intravenously are relatively normal people who cannot take orally what they require for maintenance. Box 14–6 shows that the range of tolerance for water and electrolytes (homeostatic limits) permits reasonable latitude in therapy, provided normal renal function exists to accomplish the final regulation of volume and concentration (Methany, 1996; Zerwekh, 1997).

An average adult whose entire intake is parenteral would require for maintenance 2,500 to 3,000 mL of 5% dextrose in 0.2% saline solution (34 mEq Na^+ plus 34 mEq Cl^-/L). To each liter, 30 mEq of potassium chloride could be added. In 3 L, the total chloride intake would be 192 mEq, which is homeostatically compatible. Box 14–7 details daily requirements of essential electrolytes in a noncompromised adult; Box 14–8 lists the electrolyte concentrations of crystalloid solutions.

ASSOCIATED NURSING DIAGNOSES AND OUTCOMES

Each set of symptoms assessed during care requires a plan to implement appropriate activities for Fluid Management. There must be precise nursing diagnostic categories when identifying interventions to correct the fluid and electrolyte imbalances. Just as an organized assessment, clearly documented, can assist in identifying the cause of the imbalance, an accurate nursing diagnostic category

Box 14–7 Daily Maintenance for Average Adult (60–100 kg) Requiring Parenteral Fluids

Glucose	100–200 g
Sodium	80–120 mEq
Potassium	80–120 mEq
Water	2,500 mL

Box 14–8   Electrolyte Concentrations of Crystalloid Solutions

	Osmolality (mOsm/kg H₂O)	Na⁺ (mEq/L)	Cl⁻ (mEq/L)	Glucose (g/L)
Isotonic				
0.9% saline	308	154	154	0
D50.9% saline	560	154	154	50
Ringer's lactate	273	130	109	0
Hypotonic				
D5W (dextrose is metabolized, leaving free water)	252	0	0	50
0.45% saline	154	77	77	0
D50.45% saline	405	77	77	50

Sources: Cogan, M. (1991). *Fluid and electrolytes: Physiology and pathophysiology.* Stamford, CT: Appleton & Lange; Halperin, M., and Goldstein, M. (1994). *Fluid, electrolyte and acid-base physiology: A problem-based approach* (2nd ed.). Philadelphia: W.B. Saunders.

can assist in focusing nursing care to resolve the imbalance. The nursing diagnostic categories Fluid Volume Deficit and Fluid Volume Excess appear in the North American Nursing Diagnosis Association (NANDA) Classification. This chapter suggests that Hypernatremia and Hyponatremia should be developed as nursing diagnoses. Other diagnoses for which Fluid Management may be needed include the following:

Altered Nutrition
Decreased Cardiac Output
Impaired Gas Exchange
Ineffective Breathing Pattern
Altered Urinary Elimination
Decreased Intracranial Adaptive Capacity

The outcomes to evaluate the effectiveness of Fluid Management represent the eventual return to normal fluid balance or corrected balance at the end of a course of fluid management. Nursing Outcomes Classification (NOC) outcomes associated with Fluid Management include the following:

Fluid Balance
Hydration
Circulation Status
Electrolyte & Acid/Base Balance
Tissue Integrity: Skin & Mucous Membranes

CASE STUDY

LK is an 83-year-old, alert, noncognitively impaired woman living alone in her two-story row home in an urban area. Her ability to move around and up the stairs to her bathroom is seriously hampered because of osteoarthritis in both knees. She has battled a weight problem all her life, and within the last 2 years she was placed on oral antidiabetic agents. She has mitral valve regurgitation and takes warfarin daily. Recently, she attempted to control her weight by cutting her food intake by half. She lost 40 pounds in 3 months and was very excited to be able to move around in her home. After approximately 1 week of eating all the foods she had denied herself for 3 months, LK began to feel significant joint pain, and she noticed some swelling in her joints. After

1 week of self-medicating with nonsteroidal anti-inflammatory agents and aspirin, she made an appointment with her primary health care provider. The diagnoses of constipation, gout, hyperglycemia (nonketotic) syndrome, and congestive heart failure were made.

LK is in exteme pain, is unable to move very well, and comes to the office with a neighbor. LK is admitted to the hospital for treatment of her hyperosmolar state and constipation. She is discharged to home with diet instructions and a new oral antidiabetic agent. Her renal status is unclear, because her BUN, creatine, and creatinine clearance levels are elevated. LK is told by her provider to stop all anti-inflammatory nonsteroidal agents. Her gout is treated conservatively with allopurinol.

One week later, she is found sitting in a chair, unable to move. Her ankles, wrists, and fingers are swollen, and her speech is garbled. She has stopped cooking any meals and is unable to keep any fluids without vomiting. LK reports severe dryness but no appetite and no desire to drink or eat. She is unable to sleep and reports difficulty breathing when she lies down at night.

LK's change in mental status, anorexia, and vomiting are the most obvious signs of dehydration with a corrected hyperosmolar extracellular fluid compartment. Medical treatment of her underlying diseases contributed to her present problem. Gentle, even hydration in the form of oral rehydration solutions assists this patient in rebounding and preventing further disease debilitation.

CONLUSION

■

Nursing activities for Fluid Management require knowledge of underlying principles and knowledge of assessment factors in fluid balance. Nurses implementing Fluid Management need to monitor patients for fluid imbalances and evaluate the outcomes of the Fluid Management. The cornerstone in daily management is the intake and output record. Intelligent, organized nursing assessment and evaluation are necessary to assist patients receiving fluid therapy and avoid complications to restore patients to optimum health.

References

Adinaro, D. (1987). Liver failure and pancreatitis: Fluid and electrolyte concerns. *Nursing Clinics of North America, 22,* 843–852.

Armstrong, C., Browne, K., Armstrong-Esther, D., and Sander, L. (1996). The institutionalized elderly: Dry to the bone. *International Journal of Nursing Studies, 33,* 619–628.

Gaspar, P. (1988, July-August). Fluid intake: What determines how much patients drink? *Geriatric Nursing,* 221–224.

Gasparis, L., Murray, E., and Ursomanno, P. (1989, April). I.V. solutions: Which one is right for your patient? *Nursing, 19,* 62–64.

Halperin, M., and Goldstein, M. (1994). *Fluid, electrolyte and acid-base physiology. A problem-based approach* (2nd ed.). Philadelphia: W.B. Saunders.

Jacobs, L. (1994). Timing of fluid resuscitation in trauma. *New England Journal of Medicine, 331,* 1153–1155.

Lancaster, L. (1987). Renal and endocrine regulation of water and electrolyte balance. *Nursing Clinics of North America, 22,* 761–772.

Methany, N. (1996). *Fluid and electrolyte balance: Nursing considerations* (3rd ed.). Philadelphia: J.B. Lippincott.

Narins, R. (Ed.) (1994). *Maxwell and Kleeman's clinical disorders of fluid and electrolyte metabolism.* New York: McGraw-Hill.

Papadakis, M. A. (1996). Fluid and electrolyte disorders. In L. M. Tierney, Jr., S. J. McPhee, and M. A. Papadakis (Eds.), *Current medical diagnosis and treatment* (pp. 768–794). Stamford, CT: Appleton & Lange.

Rinard, G. (1989). Water intoxication. *American Journal of Nursing, 89*(12), 1635–1638.

Ross Product Division. (1989, March). *Enteral nutrition handbook.* Columbus, OH: Abbott Laboratories.

Santosham, M., Fayad, I., AbuZikri, M., Hussein, A., Amponsah, A., Duggan, C., Hashem, M., el Sady, N., and Fontaine, O. (1996). A double-blind clinical trial comparing World Health Organization oral rehydration solution with a reduced osmolarity solution containing equal amounts of sodium and glucose. *Journal of Pediatrics, 128*(1), 45–51.

Solomon, S., and Kirby, D. (1990). The refeeding syndrome. *Journal of Parenteral, Enteral Nutrition, 14,* 90–97.

Stachenfeld, N., DiPietro, L., Nadel, E., and Mack, G. (1997). Mechanism of attenuated thirst in aging: Role of central volume receptors. *American Physiological Society, 272*(1Pt.2), R148–R157.

Zerwekh, J. (1997). Do dying patients really need IV fluids? *American Journal of Nursing, 97*(3), 26–31.

Airway Management

Marita G. Titler and Michele A. Alpen

Airway patency is necessary for life. Nursing activities to achieve airway patency can be traced to the early 1900s, when nurses tried several methods to maintain a tight seal between the patient's neck and the Drinker respirator. During the 1940s, nurses began to suction tracheostomies using a variety of techniques (Adler, 1979). Today, nurses use various practices to maintain airway patency.

Airway patency is achieved through the intervention of Airway Management, a necessary prerequisite to ventilatory support. Airway Management is defined as "facilitation of patency of air passages" (McCloskey & Bulechek, 1996, p. 95). Airway Management is accomplished in several ways, ranging from correct positioning of the patient to use of various artificial airway devices. This chapter focuses on Airway Management in adults.

RESEARCH AND RELATED LITERATURE

The research and related literature that undergird the intervention of Airway Management are clustered in the areas of monitoring, positioning, insertion and management of artificial airways, and secretion removal. These four areas encompass specific activities nurses do to carry out the intervention. Pharmacological interventions used to assist with Airway Management are beyond the scope of this chapter, and the reader is referred to Henneman (1996) for a summary of pharmacological agents used in managing airway patency.

Monitoring

Monitoring for early signs of airway obstruction is an essential part of Airway Management. Indications of complete and partial airway obstruction are listed in Table 15–1. Monitoring the patient's ability to clear secretions is also an important part of Airway Management. This includes monitoring the patient's ability to take a deep breath and to generate high expiratory air flows and velocities (Cosenza & Norton, 1986; Traver, 1985). Slow vital capacity and maximal inspiratory force (MIF) are useful to determine deep-breathing ability. Normal vital capacity is dependent on the patient's age, size, and gender, with 15 mL/kg recommended for maintaining spontaneous ventilation. MIF, the amount of negative pressure the patient can generate, is usually -60 cm H_2O in a healthy adult, but an MIF of at least -20 cm H_2O is needed to maintain effective spontaneous ventilation (Traver, 1985). Forced expiratory volume in 1 second (FEV_1) and the ratio of FEV_1 to forced vital capacity (FVC) help determine the patient's ability to generate high air flow and velocities needed for effective coughing. Markedly reduced FEV_1 and FEV_1/FVC (normally reductions of more than 70%) suggest that the patient may have difficulty generating and conducting air flow (Traver, 1985).

Monitoring the need for suctioning is an important part of managing the airway. The ritual of suctioning every 2 hours should be avoided because of adverse consequences of microatelectasis, tissue damage, hemoptysis, brochospasm, hypoxia, cardiac arrhythmias, and even death (Alpen, 1993; Branson, Campbell, Chatburn, & Covington, 1993; Henneman, 1996; Knipper, 1986; Riegel & Forshee, 1985). Instead, suctioning should be based on individual patient indicators that suggest the need for suctioning. Auscultation of adventitious sounds (crackles and ronchi) over the large airways is associated with significant amounts of secretion retrieval and is a reliable indicator for tracheal suctioning (Amborn, 1976; Knipper, 1986; Smith, 1983; Titler, Bulechek, Knipper, & Alpen, 1992). Other indicators include inability of the patient to generate an effective spontaneous cough, coughing and increased peak inspiratory pressures during volume-controlled mechanical ventilation or decreased tidal volume during pressure-controlled ventilation, visible secretions in the artificial airway, changes in the monitored flow and pressure graphics of the mechanical ventilator, suspected aspiration, deterioration of arterial blood gases, and radiological changes (e.g.,

---

Table 15–1 Indications of Partial or Complete Airway Obstruction

- Inability to speak
- Debris or foreign matter in the mouth or pharynx
- Lack of chest movement
- Absence of breath sounds
- Absence of air movement
- Cyanosis
- Abnormal breath sound (e.g., crowing, wheezing, stridor)
- Nasal flaring
- Coarse breath sounds
- Prolonged expiration
- Pharyngeal gurgle
- Supraclavicular and intercostal retractions
- Increased restlessness or anxiety
- Air hunger or dyspnea
- Increased ventilatory system pressures and decreased tidal volume in the mechanically ventilated patient
- Cough and sputum production

Source: Data from: Titler, M. G., and Jones, G. A. (1992). Airway management. In G. M. Bulechek and J. C. McCloskey (Eds.), Nursing interventions: Essential nursing treatments (2nd ed., pp. 512–530). Philadelphia: W. B. Saunders.

atelectasis) consistent with retention of pulmonary secretions (Baker, 1996; Boggs, 1993; Branson et al., 1993; Hilling et al., 1992; Hoffman & Maszkiewicz, 1987).

Arterial blood gases, capnography or capnometry, and pulse oximetry are used clinically for monitoring airway patency. These physiological indices of oxygenation are also influenced, however, by ventilation and oxygen transport (Ahrens, 1996; Baker, 1996).

ARTERIAL BLOOD GASES

Arterial blood gas (ABG) analysis is used for a variety of clinical conditions including acute respiratory failure, airway occlusion, and acid-base imbalance (Ahrens, 1996; Baker, 1996; Henneman, 1996). One cause of increased partial pressure of arterial carbon dioxide ($PaCO_2$) is the inability to eliminate carbon dioxide (CO_2) through the respiratory system secondary to airway obstruction. This results in hypercapnia. A low level of arterial oxygenation (PaO_2) occurs from a variety of conditions including low inspired oxygen secondary to airway obstruction. This results in hypoxemia. Acute airway obstruction results in a high $PaCO_2$, a low PaO_2, and a low pH. Signs and symptoms of hypoxemia and hypercapnia are in Table 15–2, and the reader is referred to Ahrens (1996), Baker (1996), and Henneman (1996) for a comprehensive discussion of oxygenation and ABG analysis.

CAPNOGRAPHY/CAPNOMETRY

Capnography is the continuous analysis and recording of CO_2 concentrations in respiratory gases. The terms *capnography* and *capnometry* are used synonymously, but, technically, capnography is documentation of the waveform as well as the numeric reading, and capnometry is analysis of the numerical measure alone.

Although continuous end-tidal carbon dioxide ($PETCO_2$ mm Hg) measurements may permit early detection of alveolar hypoventilation, apnea, and airway obstruction, technical difficulties preclude widespread clinical use in patients breathing spontaneously without artificial airways. Capnography by nasal cannula appears to be a useful monitoring device during conscious sedation, but further research is required before routine clinical use can be recommended (Wright, 1992). Devices such as the naso-oral discriminate sampling system have

Table 15–2 Signs and Symptoms of Hypoxemia and Hypercapnia

Hypoxemia/Low PaO_2*	Hypercapnia/Elevated $PaCO_2$†
• Restlessness	• Headache
• Anxiety	• Decreased level of consciousness
• Confusion	• Coma
• Poor judgment	• Hypotension
• Coma	• Dysrhythmias
• Tachycardia	• Decreased peripheral perfusion
• Hypertension (initially)	
• Hypotension (late)	
• Cyanosis	
• Dyspnea	
• Tachypnea	

*Normal PaO_2 = 60–100 mm Hg.
†Normal $PaCO_2$ = 35–45 mm Hg.
Source: Data from Henneman, E. A. (1996). Patients with acute respiratory failure. In J. M. Clochesy, C. Breu, S. Cardin, A. A. Whittaker, and E. B. Rudy (Eds.), *Critical care nursing* (2nd ed., pp. 630–648). Philadelphia: W. B. Saunders.

been tested and show promise for possible use in spontaneously breathing patients without artificial airways (Derrick, Waters, Kang, Cwalina, & Simmons, 1993).

Capnography is considered a standard of care during anesthesia, and the Society of Critical Care Medicine has suggested that capnography be available in every intensive care unit (ICU) (Campbell, Branson, Burke, Covington, & Graybeal, 1995). Capnography is used for monitoring during weaning trials, changes in mechanical ventilation, cardiopulmonary resuscitation, endotracheal intubation, and dead space analysis (Aherns, 1996). $PETCO_2$ measurements are usually less than $PaCO_2$ measurements but can be used to approximate $PaCO_2$ values (Ahrens, 1996) as demonstrated by some investigators (Hess & Agarwal, 1992; Hess, Schlottag, Levin, Mathai, & Rexrode, 1991; Saura et al., 1996). Although analysis of published research on use of bedside capnometry in critical care resulted in discouraging the routine use of bedside capnometry (Technology Subcommittee of the Working Group on Critical Care, Ontario Ministry of Health, 1992), other investigators have demonstrated the value of capnometry for monitoring CO_2 elimination during a variety of invasive procedures (Baraka et al., 1994; Magnan et al., 1993; Nyarwaya, Mazoit, & Samii, 1994; Thrush, Mentis, & Downs, 1991). Kerr, Zempsky, Sereika, Orndoff, and Rudy (1996) found a low correlation between $PaCO_2$ and $PETCO_2$ and thus question the clinical usefulness of $PETCO_2$, particularly in mechanically ventilated patients with irregular spontaneous respirations and in patients with pulmonary dysfunction (positive end-expiratory pressure [PEEP] > 5 cm H_2O; low PaO_2/FIO_2 ratios). Practice guidelines for use of capnography are available from the American Association of Critical Care Nurses (AACN) and the American Association of Respiratory Care (AARC) (Campbell et al., 1995; St. John, 1996).

PULSE OXIMETRY

Pulse oximetry is used frequently in clinical practice as one indicator of ventilation and airway patency. It is used in transport of critically ill patients (Evans & Winslow, 1995), to monitor functional activity (Hogan, 1995), for bedside monitoring of critically ill adult patients (Hess & Agarwal, 1992; Szaflarski & Cohen, 1989; Technology Subcommittee of the Working Group on Critical Care, Ontario Ministry of Health, 1992), for weaning patients from oxygen or mechanical ventilation (Berels & Marz, 1991; Noll & Byers, 1995; Thrush et al., 1991), during conscious sedation in the emergency department (Wright, 1992), and during surgery, cardiac catheterization, and coronary angioplasty (Amar, Greenberg, Menegus, & Breitbart, 1994; Baraka et al., 1994; Nyarwaya, Mazoit, & Samii, 1994). These investigators and clinicians report that pulse oximetry is clinically useful but should not be the sole indicator of airway patency. Ahrens (1996) notes that the most practical use of pulse oximetry is for continual monitoring of the patient during tapering of the amount of oxygen (FIO_2) while avoiding the need to measure ABGs. As a guide, FIO_2 levels can be tapered until a desired pulse oximetry (SpO_2) is reached—usually 93%. SpO_2 of less than 90% reflects desaturation, with one possible cause being ineffective airway clearance (Grap, 1996).

The use of pulse oximetry requires correct application of the device, overcoming common problems that arise, and correct interpretation of the results, keeping in mind the importance of the oxyhemoglobin disassociation curve (Ahrens, 1996; Hess & Agarwal, 1992; Jones, 1995; Rotello, Warren, Jastremski, & Milewski, 1992). Bowton, Scuderi, Harris, and Haponik (1991) found that 75% of noncritical care patients had at least one episode of desaturation detected by pulse oximetry, but episodes of less than 90% were documented only 33% of the time in nursing notes and 7% of the time in physician notes. Changes in respiratory therapy (e.g., changes in FiO_2, changes in delivery mode) occurred in 20% of those who desaturated to less than 90% and in 26% of those who desaturated to less than 85%. Wiklund, Hok, Stahl, and Jordeby-Johnson (1994) found during a 100-minute observation period that patient pulse oximetry devices set off an alarm every 8 minutes, with 77% of them being false alarms. Practice guidelines for use of pulse oximetry are available from the AACN (Grap, 1996) and the AARC (Shrake et al., 1991).

Positioning

Relaxation of the oropharyngeal muscles allows the tongue to block the airway, a common cause of airway obstruction (Hurn & Hartsock, 1994). According to the American Heart Association (AHA) (1994), the head tilt, assisted by the chin lift, is the most important step in opening the airway in an adult. If cervical spine injury is suspected, the jaw thrust technique is recommended instead of the head-tilt chin-lift method. If positioning is unsuccessful in opening the airway, or if the patient is unable to maintain a patent airway following this acute action, artificial means of maintaining airway patency must be considered.

Positioning is also helpful to optimize oxygenation. For years researchers have advocated positioning with the healthy lung down (HLD) in patients with unilateral lung disease (Dhainaut, Bons, Bricard, & Monsailler, 1980; Doering, 1993; Fontaine & McQuillan, 1989; Piehl & Brown, 1976; Remolina, Khan, Santiago, & Edelman, 1981; Seaton, Lapp, & Morgan, 1979; Zack, Pontoppidan, & Kazemi, 1974). Use of this positioning maneuver has been shown to produce elevations in PaO_2 through better ventilation-perfusion (V/Q) matching. HLD positioning allows the best-ventilated areas to come in contact with the best-perfused areas of the lung, thereby allowing maximum exchange of CO_2 for oxygen in the alveoli.

In a study of 39 patients with stable unilateral lung disease (Yeaw, 1996), oxygen saturation and systolic blood pressure did not differ by positioning the healthy lung up or down. These results suggest the need for more research and the need to individualize patient care based on the patient's response to treatment.

A growing body of scientific evidence demonstrates that oxygenation frequently improves when patients with acute lung insufficiency are rotated from the supine to the prone position (Gattinoni, Tognoni, Brazzi, & Latini, 1997; Langer, Mascheroni, Marcolin, & Gattinoni, 1988; Murse, Martling, & Lindahl, 1997; Piehl & Brown, 1976; Schmitz, 1991; Vollman & Bander, 1996). Murse et al. (1997) demonstrated in 13 patients suffering from severe acute lung insufficiency that the prone position significantly improved impaired gas exchange in 12 of 13 patients. The oxygenation index increased significantly ($p < .0002$), and the alveolar-arterial oxygen gradient decreased dramatically ($p < .0001$) in the prone position.

Compared with the use of nitric oxide or extracorporeal membrane oxygenation (ECMO), treatments often required in severe pulmonary insufficiency, prone positioning is a relatively noncomplex mode of therapy. Albert (1997) notes that severe complications from using prone positioning occur infrequently. Techniques for prone positioning with and without an assistive device are described in detail by Vollman (1997).

Artificial Airway Insertion and Management

When it becomes apparent that a patient is experiencing problems with airway obstruction, possible aspiration, the need for tracheal suctioning, or mechanical ventilatory support, a decision is made to use one or more airway management tools. Many devices are available, and the choice of methods depends on the nature of the airway obstruction, the hemodynamic status of the patient, the skills and expertise of available personnel, the supplies and devices available, and the presence of facial or cervical spine injuries.

Cannulation of the trachea can result in various injuries, including airway trauma, pulmonary infection, laryngeal edema, tracheal stenosis, dilatation, necrosis, tracheomalacia, tracheoesophageal fistula, and tracheo-innominate artery fistula (Barnes, Boudin, Durbin, Fluck, & Malinowski, 1995; Bishop, 1989; Heffner, 1990; Heffner, Miller, & Sahn 1986a, 1986b; Lane, 1990; Mackenzie, 1983; Marsh, Gillespie, & Baumgartner, 1989; Shekleton & Nield, 1987). A variety of nursing activities are used to manage patients with artificial airways in an effort to minimize these complications. These include facilitating insertion of endotracheal (ET) tubes, tracheostomy tubes, and other devices; stabilizing artificial airways; administering hydration; managing cuff pressures; and providing tracheostomy tube care.

INSERTING ARTIFICIAL AIRWAYS

Nasopharyngeal and *oropharyngeal airways* enhance nasotracheal suctioning and prevent obstruction of the posterior pharynx by the tongue (Boggs, 1993). Nurses routinely insert oral and nasopharyngeal airways, which come in a variety of sizes. An oral airway is inserted into the mouth either right side up or upside down and then rotated downward to pull the tongue forward. Care must be taken to ensure that the tongue is not pushed back, thus obstructing rather than opening the airway. Oral airways should not be used in awake patients, as they may induce vomiting, aspiration, or laryngospasm (Kharasch & Graff, 1995). Oral airways facilitate suctioning of the pharynx and can be used to prevent patients from biting their tongues and occluding endotracheal and gastric tubes (Boggs, 1993).

Nasopharyngeal airways are flexible rubber devices that are inserted into the nostril and should fit comfortably, extending from the external naris to the base of the tongue. This airway adjunct is most commonly used to facilitate nasotracheal suctioning and is tolerated better by more alert patients (Boggs, 1993). Care should be taken to prevent injuring the mucosa with insertion; this airway is best avoided in patients with bleeding disorders or basilar skull fracture (Boggs, 1993; Kharasch & Graff, 1995).

ET intubation is indicated for impending or actual airway compromise, for respiratory failure, and when there is a need to protect the airway (Barnes et al., 1995). ET tubes can be placed via the oral or nasotracheal route and come in a variety of sizes. Most are made of polyvinyl chloride or silicone rubber and are disposable. Factors that must be considered when selecting an ET tube are the size of the patient, cannulation route, and reason for insertion. There are various guides available to help in selection of the correct ET tube size, but a quick rule of thumb is to select a tube with an outside diameter that matches the diameter of the patient's little finger (Boggs, 1993; Klein, 1996).

Table 15–3 lists the advantages and disadvantages of the two routes for ET intubation. The oral route provides quick and certain airway control in emergent situations. Nasotracheal intubation provides airway access in patients with oral

Table 15–3 Advantages and Disadvantages of Orotracheal versus Nasotracheal Intubation

Type	Advantages	Disadvantages
Orotracheal Tube	• Earlier to insert during airway emergencies • More apt to be able to use larger-diameter tube, thus decreasing the work of breathing • Easier to suction than nasotracheal tube • Facilitates secretion management and passage of a fiberoptic bronchoscope	• Requires direct laryngoscopy to insert • Occludes easily by patient biting • More easily dislodged by tongue or by other means • More difficult to secure and stabilize • Oral hygiene more difficult • More difficult to communicate by lip reading • Impairs ability to swallow • Can cause laryngeal injury
Nasotracheal Tube	• Inserted blindly • More easily secured • Allows better oral hygiene • Easier for patient to communicate • Perceived to be better tolerated	• More difficult to insert • Unable to use larger tube diameter, thus increases resistance • May cause less laryngeal injury than oral route • Increased incidence of sinusitis and otitis media due to inability to drain sinuses and eustachian tubes • Increased risk of nasal necrosis • Can cause nasal bleeding or hemorrhaging

trauma and is purported to be more comfortable than the oral route. However, a study of postoperative cardiac surgery patients demonstrated no difference in the degree of discomfort or amount of sedation required in the orotracheal and nasotracheal groups (Fletcher, Olsson, Helbo-Hansen, Nihlson, & Hedestrom, 1984). Although the nasotracheal route is believed to cause less laryngotracheal injury, this is not supported by research (El-Naggar, Sadagopa, Levin, Kantor, & Collins, 1976; Rashkin & Davis, 1986; Stauffer, Olson, & Petty, 1981; Via-Reque & Rattenburg, 1981).

Techniques of ET tube insertion are reviewed elsewhere (Boggs, 1993; Deem & Bishop, 1995). Insertion of ET tubes is limited to those who are trained and credentialed (Barnes et al., 1995; Plummer & Gracey, 1989). Nurses either insert or assist with insertion of an ET tube by preparing the necessary equipment (i.e., laryngoscope, ET tube, stylet, oxygen source, suction), ensuring optimal positioning of the patient, informing the patient about the procedure, administering appropriate medications as ordered, and monitoring for complications during insertion (e.g., cardiac arrhythmias, esophageal intubation, hemodynamic instability). Auscultation of the chest and epigastrium, observation of rise and fall of the chest, presence of humidity in the ET tube, detection of CO_2 via capnometry, and postintubation radiographs are necessary to ensure correct placement of the tube. The tip of the endotracheal tube should be 2 to 4 cm above the carina (Chulay, Connolly, & Parr, 1997). In women that equates to approximately 21 cm at the teeth and in males to approximately 23 cm at the teeth (Deem & Bishop, 1995).

Unsuccessful intubation efforts in the nonapneic, awake, or semiawake patient most frequently result from insufficient administration of topical anesthesia, general sedation, or muscle-paralyzing agents. Patients with increased intracranial pressure, increased anxiety, extreme sensitivity to airway stimulation, or agitation benefit from receiving general sedation with or without muscle paralysis. Drugs commonly used for intubation include short-acting barbiturates (thiopental), narcotic analgesics (fentanyl), benzodiazepines (midazolam), and neuromuscular blocking agents (succinylcholine, pancuronium, vecuronium). Ensuring that adequate ventilation can be maintained by face mask is extremely important before administering paralyzing agents (Heffner, 1990; Kharasch & Graff, 1995).

Following insertion, validation of placement, and stabilization of the tube, the nurse marks the ET tube at the centimeter markings corresponding to the position of the lips or naris. The practitioner can then tell at a glance whether the tube has slipped farther into the trachea or has become dislodged (Boggs, 1993; Hoffman & Maszkiewicz, 1987; Stauffer & Silvestri, 1982).

Tracheostomy tubes are used to prevent or reverse upper airway obstruction, facilitate secretion removal, and cannulate the airway for long-term mechanical ventilation (Boggs, 1993; Heffner, 1990; Tayal, 1994). Single-lumen, double-lumen, and fenestrated tracheostomies are among the most commonly used. Depending on the manufacturer, tracheostomies can vary in design, type of neck flange, size, length, and cuff design (Wilson, 1996). Like ET tubes, tracheostomy tube cuffs are designed with low-pressure, high-volume (soft) cuffs to minimize tracheal wall trauma (Boggs, 1993; Wilson, 1996).

Insertion of a tracheostomy tube is most valuable when done as an elective surgical procedure. Emergent tracheostomy has a fivefold increased rate of complications and should be avoided in preference of cricothyroidotomy if immediate surgical airway access is required (Deem & Bishop, 1995; Heffner, 1990). Many patients are switched from an ET tube to a tracheostomy to improve airway suctioning, to promote patient comfort and mobility, to facilitate rapid reintubation following spontaneous decannulation, to maximize the potential for fewer ventilator days, and to clear the mouth for speech, eating, and hygiene (Heffner, 1990; Hoffman, 1994; Wilson, 1996). Because standard tracheostomies are preferentially inserted as an elective surgical procedure in the operating room, nursing responsibilities focus on assisting with performance of emergent tracheostomies and monitoring for complications following completion of the procedure (Boggs, 1993).

Percutaneous dilatational tracheostomy (PDT) is an alternative method of providing a tracheostomy. PDT has received increasing attention as a viable option for patients requiring long-term airway support. PDT is a technique that can be performed at the patient's bedside versus the operating room and has been reported to cause fewer complications, be less expensive, and take a shorter period of time to place (Deem & Bishop, 1995; Hill et al., 1996). Before the procedure, nurses need to ensure that all appropriate personnel and supplies are in place, that the patient understands what is happening, and that the patient's pulmonary assessment and relevant laboratory test results have not changed. During the procedure, the patient is closely monitored to ensure that any problems are detected early and that the patient receives sedation along with narcotics or benzodiazepines for the procedure. Postoperative care of the PDT is not different from that of a standard tracheostomy, and the tube can safely be changed after approximately 1 week (Zavotsky & D'Amelio, 1995).

The length of time that an ET tube can be left in place before performing a tracheostomy has been the point of lively conversation among researchers and clinicians for years (Heffner, 1990; Hoffman, 1994; King, 1988; Marsh et al., 1989; Stauffer et al., 1981; Sugerman et al., 1997). Experts attending a consensus conference initiated by the National Association of Medical Directors of Respiratory Care recommended that an ET tube be used when the anticipated length of time for an artificial airway is 10 days or less. If the anticipated need for an artificial airway is more than 21 days, a tracheostomy is preferred. When the length of time for artificial airway management is unclear, ongoing monitoring is required to determine whether conversion to a tracheostomy is indicated (Hoffman, 1994; Plummer & Gracey, 1989).

Several studies provide evidence that early tracheostomy may, in fact, be beneficial. Rodriguez et al. (1990) were able to show in 106 trauma patients randomized to tracheostomy on day 7 or earlier, versus day 8 or later, that patients were weaned more quickly from the ventilator. The average number of ventilator days for the early group was 12 (SD 18 days), versus 37 (SD 3 days) for the late group. Likewise, in a second study involving early tracheostomy (within 4 days of intubation) in trauma patients (Lesnik, Rappaport, Fulginiti, & Witzke, 1992), researchers were able to start weaning patients with early tracheostomy within 6 days, versus 20.6 days in patients who received tracheostomies later. The incidence of nosocomial pneumonias was also significantly less in those patients who underwent early tracheostomy. A study by Sugerman et al. (1997) was unable to confirm these results.

Despite these recommendations, researchers continue to question the value of a tracheostomy when an artificial airway is required for periods as long as 3 weeks (Marsh et al., 1989; Stauffer et al., 1981). Thus, there does not seem to be an absolute time limit for converting an ET tube to a tracheostomy (Heffner, 1990; Marsh et al., 1989).

Management of the difficult airway must always be a top concern for all practitioners involved in Airway Management. In 1993, a task force formed by the American Society of Anesthesiologists (ASA) produced practice guidelines for management of the difficult airway (ASA, 1993). These guidelines and algorithms help clinicians focus their efforts on assessment of the likelihood of a difficult airway, management choices, and development of alternative strategies for airway management. Alternative nonsurgical strategies may involve use of newer airway options such as the Esophageal-Tracheal Double Lumen Airway or Combitube (Kendall Sheridan, Argyle, NY) and the Laryngeal Mask Airway (LMA).

The Esophageal-Tracheal Double Lumen Airway or Combitube is an option for airway control when an ET tube cannot be placed for reasons of difficulty or lack of training or skill. It is most effective in patients over 5 feet tall and is contraindicated in responsive patients with a gag reflex and known esophageal disease. It should be used cautiously in patients with burns and evidence of inhalation injury. This device is inserted blindly into either the esophagus or the trachea, and, based on location, ventilation is achieved through one of the two lumina (Deem & Bishop, 1995; Gonzalez, Herlich, Krohner, Boerner, & Schaefer, 1996). Once inserted, a large proximal cuff that holds 100 mL of air is inflated and rests in the pharynx. A second cuff located at the distal end of the device is inflated with 15 mL of air. After placement, a series of assessments must be performed quickly to establish location and proper ventilation. Successful use of the Combitube has been reported in cardiopulmonary resuscitation and in ICUs and operating rooms (Deem & Bishop, 1995). Because this airway is also rapidly replacing the esophageal obturator airway in the prehospital setting, nurses receiving these patients need to be familiar with this device and able to deal with airway concerns that may arise. Frequently, once patients are stabilized, they are switched to oral ET tubes.

The *Laryngeal Mask Airway (LMA)* is a general-purpose airway available in six sizes that consists of a large-bore tube (like an ET tube) with an inflatable oval mask at one end. The mask is designed to produce a seal around the laryngeal aperture once the airway is inserted and the mask is inflated. It is used for airway control primarily in the operating room but may be helpful in difficult airway situations because it does not require direct laryngoscopy for insertion. The main concerns with this airway are lack of protection of the lungs from aspiration and ineffectiveness in prolonged positive pressure ventilation (Brimacombe, 1992; Deem & Bishop, 1995; Gonzalez et al., 1996).

STABILIZING ARTIFICIAL AIRWAYS

Movement of ET and tracheostomy tubes causes abrasions to tracheal mucosa and contributes to laryngeal injury (Bishop, 1989; Mackenzie, 1983). Nasopharyngeal and oropharyngeal airways are taped in place to prevent them from becoming dislodged and obstructing the posterior pharynx (Elpern & Bone, 1990). ET tubes can be secured with commercially available ET tube holders, twill ties, or adhesive tape (Boggs, 1993; Dunleap, 1987; Hoffman & Maszkiewicz, 1987). Tapes and ties are changed daily, and oral ET tubes are moved to the other side of the mouth to prevent tissue necrosis. It is important to minimize motion between the tube and patient, administer meticulous mouth care, and monitor the integrity of oral mucous membranes during this process. Tube holders are loosened at least daily, and skin care is administered. Breath sounds are noted after the tape or twills are changed.

Tracheostomy tubes are stabilized with twill tape. According to one author, this is an unappreciated aspect of caring for patients with tracheostomies (Dunleap, 1987). It is recommended that (1) tapes be changed every 24 hours and/or following performance of routine tracheostomy care; (2) old tapes be left in place while new tapes are inserted; (3) tapes be tied at the side of the neck, with a piece of gauze or foam placed between the patient's skin and the tie; and (4) tapes be tied snugly enough to prevent slippage of the tracheostomy but loose enough to prevent neck irritation and erosion (one to two fingers should fit between the ties and the patient's skin) (Boggs, 1993; Dunleap, 1987). Specific procedures for changing ties are published elsewhere (Boggs, 1993; Dunleap, 1987).

Leverage and traction on ET and tracheostomy tubes should be minimized by suspending the ventilator tubing from overhead supports, using flexible catheter mounts and swivels, and supporting tubes during turning, suctioning, and ventilator disconnection and reconnection (Boggs, 1993; Heffner et al., 1986b; Mackenzie, 1983; Stauffer & Silvestri, 1982). A unique procedure for securing the ventilator tubing of tracheostomized patients has been described (Hravnak, 1984). Prolonged coughing, breathing out of phase with the ventilator, agitation, and decerebrate or decorticate posturing cause trauma to the tracheal mucosa and should be avoided by rectifying the cause, providing sedation, and, if necessary, administering muscle relaxants for mechanically ventilated patients (Heffner et al., 1986b; Mackenzie, 1983). Precautions should be taken to avoid unintentional extubation and spontaneous dislocation of airways. Use of arm restraints, appropriate sedation, tube fixation devices, and maintenance of appropriate cuff inflation and tube length are some of the nursing activities reported to prevent unintentional extubation (Kaplow & Bookbinder, 1994; Pesiri, 1994; Tominaga, Rudzwick, Scannell, & Waxman, 1995).

HYDRATION

Bypassing upper airways with an artificial device causes mucosal drying, interferes with the mucociliary transport system, diminishes the cough reflex, and creates dry, thick secretions that are difficult to remove (Clarke, 1995; Lane, 1990; Shekleton & Nield, 1987; Wanner, 1977, 1986). Warming and humidifying inspired air or oxygen with sterile water or hypotonic, isotonic, or hypertonic saline is necessary to minimize these complications (Branson, Campbell, Chatburn, & Covington, 1992; Nilsestuen, Fink, Stoller, Volpe, & Witek, 1993). During mechanical ventilation, the heated humidifier should be set to provide a minimum of 30 mg H_2O/L of delivered gas with an inspired gas temperature of 33°C to 37°C (Branson et al., 1992; Wright, Doyle, & Yoshihara, 1996). Cool aerosol therapy is used with upper airway edema such as laryngeotracheobronchitis, subglottic edema, and postextubation edema (Nilsestuen et al., 1993).

Nebulizers create a vapor mist and are used when inspired air or gas is delivered via a T-piece or tracheostomy mask (Shekleton & Nield, 1987). Controversy exists regarding the efficacy of mist therapy and ultrasonic nebulizers (USNs) (Cosenza & Norton, 1986; Nilsestuen, Fink, Witek, & Volpe, 1992; Shekleton & Nield, 1987). Efficacy of aerosol delivery devices is design dependent and user dependent (Nilsestuen et al., 1992). Guidelines for humidification and aerosol delivery are available from the AARC (Branson et al., 1992; Nilsestuen et al., 1992, 1993).

The efficacy of intermittent or continuous use of aerosol as a mucoevacuant has not been established, and it is not a substitute for systemic hydration. Adequate hydration is one of the most reliable ways to reduce the risk of inspissation of mucus production (Cosenza & Norton, 1986; Nilsestuen et al., 1992; Shekleton & Nield, 1987). Rehydration of dehydrated patients has been demonstrated to increase mucociliary clearance rates (Chopra, Talpin, & Simmons, 1977; Hirsh, Tokayer, & Robinson, 1975). Therefore, oral and intravenous fluid administration is needed to maintain systemic fluid balance in patients with ineffective airway clearance.

MANAGING CUFF PRESSURES

Because tracheal mucosa capillary perfusion pressure is about 20 to 30 mm Hg, cuff pressures should be maintained at a volume just high enough to prevent a leak from occurring (Goodnough, 1988; Heffner, 1990; Lane, 1990; Wilson, 1996). The most widely used cuffs are high-volume, low-pressure cuffs that allow a large surface area to come into contact with the tracheal wall, thus distributing the pressure over a much greater area (Boggs, 1993; Wilson, 1996).

Two methods are used for placing the optimal volume of air into the cuff (Lane, 1990; Snowberger, 1986). The minimal occlusive volume (MOV) technique is achieved by injecting air slowly during the inspiratory phase of ventilation until the patient receives the prescribed tidal volume on the ventilator or until an air leak cannot be auscultated over the trachea. The pressure in the cuff is measured and should not exceed 20 to 30 mm Hg. Most tubes will seal at about 20 mm Hg. The minimal leak technique is like the MOV technique, but 0.1 mL to 0.5 mL of air is withdrawn following insertion of the minimal occlusive volume to allow a small leak auscultated over the trachea during the end of the inspiratory phase of a positive-pressure breath (Hoffman & Maszkiewicz, 1987; Wilson, 1996).

Cuff pressures are monitored during expiration every 4 to 8 hours, using a three-way stopcock that is simultaneously connected to the cuff, a calibrated syringe, and a mercury manometer or commercially available pressure manometer. Cuff pressures are also checked after general anesthesia to minimize the effect of nitrous oxide diffusion into the cuff. Complications from cuff pressures exceeding tracheal perfusion pressure include tracheal stenosis, tracheoesophageal fistulas, and tracheomalacia. Procedures for inflating and measuring cuff pressures are described in detail by several experts (Goodnough, 1985, 1988; Lane, 1990; Wilson, 1996).

TRACHEOSTOMY CARE

Meticulous tracheostomy care is necessary to minimize accompanying complications, such as infection, skin breakdown, and airway obstruction. Although procedures for tracheostomy care are readily available in the literature (Boggs, 1993; Clarke, 1995; Hooper, 1996; Provine, 1996; Rudy, 1997), little research exists on the best method of tracheostomy care. Generally, care includes keeping the area around the stoma clean, dry, and open to air; preventing traction on the tubing; and cleaning the inner cannula as often as necessary to prevent buildup of secretions. Sterile technique is recommended for hospitalized patients to decrease the risk of infection. Tracheostomy ties are changed following cleansing of the stoma site and inner cannula. A tracheostomy dressing is not used unless there is an excessive amount of exudate, because wet dressings promote infections and tissue breakdown. If the area around the stoma is not infected, but irritation and redness are present, an occlusive dressing can be used on the area to protect the skin (Boggs, 1993; Wilson, 1996).

Secretion Removal

Removal of secretions, an important component of Airway Management, is accomplished by endotracheal and nasotracheal suctioning and chest physical therapy (chest percussion, postural drainage, chest vibration, and cough).

ENDOTRACHEAL SUCTIONING

Various methods of endotracheal suctioning (ETS) have been investigated in an attempt to prevent or reverse side effects, particularly suction-induced hypoxemia (SIH) and hemodynamic compromise. These methods include preoxygenation, hyperventilation, hyperinflation, manual inflation, and oxygen insufflation. Using these terms interchangeably and without conceptual clarity has led to confusion and variation in research findings. These terms, as defined by Barnes and Kirchhoff (1986) and Mancinelli-Van Atta and Beck (1992), are listed in Table 15–4 to provide a common ground for discussion of ETS activities.

Universal precautions are recommended as part of the suction protocol, particularly with high-risk patients. According to the Centers for Disease Control and Prevention (CDC) guidelines, universal precautions apply to blood and other body fluids containing visible blood (CDC, 1988). Because suctioning may result in blood-tinged secretions and it is difficult to predict when this will happen, wearing gloves and goggles for protection is recommended.

Sterile suction equipment is used in the hospital for each suction procedure. The ratio of the catheter diameter to the internal diameter of the tube should be less than 0.5 to prevent excessive negative pressure and atelectasis (Baier, Begin, & Sackner, 1976; Rosen & Hillard, 1962). The magnitude of negative pressure applied to the catheter affects the amount of hypoxemia, secretion recovery, endotracheal mucosal damage, and negative airway pressure (Kuzenski, 1978; Pardowsky & Guthrie, 1983; Plum & Dunning, 1956; Polacek & Guthrie, 1981; Sackner, Landa, Greeneltch, & Robinson, 1973). A negative pressure setting of 100 to 120 mm Hg is recommended. High negative airway pressure may result in removal of intrapulmonary gas and airway collapse (Bradstater & Muallem, 1969; Rosen & Hillard, 1962).

Table 15–4 Terms and Techniques Used to Reduce Suctioning-Induced Hypoxemia

Term	Definition	Technique
Manual inflation	Lung inflation by means of a resuscitation bag; does not imply an increase in percentage of oxygen and/or pressure	Bagging
Preoxygenation	Administration of oxygen before suctioning; does not imply an increase in percentage of oxygen and/or pressure	Bagging Change in ventilation rate Mechanical sigh
Insufflation	Delivery of oxygen through the double lumen of a suction catheter or the sidearm of an endotracheal tube adapter; allows oxygen to be administered simultaneously with suctioning	
Hyperoxygenation	Administration of oxygen at an FiO_2 greater than the patient is receiving or is usually required; may be performed before, during, and/or after suctioning	Bagging with supplemental O_2 Increasing the ventilator FiO_2
Hyperinflation	Lung inflation by means of a resuscitation bag or ventilator; may be at a volume equivalent to the ventilator setting or as much as one and one-half times the preset ventilator value; does not imply a change in oxygen concentration	Bagging Mechanical sigh
Hyperventilation	An increase in rate of ventilation; does not imply an increase in volume or oxygen concentration	Bagging Increasing the ventilator rate
Open system suctioning (OSS)	ETS requiring opening of the ventilatory circuit	Conventional sterile suction catheter Suction source
Closed system suctioning (CSS)	ETS through an intact ventilator circuit that does not require disconnection	Use of a plastic-covered suction catheter attached to the ventilator via an adapter Suction source

Source: Data from Barnes, C., and Kirchhoff, K. (1986). Minimizing hypoxemia due to endotracheal suctioning: A review of the literature. *Heart and Lung, 15,* 164–176; Mancinelli-Van Atta, J., and Beck, S. L. (1992). Preventing hypoxemia and hemodynamic compromise related to endotracheal suctioning. *American Journal of Critical Care, 1*(3), 62–79.

Research has consistently shown that some type of hyperoxygenation before, during, and after each suctioning episode should be standard practice in order to avoid the possible negative effects of hypoxemia (Barnes & Kirchhoff, 1986; Branson et al., 1993; Mancinelli-Van Atta & Beck, 1992; Riegel & Forshee, 1985; Stone, 1990; Stone & Turner, 1988; Wainwright & Gould, 1996). The appropriate method for hyperinflation and hyperoxygenation before, during, and after the passage of a suction catheter remains controversial. Most clinicians use either the manual resuscitation bag (MRB) or the ventilator to deliver additional oxygen and volume. Research indicates that both manual and ventilator techniques prevent deoxygenation; however, the ventilator appears to be more effective (Glass, Grap, Corley, & Wallace, 1993; Grap, Glass, Corley, & Parks, 1996; Stone, 1990). Hyperoxygenation and hyperinflation by the ventilator result in lower peak inspiratory pressures and comparable, if not higher, PaO_2 levels. Both manual and ventilator-delivered hyperoxygenation-hyperinflation breaths produce hemodynamic consequences, primarily increases in mean arterial pressure (MAP), cardiac output (CO), and heart rate (HR) (Stone, 1990). Researchers have found that even under ideal conditions it is difficult to deliver adequate tidal volumes and 100% FiO_2 levels using MRBs (Glass et al., 1993; McCabe & Smeltzer, 1993).

Hemodynamic changes associated with hyperoxygenation and hyperinflation followed by ETS include increased airway pressure, increased MAP, and increased CO (Preusser et al., 1988; Stone, Preusser, Groch, Karl, & Gonyon, 1991). This is dangerous for people with new grafts and for those with increased intracranial pressure (Rudy, Baun, Stone, & Turner, 1986), particularly when these findings are combined with the results of Walsh, Vanderwarf, Hoscheit, and Fahey (1989) indicating a 27% mean increase in oxygen consumption during ETS.

Although further research is required to determine the optimal methods for hyperoxygenation and hyperinflation for ETS, current data suggest hyperoxygenation of the patient with the ventilator FiO_2 setting at 1.0 (100%) and hyperinflation with the ventilator set at one and a half times the preset tidal volume. Rogge, Bunde, and Baun (1989) found that oxygenation at 20% above baseline in addition to 150% tidal volume produced no significant differences in oxygen saturation, blood pressure, HR, or rhythm compared with 100% hyperoxygenation in patients with chronic obstructive pulmonary disease. This is the only study investigating the effects of less than 100% oxygen.

It can take up to 3 minutes for oxygen delivered to reach 100% following an increase in ventilator FiO_2 to 1.0 (Hess & Easter, 1986). This washout time is variable and depends on the rate, flow, and tidal volume settings on the ventilator, as well as the length and diameter of the ventilator tubing (Stone & Turner, 1988). Newer-generation ventilators achieve 100% FiO_2 nearly immediately. If the nurse decides to use an MRB, the patient may receive less than 100% oxygen (Barnes & Watson, 1982, 1983; Glass et al., 1993). It is recommended that the oxygen flow rate to the reservoir be set to flush, a reservoir of between 1,000 mL and 2,600 mL be used, and sufficient time be allowed to refill the MRB from the reservoir (Preusser, 1985; Stone, 1989).

Ten to 15 seconds is the recommended duration for each suction pass (Lane, 1990). An observational study of clinical practice revealed a 7-second mean suction duration, with the majority of fall in PaO_2 occurring during the first 5 seconds. Suction durations of 10 seconds and 15 seconds did not significantly increase the fall in PaO_2 occurring during the first 5 seconds (Rindfleisch & Tyler, 1983).

The number of consecutive suction passes seems to have an insignificant effect on tidal volume and hypoxemia, with the greatest fall occurring after the first suction pass (Hipenbecker & Guthrie, 1981). However, if the MRB is being used for hyperinflation, increases in mean arterial pressure seem to be cumulative and thus increase from one hyperinflation-suction sequence to the next (Stone, Vorst, Lanham, & Zahn, 1989). Although further research is indicated, it seems that the number of suction passes is insignificant if the ventilator is used for hyperinflation.

Normal saline instillation (NSI) is often used with suctioning to facilitate secretion retrieval. The main rationales cited for use of NSI include loosening, thinning, or mixing of secretions; stimulating a cough; lubricating the suction catheter; and bronchial lavage (Ackerman, Ecklund, & Abu-Jumah, 1996). This practice, however, is receiving increased scrutiny, with suggestions that NSI may have little advantage and may actually be harmful (Ackerman, 1993; Ackerman et al., 1996; Briening, 1996; Hagler & Traver, 1994; Raymond, 1995).

Use of saline has been found to increase the release of viable bacteria from the ET tube into the lower airways, raising concerns over increased risk of infection (Hagler & Traver, 1994). The effect of NSI on oxygenation is inconclusive. In one study, SpO$_2$ was lower in patients when NSI was used (Ackerman, 1993).

Research recommendations clearly suggest that NSI should not be routine practice with suctioning. Instead, clinicians should focus efforts on ensuring adequate systemic hydration of patients and proper humidification of airways through ventilator circuits (Ackerman et al., 1996; Raymond, 1995).

Inline Suctioning Devices   Use of suction devices that permit patients to remain on the ventilator during suctioning (closed tracheal suctioning systems [CTSS]) may reduce complications associated with suctioning procedures. Many independent and dependent variables related to CTSS have been researched and are reviewed elsewhere (DePew & Noll, 1994; Ochsenreither, 1995). CTSS compared with open system suctioning (OSS) generally results in less oxygen desaturation even in the absence of hyperoxygenation (DePew & Noll, 1994; Harshbarger, Hoffman, Zullo, & Pinsky 1992). At this time, the major advantages of such systems are for patients on greater than 10 cm H$_2$O of PEEP. Carlon, Fox, and Ackerman (1987) found that the mean PaO$_2$ drop for patients on PEEP of greater than 10 cm H$_2$O was 7.7% with the CTSS versus 19.5% with OSS.

Cost-effectiveness of the CTSS remains controversial (DePew, Moseley, Clark, & Morales, 1994; Johnson et al., 1994; Noll, Hix, & Scott, 1990). Because of the cost of CTSS catheters, it is recommended that their use be limited to patients with frequent need of suctioning, presence of bloody secretions, PEEP of 10 cm H$_2$O or higher, highly contagious respiratory infections, and evidence of cardiopulmonary compromise during suctioning (Chulay et al., 1997).

One of the chief complaints regarding CTSS is the perception of less effective secretion retrieval. Witmer, Hess, and Simmons (1991) compared the quantity of secretions retrieved with OSS versus CTSS and found no significant difference (median 1.7 g with CTSS versus median 1.9 g with OSS). Further research is needed in this area.

Use of a catheter repeatedly over a 24-hour period has raised concerns about infections. Studies examining this issue report increased colonization rates of CTSS versus OSS but no significant differences in rates of nosocomial pneumonia (Conrad, George, Romers, & Owens, 1989; Deppe et al., 1990; Johnson et al., 1994).

Suctioning the Head-Injured Patient   ETS is especially challenging for the nurse caring for the head-injured patient. Significant increases in intracranial pressure (ICP) have been caused by the ETS procedure and put these patients at risk of intracranial hypertension and cerebral ischemia (Kerr, Rudy, Brucia, & Stone, 1993; Rudy et al., 1986; Rudy, Turner, Baun, Stone, & Brucia, 1991). Rudy et al. (1991) found cumulative increases in MAP, ICP, and cerebral perfusion pressure (CPP) with successive passes of the suctioning catheter. Brucia and Rudy (1996) found that just inserting a suction catheter and causing tracheal stimulation significantly increase ICP, MAP, and CPP. Future research needs to address ways to abate or blunt the deleterious effects of ETS in the head-injured adult (Kerr et al., 1997). Based on the research to date, several suggestions for suctioning the head-injured patient are listed in Table 15–5.

In summary, most studies on ETS have used convenience samples, acutely ill but stable patients, and patients who had undergone open heart surgery with minimal pulmonary complications. Studies report improved oxygenation of most patients with use of a certain suction procedure but also list outliers whose oxygenation was decreased using the same technique (Bodai, Walton, Briggs, & Goldstein, 1987; Chulay, 1988). Individual patient variables reported as contributing to SIH are positive smoking history, elderly (older than 70 years), presence of arrhythmias before ETS, PaO_2 less than 70 mm Hg, a wide alveolar to arterial (A-a) gradient, acid-base imbalances, and cardiovascular instability (Chulay, 1988; Chulay & Graber, 1988; Fell & Cheney, 1971; Jones, 1989; Lane, 1990).

Responses to ETS vary based on types of patients studied; therefore, the nurse must monitor and evaluate each patient's oxygen (SpO_2, oxygen saturation in arterial blood [SaO_2], venous oxygen saturation [SvO_2], and respiratory rate [RR]), hemodynamic status (MAP, cardiac rate and rhythm, ICP, CPP), and subjective response immediately before, during, and after suctioning. If adverse consequences occur during suctioning, the suction procedure is terminated, and supplemental oxygen is administered. Suctioning techniques should be varied, based on the clinical response of the patient. The amount and type of secretions retrieved are noted. Steps for carrying out ET suctioning are summarized in Table 15–5.

Table 15–5 Recommendations for Suctioning through an Artificial Airway

1. Determine the need for suctioning. Clinical indicators of the need for suctioning include the following:
   - Coughing
   - Increase in ventilator airway pressures
   - Decreased tidal volume during pressure-controlled ventilation
   - Changes in the monitored flow and pressure graphics of the mechanical ventilator
   - Respiratory distress (e.g., dyspnea, increased RR, air hunger, increased anxiety)
   - Decrease in arterial oxygen levels
   - Decreased breath sounds
   - Adventitious sounds over large airways during chest auscultation
   - Noisy respirations
   - Visible secretions in the artificial airway
2. Hyperoxygenate with 100% oxygen using the MRB or ventilator before and after each suction pass. Assess each patient's response to ETS before deciding if hyperinflation is also indicated. If using an MRB, optimize oxygen delivery by ensuring that the reservoir is fully expanded, the oxygen flow to the bag is 15 L/min or greater, and hand-to-forearm or two-handed technique is used.
3. Limit suction passes to two or three at most, with suction duration limited to 10 sec or less, and negative suction pressure of 100 to 120 mm Hg. Use sterile technique in hospitalized patients. Refrain from using catheters that occlude more than one half of the ET tube.
4. Continuously monitor the patient's response to suctioning (cardiac rhythm, SaO_2, color, heart rate, respiratory rate, MAP, ICP, and the patient's subjective response). Stop suctioning and hyperoxygenate immediately if signs of intolerance occur.
5. Once the airway is cleared, document the patient's tolerance of the procedure along with a description of the secretions removed.

Special Considerations for Head-Injured Patients
- Use hyperventilation with caution to avoid CO_2 levels below 25 mm Hg.
- Try to limit suctioning passes to 1–2.
- Avoid rotating the head, which may increase ICP.

NASOTRACHEAL SUCTIONING

Nasotracheal suctioning (NTS) refers to the insertion of a suction catheter through the nasal passage and pharynx into the trachea to aspirate accumulated secretions or foreign material (Hilling et al., 1992). NTS is indicated in patients with coarse breath sounds over large airways who are unable to cough effectively to remove secretions but do not have an ET tube or tracheostomy tube in place. Many of the same principles of ETS apply to NTS. Hyperoxygenation and hyperinflation are necessary before, during, and after each suction pass. These maneuvers can be accomplished with an MRB or by instructing the patient to take deep breaths through an oxygen delivery system.

It is important to elicit the cooperation of the conscious patient before insertion of the catheter. Instructing the patient to take slow, deep breaths reduces the gag reflex and feelings of suffocation and helps retract the epiglottis, thereby facilitating catheter passage through the vocal cords into the trachea (Elpern & Bone, 1990; Hilling et al., 1992). Practice guidelines for NTS are available from the AARC (Hilling et al., 1992).

CHEST PHYSIOTHERAPY

Chest physiotherapy (CPT) is designed to improve the mobilization of bronchial secretions, the matching of ventilation and perfusion, and the normalization of functional residual capacity based on the effects of gravity and external manipulation of the thorax. This includes postural drainage, chest percussion, chest vibration, and cough, all directed at improving mucus and sputum clearance from the airways (Ciesla, 1996; Hilling et al., 1990a, 1990b; Kirilloff, Owens, Rogers, & Mazzocco, 1985; Lane, 1990; Shekelton & Nield, 1987; Silverberg, Johnson, Gorga, Nagler, & Goodwin, 1995).

CPT is a well-entrenched standard in pulmonary care and has been used with a variety of acute and chronically ill populations, but the efficacy of CPT is questionable. It has been used excessively and in patients for whom it is not indicated (Hilling et al., 1990a, 1990b; Kirilloff et al., 1985; Poelaert et al., 1991). CPT appears to be beneficial for acutely ill patients who have large volumes of secretions and patients with lobar atelectasis. It is not efficacious in people with exacerbations of chronic bronchitis, patients with pneumonia who have limited amounts of secretions, and status asthmaticus. CPT used in acutely ill patients is associated with increased oxygen consumption, bronchoconstriction, hypoxemia, tachycardia, increased intracranial pressure, acute hypotension, dysrhythmias, and other adverse events (Harding, Kemper, & Weissman, 1995; Weissman & Kemper, 1993). It is contraindicated in patients with seizures, resectable carcinoma, recent hemoptysis, severe hypertension, unstable hemodynamics, and increased intracranial pressure (Lane, 1990). CPT should not be performed within 1 hour after eating because of the increased risk of regurgitation and aspiration.

Postural drainage is performed by positioning the patient with the lung segment to be drained in the uppermost position. This facilitates movement of secretions toward major bronchi for clearance (Norton & Conforti, 1985; Techlin, 1979).

Percussion is done with cupped hands held rigid so that a hollow sound is produced when an area of the chest wall is clapped. The purpose is to loosen and dislodge secretions from the airways. The amount of force used is relative to the person's body physique.

Chest vibration is the delivery of vibratory movements to the chest wall as the patient exhales. It can be delivered with the nurse's flat hand or with a machine (Lane, 1990). Mechanical vibratory devices have not been sufficiently evaluated to reach a conclusion about their efficacy (Kirilloff et al., 1985). Although percussion and vibration are used widely, empirical evidence demonstrates little efficacy in their use (Hilling et al., 1990a, 1990b; Kirilloff et al., 1985).

Directed cough is a critical part of CPT. Several important points necessary to promote effective coughing are reviewed here (Consenza & Norton, 1986; Hilling et al., 1993; Traver, 1985). The first activity in promoting an effective cough is encouraging the patient to take a deep breath. Firm placement of the nurse's hands on the lateral basal area of the chest wall is used to encourage deep breathing. The nurse should be careful to avoid restricting chest movement with the hands; rather, the hands are placed to encourage the individual to push them out as far as possible with each inspiration. Several deep breaths are taken before the actual cough maneuver, and the individual is given positive feedback with each deep breath. Incentive spirometers can also be used to encourage deep breathing (Hilling et al., 1993b; Hilling et al., 1993).

Several cough techniques are used to stimulate a cough. To elicit a cascade (normal) cough, the nurse instructs the patient to take a deep breath, followed by a succession of three to four coughs until almost all the air is out of the lungs. Cascade coughing moves secretions from the periphery of the lungs to the central airways (Cosenza & Norton, 1986; Janson-Bjerklie, 1983; Oldenburg, Dolovich, Montgomery, & Newhouse, 1979).

The huff cough (forced expiration technique) is a simple modification of the cascade cough. The patient inhales deeply, bends forward slightly, and then performs a series of three to four huffs against an open glottis (Hilling et al., 1993). The goal of this technique is to clear bronchial secretions with less airway compression than occurs with a cascade cough. Investigators have found a significant amount of secretion expectoration using this maneuver (Pryor, Webber, Hodson, & Batten, 1979; Sutton et al., 1983).

The end-expiratory cough is a modification used for patients with bronchiectasis (Traver, 1985). The patient inhales deeply several times, followed by a prolonged slow exhalation. On the third or fourth breath, the patient exhales to a lung volume below normal resting lung volumes and then coughs without inhaling. This empties mucus from bronchiectatic dilations of the airways (Traver, 1985).

Augmented or manually assisted cough is used in patients who are unable to generate sufficient expiratory muscle force. Mechanical pressure is applied to the epigastric region or thoracic cage during the expiratory phase of the cough maneuver (Hilling et al., 1993).

After coughing, a voluntary maximal inhalation of 3 to 10 seconds is necessary to aid in reinflating collapsed alveoli. Maximal inhalation following coughing helps avoid complications of pooled mucus, decreased oxygenation, and increased risk of infection. The use of an incentive spirometer for these inspiratory efforts is helpful in encouraging maximal inhalation (Hilling et al., 1990b).

THE INTERVENTION

Airway Management is broad in scope and critical to life. Nursing activities to carry out the Nursing Interventions Classification (NIC) intervention of Airway Management focus on respiratory monitoring; positioning; insertion, stabilization, and management of artificial airways; and secretion removal (Table 15–6). The activity list of Airway Management refers to other interventions in the NIC. For example, the Airway Management activity of *monitor respiratory and oxygenation status, as appropriate* might be adequate, or the NIC intervention of Respiratory Monitoring may be needed. Depending on the patient situation, the

Table 15–6 Airway Management

DEFINITION: Facilitation of patency of air passages.

ACTIVITIES:

Open the airway, using the head tilt, chin lift, or jaw thrust technique, as appropriate

Position patient to maximize ventilation potential

Identify patient requiring actual/potential airway insertion

Insert oral or nasopharyngeal airway, as appropriate

Perform chest physical therapy, as appropriate

Remove secretions by encouraging coughing or suctioning

Encourage slow, deep breathing; turning; and coughing

Instruct how to cough effectively

Assist with incentive spirometer, as appropriate

Auscultate breath sounds, noting areas of decreased or absent ventilation and presence of adventitious sounds

Perform endotracheal or nasotracheal suctioning, as appropriate

Administer bronchodilators, as appropriate

Teach patient how to use prescribed inhalers, as appropriate

Administer aerosol treatments, as appropriate

Administer ultrasonic nebulizer treatments, as appropriate

Administer humidified air or oxygen, as appropriate

Regulate fluid intake to optimize fluid balance

Position to alleviate dyspnea

Monitor respiratory and oxygenation status, as appropriate

Source: McCloskey, J. C., and Bulechek, G. M. (1996). *Nursing interventions classification (NIC)* (2nd ed., p. 95). St. Louis: Mosby–Year Book.

more global intervention of Airway Management may be sufficient, or, in other situations, a more specific intervention such as Respiratory Monitoring or Airway Suctioning may be more appropriate or used in conjunction with the intervention of Airway Management. The selection of nursing interventions for use with an individual patient is part of the clinical decision making of the nurse (McCloskey & Bulechek, 1996).

A critical first step in Airway Management is positioning the patient to maintain an open airway, minimize dyspnea, and maximize ventilation. This activity is particularly important for patients who are unconscious, sedated, or recovering from anesthesia. The NIC needs an intervention on Positioning: Respiratory to reflect this essential part of respiratory care. Positioning: Respiratory includes nursing activities specific to positioning patients to open or protect their airway and to promote matching of ventilation and perfusion in the lung.

Identifying persons at risk for ineffective airway clearance is equally important in order for an artificial airway to be inserted as necessary. Persons at risk for airway obstruction include those with head and cervical spine injuries, patients receiving conscious sedation or anesthesia, and those with acute or chronic lung disease.

Use of nebulizers and inhalers by patients is also a component of Airway Management. A variety of bronchodilators are used to open airways, and some of these are administered via an inhaler. Patients and family members must be educated about the appropriate use of inhalers and other pharmacological agents that have a bronchodilatory effect.

The nursing activities of monitoring respiratory status and monitoring oxygenation status are critical to ensuring that medical and nursing treatments are effective and to preventing complications associated with their use. Signs and symptoms of airway obstruction are listed in Table 15–1. It is important that nurses are knowledgeable of these signs and symptoms and that they identify early those patients who may need an artificial airway inserted. The NIC intervention of Respiratory Monitoring, defined as "collection and analysis of patient data to ensure airway patency and adequate gas exchange" (McCloskey & Bulechek, 1996, p. 473), is an adjunct to Airway Management.

Insertion and stabilization of an artificial airway are indicated when a patient is unable to maintain an open airway or needs mechanical ventilatory support. The NIC intervention of Airway Insertion and Stabilization, defined as "insertion or assisting with insertion and stabilization of an artificial airway" (McCloskey & Bulechek, 1996, p. 94), may be used. Following insertion and stabilization of artificial airways, a number of nursing activities are essential to prevent complications associated with use of artificial airways. These activities include administering aerosol, nebulizer, or humidified air or oxygen as indicated. All patients who have an artificial airway need humidification and warming of inspired air or oxygen to minimize mucosal drying, interference with the mucociliary transport system, and creation of dry, thick secretions that are difficult to remove. In addition, systemic fluid balance must be optimized, because adequate hydration is among the most reliable ways to reduce the risk of inspissation of mucus production (Nilsestuen et al., 1992). Artificial Airway Management, defined as "maintenance of endotracheal and tracheostomy tubes and preventing complications associated with their use" (McCloskey & Bulechek, 1996, pp. 112–113), is an adjunct intervention for patients with artificial airways.

Nursing activities to remove secretions or foreign debris from the airway are a critical part of Airway Management. Secretion removal can be achieved through endotracheal and nasotracheal suctioning, chest physiotherapy, and promotion of coughing and deep breathing. Vigilance in monitoring the patient's ability to clear secretions from the airway is an important nursing activity, particularly in high-risk patients. NIC interventions to consider using for secretion removal are as follows:

- Airway Suctioning—"removal of airway secretions by inserting a suction catheter into the patient's oral airway and/or trachea" (McCloskey & Bulechek, 1996, pp. 96–97)
- Chest Physiotherapy—"assisting the patient to move airway secretions from peripheral airways to more central airways for expectoration and/or suctioning" (McCloskey & Bulechek, 1996, p. 171)
- Cough Enhancement—"promotion of deep inhalation by the patient with subsequent generation of intrathoracic pressures and compression of underlying lung parenchyma for the forceful expulsion of air" (McCloskey & Bulechek, 1996, p. 189)

Table 15–5 outlines steps for suctioning through an artificial airway.

NURSING DIAGNOSES AND APPROPRIATE PATIENT GROUPS

Airway Management is used with patients who have any of the following nursing diagnoses:

- Ineffective Airway Clearance—"a state in which an individual is unable to clear secretions or obstructions from the respiratory tract to maintain airway patency" (North American Nursing Diagnosis Association [NANDA], 1994, p. 26)

- Impaired Gas Exchange—"the state in which the individual experiences a decreased passage of oxygen and/or carbon dioxide between the alveoli of the lungs and the vascular system" (NANDA, 1994, p. 26)
- Ineffective Breathing Pattern—"a state in which an individual's inhalation and/or exhalation pattern does not enable adequate pulmonary inflation or emptying" (NANDA, 1994, p. 27)
- Inability to Sustain Spontaneous Ventilation—"a state in which the response pattern of decreased energy reserves results in an individual's inability to maintain breathing adequate to support life" (NANDA, 1994, p. 27)
- Dysfunctional Ventilatory Weaning Response—"a state in which a patient cannot adjust to lowered levels of mechanical ventilator support, which interrupts and prolongs the weaning process" (NANDA, 1994, p. 28)
- Risk for Aspiration—"the state in which an individual is at risk for entry of gastrointestinal secretions, oropharyngeal secretions, or solids or fluids into tracheobronchial passages" (NANDA, 1994, p. 33)

Patients with Ineffective Airway Clearance, Risk for Aspiration, Inability to Sustain Spontaneous Ventilation, and Dysfunctional Ventilatory Weaning Response need the intervention of Airway Management to ensure an open airway, decrease the risk for aspiration into the tracheobronchial tree, and manage artificial airways associated with mechanical ventilation. Patients with Impaired Gas Exchange and Ineffective Breathing Pattern may have Airway Management in their treatment plan depending on the underlying cause of their nursing and medical diagnoses. For example, a patient with Impaired Gas Exchange may benefit from Airway Management if the major cause is impaired ventilation secondary to airway occlusion or secretion retention. Patient populations that also need Airway Management are comatose patients, those receiving conscious sedation or anesthesia, and patients with gastrointestinal hemorrhage. These patients are at Risk for Aspiration.

OUTCOMES

Critical outcomes of effective Airway Management are freedom from airway obstruction (see Table 15–1) and adequate ventilation (lack of hypoxemia and hypercapnia; see Table 15–2). The two major outcomes from the Nursing Outcomes Classification (NOC) that are applicable for measuring the effectiveness of Airway Management are as follows:

- Respiratory Status: Ventilation—"movement of air in and out of the lungs" (Johnson & Maas, 1997, p. 241)
- Respiratory Status: Gas Exchange—"alveolar exchange of CO_2 or O_2 to maintain arterial blood gas concentrations" (Johnson & Maas, 1997, p. 240)

Respiratory Status: Ventilation is the primary outcome. If this outcome is not achieved, gas exchange is likely to be impaired; that is, alveolar exchange of O_2 and CO_2 to maintain arterial blood gas concentration will be compromised. Table 15–7 summarizes the relationships among the nursing diagnoses and examples of specific patient populations, nursing interventions, and patient outcomes.

Table 15–7 Nursing Diagnoses, NIC Interventions, and Patient Outcomes for Airway Management

Nursing Diagnoses	Examples of Patient Populations	NIC Interventions to Consider in Addition to Airway Management	Patient Outcomes
Ineffective Airway Clearance	• Pneumonia • Cystic fibrosis bronchiectasis • Asthma • Atelectasis	• Respiratory Monitoring • Positioning: Respiratory • Cough Enhancement • Chest Physiotherapy • Airway Suctioning • Fluid Management	Respiratory Status: Ventilation
Risk for Aspiration	• GI hemorrhage • Postanesthesia • Decreased level of consciousness	• Positioning: Respiratory • Aspiration Precautions • Airway Insertion and Stabilization	Respiratory Status: Ventilation
Inability to Sustain Spontaneous Ventilation	• Cervical-spine fracture • Guillain-Barré syndrome • COPD* with pneumonia • Head injury • Pulmonary infection	• Airway Insertion and Stabilization • Artificial Airway Management • Mechanical Ventilation • Airway Suctioning • Respiratory Monitoring • Fluid Management	Respiratory Status: Ventilation
Dysfunctional Ventilatory Weaning Response	• End-stage COPD • Cardiac failure • Interstitial lung disease	• Artificial Airway Management • Mechanical Ventilatory Weaning • Airway Suctioning • Fluid Management • Nutrition Therapy	Respiratory Status: Ventilation Respiratory Status: Gas Exchange
Impaired Gas Exchange	• Pneumonia • Sepsis • ARDS† • Chest trauma	• Respiratory Monitoring • Cough Enhancement • Positioning: Respiratory • Oxygen Therapy	Respiratory Status: Gas Exchange
Ineffective Breathing Pattern	• COPD • Chest trauma • Neuromuscular defects • Postoperative complications	• Respiratory Monitoring • Ventilation Assistance • Positioning: Respiratory • Oxygen Therapy	Respiratory Status: Ventilation

*COPD: chronic obstructive pulmonary disease.
†ARDS: acute respiratory distress syndrome.

CASE STUDY

SB, a 45-year-old man, was driving his family across Iowa to a family reunion. On the interstate, they were involved in a motor vehicle crash when a driver heading eastbound crossed the median and hit SB's van on the driver's side at interstate speeds. SB's son, who was the backseat passenger on the driver's side, was dead at the scene. His wife was uninjured, and a second son suffered a fractured ankle. Triage at the scene designated SB for transport by helicopter to a Level I trauma center. Upon arrival, he was complaining of shortness of breath and severe pain in his chest, pelvis, and flank. Workup included bony films, head and abdominal computed tomography (CT) scans, aortogram, and laboratory studies.

These tests revealed a left hemopneumothorax relieved by chest tube placement with 600 mL of blood returned; a left pulmonary contusion; fractured ribs 3, 4, 5, and 6 on the left side; a left superior-inferior ramus fracture minimally displaced; a probable right renal contusion; hemoglobin (HgB) 9.1, hematocrit (Hct) 28%, sodium (Na) 136, potassium (K) 4.8, blood urea nitrogen (BUN) 27, creatinine 1.3; and ABGs on 4 L nasal cannula—pH 7.38, PaO_2 79 torr, $PaCO_2$ 37 torr, HCO_3 23, base excess (BE) −2. SB was admitted to the surgical intensive care unit (SICU), where he was started on morphine via patient-controlled analgesia. His respiratory rate on admission to SICU was 40 breaths per minute, which gradually decreased over the next several hours following pain control.

Over the next 36 hours, SB's pulmonary status worsened. He developed crackles throughout both lung fields, with diminished breath sounds in the left lower lobe. Chest x-ray (CXR) revealed bilateral pleural effusions, left lower lobe consolidation, and right lower lobe atelectasis. SB was unable to cough because of the pain induced with deep breathing and coughing. Therefore, the pain service inserted an epidural catheter with hydromorphone and bupivacaine. Throughout day 3, SB's oxygen delivery was adjusted, with an FiO_2 ranging between 50% and 100% via face mask.

By day 5, it was clear that SB was working hard to breathe and was unable to cough effectively. When his face mask oxygen was removed for any reason, oxygen saturations as measured by pulse oximetry dropped below 90%. His CXR was not improving, despite aggressive attempts at coughing and deep breathing. His white blood cell count elevated to 18.1, Hct dropped to 27%, and he was given one unit of packed red blood cells to optimize his oxygen-carrying capacity. Meanwhile, pastoral care, social services, and a psychiatric clinical nurse specialist were providing support to SB and his family as they dealt with a critically injured father and preparing for their loved one's funeral. By the afternoon, SB agreed with the ICU staff that he needed assistance with breathing, and he was intubated with an 8.0 mm oral ET tube and placed on pressure-regulated volume-controlled mechanical ventilation with an FiO_2 of 65%. End-tidal CO_2 monitoring was also initiated, with values ranging from 32 to 35 mm Hg. ABGs obtained shortly after intubation were pH 7.45, PaO_2 68, $PaCO_2$ 39, HCO_3 26, BE +3. The FiO_2 was increased to 70% and then 80%. SB initially required ET suctioning every 1 to 2 hours because of copious secretions. By the end of the day, however, frequency of suctioning decreased

to every 3 to 4 hours, and the FiO_2 was decreased to 40%.

Over the next 4 days, SB remained on the ventilator, which required the interventions of Artificial Airway Management, Airway Suctioning, and Fluid Management to promote airway patency. The mode of mechanical ventilation was changed to synchronized intermittent mandatory ventilation (SIMV) with pressure control, and weaning was initiated on day 7, but SB's PaO_2 dropped to 67 torr. On day 8, his chest tube was discontinued, and he was started on trials of pressure support versus periods of rest on SIMV. On day 10, SB was weaned from mechanical ventilation, extubated, and placed on 40% FiO_2 via face mask. SB was encouraged to cough and use the incentive spirometer every 2 hours; he expectorated 50 to 100 mL of secretions per day. Antibiotic coverage was changed to nafcillin 2 g IV every 4 hours. By day 11, he was transferred to a monitored stepdown unit where aggressive physical therapy was undertaken. On day 13, SB was transferred via ground ambulance to a hospital in his hometown to be closer to his family and home.

This case highlights numerous aspects of Airway Management. From the time of his accident, SB's respiratory status was closely monitored by oximetry, capnometry, ABGs, electrocardiography, and physical assessment. During the period of time when SB's pulmonary status was borderline, nursing interventions included Positioning to facilitate oxygenation, Airway Management, and aggressive Chest Physiotherapy. When it became clear that SB would need mechanical ventilatory support, nurses prepared for and assisted with insertion and stabilization of an oral endotracheal tube—Airway Insertion and Stabilization. During the ensuing days, they managed his airway through Respiratory Monitoring, Artificial Airway Management, Airway Suctioning, Positioning, Chest Physiotherapy, and administration of nebulizer treatments. SB achieved the outcome of Respiratory Status: Ventilation.

SUMMARY
■

Airway Management is a direct care intervention that is applicable in a variety of clinical situations with a number of different patient populations. It is an intervention that is global in nature but critical for survival. Nursing activities of Airway Management encompass monitoring, positioning, insertion and management of artificial airways, and secretion removal. Critical outcomes of effective Airway Management are Respiratory Status: Ventilation and Respiratory Status: Gas Exchange.

References

Ackerman, M. H. (1993). The effect of saline lavage prior to suctioning. *American Journal of Critical Care, 2*, 326–330.

Ackerman, M. H., Ecklund, M. M., and Abu-Jumah, M. (1996). A review of normal saline instillation: Implications for practice. *Dimensions of Critical Care Nursing, 15*(1), 31–38.

Adler, D. C. (1979). Pulmonary nursing, 1900–1979, and future projections. *Heart and Lung, 8*, 882–890.

Ahrens, T. (1996). Respiratory monitoring. In J. M. Clochesy, C. Breu, S. Cardin, A. A. Whittaker, and E. B. Rudy (Eds.), *Critical care nursing* (2nd ed., pp. 245–261). Philadelphia: W.B. Saunders.

Albert, R. (1997). The prone position in acute respiratory distress syndrome: Where we are, and where do we go from here? *Critical Care Medicine, 25*, 1453–1454.

Alpen, M. A. (1993). *Variables influencing secretion retrieval with endotracheal suctioning.* Unpublished master's thesis, University of Iowa, Iowa City.

Amar, D., Greenberg, M. A., Menegus, M. A., and Breitbart, S. (1994). Should all patients undergoing cardiac catheterization or percutaneous transluminal coronary angioplasty receive oxygen? *Chest: the Cardiopulmonary Journal, 105*, 727–732.

Amborn, S. A. (1976). Clinical signs associated with the amount of tracheobronchial secretions. *Nursing Research, 25*, 121–126.

American Heart Association. (1994). Adjuncts for airway control, ventilation, and oxygenation. In *Textbook of advanced cardiac life support* (pp. 2-1–2-17). Dallas: Author.

American Society of Anesthesiologists task force on management of the difficult airway: Practice guidelines for management of the difficult airway. (1993). *Anesthesiology, 78*, 597–602.

Baier, G., Begin, R., and Sackner, M. (1976). Effect of airway diameter, suction catheter, and the bronchofiberscope on airflow in endotracheal and tracheostomy tubes. *Heart and Lung, 5*, 235–238.

Baker, C. E. (1996). Acid-base physiology. In J. M. Clochesy, C. Breu, S. Cardin, A. A. Whittaker, and E. B. Rudy (Eds.), *Critical care nursing* (2nd ed., pp. 583–600). Philadelphia: W.B. Saunders.

Baraka, A., Jabbour, S., Hammoud, R., Aouad, M., Najjar, F., Khoury, G., and Sibai, A. (1994). Can pulse oximetry and end-tidal capnography reflect arterial oxygenation and carbon dioxide elimination during laparoscopic cholecystectomy? *Surgical Laparoscopy and Endoscopy, 4*, 353–356.

Barnes, C., and Kirchhoff, K. (1986). Minimizing hypoxemia due to endotracheal suctioning: A review of the literature. *Heart and Lung, 15*, 164–176.

Barnes, R., and Watson, M. (1982). Oxygen delivery performance of four adult resuscitation bags. *Respiratory Care, 27*, 139–146.

Barnes, R., and Watson, M. (1983). Oxygen delivery performance of old and new designs of the Laerdal, Vitalograph, and AMBU adult manual resuscitators. *Respiratory Care, 28*, 1121–1128.

Barnes, T. A., Boudin, K. M., Durbin, C. G., Fluck, R. R., and Malinowski, C. (1995). American Association of Respiratory Care. Clinical practice guideline: Management of airway emergencies. *Respiratory Care, 40*, 749–760.

Berels, D. J., and Marz, M. S. (1991). SaO_2 monitoring in the postanesthesia care unit. *Journal of Post Anesthesia Nursing, 6*, 394–401.

Bishop, M. J. (1989). Mechanisms of laryngotracheal injury following prolonged tracheal intubation. *Chest, 96*, 185–186.

Bodai, B. T., Walton, C. B., Briggs, S., and Goldstein, M. (1987). A clinical evaluation of an oxygen insufflation/suction catheter. *Heart and Lung, 16*, 39–46.

Boggs, R. L. (1993). Airway management. In R. L. Boggs and M. Wooldridge-King (Eds.), *AACN procedure manual for critical care* (pp. 1–65). Philadelphia: W.B. Saunders.

Bowton, D. L., Scuderi, P. E., Harris, L., and Haponik, E. F. (1991). Pulse oximetry monitoring outside the intensive care unit: Progress or problem? *Annals of Internal Medicine, 115*, 405–454.

Bradstater, B., and Muallem, M. (1969). Atelectasis following tracheal suction in infants. *Anesthesiology, 31*, 468–473.

Branson, R. D., Campbell, R. S., Chatburn, R. L., and Covington, J. (1992). AARC clinical practice guideline: Humidification during mechanical ventilation. *Respiratory Care, 37*, 887–890.

Branson, R. D., Campbell, R. S., Chatburn, R. L., and Covington, J. (1993). AARC clinical practice guideline: Endotracheal suctioning of mechanically ventilated adults and children with artificial airways. *Respiratory Care, 38*, 500–504.

Briening, E. P. (1996). The effects of saline instillation prior to endotracheal suctioning. *Online Journal of Knowledge Synthesis for Nursing, 3* (Doc 9, Online #33), 1–9.

Brimacombe, J. R. (1992). AANA journal course: Update for nurse anesthetists—The laryngeal mask airway: A review for the nurse anesthetist. *Journal of the American Association of Nurse Anesthetists, 60*, 490–499.

Campbell, R. S., Branson, R. D., Burke, W., Covington, J., and Graybeal, J. (1995). AARC clinical practice guideline: Capnography/capnometry during mechanical ventilation. *Respiratory Care, 40*, 1321–1324.

Carlon, G. C., Fox, S. J., and Ackerman, N. J. (1987). Evaluation of a closed-tracheal suction system. *Critical Care Medicine, 15*, 522–525.

Centers for Disease Control and Prevention (CDC). (1988). Update: Universal precautions for prevention of transmission of human immunodeficiency virus, hepatitis B virus, and other bloodborne pathogens in healthcare settings. *Morbidity and Mortality Weekly Report, 37*, 377–382.

Chopra, S., Talpin, G., and Simmons, D. (1977). Effects of hydration and physical therapy on tracheal transport velocity. *American Review of Respiratory Diseases, 115*, 1009–1014.

Chulay, M. (1988). Arterial blood gas changes with a hyperinflation and hyperoxygenation suctioning intervention in critically ill patients. *Heart and Lung, 17*, 654–661.

Chulay, M., Connolly, M. A., and Parr, M. (1997). Airway and ventilatory management. In M. Chulay, C. Guzzetta, and B. Dossey (Eds.), *AACN handbook of critical care nursing* (pp. 119–153). Stamford, CT: Appleton & Lange.

Chulay, M., and Graber, G. M. (1988). Efficacy of hyperinflation and hyperoxygenation suctioning intervention. *Heart and Lung, 17,* 15–22.

Ciesla, N. (1996). Chest physical therapy for patients in the intensive care unit. *Physical Therapy, 76,* 609–625.

Clarke, L. (1995). A critical event in tracheostomy care. *British Journal of Nursing, 4,* 677–681.

Conrad, S. A., George, R. B., Romers, M. W., and Owens, M. W. (1989). Comparison of nosocomial pneumonia rates in closed and open tracheal suction systems. *Chest, 96,* 1845.

Cosenza, J., and Norton, L. (1986). Secretion clearance: State of the art from a nursing perspective. *Critical Care Nurse, 6*(4), 23–27.

Deem, S., and Bishop, M. (1995). Evaluation and management of the difficult airway. *Critical Care Clinics, 11*(1), 1–27.

DePew, C. L., and Noll, M. L. (1994). Inline closed-system suctioning: A research analysis. *Dimensions of Critical Care Nursing, 13*(2), 73–83.

DePew, C. L., Moseley, M. J., Clark, E. G., and Morales, C. C. (1994). Open versus closed system endotracheal suctioning: A cost comparison. *Critical Care Nurse, 4*(1), 94–100.

Deppe, S. A., Kelly, J. W., Thoi, L. L., Chudy, J. H., Longfield, R. N., Ducey, J. P., Truiwit, C. L., and Antopal, M. R. (1990). Incidence of colonization, nosocomial pneumonia, and mortality in critically ill patients using a trach care closed suction system versus an open-suction system: prospective randomized study. *Critical Care Medicine, 18,* 1389–1393.

Derrick, S. J., Waters, H., Kang, S. W., Cwalina, T. F., and Simmons, W. (1993). Evaluation of a nasal/oral discriminate sampling system for capnographic respiratory monitoring. *AANA Journal, 61,* 509–520.

Dhainaut, J., Bons, J., Bricard, C., and Monsailler, J. (1980). Improved oxygenation in patients with extensive unilateral pneumonia using lateral decubitus position. *Thorax, 35,* 792–793.

Doering, L. (1993). The effect of positioning on hemodynamics and gas exchange in the critically ill: A review. *American Journal of Critical Care, 2,* 208–211.

Dunleap, E. (1987, August). Safe and easy ways to secure breathing tubes. *RN, 50,* 26–27.

El-Naggar, M., Sadagopa, S., Levin, H., Kantor, H., and Collins, V. J. (1976). Factors influencing choice between tracheostomy and prolonged translaryngeal intubation in acute respiratory failure: A prospective study. *Anesthesia Analog, 55,* 195–201.

Elpern, E., and Bone, R. (1990). The technique of nasotracheal suctioning. *Journal of Critical Illness, 5,* 993–999.

Evans, A., and Winslow, E. H. (1995). Oxygen saturation and hemodynamic response in critically ill, mechanically ventilated adults during intrahospital transport. *American Journal of Critical Care, 4*(2), 106–111.

Fell, T., and Cheney, F. W. (1971). Prevention of hypoxia during endotracheal suction. *Annals of Surgery, 174,* 24–28.

Fletcher, R., Olsson, K., Helbo-Hansen, S., Nihlson, C., and Hedestrom, P. (1984). Oral or nasal intubation after cardiac surgery? A comparison of effects on heart rate, blood pressure, and sedation requirements. *Anaesthesia, 39,* 376–378.

Fontaine, D., and McQuillan, K. (1989). Positioning as a nursing therapy in trauma care. *Critical Care Nursing Clinics of North America, 1*(1), 105–112.

Gattinoni, L., Tognoni, G., Brazzi, L., and Latini, R. (1997). Ventilation in the prone position. The prone-supine study collaborative group [Letter]. *Lancet, 350,* 815.

Glass, C., Grap, M., Corley, M. C., and Wallace, D. (1993). Nurses' ability to achieve hyperinflation and hyperoxygenation with a manual resuscitation bag during endotracheal suctioning. *Heart and Lung, 22*(2), 158–165.

Gonzalez, R., Herlich, A., Krohner, R., Boerner, T., and Schaefer, J. (1996). Recent advances in airway management in anesthesiology: An update for otolaryngologists. *American Journal of Otolaryngology, 17*(3), 145–160.

Goodnough, S. (1985). The effects of oxygen and hyperinflation on arterial oxygen tension after endotracheal suctioning. *Heart and Lung, 14,* 11–17.

Goodnough, S. (1988). Reducing tracheal injury and aspiration. *Dimensions of Critical Care Nursing, 7,* 324–332.

Grap, M. J. (1996). Pulse oximetry. In M. Chulay and S. Burns (Eds.), *Protocols for practice: Non invasive monitoring series.* Aliso Viejo, CA: American Association of Critical-Care Nurses.

Grap, M. J., Glass, C., Corley, M., and Parks, T. (1996). Endotracheal suctioning: Ventilator vs. manual delivery of hyperoxygenation breaths. *American Journal of Critical Care, 5*(3), 192–197.

Hagler, D. A., and Traver, G. A. (1994). Endotracheal saline and suction catheters: Sources of lower airway contamination. *American Journal of Critical Care, 3,* 444–447.

Harding, J., Kemper, M., and Weissman, C. (1995). Pressure support ventilation attenuates the cardiopulmonary response to an acute increase in oxygen demand. *Chest, 107,* 1665–1172.

Harshbarger, S. A., Hoffman, L. A., Zullo, T. G., and Pinsky, M. R. (1992). Effects of a closed tracheal suction system on ventilatory and cardiovascular parameters. *American Journal of Critical Care, 1*(3), 57–61.

Heffner, J. E. (1990). Airway management in the critically ill patient. *Critical Care Clinics, 6,* 533–550.

Heffner, J. E., Miller, S., and Sahn, S. A. (1986a). Tracheostomy in the intensive care unit. Part I. *Chest, 90,* 269–274.

Heffner, J. E., Miller, S., and Sahn, S. A. (1986b). Tracheostomy in the intensive care unit. Part II. *Chest, 90,* 430–436.

Henneman, E. A. (1996). Patients with acute respiratory failure. In J. M. Clochesy, C. Breu, S. Cardin, A. A. Whittaker, and E. B. Rudy (Eds.), *Critical care nursing* (2nd ed., pp. 630–648). Philadelphia: W.B. Saunders.

Hess, D., and Agarwal, N. N. (1992). Variability of blood gases, pulse oximeter saturation, and end-tidal carbon dioxide pressure in stable, mechanically ventilated trauma patients. *Journal of Clinical Monitoring, 8*(2), 111–115.

Hess, D., and Easter, G. (1986). Delivery 100% oxygen with a ventilator. A study of lag time. *Respiratory Therapy, 31,* 17–21, 39.

Hess, D., Schlottag, A., Levin, B., Mathai, J., and Rexrode, W. O. (1991). An evaluation of the usefulness of end-tidal PCO_2 to aid weaning from mechanical ventilation following cardiac surgery. *Respiratory Care, 36,* 837–843.

Hill, B. B., Zweng, T. N., Maley, R. H., Charash, W. E., Toursarkissian, B., and Kearney, P. (1996). Percutaneous dilational tracheostomy: Report of 356 cases. *Journal of Trauma, 41,* 238–243.

Hilling, L., Bakow, E., Fink, J., Kelly, C., Sobush, D., and Southorn, P. A. (1990a). AARC clinical practice guideline: Postural drainage therapy. *Respiratory Care, 36,* 1418–1426.

Hilling, L., Bakow, E., Fink, J., Kelly, C., Sobush, D., and Southorn, P. A. (1990b). AARC clinical practice guideline: Incentive spirometry. *Respiratory Care, 36,* 1402–1405.

Hilling, L., Bakow, E., Fink, J., Kelly, C., Sobush, D., and Southorn, P. A. (1992). AARC clinical practice guideline: Nasotracheal suctioning. *Respiratory Care, 37,* 898–901.

Hilling, L., Bakow, E., Fink, J., Kelly, C., Sobush, D., and Southorn, P. (1993). AARC clinical practice guideline: Directed cough. *Respiratory Care, 38,* 495–499.

Hipenbecker, D., and Guthrie, M. (1981). The effects of negative pressure generated during suctioning on lung volumes and pulmonary compliance. *American Review of Respiratory Diseases, 123,* 120–122.

Hirsch, J., Tokayer, J., and Robinson, M. (1975). Effect of dry air and subsequent humidification on tracheal mucous velocity in dogs. *Journal of Applied Physiology, 39,* 242–246.

Hoffman, L. (1994). Timing of tracheotomy: What is the best approach? *Respiratory Care, 39,* 378–385.

Hoffman, L. A., and Maszkiewicz, R. C. (1987). Airway management. *American Journal of Nursing, 87,* 40–53.

Hogan, B. M. (1995). Pulse oximetry for an adult with a pulmonary disorder. *American Journal of Occupational Therapy, 49,* 1062–1064.

Hooper, M. (1996). Nursing care of the patient with a tracheostomy. *Nursing Standard, 10*(34), 40–43.

Hravnak, M. (1984). Ventilator tubing stabilization for the tracheostomized patient. *Critical Care Nurse, 4*(5), 20–21.

Hurn, P. D., and Hartsock, R. L. (1994). Thoracic injuries. In V. D. Cardona, P. D. Hurn, P. J. Mason, A. M. Scanlon, and S. W. Veise-Berry (Eds.), *Trauma nursing from resuscitation through rehabilitation* (pp. 466–511). Philadelphia: W.B. Saunders.

Janson-Bjerklie, S. (1983). Defense mechanisms protecting the healthy lung. *Heart and Lung, 12,* 643–649.

Johnson, K. L., Kearney, P. A., Johnson, S. B., Niblett, J. B., MacMillan, N. L., and McClain, R. E. (1994). Closed versus open endotracheal suctioning: Costs and physiologic consequences. *Critical Care Medicine, 22,* 658–666.

Johnson, M., and Maas, M. (Eds.). (1997). *Iowa outcomes project: Nursing outcomes classification (NOC).* St. Louis: Mosby-Year Book.

Jones, G. (1989). *Effectiveness of two suction methods.* Unpublished master's thesis, University of Iowa, Iowa City.

Jones, S. E. (1995). Getting the balance right: Pulse oximetry and inspired oxygen concentration. *Professional Nurse, 10,* 368–373.

Kaplow, R., and Bookbinder, M. (1994). A comparison of four endotracheal tube holders. *Heart and Lung, 1,* 59–66.

Kerr, M. E., Rudy, E. B., Brucia, J., and Stone, K. S. (1993). Head-injured adults: Recommendations for endotracheal suctioning. *Journal of Neuroscience Nursing, 25*(2), 86–91.

Kerr, M. E., Rudy, E. B., Weber, B. B., Stone, K. S., Turner, B. S., Orndoff, P. A., Sereika, S. M., and Marion, D. W. (1997). Effect of short-duration hyperventilation during endotracheal suctioning on intracranial pressure in severe head-injured adults. *Nursing Research, 46,* 195–201.

Kerr, M. E., Zempsky, J., Sereika, S., Orndoff, P., and Rudy, E. (1996). Relationship between arterial carbon dioxide and end-tidal carbon dioxide in mechanically ventilated adults with severe head trauma. *Critical Care Medicine, 24,* 785–790.

Kharasch, M., and Graff, J. (1995). Emergency management of the airway. *Critical Care Clinics, 11*(1), 53–56.

King, E. G. (1988). Respiratory failure in the critically ill. In W. Sibbald (Ed.), *Synopsis of critical care* (3rd ed.). Baltimore: Williams & Wilkins.

Kirilloff, L. H., Owens, G. R., Rogers, R. M., and Mazzocco, M. C. (1985). Does chest physical therapy work? *Chest, 88,* 436–444.

Klein, D. G. (1996). Patients with trauma. In J. M. Clochesy, C. Breu, S. Cardin, A. A. Whittaker, and E. B. Rudy (Eds.), *Critical care nursing* (2nd ed., pp. 1335–1358). Philadelphia: W.B. Saunders.

Knipper, J. S. (1986). Minimizing the complications of tracheal suctioning. *Focus on Critical Care, 13*(4), 23–26.

Kuzenski, B. (1978). Effect of negative pressure on tracheobronchial trauma. *Nursing Research, 27,* 260–263.

Lane, G. H. (1990). Pulmonary therapeutic management. In L. A. Thelan, J. K. Davie, and L. D. Urden (Eds.), *Textbook of critical care nursing: Diagnosis and management* (pp. 444–471). St. Louis: C.V. Mosby.

Langer, M., Mascheroni, D., Marcolin, R., and Gattinoni, L. (1988). The prone position in ARDS patients: A clinical study. *Chest, 94*(1), 103–107.

Lesnik, I., Rappaport, W., Fulginiti, J., and Witzke, D. (1992). The role of early tracheostomy in blunt, multiple organ trauma. *American Surgeon, 58,* 346–349.

Mackenzie, C. F. (1983). Compromises in the choice of orotracheal or nasotracheal intubation and tracheostomy. *Heart and Lung, 12,* 485–492.

Magnan, A., Philip-Joet, F., Rey, M., Reynaud, M., Porri, F., and Arnaud, A. (1993). End-tidal CO_2 analysis in sleep apnea syndrome. Conditions for use. *Chest, 103*(1), 129–131.

Mancinelli-Van Atta, J., and Beck, S. L. (1992). Preventing hypoxemia and hemodynamic compromise related to endotracheal suctioning. *American Journal of Critical Care, 1*(3), 62–79.

Marsh, H. M., Gillespie, D. J., and Baumgartner, A. E. (1989). Timing of tracheostomy in the critically ill patient. *Chest, 96,* 190–193.

McCabe, S. M., and Smeltzer, S. C. (1993). Comparison of tidal volumes obtained by one-handed and two-handed ventilation techniques. *American Journal of Critical Care, 2,* 467–473.

McCloskey, J. C., and Bulechek, G. M. (Eds.). (1996). *Nursing interventions classification (NIC)* (2nd ed.). St. Louis: Mosby-Year Book.

Mure, M., Martling, C., and Lindahl, S. (1997). Dramatic effect on oxygenation in patients with severe acute lung insufficiency treated in the prone position. *Critical Care Medicine, 25,* 1539–1544.

North American Nursing Diagnosis Association. (1994). *Nursing diagnoses: Definitions and classification 1995–1996.* Philadelphia: Author.

Nilsestuen, J., Fink, J., Witek, T., and Volpe, J. III. (1992). AARC clinical practice guideline: Selection of aerosol delivery device. *Respiratory Care, 37,* 891–897.

Nilsestuen, J., Fink, J. B., Stoller, J. K., Volpe, J., and Witek, T., Jr. (1993). AARC clinical practice guideline: Bland aerosol administration. *Respiratory Care, 38,* 1196–1200.

Noll, M. L., and Byers, J. F. (1995). Usefulness of measures of SvO_2, SpO_2, vital signs and derived dual oximetry parameters as indicators of arterial blood gas variables during weaning of cardiac surgery patients from mechanical ventilation. *Heart and Lung, 24,* 220–227.

Noll, M., Hix, C., and Scott, G. (1990). Closed tracheal suction systems: Effectiveness and nursing implications. *AACN Clinical Issues, 1,* 318–328.

Norton, L., and Conforti, C. (1985). The effects of body position on oxygenation. *Heart and Lung, 14,* 45–52.

Nyarwaya, J. B., Mazoit, J. X., and Samii, K. (1994). Are pulse oximetry and end-tidal carbon dioxide tension monitoring reliable during laparoscopic surgery? *Anaesthesia, 49,* 775–778.

Ochsenreither, J. M. (1995). Closed tracheal suctioning: Advantages, drawbacks, and research recommendations. *Online Journal of Knowledge Synthesis for Nursing, 2*(Doc 2, Online #14), 1–8.

Oldenburg, F. A., Dolovich, M. B., Montgomery, J. M., and Newhouse, M. T. (1979). Effects of postural drainage, exercise and cough on mucous clearance in chronic bronchitis. *American Review of Respiratory Diseases, 120,* 739–745.

Pardowsky, B. J., and Guthrie, M. M. (1983). Negative airway pressure during endotracheal suctioning. *American Review of Respiratory Diseases, 127,* 147–151.

Pesiri, A. J. (1994). Two-year study of the prevention of unintentional extubation. *Critical Care Nursing Quarterly, 17*(3), 35–39.

Piehl, M. A., and Brown, R. S. (1976). Use of extreme position changes in acute respiratory failure. *Critical Care Medicine, 4*(1), 13–14.

Plum, F., and Dunning, M. F. (1956). Techniques for minimizing trauma to the tracheobronchial tree after tracheostomy. *New England Journal of Medicine, 254,* 193–200.

Plummer, A. L., and Gracey, D. R. (1989). Consensus conference on artificial airways in patients receiving mechanical ventilation. *Chest, 96,* 178–180.

Poelaert, J., Lannoy, B., Vogelaers, D., Everaert, J., Decruyenaere, J., Capiau, P., and Colardyn, F. (1991). Influence of chest physiotherapy on arterial oxygen saturation. *Acta Anaestheiologica Belgica, 42*(3), 165–170.

Polacek, L., and Guthrie, M. M. (1981). The effect of suction catheter size and suction flow rate on negative airway pressure and its relationship to the fall in arterial oxygen tension. *American Review of Respiratory Diseases, 123,* 120–122.

Preusser, B., Stone, K., Gonyon, D., Winningham, M. L., Groch, K. F., and Karl, J. E. (1988). Effects of two methods of preoxygenation on mean arterial pressure, cardiac output, peak airway pressure, and postsuctioning hypoxemia. *Heart and Lung, 17,* 290–299.

Preusser, B. A. (1985). The efficiency of commercially available manual resuscitation bags. *Focus on Critical Care, 12,* 59–61.

Provine, B. (1996). Consultation corner. Education about tracheostomy care. *Perspectives in Respiratory Nursing, 7*(2), 6.

Pryor, S., Webber, B., Hodson, M., and Batten, J. (1979). Evaluation of the forced expiration technique as an adjunct to postural drainage in treatment of cystic fibrosis. *British Medical Journal, 2,* 417–418.

Rashkin, M. C., and Davis, T. (1986). Acute complications of endotracheal intubation. *Chest, 89,* 165–167.

Raymond, S. J. (1995). Normal saline instillation before suctioning: Helpful or harmful? A review of the literature [Review]. *American Journal of Critical Care, 4,* 267–271.

Remolina, C., Khan, A., Santiago, T., and Edelman, N. (1981). Positional hypoxemia in unilateral lung disease. *New England Journal of Medicine, 304,* 523–525.

Riegel, B., and Forshee, T. (1985). A review of the literature on preoxygenation for endotracheal suctioning. *Heart and Lung, 14,* 507–518.

Rindfleisch, S., and Tyler, M. (1983). Duration of suctioning: An important variable. *Respiratory Care, 28,* 457–459.

Rodriguez, J. L., Steinberg, S. M., Luchetti, F. A., Gibbons, K. J., Taheri, P. A., and Flint, L. M. (1990). Early tracheostomy for primary airway management in the surgical critical care setting. *Surgery, 108,* 655–659.

Rogge, J., Bunde, L., and Baun, M. (1989). Effectiveness of oxygen concentrations of less than 100% before and after endotracheal suction in patients with chronic obstructive pulmonary disease. *Heart and Lung, 18,* 64–71.

Rosen, M., and Hillard, E. K. (1962). The effects of negative pressure during tracheal suction. *Anesthesia Analgesia, 41,* 322–325.

Rotello, L. C., Warren, J., Jastremski, M. S., and Milewski, A. (1992). A nurse-directed protocol using pulse oximetry to wean mechanically ventilated patients from toxic oxygen concentrations. *Chest: The Cardiopulmonary Journal, 102,* 1833–1835.

Rudy, E., Baun, M., Stone, K., and Turner, B. (1986). The relationship between endotracheal suctioning and changes in intracranial pressure. A review of the literature. *Heart and Lung, 15,* 488–494.

Rudy, E. B., Turner, B. S., Baun, M., Stone, K. S., and Brucia, J. (1991). Endotracheal suctioning in adults with head injury. *Heart and Lung, 20,* 667–674.

Rudy, S. F. (1997). Review of tracheostomy videos for staff education. *ORL-Head and Neck Nursing, 15*(1), 15–16, 18–19.

Sackner, M. A., Landa, J. F., Greeneltch, N., and Robinson, M. J. (1973). Pathogenesis and prevention of tracheobronchial damage with suction procedures. *Chest, 64,* 284–290.

St. John, R. E. (1996). *End-tidal CO_2 monitoring.* Aliso Viejo, CA: American Association of Critical-Care Nurses.

Saura, P., Blanch, L., Lucangelo, U., Fernandez, R., Mestre, J., and Artigas, A. (1996). Use of capnography to detect hypercapnic episodes during weaning from mechanical ventilation. *Intensive Care Medicine, 22,* 374–381.

Schmitz, T. M. (1991). The semi-prone position in ARDS: Five case studies. *Critical Care Nurse, 11*(5), 22–30.

Seaton, D., Lapp, N. C., and Morgan, K. C. (1979). Effect of body position on gas exchange after thoracotomy. *Thorax, 34,* 518–522.

Shekleton, M. E., and Nield, M. (1987). Ineffective airway clearance related to artificial airway. *Nursing Clinics of North America, 22,* 167–177.

Shrake, K., Blonshine, S., Brown, R., Crapo, R., Martineau, R., Ruppell, G., and Wanger, J. (1991). AARC clinical practice guideline: Pulse oximetry. *Respiratory Care, 36,* 1406–1409.

Silverberg, R., Johnson, J., Gorga, D., Nagler, W., and Goodwin, C. (1995). A survey of the prevalence and application of chest physical therapy in U.S. burn centers. *Journal of Burn Care and Rehabilitation, 16*(2 Pt. 1), 154–159.

Smith, A. E. (1983, January). Endotracheal suctioning. Are we harming our patients? *Critical Care Update,* 29–31.

Snowberger, P. (1986). Decreasing tracheal damage due

to excessive cuff pressures. *Dimensions of Critical Care Nursing, 5,* 136–142.

St. John, R. E. (1996). End-tidal carbon dioxide monitoring. In M. Chulay and S. Burns (Eds.), Protocols for practice: non-invasive monitoring series. Aliso Viejo, CA: AACN Publications.

Stauffer, J. L., Olson, D. E., and Petty, T. L. (1981). Complications and consequences of endotracheal intubation and tracheostomy. A prospective study of 150 critically ill adult patients. *American Journal of Medicine, 70,* 65–68.

Stauffer, J. L., and Silvestri, R. C. (1982). Complications of endotracheal intubation, tracheostomy, and artificial airways. *Respiratory Care, 27,* 417–433.

Stone, K. (1989). Endotracheal suctioning in the critically ill. *Critical Care Nursing Currents, 7*(2), 5–8.

Stone, K., and Turner, B. (1988). Endotracheal suctioning. *Annual Review of Nursing Research, 7,* 27–49.

Stone, K., Vorst, E., Lanham, B., and Zahn, S. (1989). Effects of lung hyperinflation on mean arterial pressure and postsuctioning hypoxemia. *Heart and Lung, 18,* 377–385.

Stone, K. S. (1990). Ventilator versus manual resuscitation bag as the method for delivering hyperoxygenation before endotracheal suctioning. *AACN Clinical Issues, 1,* 289–299.

Stone, K. S., Preusser, B. A., Groch, K. F., Karl, J. I., and Gonyon, D. S. (1991). The effect of lung hyperinflation and endotracheal suctioning on cardiopulmonary hemodynamics. *Nursing Research, 40*(2), 76–80.

Sugerman, H., Wolfe, L., Pasquale, M., Rogers, F., O'Malley, K., Knudson, M., DiNardo, L., Gordon, M., and Schaffer, S. (1997). Multicenter, randomized, prospective trial of early tracheostomy. *Journal of Trauma, 43,* 741–747.

Sutton, P., Parker, R., Webber, B., Newman, S., Garland, N., Lopez-Vidriero, M., Pavia, D., and Clark, S. W. (1983). Assessment of forced expiration technique, postural drainage and directed coughing in chest physiotherapy. *European Journal of Respiratory Disease, 64,* 62–68.

Szaflarski, N. L., and Cohen, N. H. (1989). Use of pulse oximetry in critically ill adults. *Heart and Lung, 18,* 444–452.

Tayal, V. S. (1994). Tracheostomies. *Emergency Medicine Clinics of North America, 12,* 707–727.

Techlin, J. S. (1979). Positioning, percussing and vibrating patients for effective bronchial drainage. *Nursing, 79,* 64–71.

Technology Subcommittee of the Working Group on Critical Care, Ontario Ministry of Health. (1992). Noninvasive blood gas monitoring: A review for use in the adult critical care unit [Review]. *Canadian Medical Association Journal, 146,* 703–712.

Thrush, D. N., Mentis, S. W., and Downs, J. B. (1991). Weaning with end-tidal CO_2 and pulse oximetry. *Journal of Clinical Anesthesia, 3,* 456–460.

Titler, M., Bulechek, G., Knipper, J., and Alpen, M. (1992). Coarse breath sounds as an indicator for tracheal suctioning. In S. R. Clark and J. Boller (Eds.), *Proceedings of the 1992 National Teaching Institute* [Abstract] (p. 385). Aliso Viejo, CA: American Association of Critical-Care Nurses.

Tominaga, G. T., Rudzwick, H., Scannell, G., and Wax-man, K. (1995). Decreasing unplanned extubations in the surgical intensive care unit. *American Journal of Surgery, 170,* 586–590.

Traver, G. (1985). Ineffective airway clearance: Physiology and clinical application. *Dimensions in Critical Care Nursing, 4,* 198–208.

Via-Reque, E., and Rattenburg, C. (1981). Prolonged oro-or nasotracheal intubation. *Critical Care Medicine, 9,* 37–42.

Vollman, K. (1997). Prone positioning for the ARDS patient. *Dimensions of Critical Care Nursing, 16*(4), 184–193.

Vollman, K. M., and Bander, J. J. (1996). Improved oxygenation utilizing a prone positioner in patients with acute respiratory distress syndrome. *Intensive Care Medicine, 22,* 1105–1111.

Wainwright, S. P., and Gould, D. (1996). Endotracheal suctioning: An example of the problems of relevance and rigour in clinical research. *Journal of Clinical Nursing, 5,* 389–398.

Walsh, J. M., Vanderwarf, C., Hoscheit, D., and Fahey, P. J. (1989). Unsuspected hemodynamic alterations during endotracheal suctioning. *Chest, 95,* 162–165.

Wanner, A. (1977). Clinical aspects of mucociliary transport. *American Review of Respiratory Diseases, 116,* 73–125.

Wanner, A. (1986). Mucociliary clearance in trachea. *Clinical Chest Medicine, 7,* 247–258.

Weissman, C., and Kemper, M. (1993). Stressing the critically ill patient: The cardiopulmonary and metabolic responses to an acute increase in oxygen consumption. *Journal of Critical Care, 8*(2), 100–108.

Wiklund, L., Hok, B., Stahl, K., and Jordeby-Johnson, A. (1994). Postanesthesia monitoring revisited: Frequency of true and false alarms from different monitoring devices. *Journal of Clinical Anesthesia, 6,* 182–188.

Wilson, D. (1996). Care of the chronic mechanically ventilated patient. In J. M. Clochesy, C. Breu, S. Cardin, A. A. Whittaker, and E. B. Rudy (Eds.), *Critical care nursing* (2nd ed., pp. 689–705). Philadelphia: W.B. Saunders.

Witmer, M. T., Hess, D., and Simmons, M. (1991). An evaluation of the effectiveness of secretion removal with the Ballard closed-circuit suction catheter. *Respiratory Care, 36,* 844–848.

Wright, J., Doyle, P., and Yoshihara, G. (1996). Mechanical ventilation: Current uses and advances. In J. M. Clochesy, C. Breu, S. Cardin, A. A. Whittaker, and E. B. Rudy (Eds.), *Critical care nursing* (2nd ed., pp. 262–288). Philadelphia: W.B. Saunders.

Wright, S. W. (1992). Conscious sedation in the emergency department: The value of capnography and pulse oximetry. *Annals of Emergency Medicine, 21,* 551–555.

Yeaw, E. (1996). The effect of body positioning upon maximal oxygenation of patients with unilateral lung pathology. *Journal of Advanced Nursing, 23,* 55–61.

Zack, M. B., Pontoppidan, H., and Kazemi, H. (1974). The effect of lateral position on gas exchange in pulmonary disease. *American Review of Respiratory Disease, 110,* 49–55.

Zavotsky, K. E., and D'Amelio, L. F. (1995). Bedside percutaneous tracheostomy: Implications for critical care nurses. *Critical Care Nurse, 15*(5), 37–38, 40–43.

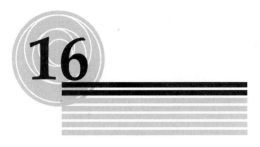

Chemotherapy Management

Mary H. Wegenka

Chemotherapy is the administration of antineoplastic agents to treat systemic cancer. The goals of treatment are cure of disease, control of disease with remission or increased survival, and palliation of symptoms. Chemotherapy is used as adjuvant therapy in combination with other treatment modalities such as surgery and radiation or as neo-adjuvant therapy before another treatment modality.

Chemotherapy protocols are often complex, requiring combinations of multiple chemotherapeutic agents and medications to prevent toxicity and manage the side effects of the agents. Side effects and toxicities are specific to each chemotherapeutic agent. Cyclic treatments continued over months are administered in a variety of settings including the hospital, ambulatory clinic or doctor's office, and home.

The trend toward outpatient chemotherapy and shortened hospital stay places much of the responsibility for side effect management on the patient and family. It is imperative that patients and their families be prepared to monitor and respond when side effects occur.

Effective nursing interventions for Chemotherapy Management include nursing activities to ensure safe administration of chemotherapy, monitor for toxicities, and prepare patients to manage the self-care activities needed to prevent and respond to the side effects and toxicities of chemotherapy.

REVIEW OF THE LITERATURE

Guidelines for Practice

Guidelines or standards regarding chemotherapy administration have been developed by the Oncology Nursing Society (ONS), Intravenous Nurses Society

(INS), American Society of Hospital Pharmacists (ASHP), and Occupational Safety and Health Administration (OSHA) (ASHP, 1990; ONS, 1984, 1988, 1991, 1996; OSHA, 1995; Rutherford, 1992).

The INS (Rutherford, 1992) and the ONS (1991) have published position statements regarding administration of chemotherapy and preparation of the nurse. The ONS (1988, 1996) published a course outline for education of nurses administering chemotherapy.

Antineoplastic drugs are known to be mutagenic, teratogenic, and carcinogenic. Safety measures are incorporated in the process of Chemotherapy Management to minimize exposure and untoward effects of chemotherapy to the environment and to the patient, family, health care team, and others involved with the handling and disposal of cytotoxic agents (ASHP, 1990; ONS, 1988, 1996; OSHA, 1995). Research has shown that cytotoxic drugs and metabolites are eliminated through the digestive and renal systems; therefore, safe handling of body waste must continue after the administration. Patients and families must be taught safe handling of body waste at home for 48 hours after administration.

Preparing the Patient

Chemotherapy Management begins with preparing the patient for the treatment. Patient education before receiving chemotherapy is both informational and supportive. The purpose is to reduce anxiety, empower the patient to make decisions, and prepare the patient and family to manage self-care. Teaching patients about their treatment reduces fear, improves compliance, and enhances participation in self-care (Dodd, 1982; Fernsler, 1991; Goodman, 1989).

Administration Issues: Intravenous Access and Extravasation

The frequency and intensity of treatment, the long-term nature of treatment, the vesicant potential of many chemotherapy drugs, and the potential sclerosing effect on veins of frequent venous access require the nurse to assess the need for long-term venous access for the patient. The most commonly used types of long-term venous access devices (VADs) are tunneled catheters, implanted ports, and peripherally inserted central catheters (PICCs). Selection of a long-term VAD is determined by the type of therapy and by patient characteristics. After identifying the need for a VAD, the nurse uses knowledge of the use, features, cost, insertion, and maintenance requirements of each type of VAD to facilitate the selection of the most appropriate VAD for the particular therapy and patient (Reymann, 1993; Winslow, Trammell, & Camp-Sorrell, 1995).

Many chemotherapy agents are classified as vesicants—that is, having the potential to cause tissue necrosis if infiltrated into the subcutaneous tissue. Chemotherapy Management requires the nurse to identify the potential for vesicant extravasation and to administer vesicant medications following safety guidelines and with constant vigilance (Bender, 1992; ONS, 1996; Reymann, 1993). Vesicant administration also requires the cooperation of the patient, who has been instructed to report any symptoms of pain, burning, or change in sensation. Even with the safest techniques, some agents have the potential to cause late signs of extravasation. Because early intervention can decrease morbidity, the patient must be instructed to report any signs of extravasation to the health care provider (Boyle & Engelking, 1995).

SIDE EFFECT AND SYMPTOM MANAGEMENT

Antineoplastic agents are not specific to cancer cells. Other rapidly dividing cells are damaged in differing degrees. Cells most rapidly dividing are those of the bone marrow, lining of the gastrointestinal (GI) tract, hair, skin, and nails. Symptoms may be mild or severe, early or late. Failure to manage symptoms can have a negative outcome on patients' quality of life, cause patients to discontinue therapy (Rhodes & Watson, 1987), require reduction of optimal doses, and cause morbidity, hospitalization, or even death (Musci & Dodd, 1990). If symptom management is not identified, there is the possibility that patients will rely on their own management and that symptoms will be unreported or poorly managed (University of California, San Francisco School of Nursing Symptom Management Group, 1994). Dodd (1997) identified that family members or caregivers needed skills and knowledge to manage symptoms or they could feel guilty or responsible for poor patient outcomes. Dodd (1997) concluded that nurses need to be proactive and anticipate needed information rather than expect the family or caregiver to seek information.

In a review of the literature, Camp-Sorrell (1993) identified fatigue, nausea, vomiting, alopecia, anorexia, and mouth sores as the most distressing side effects to the patients. In a study of patients receiving inpatient chemotherapy, respondents identified alopecia, fatigue, nausea, taste change, appetite loss, sleeping difficulty, and constipation as the most frequently occurring and severe side effects of chemotherapy (Foltz, Gaines, & Gullatte, 1996). In an effort to identify effective interventions, Nail, Jones, Greene, Schipper, and Jensen (1991) and Foltz, Gaines, and Gullatte (1996) used patient self-report to identify effective and ineffective self-care actions for side effect management.

Based on knowledge of each individual chemotherapeutic agent's toxicity profile, and with knowledge of influencing or precipitating patient-related factors, the nurse can develop effective self-care activities for the patient's management of side effects and symptoms related to chemotherapy.

Myelosuppression

Bone marrow suppression, myelosuppression, is a common and dose-limiting side effect of most chemotherapeutic agents. It affects hematopoiesis of leukocytes, erythrocytes, and platelets. The *nadir* is the point after chemotherapy when myelosuppression is the greatest and the blood count is at its lowest. The degree of myelosuppression and the nadir vary with the agent and dose (Rostad, 1990; Tenenbaum & Leshin, 1994).

Leukopenia is a reduction in the total number of white cells. Neutropenia is a reduction in the neutrophil count. Neutropenia puts the patient at risk for bacterial infection because the body is unable to mount an adequate inflammatory response to bacterial infection. Because the inflammatory response is suppressed, the ordinary signs and symptoms of infection may be absent, and fever may be the only sign of infection (Brandt, 1990; Rostad, 1990). Infection in the neutropenic patient occurs from both exogenous and endogenous sources. As much as 50% to 80% of infections result from endogenous sources such as normal flora of the skin or gastrointestinal (GI) tract (Brandt, 1990; Carter, 1994). Risk of infection is further increased when other side effects of chemotherapy include an assault on the body's first line of defense, the skin and mucous membranes.

The use of colony-stimulating factors to decrease the nadir have helped reduce some of the risk of infection. These medications are given subcutaneously over a period of time after chemotherapy. Patients and families are taught to self-inject the medicine.

Thrombocytopenia, decreased platelet count, can predispose to superficial or internal bleeding. The degree of thrombocytopenia dictates the need for medical intervention. A severe decrease in platelets may require hospitalization and platelet transfusions.

Anemia is a side effect of some chemotherapy, but it is more disease related than treatment related. Side effects affecting nutrition can also affect anemia.

Nausea and Vomiting

Nausea, vomiting, and retching have been described by patients as the most feared side effects of chemotherapy treatment (Rhodes, Johnson, & McDaniel, 1995). Most chemotherapeutic agents have some emetic potential. The degree, intensity, onset, and duration are specific to each agent. The pathophysiology of nausea, vomiting, and retching involves stimulation of complex pathways involving areas of the brain and the GI tract. Antiemetic therapy is aimed at interrupting these pathways. One method is blocking specific chemical neurotransmitter receptors to prevent stimulation of the vomiting center (VC) and the chemoreceptor trigger zone (CTZ) in the brain.

Nausea, vomiting, and retching are separate conditions. Nausea is a subjective, unpleasant experience. It is the desire to vomit. Vomiting is forceful expulsion of the contents of the stomach. Retching is a forceful movement of the diaphragm and abdominal muscles, often referred to as "dry heaves." Nausea and vomiting can be acute, occurring within hours of chemotherapy and ending within 24 hours. They can also be delayed, developing 24 hours after chemotherapy (Camp-Sorrell, 1993; Rhodes et al., 1995). Management of nausea and vomiting is inconsistent (Johnson, Moroney, & Gay, 1997). Pharmacological management should be based on the emetic profile of the chemotherapy, patient characteristics, and history of previous chemotherapy and response to antiemetics. Nonpharmacological methods include use of relaxation techniques, music therapy (see Chapter 28), and hypnosis.

Alopecia

Alopecia can affect a person's self-image, relationships, and mental well-being. It is a visible sign to the world of the diagnosis of cancer (Pickard-Holley, 1995). Many, but not all, chemotherapy agents cause alopecia. Hair follicles are in active cell division most of the time, and division is the stage affected by chemotherapy. Chemotherapy can damage the hair shaft, causing the hair to break, or damage the root follicle, causing the hair to fall out.

Alopecia occurs about 2 to 3 weeks after chemotherapy, so the patient needs to be assisted at the first treatment. Patient surveys by Ehmann, Sheen, and Decker (1991) indicated that patients wanted nurses to take a proactive role in assisting them to manage alopecia.

Results of hair preservation studies using hypothermia and scalp tourniquets to reduce circulation to the scalp have had inconclusive results (Pickard-Holley, 1995). In addition, there is a risk in preventing chemotherapy from reaching the skin in cancers where skin metastasis and tumor cell sanctuary are possibilities (ONS, 1996).

Nursing activities should focus on helping the patient adjust to hair loss.

Teach the patient that hair loss is not permanent. Encourage selection and use of head coverings such as caps, scarves, toupees, or wigs. Assist the patient in finding sources of head coverings by preparing a list of community resources. Refer to programs such as the American Cancer Society's program "Look Good. Feel Better."

Stomatitis

Stomatitis, inflammation of the oral cavity, is a potential side effect of cancer chemotherapy. It is estimated that 400,000 patients per year develop this complication (Dodd, Larson, et al., 1996; Dose, 1995). The prevalance of stomatitis is reported to be from 30% to 39% and as high as 75% with fluorouracil (Dodd, Facione, Dibble, & MacPhail, 1996). Stomatitis can be mild, moderate, or severe, ranging from erythema and sensitivity to sloughing and ulceration, and can affect nutritional intake, comfort level, and ability to communicate and increase the risk of infection. Severe stomatitis can be dose limiting, causing chemotherapy doses to be reduced.

Frequent monitoring of the oral cavity is used to detect early changes in the mucosa. Patients are taught to monitor voice, swallow, lips, tongue, oral mucosa, teeth or dentures, and saliva (Beck, 1992). Oral hygiene is performed to promote cleanliness, provide comfort, and prevent infection (Madeya, 1996). If stomatitis occurs, treatment is determined by the degree of severity. Swabs can be used for cleaning if the mouth is too sore for brushing with a soft toothbrush or if there is bleeding. Analgesic rinses can be used to promote comfort. Oral or systemic medication is required for any signs of bacterial, fungal, or viral infection (Beck, 1992). A person experiencing severe stomatitis can require hospitalization with intravenous (IV) antibiotics, IV fluid and nutritional support, and opiate medication for pain control.

Anorexia

Anorexia is often associated with cancer and complications of cancer. In addition, chemotherapy can cause taste alterations that contribute to anorexia (Ropka, 1994). Certain drugs, such as cyclophosphamide, methotrexate, and cisplatin, cause metallic taste when infused (ONS, 1996).

Treatment for anorexia begins by treating the underlying disease and related symptoms, such as nausea and vomiting, pain, diarrhea, or constipation. Research continues to determine the efficacy of medication for appetite stimulation. Megestrol acetate, cannabinoids, and corticosteroids appear to influence appetite and weight gain. Metoclopramide can be beneficial to patients who experience early satiety (Grant & Rivera, 1995).

Altered Elimination

Constipation is a possible side effect of chemotherapy drugs known as vinca alkaloids, which have a neurotoxic effect, decreasing peristalsis or causing paralytic ileus. Vinca alkaloids are vincristine, vinblastine, and vinorelbine. Frequency of constipation varies with drug, dose, and administration schedule. Other contributing factors may be the use of other medications such as opioids or antiemetics used with chemotherapy, especially the serotonin receptor antagonists (Wright & Thomas, 1995).

The effect of chemotherapy on the GI mucosa can cause diarrhea (ONS, 1996).

The degree and duration depend on the agent, dose, administration route, and schedule. The antimetabolites are most commonly associated with diarrhea. Fluorouracil is the most common antimetabolite agent causing diarrhea (Clark, McGee, & Preston, 1992).

Fatigue

Although the cause is unknown, patients receiving chemotherapy experienced fatigue cyclic in relation to chemotherapy. They reported less fatigue before treatment and more mid-cycle (Graydon, Bubela, Irvine, & Vincent, 1995; Winningham et al., 1994). Research-based nursing activities recommended by Winningham et al. (1994) are focused on education to alter perception of fatigue, exercise, and activities intended to restore attentional capacity.

Secondary Malignancies

Some cytotoxic drugs are known to be carcinogenic. Secondary malignancies have occurred months to years after treatment for primary cancer. Both leukemias and solid tumors have been reported. Alkylating agents, anthracyclines, and etoposide are most often involved in secondary malignancies (Bender, 1992; ONS, 1996). The relative risk is related to specific protocols, but the benefit of primary curative therapy is said to outweigh the risk (Camp-Sorrell, 1993).

Reproduction

Chemotherapy drugs can affect the reproductive system. Reproductive impact varies by agent and by dose. Effects on women may include low sexual desire, infertility, and sterility (Beck, 1992). Women may experience early menopause and related symptoms (Dow, 1995). Men may experience low sexual desire, infertility, or sterility (Beck, 1992).

Treatment includes providing information related to the side effects of the medication and discussing the patient's desire for children. Men need information about sperm banking (Koeppel, 1995).

Organ Toxicities

The potential for organ toxicities related to chemotherapy has implications for Chemotherapy Management by nurses. Toxicities are specific for agents. Patient preparation for treatment and instruction for continued monitoring incorporate information specific to each drug or combination of drugs.

Systematic monitoring after each treatment and before the next treatment is based on the toxicity profile of specific cytotoxic agents. Protocols for drug administration incorporate procedures to prevent or decrease toxicity (Cooley, Davis, & Abraham, 1994; Cooley, Davis, DeStefano, & Abraham, 1994; Evans, 1990; Lubejko & Sartorius, 1993).

Information about toxicities is readily available in pharmocology books and in the medical oncology and nursing oncology literature. Any nurse using the Chemotherapy Management intervention must acquire this information. Chemotherapy Management incorporating knowledge of toxicities will be demonstrated in the case studies.

CHEMOTHERAPY MANAGEMENT: TOOLS AND PROTOCOLS

The Nursing Interventions Classification (NIC) intervention Chemotherapy Management with associated activities is shown in Table 16–1. Intervention tools are developed to support patient teaching for side effect and symptom management.

Table 16–1 Chemotherapy Management

DEFINITION: Assisting the patient and family to understand the action and minimize side effects of antineoplastic agents.

ACTIVITIES:

Monitor for side effects and toxic effects of chemotherapeutic agents

Provide information to patient and family on how antineoplastic drugs work on cancer cells

Teach patient and family about the effects of chemotherapy on bone marrow functioning

Instruct patient and family on ways to prevent infection, such as avoiding crowds and using good hygiene and handwashing techniques

Instruct patient to promptly report fevers, chills, nosebleeds, excessive bruising, and tarry stools

Instruct patient and family to avoid the use of aspirin products

Institute neutropenic and bleeding precautions

Determine the patient's previous experience with chemotherapy-related nausea and vomiting

Administer antiemetic drugs for nausea and vomiting

Minimize stimuli from noises, light, and odors, especially food

Teach the patient relaxation and imagery techniques to use before, during, and after treatments, as appropriate

Offer the patient a bland and easily digested diet

Administer chemotherapeutic drugs in the late evening, so the patient may sleep at the time emetic effects are greatest

Ensure adequate fluid intake to prevent dehydration and electrolyte imbalance

Monitor the effectiveness of measures to control nausea and vomiting

Teach patient and family to monitor for signs and symptoms of stomatitis

Instruct patient on proper oral hygiene techniques

Teach patient to use oral nystatin suspension to control fungal infection, as appropriate

Teach patient to avoid temperature extremes and chemical treatments of the hair while receiving chemotherapy

Teach patient to comb hair gently and to sleep on a silk pillow case to minimize hair loss

Inform patient that hair loss is expected, as determined by type of chemotherapeutic agent used

Assist patient in obtaining a wig or other head-covering device, as appropriate

Offer six small feedings daily, as tolerated

Instruct patient to avoid hot, spicy foods

Provide nutritious, appetizing foods of patient's choice

Monitor nutritional status and weight

Teach patient and family to monitor for organ toxicity, as determined by type of chemotherapeutic agent used

Discuss with patient the possibility of sterility and other reproductive system impairments, as appropriate

Instruct long-term survivors and their families of the possibility of second malignancies and the importance of reporting increased susceptibility to infection, fatigue, or bleeding

Follow recommended guidelines for safe handling of parenteral antineoplastic drugs during drug preparation and administration

Source: McCloskey, J. C., and Bulechek, G. M. (1996). *Nursing interventions classification (NIC).* St. Louis: Mosby–Year Book.

Individual hospitals and agencies usually develop these tools. The following are examples of available tools to facilitate the use of the activities.

The most frequent monitors used in chemotherapy are laboratory results and physical assessment. Because treatments are cyclic, flow sheets enable the clinician to monitor continued progress and detect trends in patient response to treatment.

Community and government agencies are a source of information for patients receiving chemotherapy. The National Cancer Institute and the American Cancer Society have developed resources used by nurses in cancer care. Two books used at the beginning of therapy to reinforce information about chemotherapy that are available from the National Cancer Institute are *What You Need to Know about Cancer* and *Chemotherapy and You; A Guide to Self Help during Treatment*. It also offers supplemental information about nutrition and anorexia in *Eating Hints: Recipes & Tips for Better Nutrition during Cancer Treatment*. The American Cancer Society offers two books to use when discussing reproductive and sexual matters: *Sexuality and Cancer: For the Woman Who Has Cancer and Her Partner* and *Sexuality and Cancer: For the Man Who Has Cancer and His Partner*.

Patient Instructions for Oral Hygiene

Steps for keeping your mouth healthy are as follows:

1. Look into your mouth every day. Use a good light and look at your lips, gums, tongue, under your tongue, the roof of your mouth, and under your dentures. Look for red, white, or broken spots.
2. Keep your mouth clean. Use a soft toothbrush and toothpaste to brush your teeth or dentures after every meal and at bedtime.
3. Keep your mouth moist. Rinse your mouth with a low-alcohol mouthwash or use plain salt water.
4. Keep your lips moist. Use Vaseline or any lip moisturizer.

If your mouth becomes sore, follow these steps:

1. Continue to keep your mouth very clean. Use a sponge-tipped swab (toothette) if your mouth is too sore to brush or if you have bleeding when you brush.
2. Do not use mouthwash with alcohol if it causes discomfort. Instead, rinse your mouth every 2 to 4 hours with a solution of 1/2 tsp baking soda and 1/2 tsp salt dissolved in a cup of warm water. Make new salt-soda solution frequently.
3. Do not eat foods that can irritate your mouth such as spicy, hot, or acidic foods (e.g., oranges, grapefruit).

Call your doctor if any of the following occur:

1. Your mouth is too sore and you cannot eat. You might need to use another mouth rinse to help with the pain; your doctor can order it for you.
2. You see white or yellow spots in your mouth. You may need some medicine to treat or prevent infection.

Patient Instructions for Neutropenic Precautions

1. *Handwashing is the most important way to prevent infection.*
2. Perform oral care as instructed.
3. Keep your skin very clean. Pay special attention to skin folds and to your rectal area. Use moisturizer to prevent dry, cracking skin.

4. Limit your exposure to crowded areas when your counts are at their lowest.
5. Be aware of signs of illness or infection, such as swelling, pain, or pus at the site of an injury; cough, oral pain, back pain, urinary pain, burning, or urgency; and rectal discomfort.
6. Call your doctor if you experience any fever, chills, or rigors.

Patient Instructions for Thrombocytopenia

1. Do not take aspirin, drugs containing aspirin, or nonsteroidal anti-inflammatory drugs without first talking to your doctor.
2. Avoid physical injury.
3. Use electric razors.
4. Maintain good oral hygiene.
5. Keep your rectal area clean. Be very gentle when wiping or cleaning the rectal area. Do not use suppositories.
6. Avoid constipation.
7. Avoid straining.

ASSOCIATED NURSING DIAGNOSES AND CLIENT GROUPS

The *client group* is any patient receiving chemotherapy. The following nursing diagnoses could apply to this client group at any point in the process of receiving chemotherapy.

Anxiety—related to the diagnosis, treatment, and side effects
Body Image Disturbance—related to alopecia and long-term IV access
Caregiver Role Strain, Risk for—related to assumption of caregiver role because of chronic illness
Constipation—possible side effect
Diarrhea—possible side effect
Fatigue—possible side effect
Fear—about the disease, treatment, and outcome
Home Maintenance Management, Impaired—related to side effects
Individual Management of Therapeutic Regimen, Effective—related to continuing treatment and symptom management
Infection, Risk for—side effect
Knowledge Deficit—chemotherapy, symptom management
Nutrition, Less Than Body Requirements, Altered—side effect
Oral Mucous Membrane, Altered—side effect
Peripheral Neurovascular Dysfunction, Risk for—toxicity
Protection, Altered—assault from chemotherapy
Role Performance, Altered—related to schedule of treatment, side effects, and fatigue
Sexual Dysfunction—side effect
Skin Integrity, Risk for Impaired—side effect

ASSOCIATED PATIENT OUTCOMES

Adherence Behavior
Body Image
Bowel Elimination
Caregiver Performance: Indirect Care
Compliance Behavior

Coping
Health Beliefs: Perceived Ability to Perform
Health Beliefs: Perceived Control
Health Promoting Behavior

Health Seeking Behavior
Immune Status
Infection Status
Information Processing
Knowledge: Disease Process
Knowledge: Health Behaviors
Knowledge: Infection Control
Knowledge: Medication
Knowledge: Treatment Procedure(s)
Knowledge: Treatment Regimen

Nutritional Status: Food and Fluid Intake
Oral Health
Role Performance
Self-Care: Non-Parenteral Medication
Self-Care: Oral Hygiene
Self-Care: Parenteral Medication
Symptom Control Behavior
Symptom Severity
Treatment Behavior: Illness or Injury

CASE STUDY

ML is a 38-year-old woman with breast cancer. She has come to the outpatient infusion center for her first course of intravenous Cytoxan, Adriamycin, and 5-fluorouracil (CAF). The plan is for treatment every 3 weeks for eight courses. She had a lumpectomy of her right breast 8 weeks ago and has just completed radiation therapy to the right axillary nodes. The incision is healed, and the radiation site is benign. She is 5 feet tall and weighs 165 pounds. Results of laboratory work are within normal limits.

ML has no previous knowledge of chemotherapy. She is accompanied by her husband, who is supportive but visibly anxious. She reports that she would like to return to work. She works as a hair stylist and has been out of work since the surgery. She has the opportunity to work part-time. Her children are in high school, and she is alone at home during the day.

Using the Chemotherapy Management intervention, the nurse selects the following activities: Provide information to patient and family on how antineoplastic drugs work. Describe the process for administration. Monitor for side effects and toxic effects of drugs.

The specific side effects will determine which activities are needed for this intervention. The side effects of Cytoxan are hemorrhagic cystitis, nausea, alopecia, myelosuppression (nadir, days 8 to 14), amenorrhea, and sterility. Patients may also experience nasal stuffiness and metallic taste with infusion. The side effects of Adriamycin, a vesicant drug, are alopecia, myelosuppression (nadir, days 10 to 14), nausea and vomiting, stomatitis, dose-limiting cardiotoxicity, radiation recall, photosensitivity, hyperpigmentation of skin and nail beds, and the drug excreted red in urine. The side effects for 5-fluorouracil are myelosup-

pression (white blood cells, days 9 to 14; platelets, days 7 to 14), nausea and vomiting, diarrhea, stomatitis, alopecia, photosensitivity, and hand-foot syndrome.

Activities specific to these drugs are as follows: Instruct ML to drink 2 to 3 L of fluid to prevent hemorrhagic cystitis from the Cytoxan. If nausea or vomiting causes her to be unable to get necessary fluids, she needs to call the doctor. Because Adriamycin is a vesicant, ML is moderately obese, and she had surgery and radiation on the right side, consider whether she may benefit from a long-term IV access device. Begin documentation to monitor total Adriamycin dose to prevent cardiotoxicity.

Activities are needed to address myelosuppression and infection prevention. The nurse will teach ML and her family about the effects of chemotherapy on bone marrow functioning, ways to prevent infection, and avoidance of aspirin-containing medications and to report signs of infection or bleeding.

Activities are used to alleviate nausea and vomiting. Determine past experience with nausea and vomiting, administer antiemetic drugs, and instruct the patient on how to use them at home. Modify the environment to reduce stimuli.

Instruct the patient on oral hygiene measures. Prepare her for alopecia, which will surely occur with this combination of drugs, and instruct the patient in skin care. Teach her to protect the skin from sunlight, use sun block, cover her head when outdoors. Observe the palms of her hands and soles of her feet for peeling or cracking.

Instruct the patient about the possible bowel changes from the chemotherapy and discuss with her the possibility of sterility and other reproductive impairments. Instruct the patient in safety measures at home, such as flushing the toilet twice at each use for 2 days. Instruct her to wash her hands immediately after wiping. ML is ambulatory, so there is unlikely to be a need for her family to handle linens soiled with urine or stool, but should that occur, the family needs to wear latex gloves (unless they are allergic to latex).

This information is written down for ML and her husband. They are given a telephone number to call with any questions. Ideally, treatment should be followed by a telephone call in a couple of days.

ML can return to work, depending on how she feels. Her first cycle will be an indication of how she will experience myelosuppression and nausea. Supportive therapy can be modified for more satisfactory results. Good communication about symptoms can make management of side effects more effective and enable this patient to get on with her life while continuing her chemotherapy treatment.

References

American Society of Hospital Pharmacists. (1990). *Safe handling of cytotoxic and hazardous drugs study guide.* Bethesda, MD: Author.

Beck, S. L. (1992). Prevention and management of oral complications in the cancer patient. In S. M. Hubbard, P. E. Greene, and M. T. Knobf (Eds.), *Current issues in cancer nursing updates* (pp. 1–12). Philadelphia: J.B. Lippincott.

Bender, C. (1992). Implications of antineoplastic therapy for nursing. In J. C. Clark and R. F. McGee (Eds.), *Core curriculum for oncology nursing* (2nd ed., pp. 329–345). Philadelphia: W.B. Saunders.

Boyle, D. M., and Engelking, C. (1995). Vesicant extravasation: Myths and realities. *Oncology Nursing Forum, 22,* 57–67.

Brandt, B. (1990). Nursing protocol for the patient with neutropenia. *Oncology Nursing Forum, 17*(1 Suppl.), 9–15.

Camp-Sorrell, D. (1993). Chemotherapy: Toxicity management. In S. L. Groenwald, M. H. Frogge, M. Goodman, and C. H. Yarbro (Eds.), *Cancer nursing: Principles and practice* (3rd ed., pp. 331–365). Boston: Jones and Bartlett.

Carter, L. W. (1994). Bacterial relocation: Nursing implications in the care of patients with neutropenia. *Oncology Nursing Forum, 21,* 857–865.

Clark, J. C., McGee, R. F., and Preston, R. (1992). Nursing management of responses to the cancer experience. In J. C. Clark and R. F. McGee (Eds.), *Core curriculum for oncology nursing* (2nd ed., pp. 67–155). Philadelphia: W.B. Saunders.

Cooley, M. E., Davis, L. E., and Abraham, J. (1994). Cisplatin: A clinical review: Part 2—Nursing assessment and management of side effects of cisplatin. *Cancer Nursing, 17,* 283–293.

Cooley, M. E., Davis, L. E., DeStefano, M., and Abraham, J. (1994). Cisplatin: A clinical review: Part 1—Current uses of cisplatin and administration guidelines. *Cancer Nursing, 17,* 173–184.

Dodd, M. (1982). Cancer patients' knowledge of chemotherapy: Assessment and informational interventions. *Oncology Nursing Forum, 9,* 39–44.

Dodd, M. J. (1997). Self-care: Ready or not. *Oncology Nursing Forum, 24,* 983–990.

Dodd, M. J., Facione, N. C., Dibble, S. L., and MacPhail, L. (1996). Comparisons of methods to determine the prevalance and nature of oral mucositis. *Cancer Practice, 4,* 312–318.

Dodd, M. J., Larson, P. J., Dibble, S. L., Miaskowski, C., Greenspan, D., MacPhail, L., Hauck, W. W., Paul, S. M., Ignoffo, R., and Shiba, G. (1996). Randomized clinical trial of chlorhexidine versus placebo for prevention of oral mucositis in patients receiving chemotherapy. *Oncology Nursing Forum, 23,* 921–927.

Dose, A. M. (1995). The symptom experience of mucositis, stomatitis, and xerostoma. *Seminars in Oncology Nursing, 11,* 248–255.

Dow, K. H. (1995). A review of late effects of cancer in women. *Seminars in Oncology Nursing, 11,* 128–136.

Ehmann, I. L., Sheen, A., and Decker, G. M. (1991). Intervening with alopecia: Exploring an entrepreneurial role for oncology nurses. *Oncology Nursing Forum, 18,* 769–773.

Evans, S. (1990). Nursing measures in the prevention and treatment of renal cell damage associated with cisplatin administration. *Cancer Nursing, 14,* 91–97.

Fernsler, J. I., and Cannon, C. A. (1991). The whys of patient education. *Seminars in Oncology Nursing, 7,* 79–86.

Foltz, A. T., Gaines, G., and Gullatte, M. (1996). Recalled side effects and self care actions of patients receiving chemotherapy. *Oncology Nursing Forum, 23,* 679–683.

Goodman, M. (1989). Managing the side effects of chemotherapy. *Seminars in Oncology Nursing, 5*(2 Suppl.), 29–52.

Grant, M. M., and Rivera, L. M. (1995). Anorexia, cachexia, and dysphagia: The symptom experience. *Seminars in Oncology Nursing, 11,* 266–271.

Graydon, J. E., Bubela, N., Irvine, D., and Vincent, L. (1995). Fatigue reducing strategies used by patients receiving treatment for cancer. *Cancer Nursing, 18,* 23–28.

Johnson, M. H., Moroney, C. E., and Gay, C. F. (1997). Relieving nausea and vomiting in patients with cancer: A treatment algorithm. *Oncology Nursing Forum, 24,* 51–57.

Koeppel, K. M. (1995). Sperm banking and patients with cancer, issues concerning patients and healthcare professionals. *Cancer Nursing, 18,* 306–312.

Lubejko, B. G., and Sartorius, S. E. (1993). Nursing considerations in paclitaxel (Taxol) administration. *Seminars in Oncology, 20*(Suppl. 3), 26–30.

Madeya, M. L. (1996). Oral complications from cancer therapy: Part 2—Nursing implications for assessment and treatment. *Oncology Nursing Forum, 23,* 801–819.

Musci, E. C., and Dodd, M. J. (1990). Predicting self-care with patients' and family members' affective states and family functioning. *Oncology Nursing Forum, 17,* 394–400.

Nail, L. M., Jones, L. S., Greene, D., Schipper, D. L., and Jensen, R. (1991). Use and perceived efficacy of self-care activities in patients receiving chemotherapy. *Oncology Nursing Forum, 18,* 883–887.

Occupational Safety and Health Administration. (1995). *Controlling occupational exposure to hazardous drugs* (OSHA Instruction CPL 2-2.20B). Washington, DC: Author.

Oncology Nursing Society. (1984). *Cancer chemotherapy guidelines and recommendations for nursing education and practice.* Pittsburgh, PA: Author.

Oncology Nursing Society. (1988). *ONS cancer chemotherapy guidelines, modules I–IV.* Pittsburgh, PA: Author.

Oncology Nursing Society. (1991). *Position statement—Preparation of the professional registered nurse who administers and cares for the individual receiving chemotherapy.* Pittsburgh, PA: Author.

Oncology Nursing Society. (1996). *Cancer chemotherapy guidelines and recommendations for practice.* Pittsburgh, PA: Author.

Pickard-Holley, S. (1995). The symptom experience of alopecia. *Seminars in Oncology Nursing, 11,* 235–238.

Reymann, P. E. (1993). Chemotherapy: Principles of administration. In S. L. Groenwald, M. H. Frogge, M. Goodman, and C. H. Yarbro (Eds.), *Cancer nursing: Principles and practice* (3rd ed., pp. 293–330). Boston: Jones and Bartlett.

Rhodes, V. A., Johnson, M. H., and McDaniel, R. W. (1995). Nausea, vomiting, and retching: The management of the symptom experience. *Seminars in Oncology Nursing, 11,* 256–265.

Rhodes, V. A., and Watson, P. M. (1987). Symptom distress—The concept: Past and present. *Seminars in Oncology Nursing, 3,* 242–247.

Ropka, M. E. (1994). Nutrition. In J. Gross and B. L. Johnson (Eds.), *Handbook of oncology nursing* (2nd ed., pp. 329–372). Boston: Jones and Bartlett.

Rostad, M. E. (1990). Management of myelosuppression in the patient with cancer. *Oncology Nursing Forum, 17*(1 Suppl.), 4–8.

Rutherford, C. (1992). Position paper—Administration of antineoplastic agents. *Journal of Intravenous therapy, 15,* 8–9.

Tenenbaum, L., and Leshin, D. (1994). Hematopoietic alterations associated with chemotherapy and biotherapy. In L. Tenenbaum (Ed.), *Cancer chemotherapy and biotherapy, a reference guide* (2nd ed., pp. 223–239). Philadelphia: W.B. Saunders.

University of California, San Francisco, School of Nursing Symptom Management Group. (1994). A model for symptom management. *Image, 4,* 272–276.

Winningham, M. L., Nail, L. M., Burke, M. B., Brophy, L., Cimprich, B., Jones, L. S., Pickard-Holley, S., Rhodes, V., Mooney, K. H., and Piper, B. (1994). Fatigue and the cancer experience: The state of the knowledge. *Oncology Nursing Forum, 21,* 23–35.

Winslow, M. N., Trammell, L., and Camp-Sorrell, D. (1995). Selection of vascular access devices and nursing care. *Seminars in Oncology Nursing, 11,* 167–173.

Wright, P. S., and Thomas, S. L. (1995). Constipation and diarrhea: The neglected symptoms. *Seminars in Oncology Nursing, 11,* 289–297.

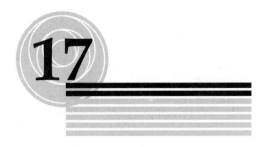

Conscious Sedation

Steven J. Somerson, Susan W. Somerson,
and Michael R. Sicilia

The number of procedures that can be performed using infiltration of local anesthetics and titration of intravenous (IV) narcotics and sedatives for patient cooperation and comfort has substantially increased since the late 1980s. Along with this increase in types of procedures has been an increase in the variety of locations in which they can be performed. As a result of these recent developments, registered nurses (RNs) in various specialties have been learning administration and monitoring techniques for Conscious Sedation.

Administration of Conscious Sedation medications and subsequent monitoring skill and technique have continued to be the focus of much attention of nurses involved in specialties that provide care for patients undergoing numerous invasive procedures (Batson, 1993). It is generally acknowledged through nurse practice acts and position statements that it is considered within the scope of practice for nurses to administer Conscious Sedation medications and monitor patients if appropriate criteria have been met (American Association of Nurse Anesthetists [AANA], 1991; Association of Operating Room Nurses [AORN], 1992; Murphy, 1993). Nurses involved with procedures performed under Conscious Sedation must acquire the skills and knowledge to provide conscientious and appropriate care (Murphy, 1988, 1993).

Classification of progressive sedation levels is as follows: light or preoperative sedation, conscious sedation, deep sedation, and general anesthesia. Conscious Sedation may progress rapidly to a state of deep sedation or loss of consciousness, depending on medication dosage and sensitivities, the patient's physical condition, and the lack of recovery period stimulation (AANA, 1991; AORN, 1992; Kaller, 1991).

A patient under light sedation or Conscious Sedation is capable of responding to verbal stimuli and can capably maintain protective reflexes (cough, gag, laryngeal). The patient may be lethargic but is easily aroused. Deep sedation progressively causes the patient's reflexes to become weak or absent. The patient becomes considerably more lethargic and more difficult to arouse, and there may be inconsistent response to painful stimuli. General anesthesia renders the patient insensible to all stimuli. In this completely unconscious state, protective reflexes are usually lost (Eichorn et al., 1986; Stoelting, 1991; Waugaman et al., 1988).

Conscious Sedation, provided during minor diagnostic and surgical procedures, is directed toward minimizing the patient's fear during the procedure. Psychological preparation is important, because many patients face thoughts of death and are often experiencing multiple life alterations and stressors when scheduled for surgery or other invasive procedures (Watson & James, 1990; Zambricki, 1988). Thorough preparation and reassurance contribute to effective sedation and may reduce the need for additional medication. Sedation objectives within this setting are mood alteration, maintenance of consciousness and cooperation, pain threshold elevation with minimal vital sign variation, partial amnesia, and a prompt, safe return to ambulation and discharge (AANA, 1991; Watson & James, 1990). Goals of Conscious Sedation during a procedure consist of reinforcing patient cooperation and compliance through relief of anxiety and pain control, in addition to maintaining continual patient safety (Proudfoot, 1995).

Conscious Sedation has been successfully used for many inpatient and outpatient diagnostic procedures, including eye and dental surgery, endoscopies, cardioversion and angiography, computed tomography (CT) scans, bone marrow biopsies, and painful dressing changes. In invasive or operative procedures, Conscious Sedation is used to minimize discomfort during administration of local anesthesia and as an anxiety-reducing adjunct during the procedure. Local anesthesia, in many circumstances, does not always produce a pain-free or anxiety-free procedure. There are often associated sensations of pressure, pulling, or tissue spreading at or adjacent to the operative site (AORN, 1992; Batson, 1993; Watson & James, 1990).

Lengthy and invasive procedures are often best managed under general anesthesia. Patients who are not motivated to have procedures conducted with local anesthesia and Conscious Sedation may prove to be managed more safely under general anesthesia. Medications must always be carefully titrated, and the patient must always be closely and continuously monitored, but the nurse may frequently be confronted with the subtle distinctions between Conscious Sedation and the onset of deep sedation or general anesthesia. The definitions of Conscious Sedation and deep sedation further emphasize the necessity of continually monitoring cardiorespiratory parameters. Sedation is more thoroughly characterized as a continuum, ranging from simple anxiety reduction with a minimal level of consciousness interference to deeper states that may produce general anesthesia and profoundly affect airway and protective reflexes. All sedatives are capable of producing general anesthesia and cardiorespiratory compromise. The nurse performing the intervention of Conscious Sedation is confronted with the challenge of agent selection and administration for a procedure that will produce adequate sedation and minimize potential adverse effects (Proudfoot, 1995).

REVIEW OF MEDICATIONS CURRENTLY USED FOR INTRAVENOUS CONSCIOUS SEDATION

Narcotics and sedatives are the medications routinely administered to provide IV Conscious Sedation. Dosage, onset and duration of action, and precautions for each medication are reviewed in Table 17–1. Medications and dosages ordered depend on a wide variety of variables, including the procedure's duration and the patient's pain control requirements, anxiety level, age, physical condition, allergies, and previous experience with Conscious Sedation. Medication costs and preferences are additional factors that must be considered (Proudfoot, 1995; Tanaka, 1988).

Frequently used narcotics include morphine, meperidine, fentanyl, and alfentanil. These narcotics are used to render analgesia, which can usually be produced without disturbing other central nervous system functions (Tanaka, 1988). Clinically, the pain threshold is raised, and the perception of pain is blunted. The painful stimulus may be noted but is not perceived as painful. Most types of pain are relieved by narcotics, but dull, continuous pain is more often effectively relieved than sharp, intermittent pain. Analgesia usually occurs without loss of consciousness, but sedation and drowsiness become more prominent as the dose is increased. Therapeutic narcotic doses usually produce minimal sedative effects, but larger amounts can create effects ranging from sedation to coma. Onset of sedation is slower than the onset of analgesia, but its duration is longer. Although narcotics afford excellent analgesia, they do not always produce sedation when used alone (*Physicians' Desk Reference* [PDR], 1997; Tanaka, 1988; Tung & Rosenthal, 1995).

The most common serious adverse effect of narcotics is respiratory depression progressing to apnea, which can occur even in arousable, responsive patients. If not promptly recognized and treated, this condition could result in respiratory or cardiac arrest. Other associated reactions include nausea and vomiting from stimulation of the chemoreceptor trigger zone, histamine release with hypotension, euphoria or dysphoria with hypertension, dizziness, blurred vision, diaphoresis, biliary colic, and urinary retention (*PDR*, 1997).

Narcotics should be given with greater caution to patients with acute asthma, chronic obstructive pulmonary disease, or significantly decreased respiratory reserve. Elderly or debilitated patients also require more cautious and careful observation, particularly those presenting with lung disease, hepatic and renal impairment (because of the importance of these organs in metabolism or excretion), or Addison's disease (*PDR*, 1997).

Sedatives are medications used to create sedation, reduction of anxiety, and amnesia. Those most often used for IV Conscious Sedation are the benzodiazepines diazepam (Valium) and midazolam (Versed). Concomitantly administered narcotics usually reduce the required amount of benzodiazepine. The benzodiazepines, however, are not analgesic in action and do not directly enhance the action of narcotics, although the anti-anxiety effect combined with narcotic-induced sleep may appear to produce analgesia (*PDR*, 1997; Ramoska et al., 1991; Ringler, 1995; Tanaka, 1988; Watson & James, 1990).

Diazepam has been found to act on parts of the limbic system, specifically the thalamus and hypothalamus, inducing calming effects. There is considerable individual variation in the response to diazepam, but amnestic actions have been found to be most prominent when sedation is produced. Patients often respond appropriately to questions or commands, but there is noticeable suppression of recall. Slurred speech and nystagmus frequently precede onset of sleep. These two signs are often used as end points when titrating doses (*PDR*, 1997; Ramoska et al., 1991; Ringler, 1995; Tanaka, 1988; Watson & James, 1990).

The most common serious warnings regarding diazepam involve venous thrombosis, phlebitis, and local irritation and swelling. Serious vascular impairment is rare, although thrombotic and phlebitic problems have been encountered

Table 17-1 Medications Used for Conscious Sedation (Adult Dosage)

Drug	Classification	Dose	Onset	Duration	Comments
Morphine Sulfate	Opiate	1–2 mg increments	1–3 min	4 hr	Standards against which all other opiates are measured. Monitor respiratory rate and depth continuously; pulse oximetry may show oxygen desaturation before overt signs of distress. Be prepared to assist ventilation with bag-valve mask and supplemental oxygen. Hypotension, particularly if there is a pre-existing hypovolemia. Nausea and vomiting; lethargic patients may need suctioning to clear airway.
Meperidine HCl (Demerol)	Opiate	10 mg increments titrated to response	1–3 min	1–3 hr	1/10th as potent as morphine. Same as for morphine but greater potential for nausea and vomiting.
Fentanyl (Sublimaze)	Opiate	1.0–2.0 μg/kg, titrated to response	1–3 min	30–60 min	Analgesia may not be effective until several minutes after the onset of sedative effect. Respiratory depression may persist for more than 1 hr unless reversal agent is used. 100 times as potent as morphine. Same as for morphine
Alfentanil (Alfenta)	Opiate	8–20 μg/kg, titrated	1–2 min	30 min	Same as for morphine.
Diazepam (Valium)	Benzodiazepine	2.5–10 mg Reduce dose by 1/3 when an opioid is being used concomitantly	30 sec to 2 min	2–4 hr	Slurred speech and nystagmus precede onset of sleep. Contraindications include untreated narrow angle glaucoma. Solution is irritating to vein; may cause phlebitis, thrombosis, swelling, local irritation. Should not be used when venous access is through small hand or wrist veins. Response varies greatly. Titration based on individual response is essential.

Drug	Classification	Dosage	Onset	Duration	Comments
Midazolam (Versed)	Benzodiazepine	Initial dose of 0.5–1 mg; should not exceed 2.5 mg. Titrate to effect, allowing at least 2 min between dosing to evaluate full effect of drug. Maintenance dose of 0.25–1 mg; titrate to effect.	3–5 min	Peak effect at 5 min; gradual decline over 30–40 min. Gross recovery within 2 hr; effects may last 6 hr.	May potentiate adverse effects of opioids (including respiratory depression) when used concomitantly. Reduce dosage in the elderly, debilitated, and those with compromised renal function. Also produces amnestic effects. May be given oral, or nasal, or rectal using different dosing guidelines or regimens.
Lorazepam (Ativan)	Benzodiazepine	0.044 mg/kg up to 2 mg	1–5 min	6–8 hr	
Ketamine (Ketalar)	Phencyclidine	1 mg/kg	5–6 min	2 hr	Produces a cataleptic state (patient may appear awake but disconnected from events in the immediate environment). Increases blood pressure, heart rate, cardiac output, intracranial pressure, and airway secretions. May produce laryngospasm. Contraindications include children <3 months or >10 years, head injury, psychiatric illness. May produce vomiting and emergence hallucinations (control with benzodiazepine). May be given orally or rectally using different dosage.
Naloxone (Narcan)	Narcotic antagonist	0.1–0.2 mg, titrated to patient response	2–3 min	Varies with dose and route administered. May need to repeat dosing after 1–2 hr.	Effects of opioids may last longer than effects of naloxone; repeated doses may be necessary.
Flumazenil (Romazicon)	Benzodiazepine antagonist	0.2 mg given over 15 sec; after waiting 45 sec, additional dose of 0.2 mg can be given. May be repeated at 60 sec intervals up to 1.0 mg	Effect evident within 1–2 min; peak 6–10 min	Duration 30–60 min	Duration of most benzodiazepines exceeds duration of flumazenil; careful monitoring must continue for 1 hr after reversal is initiated. Treatment of resedation: after 20 min, 1.0 mg may be given in 0.2 mg/min increments until desired effect achieved. No more than 3 mg/hr is recommended. Patients on long-term benzodiazepine therapy may develop seizures when flumazenil is administered.

with small hand or wrist veins. It is safest to slowly inject the medication in large veins. Confusion, drowsiness, hypotension, and apnea are always possible complications (*PDR*, 1997).

Lorazepam (Ativan) is also a commonly used benzodiazepine. It is preferred for some procedures, because it usually produces a greater level of analgesia than diazepam or midazolam. The duration of action (6 to 8 hours), however, is considerably longer than that of the other benzodiazepines. Lorazepam must be prepared with an equal amount of compatible diluent before IV administration and, to achieve the maximum amnestic effect, should be given 15 to 20 minutes before the procedure (*PDR*, 1997; Ringler, 1995).

Midazolam (Versed) is a short-acting, water-soluble benzodiazepine, approximately three times more potent than diazepam and currently available in 1 mg/mL or 5 mg/mL concentrations. The 1 mg/mL formulation is recommended for Conscious Sedation and may be further diluted in 0.9% sodium chloride or 5% dextrose in water. Midazolam is regarded as clinically superior to diazepam or lorazepam for conscious sedation and amnesia because of its rapid onset of action and metabolism. Additionally, intravenous midazolam has not been associated with the venous irritation characteristic of diazepam (*PDR*, 1997). This medication should be slowly titrated until the patient's speech becomes slurred or nystagmus becomes evident, although individual responses are somewhat variable. Onset time is directly affected by the amount injected and by concurrent use of a narcotic. Time should be allowed (2 minutes or more after the initial dose) to evaluate the sedative effect, because response is highly individualistic (*PDR*, 1997; Tanaka, 1988; Watson & James, 1990).

Reduced doses of all benzodiazepines and longer evaluation periods are certainly indicated for patients older than 60 years and whenever other central nervous system depressants are used. The total amount of the initial dose should be reduced by one third when administered with a narcotic. Older or chronically ill patients are at greater risk for hypoventilation and apnea, especially if the patient has chronic obstructive lung disease or compromised renal function (*PDR*, 1997).

Ketamine is a phencyclidine that has analgesic, sedative, and amnestic properties. It is a dissociative anesthetic agent that produces a cataleptic state that interferes with sensory perception of painful stimuli and memory. The eyes remain open with a slow nystagmic gaze. Corneal and light reflexes remain intact. A functional dissociation is created between the cortical and limbic systems of the brain. Patients appear awake but disconnected. There is occasional random, tonic extremity movement. Ketamine increases blood pressure, heart rate, cardiac output, and intracranial pressure. It also increases airway secretions; it has caused laryngospasm. Ketamine produces limited depression on airway reflexes but has increased flow of saliva. Pretreatment with atropine is usually necessary. Contraindications include children younger than 3 months or older than 10 years, upper respiratory illness, or psychiatric illness. Recovery may be prolonged (up to 2 hours). There may be postsedation emesis and emergence hallucinations. Emergence reactions may be effectively prevented by co-administering a small dose of benzodiazepine. Use of this drug requires training and thorough understanding regarding its clinical consequences (*PDR*, 1997; Proudfoot, 1995; Tung & Rosenthal, 1995).

Naloxone hydrochloride (Narcan), a narcotic antagonist, and flumazenil (Romazicon), a benzodiazepine antagonist, are the currently available reversal agents. Naloxone is a synthetic congener of oxymorphone, available in 0.02, 0.4, and 1 mg/mL concentrations. Naloxone antagonizes specific opioid effects:

respiratory depression, sedation, hypotension, and analgesia. This medication is a pure antagonist; it possesses no narcotic properties and does not appear to exert any pharmacological activity in the absence of narcotics. Small increments of the medication (0.1 to 0.2 mg IV) should be titrated to the patient's response at 2- to 3-minute intervals. Desirable reversal is characterized by alertness and adequate ventilation without discomfort. Early intervention with naloxone can eliminate problematic side effects without complete loss of analgesia. Repeated doses may be required, because narcotic half-life and duration exceed that of naloxone. An additional intramuscular dose offers a more prolonged effect. Reversal brought on too rapidly may cause nausea, sweating, and hypertension (*PDR*, 1997; Watson & James, 1990).

Flumazenil (Romazicon) antagonizes benzodiazepine action on the central nervous system and is indicated for partial or complete reversal of benzodiazepine sedative effects. The majority of patients respond to a cumulative IV dose of .6 to 1 mg within 1 to 2 minutes after the medication is injected. Resedation is a serious risk, as benzodiazepine duration often exceeds that of flumazenil. Resedation may be treated after a 20-minute waiting period with an additional dose of 1 mg given intravenously in increments of 0.2 mg/min. No more than 3 mg is advised to be given in any 1-hour period. Patients who have received benzodiazepines for long-term therapy are at risk for seizures when given flumazenil. Medication doses often vary considerably, depending on the patient's physiological and psychological requirements (*PDR*, 1997; Watson, 1993).

DESCRIPTION OF THE INTERVENTION

The definition and activities for the intervention Conscious Sedation appear in Table 17–2. Patients selected to receive IV Conscious Sedation must be thoroughly assessed physiologically and psychologically before undergoing any procedure. Comprehensive risk factor assessment includes physical evaluation, possibility of pregnancy, current medications, medication allergies and sensitivities, smoking history, chief complaint and pertinent medical history, age, height, weight, baseline vital signs, NPO (nothing by mouth) status, level of consciousness and emotional state, ability to communicate, and perceptions concerning the procedure or method of sedation (Kaller, 1991; Watson & James, 1990; Zambricki, 1988).

Patient selection should be determined by established practice criteria such as the classification established by the American Society of Anesthesiologists. Physiologically or psychologically limited patients may not be acceptable candidates for local anesthesia and monitored sedation. These patients often require deep sedation or general anesthesia in combination with more invasive monitoring. Careful identification of these patients is best accomplished in consultation with anesthesia, surgical, and nursing representatives (AANA, 1991; AORN, 1992; Murphy, 1988; Zambricki, 1988).

Conscious Sedation should be provided by nurses who have become qualified to safely administer the required medications and who have learned effective patient monitoring and management of potential complications—specifically, airway management, intubation, and resuscitation. A nurse administering Conscious Sedation must be constantly vigilant to patient response, recognize the occurrence of untoward events or complications, and intervene immediately should these events occur. Provisions must also be in place for notification of personnel regarded as experts in airway management, endotracheal intubation,

Table 17–2 Conscious Sedation

DEFINITION: Administration of sedatives, monitoring of the patient's response, and provision of necessary physiological support during a diagnostic or therapeutic procedure.

ACTIVITIES:

Review patient's health history and results of diagnostic tests to determine whether patient meets agency criteria for conscious sedation by a registered nurse

Ask patient or family about any previous experiences with conscious sedation

Check for drug allergies

Verify that patient has complied with dietary restrictions, as determined by agency criteria

Review other medications patient is taking and verify absence of contraindications for conscious sedation

Instruct the patient and/or family about effects of sedation

Evaluate the patient's level of consciousness and protective reflexes before conscious sedation

Obtain baseline vital signs

Obtain baseline oxygen saturation and EKG rhythm, as appropriate

Initiate an IV line, as appropriate

Administer medication as per physician's order or protocol, titrating carefully according to patient's response

Monitor the patient's level of consciousness and vital signs, as per agency protocol

Monitor oxygen saturation, as appropriate

Monitor the patient's EKG, as appropriate

Monitor the patient for adverse effects of medication, including agitation, respiratory depression, undue somnolence, hypoxemia, arrhythmias, apnea, or exacerbation of a preexisting condition

Restrain the patient, as appropriate

Ensure availability of and administer benzodiazepine receptor antagonist (flumazenil), as appropriate per physician's order or protocol

Ensure availability of and administer narcotic antagonists, as appropriate per physician's order or protocol

Determine whether the patient meets discharge or unit transfer criteria

Discharge or transfer patient, as per agency protocol

Document actions and patient response, as per agency protocol

Source: Bulechek, G. M., and McCloskey, J. C. (1995). *Nursing interventions classification (NIC)*. St. Louis: Mosby–Year Book.

and advanced techniques of cardiopulmonary resuscitation (AANA, 1988, 1991; AORN, 1992; Eichorn, 1986; Murphy, 1988; Watson & James, 1990).

After comprehensive screening, a patent, reliable IV access line must be obtained and continually maintained until the patient is considered fully recovered. Electrocardiogram, blood pressure, and pulse oximetry monitors are then systematically placed, and baseline measurements are obtained and recorded. A baseline oxygen saturation level is particularly important. Desaturation can occur rapidly after injection of IV narcotics or sedatives. Observations must also be made as to the patient's respiratory rate and rhythm in conjunction with the baseline room air oximetry reading. Supplemental oxygen is then provided for the patient via nasal cannulas or masks before the administration of any narcotics or sedatives. Before the administration of medications, the patient must be properly positioned to prevent injury during the procedure. The nurse must ensure that pressure areas such as the elbows and heels are comfortably padded. Arms must be either tucked or positioned on armboards that are placed at less than 90 degrees abduction. Legs should be uncrossed to prevent circulatory compromise (alteration of tissue perfusion) and possible nerve injury. A safety strap should be placed above the patient's knees (AANA, 1991; American Nurses Association [ANA], 1991; AORN, 1992; Eichorn, 1986; Ringler, 1995; Zambricki, 1988).

Every clinical area where Conscious Sedation is performed must have immediate access to emergency resuscitative equipment, specifically airway and ventilatory adjuncts, a source for delivery of 100% oxygen, emergency resuscitative medications, and a defibrillator. Procedure rooms must be furnished with a 100% oxygen supply, a positive-pressure breathing device (i.e., self-inflating bag-valve-mask system, or one-way valve pocket mask that can be connected to oxygen), and oropharyngeal and nasopharyngeal airways. Expert emergency support personnel must be immediately available in the event of complications (AANA, 1991; AORN, 1992).

Although there has been some controversy, the authors and most of nursing specialty organizations acknowledge that the RN managing the care of a patient receiving IV Conscious Sedation must have no other responsibilities during the procedure that would entail leaving the patient unattended and compromise continuous monitoring. Leaving the patient unobserved may delay recognition of an adverse response to the local anesthetic, narcotic, or sedative being administered. Maximum safety dictates that an RN should be assigned to exclusively monitor the patient in order to avoid the risk inherent in providing less than ideal care (AANA, 1988, 1991; AORN, 1992; Eichorn, 1986; Murphy, 1988, 1993; Watson & James, 1990).

Administration and management of IV Conscious Sedation by an RN must be performed in compliance with patient-specific written orders. Many current provisions state that specific doses of medication must be ordered in writing by a licensed physician and that a physician must be present in the room while the medication is being given. After the initial doses of narcotic, sedative, or medication combinations have been given, several minutes should be taken to observe the patient's response. Rapid onset of sedation occurs when narcotics or sedatives are given intravenously, particularly in combination. It cannot be emphasized strongly enough that careful titration and control must be maintained to prevent deep sedation or general anesthesia (AANA, 1991; AORN, 1992; Kaller, 1991; Tanaka, 1988).

Development of a functionally therapeutic sedation plan depends on attentive, continual patient assessment to determine potential complications and stress responses. Overdosage or untoward reactions to the procedure or medication may occur at any time. Observations and measurements regarding the patient's respiratory rate and quality, pulse heart rate and rhythm, blood pressure, and oxygen saturation must be assessed and documented at least every 5 minutes. Continuous assessments must be performed more frequently during the initial medication titration and if dictated by changing parameters in the patient's condition (AANA, 1991; AORN, 1992; Eichorn, 1986; Murphy, 1988, 1993).

Mood alteration, maintenance of consciousness and cooperation, pain threshold elevation with minimal vital sign variation, some degree of amnesia, and a safe, timely return to ambulation and discharge constitute effective and successful Conscious Sedation. The nurse must attempt to maintain the patient in a relaxed, arousable, cooperative state with intact, protective reflexes. Vigilance must continually be directed toward the detection of adverse reactions such as agitation or combativeness, unarousable sleep and hypotension, or respiratory depression and hypoventilation that progresses to airway obstruction and apnea. Hypovolemia may be caused by blood loss or may be pre-existing and unmasked by sedation (AANA, 1991; AORN, 1992; Eichorn, 1986; Murphy, 1988, 1993; Watson & James, 1990).

Should untoward reactions or complications occur, the nurse must initiate necessary supportive measures, which may include maintenance of a patent airway using the head-tilt–chin-lift maneuver, ventilatory support with application of positive pressure, or provision of cardiopulmonary resuscitation. In order to ensure airway safety for a sedated, vomiting patient, the bed must be capable of being placed in Trendelenburg (head down) position. Nurse-initiated interventions for hypotension may include an appropriate IV fluid challenge, leg elevation or Trendelenburg position, and judicious use of vasopressors, naloxone, or flumazenil, covered by standing physician orders. All patient responses, incidents, and interventions should be accurately documented and properly reported to the supervising physician (AANA, 1991; AORN, 1992; Eichorn, 1986; Murphy, 1988, 1993; Watson & James, 1990).

Patient record documentation should reflect ongoing, conscientious assessment, implementation, and evaluation of patient care. Time, dosage, route, and effect of all administered medications should be recorded. Obligatory interventions, such as oxygen therapy, ventilation, or IV therapy, should be indicated, with specific reference to untoward reactions and their resolutions. Meticulous documentation provides an accurate medicolegal record, establishes a retrospective procedure review, and indicates a reliably safe and controlled, continuously monitored environment. It also guides the choice of appropriate medications and timing of maintenance doses (AANA, 1991; AORN, 1992; Eichorn, 1986; Murphy, 1988, 1993; Watson & James, 1990).

Postprocedure care, monitoring, and specific discharge criteria vary according to the procedure, the type and amount of sedation, and the location and characteristics of the patient care unit. Vigilant monitoring must continue throughout recovery, until the patient is considered stable and discharged by an on-site, qualified professional authorized to discharge in accordance with established institutional criteria. Discharge guidelines emphasize criteria that evaluate a patient's return to safe physiological function. This is indicated by stable vital signs, alert level of consciousness, airway patency, mobility, intact protective reflexes, satisfactory surgical site and dressing condition, absence of protracted nausea or vomiting, and ability to urinate. Release of the patient from a short procedure unit to a responsible adult is often required (AANA, 1991; American Society of Post Anesthesia Nurses [ASPAN], 1991; AORN, 1992; Kaller, 1991; Murphy, 1988, 1993; Watson & James, 1990).

Patients and their families and significant others should be given written discharge instructions that emphasize warnings specifically pertaining to use of alcohol or operation of machinery and motor vehicles until the following day. Patients and family members should be able to verbalize these instructions. Presenting them in writing is particularly important, because Conscious Sedation medications may cause significant amnesia that directly affects recall ability (ASPAN, 1991; Kaller, 1991; Murphy, 1988, 1993; Watson & James, 1990).

Should the patient be admitted to a general medical or surgical unit, frequent monitoring should continue for 1 to 3 hours. Observation should be directed to an acceptable level of consciousness, airway patency, continued provision of supplemental oxygen if required, and stable vital signs. Minimum standards that have been established for monitoring specify use of a cardiac monitor, assessment of respiratory rate, observation of oxygen saturation by pulse oximetry, and regularly measured blood pressure readings by a manual or automatic cuff. The patient's level of consciousness is evaluated by observation and communication. Monitoring time frames can vary from once per minute following medication administration to every 15 minutes during the recovery period. On average, the patient should be monitored and measurements and observations recorded every 3 to 5 minutes during the procedure. Children and elderly patients have a less predictable response to the medications and should be monitored more frequently, depending on reactions to the procedure (AANA, 1991; AORN, 1992; ASPAN, 1991; Eichorn, 1986; Kaller, 1991; Murphy, 1988, 1993; Watson & James, 1990).

ADMINISTRATIVE IMPLICATIONS

Policies pertaining to monitoring patients receiving IV Conscious Sedation should be written, annually reviewed, and readily available within the practice setting. Effective written policies should delineate patient selection criteria, extent and responsibility for monitoring, methods of recording detailed patient data, frequency of physiological data documentation, medications that may be administered by an RN, and relevant discharge criteria. Written guidelines should definitively identify authority, responsibility, and accountability to enhance quality assurance. They are also essential for minimizing risk factors and standardization of accepted practice. These policies should be devised from interdisciplinary collaboration among nursing, anesthesia, pharmacy, and surgery departments. This ensures construction of a policy responsive to the patient, physician, and institution and cognitive of patient safety and nursing integrity (AANA, 1991; AORN, 1992; Murphy, 1988, 1993; Watson & James, 1990).

All staff members responsible for administering IV Conscious Sedation should receive formal education regarding applicable medications and monitoring equipment. Constructive inservice education should be conducted in conjunction with the pharmacy and anesthesia departments and should emphasize proper dosages, administration techniques, and characteristics of adverse reaction and overdosage. An educational or credentialing mechanism related to the practice of IV Conscious Sedation should be in place in every institution or practice setting. Evaluation and competence documentation should be periodically conducted, incorporating guidelines addressing monitoring modalities, emergency medications and equipment, and availability of expert personnel (AANA, 1991; AORN, 1992; Murphy, 1988, 1993; Spry, 1990; Watson & James, 1990).

Nurses accepting responsibility for the practice of Conscious Sedation must acquire the knowledge and practical skill to provide prudent and responsible patient care. They must learn to anticipate and recognize potential complications and subsequently assess, diagnose, and effectively intervene when these complications occur. These fundamental skills depend on thorough preparation in anatomy, physiology, pharmacology, dysrhythmia recognition, and complications related to the characteristics of Conscious Sedation. Comprehensive knowledge is also necessary concerning IV therapy, oxygen delivery devices, and airway and resuscitative management. Advanced cardiac life support (ACLS) course completion, although not always required, is recommended for physicians and nurses responsible for the care of patients receiving IV Conscious Sedation. The focal skills of ACLS training include airway management, dysrhythmia recognition, review of emergency resuscitative medications, and management of cardiac arrest. Practitioners familiar with these skills can more confidently anticipate emergency situations and more effectively stabilize patients until expert personnel, additional medications, and equipment can be obtained (AANA, 1991; AORN, 1992; Kaller, 1991; Murphy, 1988, 1993; Spry, 1990; Watson & James, 1990; Zambricki, 1988).

Nurses must thoroughly recognize and understand the legal ramifications of the practice of IV Conscious Sedation, especially the responsibilities and liabilities in the event of an untoward reaction or life-threatening complication. Important areas of legal concern involve licensure and the potential for malpractice liability. If administration and monitoring of IV sedation are considered outside the legal scope of nursing practice in a region where practice occurs, participating nurses risk licensure discipline. When in doubt, nurses should consult the state nurse practice act, administrative regulations of the particular nursing board, and, possibly, representatives of the nursing board staff. Nurse practice acts are often broad in scope and may not specifically address the practice of IV Conscious Sedation. There may be general provisions that allow or prohibit this practice. Administration and monitoring of IV Conscious Sedation may be permitted by inclusion under the general rules applying to all nurses accepting and performing medically delegated acts (Murphy, 1988, 1993; Watson & James, 1990).

ASSOCIATED NURSING DIAGNOSES AND OUTCOMES

The nursing diagnoses of Pain, Risk for Injury, and Fear may be appropriately treated using conscious sedation. Complications following administration of Conscious Sedation involve nursing diagnoses related to airway management and shock. Airway management diagnoses are Ineffective Airway Clearance, Impaired Gas Exchange, and Ineffective Breathing Pattern. Diagnoses applicable to shock include Altered Level of Consciousness, Fluid Volume Deficit, Decreased Cardiac Output, and Altered Tissue Perfusion. Initiating the intervention of Conscious Sedation involves potential risks that may also lead to Risk for Injury, Risk for Aspiration, Impaired Tissue Integrity, Altered Nutrition: Less Than Body Requirements, Risk for Altered Oral Mucous Membrane, Impaired Swallowing, Body Image Disturbance, and Impaired Verbal Communication. Associated nurse-sensitive patient outcomes include Pain Level, Vital Signs Status, Fear Control, and Comfort Level. Should complications occur, other outcomes related to respiration and circulation would need to be addressed. The nurse administering Conscious Sedation must be able to recognize and treat all these diagnoses.

CASE STUDY

PT, a 23-year-old man, presents to the triage nurse in the emergency department. His history includes a fall onto his left shoulder while playing basketball that occurred just before arrival. He is quite agitated, complaining of considerable pain in his left shoulder, and supports his left forearm with his right hand. Additional history reveals no similar injuries in the past, no medical problems, and no medication use or allergies. Attempts at gentle palpation of the shoulder cause PT to scream in pain; the triage nurse is able to palpate a radial pulse.

The patient is immediately moved to a bed in the treatment area, and his shirt is cut away, revealing an obvious anterior deformity of the humeral head. A physician is called to the bedside while the nurse obtains baseline vital signs: Blood pressure of 120/84, pulse of 84/minute, and respiratory rate of 20/minute. The nurse then inserts an IV catheter and initiates an IV line of normal saline solution (NSS) at keep-vein-open rate in the right arm. Anticipating the need for Conscious Sedation to reduce a shoulder dislocation, the nurse administers low-flow oxygen via nasal cannula, attaches the patient to the cardiac monitor and pulse oximeter, and applies the cuff of the noninvasive blood pressure machine. Morphine 2 mg IV is ordered to provide some pain relief during the x-ray. The patient is maintained in a semi-Fowler position, because he has identified that as the position of comfort.

While a portable left shoulder x-ray is obtained, PT's nurse gives a brief report on the status of her other patients to the charge nurse, so that the charge nurse can assume responsibility for the other patients during the Conscious Sedation procedure.

PT's nurse returns to the bedside and provides a

simple description of the intended procedure, assuring the patient that the team will strive to ensure his comfort and safety. Wall suction is checked to make sure it is functional. A technician positions the code cart outside the room and then stays to assist the physician in the manual reduction. Once the physician is at the bedside, morphine 4 mg and Versed 2 mg are administered over 2 minutes. PT's nurse begins surveillance of the following patient parameters: level of consciousness, respiratory rate and effort, pulse oximetry, pulse, and blood pressure. Assessment of these parameters is recorded every 5 minutes. Additionally, the nurse continually monitors the patient's level of consciousness, airway patency, and respiratory effort.

Approximately 5 minutes after administration of the medications, the physician attempts to reduce the shoulder. The patient is awake and is quiet when the shoulder is touched. However, as the physician attempts to move the arm, the patient screams with pain and begins sobbing. Assessment parameters are as follows: Blood pressure of 136/74, pulse of 110/minute, respiratory rate of 24, and pulse oximetry 100%. An additional 2 mg of morphine IV is ordered by the physician and given by the nurse. The nurse then resumes surveillance of the patient's parameters. Approximately 3 minutes after the last dose of morphine, the patient begins to complain of feeling dizzy, stating that he is "going to be sick." The nurse notes that the patient is pale and diaphoretic and then lowers the head of the bed and cycles a blood pressure on the machine. The cardiac monitor shows sinus rhythm at a rate of 50, with a reported blood pressure of 98/56. An IV bolus of 500 mL of NSS wide open is ordered and administered. The nurse increases the frequency of recording vital signs and parameters to every 3 minutes. The patient remains responsive throughout but has his eyes closed when not stimulated. The patient starts to respond after 400 mL of NSS has been absorbed, and the patient's color is again pink, with warm, dry skin. Pulse oximetry remains constant at 100%, with a

pulse of 95 and blood pressure of 116/64. With help from the technician, the physician again attempts shoulder reduction and is successful. The patient complains of discomfort at the moment of reduction but quickly becomes silent. A shoulder immobilizer is applied to prevent recurrence of the dislocation, and a postreduction x-ray is ordered.

The nurse remains with the patient, monitoring parameters every 5 minutes. PT dozes but awakens to voice and maintains stable vital signs with good oximetry levels. Approximately 30 minutes after the final dose of morphine, he is no longer dozing and remains awake, talking with his family. He reports that his shoulder feels much better and recalls nothing of the reduction procedure. The nurse continues to monitor his parameters but now does so every 15 minutes. She again assumes responsibility for those patients handed off during the Conscious Sedation process.

PT remains in the emergency department for another hour, while the nurse watches for any signs of resedation. After ensuring orthopedic follow-up and discharge instructions related to the care of his injury, the nurse reviews discharge instructions pertinent to the Conscious Sedation procedure. PT is not permitted to drive home and is released only to another adult who can ensure continued monitoring for the next 24 hours. He is further instructed to remain at home for the next 24 hours and to avoid any activity that demands full alertness. He is advised to refrain from alcohol consumption and to use only the pain medicine prescribed by the physician in the doses ordered. Finally, PT is advised not to sign any contracts or make major decisions for at least 24 hours after the Conscious Sedation procedure.

The nurse's role of constant vigilance in this case allowed early identification and rectification of a vasovagal-hypotensive event. Knowledgeable practice and preparedness contribute to the successful outcome of procedures performed using Conscious Sedation.

SUMMARY

Registered professional nurses who are not Certified Registered Nurse Anesthetists must obtain documented evidence of appropriate training in order to safely participate in the administration and monitoring of IV Conscious Sedation.

Organizational policies and procedures must be in place within the institution that include guidelines for medication administration, patient monitoring during and after the procedure, and protocols applicable to the development of potential complications or emergency situations. Prudent, responsible, and effective patient care provided in the practice of IV Conscious Sedation depends on the nurse's comprehension of pharmacology and potential adverse medication reactions and mastery of appropriate emergency intervention skills.

References

American Association of Nurse Anesthetists. (1988). Separation of operator-anesthetist responsibilities. *American Association of Nurse Anesthetists Position Statements*, 2.3. Park Ridge, IL: Author.

American Association of Nurse Anesthetists. (1991). Qualified providers of conscious sedation. *American Association of Nurse Anesthetists Position Statements*, 2.2. Park Ridge, IL: Author.

American Nurses Association. (1991). *Position statement on the role of the registered nurse (RN) in the management of patients receiving intravenous conscious sedation.* Washington, DC: Author.

American Society of Post Anesthesia Nurses. (1991). *Standards of post anesthesia nursing practice* (pp. 26–29). Richmond, VA: Author.

Association of Operating Room Nurses. (1992). Proposed recommended practice: Monitoring the patient receiving IV conscious sedation. *AORN Journal, 56,* 316–324.

Batson, V. D. (1993). Conscious sedation: Implications for perioperative nursing practice. *Seminars in Perioperative Nursing, 2*(1), 45–47.

Eichorn, J. H., Cooper, J. B., Cullen, D. J., Maier, W. R., Philip, J. H., and Seeman, R. G. (1986). Standards for patient monitoring during anesthesia at Harvard Medical School. *JAMA, 256,* 1017–1020.

Kaller, S. (1991). Conscious sedation in ambulatory surgery. *Anesthesiology Review, 18*(1), 9–12.

Murphy, E. K. (1988). Legal considerations in RN monitoring of intravenous sedation. *AORN Journal, 48,* 1184–1187.

Murphy, E. K. (1993). Monitoring IV conscious sedation, the legal scope of practice. *AORN Journal, 57,* 512–514.

Physicians' desk reference (51st ed.). (1997). Montvale, NJ: Medical Economics Company.

Proudfoot, J. (1995). Analgesia, anesthesia, and conscious sedation. *Emergency Medical Clinics of North America, 13,* 357–370.

Ramoska, E. A., Linkenheimer, R., and Glasgow, D. (1991). Midazolam use in the emergency department. *Journal of Emergency Medicine, 9,* 247–250.

Ringler, J. D. (1995). The use of diazepam and ketamine for IV conscious sedation in outpatient settings. *AORN Journal, 62,* 638–645.

Spry, C. C. (1990). Perioperative nurses should keep monitoring within their specialty. *AORN Journal, 51,* 1071–1072.

Stoelting, R. K. (1991). *Pharmacology and physiology in anesthetic practice* (2nd ed., 71–74, 84–87, 118–133). Philadelphia: J.B. Lippincott.

Tanaka, D. J. (1988). Intravenous anesthetics. In W. R. Waugaman, B. M. Rigor, L. E. Katz, H. W. Bradshaw, and J. F. Garde, *Principles and practice of nurse anesthesia* (pp. 187–216). Norwalk, CT: Appleton & Lange.

Tung, A., and Rosenthal, M. (1995). Patients requiring sedation. *Critical Care Clinics, 11,* 791–801.

Watson, D. S., and James, D. S. (1990). Intravenous conscious sedation: Implications of monitoring patients receiving local anesthesia. *AORN Journal, 51,* 1512–1522.

Watson, D. S. (1993). The use of the benzodiazepine antagonist flumazenil. *AORN Journal, 57,* 497–502.

Waugaman, W. R., Rigor, B. M., Katz, L. E., Bradshaw, H. W., and Garde, J. F. (Eds.). (1988). *Principles and practice of nurse anesthesia* (pp. 139–150). Norwalk, CT: Appleton & Lange.

Zambricki, C. S. (1988). Preoperative preparation and evaluation. *In* W. R. Waugaman, B. M. Rigor, L. E. Katz, H. W. Bradshaw, and J. F. Garde, *Principles and practice of nurse anesthesia* (pp. 139–150). Norwalk, CT: Appleton & Lange.

Zambricki, C. S. (1988). Intubation and airway management. *In* W. R. Waugaman, B. M. Rigor, L. E. Katz, H. W. Bradshaw, and J. F. Garde, *Principles and practice of nurse anesthesia* (pp. 151–166). Norwalk, CT: Appleton & Lange.

Shock Management

Meg Gulanick and Carol Ruback

Shock is a pathogenic condition resulting from the inability of the circulatory system to maintain adequate tissue perfusion. Although complication and mortality rates remain persistently high for patients in shock, especially those in cardiogenic shock, chances for a successful outcome are contingent on early recognition and prompt aggressive therapy. Nurse monitoring of sometimes subtle changes in the patient's hemodynamic status, followed by immediate and appropriate intervention, can improve patients' chance of survival.

The acute care nurse providing care for the challenging shock patient must have an armamentarium of knowledge and skills: sound understanding of the pathophysiology of shock and its potential complications, the ability to assess multiple parameters simultaneously, understanding of current treatment modalities and their rationale, and the ability to provide rapid emergency care in a calm, deliberate manner. Shock Management entails a variety of nursing actions—independent as well as collaborative. The essential concepts the nurse uses to assist the patient to maintain his or her integrity in this process of survival include providing surveillance, improving oxygenation, maintaining tissue perfusion, regulating vital body functions, and providing emotional support. This chapter focuses on the general Nursing Interventions Classification (NIC) intervention Shock Management as displayed in Table 18–1. However, because many of the interventions are directed at the underlying pathophysiology of shock, the reader is also referred to additional NIC interventions: Shock Management: Cardiac, Shock Management: Vasogenic, and Shock Management: Volume (McCloskey & Bulechek, 1996).

Table 18–1 Shock Management

DEFINITION: Facilitation of the delivery of oxygen and nutrients to systemic tissue with removal of cellular waste products in a patient with severely altered tissue perfusion.

ACTIVITIES:

Inspect for bleeding from mucous membranes, bruising after minimal trauma, oozing from puncture sites, and presence of petechiae

Monitor trends in blood pressure and hemodynamic parameters, if available (e.g., central venous pressure and pulmonary capillary/artery wedge pressure)

Promote bed rest and limit activity

Note tachycardia, decreased blood pressure, or abnormally low systemic arterial pressure, as well as pallor, decreased capillary refill, and diaphoresis

Monitor fetal heart rate for bradycardia (less than 110 beats per minute) or tachycardia (greater than 160 beats per minute) lasting longer than 10 min, if appropriate

Observe extremities for color, warmth, swelling, pulses, texture, edema, and ulcerations

Monitor for cerebral ischemia or indications of insufficient cerebral blood flow or cerebral perfusion pressure

Monitor renal function (e.g., BUN and Cr levels), if appropriate

Administer vasoactive medications

Insert urinary catheter, if appropriate

Monitor fluid status, including intake and output, as appropriate

Monitor serum glucose and treat abnormal levels, as appropriate

Monitor neurological functioning

Monitor coagulation studies and complete blood count (CBC) with WBC differential

Draw arterial blood gases and monitor tissue oxygenation

Use arterial line monitoring to improve accuracy of blood pressure readings, if appropriate

Provide oxygen therapy and/or mechanical ventilation, if necessary

Insert nasogastric tube to suction and monitor secretions, if appropriate

Monitor orthostatic vital signs, including blood pressure

Maintain patient IV access

Encourage realistic expectations for the patient and family

Monitor determinants of tissue oxygen delivery (e.g., low PaO_2, SaO_2, and hemoglobin levels and cardiac output), if available

Monitor for symptoms of inadequate tissue oxygenation (e.g., pallor, cyanosis, and sluggish capillary refill)

Monitor for symptoms of respiratory failure (e.g., low PaO_2 and elevated $PaCO_2$ levels and respiratory muscle fatigue)

Monitor lab values for changes in oxygenation or acid-base balance, as appropriate

Evaluate effects of fluid therapy

Protect from trauma

Administer fluids to maintain blood pressure and cardiac output, as appropriate

Position the patient for optimal perfusion

Position for peripheral perfusion

Offer emotional support to the patient and family

Monitor gastrointestinal functioning (e.g., distension and bowel sounds)

Monitor peripheral perfusion

Promote stress reduction

Source: McCloskey, J. C., and Bulechek, G. H. (1996). *Nursing interventions classification (NIC)* (pp. 498–499). St. Louis: Mosby–Year Book.

TYPES OF SHOCK

The circulatory system is made up of the chambers of the heart and the blood vessels. To function properly, there must be adequate blood to fill this system (blood volume), the heart muscle must pump efficiently to keep the blood circulating, and the blood vessels must dilate or constrict appropriately to channel the blood to all vital tissues. If there is significant failure anywhere within this system, and perfusion to one vital organ is reduced, a myocardial infarction, stroke, or renal failure may occur. If perfusion to several vital organs is compromised, shock occurs (Bordicks, 1980).

Shock as a clinical entity represents inadequate tissue perfusion resulting in metabolic changes at the cellular level. The subsequent metabolic derangements are most crucial in the cells of the vital organs: the brain, the heart, and the kidneys (Guyton, 1996). Shock can be classified in several different ways. For our purposes, shock is classified according to its cause as cardiac, volume, or vasogenic (Chulay, Guzzetta, & Dossey, 1997).

In cardiogenic shock, cardiac dysfunction (inability of the heart to pump blood efficiently) is the primary problem. It can result from mechanical, structural, or electrical problems with the heart (Weeks, 1986) and can also be classified according to coronary and noncoronary etiologies (Rice, 1991a). It is a self-perpetuating condition, because the early compensatory mechanism of increased arterial vasoconstriction later becomes a liability for the failing pump. To compensate for the increased afterload, the heart must pump harder, which requires additional coronary artery blood flow. But because the shock has reduced coronary blood flow, the myocardium now becomes even more ischemic, causing further ventricular dysfunction and ischemia (Bordicks, 1980). The mortality rate for cardiogenic shock often exceeds 80%.

Hypovolemic shock occurs from decreased intravascular fluid volume due to either internal fluid shifts or external fluid loss. It is associated with a blood volume deficit of at least 15% to 30% (American College of Surgeons [ACS], 1993). Elderly patients may exhibit signs of shock with smaller losses of fluid volume because of their compromised ability to compensate for fluid changes.

Vasogenic shock is due to excessive dilation of the blood vessels, resulting in pooling of blood in the peripheral vessels. This category encompasses three types of shock: septic, anaphylactic, and neurogenic.

Whatever the initiating cause of the shock state, the ultimate defect involved is the inadequacy of cardiac output to perfuse vital organs. This results in a chain reaction, beginning with impaired tissue perfusion, anaerobic metabolism, and metabolic acidosis that leads to increased capillary permeability, cell membrane deterioration, cell death, and organ failure. The body has homeostatic mechanisms to meet this crisis. Initially, as the sympathetic system is stimulated, the heart's rate and force of contraction increase in an attempt to correct the drop in blood pressure and cardiac output. The peripheral blood vessels constrict in order to redistribute blood to priority tissue areas. Both effects may be immediately useful; however, they increase oxygen demands on the heart itself, which may interfere with its normal functioning (Rice, 1991b; Weil, von Planta, & Rackow, 1992).

NURSING DIAGNOSES AND OUTCOMES

Regardless of the primary culprit in shock, the adult patient is at risk for several nursing diagnoses: Fluid Volume Deficit, Decreased Cardiac Output, and Altered Tissue Perfusion. As the shock state progresses, disturbances in ventilatory status, such as Impaired Gas Exchange or Ineffective Breathing Pattern and coping difficulties such as Anxiety, Fear, Altered Level of Consciousness, Risk for Impaired Skin Integrity, and Altered Nutrition, may likewise be diagnosed. In septic shock, Risk for Infection and Hyperthermia will be evident.

The following patient outcomes can be expected from the shock management interventions: Tissue Perfusion (Abdominal Organs, Cardiac, Cerebral, Peripheral, and Pulmonary), Cardiac Pump Effectiveness, Circulation Status, and Fluid Balance.

The focus of this chapter is the intervention Shock Management. However, the nurse must also be aware of the importance of preventing shock in high-risk patients, as described in a related NIC intervention: Shock Prevention. Through prevention, patients have the greatest chance for successful resolution of their problem.

DESCRIPTION OF THE INTERVENTION

The immediate goal in treating shock is to improve tissue perfusion in an effort to maintain vital organ function (Rice, 1991c). Table 18–1 provides a general overview of Shock Management that incorporates a wide range of nursing activities corresponding to a general approach to Shock Management (McCloskey & Bulechek, 1996). For discussion purposes, the activities displayed in the table are grouped into the following categories: providing surveillance, maintaining tissue perfusion, regulating vital organ functions, and providing emotional support.

Providing Surveillance

The classic shock patient—hypotensive, oliguric, with rapid weak pulse and cold clammy skin, restless, and anxious—is easy to recognize. By the time most patients reach this stage, their chances for a successful recovery are limited. Therefore, the nurse needs to be skilled at assessing the earlier signs of shock—those subtle trends and changes that signal potential problems with tissue perfusion (Rice, 1991d).

Because the patient is changing constantly, the nurse in attendance has a primary role in ongoing monitoring or surveillance (Laurent-Bopp & Shinn, 1995). Knowing what to look for and when and how to look are basic characteristics of surveillance. Ongoing monitoring involves not only the observation of the relevant parameters but also the complex process of integrating the information in a meaningful way so as to be useful in guiding nursing actions. There are several specific parameters for surveillance in shock.

Monitor Skin Color and Moisture and Body Temperature   One of the most immediate, simple, and extremely useful assessments the nurse makes is that of peripheral skin color, temperature, and moisture. The nurse should check the nail beds for blanching, because a quick return of color (<2 sec) suggests adequate tissue oxygenation. In cardiogenic and hypovolemic shock, blood is initially shunted to the vital organs at the expense of the skin. The profound vasoconstriction that occurs causes the skin to be pale, cool, and diaphoretic. These changes reflect inadequate tissue oxygenation. Cyanosis is a late sign in the shock state. Persistently cold, clammy skin despite fluid and pharmocological treatment signals to the nurse the need for reevaluation of therapy. In contrast, early septic shock due to generalized vasodilation commonly finds the patient to be warm, pink, and dry (Rice, 1991d).

Core body temperature should be assessed intermittently by using a temperature probe inserted into the ear, by continuously using a rectal probe, or by using a probe in the bladder as part of an indwelling catheter. In septic shock, core body temperature can increase above 38°C and be associated with chills that often precede temperature spikes.

Monitor Mentation and Neurological Functioning   Subtle changes in sensorium or level of consciousness are early manifestations of cerebral hypoxia and impending shock. This response is characterized by restlessness, irritability, and anxiety. Serial assessments are critical so the earliest changes or signs of further deterioration can be identified. As shock progresses, signs such as lethargy, confusion, and reduced response to pain may indicate insufficient cerebral blood flow or cerebral perfusion pressure. Neurological checks, including pupil size and reactivity and sensation and movement, can also be performed to detect changes in neurological status (Rice, 1991d).

Monitor Blood Pressure and Pulse Pressure   Blood pressure measurements are used to assess the status of the circulating blood volume. Blood pressure varies with the stage of shock. For example, in early septic shock, the blood pressure is relatively normal secondary to peripheral shunting. And in cardiogenic or hypovolemic shock, the alpha-stimulating effects of the sympathetic nervous system (vasoconstriction) may produce a near-normal blood pressure in the early or compensatory stage of shock. Therefore, arterial hypotension may or may not be an early manifestation of shock. Orthostatic hypotension may be especially evident with hypovolemic shock.

Auscultatory blood pressure measurement may be unrealiable secondary to peripheral vasoconstriction either from physiological compensatory mechanisms or from vasopressor drug treatment (Rice, 1991d; Robenson-Piano, Holm, & Powers, 1987). Therefore, it can be risky for nurses to rely only on cuff pressures to guide titration of inotropic and vasopressor drug treatment. Direct intra-arterial monitoring of pressures should be instituted as soon as possible. Once initiated, the nurse needs to monitor the patient for the potential hazards associated with such hemodynamic monitoring: infection, bleeding, and air embolism.

Several important measurements can be derived from an accurate blood pressure reading. The mean arterial pressure provides information about the overall perfusion pressure to the tissues and organs. The pulse pressure (the difference between systolic and diastolic pressures) provides an estimate of the heart's stroke volume or pumping ability. Pulse pressure generally narrows in shock because the systolic pressure falls more rapidly than the diastolic pressure. In fact, diastolic pressure initially increases secondary to vasoconstriction. The body generally needs a systolic pressure of 80 to 90 mm Hg for optimal perfusion. During the later stages of shock, both systolic and diastolic pressures fall, leading to cardiovascular collapse. A fall below 80 mm Hg generally indicates inadequate coronary blood flow.

Monitor Heart Rate   The heart rate of hypotensive patients is usually rapid—an adaptive mechanism to optimize cardiac output. However, significant and persistent tachycardia reduces the filling time of the heart and increases myocardial oxygen demands—both of which can lead to reduced cardiac output and subsequent inadequate tissue perfusion if left unchecked.

The nurse must evaluate both central and peripheral pulses regularly to detect critical changes in the patient's hemodynamic status. Palpation of the central pulses (femoral, carotid) provides valuable information about stroke volume and arterial pressure. Weak, thready pulses require treatment. Assessment of peripheral pulses provides data on the amount of vasoconstriction, which indicates impaired peripheral perfusion. The need for early detection of subtle changes is vitally important. At the later stages of refractory shock, a progressive slowing of the heart rate may be noted. Elderly patients have a reduced response to catecholamines; thus, their response to reduced cardiac output may be blunted, with less rise in heart rate.

The pulses need to be monitored for at least 30 seconds to determine the presence of dysrhythmias, and the patient should be placed on continuous electrocardiogram (ECG) monitoring as soon as possible. Cardiac dysrhythmias may occur from low perfusion states, acidosis, or hypoxia. Tachycardia or bradycardia and frequent ectopic beats can compromise cardiac output further and must be treated promptly according to medical orders or protocols (Guidelines, 1992).

The nurse also should take routine 12-lead ECGs to monitor for signs of myocardial ischemia (ST-T wave changes) or frank infarction patterns (Q waves) occurring from reduced coronary blood flow.

Monitor Renal Function and Urine Output The shock state is associated with reduced renal blood flow and the subsequent decrease in urine formation. Inadequate renal perfusion is reflected in oliguria (less than 30 mL/hr of urine). Even when vital signs return to normal, it is important for the nurse to continue monitoring urine output, because continuing oliguria is a feature of impending renal shutdown. Accurate measurement of intake and output is essential in detecting negative fluid balance and determining adequacy of fluid replacement. It is imperative that the nurse insert a Foley catheter early so that hourly trends in urine output can be monitored.

Laboratory studies are indicated to further assess renal function. Urine specific gravity and osmolality are reduced because of the inability of the kidneys to reabsorb sodium. Fixed specific gravity indicates renal dysfunction or failure. Elevated levels of blood urea nitrogen (BUN) (>20 mg/dL) and creatinine (>1.5 mg/dL) indicate renal dysfunction. In later stages of shock, renal failure and anuria occur. Urinalysis reports, as well as color and opacity of urine, need to be evaluated for possible causes of septic shock.

Monitor Invasive Hemodynamic Parameters Hemodynamic monitoring is essential for accurately assessing the filling pressures of the heart (preload) in critically ill patients (Rice, 1991d; Summers, 1990). Central venous pressure (CVP) catheters inserted into the vena cava or right atrium provide information on the circulating fluid volume and thus on the ability of the right side of the heart to handle fluid challenges. Low CVP readings indicate hypovolemia. However, CVPs are not accurate indicators of left ventricular filling pressures. Although fluid challenges may be required to assess the cardiovascular response to increased fluid volume, it can be risky giving intravenous (IV) fluid therapy without first assessing the left side of the heart.

Fortunately, flow-directed balloon-tipped (Swan-Ganz) catheters, which can be positioned in the pulmonary artery, can be easily inserted at the bedside. The nurse needs to anticipate their use and be prepared to promptly assist with their insertion (Woods, 1976). These catheters monitor pulmonary artery end diastolic pressures, as well as pulmonary capillary wedge pressures (PCWP). In the absence of mitral valve disease, these measurements provide the most accurate evaluation of the preload of the left ventricle. In healthy individuals, the normal range is 4 to 12 mm Hg. Lower values indicate hypovolemia; higher values around 30 mm Hg indicate pulmonary congestion and left ventricular impairment. However, for acutely ill patients, especially those with significant left ventricular impairment, a higher filling pressure, or wedge pressure of at least 14 to 18mm Hg, is usually required for maintaining an optimal cardiac output (Laurent-Bopp & Shinn, 1995).

Swan-Ganz catheters also provide indirect determination of cardiac output, cardiac index, and systemic vascular resistance, information that can be most useful in determining the cause of shock and evaluating response to therapeutic measures (Rice, 1991d; Summers, 1990). For example, in early stages of septic shock, the cardiac output is increased and the systemic vascular resistance is reduced. In cardiogenic shock, systemic vascular resistance is increased as a result of compensatory vasoconstriction.

Monitor Arterial Tissue Oxygenation   In general, the body responds to tissue hypoxia with rapid, shallow respirations. In the presence of tachypnea, the nurse must auscultate for crackles and wheezes. In late or irreversible shock, slow, shallow respirations with often-varying patterns are noted. Skin, nail beds, and mucous membranes must be assessed for signs of pallor or cyanosis. Adult respiratory distress syndrome may also occur, resulting in hypoxemia.

Arterial oxygen saturation (SaO_2) can be continually assessed using noninvasive pulse oximetry. Measurements below 90% saturation indicate pulmonary compromise and deterioration. Measurement of arterial blood gases provides needed information about the adequacy of both gas exchange and acid-base balance. The nurse must be knowledgeable of normal parameters and report immediately any significant deviations. Hypoxemia (low PaO_2) can contribute to cardiac dysrhythmias. Metabolic acidosis (low pH) is expected because of anaerobic metabolism and lactic acid production. Metabolic or lactic acidosis impairs the contractility of the heart and inactivates most vasoactive drugs (Guidelines, 1992). Respiratory acidosis (low pH secondary to elevated $PaCO_2$) decreases the availability of oxygen to the tissues and needs to be treated with improved ventilatory methods. The pH must be maintained within the 7.35 to 7.45 range. Metabolic alkalosis (high pH) is likewise a problem, occurring usually from overzealous treatment with sodium bicarbonate or from use of citrated bank blood. Bicarbonate levels should be held within 15 to 18 mEq/L.

Monitor Gastrointestinal (GI) Status   Thirst becomes a significant sign in evaluating the progression of shock. It intensifies as hypovolemia remains untreated. As blood is shunted to other organs, bowel sounds become hypoactive, and abdominal distention and tenderness may be evident. A paralytic ileus may occur.

Monitor Complete Blood Count (CBC) and Coagulation Studies   All body orifices and puncture sites must be assessed for signs of bleeding. The hematocrit will be reduced from significant blood loss in hypovolemia. However, it will also be reduced as fluids are administered because of dilutional effects. In the setting of traumatic injury causing significant GI bleeding, the hematocrit will decrease 1% per liter of fluid replacement. Any further hematocrit drop must be evaluated as an indication of continued blood loss. Coagulation studies, including prothrombin time (PT), partial thromboplastin time (PTT), fibrinogen, fibrin split products, and platelets, are evaluated as appropriate.

Monitor Serum Glucose   Glucose may be elevated in response to the shock state and altered metabolism. It does not indicate diabetes mellitus.

Determine Emotional Status The nurse must recognize the patient's level of fear or anxiety and note signs and symptoms. Shock is an acute life-threatening illness that produces high levels of anxiety in the patient and his or her significant others. Controlling anxiety will help decrease physiological reactions that can aggravate the condition. The nurse should assess for measures the patient has used in the past to deal with stressful situations.

Maintaining Tissue Perfusion

The basic defect in shock from any cause is a decrease in tissue perfusion; therefore, many of the nursing activities used to treat shock are the same despite different causes.

Position The nurse promotes bed rest and limits the patient's activity in order to reduce oxygen demand. The patient is placed into a position that will facilitate both perfusion to vital organs and ventilation. The ideal position is supine. This position provides adequate blood flow to the brain and promotes venous return from the brain to the heart. If the patient is hypovolemic, the nurse may elevate the patient's legs slightly in order to mobilize fluids. However, the patient should not be placed in the Trendelenburg position because, although blood flow to the brain will be increased, venous return of blood to the heart will be impeded. This causes the blood to pool in the brain, resulting in tissue hypoxia. Additionally, the Trendelenburg position can interfere with ventilation, because gravity will push the abdominal organs upward against the diaphragm. For the patient experiencing respiratory distress, the nurse can elevate the head of the bed slightly to facilitate ventilation. Turning the patient frequently prevents pooling of secretions and also improves ventilation. The nurse must determine the priority needs of the patient: ventilation or perfusion.

Ventilation and Oxygenation Shock results in hypoperfusion of cells and resultant tissue hypoxia. The nurse intervenes promptly to optimize the patient's state of oxygenation, positioning as described, suctioning to remove secretions, and inserting a nasogastric tube into the patient's stomach to prevent aspiration of stomach contents.

Once the airway has been established, supplemental oxygen must be administered. The patient in shock has an increased need for oxygen to offset the hypoperfusion and increased metabolic state. If previous actions are not effective, the patient may require tracheal intubation and mechanical ventilation to maintain oxygenation.

Volume Replacement The patient in hypovolemic shock needs fluid replacement immediately, and restoring blood volume is the priority. The physician determines the appropriate fluid for replacement based on the source of fluid loss and the patient's clinical condition. Only isotonic fluids should be used for resuscitation, because there are no net osmotic forces moving water into or out of the intracellular compartment (Bongard & Sue, 1994). When isotonic solutions are used for resuscitation, administration of three to four times the actual deficit is required to account for fluid shifts into the extracellular spaces (ACS, 1993; Bongard & Sue, 1994). Two large-bore IV catheters should be inserted, and a balanced isotonic solution such as Ringer's lactate should be rapidly infused. One-half normal saline solution and dextrose solution should never be given to the hypovolemic patient, because they are hypotonic solutions and may lead to water intoxication (Bordicks, 1980; Lanros, 1988). Colloid volume expanders such as albumin, dextran, and hetastarch are effective hypertonic solutions. They may be useful in the patient with normal or excessive total body water but intravascular dehydration. These fluids increase the osmolality of intravascular fluid, drawing interstitial fluid into the vascular space. As a result, the circulating blood volume is expanded, but extracellular fluid volume decreases (Shires, Barber, & Illner, 1995).

The volume replacement of choice in the hemorrhagic patient with a hematocrit level of less than 35% is blood and blood components. Type-specific cross-matched packed red blood cells (PRBC) are preferred. Universal-donor blood type O can be given emergently and is relatively safe (Lanros, 1988). PRBC are preferred over whole blood in both type-specific and universal donor transfusion, because they reduce the risk of transfer of donor antibodies.

When transfusing large amounts of blood, warming the blood before transfusion is generally recommended (Lanros, 1988). Multiple transfusions of unwarmed blood are associated with cardiac dysrhythmias.

PRBC do not contain the normal clotting factors; when multiple transfusions are given, the patient's own clotting factors are diluted. Properly crossmatched fresh frozen plasma and packed platelets should be given to patients receiving more than 10 units of PRBC to prevent coagulopathy (Lanros, 1988).

It is essential for the nurse to have an understanding of the character of the prescribed fluid therapy and its effects in order to evaluate the patient's response to treatment (see Chapter 14). The nurse carefully records the type and amount of fluid and the effect on the patient.

Once blood volume replacement has been initiated, the source of the bleeding or fluid loss should be found and stopped. When external bleeding is found, direct pressure over the site should be applied. If no obvious bleeding points are found, occult bleeding must be considered, especially with patients with pelvic and femur fractures and those having undergone invasion of a major vessel for any reason (e.g., cardiac catheterization procedure).

In septic shock, restoration of adequate circulating blood volume with a crystalloid is important. Ongoing capillary leakage will require continued aggressive fluid replacement.

Medication Therapy   Several types of drugs are used to treat shock. The nurse assumes responsibility for titrating the administration of these powerful medications to regulate vital signs within established parameters.

1. Inotropic agents.   In the normovolemic patient in shock, the physician may order an inotropic agent such as dobutamine, amrinone or milrinone, or low-dose dopamine to optimize cardiac output and hence oxygen delivery (Shoemaker, Kram, & Appel, 1990) (Table 18–2). These agents are one of the main therapies for patients in cardiogenic shock associated with reduced myocardial contractility. The acute care nurse should use caution when administering these agents to patients with minimal cardiac reserve or coronary artery disease, because these medications increase the myocardial oxygen demand (Underhill, Woods, Froelicher, & Halpenney, 1990).

Additionally, the use of these agents can be disastrous in the hypovolemic patient, because they cause vasodilatation, which can lead to dangerous hypotension. This reaction can be prevented as well as reversed with administration of fluid.

2. Diuretics.   Diuretics may be helpful in maintaining renal function once blood volume deficits are corrected. Diuretics also are used to remove excess extravascular fluid associated with heart failure in cardiogenic shock.

Table 18–2 Effects of Inotropic Agents

Dobutamine: Dobutamine has a positive inotropic effect that increases stroke volume and cardiac output. Dobutamine also has the additional beneficial effect of reducing afterload by decreasing peripheral vasoconstriction, also resulting in higher cardiac output.

Dopamine: In low- and medium-range doses, dopamine has a positive inotropic and chronotropic effect on the heart that improves stroke volume and cardiac output. Low-dose dopamine also enhances renal blood flow, thus improving renal output. Dopamine, however, greatly increases myocardial demand for oxygen. High doses of dopamine can cause peripheral vasoconstriction and can be arrhythmiogenic.

Amrinone: Amrinone has similar effects as dobutamine but has a different mechanism of action; therefore, some patients may respond better to amrinone than to dopamine. It has both a positive inotropic and a peripheral vasodilation effect to improve cardiac output.

Note: Drugs may be used in combination for enhanced effect.

3. Vasopressors. The patient should receive vasopressors only as a last resort (Lanros, 1988; Shoemaker et al., 1990). When the patient is in shock, compensatory neurohormonal mechanisms are maximally activated to produce vasoconstriction, which maintains blood pressure, and to shunt blood away from nonessential tissues to the heart, brain, and working muscles. As this maldistribution of blood flow continues, and tissues become anoxic, the shock state worsens and becomes irreversible. The use of vasopressors hastens and worsens this process. Exceptions to the precaution of vasopressors include patients with compromised coronary or cerebral blood flow secondary to atherosclerosis (Lanros, 1988; Shoemaker et al., 1990). These individuals may benefit from the increased perfusion pressure produced by a vasopressor.

4. Vasodilators. Vasodilators increase cardiac output by decreasing the resistance (afterload) to ejection of blood from the left ventricle. They may therefore be beneficial in the treatment of shock by improving the delivery of oxygen to anoxic tissues. For patients in cardiogenic shock, the use of vasodilators in conjunction with inotropic agents will enhance the pumping ability of the heart. Vasodilators must be used cautiously in the hypotensive patient, however, and any hypovolemia should be corrected before administration.

The nurse has a critical role in maintaining parameters at prescribed levels. According to protocols and based on assessments and judgments, the nurse may titrate inotropic, vasodilator, or diuretic medications along with fluid challenges to maintain the fragile balance between overhydration and underhydration.

5. Antidysrhythmics. Although cardiac dysrhythmias are not usually the precipitating cause of shock, they can severely aggravate an already existing low output state. Therefore, the nurse needs to appropriately intervene to correct the dysrhythmia according to unit protocol.

6. Antibiotics. For the septic patient, antibiotics must be initiated to treat the infection, usually caused by the release of gram-negative bacilli into the blood. The nurse collects specimens for culturing and drug sensitivities and monitors the patient for drug reactions. The nurse should, if indicated, also anticipate the removal of the source of infection either surgically or at the bedside.

7. Additional medication. Dyphenhydramine and epinephrine are used in the treatment of anaphylactic shock to counteract the massive effects of histamine and bradykinin release resulting in bronchospasm and dilation of peripheral blood vessels.

The use of steroids in large doses is not indicated except in patients taking steroids for immunosuppression, anti-inflammatory purposes, or hypoadrenalism (Shires et al., 1995).

Circulatory Assist Devices   Several types of invasive mechanical devices can be used to support circulation when the impaired left ventricle cannot generate an effective cardiac output (Laurent-Bopp & Shinn, 1995). The most common is the intra-aortic balloon pump. It provides partial support to a compromised left ventricle by decreasing left ventricular workload and increasing coronary artery perfusion. Its use is confined to critical care units because of the high degree of technical monitoring and skill required. In patients whose ventricular function is severely compromised, a left ventricular assist device (LVAD) can be implanted at some tertiary care centers. This device assumes the total workload of the left ventricle, replacing its pumping function. Pulsatile pumps may be air-driven or electric. In the future, the electrically driven pump has the potential to be totally implantable for chronic use.

Regulating Vital Body Functions

Temperature   Typically, in shock the body's compensatory mechanisms are fully activated, causing peripheral vasoconstriction and resultant cool skin. However, the nurse should never apply external heat to such a patient. Applying heat will cause vasodilatation, which will lead to a decrease in blood pressure. Additionally, an elevation of body temperature of 1°C will increase the body metabolism by 7%. Any increase in metabolism will increase the need for oxygen and the production of carbon dioxide, thus worsening the state of shock. However, in situations where the patient is shivering (the body's way of increasing internal temperature by muscle contractions), the nurse *should* apply heat. External heat, such as a lightweight blanket, will not increase the metabolic rate as much as shivering. In the septic febrile patient, the nurse administers antipyretics to maintain normothermia and prevent the hypermetabolism caused by fever.

Nutrition   The nurse acts to ensure that the patient's nutritional needs are met. The patient in shock requires supplemental nutrition because of the hypermetabolism and increased catabolism that occur. The patient needs 3,000 to 4,000 calories a day to prevent malnutrition (Rice, 1991c). However, the patient will not be able to consume or digest food normally. The preferred route of supplemental nutrition in all cases of shock is enteral rather than parenteral (Kuhn, 1990). Enteral nutrition maintains the structure and function of the GI tract and prevents the translocation of GI flora, which can lead to septicemia. Another advantage of enteral alimentation is the avoidance of the risk of infection associated with the IV catheter necessary for parenteral nutrition. If the patient cannot take nutrients orally, a nasoduodenal feeding tube can be placed for short-term use, or a jejunostomy tube can be placed for long-term use (Kuhn, 1990). However, if the GI tract cannot be used, parenteral nutrition may be necessary. The patient should begin to receive supplemental nutrition via either route upon admission.

Providing Emotional Support

The priority in caring for the patient in actual or impending shock is prompt recognition and diagnostic investigation of inadequacies in vital organ perfusion, and then implementation of appropriate therapeutic modalities. The acute care nurse must also understand how critical it is to focus on the whole patient—to render "emergency care" to patients' emotional and spiritual needs, as well as to those of their significant others. This can be accomplished in several ways. Nurses need to display intelligent nursing action in a calm, confident manner so both patients and family feel secure in the care rendered during this stressful time. If the patient is alert, the nurse needs to acknowledge the fear and anxiety that is being experienced and explain that this is a normal and appropriate response to the situation. It is important to explain the purpose for the myriad tubes, monitors, and machines that may suddenly be attached to the patient, as well as to remove any unnecessary equipment from the immediate environment. Finally, the patient must be assured that the close continuous monitoring that is being provided ensures prompt action. When specific procedures are undertaken (e.g., tracheal intubation, invasive monitoring), the nurse must discuss the rationale for these procedures, as appropriate. Health professionals should avoid unnecessary technical conversations about equipment and therapeutics when near the patient so as not to increase the patient's apprehension.

Emotional needs can be addressed by identifying and using support systems available to the patient (family, significant other, clergy, psychiatric liaison staff). When the patient is hemodynamically stable, staff should encourage selective visiting by family members and significant others, which may assist the patient in coping with this stressful situation.

Stress reduction and self-calming techniques should be used as appropriate to reduce fear or make it more manageable. These may include breathing modification to reduce the physiological response to fear, exercises in meditation or guided imagery, music therapy (see Chapter 28), massage, and the use of affirmations and calming self-talk to enhance the patient's sense of reassurance.

Nurses also need to be cognizant of the special needs of family members, such as honest and frequent information about the patient's status and prognosis, recognition of the need for realistic expectations, mechanisms by which they can contact physicians and nurses, and reassurances that their family member is receiving optimal care (Hall, 1995; Hickey, 1990).

CASE STUDY

Mr. H is a 70-year-old man recovering in the coronary care unit from an acute anterior myocardial infarction that occurred 1 day ago. He suddenly complains of chest pressure and shortness of breath. The nurse notes that he is pale and that his skin is cool and damp. His blood pressure is 94/76 mm Hg (normal blood pressure for him is 140/70 mm Hg); his pulse is weak at 120 beats per minute and irregular. The ECG monitor shows premature ventricular beats and S-T segment elevation in the anterior V leads. His breathing is rapid at 32 breaths per minute; new crackles are heard upon auscultation. The nurse administers supplemental oxygen at 4 L/min, positions him supine with the head of the bed slightly elevated, and calls for assistance. Next the nurse inserts a large-bore IV catheter and infuses fluids at a keep-vein-open rate in anticipation of medication administration.

This nurse correctly identifies Mr. H's problem as myocardial ischemia causing pump failure and impending cardiogenic shock, a situation requiring immediate action. The nurse intervened in the early stages of shock by positioning Mr. H for optimal tissue perfusion and ventilation, administering supplemental oxygen to enhance oxygen delivery to the peripheral tissues and myocardium, and initiating IV fluids.

Next, the nurse mobilizes the health care team; the decision is made to stabilize and then transfer Mr. H to a tertiary care center for further management. Before transfer, Mr. H continues to complain of chest pain. His blood pressure is now 90/60 mm Hg, and a 12-lead ECG confirms extension of his myocardial infarction. He is given the prescribed analgesic. Mr. H is very anxious and concerned about what is happening. The critical care nurse intervenes by maintaining a calm professional manner and explaining the need for specialized equipment and procedures. The nurse tries to relieve Mr. H's anxiety as much as possible, because anxiety will cause further catecholamine release and vasoconstriction, which would increase his cardiac demands. Next, the nurse hangs a continuous dobutamine infusion to optimize cardiac output and inserts a Foley catheter to monitor his urine output. Low-dose dopamine also is started to improve renal perfusion. The critical care nurse assists with insertion of a Swan-Ganz catheter, used to evaluate the filling pressures in the heart. On insertion, Mr. H's pressures are markedly elevated (PCWP = 26 mm Hg). The nurse therefore titrates his dose of dobutamine upward, and amrinone is added in an effort to further increase his cardiac output. IV furosemide is also given to promote diuresis of excessive pulmonary extravascular fluid. Mr. H responds to these measures with lower pulmonary artery and capillary wedge pressures and an increase in his urinary output. However, despite optimal pharmacological therapy, Mr. H remains hypotensive, with cool extremities, and continues to complain of chest pain. Therefore, the cardiologist elects to insert an intra-aortic balloon. Once the nurse connects it to the pump, Mr. H's chest pain is relieved, and his vital signs stabilize. Because Mr. H's condition has improved, the nurse starts to titrate the inotropic agents downward so that the myocardial oxygen demand will be reduced. The nurse prepares the patient for transfer.

In collaboration with the physician and other members of the health team, the nurse in this situation used both assessment skills and expert judgment in correctly identifying critical interventions needed to treat Mr. H. Such prompt aggressive treatment improved Mr. H's chance of survival.

CONCLUSION
■

Shock is a devastating syndrome with dire consequences. This condition may be reversible if an accurate diagnosis is made early and aggressive shock management is implemented immediately. Because of their constant presence at the bedside, acute care nurses play a prominent role in providing surveillance, alerting the health team members when indicated, and initiating further Shock Management modalities as needed. At the same time, these nurses attend to the psychosocial needs of both critically ill patients and their significant others. Shock Management presents a true challenge to the professional nurse.

References

American College of Surgeons Committee on Trauma. (1993). *Advanced trauma life support (ATLS)*. Chicago: Author.

Bongard, F., and Sue, D. (Eds.). (1994). *Current critical care diagnosis and treatment*. Norwalk, CT: Appleton & Lange.

Bordicks, K. (1980). *Patterns of shock: Implications for nursing care* (2nd ed.). New York: Macmillan.

Chulay, M., Guzzetta, C., and Dossey, B. (1997). *AACN handbook of critical care nursing*. Stamford, CT: Appleton & Lange.

Guidelines for cardiopulmonary resuscitation and emergency care. (1992). *JAMA, 286*, 2171–2302.

Guyton, A. (Ed.). (1996). *The textbook of medical physiology*. Philadelphia: W.B. Saunders.

Hall, P. (1995). Psychosocial support for the patient's family and significant others. In P. Swearingen and J. Keen (Eds.), *Manual of critical care nursing* (3rd ed.). St. Louis: Mosby-Year Book.

Hickey, M. (1990). What are the needs of families of critically ill patients? A review of the literature since 1976. *Heart and Lung, 19*, 401–415.

Kuhn, N. (1990). Nutritional support for the shock patient. Review article. *Critical Care Nursing Clinics of North America, 2*, 201–220.

Lanros, N. (1988). *Assessment and intervention in emer-*

gency nursing (3rd ed.). Norwalk, CT: Appleton & Lange.

Laurent-Bopp, D., and Shinn, J. (1995). Shock. In S. Woods, E. Froelicher, C. J. Halpenny, and S. Motzer (Eds.), *Cardiac nursing* (3rd ed.). Philadelphia: J.B. Lippincott.

McCloskey, J., and Bulechek, G. (Eds.). (1996). *Nursing interventions classification (NIC)* (2nd ed.). St. Louis: Mosby-Year Book.

Rice, V. (1991a). Shock, a clinical syndrome: An update. Part 1: Overview of shock. *Critical Care Nurse, 11*(4), 20–27.

Rice, V. (1991b). Shock, a clinical syndrome: An update. Part 2: The stages of shock. *Critical Care Nurse, 11*(5), 74–82.

Rice, V. (1991c). Shock, a clinical syndrome: An update. Part 3: Therapeutic management. *Critical Care Nurse, 11*(6), 34–39.

Rice, V. (1991d). Shock, a clinical syndrome. Part 4: Nursing intervention. *Critical Care Nurse, 11*(7), 28–40.

Robenson-Piano, M., Holm, K., and Powers, M. (1987). An examination of the differences that occur between direct and indirect blood pressure measurement. *Heart and Lung, 16,* 285–294.

Shires, G., Barber, A., and Illner, H. (1995). Current status of resuscitation: Solutions including hypertonic saline. *Advances in Surgery, 28,* 133–170.

Shoemaker, W., Kram, H., and Appel, P. (1990). Therapy of shock based on pathophysiology, monitoring, and outcome prediction. *Critical Care Medicine, 18,* S19–25.

Summers, G. (1990). The clinical and hemodynamic presentation of the shock patient. *Critical Care Nursing Clinics of North America, 2*(2), 161–166.

Underhill, S., Woods, S., Froelicher, E., and Halpenney, C. J. (1990). *Cardiovascular medications for cardiac nursing.* Philadelphia: J.B. Lippincott.

Weeks, L. (1986). Heart failure. In L. Weeks (Ed.), *Advanced cardiovascular nursing.* Boston: Blackwell Scientific Publications.

Weil, M., von Planta, M., and Rackow, E. (1992). Acute circulatory failure (shock). In E. Braunwald (Ed.), *Heart disease.* Philadelphia: W.B. Saunders.

Woods, S. (1976). Monitoring pulmonary artery pressures. *American Journal of Nursing, 76,* 1765–1771.

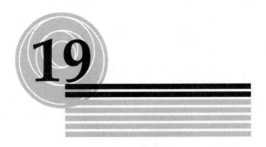

Hypoglycemia Management

Vicki L. Kraus

Hypoglycemia occurs when the blood glucose level is below normal. Its most frequent cause is the treatment of diabetes mellitus. Hypoglycemia is a potential acute complication for all persons with Type 1 diabetes and for some persons with Type 2 diabetes who are treated with insulin or oral sulfonylureas. Persons with Type 1 diabetes have an average of one to two episodes of symptomatic hypoglycemia per week, and, in a given year, 10% to 20% have an episode of severe hypoglycemia that is, at minimum, temporarily disabling and may cause seizure or coma. Hypoglycemia has been identified as the cause of death in 4% of persons with Type 1 diabetes (Cryer & Gerich, 1990).

The morbidity caused by hypoglycemia may be physical or psychosocial. Physical morbidity is largely neurological and ranges from unpleasant symptoms to focal neurological deficits. These effects all clear promptly when the blood glucose level is raised. It has yet to be proven that recurrent hypoglycemia causes permanent impairment of brain function over time (Cryer, Fisher, & Shamoon, 1994). In the recently completed Diabetes Control and Complications Trial (DCCT), despite the increased frequency of severe hypoglycemia in persons in the intensive therapy group, there was no evidence of worsening of neuropsychological or cognitive functioning over time. The neurocognitive test scores of the intensive and conventional therapy groups did not differ significantly at the end of the study (DCCT Research Group, 1996).

Fear of hypoglycemia may cause recurrent or even persistent psychosocial problems that can interfere with efforts to normalize blood glucose levels (Cox, Irvine, Gonder-Frederick, Nowacek, & Butterfield, 1987; Cryer & Gerich, 1990;

Pramming, Thorsteinsson, Bendtson, & Binder, 1991). Pramming et al. (1991) found that although mild hypoglycemic episodes did not cause much worry in persons with diabetes, anxiety related to severe hypoglycemia was almost equal to concern related to the risk of eye and kidney complications.

In the daily management of diabetes, blood glucose levels defined as hypoglycemia are individually determined. A blood glucose level of 50 mg/dL or less is always too low and requires treatment in all persons with diabetes; however, in some persons a level of 60 mg/dL, 70 mg/dL, or even higher may prompt treatment as well as a decision to adjust the diabetes regimen, that is, reduce insulin or oral sulfonylurea dose to prevent recurrence. Hypoglycemia is documented on the basis of the following sequence of events: there are symptoms of hypoglycemia; the blood glucose level is found to be low; and symptoms are relieved and the blood glucose level is raised after carbohydrate is ingested (Cryer et al., 1994).

Attention to hypoglycemia as a serious complication of the treatment of diabetes has increased as efforts to normalize blood glucose levels have intensified. The large multicenter DCCT demonstrated that maintaining blood glucose levels as close to normal as possible in persons with Type 1 diabetes using intensive insulin therapy had beneficial effects in preventing or delaying the onset of major complications or in slowing their progression. The intensive therapy group had significantly reduced risks of retinopathy, nephropathy, and neuropathy as compared with the conventional therapy group (DCCT Research Group, 1993). There is evidence to support the benefits of normalizing blood glucose levels in persons with Type 2 diabetes as well. In a smaller randomized trial involving persons with Type 2 diabetes, improved blood glucose control reduced the incidence of microvascular and neurological complications (Ohkubo et al., 1995).

Recommendations for blood glucose control established by the American Diabetes Association (ADA) are based on the evidence that normalization of blood glucose levels in persons with Type 1 and Type 2 diabetes reduces the risk of long-term complications. These recommendations are for blood glucose levels of 80 to 120 mg/dL before meals and 100 to 140 mg/dL at bedtime and hemoglobin A_{1c} levels of 7% or below. These targets should be adjusted for individuals with a history of severe hypoglycemia or hypoglycemia unawareness who do not have the capacity to understand and carry out an intensified treatment regimen or who have factors present that increase the risk or decrease the benefit of normalization of blood glucose levels, such as very young or very old age or presence of advanced diabetes complications (ADA, 1997b). As efforts are made to normalize blood glucose levels with intensified regimens, there will be an increase in the frequency and severity of hypoglycemia, necessitating immediate and effective management.

Hypoglycemia Management is defined as preventing and treating below-normal blood glucose levels. It is a direct care intervention (i.e., a treatment that is performed through interaction with a patient and involves both physiological and psychosocial nursing actions) (McCloskey & Bulechek, 1996). Hypoglycemia Management is initiated by nurses in all health care settings to prevent and treat hypoglycemia.

RELATED LITERATURE

Normal brain function is dependent on blood glucose. The brain cannot synthesize or store glucose, which makes it dependent on a constant exogenous supply.

In a person without diabetes, a fall in brain glucose levels results in the suppression of insulin secretion and a series of physiological counterregulatory responses that return blood glucose levels to normal. Glucagon is the major counterregulatory hormone, but epinephrine also has a significant effect. Growth hormone and cortisol are other counterregulatory hormones; they are released more slowly and therefore become important when hypoglycemia is prolonged. The counterregulatory hormones raise blood glucose levels by stimulating the synthesis and release of glucose by the liver, by breaking down fat and protein to provide precursors for glucose synthesis in the liver, and by inhibiting glucose uptake and use in the peripheral tissues (ADA, 1994; Amiel & Gale, 1993; Cryer et al., 1994).

Hypoglycemia occurs when the rate of glucose removal from the circulation exceeds the rate of glucose entry into the circulation. In persons with diabetes, this imbalance is most often due to a relative or absolute insulin excess. The risk factors for relative or absolute insulin excess include wrong type, excessive, or ill-timed insulin doses; decreased or delayed food intake; increased level of exercise; alcohol intake; increased sensitivity to insulin related to intensive therapy, vigorous exercise, or hypopituitarism or primary adrenocortical insufficiency; and decreased insulin clearance due to renal insufficiency (ADA, 1994; Cryer et al., 1994; Levandoski, 1993; Santiago, Levandoski, & Bubb, 1994). A relative or absolute insulin excess decreases the rate of glucose entry into the circulation and increases the rate of glucose removal from the circulation. The production and release of glucose from the liver is inhibited, or glucose use by muscle and adipose tissue is stimulated, or both (ADA, 1994; Levandoski, 1993).

In persons with Type 1 diabetes, glucose counterregulatory responses are defective. There is a persistent insulin effect even when the blood glucose level is falling, because circulating insulin levels are dependent on the timing and nature of the insulin that has been injected. The glucagon response to hypoglycemia becomes impaired in persons with diabetes a few years after its onset. The epinephrine and sympathetic responses to hypoglycemia are also lost in a significant number of persons with long-standing diabetes, placing them at special risk because of reduced warning symptoms of hypoglycemia and failure of hormone-mediated recovery (Amiel & Gale, 1993; Cryer et al., 1994). The loss of neurogenic warning symptoms of low blood glucose levels is called *hypoglycemia unawareness* (Cryer, 1993).

Hypoglycemia is most commonly self-diagnosed by persons with diabetes, so the detection of symptoms is critical to its recognition and treatment. In addition, family members, friends, coworkers, and health professionals are able to recognize signs of hypoglycemia. Each person with diabetes usually has a symptom or symptom complex that most reliably provides a warning of developing hypoglycemia and the need for immediate treatment. In addition to symptom recognition, persons with diabetes are encouraged to use self-monitoring of blood glucose to estimate the plasma blood glucose level (Cryer et al., 1994).

The symptoms of hypoglycemia are usually divided into two categories. Neurogenic symptoms are those that result from autonomic nervous system discharge mediated by catecholamines and acetylcholine. These symptoms include shakiness, sweating, and palpitations. Neuroglycopenic symptoms are those that result from the low glucose levels in the brain. These symptoms are primarily cognitive and behavioral and include loss of consciousness and seizures (Cryer et al., 1994). Symptoms of hypoglycemia are similar in Type 1 and Type 2 diabetes (Hepburn, MacLeod, Pell, Scougal, & Frier, 1992). In children, neurogenic and neuroglycopenic symptoms are generated at similar blood glucose levels, and behavior changes—acting aggressive, argumentative, irritable, and naughty—are the primary signs (McCrimmon, Gold, Deary, Kelnar, & Frier, 1995). The symptoms of hypoglycemia and their classifications are listed in Table 19–1.

Hypoglycemia can be classified as mild, moderate, or severe on the basis of symptoms. This classification is helpful in understanding the clinical presentations of hypoglycemia but does not necessarily mean that hypoglycemia will progress in a linear order (Cox, Gonder-Frederick, Antoun, Cryer, & Clarke, 1993). Mild hypoglycemia is characterized by tremors, palpitations, sweating, and hunger. These symptoms are mainly neurogenic and usually not accompanied by any cognitive impairment. Moderate hypoglycemia is characterized by neurogenic and neuroglycopenic symptoms, such as headache, irritability, impaired thinking, and drowsiness. Because some cognitive impairment is present, assistance with treatment may be necessary. Moderate hypoglycemia tends to last longer, produces more severe symptoms, and requires more simple carbohydrate intake for effective treatment (ADA, 1994). Severe hypoglycemia is characterized by neurological impairment that prevents self-treatment and places the person with diabetes at risk for injury to self or others (DCCT Research Group, 1991, 1997).

Severe hypoglycemia was the most common adverse event in the DCCT, occurring three times more often in the intensive therapy group (DCCT Research Group, 1995). There were 1,441 patients with Type 1 diabetes in the DCCT who were followed an average of 6.5 years. There were 3,788 episodes of severe hypoglycemia (requiring assistance), and, of those episodes, 1,027 were associated with seizure or coma. Sixty-five percent of the patients in the intensive therapy group, as compared with 35% of the patients in the conventional therapy group, had at least one episode of severe hypoglycemia by the end of the study. The overall rates of severe hypoglycemia were 61.2 per 100 patient-years in the intensive therapy group, as compared with 18.7 per 100 patient-years in the

Table 19–1 Signs and Symptoms of Hypoglycemia

Neurogenic	Neuroglycopenic
Shakiness/tremor	Headache
Sweating	Fatigue/drowsiness
Nervousness	Weakness
Anxiety	Warmth
Irritability	Dizziness/faintness
Impatience	Blurred vision
Tachycardia/palpitations	Nightmares/crying out during sleep
Chills/clamminess	Amnesia
Light-headedness	Paresthesias
Pallor	Difficulty concentrating
Hunger	Difficulty speaking
Nausea	Uncoordination
	Behavior change
	Confusion
	Coma
	Seizure
	Death

Sources: Cryer, P. E., Fisher, J. N., and Shamoon, H. (1994). Hypoglycemia. *Diabetes Care, 17,* 734–755; Field, J. B. (1989). Hypoglycemia. Definition, clinical presentations, classification, and laboratory tests. *Endocrinology and Metabolism Clinics of North America, 18*(1), 27–43; American Diabetes Association (1996a). *American Diabetes Association complete guide to diabetes.* Alexandria, VA: Author.

conventional therapy group. This increased risk of severe hypoglycemia with intensive therapy persisted over the duration of the study (DCCT Research Group, 1997).

Early in the DCCT, investigators analyzed 714 episodes of severe hypoglycemia that had occurred in 216 of the study participants. Over half the episodes (55%) had occurred during sleep. There were no warning symptoms in 36% of the episodes that occurred during times of wakefulness. Although the intensive therapy group had more episodes of severe hypoglycemia, the proportion of persons experiencing hypoglycemia during sleep and without warning was the same in both groups. A missed meal was the only conventional hypoglycemia risk factor that occurred significantly more often on a hypoglycemia day as compared with a nonhypoglycemia day. Five significant risk factors for severe hypoglycemia were identified: previous severe hypoglycemia, longer duration of diabetes, lower recent hemoglobin A_{1c}, higher baseline hemoglobin A_{1c}, and higher baseline insulin dose. The most powerful predictor was previous severe hypoglycemia (DCCT Research Group, 1991). These risk factors have not been found to be sufficiently sensitive or specific for the selection of persons with diabetes at higher risk and consequently for the reduction of the occurrence of severe hypoglycemia. The most effective approach to reducing the risk of severe hypoglycemia is the modification of the goal for blood glucose control. There is no hemoglobin A_{1c} threshold to use as a marker for reduction of risk of severe hypoglycemia; instead, this risk appears to be continuously and inversely related to the hemoglobin A_{1c} level (ADA, 1995).

The efficacy of carbohydrate sources in raising blood glucose levels in persons with diabetes has been studied and provides evidence on which to base hypoglycemia treatment. A 20 g dose of glucose has been recommended and may be taken in the form of glucose or carbohydrate-containing foods. The greatest blood glucose response from this amount of glucose occurs in 15 minutes and lasts for about 45 minutes. After 60 minutes, the glucose level begins to fall, making additional food intake necessary to prevent recurrent hypoglycemia (Brodows, Williams, & Amatruda, 1984; Slama et al., 1990; Wiethrop & Cryer, 1993).

Current ADA recommendations for hypoglycemia treatment are to use 15 g of simple carbohydrate at 15-minute intervals until hypoglycemia is relieved and a follow-up snack if a meal or snack is not scheduled within 30 minutes (ADA, 1996a, 1997a, 1997b). Typically, with mild hypoglycemia, one treatment with 15 g of carbohydrate is effective. With moderate hypoglycemia, a repeat treatment of 15 g of carbohydrate will probably be necessary (ADA, 1994). Fifteen-gram carbohydrate sources for treatment of hypoglycemia are listed in Table 19–2.

Severe hypoglycemia may be able to be treated with oral carbohydrate if it is provided with the assistance of another person; however, usually parenteral glucagon or intravenous glucose is necessary (DCCT Research Group, 1991). Alterations in consciousness place a person at risk for aspiration if given oral carbohydrate; however, use of glucose gels between the cheek and gum may work if no other treatment is immediately available. Glucagon can be administered by a spouse, family member, friend, or coworker and is the treatment of choice for severe hypoglycemia outside the hospital setting. Glucagon stimulates production and release of glucose by the liver and results in an increase in the blood glucose level and recovery of normal mental function within 10 to 15 minutes. The dose of glucagon for a child younger than 5 years is 0.25 to 0.50 mg; for a child 5 to 10 years old, 0.50 to 1 mg; and for a child older than 10

Table 19–2   Fifteen-Gram Carbohydrate Sources for Treatment of Hypoglycemia

- 4 oz (½ cup) orange, apple, pineapple, or grapefruit juice
- 3 oz (⅓ cup) grape, prune, or cranberry juice
- 4–6 oz (½ can) nondiet soft drink
- ½ cup nondiet prepared gelatin
- 2 Tbsp raisins
- 5 Lifesavers
- 5 small gumdrops
- 6 jellybeans
- 1 c skim milk
- 3–5 glucose tablets or a tube of glucose gel (per manufacturer's directions)
- 3–4 tsp sugar
- 1 Tbsp honey or corn syrup
- 1 tube (0.68 oz) Cake Mate decorator gel

Sources: ADA. (1997a). Answers to frequently asked questions about low blood glucose. *Diabetes Spectrum 10*(1), 71–72; ADA. (1997b). Standards of medical care for patients with diabetes mellitus. *Diabetes Care 20*(Suppl. 1), S5–S13; American Diabetes Association (1996a). *American Diabetes Association complete guide to diabetes.* Alexandria, VA: Author; Pennington, J. A. T. (1994). *Bowes' and Church's food values of portions commonly used* (16th ed.). Philadelphia, J. B. Lippincott.

years and for adults, 1 mg. Intravenous glucose is the treatment of choice for severe hypoglycemia in the hospital setting. The usual dose is 10 to 25 g of 50% dextrose given over 1 to 3 minutes. Once this bolus dose is given, 5 to 10 g of glucose should be given per hour by continuous intravenous infusion. Following treatment with glucagon or intravenous glucose, the person with diabetes should be given oral carbohydrate once consciousness is regained (ADA, 1994).

Activities designed to prevent hypoglycemia are a critical component of hypoglycemia management. Insulin regimens that simulate insulin levels present in persons without diabetes should be used in the management of diabetes (e.g., multiple daily injections, continuous subcutaneous insulin infusion therapy, use of the fast-acting insulin analogue lispro) (Ahern & Tamborlane, 1997). The result is reduction of instances of insulin excess and, consequently, reduced frequency of hypoglycemia. In addition, instruction about the interaction of insulin, food intake, and exercise will help patients make anticipatory adjustments in insulin taken and food eaten to prevent hypoglycemia (ADA, 1994; Levandoski, 1993). The information required to make these adjustments includes insulin action patterns, the carbohydrate content of foods, and the immediate and delayed effects of exercise on blood glucose levels (Havlin & Cryer, 1988).

Self-monitoring of blood glucose levels is of critical importance in both the prevention and the detection of hypoglycemia (Ahern & Tamborlane, 1997; Levandoski, 1993). When the treatment of diabetes is intensified, the frequency of self-monitoring of blood glucose levels should be increased and should be done, at minimum, four times daily—before meals and at bedtime—as well as after meals, during the night, before and after exercise, and before driving. The results are used to improve control and reduce the risk of hypoglycemia (ADA, 1995). In addition, measurement of the blood glucose level when hypoglycemia is suspected (Levandoski, 1993) or to evaluate the effectiveness of treatment is recommended.

Persons with diabetes and members of their household, family members, and close friends should be instructed on signs, symptoms, risk factors, and treatments of hypoglycemia (Ahern & Tamborlane, 1997; Havlin & Cryer, 1988; Levandoski, 1993). Carbohydrate sources should be carried at all times, and family members and close associates should be instructed on the use and administration of glucagon (Havlin & Cryer, 1988; Levandoski, 1993). This instruction should be initial and ongoing and should be repeated at key times, such as when the treatment regimen is intensified or when an anticipated event may increase the risk for hypoglycemia (Levandoski, 1993). When intensive therapy is initiated, persons with diabetes should be warned that the incidence of hypoglycemia increases, that symptoms of hypoglycemia may change, and that the glucose threshold at which symptoms occur often also changes (ADA, 1995; Ahern & Tamborlane, 1997). Instruction should include the advice to provide immediate treatment of hypoglycemia when neuroglycopenic symptoms occur (Ahern & Tamborlane, 1997). Persons with diabetes should be instructed to carry an identification card or wear medical identification jewelry to alert others to the fact that they have diabetes and take insulin (Levandoski, 1993) or medication to lower the blood glucose level.

Ongoing contact with the diabetes care team for assistance in making adjustments in the treatment regimen is essential in preventing or reducing the incidence of hypoglycemia. This is especially important when intensive therapy is initiated (Ahern & Tamborlane, 1997). After an episode of hypoglycemia, problem solving to identify potentially remediable risk factors is indicated to allow appropriate changes in self-management behaviors (ADA, 1995; Havlin & Cryer, 1988), and positive feedback should be given when good judgment was used to prevent or treat hypoglycemia. Hypoglycemia that is occurring on a daily basis mandates an adjustment in the diabetes treatment regimen (Levandoski, 1993).

For persons at risk for severe hypoglycemia, such as those with hypoglycemia unawareness, goals for blood glucose control should be modified (ADA, 1995). There is evidence that rigorous avoidance of hypoglycemia (Cranston, Lomas, Maran, MacDonald, & Amiel, 1994; Dagago-Jack, Rattarasarn, & Cryer, 1994) and intensive blood glucose awareness training (Cox et al., 1995) can improve awareness of hypoglycemia symptoms (ADA, 1995; Ahern & Tamborlane, 1997). Hypoglycemia avoidance has been found to require substantial time and effort by both the person with diabetes and the diabetes care team. Important features of hypoglycemia avoidance are clear understanding of the need to avoid low blood glucose levels, reductions in overnight insulin doses following vigorous exercise, between-meal and bedtime snacks, re-education to overcome fear of hypoglycemia, and weekly contact to facilitate recognition of blood glucose patterns (Cranston et al., 1994).

INTERVENTION

The Nursing Interventions Classification (NIC) intervention Hypoglycemia Management is shown in Table 19–3. Hypoglycemia Management activities are of two types: those that a nurse performs to monitor for signs and symptoms of hypoglycemia and to provide treatment and those that a nurse performs to prevent hypoglycemia and ensure its appropriate treatment by persons with diabetes or their significant others.

A critical first step in the management of hypoglycemia is the identification of persons with diabetes who are at risk for its development. This includes all persons with Type 1 diabetes and those persons with Type 2 diabetes who are treated with insulin or an oral sulfonylurea, such as glyburide, glipizide, or glimepiride. Persons with diabetes who are at risk should be monitored for signs and symptoms of hypoglycemia at intervals that are appropriate to the situation. This includes monitoring blood glucose levels using a meter, observing persons for signs of hypoglycemia, and querying them about the presence of symptoms.

Table 19–3 Hypoglycemia Management

DEFINITION: Preventing and treating low blood glucose levels.

ACTIVITIES:

Identify patient at risk for hypoglycemia

Determine hypoglycemia awareness/unawareness

Monitor blood glucose levels, as indicated

Monitor for signs and symptoms of hypoglycemia, e.g., shakiness, tremor, sweating, nervousness, anxiety, irritability, impatience, tachycardia, palpitations, chills, clamminess, light-headedness, pallor, hunger, nausea, headache, tiredness, drowsiness, weakness, warmth, dizziness, faintness, blurred vision, nightmares, crying out in sleep, paraesthesias, difficulty concentrating, difficulty speaking, incoordination, behavior change, confusion, coma, seizure

Provide simple carbohydrate, as indicated

Provide complex carbohydrate and protein, as indicated

Administer glucagon, as indicated

Contact emergency medical services, as necessary

Administer intravenous glucose, as indicated

Maintain IV access, as appropriate

Maintain patent airway, as necessary

Protect from injury, as necessary

Review events prior to hypoglycemia to determine probable cause

Provide feedback regarding appropriateness of self-management of hypoglycemia

Instruct patient and significant others on signs and symptoms, risk factors, and treatment of hypoglycemia

Instruct patient to have simple carbohydrate available at all times

Instruct patient to obtain and carry/wear appropriate emergency identification

Instruct significant others in the use and administration of glucagon, as appropriate

Instruct in interaction of diet, insulin, and exercise

Provide assistance in making self-care decisions to prevent hypoglycemia, e.g., reducing insulin or increasing food intake for exercise

Encourage self-monitoring of blood glucose levels

Encourage ongoing telephone contact with diabetes care team for consultation regarding adjustments in treatment regimen

Collaborate with patient and diabetes care team to make changes in insulin regimen, e.g., multiple daily injections, as indicated

Modify blood glucose goals for hypoglycemia unawareness

Inform patient of increased risk of hypoglycemia with intensive therapy and normalization of blood glucose levels

Instruct patient regarding probable changes in hypoglycemia symptoms with intensive therapy and normalization of blood glucose levels

Source: McCloskey, J. C., and Bulechek, G. M. (1996). *Nursing interventions classification (NIC)* (2nd ed.). St. Louis: Mosby–Year Book.

When hypoglycemia is suspected, blood glucose levels should be measured to verify its presence; however, treatment should not be delayed for a blood glucose measurement if one is not immediately available. As soon as hypoglycemia is identified, 15 g of simple carbohydrate should be given as treatment. Every 15 minutes another 15 g of carbohydrate should be given if the blood glucose is not in the target range or if the person continues to have symptoms of hypoglycemia. The amount of carbohydrate given may be increased or decreased based on consideration of several factors, including the level of the blood glucose, the goals for blood glucose control, the planned activity, and the proximity of the hypoglycemic episode to the next meal. Once the symptoms are relieved and the blood glucose is back in the target range, an additional snack consisting of complex carbohydrate and protein should be given if a snack or meal is not scheduled to be eaten within 30 minutes. This is to ensure prevention of a recurrence of hypoglycemia before the next time food is eaten.

If hypoglycemia is severe, glucagon or intravenous dextrose should be administered. Glucagon should be administered by a family member or significant other, and emergency medical services should be contacted. Intravenous dextrose is always the treatment of choice when emergency medical services are available. Severe hypoglycemia in the hospitalized person with diabetes may require continuous infusion of dextrose-containing fluids and, consequently, maintenance of intravenous access. A person who is unconscious or having seizures because of severe hypoglycemia requires maintenance of a patent airway and protection from injury.

After an episode of hypoglycemia, the events that preceded it should be reviewed in an effort to determine what may have been the cause. This review may help prevent hypoglycemia in the future, and it also provides instruction on diabetes self-management. Providing feedback regarding the appropriateness of self-management of hypoglycemia serves to enhance the person's feelings of competence in performing self-care.

Instructions about signs and symptoms, risk factors, and treatment of hypoglycemia are needed by persons with diabetes and by their families, significant others, and associates when treatment is initiated, and instructions should be repeated when a need for review and reinforcement is identified. Instructions should emphasize the need to have a simple carbohydrate available at all times and to wear medical identification indicating the potential for hypoglycemia. Family members and others should be instructed in the use and administration of glucagon. In addition, instruction on the interaction of diet, insulin, and exercise is fundamental to making self-care decisions that prevent hypoglycemia. Persons with diabetes often need assistance in making these self-care decisions on an ongoing basis. Self-monitoring of blood glucose levels is necessary for all persons with diabetes, and more frequent monitoring is indicated for persons who are at risk for hypoglycemia. Ongoing telephone contact with the diabetes care team to review blood glucose monitoring results and discuss indicated adjustments in the treatment regimen is directed at reducing the frequency and severity of hypoglycemia.

Frequent or severe hypoglycemia may indicate that the insulin regimen should be changed. The decision to make this change should be collaborative, with the risks and benefits of proposed regimens clearly described. When persons with diabetes have hypoglycemia unawareness, the goals for blood glucose control should be modified to reduce the risk of hypoglycemia. If the therapy is being intensified in an effort to normalize blood glucose levels, persons with diabetes should be informed that the risk of hypoglycemia is higher and that symptoms that warn of its occurrence may change—that is, neuroglycopenic symptoms may predominate.

NURSING DIAGNOSES AND APPROPRIATE PATIENT GROUPS

The North American Nursing Diagnosis Association (NANDA) has no diagnoses that can be linked with the NIC intervention Hypoglycemia Management (McCloskey & Bulechek, 1996; NANDA, 1994). Hypoglycemia is a medical diagnosis or an adverse effect of the treatment of diabetes and consequently is not included as a NANDA diagnosis at the present time. A nursing diagnosis is "a clinical judgment about individual . . . responses to actual and potential health problems" (NANDA, 1994, p. 7). The identification of actual or potential hypoglycemia is a clinical judgment. Hypoglycemia should be developed as a nursing diagnosis within the NANDA classification.

Hypoglycemia Management is an intervention that may be needed by all persons with Type 1 diabetes and by some persons with Type 2 diabetes. Most persons with diabetes have one of two clinical types: Type 1, which is caused primarily by pancreatic islet β-cell destruction stemming from autoimmune causes, and Type 2, which results from insulin resistance and a defect in insulin secretion (Expert Committee on the Diagnosis and Classification of Diabetes Mellitus, 1997). The treatment of Type 1 diabetes always consists of insulin, diet, and exercise. The treatment of Type 2 diabetes may include insulin or oral agents and always includes diet, weight reduction as needed, and an exercise program. Approximately 43% of adults with diabetes use insulin, and about the same proportion use oral agents (ADA, 1996b). Self-monitoring of blood glucose is done by all persons with diabetes to evaluate the effectiveness of and make adjustments in the treatment regimen (ADA, 1997c).

There are approximately 8 million persons with known diabetes in the U.S. population. The estimated prevalence of Type 1 diabetes is nearly 675,000, with approximately 127,000 of these cases occurring in children. Approximately 90% to 95% of persons with diabetes who are older than age 20 have Type 2 diabetes (ADA, 1996b).

OUTCOMES

The critical and most definitive outcome in evaluating the effectiveness of Hypoglycemia Management is that the blood glucose level is raised to normal or to within the target range. Relief of symptoms is also used to evaluate the effectiveness of Hypoglycemia Management when persons are aware of hypoglycemia symptoms. In addition, two outcomes in the Nursing Outcomes Classification (NOC) could be selected to evaluate the impact of Hypoglycemia Management: Symptom Control Behavior and Compliance Behavior. Symptom Control Behavior is defined as "personal actions to minimize perceived adverse changes in physical and emotional functioning" (Johnson & Maas, 1997, p. 287). Indicators for this outcome are related to self-care behaviors that persons with diabetes would have to carry out to effectively prevent, detect, and treat hypoglycemia. Compliance Behavior is defined as "actions taken on the basis of professional advice to promote wellness, recovery, and rehabilitation" (Johnson & Maas, 1997, p. 132). Indicators for this outcome are related to following the diabetes treatment regimen and making appropriate modifications that may be necessary for the prevention of hypoglycemia.

CASE STUDY

EB is a 36-year-old woman who has had Type I diabetes for 24 years. Her insulin regimen consists of Ultralente Insulin taken twice daily and Regular Insulin taken three times daily, before each meal. She also uses supplemental Regular Insulin for blood glucose levels that are over 200 mg/dL. She does not follow her 1,900-calorie ADA diet, and currently she does not exercise regularly. Her diabetes control has not been ac-

ceptable; a recent hemoglobin A_{1c} of 9.3% translates to an average blood glucose level of 224 mg/dL. In addition, her record of self-monitoring of her blood glucose level indicates highly variable blood glucose levels and at least four to five hypoglycemia episodes per week. She is aware of hypoglycemia symptoms; the most common ones for her are sweating and palpitations when her blood glucose level is in the 50s or 60s and numbness and tingling of her tongue and nose when her blood glucose level is in the 40s.

EB stopped by the diabetes clinic to have her prescriptions rewritten on a day she did not have an appointment. It was late in the afternoon, and she had been at the medical center most of the day for appointments in other clinics. After the prescriptions were written, they were taken to EB by the clinic secretary. He informed the advanced practice nurse that EB needed something else but was unable to describe what it was and that she was crying. The advanced practice nurse went to the waiting room and found the patient crying, perspiring profusely, and having difficulty speaking. EB was immediately given 6 ounces of orange juice, and her blood glucose level was measured and found to be 36 mg/dL. EB said that she had not taken the time to finish her lunch because of all the appointments she had and instead had taken small snacks throughout the day. She had taken her noon Regular Insulin. She had done more walking than usual to go to the various clinics where she had appointments. Because EB had not eaten lunch, she was also given three graham crackers.

After 15 minutes, EB's blood glucose level was again measured; it was 48 mg/dL. She said that her symptoms were beginning to diminish, and she had stopped crying and was speaking more clearly. She was given an additional 6 ounces of orange juice. After another 15-minute interval, another blood glucose level measurement gave a result of 82 mg/dL. She was going to be driving home and would not be eating her evening meal for 1 to 2 hours. Consequently, she was given 8 ounces of skim milk and 3 additional graham crackers.

When EB's blood sugar was >80 mg/dL, and her symptoms of hypoglycemia had been relieved, the events leading up to this episode of severe hypoglycemia were reviewed. She had taken her noon Regular Insulin and had not eaten, and she had had an increased exercise level. She had an excess of insulin that caused her to have hypoglycemia. Options for preventing this situation in the future were discussed, including reducing the amount of her noon Regular Insulin or eliminating it when she was not planning to eat her usual meal, and eating more food to compensate for the increase in her exercise level. She was given instructions to begin calling the advanced practice nurse to report blood glucose results and make any indicated adjustments in her insulin regimen.

SUMMARY

Efforts to normalize blood glucose levels to reduce the risk of long-term complications of diabetes have resulted in an increase in the frequency and severity of hypoglycemia. Hypoglycemia Management is a direct care intervention that is implemented by nurses in all health care settings to prevent and treat hypoglycemia. It includes activities directed at monitoring for signs and symptoms, providing treatment, and preventing or reducing the frequency and severity of hypoglycemia.

References

Ahern, J., and Tamborlane, W. V. (1997). Steps to reduce the risks of severe hypoglycemia. *Diabetes Spectrum, 10*(1), 39–41.

American Diabetes Association. (1994). *Medical management of insulin-dependent (type I) diabetes* (2nd ed.). Alexandria, VA: Author.

American Diabetes Association. (1995). *Intensive diabetes management.* Alexandria, VA: Author.

American Diabetes Association. (1996a). *American Diabetes Association complete guide to diabetes.* Alexandria, VA: Author.

American Diabetes Association. (1996b). *Diabetes 1996: Vital statistics.* Alexandria, VA: Author.

American Diabetes Association. (1997a). Answers to frequently asked questions about low blood glucose. *Diabetes Spectrum, 10*(1), 71–72.

American Diabetes Association. (1997b). Standards of medical care for patients with diabetes mellitus. *Diabetes Care, 20*(Suppl. 1), S5–S13.

American Diabetes Association. (1997c). Tests of glycemia in diabetes. *Diabetes Care, 20*(Suppl. 1), S18–S20.

Amiel, S. A. (1994). R. D. Lawrence lecture 1994. Limits of normality: The mechanisms of hypoglycaemia unawareness. *Diabetic Medicine, 11*, 918–924.

Amiel, S. A., and Gale, E. (1993). Physiologic responses to hypoglycemia. *Diabetes Care, 16*(Suppl. 3), 48–55.

Brodows, R. G., Williams, C., and Amatruda J. M. (1984).

Treatment of insulin reactions in diabetics. *JAMA, 252,* 3378–3381.

Cox, D. J., Gonder-Frederick, L., Antoun, B., Cryer, P. E., and Clarke, W. L. (1993). Perceived symptoms in the recognition of hypoglycemia. *Diabetes Care, 16,* 519–527.

Cox, D. J., Gonder-Frederick, L., Polonsky, W., Schlundt, D., Julian, D., and Clarke, W. (1995). A multicenter evaluation of blood glucose awareness training—II. *Diabetes Care, 18,* 523–528.

Cox, D. J., Irvine, A., Gonder-Frederick, L., Nowacek, G., and Butterfield, J. (1987). Fear of hypoglycemia: Quantification, validation, and utilization. *Diabetes Care, 10,* 617–621.

Cranston, I., Lomas, J., Maran, A., MacDonald, P. I., and Amiel, S. A. (1994). Restoration of hypoglycemia awareness in patients with long-duration insulin-dependent diabetes. *Lancet, 344,* 283–287.

Cryer, P. E. (1993). Hypoglycemia unawareness in IDDM. *Diabetes Care, 16*(Suppl. 3), 40–47.

Cryer, P. E., Fisher, J. N., and Shamoon, H. (1994). Hypoglycemia. *Diabetes Care, 17,* 734–755.

Cryer, P. E., and Gerich J. E. (1990). Hypoglycemia in insulin-dependent diabetes mellitus: Insulin excess and defective glucose counterregulation. In H. Rifkin and D. Porte (Eds.), *Ellenberg and Rifkin's diabetes mellitus. Theory and practice.* (4th ed., pp. 526–526). New York: Elsevier.

Dagago-Jack, S., Rattarasarn, C., and Cryer, P. E. (1994). Reversal of hypoglycemia unawareness, but not defective glucose counterregulation, in IDDM. *Diabetes, 43,* 1426–1434.

Diabetes Control and Complications Trial Research Group. (1991). Epidemiology of severe hypoglycemia in the Diabetes Control and Complications Trial. *American Journal of Medicine, 90,* 450–459.

Diabetes Control and Complications Trial Research Group. (1993). The effect of intensive treatment of diabetes on the development and progression of long-term complications in insulin-dependent diabetes mellitus. *New England Journal of Medicine, 329,* 977–986.

Diabetes Control and Complications Trial Research Group. (1995). Adverse events and their association with treatment regimens in the Diabetes Control and Complications Trial. *Diabetes Care, 18,* 1415–1427.

Diabetes Control and Complications Trial Research Group. (1996). Effects of intensive diabetes therapy on neuropsychological function in adults in the Diabetes Control and Complications Trial. *Annals of Internal Medicine, 124,* 379–388.

Diabetes Control and Complications Trial Research Group. (1997). Hypoglycemia in the Diabetes Control and Complications Trial. *Diabetes, 46,* 271–286.

Expert Committee on the Diagnosis and Classification of Diabetes Mellitus. (1997). Report of the Expert Committee on the Diagnosis and Classification of Diabetes Mellitus. *Diabetes Care, 20,* 1184–1185.

Field, J. B. (1989). Hypoglycemia. Definition, clinical presentations, classification, and laboratory tests. *Endocrinology and Metabolism Clinics of North America, 18*(1), 27–43.

Havlin, C. E., and Cryer, P. E. (1988). Hypoglycemia: The limiting factor in the management of insulin-dependent diabetes mellitus. *Diabetes Educator, 14,* 407–411.

Hepburn, D. A., MacLeod, K. M., Pell, A. C., Scougal, I. J., and Frier, B. M. (1992). Frequency and symptoms of hypoglycaemia experience by patients with type 2 diabetes treated with insulin. *Diabetic Medicine, 10,* 231–237.

Johnson, M., and Maas, M. (Eds.). (1997). *Nursing outcomes classification (NOC).* St. Louis: Mosby.

Levandoski, L. A. (1993). Hypoglycemia. In V. Peragallo-Dittko (Ed.), *A core curriculum for diabetes education* (pp. 351–372). Chicago: American Association of Diabetes Educators and AADE Education and Research Foundation.

McCloskey, J. C., and Bulechek, G. M. (Eds.). (1996). *Nursing interventions classification (NIC)* (2nd ed.). St. Louis: Mosby.

McCrimmon, R. J., Gold, A. E., Deary, I. J., Kelnar, C. J. H., and Frier, B. M. (1995). Symptoms of hypoglycemia in children with diabetes. *Diabetes Care, 18,* 858–861.

North American Nursing Diagnosis Association. (1994). *NANDA nursing diagnoses: Definitions and classification, 1995–1996.* Philadelphia: Author.

Ohkubo, Y., Kishikawa, H., Araki, E., Miyata, T., Isami, S., Motoyoshi, S., Kojima, Y., Furuyoshi, N., and Shichiri, M. (1995). Intensive insulin therapy prevents the progression of diabetic microvascular complications in Japanese patients with non–insulin-dependent diabetes mellitus: A randomized prospective 6-year study. *Diabetes Research and Clinical Practice, 28,* 103–117.

Pennington, J. A. T. (1994). *Bowes' and Church's food values of portions commonly used* (16th ed.). Philadelphia: J. B. Lippincott.

Pramming, S., Thorsteinsson, B., Bendtson, I., and Binder, C. (1991). Symptomatic hypoglycemia in 411 type I diabetic patients. *Diabetic Medicine, 8,* 217–222.

Santiago, J. V., Levandoski, L. A., and Bubb, J. (1994). Hypoglycemia in patients with type I diabetes. In H. E. Lebovitz (Ed.), *Therapy for diabetes mellitus and related disorders* (2nd ed., pp. 170–177). Alexandria, VA: American Diabetes Association.

Slama, G., Traynard, P., Desplanque, N., Pudar, H., Dhunputh, I., Letanoux, M., Bornet, F. R. J., and Tchobroutsky, G. (1990). The search for an optimized treatment of hypoglycemia. *Archives of Internal Medicine, 150,* 589–593.

Wiethrop, B. V., and Cryer, P. E. (1993). Alanine and terbutaline in the treatment of hypoglycemia in IDDM. *Diabetes Care, 16,* 1131–1136.

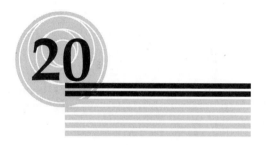

Intracranial Pressure Monitoring

Mary Kay Bader and Linda Littlejohns

Increased intracranial pressure (ICP) is an abnormal state of high pressure inside the cranium that results from an increase in blood, cerebrospinal fluid (CSF), tissue, or water content. In addition, increased ICP may occur as a result of premature closure of sutures or fontanels of the skull. It occurs in individuals across the life span. Intracranial Pressure Monitoring is used to assist the health care team in assessing the dynamics of the cranium and directing activities to regulate ICP.

Monitoring ICP requires nurses to be knowledgeable in many aspects of care. Nurses use a focused neurological assessment to monitor and detect clinical changes indicative of increased ICP. The various types of ICP monitoring tools require personnel capable of maintaining the system and using the data from the monitor to direct care. By understanding the pathophysiological changes of this clinical state, nurses plan care activities to optimize the patient's status. Strategies used by nurses to reduce ICP and optimize perfusion to the brain are both independent and interdependent. Clinical research related to this topic is evolving, and guidelines are available to direct nursing action.

BACKGROUND

There is a natural balance within the cranium. Normally, the contents of the adult cranium include 1,400 mL of brain tissue, 150 mL of blood, and 150 mL of CSF (Hickey, 1997). These three major substances exist in a state of equilibrium inside a closed, rigid box. If one of the three increases in content, one or both of the other components must decrease in content in order for the cranium to remain in balance. In situations where there is an increase in one but no substantial decrease in another component of the cranium, an increase in ICP results (Hickey, 1997). Normal ICP ranges from 0 to 10 mm Hg. ICPs greater than 20 mm Hg are considered elevated (Lang & Chesnut, 1994).

The causes of increased ICP can be divided into five major categories:

1. Increases in blood volume occur as a result of hemorrhage inside the cranium; cerebrovasodilation of blood vessels secondary to hypoxia, hypercapnia, and hyperthermia; or decreased venous return from the cranium to the heart.

2. Increases in tissue volume or brain water content result from tumors, abscesses, or cerebral edema secondary to ischemic stroke, trauma, or hypoxic injuries.

3. Increases in CSF volume occur in hydrocephalus and choroid plexus tumors, resulting in an overproduction of CSF.

4. Congenital causes that may result in increased ICP include Arnold-Chiari malformation, craniosynostosis, myelomeningocele, and congenital cysts.

5. Metabolic imbalances such as inappropriate antidiuretic hormone (ADH), hypertonic states, acidosis, hypoxia, hypercapnia, hyperthermia, and drug or lead poisoning can lead to states of increased ICP (American Association of Neuroscience Nurses [AANN], 1996).

Indications for ICP monitoring are based on clinical and radiographic evaluation (Lang & Chesnut, 1994). The most common indication for ICP monitoring is traumatic brain injury. According to the published Guidelines for the Management of Severe Head Injury, ICP monitoring is appropriate when patients present with severe head injury, defined as a score on the Glasgow Coma Scale (GCS) of between 3 and 8 after cardiopulmonary resuscitation and concurrent abnormal computed tomography (CT) scan of the brain (Bullock et al., 1995). In addition, the document identifies patients with severe head injury and normal CT scans as candidates for ICP monitoring if two or more of the following factors are present: (1) age older than 40 years, (2) unilateral or bilateral motor posturing, and (3) systolic blood pressure (BP) less than 90 mm Hg (Bullock et al., 1995).

There are other clinical situations that call for ICP monitoring. Patients with the following diagnoses are candidates for monitoring: ruptured cerebral aneurysm, extensive surgical manipulation during a craniotomy, hydrocephalus, Reye's syndrome, stroke, hypoxic insults, primary or metastatic tumors, encephalitis, and encephalopathic states (AANN, 1996; Lang & Chesnut, 1994; Marshall, Marshall, Vos, & Chesnut, 1990; McQuillan, 1991). Contraindications to monitoring include the presence of a coagulopathy and immunosuppression states (Lang & Chesnut, 1994).

Care must be taken to ensure that the clinical examination of the patient is not diminished or overlooked. The examination must be complete, comprehensive, and continuous; it is the basis of Intracranial Pressure Monitoring. An understanding of neuroanatomy and potential changes in patients in the presence of increased ICP is essential to the successful management of this patient population.

Intracranial hypertension is present in the majority of patients with severe head injury and if untreated can result in herniation of brain tissue through the foramen magnum or the incisura or under the falx, causing damage to vital structures. Although we have difficulty obtaining data on regional blood flow and perfusion in the microvasculature, the fundamental goal of ICP management remains to eliminate secondary injury resulting from ischemia. The focus has therefore shifted from ICP to cerebral perfusion pressure (CPP), and many treatment modalities have become outdated because of their potential to increase cerebral ischemia. In the face of this change in thinking, we have become increasingly aware that each patient warrants individual evaluation and targeted therapy (Chesnut, 1996).

As the volume increases within the cranial vault, pressure is exerted on exquisitely sensitive regions of the brain, causing the associated impairment in function. It is well accepted that the respiratory pattern allows for recognition of evolving cerebral insults, and changes in its rate, rhythm, and depth must be noted. Potential patterns include Cheyne-Stokes respiration, central neurogenic hyperventilation, and apneustic, cluster, and ataxic breathing patterns (Hickey, 1997; Plum & Posner, 1980).

Cardiovascular regulation in the medulla and hypothalamus provides rapid adjustments of heart rate and blood pressure in response to certain traumas and intracranial hypertension (Hickey, 1997). The Cushing response, which is characterized by a widened pulse pressure and a concomitant slowing of the pulse, is a late finding and a compensatory attempt to maintain blood flow (Cushing, 1902; Marshall et al., 1990). This finding indicates imminent brain herniation and may prove to be of minimal value as a warning of impending catastrophe. Severe head injury may be accompanied by hypertension and tachycardia related to the catecholamine release. Hypotension accompanied by tachycardia is rarely seen in head injury and may signal irreversible shock in the multiple-trauma patient (Aumick, 1991). Electrocardiogram (ECG) monitoring is required to observe changes in the pattern or waveform, which are frequently seen in subarachnoid hemorrhage and severe head injury (Hickey, 1997; Plum & Posner, 1980).

A triad of symptoms, including a deteriorating level of consciousness, pupillary dilation, and hemiparesis, has been suggestive of a hemispheric lesion causing transtentorial herniation (Kelly, Doberstein, & Becker, 1996). Altered level of consciousness is one of the first indicators of declining neurological status, and patient evaluation requires a systematic approach. The degree of arousal and content processing can be measured on the GCS, the most widely used monitoring tool, which was developed by Teasdale and Jennet in 1974. Consciousness is determined by the appropriateness of eye opening, verbal response, and orientation to questions and the ability to perform motor activities. Scoring is based on the best response, and the postresuscitation GCS is one of the strongest predictors of long-term outcome following craniocerebral trauma (Kelly et al., 1996).

Cranial nerve (CN) functions are evaluated with specific note made of pupillary function and extra-ocular movements, because the eyes are governed by both voluntary and involuntary mechanisms. Changes in the pupil shape can be indicative of early elevation of ICP and will return to normal if the ICP can be controlled. If, however, an increasing lesion is present, changes in pupil shape and size are usually representative of CN III compression due to transtentorial herniation. In this situation, the response to direct or consensual light is usually reduced or absent because of CN III compression or midbrain injury (Marshall et al., 1990).

The motor response is the third element of a triad of symptoms seen in head-injured patients with deteriorating levels of consciousness. Comparison of function between both sides and detailed documentation of each extremity must be noted. On the GCS, only the best motor response is recorded. Patients who have increasing lesions deteriorate from obeying commands to move extremities to localizing, withdrawing from pain, abnormal flexion and extension, and, finally, flaccidity of extremities. True flaccidity is defined as the absence of movement and tone in any extremity in response to deep, painful stimuli (Marshall et al., 1990).

It should be noted that these signs may be absent in the presence of diffuse brain injury, and other causes of decreased consciousness must also be considered (Wilberger, Rothfus, Tabas, Goldberg, & Deeb, 1990). Ongoing serial evaluation is essential in the head-injured population to achieve optimal outcomes. A study analyzing outcomes of 7,900 head trauma patients from 41 hospitals concluded that the excessive mortality demonstrated in some centers was probably due to inadequate observation of the less severely injured patients (Klauber et al., 1989).

Monitoring and aggressive treatment of elevated ICP have become routine procedures in severely head-injured patients, according to a review of the literature by Unterberg, Kiening, Schmiedek, & Lanksch in 1993. Use of ICP monitoring allows the health care team to review data trends and pulse waveforms to plan care, initiate interventions, and predict outcomes in this difficult patient population (Lang & Chesnut, 1994).

ICP MONITORING TOOLS

Selection of the device and technique to be used for monitoring depends on several factors, including the desire to drain CSF, risk factors associated with the patient and the device, clinical situation, ease of insertion, available systems, surgeon preference and familiarity, and cost (Lang & Chesnut, 1994). Additionally, as newer technology becomes available, there may be the desire to measure multiple parameters such as blood flow, oxygen, and temperature simultaneously with ICP. Historically, when determining the accuracy of a given sensor, it has been customary to compare it to the "gold standard,"—the ventricular catheter (Miller, Piper, & Stathan, 1996).

Selection of the monitoring device usually depends on the site chosen for monitoring ICP, including epidural, subdural, parenchymal, and ventricular. In studies in which both parenchymal and ventricular pressure have been measured simultaneously, significantly different pressures have been noted between the two systems, with the parenchymal being the higher of the two (Wolfa, Luerssen, Bowman, & Putty, 1996). Other sources have questioned the reliability of these findings, citing equal pressures in bilateral frontal lobes during monitoring (Yano, Ikeda, Kobayashi, & Otsuka, 1987). This information suggests that ICP alone is limited in its ability to reflect a patient's condition, and all clinical parameters should be considered in treatment decisions.

Epidural/Subdural

Epidural monitors are placed between the dura and skull (Fig. 20–1) and for this reason should not be considered a direct measure of ICP. Both fiberoptic and strain-gauge catheters are available, but care should be exercised to ensure that the pressure exerted by the skull is not directed over the monitoring sensor. An increase in pressure that places undue stress on the sensor could produce inaccurate readings. Any suction device or draining catheter in the same compartment can also adversely affect the accuracy of the reading. The advantage of measurement in the extradural space is that it is the least invasive of the

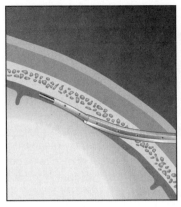
Epidural/subdural device

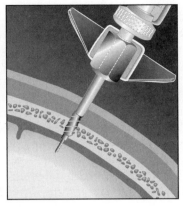
Intraparenchymal device

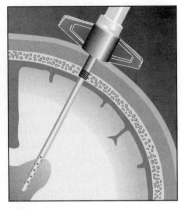
Ventricular device with drainage

Figure 20–1 Types of IPC tools. (Courtesy of Neurocare Group, Camino, San Diego, CA.)

monitoring techniques, but the accuracy should be carefully considered (Germon, 1994).

Monitoring in the subdural space usually occurs after an open craniotomy, with the catheter placed beneath the dura at the operative site before closing (see Fig. 20–1). A fiberoptic device with a sensor in the tip offers the most reliable information. Although fluid-filled catheters are sometimes used in the subdural space, they can become compressed by increasing brain edema and produce a resulting dampened waveform and inaccurate pressure reading. The advantage of this technique is the ease of placement postoperatively, but the limitation relates to the inability to drain CSF. Accuracy remains questionable (Germon, 1994; Lang & Chesnut, 1994).

Parenchymal

Parenchymal monitoring may be done through a bolt in the skull with a fiberoptic catheter. The catheter can also be placed by tunneling under the scalp and passing the catheter through a burr hole, as in the strain-gauge device or the fiberoptic catheter. The catheter routinely is placed within the parenchyma to a depth of 1 to 1.5 cm; this is quick and easier to accomplish in patients who have intracranial hypertension and slitlike ventricles.

The advantages of these catheters are the ease of placement and the minimal penetration of the brain. Because of the smaller diameter of the catheters, they are also more appropriate in the pediatric population and in the case of head injury in which the status of the coagulation cascade may be questionable (Lang & Chesnut, 1994). The disadvantage is that CSF cannot be drained, but it is not uncommon for a ventricular catheter to be placed subsequently when the results of the CT scan and laboratory studies are known.

Ventricular

The ventricular catheter is usually placed in the nondominant, frontal horn of the lateral ventricle and is considered the gold standard of ICP measurement (see Fig. 20–1). The crisp waveform generated by the ventricular catheter reflects the dynamic pressure generated by the choroid plexus and is best transmitted by a sensor in the tip of the catheter at the pressure source (Miller et al., 1996).

The additional advantage of monitoring in the ventricle is the access and the ability to drain CSF, reduce ICP, and remove bloody CSF (Bullock et al., 1995).

The disadvantage of ventricular monitoring is related to the diameter of the catheter, which is larger than the parenchymal version, and the potential difficulty in locating the ventricles in a patient with intracranial hypertension and displacement of the ventricular system. There is additional cause for concern because of the external transducer, which requires the system to be opened for periodic zeroing, and the potential for CSF leakage. A higher incidence of ventriculitis has been reported with ventricular catheter use, and a catheter change at 5 days was suggested (Mayhall et al., 1984). These statistics were negated in a study in which strict adherence to aseptic technique, vigilant management of the system, and prophylactic antibiotics allowed the use of ventricular draining for 14 days with no associated infections (Bader, Littlejohns, & Palmer, 1995). Holloway et al., (1996) agreed that there appears to be no benefit from changing the catheter nor any need to do so but that it should be removed as soon as possible. Also, the externally transduced ventricular monitoring system requires the most nursing time for monitoring and management (Kunkel & Webb, 1997).

Management of the monitoring system includes developing a standard of nursing care for this population and competency-based practice (Allan, 1989). A closed fiberoptic system requires less manipulation and less nursing time in addition to allowing the transducer to be placed within the cranial vault, ensuring accurate data readings at the source. Care must be exercised to avoid breaking the fiberoptic catheter. Although considered the gold standard, the fluid-filled, externally transduced system has the potential to display inaccurate readings if the transducer is not correctly placed. It cannot monitor and drain simultaneously. Regular rezeroing entails a break in the system, and scrupulous care must be taken to ensure aseptic technique.

DESCRIPTION OF THE INTERVENTION

The Nursing Interventions Classification (NIC) defines Intracranial Pressure Monitoring as the "measurement and interpretation of patient data to regulate intracranial pressure" and includes activities to implement the intervention (Table 20–1). The activities used to care for patients with ICP monitoring fall into six main categories: (1) preparation and monitoring, (2) airway management, (3) cerebral perfusion management, (4) positioning, (5) stimulation and regulation of environment, and (6) thermoregulation.

Preparation and Monitoring

In preparation for ICP monitoring, nursing management includes informing the family and significant others of the plan of care and the progress of the patient, obtaining consent according to hospital procedure, and preparing for the placement of a monitoring device. The device must be calibrated and prepared according to the manufacturer's directions and, if fluid-filled and externally transduced, the tubing and drainage system must be flushed and assembled using aseptic technique. The nurse is responsible for positioning the patient, administering sedation as ordered, and restraining the extremities to avoid injury or contamination of the field (Kunkel & Webb, 1997).

Parameters to monitor include the catheter insertion site, the device, the reliability of the displayed data, and the waveform. Baseline data from before

Table 20–1   Intracranial Pressure (ICP) Monitoring

DEFINITION: Measurement and interpretation of patient data to regulate intracranial pressure.

ACTIVITIES:

Assist with (ICP) monitoring device insertion

Provide information to family/significant others

Calibrate and level the transducer

Irrigate flush system

Set alarms

Obtain cerebrospinal fluid (CSF) drainage samples, as appropriate

Record ICP pressure readings and analyze waveforms

Monitor cerebral perfusion pressure (CPP)

Note patient's change in response to stimuli

Monitor patient's ICP and neurological response to care activities

Monitor amount/rate of cerebrospinal fluid drainage

Monitor intake and output

Restrain patient as needed

Monitor pressure tubing for bubbles

Change transducer/flush system

Change or reinforce insertion site dressing, as necessary

Monitor insertion site for infection

Monitor temperature and white blood cell (WBC) count

Check patient for nuchal rigidity

Administer antibiotics

Position the patient with head of bed elevated 30 to 45 degrees with neck in neutral position

Minimize environmental stimuli

Space nursing care to minimize ICP elevation

Alter suctioning procedure to minimize increase in ICP with catheter introduction (e.g., give lidocaine and limit number of suction passes)

Maintain controlled hyperventilation, as ordered

Maintain systemic arterial pressure within specified range

Administer pharmacological agents to maintain ICP within specified range

Notify physician of elevated ICP that does not respond to treatment protocols

Source: Iowa Intervention Project. (1996). Intracranial pressure monitoring. In J. C. McCloskey and G. M. Bulechek (Eds.), *Nursing interventions classification (NIC)* (2nd ed., p. 345). St. Louis: Mosby–Year Book.

and after device insertion must be compared and documentation of the patient's response to the procedure noted in the record. The ICP, CPP, waveform, or drainage status changes must be communicated to the physician, particularly if the information is outside the set parameters. Monitoring of the insertion site for hematoma formation and observation for signs of infection, including nuchal rigidity, positive CSF cultures, drainage, and fever, are fundamental and must be documented and reported to the physician (Kunkel & Webb, 1997).

Management of all monitoring systems requires knowledge of the system and ability to troubleshoot. Monitor alarms must be set to the ordered parameters. The presence of a dampened or lost waveform may indicate loose connections, occlusion of the tubing with blood or tissue, incorrectly positioned stopcocks, or bubbles in an external transducer. The fiberoptic catheter may have broken if this is the system in use (Kunkel & Webb, 1997). Caution should be exercised to avoid overdrainage of CSF and the physician notified if changes are noted in the amount or character of the drainage. Specimen collection varies with the institution, but a sample or the changed bag should be sent every 48 hours to monitor for infection (Bader et al., 1995).

Other nursing responsibilities include interpretation of the ICP recordings, waveform analysis, and documentation. The normal pulse waveform has three components, P_1, P_2, and P_3, descending in a sawtoothed manner and corresponding to each heartbeat (Fig. 20–2). These components can be measured using any device but are best seen with the transducer in the ventricular system where the waveform is generated. P_1, the percussion wave, originates with the pulsation of the choroid plexus; P_2, the tidal wave, is the most variable; and P_3, the dicrotic wave, tapers down to the diastolic position. As mean ICP rises, a progressive rise in P_2 can be seen, causing the appearance of a peak and indicating a loss of compliance (Germon, 1994). Because patients are unique in their compensatory abilities, pulse waveform analysis is a key to understanding each individual (Germon, 1988). Cardoso, Rowan, and Galbraith (1983) demonstrated a change in the P_1/P_2 relationship of the waveform associated with hyper- or hypoventilation, and this has been anecdotally identified by many professionals at the bedside (Fig. 20–3).

The trending of the waveform over a period of hours allows the bedside nurse to plan activities according to the patient's ability to tolerate the care.

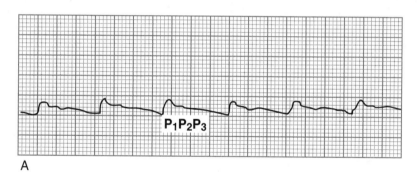

A

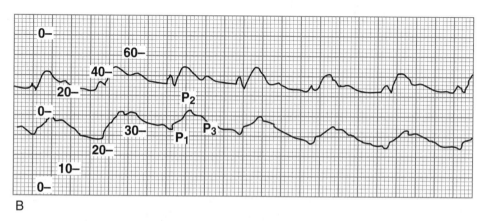

B

Figure 20–2 ICP pulse waveform. *A*, Demonstration of normal ICP P_1, P_2, P_3. *B*, Abnormal waveform with elevated P_2 demonstrating loss of compliance.

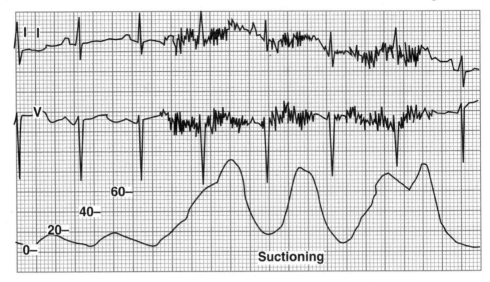

Figure 20–3 Waveform with increased ICP during suctioning.

Changes in ICP pressures during suctioning, sedation administration, CSF drainage, and lowered head of the bed during transport and CT scan are clearly demonstrated graphically on a trend waveform (Fig. 20–4). Technology is exciting and is expanding, but nurses must not use these data in isolation and should be ever conscious of the total clinical picture.

Airway Management

If the patient is unable to maintain patency of the airway, intubation should be considered. Tracheal intubation, while maintaining the patency of the airway,

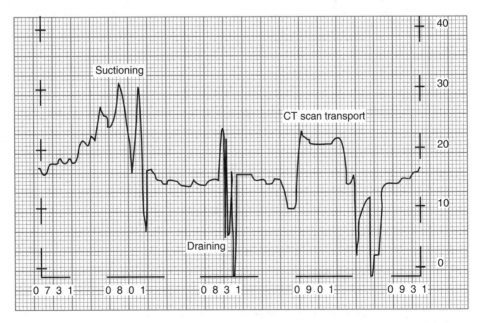

Figure 20–4 Trend with suctioning, sedation, draining, and lowered head of bed during CT scan transport.

also protects the patient from aspiration and allows for the removal of secretions (see Chapter 15). Hypoxia during resuscitation was documented in 46% of patients in the Trauma Coma Data Bank, and it indicated poor patient outcome (Chesnut et al., 1993). Evolving cerebral insult can be identified on the basis of respiratory rate and pattern and, if not identified, may further affect secondary brain injury (Plum & Posner, 1980).

To ensure adequate oxygenation, any patient with a GCS score of 8 or less should be intubated and oxygenated with an FIO_2 of 80% to 100% (Chesnut, 1996). Titration of the FIO_2 should occur as soon as tolerated to maintain oxygen saturation at 95% or higher. This may be accomplished with a tidal volume of 10 to 12 mL/kg and a rate of 12 and adjusted as tolerated. Pulse oximetry to monitor oxygen saturation, arterial blood gases, and end-tidal carbon dioxide readings is used to maintain the proper ventilatory parameters and avoid hypoxia. Chest x-ray examinations must be performed initially to exclude barotrauma and at least daily to check for new infiltrates, atelectasis, effusions, and placement of tubes.

Aggressive hyperventilation (arterial $PCO_2 \leq 25$) has been considered the desirable management of severe head injury because of the associated rapid decrease in blood flow and therefore ICP. However, because most head-injured patients experience a 50% reduction in cerebral blood flow during the immediate postinjury phase, the risk for cerebral ischemia is high in the presence of aggressive hyperventilation. It is now known that acute hyperventilation, through its effect on extracellular pH, produces vasoconstriction, reducing cerebral blood flow and cerebral blood volume (Muizelaar et al., 1991). Vascular reactivity, or the sensitivity of the ICP to changes in PCO_2, in head-injured patients has been used as a prognosticator for outcome (Yoshihara, Bandoh, & Marmarou, 1995).

The Guidelines for Management of Severe Head Injury (Bullock et al., 1995) suggest that chronic prophylactic hyperventilation therapy should be avoided during the first 5 days after injury. Moderate hyperventilation therapy, with a $PaCO_2$ of 35 mm Hg, showed a significantly better outcome and is the suggested range of therapy (Muizelaar et al., 1991).

Because endotracheal suctioning (ETS) is necessary to clear secretions and maintain adequate oxygenation, careful planning and evaluation of a patient's responses are important. Suctioning is one of the most noxious stimuli to a patient with an intact gag and cough reflex and can adversely affect the ICP (Boortz-Marx, 1985; Shalit & Umansky, 1977; Snyder, 1983). To reduce the risk of increased ICP during suctioning, the patient should be hyperoxygenated with 100% oxygen, and suctioning should be limited to one or two quick passes with the suction catheter. The administration of lidocaine via the trachea or intravenously is thought to blunt the ICP response to ETS (Brucia, Owen, & Rudy, 1992) but should not be used more than once per hour (Lang & Chesnut, 1994). The use of sedation before suctioning is essential, and morphine sulfate is known to depress airway reflexes (Lang & Chesnut, 1994).

The importance of early airway protection and close monitoring of oxygen delivery cannot be overstressed if hypoxia ($PaO_2 < 60$ mm Hg) is to be avoided. The role of nursing in monitoring and ensuring patient safety in this area of management can have a huge impact on ICP, as each patient requires individual therapy to allow for optimal ventilation.

Cerebral Perfusion Management

Cerebral perfusion incorporates actions to optimize blood delivery to the brain. It includes activities related to monitoring the perfusion pressure, regulating and delivering intravascular volume, administering pharmacological agents, and adjusting ventilatory rates and carbon dioxide.

Cerebral perfusion pressure (CPP) is one assessment parameter clinicians use in the clinical setting to monitor perfusion to the brain. CPP requires continuous assessment of the mean arterial pressure (MAP) and ICP. CPP equals the MAP minus the ICP. In the normal adult, the lowest acceptable level of CPP is 50 mm Hg (Chesnut, 1996; Lang & Chesnut, 1994). If CPP falls below 50 mm Hg, cerebral blood flow rapidly falls, and cerebral ischemia results. Optimal CPP management is key in patients with increased ICP. When CPP ranges are on the lower end of normal (50 to 70 mm Hg), cerebral blood vessels dilate, increasing blood flow to the brain to maintain adequate perfusion (Chesnut, 1996; Rosner, Rosner, & Johnson, 1995). This increase in blood flow results in an increase in ICP. As CPP climbs above 70 to 80 mm Hg, the cerebral vessels constrict, reducing excess blood flow and ICP (Chesnut, 1996; Prociuk, 1995). A CPP threshold of 70 to 80 mm Hg has been cited as the minimum acceptable level in patients with increased ICP related to head injury (Bouma & Muizelaar, 1990; Bouma, Muizelaar, Bandoh, & Marmarou, 1992; McGraw, 1989; Rosner & Daughton, 1990; Rosner et al., 1995). The minimum threshold for CPP varies depending on the autoregulatory status and must be individualized to the specific clinical situation. Vigilant monitoring of both the MAP and ICP levels and calculating CPP will direct the interventions needed to maintain CPP above 70 mm Hg.

When ICP is elevated despite interventions to reduce it, such as CSF drainage, then activities related to raising MAP and maintaining euvolemia are critical to maintain an adequate CPP. Systemic arterial blood pressure is maintained at a prescribed level. Increasing MAP is accomplished by establishing euvolemia through the administration of intravenous fluids to achieve a central venous pressure of 10 to 12 mm Hg or pulmonary capillary wedge pressures of 14 to 16 mm Hg (Lang & Chesnut, 1994). Monitoring intake and output assists the nurse in tracking fluid volume balance. If MAP needs further enhancement, intravenous vasopressors are used to titrate the MAP to the desired level (Rosner et al., 1995). Close monitoring of the MAP with an invasive arterial catheter is necessary to evaluate changes with titration of the vasopressors.

When CPP falls below 70 mm Hg in the presence of ICP levels above 20 mm Hg despite aggressive fluid and vasopressor management, the use of intravenous mannitol increases cerebral perfusion and oxygen delivery to the brain by expanding the plasma volume (Bullock et al., 1995; Paczynski, 1997). The hemodynamic actions of mannitol are related to the increase in preload, enhancement of myocardial contractility, decrease in blood viscosity, and shrinkage and dehydration of blood cells, resulting in improved delivery of oxygenated hemoglobin (Paczynski, 1997). Mannitol is given as a bolus, which has the dramatic effect of lowering ICP within 20 to 40 minutes (Bullock et al., 1995; Paczynski, 1997). The osmotic diuretic effects eventually reduce intravascular volume, requiring replacement of the fluid to prevent dehydration.

The regulation of carbon dioxide and ventilation is critical to maintain blood flow to the brain. Hypocapnia reduces blood flow and the amount of oxygen available to be extracted by cerebral tissues. Regulation of the $PaCO_2$ level has been accomplished historically by watching for a decline in the elevated ICP. Some literature supports the use of jugular bulb oxygen saturation monitoring to calculate the difference between arterial and jugular saturation and cerebral extraction of oxygen (Feldman & Robertson, 1997; Kerr, Lovasik, & Darby, 1995; Prociuk, 1995; Sikes & Segal, 1994).

Because of the uniqueness of each patient's injury or clinical situation, individualization of the nursing activities will assist in reducing increased ICP while maintaining cerebral perfusion. The NIC interventions Cerebral Edema Management and Cerebral Perfusion Promotion can provide additional information.

Positioning

The position of the patient's body, neck, and head affects venous drainage from the cranium. As mentioned in the beginning of the chapter, the cranium's three major components exist in a state of equilibrium. The patient with increased ICP is in a compromised state as an increase in the blood volume inside the brain affects ICP.

The internal jugular veins are the major routes of venous drainage from the brain (Lipe & Mitchell, 1980). Watson (1974) studied the effects of head rotation and venous drainage in the internal jugular veins. Ipsilateral turning of the head 45 degrees caused decreased venous flow and return from the cranium. When the head was rotated 90 degrees, there was complete occlusion of the ipsilateral internal jugular vein in 41 of 60 infants and children. Lipe and Mitchell (1980) studied 15 healthy adults and found that 90-degree rotation of the head affected venous outflow drainage from the brain by partially or totally occluding the internal jugular vein.

Research on neurosurgery patients with ICP monitoring suggests neck rotation and turning of patients adversely affect ICP. One of the earliest nursing research studies of patients with head injury found that ICP increased significantly with rotation of the head to the right or left (Shalit & Umansky, 1977). Mitchell and Mauss's study (1978) noted an increase in CSF drainage from the lateral ventricles when some of the patients were turned to the lateral position. These results were consistent with further research involving 18 neurosurgical patients; increased ICP was noted in some patients when they were turned to the left or right while in the supine position (Mitchell, Ozuna, & Lipe, 1981). Lee's research (1989) involving 30 patients with head injury suggested that turning patients to a three-fourths prone or supine position increased ICP. Williams and Coyne (1993) investigated the effects of neck turning and flexion in 10 patients with ICP monitoring. Rotation of the neck to the right and left and flexing the neck resulted in higher ICP readings than those of the same patients with their necks in the neutral position or extended.

Elevation of the head of the bed to 30 or 45 degrees for patients with ICP monitoring has been investigated. In a study of 26 neonates with ICP monitoring in place, investigators found that elevation of the head of the bed to 30 degrees resulted in a decrease in ICP. Further study of the neonates involved turning the patient's head 90 degrees when the bed was in the flat position and when the head of the bed was raised 30 degrees. The study resulted in higher ICP readings with neck rotation (Goldberg, Joshi, Moscoso, & Castillo, 1983). Researchers examined the effect of head elevation in 22 head-injured adult patients. They compared ICP, CPP, and cerebral blood flow with the head of the bed positioned flat and at 30 degrees. ICP was lower in the majority of patients at the 30-degree head elevation than when these same patients were flat (Feldman et al., 1992).

The research studies suggest that positioning can enhance venous outflow from the brain. Nurses should position the patient with the head of the bed elevated 30 to 45 degrees, with the neck maintained in a neutral position. Turning patients should be accomplished by keeping the neck in neutral alignment.

Reassessment of the patient's ICP should guide the evaluation of the patient's tolerance to turning and repositioning.

Stimulation and Environmental Factors

The activities nurses implement related to hygiene, elimination, and invasive procedures may affect a patient's ICP. Stimulation and regulation of the environment create a variety of stimuli for a patient and have been investigated to determine their effects on ICP. Activities such as coughing, chewing, use of the bedpan, and restless movements were found to increase ventricular fluid drainage in neurosurgical patients (Mitchell & Mauss, 1978). Boortz-Marx's descriptive study (1985) of four severely head-injured patients found that turning, suctioning, bathing, conducting a physical assessment, and coughing increased ICP, whereas talking to or about the patient, touching, and environmental noises did not raise ICP. Bathing did not cause changes in ICP, according to another study (Mitchell & Mauss, 1978). Invasive procedures, such as intramuscular injections, venipuncture, lumbar punctures, and caloric examinations, produced increases in ICP in almost half of the observed occurrences (Snyder, 1983). The elevations related to invasive procedures produced increases in ICP lasting 6 to 8 minutes (Snyder, 1983). Range-of-motion activities of the extremities were tolerated by neurosurgical patients as evidenced by no significant change in ICP or ventricular fluid pressures in one study, but opposite results were found in another study (Mitchell et al., 1981; Snyder, 1983).

The spacing of activities with rest periods has been advocated to decrease adverse responses in critically ill patients. Bruya (1981) found no significant difference between two groups of neurosurgical patients when activities were spaced 10 minutes apart in one group and the same activities were followed by a rest period in the other group. The author noted that 10 minutes may not have been an adequate rest time between activities.

Environmental factors, therapeutic touch, and family presence may affect a patient in a positive or negative way. Environmental noise was investigated in one research study and found not to increase ICP (Boortz-Marx, 1985). Studies have discovered that a patient's ICP increased when conversation about the patient's condition was held over the patient's bed (Mitchell & Mauss, 1978; Snyder, 1983). Purposeful touch involving stroking the patient's hand or face lowered ICP in 25 of 30 patients (Walleck, 1983). The effects of family presence and conversation at the patient's bedside were evaluated by researchers to determine whether their presence affected ICP. Hendrickson (1987) evaluated 24 neurosurgical patients' responses to family presence and found that in the majority of patients, ICP did not rise significantly. In seven of the patients, the ICP decrease ranged from 1.41 to 4.24 mm Hg (Hendrickson, 1987). No significant differences in ICP before, during, or after family visits of 10 minutes or more were found in 15 neurosurgical patients, supporting the practice of allowing more permissive visiting policies (Prins, 1989). Familiar and unfamiliar voice recordings used on 12 head-injured patients caused little change in ICP (Treloar, Nalli, Guin, & Gary, 1991).

Monitoring a patient's ICP and response to nursing care activities will serve as the best guide in determining tolerance and response. The use of sedation, anesthetic agents, and narcotics for pain control should be considered when a patient's ICP increases during procedures or nursing activities (Bullock et al., 1995; Lang & Chesnut, 1994; McQuillan, 1991; Mitchell, 1986). Minimizing environmental stimuli should be based on the individual patient's responses to the different types of stimulation. Noting the patient's reaction to family presence, conversation, and touch helps in facilitating activities that decrease ICP. Spacing nursing care with the goal of minimizing ICP elevations should be based on a patient's individual responses.

Thermoregulation

The use of mild to moderate hypothermia in the treatment of severely head-injured patients has shown a trend toward improved outcomes in preliminary studies (Clifton et al., 1993; Marion et al., 1997). Conversely, hyperthermia in this population is associated with detrimental results related to the release of free radical compounds within the brain (Kader, Frazzini, Baker, Solomon, & Trifiletti, 1994). For every degree (centigrade) of rise in temperature, the metabolic rate of the body is increased by 7% to 10% (Marshall et al., 1990). The use of moderate hypothermia in a study by Metz et al. (1996) showed a reduction in cerebral oxygen consumption of approximately 45%, improving the cerebral oxygen supply-demand relationship. This resulted in a reduction of cerebral ischemia and a decline in lactate production to normal. Marion et al. (1997) demonstrated a reduction of ICP (40%) and CSF (26%) during moderate hypothermia. Cooling measures used include acetaminophen, cooling blankets, ice water lavage, and neuromuscular blockers to achieve normothermia. Because higher brain temperatures increase the severity of secondary brain injury, optimal thermoregulation in head injury may best be achieved by monitoring brain temperature directly (Crowder et al., 1996; Kelly et al., 1996; Mellegard, 1992).

Studies have concluded that moderate therapeutic hypothermia is safe and may positively affect outcomes, but nurses must remain vigilant for potential side effects, which may include cardiac arrhythmias, coagulopathies, infections, and pulmonary complications. Close monitoring of cardiac function and laboratory results for changes in blood counts, chemistry, and coagulation studies is necessary.

NURSING DIAGNOSES

Nursing diagnoses related to ICP monitoring include actual and potential diagnoses. The actual diagnoses are Intracranial Adaptive Capacity, Decreased and Tissue Perfusion, Altered: Cerebral. The potential diagnoses include Injury, Risk for; Skin Integrity, Impaired; Disuse Syndrome, Risk for; Infection, Risk for; and Sensory/Perceptual Alterations.

PATIENT OUTCOMES

Nursing-sensitive patient outcomes being developed by the University of Iowa nursing research team that are associated with Intracranial Pressure Monitoring include the following:

Infection Status
Neurological Status
Neurological Status: Central Motor Control
Neurological Status: Consciousness
Neurological Status: Cranial
    Sensory/Motor Functions
Neurological Status: Spinal
    Sensory/Motor Functions

Thermoregulation
Tissue Perfusion: Cerebral

CASE STUDY

Scene and Resuscitation Phase

AP, a 17-year-old boy, was on a skateboard being pulled by a golf cart when he fell and landed on the back of his head. He experienced a loss of consciousness for 20 minutes. Paramedics responded to the scene, and AP became intermittently responsive and combative. En route to the hospital, the paramedics noted AP's heart rate had decreased to 40, his BP had widened to 180/ 60, and his respirations had decreased to six per minute and become shallow in character. AP went from combative to comatose. The paramedics assisted respirations with a bag-valve-mask delivering 100% oxygen and noted that AP became combative once bagging was initiated.

On arrival at the trauma center, AP was combative while paramedics assisted ventilation. He was able to open his eyes to pain, follow simple commands, move all four extremities purposefully, and state his name. Once assisted ventilations were halted, AP became unresponsive again and did not respond to deep painful stimuli. His pupils were 5 mm on the right and 4 mm on the left with sluggish reaction to light. AP had a gaze preference to the right. Because of the change in his neurological status, AP was intubated with an endotracheal tube. Ventilations were increased to 16 breaths per minute with an end-tidal carbon dioxide level of 30 mm Hg. Oxygen was administered to maintain an arterial saturation of 100% with a resulting PaO_2 of 158 mm Hg. AP became combative once respirations were maintained, so he was chemically paralyzed with Zemuron. He received midazolam and morphine sulfate for sedation and pain management. Following insertion of a Foley catheter and a second intravenous line, AP underwent a CT scan of the brain.

The CT scan of the brain revealed basilar cerebral edema with effacement of the basilar cisterns, bilateral contusions of the frontal lobes, left basilar skull fracture, left parietal occipital calvarial fracture, and left posterior fossa pneumocephalus. The consulting neurosurgeon reviewed the incident, the patient status in the emergency department, and the CT scan. Because of the exten-

sive brain-stem edema compromising the basilar cisterns, AP underwent emergent placement of a fiberoptic ventricular ICP monitoring system. AP's opening ICP pressure was 34 mm Hg. Hyperventilation had been used initially to control ICP; the neurosurgeon's goal was to lower the ventilation rate and implement other strategies. AP received a bolus of intravenous mannitol, sedation, and CSF drainage to reduce the ICP to below 20 mm Hg. Because of the severity of the injury, the neurosurgeon and trauma surgeon elected to place a jugular bulb oximetric catheter (SjO_2) in the internal jugular vein to measure the venous saturation of blood leaving the cranial vault. This catheter would assist the team in balancing and guiding therapy to reduce AP's ICP and maintain cerebral oxygen delivery. He was transported to the pediatric intensive care unit (PICU) for stabilization.

Evaluation Point #1:

The activities initiated in the resuscitation phase of this case began with a quick but thorough assessment of the patient's neurological status. The examination revealed obvious brain-stem compression as evidenced by the change in vital signs and responsiveness. Assisting ventilations with a bag-valve-mask reduced the patient's $PaCO_2$ levels and vasoconstricted the cerebral arteries, producing more room for his swollen brain. The patient's response to supporting ventilations was to become combative and agitated. Using paralyzing agents with concurrent sedation and pain control decreased the body's and the brain's metabolic usage of oxygen and energy. Once the ICP monitor was placed, CSF drainage was used in the operating room to reduce the ICP. Sedation and a bolus of intravenous mannitol brought the ICP down to 20 mm Hg in the postanesthesia care unit.

STABILIZATION: THE FIRST 12 HOURS IN PICU

AP was positioned in bed with the head of the bed elevated to 30 degrees and the neck maintained in a neutral position. Several times when the patient's neck rotated to one side, his ICP increased 6 to 10 mm Hg. Turning his head and neck back to the neutral position returned the ICP to approximately 15 to 20 mm Hg. The nurses used CSF drainage to manage his ICP. Two hours after arriving in the PICU, AP's ICP increased to 30 mm Hg. Drainage of CSF was slow, and the team was not able to control the ICP with drainage alone. Intravenous mannitol was administered, with improvement in ICP for 60 minutes. AP began bucking the ventilator, and ventilations became harder to deliver. He received additional doses of vecuronium bromide, midazolam, and morphine sulfate to control ventilations and maintain sedation. The PICU room lights were dimmed, and external stimulation was decreased. The nurse noted that AP's temperature increased to 38.8°C. Interventions to cool him were immediately initiated and included acetaminophen, ice bags, and a fan.

As the ICP increased, AP's MAP of 80 was not high enough to maintain a CPP of 70 mm Hg. Because his fluid balance was negative, 500 mL of 5% albumin was administered. His MAP increased to 86 but still needed further enhancement. A continuous drip of dopamine was initiated and titrated to achieve a MAP between 90 and 100 mm Hg. Mannitol was administered to increase perfusion to the brain when CPP fell below 70 mm Hg. With fluids and vasopressors, his CPP was pushed past 70 mm Hg.

The SjO_2 catheter was reading 65%; normal saturation is between 55% and 70%. The physicians elected to increase his ventilator breaths to 18 per minute, which decreased the $PaCO_2$ to 26 mm Hg. The SjO_2 decreased to 60%, and the ICP decreased to 20 mm Hg. At this point AP was 12 hours postinjury. The interventions implemented by the nurses achieved a balance of CPP, ICP, and oxygen delivery. AP was "in the zone."

Evaluation Point #2:
During the initial stabilization period in the PICU, nurses performed many physician-ordered interventions as well as independent nursing actions. More important, nurses used repeated assessments of hemodynamics, ventilatory status, and ICP to achieve a balance in the cranium. The first 12 hours were only the beginning of a 12-day battle to maintain ICP, CPP, and oxygen delivery.

DAYS 1 THROUGH 17
For 12 days, nurses worked in pairs to control AP's ICP and maintain an adequate CPP. CSF

drainage was only minimally effective because of small lateral ventricles and increased pressure within the cranial vault. AP's neck and head were kept at a 30-degree elevation and in the neutral position. Stimulation was kept to a minimum. His family were allowed liberal visiting opportunities and stayed quietly at his bedside for hours. His ventilator settings were adjusted according to his SjO_2 levels, and calculations were related to his cerebral extraction of oxygen. Suctioning of the endotracheal tube was done only when absolutely necessary and was preceded by hyperinflation with 100% oxygen, an in-line suction catheter, and increased sedation. His sedation was maintained with 15 mg of midazolam per hour and 15 mg of morphine sulfate per hour. CPP was maintained between 70 and 90 mm Hg with enhancement of BP using vasopressors and maintenance of euvolemia. Mannitol was administered as needed when CPP fell below 70 mm Hg. Fluid replacement was given to maintain euvolemia. His sodium level ranged between 140 and 149 mEq, with a corresponding serum osmolality between 290 and 310 mOsm/L.

Four days into the hospital course, AP's ICP increased, and he seemed more sensitive to nursing activities and noise. A decision was made to use intravenous propofol to increase sedation. A bolus of propofol was administered, and he was placed on a drip of 75 μg/kg/min. The ICP immediately fell from 34 to 18 mm Hg with the increased sedation. The propofol was titrated throughout the next 9 days to achieve optimal sedation. Throughout the hospitalization, the CPP was maintained higher than 70 mm Hg even when the ICP increased to 30 mm Hg. The SjO_2 saturations were kept between 58% and 70%, and actions were taken by the nurses whenever levels approached abnormal boundaries.

By day 11, AP's condition had stabilized. He required less drainage of his ICP. He was weaned from vecuronium bromide. AP began moving spontaneously when the vecuronium bromide was stopped. His actions were purposeful. A decision was made to normalize his $PaCO_2$ and slowly titrate off the propofol. This was accomplished over 48 hours. His dopamine drip was titrated off. The morphine and midazolam drips were slowly eliminated over several days. AP was able to follow simple commands and hold up two fingers on command. He opened his eyes spontaneously and watched the nurses move around the bed. He responded with increased agitation at times but was calmed down by his parents and the nurses. On day 13, the ICP catheter was removed. AP was extubated on day 14. After being oriented to his surroundings and the date, AP was able to answer orientation questions correctly. He could accurately answer questions regarding his school, water polo team, and family. Sixteen days after his accident, AP walked five steps from his bed to the chair. He did not have any measurable motor deficit except for "noodle legs," as he referred to his extremities the first time he got out of bed. He began oral feedings following a swallow evaluation. AP was doing so well by day 17 that he was transferred to the acute rehabilitation unit. Three months after his injury, AP returned for his junior year of high school.

CONCLUSION

Nurses must continuously use their assessment skills and knowledge of the appropriate interventions to control and maintain ICP. In most patient care situations, the nursing activities identified in Table 20–1 are implemented concurrently. Nurses' actions must be guided by the use of technology, the dissemination of research into practice, and the minute-to-minute evaluation of the patient's responses to nursing care activities.

References

Allan, D. (1989). Intracranial pressure monitoring: A study of nursing practice. *Journal of Advanced Nursing, 14*(2), 127–131.

American Association of Neuroscience Nurses (AANN). (1996). *Core curriculum for neuroscience nurses* (3rd ed.). Chicago: Author.

Aumick, J. E. (1991). Head trauma: Guidelines for care. *Registered Nurse, 4,* 27–31.

Bader, M., Littlejohns, L. R., and Palmer, S. (1995). In search of a 0% infection rate: A study of ventriculostomy infection. *Heart & Lung, 24,* 166–172.

Boortz-Marx, R. (1985). Factors affecting intracranial pressure: A descriptive study. *Journal of Neuroscience Nursing, 17* (2), 89–94.

Bouma, G. J., and Muizelaar, J. P. (1990). Relationship between cardiac output and cerebral blood flow in patients with intact and with impaired autoregulation. *Journal of Neurosurgery, 73,* 368–374.

Bouma, G. J., Muizelaar, J. P., Bandoh, K., and Marmarou, A. (1992). Blood pressure and intracranial pressure-volume dynamics in severe head injury: Relationship with cerebral blood flow. *Journal of Neurosurgery, 77,* 15–19.

Brucia, J. J., Owen, D. C., and Rudy, E. B. (1992). The effects of lidocaine on intracranial hypertension. *Journal of Neuroscience Nursing, 24,* 205–214.

Bruya, M. A. (1981). Planned periods of rest in the intensive care unit: Nursing care activities and intracranial pressure. *Journal of Neurosurgical Nursing, 13,* 184–194.

Bullock, R., Chesnut, R. M., Clifton, G., Ghajar, J., Marion, D., Narayan, R., Newell, D. W., Pitts, L. H., Rosner, M. J., and Wilberger, J. E. (1995). *Guidelines for the management of severe head injury* (pp. 4-1–4-11, 5-1–5-29, 6-1–6-6, 8-1–8-10, 9-1–9-10, 10-1–10-12). Park Ridge, IL: Brain Trauma Foundation and American Association of Neurological Surgeons.

Cardoso, E. R., Rowan, J. O., and Galbraith, S. (1983). Analysis of cerebrospinal fluid pulse wave in intracranial pressure. *Journal of Neurosurgery, 59,* 817–821.

Chesnut, R. M. (1996). Treating raised intracranial pressure in head injury. In R. K. Narayan, J. E. Wilberger, and J. T. Povilshock (Eds.), *Neurotrauma* (pp. 445–469). New York: McGraw-Hill.

Chesnut, R. M., Marshall, L. F., Klauber, M. R., et al. (1993). The role of secondary brain injury in determining outcome from severe head injury. *Journal of Trauma, 34,* 216–222.

Clifton, G. L., Allen, S., Barrodale, P., Plenger, P., Berry, J., Koch, S., Fletcher, J., Hayes, R. L., and Choi, S. C. (1993). A phase II study of moderate hypothermia in severe brain injury. *Journal of Neurotrauma, 10,* 263–271.

Crowder, C. M., Tempelhoff, R., Theard, A., Cheng, M. A., Todorov, A., and Dacey, R. G., Jr. (1996). Jugular bulb temperature: Comparison with brain surface and core temperatures in neurosurgical patients during mild hypothermia. *Journal of Neurosurgery, 85,* 98–103.

Cushing, H. (1902). Some experimental and clinical observations concerning states of increased intracranial tension. *American Journal of the Medical Sciences, 124,* 375–400.

Feldman, Z., Kanter, M. J., Robertson, C. S., Contant, C. F., Hayes, C., Sheinberg, M. A., Villareal, C. A., Narayan, R., K., and Grossman, R. G. (1992). Effect of head elevation on intracranial pressure, cerebral perfusion pressure, and cerebral blood flow in head-injured patients. *Journal of Neurosurgery, 76,* 207–211.

Feldman, Z., and Robertson, C. S. (1997). Monitoring of cerebral hemodynamics with jugular bulb catheters. *Critical Care Clinics, 13*(1), 51–77.

Germon, K. (1988). Interpretation of ICP pulse waves to determine intracerebral compliance. *Journal of Neuroscience Nursing, 20,* 344–351.

Germon, K. (1994). Intracranial pressure monitoring in the 1990s. *Critical Care Nursing Quarterly, 17*(1), 21–32.

Goldberg, R. N., Joshi, A., Moscoso, P., and Castillo, T. (1983). The effect of head position on intracranial pressure in the neonate. *Critical Care Medicine, 11,* 428–430.

Hendrickson, S. L. (1987). Intracranial pressure changes and family presence. *Journal of Neuroscience Nursing, 19*(1), 14–17.

Hickey, J. (1997). *The clinical practice of neurological and neurosurgical nursing* (4th ed.). Philadelphia: J. B. Lippincott.

Holloway, K. L., Barnes, T., Choi, S., Bullock, R., Marshall, L. F., Eisenberg, H. A., Jane, J. A., Ward, J. D., Young, H. F., and Marmarou, A. (1996). Ventriculostomy infections: The effect of monitoring duration and catheter exchange in 584 patients. *Journal of Neurosurgery, 85,* 419–424.

Kader, A., Frazzini, V. I., Baker, C. J., Solomon, R. A., and Trifiletti, R. R. (1994). Effect of mild hypothermia on nitric oxide synthesis during focal cerebral ischemia. *Neurosurgery, 35,* 272–277.

Kelly, D. F., Doberstein, C., and Becker, D. P. (1996). General principles of head injury management. In R. K. Narayan, J. E. Wilberger, and J. T. Povilshock (Eds.), *Neurotrauma* (pp. 71–102). New York: McGraw-Hill.

Kerr, M. E., Lovasik, D., and Darby, J. (1995). Evaluating cerebral oxygenation using jugular venous oximetry in head injuries. *AACN Clinical Issues, 6*(1), 11–20.

Klauber, M. R., Marshall, L. F., Luerssen, T. G., Frankowski, R., Tabaddor, K., and Eisenberg, H. M. (1989). Determinants of head injury mortality: Importance of the low risk patient. *Neurosurgery, 24,* 31–36.

Kunkel, J., and Webb, D. (Eds.). (1997). *American Association of Neuroscience Nurses clinical guideline series: Intracranial pressure monitoring.* Chicago: AANN.

Lang, E. W., and Chesnut, R. M. (1994). Intracranial pressure: Monitoring and management. *Neurosurgery Clinics of North America, 5,* 573–605.

Lee S. T. (1989). Intracranial pressure changes during positioning of patients with severe head injury. *Heart and Lung, 18,* 411–414.

Lipe, H. P., and Mitchell, P. H. (1980). Positioning the patient with intracranial hypertension: How turning and head rotation affect the internal jugular vein. *Heart and Lung, 9,* 1031–1037.

Marion, D. W., Penrod, L. E., Kelsey, S. F., Obrist, W. D., Kochanek, P. M., Palmer, A. M., Wisniewski, S. R., and DeKosky, S. T. (1997). Treatment of traumatic brain injury with moderate hypothermia. *New England Journal of Medicine, 336,* 540–546.

Marshall, S. B., Marshall, L., Vos, H., and Chesnut, R. M. (1990). *Neurosurgical critical care: Pathophysiology and patient management* (pp. 367–368). Philadelphia: W. B. Saunders.

Mayhall, C., Archer, N., Lamb, V. A., Spadora, A. C., Baggett, J., Ward, J., and Narayan, R. (1984). Ventriculitis-related infections. A prospective epidemiologic study. *New England Journal of Medicine, 310,* 553–559.

McGraw, C. P. (1989). A cerebral perfusion pressure greater than 80 mm Hg is more beneficial. In J. T. Hoff and A. L. Betz (Eds.), *Intracranial pressure VII* (pp. 839–841). Berlin: Springer-Verlag.

McQuillan, K. A. (1991). Intracranial pressure monitoring: Technical imperatives. AACN *Clinical Issues, 2,* 623–636.

Mellegard, P. (1992). Changes in human intracerebral temperature in response to different methods of brain cooling. *Neurosurgery, 31,* 671–677.

Metz, C., Holzschuh, M., Bein, T., Woertgen, C., Frey, A., Taeger, K., and Brawanski, A. (1996). Moderate hypothermia in patients with severe head injury: Cerebral and extracerebral effects. *Journal of Neurosurgery, 85,* 533–541.

Miller, J. D., Piper, I. R., and Stathan, F. X. (1996). ICP monitoring: Indications and techniques. In R. K. Narayan, J. E. Wilberger, and J. T. Povilshock (Eds.), *Neurotrauma* (pp. 429–444). New York: McGraw-Hill.

Mitchell, P. H. (1986). Intracranial hypertension: Influence of nursing care activities. *Nursing Clinics of North America, 21*(4), 563–576.

Mitchell, P. H., Ozuna, J., and Lipe, H. P. (1981). Moving the patient in bed: Effects on intracranial pressure. *Nursing Research, 30,* 212–218.

Mitchell, P. H., and Mauss, N. K. (1978). Relationship of patient-nurse activity to intracranial pressure variations: A pilot study. *Nursing Research, 27* (1), 4–10.

Muizelaar, J. P., Marmarou, A., Ward, J. D., Kontos, H. A., Choi, S. C., Becker, D. P., Gruemer, H., and Young, H. F. (1991). Adverse effects of prolonged hyperventilation in patients with severe head injury: A randomized clinical trial. *Journal of Neurosurgery, 75,* 731–739.

Paczynski, R. P. (1997). Osmotherapy: Basic concepts and controversies. *Critical Care Clinics, 13*(1), 105–129.

Plum, F., and Posner, J. (1980). *The diagnosis of stupor and coma* (3rd ed.). Philadelphia: F. A. Davis.

Prins, M. M. (1989). The effect of family visits on intracranial pressure. *Western Journal of Nursing Research, 11,* 281–297.

Prociuk, J. L. (1995). Management of cerebral oxygen supply-demand balance in blunt head injury. *Critical Care Nurse, 15*(4), 38–45.

Rosner, M. J., and Daughton, S. (1990). Cerebral perfusion pressure management in head injury. *Journal of Trauma, 30,* 933–941.

Rosner, M. J., Rosner, S. D., and Johnson, A. H. (1995). Cerebral perfusion pressure: Management protocol and clinical results. *Journal of Neurosurgery, 83,* 949–962.

Shalit, M. N., and Umansky, F. (1977). Effect of routine bedside procedures on intracranial pressure. *Israel Medical Sciences, 13,* 881–886.

Sikes, P. J., and Segal, J. (1994). Jugular bulb oxygen saturation monitoring for evaluating cerebral ischemia. *Critical Care Nursing Quarterly, 17*(1), 9–20.

Snyder, M. (1983). Relation of nursing activities to increases in intracranial pressure. *Journal of Advanced Nursing, 8,* 273–279.

Teasdale, G., and Jennett, B. (1974). Assessment of coma and impaired consciousness: A practical scale. *Lancet 2,* 81–84.

Treloar, D. M., Nalli, B. J., Guin, P., and Gary, R. (1991). The effect of familiar and unfamiliar voice treatments on intracranial pressure in head-injured patients. *Journal of Neuroscience Nursing, 23,* 295–299.

Unterberg, A., Kiening, K., Schmiedek, P., and Lanksch, W. (1993). Long-term observations of intracranial pressure after severe head injury. The phenomenon of secondary rise of intracranial pressure. *Neurosurgery, 32*(1), 17–24.

Walleck, C. (1983). The effect of purposeful touch on intracranial pressure. *Heart and Lung, 12,* 428–429.

Watson, G. (1974). Effect of head rotation on jugular vein blood flow. *Archives of Disease in Childhood, 49,* 237–239.

Wilberger, J. E., Rothfus, W. E., Tabas, J., Goldberg, A. L., and Deeb, Z. L. (1990). Acute tissue tear hemorrhages of the brain: Computed tomography and clinicopathological correlations. *Neurosurgery, 27,* 208–213.

Williams, A., and Coyne, S. M. (1993). Effects of neck position on intracranial pressure. *American Journal of Critical Care, 2*(1), 68–71.

Wolfa, C. E., Luerssen, T. G., Bowman, R. M., and Putty, T. K. (1996). Brain tissue pressure gradients created by expanding frontal epidural mass lesion. *Journal of Neurosurgery, 84,* 642–647.

Yano, M., Ikeda, Y., Kobayashi, S., and Otsuka, T. (1987). Intracranial pressure in head-injured patients with various intracranial lesions is identical throughout the supratentorial intracranial compartment. *Neurosurgery, 21,* 688–692.

Yoshihara, M., Bandoh, K., and Marmarou, A. (1995). Cerebrovascular CO_2 reactivity assessed by ICP dynamics in severely head-injured patients. *Journal of Neurosurgery, 82,* 386–393.

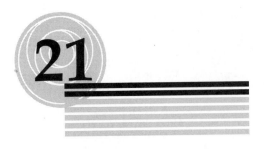

Fever Treatment

Barbara J. Holtzclaw

ever is a controlled temperature elevation above a person's usual thermoneutral range, or *set point*. Whereas normally an individual might maintain an ideal body temperature around 37°C ± .5 (98.5°F), pyrogens elevate this range to a higher level. Pyrogens need not be infectious or specifically antigenic in nature. Drugs, blood products, and foreign substances can cause release of centrally acting mediators that can elicit the febrile response. The earliest signs and symptoms of fever—chills, vasoconstriction, and shivering—reflect compensatory efforts to warm the body to the higher levels of the new set-point range. Fever should not be confused with *hyperthermia*, a pathological condition in which thermoregulatory cooling mechanisms fail (Khogali, 1997). In fever, thermoregulatory responses remain fully functional. Once internal and peripheral body temperatures reach the new set point, warming responses cease. The fact that these mechanisms remain intact in the febrile patient is important to clinical intervention and anticipated responses. For example, the tendency to chill is exaggerated during fever so that efforts to cool the patient cause shivering and compensatory warming. After several hours of elevated body temperature, falling pyrogen levels lower the set point and make the patient feel uncomfortably warm. Diaphoresis and vasodilation represent physiological responses that attempt to cool the body.

The ability to mount a fever requires some degree of immunological, metabolic, circulatory, and musculoskeletal competence. How well fever is tolerated depends on the patient's underlying health. The need to distribute body heat appropriately requires effective vasomotor activity, circulatory volume, and ability to sweat. The metabolic demands of raising the body's temperature require adequate oxygenation and caloric intake. Endocrine function is needed to maintain naturally occurring antipyresis. Finally, adequate fluid balance keeps the serum osmolality within normal range and improves the sensitivity of the thermoregulatory set point to pyrogens. Each of these demands can affect an individual's ability to self-regulate fever and provide keys to effective preventive fever-management interventions so complications can be avoided. When disease, injury, drugs, or therapy alters self-regulation competencies in fever, patients require supportive or therapeutic interventions. Although febrile temperatures are generally maintained at safe levels by the body's own endogenous antipyretics (Kluger, 1991), there is a need to assess this ability vigilantly.

THE FEBRILE RESPONSE AND HOST BENEFITS

Recognition of fever as a complex systemic response with host benefits is relatively new. Research of the last 20 years shows that mildly elevated temperatures benefit the host by creating hostile environments for several micro-organisms. Originally, it was believed that E-series *prostaglandins* (PGE) were the prime mediators (Kluger, 1991). Although they are still believed to play a major role, numerous intermediary substances have been found. These include *cytokines*, such as the interleukins, interferons, and Tumor Necrosis Factor. Interleukin-1 was at first believed to be the long-sought "endogenous pyrogen"; however, further research disclosed not one, but numerous fever-inducing substances (Kluger, 1991). Currently, there is controversy about whether PGE is necessary to evoke fever or whether PGE_2, the endogenous isoform of PGE, plays an essential role that can be mediated by noncytokine factors (Blatteis & Sehic, 1997, p. 117). The resolutions of these controversies will ultimately affect intervention, so they are of more than passing interest to nurses interested in fever care.

Cytokines are liberated by cells during infection or injury and act as cellular messengers. These substances not only raise body temperatures, but they also recruit a variety of nonspecific and antigen-specific immune factors. Some cytokines act locally on peripheral body tissues; others affect the brain and nervous system. Their pro-inflammatory actions account for some of the discomfort, appetite suppression, and general malaise experienced during fever.

Recent discoveries about cytokines and their receptor sites have clarified the pharmacodynamics of nonsteroidal anti-inflammatory drugs (NASAIDs) in fever. Drugs such as acetaminophen act on the brain and central nervous system to counteract cytokine activity and reduce fever and pain; however, they lack the anti-inflammatory action of peripherally acting aspirin or ibuprofen. The drug indomethacin appears to enhance the endogenous fever-reducing effects of arginine vasopressin in animals and may hold this potential for humans (Wilkinson & Kasting, 1993). As information about antipyretics evolves, nurses are able to make informed choices about the use and the consequences of use of antipyretics. Advances in clinical care have lagged behind rapidly evolving scientific discoveries; application to nursing care in textbooks is limited. Yet staying abreast of current literature and scientific discussion is crucial to making informed decisions in intervention.

REGULATORY MECHANISMS AFFECTED BY FEVER

In health, active and passive processes maintain a relatively narrow optimal thermoneutral range called the set point. Thermoregulatory responses react when temperature levels rise above, or fall below, the range. Body heat is constantly generated by cellular biochemical and metabolic reactions, by musculoskeletal contractions, and even by the friction of circulatory flow through vascular beds. Heat is continuously lost from the body by passive heat transference to the environment. The distribution of heat is governed primarily by vasomotor control, which determines the proximity of blood flow to skin and superficial tissues. Vasodilation promotes heat loss from the skin by conduction and radiation, whereas evaporation is promoted by sudomotor (sweating) activity. To maintain thermoneutral temperatures in cool weather, vasoconstriction conserves heat. Shivering generates heat through friction of muscle fibers and defends against falling central temperatures. Behavioral responses are active means of regulating body temperature. Changes in physical activity, dietary choices, and selection of clothing all influence the generation and conservation of heat. The notion of a thermostat is an oversimplification, but the model bears some similarities to the human body. A primary difference is that no single temperature represents the point at which thermoregulatory mechanisms are stimulated. The *integrated* input of thermosensory stimulus from central and superficial regions evokes responses that involve many coordinated systems.

During fever, the model of an elevated set point is currently used to explain the changes in body temperature (Boulant, 1997). The usual thermoregulatory mechanisms are regulated during fever, but at a higher range. For humans, thermoneutral temperatures are about 37°C ± 0.5 (98.6°F ± 1) for internal temperature and about 33.5°C ± 0.5 for skin. A pyrogen might cause the set-point limits of a person's thermoneutral range to rise from 37.5°C to 40°C. Figure 21–1 shows relationships between pyrogen levels and changes in set point. The existing body temperatures and the environment are sensed as being too cool, leading to shivering and vasoconstriction. This constitutes the *chill phase* of fever, during which patients feel miserably cold despite rising body temperature. Once body temperature reaches the set-point elevation, a *plateau phase* ensues, during which sensed temperature is more comfortable. When pyrogen levels fall, the set point returns to normal, and existing febrile temperatures are sensed as being too warm. Sweating and vasodilation characterize the *defervescence phase* of fever, during which patients complain of feeling overheated.

Of importance to activities in Fever Treatment is the recognition that skin stimulus often leads to massive thermoregulatory responses (Keatinge, Mason, Millard, & Newsstead, 1986). Sudden exposure of warm skin to cool air or

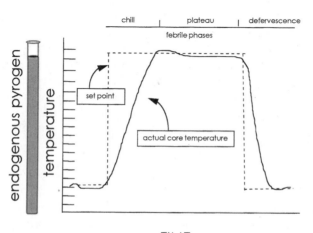

Figure 21–1 The febrile episode. Relationships between endogenous pyrogen, set-point levels, and core temperatures are shown with associated phases of the febrile episode.

TIME

surfaces triggers shivering and vasoconstriction before significant internal temperature changes occur. These principles direct action toward protection of thermosensitive regions of the skin, particularly during the chill phase of fever.

In choosing intervention activities, interrelationships between passive and active aspects of heat transfer must be considered. For example, active sweating can effectively promote passive evaporative heat loss from the skin. The subsequent rapid cooling of skin can provide a strong shivering stimulus in the febrile patient. However, the use of conductive cooling blankets to passively lower body temperature can induce such a strong thermoregulatory warming response that temperature actually rises. Similar paradoxical reactions occur when chilled liquids are given to a febrile person. The dynamic swing between the chill and hot phases of the febrile response calls for actions that promote comfort, prevent energy expenditure, maintain hydration, and allow heat loss without inducing counterproductive responses.

RELATED LITERATURE

Much emerging information about thermoregulatory responses and fever is readily applicable to patient care. Newer evidence supports interventions that are not directed at returning febrile temperatures to "normal," but at preventing dangerously high temperature levels. Temperatures above 44°C cause irreversible denaturation of proteins and sometimes fatal brain damage, but this rarely occurs with true fever. As clinicians recognize that temperature elevation is not the primary concern in fever, interventions become more comprehensive. Concern for shivering during a cooling treatment of fever has prompted some investigators to compare temperature-lowering methods. In a study of cooling blankets using four different settings, the use of higher settings reduced temperature more slowly but with less shivering and distress (Caruso, Hadley, Shukla, Frame, & Khoury, 1992). Another study found that antipyretics alone may be as effective as more aggressive means for patients not in imminent risk of hyperthermia (Morgan, 1990). Blanket "burns" caused by pressure on unperfused skin of conductive cooling pads are avoided by protecting hands, feet, and bony prominences with wraps or padding.

Sensory neurons from the skin surface become highly sensitive to the lower ambient temperature during fever (Hellon, 1981; Strom, 1960). Therefore, if surface cooling is necessary, treatment should protect sensitive regions of skin while promoting heat loss from less sensitive areas (Abbey, 1982). A greater density of heat-loss thermosensory neurons is found on skin of the hands and feet than on the trunk of the body (Keatinge et al., 1986). A protocol was developed to test the effectiveness of protecting skin surfaces of extremities with insulative wraps to prevent shivering during surface cooling (Abbey & Close, 1979). Three bath towels were placed lengthwise under arms and legs, with the sides drawn up and closed in a temporary seam by clips. Wraps were found to increase comfort and diminish shivering during induced hypothermia using conductive cooling blankets. These insulative "boots" and "mittens" conserve body heat and protect thermosensitive nerve endings on hands and feet while heat is lost from the trunk to the conductive cooling blanket (Abbey, 1982). Insulative extremity wraps can also be used when it is necessary to aggressively cool febrile patients with ice packs or convective cooling fans.

The use of insulative extremity wraps can alleviate the severity of febrile shivering during the onset of fever. The protocol is particularly effective when fever can be anticipated, as in administration of pyrogenic drugs or blood products (Holtzclaw, 1990). However, it can also be used in the early chill phase of nonspecific fever (Holtzclaw, 1992).

Studies of the role of body water and osmolality in thermoregulation show the need for better assessment and restoration of body water to prevent thermoregulatory impairment (Boulant, 1997). Fever promotes rapid water loss through metabolic consumption, sweating, and respiratory loss. In turn, water loss may cause or exacerbate fever. In chronically ill or debilitated persons, cellular destruction and metabolites require additional water for renal excretion and deplete tissue stores. Oral and intravenous fluid replacement helps to stabilize the thermoregulatory controls by normalizing serum osmolality. The subsequently improved circulatory perfusion to the skin and superficial tissues helps to dissipate heat. Fever imposes a metabolic burden on patients who are anemic or dehydrated or have poor nutritional intake.

INTERVENTION

The Nursing Interventions Classification (NIC) intervention Fever Treatment is shown in Table 21–1. The activities are of three types: those that nurses perform to detect temperature elevations and monitor febrile responses, those that are directed at stabilizing the thermoregulatory set point, and those that are performed to suppress febrile shivering.

Detecting Temperature Elevations

The measurement of body temperature seems a straightforward way to monitor thermal changes, but there is considerable confusion as to what constitutes appropriate instrumentation and technique. It is important to recognize that there is no single body temperature. Temperatures are different in various parts of the body based on the abundance of blood supply and the proximity to organs with great metabolic activity, especially the liver. Choice of thermometer type and measurement site should be based on the information being sought to direct care. In fever and hyperthermia, the primary concern is to maintain brain and neural temperatures within safe levels. Regardless of how hot skin or rectal temperatures become, the real issue is how high temperatures are in the cranial regions. Ideally, brain temperature would provide the best indicator, but the necessary instrumentation is not available for clinical use. The next best indication is pulmonary artery temperature, which approximates the temperature of blood leaving the heart and going to the brain. However, unless the patient has indwelling hemodynamic monitoring, this site, too, may be unavailable for measurement. The tympanic membrane (TM) light reflectance thermometer provides the next-closest proximity but introduces several sources of variability that can affect its reliability and accuracy (Erickson & Yount, 1991). The devices themselves vary by brand and expense in their range and accuracy when tested in laboratory conditions (Holtzclaw, 1993). The device relies on the reflectance of an infrared beam on the TM. The angle of insertion and use of an "ear tug" are some of the variations among users that can be standardized by appropriate training.

The tightly compressed ear canal of the infant makes it virtually impossible for the TM thermometer to detect anything but the temperature of the external ear canal. Rectal temperatures in infants carry risk of perforation and autonomic stimulation when thermometers are inserted to the depth necessary for accurate measurement. Full-term infant temperatures can be measured in the inguinal

Table 21–1   Fever Treatment

DEFINITION: Management of a patient with hyperpyrexia caused by nonenvironmental factors.

ACTIVITIES:

Monitor temperature as frequently as is appropriate

Monitor for insensible fluid loss

Institute a continuous core temperature monitoring device, as appropriate

Monitor skin color and temperature

Monitor blood pressure, pulse, and respiration, as appropriate

Monitor for decreasing levels of consciousness

Monitor for seizure activity

Monitor WBC, Hgb, and Hct values

Monitor intake and output

Monitor for electrolyte abnormalities

Monitor for acid-base imbalance

Monitor for presence of cardiac arrhythmias

Administer antipyretic medication, as appropriate

Administer medications to treat the cause of fever, as appropriate

Cover the patient with a sheet, only as appropriate

Administer a tepid sponge bath, as appropriate

Encourage increased intake of oral fluids, as appropriate

Administer IV fluids, as appropriate

Apply ice bag covered with a towel to groin and axilla

Increase air circulation by using a fan, as appropriate

Encourage or administer oral hygiene, as appropriate

Give appropriate medication to prevent or control shivering

Administer oxygen, as appropriate

Place patient on hypothermia blanket, as appropriate

Monitor temperature closely to prevent treatment-induced hypothermia

---

Source: McCloskey, J. C., and Bulechek, G. M. (1996). *Nursing interventions classification (NIC).* St. Louis: Mosby–Year Book.

folds, which provides a site that is safe, close to large blood vessels, and minimally influenced by environmental conditions (Bliss-Holtz, 1989).

In older children and adults, the TM thermometer is esthetically acceptable, quick, and convenient. With well-trained personnel, reliable instruments, and consistent technique, problems of measurement can be minimized. TM measurements are useful for persons in thermodynamic states who are unable to use an oral thermometer, including persons who are unconscious, in shock, hypothermic, or hyperthermic.

In thermodynamic conditions, it cannot be assumed that skin, oral, rectal, or TM temperatures are linear or vary consistently. Physiological shunting of circulation, leaving some regions hyperemic and others ischemic, creates wide gradients and regional temperature discrepancies. As long as thermoregulatory mechanisms are functional, cooling responses will strive to keep the brain cool during high temperature states, while skin and visceral temperatures rise. Such is not the case during hypothermic cooling. If conductive cooling lowers the febrile patient's core temperatures to hypothermic levels, visceral ischemia can lower rectal temperatures below those of the brain. In fever, the temperature of the oral cavity may be lower than but close to brain temperature because of the proximity of cranial and sublingual blood supplies.

The familiar mercury-in-glass thermometers are undesirable because of the risk for breakage and mercury leakage and the fact that they lose accuracy with extended shelf life. Oral electronic thermometers require electronic surveillance for periodic calibration and accuracy checks. One advantage of electronic devices over glass thermometers is their wider range of measurement and availability for continuous monitoring. Caution is needed in monitoring aggressive hypothermia treatment to be sure the lower limits of glass thermometers are sufficiently low to detect the patient's temperature.

Accurate and frequent monitoring is imperative during thermodynamic states of fever and cooling treatment. If loss of hypothalamic control impairs heat loss, body temperature, neurological signs, and hydration levels must be monitored closely to prevent secondary brain damage. Likewise, during therapy to lower hyperthermic temperature elevations, constant vigilance is necessary to forestall temperature drift, afterfall, and poikilothermia.

Stabilizing the Thermoregulatory Set Point

Ideally, interventions to treat fever are not designed to reduce body temperature directly. When possible, the offending cause is treated specifically. Infections warrant appropriate antimicrobial treatment, whereas antigenic drugs or blood products may require antihistamine or opiates to prevent shaking chills. Even antipyretic drugs alter body temperature indirectly by blocking the effects of prostaglandins and pyrogenic cytokines.

Use of antipyretic drugs has changed, with more concern being shown for comfort than for reducing mild elevations. Aspirin and other nonsteroidal anti-inflammatory agents lower febrile temperatures by blocking the production of prostaglandins and their subsequent release of cytokine mediators. NSAIDs are prescribed primarily to relieve myalgia or headache related to fever. Aspirin carries some risk of gastric irritation and interference with blood coagulation related to its antiprostaglandin activity. It has also been associated with risk for Reye's syndrome in children. Acetaminophen is not a potent prostaglandin antagonist, although it can lower febrile temperatures. Its relative safety with regard to Reye's syndrome makes it widely prescribed for children; it does not cause gastric irritation or clotting disorders, so it is useful for patients with gastric ulcers and those on anticoagulants. Despite these characteristics, acetaminophen should not be considered a harmless drug. Overdosage can lead to fatal liver toxicity, and some individuals may have idiosyncratic blood dyscrasias and allergies to the product. NSAIDs used more and more commonly for fever include ibuprofen, indomethacin, and naproxen. These drugs are better known for their anti-inflammatory activities, yet there may be other non–prostaglandin-linked mechanisms involved in fever control.

There is a close link between fluid balance and temperature regulation. Dehydration changes serum osmolality and can affect the stability of hypothalamic control, causing hyperthermia. Each 1% loss of body fluid leads to a 0.2°C gain in temperature. An aggressive oral fluid replacement regimen can be started early in the febrile episode, but intravenous infusions may be required to replace heavy loss from sweating. Supportive efforts to maintain hydration will avoid hyperthermic complications beyond those of fever. The caloric expenditure involved in thermogenesis, shivering, and negative nitrogen states of illness requires replacement in easily tolerated dietary form or parenteral supplements. Fluid by oral intake can achieve both caloric and fluid replacement. Sweetened teas and bland juices provide easily digested sources of glucose. If protein sources or supplements are tolerated orally, they should be encouraged. Room-temperature oral fluids are less likely to promote chilling and can be tolerated in larger amounts than cold ones.

Suppression of Febrile Shivering

For general supportive Fever Management, other interventions are aimed at supporting natural host responses, preventing febrile chills, and maintaining comfort. Threats to thermal balance arise from activities that promote heat generation from shivering. Care is needed during the defervescence phase when ambulating, removing damp sweaty clothing, and changing the bed. Changing to dry clothing under the bedcovers helps the patient avoid drafts and sudden cooling that can renew shivering episodes.

Pro-inflammatory mediators of fever tend to make febrile patients restless and irritable during the chill phase. During the plateau phase they are more comfortable, but defervescence makes them uncomfortably warm. Fatigue is common, and the "sick" feeling of fever has immunological origins. Consideration for a person's physiological needs during fever management must be balanced with the need for sleep and rest.

Cooling Measures

When temperatures run dangerously high and the patient's underlying condition is threatened by this hypermetabolic state, aggressive cooling measures may be warranted. One of the most effective methods of lowering febrile temperature is the conductive cooling blanket. It is effective because it overwhelms the patient's compensatory mechanisms and conducts heat away from the body to coils of circulating refrigerant. Shivering is problematic because it is aerobic activity and increases oxygen consumption and promotes lactic acidosis. Intravenous meperidine or lorazepam may attenuate shivering, but during rapid temperature fall, drugs alone are seldom effective. Use of higher settings may slow the reduction of temperature but will cause less shivering and patient distress. Blanket burns from the pressure between unperfused skin and conductive cooling pads are avoided by protecting hands, feet, and bony prominences with wraps or padding. Terrycloth towels used as extremity wraps (see case study), have been successful in diminishing shivering during surface cooling in controlled trials (Abbey et al., 1973; Abbey & Close, 1979).

A serious hazard of the conductive cooling blanket is induced hypothermia and loss of thermoregulatory competence. This condition, called poikilothermia increases the danger of uncontrolled temperature "afterdrop" once desired temperatures are reached (Giesbrecht & Bristow, 1997). Vigilant observation and temperature measurement are needed continuously throughout the procedure, using core temperature as a reference point. After the desired temperature is reached, monitoring must continue until there is stability in temperature readings for at least 1 hour.

Sponge bathing, even with tepid water, can cause defensive vasoconstriction and has not been shown to be an effective coolant during fever, and therefore should be used with caution. Compensatory shivering during sponge baths may actually raise body temperature. Alcohol sponge baths should never be used, as they liberate toxic fumes and create drastic cooling of skin. Cooling fans should be used with caution for the same reason.

Educating Colleagues and Others

The febrile response was poorly understood by the scientific community until the 1970s. From the time thermometers were given to nurses, a preponderance of nursing activity centered on measurement and recording of body temperature. Early in the 1900s, elevations in temperature were feared as the cause, rather than the effect, of an infectious illness. Interventions were aimed solely at "bringing the fever down" with aspirin and cooling measures. This simplistic and negative view of fever remains a problematic legacy today, despite growing evidence that elevated temperature is perhaps the least troublesome aspect of the febrile complex. Discoveries that symptoms of distress, headache, malaise, and aching muscles are effects of circulating cytokines and are not caused by rising temperature have brought about important changes in the way fever management is viewed. Meanwhile, education is needed to correct misdirected efforts to drastically lower body temperature by cooling measures that are often counterproductive and distressful and cause the temperature to rise even higher.

NURSING DIAGNOSES AND APPROPRIATE PATIENT GROUPS

Hyperthermia, the existing North American Nursing Diagnosis Association (NANDA) diagnosis, limits its focus to body temperature as the major alteration, rather than considering the underlying change of *altered set point*. Unfortunately, this approach tends to suggest treatment that is directed toward moving the temperature back to normal rather than toward dealing with the array of prodromal indicators and conditions that precede temperature changes. Newer views of Fever Treatment are aimed at the systemic febrile response, rather than at the temperature elevation. Even antipyretic drugs are being used more conservatively; they are given to promote comfort and relieve aching more than to reduce temperature. There are equally important needs surrounding the febrile response that are related to fluid support and suppression of febrile shivering. The diagnostic label Risk for Altered Body Temperature identifies threats to thermal balance that must be recognized, regardless of existing body temperature. Threats may involve the patient's thermal comfort level, oxygenation, energy reserves, fluid balance, or ability to tolerate compensatory mechanisms. In the elderly and the immunosuppressed, the febrile response may be blunted, and threats associated with fever are often found in parameters other than body temperature elevation. With prolonged febrile illness, fluid deficit and dehydration become increasing threats.

Fever is ubiquitous in health and illness and extends to all ages, from neonates to the elderly. It often manifests differently and has different consequences for the very young, the elderly, and those with underlying illness or injury. Fever often heralds infection, and in the immunosuppressed cancer patient can represent a life-threatening systemic infection. In the patient with human immunodeficiency virus (HIV), the chronic presence of pyrogenic cytokines may manifest itself in low-grade fever without any identifiable opportunistic infection. These same cytokines have been linked to the appetite suppression and wasting associated with HIV. Still other patients with massive tissue destruction and injury, such as those with burns or crushing injuries, may manifest a noninfection-oriented fever in response to circulating cytokines. Finally, it is not always easy to diagnose the difference between fever and hypothermia when multisystem injury or sepsis occurs and is complicated by environmentally hot conditions. In such situations, the emphasis in Fever Treatment is maintaining *safe* levels of temperature, preventing febrile shivering, and maintaining hydration.

OUTCOMES OF FEVER TREATMENT

For many years, the hallmarks of effective Fever Treatment have been the speed and magnitude of temperature decline. These outcomes may be appropriate for medical and pharmacological management of a specific infection or antigenic response, but they do not reflect the many concerns related to the febrile response. The Nursing Outcomes Classification (NOC) outcomes Thermoregulation and Thermoregulation: Neonate indicate balance among heat production, heat gain, and heat loss. Maintenance of a *safe* core body temperature (<40°C, 104°F) rather than a *normal* temperature is a desired goal throughout a febrile episode. Control of febrile shivering during all phases of fever is key to reducing heat production, energy expenditure, and distress to the patient. Restoration of fluid loss is important in maintaining thermal balance as shown by improved skin turgor, salivary moisture, urinary output, and restoration of prefebrile weight. There is need for risk control in the selection and calibration of thermometers for use in fever surveillance. Risk control in this area extends to instruction for staff, caregivers, and family members regarding fever management. Scientifically sound fever management practices, correct measurement of body temperatures, and ability to interpret temperature changes rationally are relevant.

CASE STUDY

Mr. H, age 37, was injured in a farm accident in which the tractor he was driving overturned. He sustained a concussion injury and a penetrating chest wound from the tractor gear levers. He showed signs of mild cerebral edema, although magnetic resonance imaging (MRI) studies were negative for skull fracture and hemorrhage. Frequent monitoring for increased intracranial pressure found no remarkable changes for the first 2 days. On Day 3, Mr. H continued to have oxygen by mask, chest tubes in place, and broad-spectrum intravenous antibiotics as medical treatment. His oral temperature rose suddenly to 40.6°C (105°F). Blood cultures were drawn, and a portable MRI was done to check for changes. The immediate assessment supported the view that Mr. H's fever elevation was of infectious origin, rather than from neurological injury. Physicians decided on an alternative drug treatment, but they were concerned about the effect of the rising temperature on cerebral edema. A cooling blanket was ordered.

Mr. H required immediate cooling to protect the delicate neural tissues from heat and to reduce existing cerebral edema. Although shivering is inevitable with cooling, his physician was reluctant to order meperidine or sedatives, fearing the effects of respiratory depression on his neurological and pulmonary status. His nurse recognized that shivering would further compromise his oxygenation and acid-base balance and selected a nonpharmacological intervention to prevent shivering. Extremity wraps were fashioned from 12 bath towels, 3 per extremity. Towels were stacked lengthwise, edges brought together, and seams rolled and then taped in place. A light gown and soft covering were left on Mr. H. The conductive cooling blanket was applied on top and started at 23.9°C (75°F). The cooling blanket was equipped with a rectal temperature probe and with servo controls to shut off the circulating coolant when core temperatures dropped to desired levels. The servo control was set at 38°C (100.4°F). A TM thermometer was used for monitoring every 15 minutes and to verify that servo controls remained functional. Mr. H stated that he felt cold but not uncomfortably so. He did not shiver. At 38°C (100.4°F), the cooling blanket was turned off but kept in place. Mr. H's temperature continued to fall to 37.2°C (99°F), where it stabilized for 3 hours. The cooling blanket was removed, but care was taken not to chill Mr. H during his care.

References

Abbey, J. C. (1982). Shivering and surface cooling. In C. M. Norris (Ed.), *Concept clarification in nursing* (pp. 223–242). Rockville, MD: Aspen.

Abbey, J. C., Andrews, C., Avigliano, K., Blossom, R., Bunke, B., Clark, E., Engberg, N., Healy, P., Peterson, J., Shirley, C., and Waers, C. (1973). A pilot study: The control of shivering during hypothermia by a clinical nursing measure. *Journal of Neurosurgical Nursing, 5*(2), 78–88.

Abbey, J. C., and Close, L. (1979). A study of control of shivering during hypothermia. *Communicating Nursing Research, 12*, 2–3.

Blatteis, C. M., and Sehic, E. (1997). Circulating pyrogen signaling of the brain: A new working hypothesis. In C. M. Blatteis (Ed.), *Thermoregulation: Tenth International Symposium on the Pharmacology of Thermoregulation, Annals of the New York Academy of Sciences: Vol. 813* (pp. 663–675). New York: New York Academy of Sciences.

Bliss-Holtz, J. (1989). Comparison of rectal, axillary, and inguinal temperatures in full-term newborn infants. *Nursing Research, 38*(2), 85–87.

Boulant, J. A. (1997). Thermoregulation. In P. A. Mackowiak (Ed.), *Fever: Basic mechanisms and management* (2nd ed., pp. 35–58). Philadelphia: Lippincott-Raven.

Caruso, C. C., Hadley, B. J., Shukla, R., Frame, P., and Khoury, J. (1992). Cooling effects and comfort of four cooling blanket temperatures in humans with fever. *Nursing Research, 41*(2), 68–72.

Erickson, R. S. and Yount, S. T. (1991). Comparison of tympanic and oral temperatures in surgical patients. *Nursing Research, 40*(2), 90–93.

Giesbrecht, G. G. and Bristow, G. K. (1997). Recent advances in hypothermia research. In C. M Blatteis (Ed.), *Thermoregulation: Tenth International Symposium on the Pharmacology of Thermoregulation, Annals of the New York Academy of Sciences: Vol. 813* (pp. 663–675). New York: New York Academy of Sciences.

Hellon, R. F. (1981). Neurophysiology of temperature regulation: Problems and perspectives. *Federation Proceedings, 40*, 2804.

Holtzclaw, B. J. (1990). Effects of extremity wraps to control drug-induced shivering: A pilot study. *Nursing Research, 39*, 280–283.

Holtzclaw, B. J. (1992). The febrile response in critical care: State of the science. *Heart & Lung, 2*, 482–501.

Holtzclaw, B. J. (1993). Monitoring body temperature. *AACN Clinical Issues in Critical Care Nursing, 4*(1), 44–55.

Keatinge, W. R., Mason, A. C., Millard, C. E., and Newsstead, C. G. (1986). Effects of fluctuating skin temperature on thermoregulatory responses in man. *Journal of Physiology, 378*, 241–252.

Khogali, M. (1997). Heat illness alert program: Practical implications for management and prevention. In Blatteis, C. M. (Ed.), *Thermoregulation: Tenth International Symposium on the Pharmacology of Thermoregulation, Annals of the New York Academy of Sciences: Vol. 813* (pp. 526–533). New York: New York Academy of Sciences.

Kluger, M. J. (1991). Fever: Role of pyrogens and cryogens. *Physiological Reviews, 71*(1), 93–127.

McCloskey, J., and Bulechek, G. (1995). Validation and coding of the NIC taxonomy structure. Iowa Intervention Project. Nursing Interventions Classification. *Image—the Journal of Nursing Scholarship, 27*(1), 43–49.

Morgan, S. P. (1990). A comparison of three methods of managing fever in the neurologic patient. *Journal of Neuroscience Nursing, 22*(1), 19–24.

Strom, G. (1960). Central nervous regulation of body temperature. In J. Field, H. W. Magoun, and V. E. Hall (Eds.), *Neurophysiology* (p. 1186). Washington, DC: American Physiological Society.

Wilkinson, M., and Kasting, N. (1993). Vasopressin release within the ventral septal area of the rat brain during drug-induced antipyresis. *American Journal of Physiology, 264*, R1133–1138.

Wongsurawat, N., Davis, B. B., and Morley, J. E. (1990). Thermoregulatory failure in the elderly. *Journal of the American Geriatrics Society, 38*, 899–906.

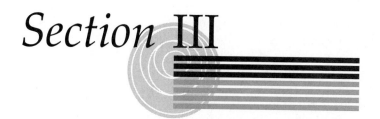

Section III

Behavioral Interventions

Overview: Care That Supports Psychosocial Functioning and Facilitates Lifestyle Changes

Gloria M. Bulechek

Joanne C. McCloskey

Nurses routinely work with clients who desire to or need to alter their lifestyles. Most people find security and comfort in their daily routines, and altering health behavior means changing familiar habits. The need for change often comes coupled with the grief and stress associated with catastrophic illness or injury. Changing behavior, especially long-term patterns, is never easy. Psychologists continue to debate about what produces individual behavioral change. Cognitive theorists believe that a change in behavior is preceded by an internal change in attitudes, values, or beliefs. On the other side of the debate are the behaviorists, who argue that behavior is shaped externally through reinforcement. The professional practitioner is forced to conclude that the theories to explain lifestyle change are inadequate. The challenge for nurses is to develop skills that will facilitate self-directed change in clients. This section of the book presents 11 interventions designed to assist with this process. The chapter authors draw from both cognitive and behaviorist theories to formulate treatments to assist clients with changes in behavior.

Reminiscence Therapy, the subject of Chapter 22, has developed to take advantage of the aged individual's normal developmental tendency to think about and relate to personally significant past experiences. The aim of the intervention is to enhance wellness in the aged client who is lonely, depressed, and withdrawn. Rebecca A. Johnson indicates that Reminiscence Therapy can be used with individual patients or with small groups. Favorable outcomes demonstrated through research include decreases in depression and in the amount of required medication and increases in socialization and self-care activities. Johnson lists the North American Nursing Diagnosis Association (NANDA) diagnoses for which this intervention may be appropriate as well as the Nursing Outcomes Classification (NOC) outcomes this intervention may produce. The chapter concludes with a case study in which the intervention is used with a group of elders in a long-term care facility.

Patient Contracting uses the principles of reinforcement to help the client achieve desired outcomes. The reinforcement is contingent on the performance of a desired behavior. It is based on the belief that all individuals have the right to self-determination and to assume responsibility for their own well-being. The intervention has been tested with multiple populations since the 1970s and is used by both nurses and other health practitioners. In Chapter 23, Margaret R. Simons uses seven steps to describe implementation of Patient Contracting. She cautions that this intervention should not be a substitute for patient teaching; the patient must have the necessary knowledge in order to comply with desired health behaviors. The chapter contains an excellent section linking the associated Nursing Interventions Classification (NIC), NOC, and NANDA terms and concludes with an illustrative case study.

Preparatory Sensory Information is an intervention that helps patients cope with stressful tests and procedures. This intervention has a strong research base, having been conducted since 1970. The majority of these studies have been done by nurses, notably Jean E. Johnson and her colleagues. In Chapter 24, Norma J. Christman, Karin T. Kirchhoff, and Marsha G. Oakley describe the studies and discuss the development of self-regulation theory. They discuss the relative benefits of subjective versus objective information as observed in the research. A case study of a woman scheduled to undergo external radiation therapy demonstrates the implementation of the intervention. Preparatory Sensory Information has low risk for the patient and takes little nursing time. Based on sound research, it is an intervention that all nurses should know how to implement.

Barbara J. Boss provides a wealth of clinical information in Chapter 25, **Communication Enhancement: Speech Deficit**. She reviews various types of communication deficits, including linguistic deficit, pragmatic deficit, and high-level language skill deficit and emphasizes the importance of complete assessment and accurate diagnosis. A table contains a list of assessment tests that the experienced nurse specialist or speech pathologist can administer to differentiate the types of communication deficits. Therapy can then be tailored to the client and may include medical management, surgery with or without prosthetic devices, and speech therapy. Communication Enhancement: Speech Deficit can be used in each of these situations. Boss organizes the application of this intervention into four parts. First, create an environment that encourages communication. Second, provide supportive actions accompanied by patience, acceptance, and recognition of the difficulty the patient is experiencing. Third, apply accepted principles regarding communication facilitation. Fourth, provide education for the patient and the patient's family. The author identifies relevant nursing diagnoses, including one she has developed. Outcomes appropriate to the intervention are identified. The chapter concludes with a case study and a helpful list of references.

Genetic Counseling is an intervention of growing importance as the mapping of the human genome constantly provides new information. In Chapter 26, Janet K. Williams and Debra L. Schutte point out that this intervention is now used across the life span and should be understood by nurses in all specialties. Multiple populations are in need of the information and support provided by this intervention. The authors link the intervention to a number of outcomes and point out that it is a fertile area for nursing research. The chapter details how to implement this intervention and shows its application in a case study of a young woman with a family history of breast cancer.

Efforts to assist clients to stop smoking have met with minimal success. In Chapter 27, Kathleen A. O'Connell and Constance A. Koerin, members of a research team studying health behavior at the University of Kansas, propose that nurses are in a key position to assist with this health-promotion goal. She asserts that efforts to stop smoking must be self-directed and require long-term support. The intervention **Smoking Cessation Assistance** provides direction to the nurse in facilitating self-change. The intervention is designed to help clients stop smoking rather than reduce it. The steps of the intervention are applied in a case study. O'Connell and Koerin offer concrete help to nurses who are working with clients who desire to or need to stop smoking.

Music has been used throughout history to relieve human suffering. In Chapter 28, Linda A. Gerdner and Kathleen C. Buckwalter call **Music Therapy** a holistic intervention and review the research, which supports the use of music in physical, psychological, social, and spiritual conditions. The extensive literature is summarized by condition and population in a table. The authors stress that individual music preferences must be determined and incorporated into the intervention. A tool to determine preferences is given, as is a tool to evaluate the impact of the intervention. A table lists the NANDA diagnoses and NOC outcomes associated with this intervention. The chapter concludes with two case studies and an extensive reference list.

In Chapter 29, Mary Lober Aquilino describes **Health Education** as an intervention that enables decision making by shaping motivation, values, attitudes, and beliefs. It emphasizes client responsibility for health and is commonly delivered to a group. The focus is health promotion and disease prevention, rather than disease treatment. It may be delivered to all age groups, from preschoolers to elders, and may cover any number of topics. The goal is to match the program with identified health risk factors for specific groups or communities. Technology is being used to help meet the demand for quality health education programs. More emphasis is being placed on effectiveness, in terms of both cost and well-being. Aquilino describes the process of implementing Health Education and identifies related NANDA diagnoses and NOC outcomes. She concludes with two case studies, one involving children and one involving adults.

Substance abuse continues to be a priority health problem for our nation. In Chapter 30, Julia Hagemaster describes the history of addictions in our society and reviews current studies that attempt to describe patterns of substance use. Multiple biological, psychological, and social risk factors make individuals of all ages vulnerable to addiction. More research on both causative factors and treatment strategies is needed. Hagemaster describes primary, secondary, and tertiary **Substance Use Prevention** and stresses that the nursing activities must be culturally relevant. She identifies NOC outcomes appropriate for this intervention and provides a table of nursing diagnoses that are common in addiction. The chapter concludes with a case study.

Nurses in all settings encounter patients with dysfunctional moods. Only a portion of this population is admitted to psychiatric settings. Agency for Healthcare Policy and Research (AHCPR) guidelines, entitled *Depression in Primary Care*, recommend pharmacotherapy, psychotherapy, electroconvulsive therapy, and light therapy. Nurses assist with these therapies, but it is the daily management of the patients that Mary Kanak describes in Chapter 31, **Mood**

Management. Mood Management is made up of nursing activities that provide safety and assist in attaining a healthier level of mental and physical functioning. Kanak describes five clusters of activities. Safety from harm to self or others is the first priority. Safety precautions are patterned according to the patient's symptoms. Self-care deficits are common in these patients, and the nurse monitors and assists while encouraging responsibility for self-care. The nurse may intervene with activities that compensate for the patient's cognitive deficits while awaiting restoration of more normal cognitive functioning. These patients often withdraw from family and friends, and the nurse can target activities to increase socialization. Patient and family knowledge is key to compliance with treatment and prevention of relapse. The intervention is appropriate for use in inpatient, outpatient, and community settings and with both adults and children. Kanak provides a table that links NANDA diagnoses and NOC outcomes associated with this intervention. The chapter concludes with a case study that illustrates the implementation of the intervention.

Kathie M. Cole is a critical care nurse and the director of the People–Animal Connection Program at the University of California, Los Angeles. Chapter 32, **Animal-Assisted Therapy**, describes a unique intervention that is becoming more widely used. There is a growing research base that documents the physiological, cognitive, physical, psychosocial, and spiritual outcomes of the intervention. Animal-Assisted Therapy can be used with both adults and children. It has been used in a variety of health care settings, including long-term care, hospital, and home. A variety of animals, including dogs, cats, fish, birds, and horses, have been used in conjunction with the intervention. Cole offers suggestions for setting up a program and preparing care plans for the use of this intervention. The chapter concludes with two case studies.

Reminiscence Therapy

Rebecca A. Johnson

> Heigh-Ho! Babyhood! Tell me where you linger!
> Let's toddle home again, for we have gone astray;
> Take this eager hand of mine and lead me by the finger
> Back to the lotus-lands of the far-away!
>
> Turn back the leaves of life—Don't read the story—
> Let's find the pictures, and fancy all the rest;
> We can fill the written pages with a brighter glory
> Than old Time, the story-teller, at his very best.
>
> *James Whitcomb Riley (1905)*

The underlying theme of this poem excerpt parallels the purpose and benefits of reminiscence. It is defined as the process of recalling past events of life, either verbally or silently. The well-being of self, self-esteem, self-actualization, or quality of life identified by many researchers may consist of a curious mixture of the joys and sorrows that make up the past. Researchers imply that a calm existence is made possible by drawing into immediate presence the individual's reminiscence of experiences and emotions.

Advice giving was one of the early uses of reminiscence, which symbolized wisdom and reverence. The themes of wisdom, purification, creativity, inspiration, gifts, and worthiness were associated with memory. Pear, in a classic book on memory, said that the "mind never photographs, it paints pictures" and that the main function of the imagery associated with memory is to convey meaning (1922, p. 44). This meaning may be either stable or shifting, but it depends on the context in which it was formed.

Pear (1922, p. 13) believed that "to good remembering, as to good art, leaving out the right things is indispensable—the art of forgetting is but the inner aspect of the art of remembering." Harriman, Greenwood, and Skinner (1942) referred to *reverie* in their discussions of daydreams, imagination, and creative thinking. They also used the terms *castle-building, musing, fantasy-making*, and *woolgathering* to designate "simple devices whereby we manage to escape from reality" (p. 206). They advocated these activities for preventing boredom and promoting recreation, and they cautioned that it was only when these activities were habitually substituted for reality that they became "detrimental to the welfare of the individual" (p. 208). Thus, whether it is called reminiscence, life review, reverie, dreaming, woolgathering, or oral history making, reminiscence is a purposeful, creative activity with the potential to bring about resolution and well-being.

The importance of reminiscence in preliterate societies was based on the need for elders to help younger members link the past with the present, providing a sense of group identity (Langness, 1965). Storytelling was important in these groups for entertainment, instruction, and admonition. Memory was the only repository of knowledge, skills, and rituals. Thus, reminiscence was a revered ability, a gift not possessed by all (Holzberg, 1984). However, the importance of reminiscing for this function probably declined sharply as communication techniques became more sophisticated. As modernization progressed, the oral method of communication dwindled in importance. "Civilized" society, with its decentralization of information sources, relegated reminiscence to a position of little value, and it was nearly lost as a recognized productive activity. It may be that at this point reminiscence became more readily recognized as an internal, individual activity rather than an important group or societal feature. Reminiscence became viewed as a negative behavior or defense mechanism predominantly present in the elderly (Brown & Cecil, 1946; Lawton, 1946; Lewis, 1943).

REMINISCENCE THERAPY DEFINED

In an early article, reminiscence was mentioned as an intervention for "mental health hazards" of the elderly (Stevenson, 1959, p. 414). This broke the previous linkage of reminiscence to senility associated with aging. The major turning point in the development of reminiscence as a basis for intervention was Butler's (1963) work coining the phrase *life review*, in which the person engages in a review of past events in order to come to an understanding and acceptance of life. According to Butler (1974), life review occurs in response to a major life event or crisis of development. Butler's work stimulated great interest in reminiscence among researchers and clinicians alike. However, in subsequent years, the process of Reminiscence Therapy has been clearly delineated as an intervention distinct from life review (Burnside & Haight, 1992; Haight & Burnside, 1993). A third process, account making, also is based on reminiscence. Accounts are stories containing a chronology of events and usually a moral or lesson learned from the events and their consideration, and they are formed as people work to gain a sense of control over their life situations (Weber, Harvey, & Stanley, 1987). They occur in response to a threatening event or may be generated over a period of years, inwardly, as people create a sense of order and purpose in life.

Reminiscence Therapy is a nursing intervention that occurs when people use recall of past events, feelings, and thoughts to facilitate pleasure, quality of life, or adaptation to present circumstances (Hamilton, 1992). It may be conducted in either a dyad or a group format. It is suitable for patients who are cognitively intact as well as for those who have some degree of cognitive impairment, as long as they are able to recall life events and express themselves (Burnside, 1988). During Reminiscence Therapy, a life history (a written account of genealogy or the major events in one's life), an autobiography, or an oral history (an audiotaped genealogy or account of one's major life events) may be created (Baum, 1980; Merrill, 1985). The goal is for the patients to share with a group their experiences of particular life events, to communicate with others, and to gain a sense of validation and reinforcement.

Life review, however, is a more in-depth psychoanalytic intervention, taking place in a dyad, in which the helping professional, by probing and guiding, encourages the patient to analyze and evaluate each phase of life. The goal is for the patient to resolve major events and stages of life in order to adjust better to the present and future, or perhaps to prepare for death.

LITERATURE RELATED TO REMINISCENCE

Before the 1980s, there was no systematic distinction made between life review and Reminiscence Therapy (Burnside & Haight, 1992; Haight & Burnside, 1993). Various authors have identified types of reminiscence (Havighurst & Glaser, 1972; Lo Gerfo, 1980; Wong & Watt, 1991). Nearly all of the published research, integrative reviews, and clinical application literature uses the two terms interchangeably. This chapter confines its discussion of the literature to works using Reminiscence Therapy. Works clearly using life review (although it may be called simply *reminiscence* by their authors) are not included insofar as it was possible to ascertain this in light of unclear definitions of concepts and delineation of methods.

During the 1980s, in a burgeoning interest in reminiscence, at least 36 studies involving reminiscence were conducted. In addition, five literature reviews were conducted (Busch, 1984; Merriam, 1980; Molinari & Reichlin, 1985; Romaniuk, 1981; Thornton & Brotchie, 1987), numerous theoretical discussion papers or book chapters were published, and a book reporting a study on reminiscence (Coleman, 1986) and another synthesizing research and clinical thinking about reminiscence (Magee, 1988) were released. Interest in reminiscence has remained strong during the 1990s, with more than 50 publications on the topic.

Reminiscence, Mood, and Well-Being

Published studies illustrate the wide diversity of variables that have received the attention of researchers. Of considerable interest are the findings suggesting that reminiscence has a positive influence on mood. This is the most commonly studied dependent variable reported in the literature. Clements (1981) made some convincing theoretical connections between reminiscence and the cure of the soul.

In two early studies, McMahon and Rhudick (1964, 1967) studied 25 noninstitutionalized Spanish-American war veterans aged 78 to 90. The studies were based on the premise that because reminiscence is so prevalent in the elderly, it must have some adaptational significance. The researchers conducted nondirective 1-hour interviews with each subject.

Reminiscing was not related to degree of intellectual deterioration or level of depression. However, in patients who were not depressed, correlations with amount of reminiscing fell just short of statistical significance (McMahon & Rhudick, 1964). Mortality data suggested that, independent of age, significantly more of those who were depressed and reminisced less at the time of interview had died at the 1-year follow-up.

Several other researchers have found Reminiscence Therapy to be related to lower levels of depression (Burnside, 1990; Dhooper, Green, Huff, & Austin-Murphy, 1993; Fallot, 1980; Fry, 1983; Merriam, 1993; Parsons, 1986; Perrotta & Meacham, 1981; Walker, 1984), to psychological well-being, or to mood (Fallot, 1980; Ferguson, 1980; Rattenbury & Stones, 1989).

Fry (1983), for example, found in his study of 162 depressed elderly that structured Reminiscence Therapy reduced self-reportings of depression and increased feelings of self-confidence and adequacy. Fry's study is particularly important because, unlike most research in this field, it used a true experimental design and careful, clear conceptualizations of both Reminiscence Therapy and depression.

Strack, Schwarz, and Gschneidinger (1985) found that recall had a positive effect on mood and, further, that vivid reminiscing had a greater effect than did nonvivid recall. Their three experiments were conducted with nonelderly students at professional schools. However, owing to the rigor of their studies and their unique findings, their work merits further discussion. In their initial experiment, they determined that recalling of present hedonic events had a positive effect on mood. However, hedonic past events were likely to produce nonhedonic mood states (Strack et al., 1985, p. 1462). In their next two experiments, they demonstrated that it is not only the hedonic quality of the reminiscences, but also the way in which they are thought about during reminiscence that influences mood. Vivid reminiscence had a greater influence on mood changes than did nonvivid reminiscence.

Some research on reminiscence and mood has not been so encouraging (Hibel, 1971). For example, Stevens-Ratchford (1992) found that reminiscence affected neither depression nor self-esteem. Similarly, Perrotta and Meacham (1981) found no improvements in either self-esteem or depression in their experimental study of 21 elderly community residents. One feature of their research that may be considered a weakness is that only three reminiscence sessions were spread over a 5-week data-collection period before postmeasurements were taken. This may not have been enough sessions, or the prolonged time lag between intervention and measurement may have influenced the findings.

Harp Scates, Randolph, Gutsch, and Knight (1986) found no pre- or posttest differences in trait anxiety in their study of 60 senior citizens after six reminiscence sessions held twice weekly. Brennan and Steinberg (1984) found that although reminiscence mediated morale and activity level, it was not significantly related to improved morale. Morale was more positively associated with level of social activity than with reminiscence. However, it may be argued that Reminiscence Therapy is a form of social activity. Finally, Arean et al. (1993) found that a problem-solving group intervention was more effective in ameliorating depression than was Reminiscence Therapy among older adults with depression.

Reminiscence and Self-Esteem

Kovach (1991) devised a model of reminiscence that posited that it enhanced self-esteem. Findings of others have supported this premise (Baker, 1985; Hamilton, 1980; Lappe, 1987; Moore, 1985; Perrotta & Meacham, 1981). A related finding of Taft and Nehrke (1990) showed that reminiscence enhanced ego integrity among their elderly nursing-home-resident subjects. McGowan (1994) found a positive effect on self-image. Rybarczyk and Auerbach (1990) found that Reminiscence Therapy significantly enhanced coping self-efficacy among elderly presurgical patients. Giltinan (1990) found that elderly female group reminiscence members developed a strong sense of belonging with one another.

Baker (1985) found that group Reminiscence Therapy allowed mentally impaired clients in her study to experience feelings of self-worth. Similarly, in her qualitative study of eight elderly community residents, Carlson (1984) found that reminiscence enabled the subjects to preserve a stability of self and identity even though they faced numerous real and potential losses.

Reminiscence and Life Satisfaction

Life satisfaction has been studied, in addition to a series of seemingly related variables such as self-actualization (Tekavec, 1982), self-acceptance (Beadleson-Baird & Lara, 1987), life justification (Revere & Tobin, 1980), and personal power (Bramlett & Gueldner, 1993). Reminiscence Therapy has been found to positively affect life satisfaction (Bennett & Maas, 1988; DeGenova, 1993; DeMotts, 1981; Haight & Bahr, 1984; Harp Scates et al., 1986), self-actualization (Beadleson-Baird & Lara, 1987; Bramwell, 1984; Eargle, 1980; Tekavec, 1982), and adjustment to present life circumstances (Coleman, 1986).

Coleman (1986), in one of the rare longitudinal studies of elderly people, found that over a 16-year period, recurring individual reminiscence assisted in the adjustment to advancing age and life circumstances. Brennan & Steinberg (1984) wrote of the "adaptiveness" of reminiscence. Berghorn and Schafer (1987) found that elderly patients in their reminiscence group who were not successfully adapting to nursing home life were more likely to be affected positively by reminiscence. Life satisfaction scores and "perceived friendliness of other residents in the home" (Berghorn & Schafer, 1987, p. 117) were affected.

Findings of DeGenova (1993), however, were conditional. Elderly subjects who had spouses present were more likely to have a significant positive response in the life satisfaction score. The opposite was true for older adults without spouses. Harp Scates et al. (1986) found no pre- and posttest differences in life satisfaction among 60 senior citizens after twice-weekly reminiscence sessions were held for 3 weeks.

Reminiscence and Functioning

Reminiscence has been found to improve behavioral, social, and cognitive functioning. In an interesting twist from the majority of reminiscence studies, Hughston and Merriam (1982) found that a structured reminiscence program resulted in improved scores of cognitive functioning in a group of 105 elderly volunteers. The study used reminiscence activities to "exercise" cognitive processes over a period of 4 weeks. Women made more considerable gains than did men. Luborsky (1987) analyzed several life histories to ascertain that the way subjects reminisced was an indicator of cognition or conceptual orientation. Namazi and Haynes (1994) found improvement in the Mini Mental State Exam scores of their elderly subjects with Alzheimer's disease, but these improvements were minimal.

Baker (1985) found that her mentally impaired female subjects engaged in more verbal interaction, leadership behavior, and active participation in their environment as a result of Reminiscence Therapy. These findings are supported by the work of David (1981) and Norris and Eileh (1982), who found that communication increased significantly in their subjects. Similarly, Orten, Allen, and Cook (1989) found that over an 8-week period, Reminiscence Therapy had a mild positive effect on social behavior among their elderly subjects.

Conversely, Brennan and Steinberg (1984) found no relationship between reminiscence, morale, and social activity level. Their findings indicated that morale was more positively associated with level of social activity than with reminiscence. Similarly, Berghorn and Schafer (1987) found no differences in attitudes or behaviors among their nursing-home-residing subjects after a Reminiscence Therapy group. Martin and Stepath (1993) found that among their subjects in a geriatric-psychiatric unit, psychodramatic techniques (enacting a theme or encounter) in combination with Reminiscence Therapy were more effective in enhancing group interaction and attention than was Reminiscence Therapy alone.

Reminiscence and the Developmental Process of Aging

Several authors have written about the role of reminiscence in facilitating the mastery of developmental tasks facing the elderly. The major task facing the elderly, according to Evans, Millicovsky, and Tennison (1984), is the gaining of a sense of integrity of their lives. Carlson (1984) emphasizes that reminiscence serves to justify the past. The premise that ego-integrity is enhanced by reminiscence was supported by the finding of Boylin, Gordon, and Nehrke (1976). The act of reminiscing about a particular event allows the reminiscer to relive the experience, together with the associated emotions. The past event can be incorporated into the individual's store of acceptable situations. Or, in the case of negatively associated events, the damaging effects of these can be examined with the added perspectives of time and distance. Butler (1980) also affirmed this function of reminiscence, explaining that it serves to help people "resolve, reorganize, and reintegrate" (p. 37) events that they find troubling or preoccupying.

Another function of reminiscence is as a means of coping with the inevitability of one's mortality. Reminiscence has been described as a mourning of old experiences; the past is gone, but mental representations of the past remain (Evans, Millicovsky, & Tennison, 1984). Reminiscence, then, serves as a connection between past and present (Castelnuovo-Tedesco, 1978). Because elderly people may be likely to experience a narrowing and increasingly small world, with lessened faculties and mobility, they are faced with the inescapability of advancing age, isolation, and death (Lappe, 1987). Life review has been found, through reflection on one's active past participation in life, to help establish a feeling of contribution to an ongoing cycle of generations (Carlson, 1984).

Related Literature and General Issues

In addition to the studies already mentioned, further research covered a range of topics within the broad themes of involvement of the elderly with the past (Revere & Tobin, 1980), functions of reminiscence (Romaniuk & Romaniuk, 1981), mental adaptability (Berghorn & Schafer, 1987), differences in memory for older versus younger people (Hyland & Ackerman, 1988), characteristics and correlates of reminiscence (Bliwise, 1982; Cones, 1987; Merriam, 1989), and reminiscence and problem solving (Parlade, 1982).

A significant body of research investigating Reminiscence Therapy is available. This is an encouraging finding; however, problems with research conducted to date include loose designs, methodological problems including unclear definitions of Reminiscence Therapy (or misidentifying it as life review), simplistic measurements with unestablished reliability and validity, and absence of linkage of variable definitions, designs, or measurement devices with theory. Readers are advised to consult the studies mentioned here for further detail to substantiate facility policy changes.

Using Reminiscence Therapy

The Nursing Interventions Classification (NIC) intervention (Table 22–1) forms the basis of the discussion of implementing Reminiscence Therapy. This interven-

Table 22–1   Reminiscence Therapy

DEFINITION: Using the recall of past events, feelings, and thoughts to facilitate adaptation to present circumstances.

ACTIVITIES:

Choose a comfortable setting

Set aside adequate time

Encourage verbal expression of both positive and negative feelings of past events

Ask open-ended questions about past events

Encourage writing of past events

Tape the reminiscence and play it back to the client, as appropriate

Ask the family to bring photo albums or scrapbooks

Help the patient to begin a family tree

Encourage the patient to write to old friends

Use communication skills—such as focusing, reflecting, and restating—to develop the relationship

Conduct group life history discussions, as appropriate

Comment on the affective quality accompanying the memories in an empathic manner

Use direct questions to refocus back to life events, if patient digresses

Encourage writing of past events (e.g., culture, traditional values, wisdom, and lessons learned)

Inform family members about the benefits of reminiscence

Gauge the length of the session by the patient's attention span

Avoid using Reminiscence Therapy with persons who are in a state of generativity or with those who are avoiding reality

Acknowledge previous coping skills

Monitor for defensiveness about the past

Repeat session weekly or more often over prolonged period

Source: McCloskey, J. C., and Bulechek, G. M. (1996). *Nursing interventions classification (NIC)* (2nd ed.). St. Louis: Mosby–Year Book.

tion is examined in relation to the literature available on particular protocols for Reminiscence Therapy.

Perhaps the most comprehensive protocol for using Reminiscence Therapy was prepared by Burnside and Haight (1994). The authors discuss both group and dyad Reminiscence Therapy and compare these to group and dyad life review. The NIC intervention list provides basic activities, but they are not specific enough to enable nurses to begin Reminiscence Therapy for the first time. It is advisable that the NIC intervention be used in tandem with protocols such as those of Burnside and Haight (1994). This will ensure that the issues not presented in the NIC can be addressed, such as identifying group size (6 to 10—fewer if clients are cognitively impaired), client characteristics for group membership, and timing and length of group sessions (1 hour—less if clients are cognitively impaired).

In addition, more detailed guidance is provided by Burnside and Haight (1994) regarding the techniques used by the group leader in facilitating Reminiscence Therapy sessions (such as use of name tags, contracts, or personal visits with members who may be reluctant to attend), together with a suggested format for sessions (holding 1-hour sessions, summarizing the previous meeting, introducing props, or thanking each member for attending). Their discussion expands on the advice of Habegger and Blieszner (1990), who stressed the importance of nurses' having considerable social interaction with group members before initiating reminiscence.

Burnside (1990) provides a thorough discussion of some of the uses of Reminiscence Therapy in health assessments, nursing care implementation, and nursing research. She also addresses some of the complexities, such as dealing with paranoid patients, those with low energy levels, and those who refuse to disclose during Reminiscence Therapy sessions.

Soltys and Coats (1995) present a model for facilitating Reminiscence Therapy. This model is not as detailed as the NIC intervention or the Burnside and Haight (1994) protocols, but it establishes the skills needed by the facilitator (listen, touch, and talk), the factors influencing the success of Reminiscence Therapy (individual autonomy, education, ethnic background, cultural perspective, health status), and the expected client outcomes (perspective, closure, gratification, and resolution).

Other protocols and resources for guiding Reminiscence Therapy are also available, such as the audiovisual training packet developed by the American Association of Retired Persons (AARP) called "Reminiscence: Finding Meaning in Memories." The packet is geared to use by nonprofessional group leaders (supported by Hogan, 1982) and may be obtained from the AARP Program Department, 1909 K Street NW, Washington, DC 20049. This packet gives concrete suggestions for operating Reminiscence Therapy groups. Another resource, a game for older adults entitled "Reminiscing!" engages two to four players in reminiscence of fads, music, radio, television, and movies. It is available from Elder Press, 731 Treat Avenue, San Francisco, CA 94110.

Those interested in Reminiscence Therapy or thinking about starting a Reminiscence Therapy program may find the newsletter entitled "Memories are Made of This" helpful. The publication gives examples of topics to stimulate Reminiscence Therapy sessions, ideas for conducting groups, and an update on events and resources related to Reminiscence Therapy. It is also available from Elder Press. Another resource, the journal *Reminiscences*, is available in bookstores nationally. It provides stories and photographs to stimulate Reminiscence Therapy.

Osborn (1989) provides a list of potential topics to guide Reminiscence Therapy sessions, including school days; favorite games; family traditions; life during the Depression; earliest childhood memories; fashion, clothes, and proper manners; weddings and raising children; and feeding the family (p. 9). This list augments the NIC intervention by providing details needed to conduct Reminiscence Therapy.

Particular guidance for conducting Reminiscence Therapy with patients who are cognitively impaired is provided by Ott (1993). Her model recommends that a technique called *milestoning* be used to guide the group toward recall of positive times in their lives via multisensory imagery. This includes providing stimulation of all five senses through props. Although this is already recommended in the NIC intervention, specific detail may be found in the Ott protocol.

Tools created to stimulate reminiscence or to assess for its presence also enhance the NIC intervention. For example, Martin (1989) presented the Personal History Form, which assesses for names of family members and friends, occupations, hobbies, pastimes, achievements, and favorite foods. This tool may be helpful to nurses initiating Reminiscence Therapy to ensure that the sessions will be meaningful for all group members. Burnside (1993) also identified themes appropriate for Reminiscence Therapy with groups of older women (first playmate, first happy memory, favorite holiday, first pet, and first job) (pp. 184–187).

A 17-item scale, the Uses of Reminiscence Scale (Merriam, 1993), may be helpful to nurses in assessing prospective Reminiscence Therapy group members. It identifies the ways in which reminiscence is used by the client. By identifying the most helpful ways reminiscence is used, the nurse may be better prepared to plan the Reminiscence Therapy sessions so as to maximize their effectiveness. Alternatively, the Reminiscence Functions Scale (Webster, 1993), a 43-item scale, also identifies how reminiscence has been used by the client over the life course. Both scales have performed favorably when subjected to considerable reliability and validity testing.

Andrada and Korte (1993) prepared one of few discussions available regarding special considerations when conducting Reminiscence Therapy with Hispanic elders. The authors suggest culturally sensitive adaptations to traditional Reminiscence Therapy approaches. This resource is invaluable for those working with Hispanic groups, and it provides a meaningful adjunct to the NIC intervention because of its cultural specificity.

In addition, there are clinical papers in which authors describe such projects as a group Reminiscence Therapy project in a nursing home (Baker, 1985; Hala, 1975; Matteson & Munsat, 1982), a retirement village (Moore, 1992), an adult day care center (King, 1982), an oral history class for elders (Perschbacher, 1984), and an oral history project spanning three generations of Jewish, Italian, and Slavic women (Krause, 1985).

ASSOCIATED NURSING DIAGNOSES AND APPROPRIATE CLIENT GROUPS

Table 22–2 lists the nursing diagnoses for which Reminiscence Therapy may be most effective, based on the existing literature. Because these were discussed in the review of literature, further elaboration is not needed.

Other nursing diagnoses may be amenable to Reminiscence Therapy, although they have not been empirically tested. It may be logically deduced, for example, that because Reminiscence Therapy has been found to facilitate self-esteem, life satisfaction, and adjustment, facilitating these variables may be helpful in the context of the grief response and among clients at risk for loneliness. Further, if during Reminiscence Therapy, clients can be helped to feel positive about themselves in light of previous life decisions, it may be that Reminiscence Therapy would be beneficial in cases of decisional conflict. Perhaps the most tenuous association may be in applying Reminiscence Therapy to the diagnoses of acute and Chronic Pain and to altered comfort. However, if Reminiscence Therapy facilitates improved mood (specifically, lessens depression and anxiety) and is known to facilitate feelings of well-being (Sherman, 1985), it may be useful as a complementary therapy for clients who have pain. Testing Reminiscence Ther-

Table 22–2 Empirically Tested Nursing Diagnoses Appropriate for Reminiscence Therapy

Impaired Adjustment	Powerlessness
Anxiety	Relocation Stress Syndrome
Diversional Activity Deficit	Chronic Low Self Esteem
Altered Family Processes	Situational Low Self Esteem
Fear	Self Concept Disturbance
Hopelessness	Social Isolation
Ineffective Individual Coping	

Table 22–3 Expected Outcomes of Reminiscence Therapy

Anxiety Control	Mood Equilibrium
Caregiver-Patient Relationship	Pain: Disruptive Effects
Caregiver Well-Being	Participation: Health Care Decisions
Comfort Level	Psychosocial Adjustment: Life Change
Communication Ability	Quality of Life
Coping	Role Performance
Decision Making	Self-Esteem
Fear Control	Social Involvement
Grief Resolution	Symptom Severity
Hope	Well-Being
Identity	Will to Live
Loneliness	

apy in these contexts may provide a fruitful line of inquiry for researchers and clinicians alike.

Clients for whom Reminiscence Therapy may be most beneficial include those who are not cognitively impaired or expressively aphasic, those who have lived long enough lives to have created a bank of memories (i.e., not young children), and those who are not so acutely ill as to require emergent intervention (e.g., Airway Management) for their primary diagnoses. However, the literature suggests that Reminiscence Therapy can be beneficial for patients in intensive care units (Jones, 1995) and in the community (Sherman & Peak, 1991) and for those with Alzheimer's disease (Crisp, 1995; Rentz, 1995) and other forms of dementia (Mills & Coleman, 1994; Orten et al., 1989).

PATIENT OUTCOMES ASSOCIATED WITH REMINISCENCE THERAPY

Table 22–3 lists the expected outcomes for Reminiscence Therapy. In most cases, they derive logically from the respective nursing diagnoses (e.g., anxiety control from the diagnosis of anxiety). However, other desired outcomes may not be as directly identifiable in relation to the diagnoses specified above. For example, Participation: Health Care Decisions may be associated with the diagnosis of Decisional Conflict and may not be a direct outcome of Reminiscence Therapy but may be facilitated through the direct outcome of strengthened self-esteem. Thus, as is the case with other interventions, the outcomes are not mutually exclusive, nor do they necessarily apply to only one diagnosis. In fact, they may be indirect results of Reminiscence Therapy in the context of several diagnoses.

Similarly, role performance may be a result of the outcome of self-esteem enhancement, as the clients are better able to perform appropriate roles once they feel better about themselves. In another example, caregiver-patient relations and, subsequently, caregiver well-being may be realized through Reminiscence Therapy as the caregiver relives happy memories of the care recipient, feels an improvement in self-esteem or life satisfaction, and subsequently is able to maintain more favorable relations with the care recipient.

CASE STUDY

Sue Smith is a registered nurse (RN) employed in a long-term care facility that houses 148 residents older than age 50. The building has been under redecoration during the past 2 months, and this will continue during the next 3 to 6 months. During this time, Sue has noticed that Mrs. M and Miss H, two long-standing residents, have been staying in their rooms more often in order to avoid the confusion of the redecoration process. At mealtimes, these residents have become less communicative, and they isolate themselves by sitting at a table away from the rest of the residents. Sue has noticed that other residents also seem to be less communicative since the redecoration began.

Sue identifies Social Isolation as the nursing diagnosis for Mrs. M and Miss H, and she would like to begin a Reminiscence Therapy program to help them and any other residents who are feeling isolated. She invites Mrs. M, Miss H, and eight other residents who are not cognitively impaired to join the Reminiscence Therapy group. At the first meeting, she administers the Personal History Form and the Uses of Reminiscence Scale to help her in planning the series of six weekly 1-hour sessions. The group members express interest in meeting to "relive old times." The group agrees that they have few opportunities to engage in pleasant conversation and that possibly the group meetings will help them with this. Sue encourages them to bring to the group meetings anything they would like to talk about that will revive memories.

Sue provides the group members with a list of possible themes for the group meetings and encourages them to add to the list any themes that are of interest to them. After reviewing these data, she plans the following schedule of themes for the sessions: Session #1, My Favorite Holiday; Session #2, My Favorite Pet; Session #3, My First Job; Session #4, My Favorite Foods When I Was Growing Up; Session #5, Things My Grandparents Taught Me; and Session #6, When I Learned to Drive. Sue brings to each session props to stimulate at least two of the five senses for each theme.

Sue schedules the meetings in the small, sunny, quiet lounge at the end of one wing of the building. The room is infrequently used and provides comfortable chairs and a sofa arranged in a circle. During the Reminiscence Therapy sessions, Sue closes the door and posts a sign indicating that a meeting is in progress. She provides coffee, water, fruit, and cookies for the members to enjoy before, during, and after the group. She also has nametags made for each member, which she collects at the end of each session and distributes at the beginning of the next session.

Sue is careful not to direct the sessions but to use an affirming, positive response to members' contributions to the discussion. She asks open-ended questions, listens attentively, and redirects the focus of the discussion when the conversation lags.

The outcomes of the six sessions are far better than Sue expected. Group members write very positive evaluations of the 6-week program. They say that they "felt better," like they "belonged to something," which they had missed since moving to the facility. After the first meeting, all members of the group brought an item to share with the rest. Mrs. M and Miss H found some new dining partners in members of the group. Because the Reminiscence Therapy group meetings were held in the morning just before lunch, the discussion from the meeting frequently carried over into the dining room. In short, discussion increased so much that other residents noticed and asked to job the "memory group." Toward that end, Sue spoke to her administrator, who provided funds for her to purchase the AARP Reminiscence Therapy packet. She trained two other RNs to use the packet to lead RT groups, and now the facility has three RT groups conducted in "semesters" of 6 weeks, three times a year. The nursing diagnosis of Social Isolation was resolved for both Mrs. M and Miss H, and their outcomes were that they showed greater communication abilities, less loneliness, and improved quality of life, according to their own reports.

References

Andrada, P., and Korte, A. (1993). En aquellos tiempos: A reminiscing group with Hispanic elderly. *Journal of Gerontological Social Work, 20*(3/4), 25–42.

Arean, P., Perri, M., Nezu, A., Schien, R., Christopher, F., and Joseph, T. (1993). Comparative effectiveness of social problem-solving therapy and reminiscence therapy as treatments for depression in older adults. *Journal of Consulting and Clinical Psychology, 61,* 1003–1010.

Baker, N. (1985). Reminiscing in group therapy for self-worth. *Journal of Gerontological Nursing, 11*(7), 21–24.

Baum, W. (1980). Therapeutic value of oral history. *International Journal of Aging and Human Development, 12*(1), 49–53.

Beadleson-Baird, M., and Lara, L. (1987). *Verbal reminiscing and the mood, ego integration and socialization of the institutionalized elderly.* Unpublished paper, Sigma Theta Tau International 29th Biennial Convention, San Francisco, CA.

Bennett, S., and Maas, F. (1988). The effect of music-based life review on the life satisfaction and ego integrity of elderly people. *British Journal of Occupational Therapy, 51,* 433–436.

Berghorn, F., and Schafer, D. (1987). Reminiscence intervention in nursing homes: What and who changes? *International Journal of Aging and Human Development, 24*(2), 113–127.

Bliwise, N. G. (1982). *Reminiscence: Presentations of the personal past in middle and late life.* Unpublished doctoral dissertation, University of Chicago.

Boylin, W., Gordon, S., and Nehrke, M. (1976). Reminiscing and ego integrity in institutionalized elderly males. *The Gerontologist, 16*(2), 118–124.

Bramlett, M., and Gueldner, S. (1993). Reminiscence: A viable option to enhance power in elders. *Clinical Nurse Specialist, 7*(2), 68–74.

Bramwell, L. (1984, October). Use of the life history in pattern identification and health promotion. *Advances in Nursing Science, 7*(1), 37–44.

Brennan, P., and Steinberg, L. (1984). Is reminiscence adaptive: Relations among social activity level, reminiscence, and morale. *International Journal of Aging and Human Development, 18*(2), 99–109.

Brown, A., and Cecil, R. (1946). *Medical nursing.* Philadelphia: W. B. Saunders.

Burnside, I. (1988). Reminiscence and other therapeutic modalities. In I. Burnside (Ed.). *Nursing and the Aged* (3rd ed.) (p. 645–685). New York: McGraw-Hill Book Co.

Burnside, I. (1990). Reminiscence: An independent nursing intervention for the elderly. *Issues in Mental Health Nursing, 11,* 33–48.

Burnside, I. (1993). Themes in reminiscence groups with older women. *International Journal of Aging and Human Development, 37,* 177–189.

Burnside, I., and Haight, B. (1992). Reminiscence and life review: Analyzing each concept. *Journal of Advanced Nursing, 17,* 855–862.

Burnside, I., and Haight, B. (1994). Reminiscence and life review: Therapeutic interventions for older people. *Nurse Practitioner, 19*(4), 55–61.

Busch, C. D. (1984). Common themes in group psychotherapy with older adult nursing home residents: A review of selected literature. *Clinical Gerontologist, 2*(3), 25–38.

Butler, R. (1963). The life review: An interpretation of reminiscence in the aged. *Psychiatry, 26*(1), 65–76.

Butler, R. (1974). Successful aging and the role of life review. *Journal of the American Geriatric Society, 22,* 529–535.

Butler, R. (1980). The life review: An unrecognized bonanza. *International Journal of Aging and Human Development, 12*(1), 35–38.

Carlson, C. (1984). Reminiscing: Toward achieving ego integrity in old age. *Social Casework: The Journal of Contemporary Social Work, 65*(2), 81–89.

Castelnuovo-Tedesco, P. (1978). "The mind as a stage": Some comments on reminiscence and internal objects. *International Journal of Psychoanalysis, 59*(19), 19–25.

Clements, W. (1981). Reminiscence as the cure of souls in early old age. *Journal of Religion and Health, 20*(1), 41–47.

Coleman, G. (1986). *Aging and reminiscence processes: Social and clinical implications.* New York: Wiley & Sons.

Cones, J. H. (1987). *Correlates of reminiscence and cognitive organization in the older adult: A construct validity study.* Unpublished doctoral dissertation, Virginia Commonwealth University, Richmond.

Crisp, J. (1995). Making sense of the stories that people with Alzheimer's tell: A journey with my mother. *Nursing Inquiry, 2,* 133–140.

David, D. D. (1981). *The uses of memory: Social aspects of reminiscence in old age.* Unpublished doctoral dissertation, University of California, Berkeley.

DeGenova, M. (1993). Reflections of the past: New variables affecting life satisfaction in later life. *Educational Gerontology, 19,* 191–201.

DeMotts, J. R. (1981). *Reminiscence in older persons as a function of the cognitive control principle of leveling-sharpening and its relationship to life satisfaction and affect.* Unpublished doctoral dissertation, California School of Professional Psychology, San Diego.

Dhooper, S., Green, S., Huff, M., and Austin-Murphy, J. (1993). Efficacy of a group approach to reducing depression in nursing home elderly residents. *Journal of Gerontological Social Work, 20*(3/4), 87–100.

Eargle, D. (1980). *Reminiscence and self-actualization: Relationship to residential setting of elderly.* Unpublished doctoral dissertation, University of Arizona, Tucson.

Evans, D., Millicovsky, L., and Tennison, C. (1984). Aging, reminiscence and mourning. *The Psychiatric Forum, 12*(1), 19–32.

Fallot, R. D. (1980). The impact on mood of verbal reminiscing in later adulthood. *International Journal of Aging and Human Development, 10,* 385–400.

Ferguson, J. D. (1980). *Reminiscence counseling to increase psychological well-being of elderly women in nursing home facilities.* Unpublished doctoral dissertation, University of South Carolina, Columbia.

Fry, P. (1983). Structured and unstructured reminiscence training and depression among the elderly. *Clinical Gerontologist, 1*(3), 15–37.

Giltinan, J. (1990). Using life review to facilitate self-actualization in elderly women. *Gerontology and Geriatrics Education, 10*(4), 75–83.

Habegger, C., and Blieszner, R. (1990). Personal and social aspects of reminiscence: An exploratory study of neglected dimensions. *Activities, Adaptation & Aging, 14*(4), 21–38

Haight, B., and Bahr, R. (1984). The therapeutic role of the life review in the elderly. *Academic Psychology Bulletin, 6,* 287–299.

Haight, B., and Burnside, I. (1993). Reminiscence and

life review: Explaining the differences. *Archives of Psychiatric Nursing, 7*(2), 91–98.

Hala, M. (1975). Reminiscence group therapy project. *Journal of Gerontological Nursing, 1*(3), 34–41.

Hamilton, D. (1992). Reminiscence therapy. In J. C. McCloskey, and G. Bulechek (Eds.), *Nursing interventions classification (NIC)* (2nd ed., pp. 292–302). St. Louis: Mosby–Year Book.

Hamilton, D. (1980). *The effects of group reminiscence on the self-esteem of aged institutionalized clients.* Unpublished master's thesis, University of Iowa, Iowa City.

Harp Scates, S., Randolph, D., Gutsch, K., and Knight, H. (1986). Effects of cognitive-behavioral, reminiscence, and activity treatments on life satisfaction and anxiety in the elderly. *International Journal of Aging and Human Development, 22*(2), 141–146.

Harriman, P., Greenwood, L., and Skinner, C. (1942). *Psychology in nursing practice.* New York: Macmillan.

Havighurst, R., and Glaser, R. (1972). An exploratory study of reminiscence. *Journal of Gerontology, 27*, 245–253.

Hibel, D. E. (1971). *The relationship between reminiscence and depression among 30 selected institutionalized aged males.* Unpublished doctoral dissertation, Boston University School of Nursing.

Hogan, M. (1982). *The use of nonprofessional volunteer leaders in reminiscing groups for the institutionalized elderly.* Unpublished master's thesis, San Jose State University Department of Nursing, San Jose, CA.

Holzberg, C. (1984). Anthropology, life histories, and the aged: The Toronto Baycrest Centre. *International Journal of Aging and Human Development, 18*(4), 255–275.

Hughston, G., and Merriam, S. (1982). Reminiscence: A nonformal technique for improving cognitive functioning in the aged. *International Journal of Aging and Human Development, 15*(2), 139–149.

Hyland, D., and Ackerman, A. (1988). Reminiscence and autobiographical memory in the study of the personal past. *Journal of Gerontology, 43*(2), 35–39.

Jones, C. (1995). "Take me away from all this" . . . Can reminiscence be therapeutic in an intensive care unit? *Intensive and Critical Care Nursing, 1*, 341–343.

King, K. S. (1982). Reminiscing psychotherapy with aging people. *Journal of Psychosocial Nursing and Mental Health Services, 20*(2), 21–25.

Kovach, C. (1991). Reminiscence: Exploring the origins, processes, and consequences. *Nursing Forum, 26*(3), 14–20.

Krause, C. (1985). *Grandmothers, mothers, and daughters: An oral history of ethnicity, mental health, and continuity of three generations of Jewish, Italian, and Slavic-American Women.* Pittsburgh: Institute on Pluralism and Group Identity of the American Jewish Committee.

Langness, L. (1965). *The life history in anthropological science.* New York: Holt, Rinehart & Winston.

Lappe, J. M. (1987). Reminiscing: The life review therapy. *Journal of Gerontological Nursing. 13*(4), 12–16.

Lawton, G. (1946). *Aging successfully.* New York: Columbia University Press.

Lenkowsky, L. (1990). The elderly are not mistreated by society. In K. Swisher (Ed.), *The elderly: Opposing viewpoints* (pp. 23–27). San Diego, CA: Greenhaven Press.

Lewis, N. D. (1943). Mental hygiene in old age. In G. Lawton (Ed.), *New goals for old age* (pp. 91–105). New York: Columbia University Press.

Lo Gerfo, M. (1980). Three ways of reminiscence in theory and practice. *International Journal of Aging and Human Development, 12*(1), 39–47.

Luborsky, M. (1987). Analysis of multiple life history narratives. *Ethos, 15*, 366–381.

Magee, J. J. (1988). *A professional's guide to older adults' life review: Releasing the peace within.* Lexington, MA: Lexington Books.

Martin, J. (1989). Expanding reminiscence therapy with elderly mentally infirm patients. *British Journal of Occupational Therapy, 52*, 435–436.

Martin, R., and Stepath, S. (1993, Winter). Psychodrama and reminiscence for the geriatric patient. *Journal of Group Psychotherapy, Psychodrama and Sociometry, 46*, 139–148.

Matteson, M., and Munsat, E. (1982). Group reminiscing therapy with elderly clients. *Issues in Mental Health Nursing, 4*, 177–189.

McGowan, T. (1994). Mentoring-reminiscence: A conceptual and empirical analysis. *International Journal of Aging and Human Development, 39*, 321–336.

McMahon A., and Rhudick, P. (1964). Reminiscing: Adaptational significance in the aged. *Archives of General Psychiatry, 10*, 292–298.

McMahon, A., and Rhudick, P. (1967). Reminiscing in the aged: An adaptational response. In S. Levin, and R. Kahana (Eds.), *Psychodynamic studies on aging: Creativity, reminiscing and dying* (pp. 64–78). New York: International Universities Press.

Merriam, S. (1980). The concept and function of reminiscence: A review of the research. *The Gerontologist, 20*, 604–608.

Merriam, S. B. (1989). The structure of simple reminiscence. *The Gerontologist, 29*, 761–767.

Merriam, S. B. (1993). Race, sex, and age-group differences in the occurrence and uses of reminiscence. *Activities, Adaptation and Aging, 18*(1), 1–18.

Merrill, E. (1985). *Oral history guide.* Salem, WI: Sheffield Publishing.

Mills, M., and Coleman, P. (1994). Nostalgic memories in dementia: A case study. *International Journal of Aging and Human Development, 38*, 203–219.

Molinari, V., and Reichlin, R. (1985). Life review reminiscence in the elderly: A review of the literature. *International Journal of Aging and Human Development, 20*(2), 81–91.

Moore, B. (1992). Reminiscing therapy: A CNS intervention. *Clinical Nurse Specialist, 6*(3), 170–173.

Moore, M. A. (1985). *Effects of reminiscence and therapeutic touch on self-esteem and morale of institutionalized elderly.* Unpublished master's thesis, San Jose State University, San Jose, CA.

Namazi, K., and Haynes, S. (1994). Sensory stimuli reminiscence for patients with Alzheimer's disease: Relevance and implications. *Clinical Gerontologist, 14*(4), 29–46.

Norris, A. and Eileh, M. (1982, August 11). Reminiscence groups. *Nursing Times 78*(32), 1368–1369.

Orten, J., Allen, M., and Cook, J. (1989). Reminiscence groups with confused nursing center residents: An experimental study. *Social Work in Health Care, 14*(1), 73–86.

Osborn, C. (1989). Reminiscence: When the past eases the present. *Journal of Gerontological Nursing, 15*(10), 6–12.

Ott, R. (1993). Enhancing validation through milestoning with sensory reminiscence. *Journal of Gerontological Social Work, 20*(1/2), 147–158.

Parlade, R. J. (1982). *Reminiscence and problem-solving approaches: A comparison study with a geriatric population.* Unpublished doctoral dissertation, University of Georgia, Athens.

Parsons, C. L. (1986). Group reminiscence therapy and levels of depression in the elderly. *Nurse Practitioner, 11*(3), 68–76.

Pear, T. H. (1922). *Remembering and forgetting.* New York: E. P. Dutton.

Perrotta, P., and Meacham, J. (1981). Can a reminiscing intervention alter depression and self-esteem? *International Journal of Aging and Human Development, 14*(1), 23–29.

Perschbacher, R. (1984). An application of reminiscence in an activity setting. *Gerontologist, 24,* 343–345.

Rattenbury, C., and Stones, M. (1989). A controlled evaluation of reminiscence and current topics discussion groups in a nursing home context. *The Gerontologist, 29,* 768–771.

Rentz, C. (1995). Reminiscence: A supportive intervention for the person with Alzheimer's disease. *Journal of Psychosocial Nursing, 33*(11), 15–20.

Revere, V., and Tobin, S. (1980). Myth and reality: The older person's relationship to his past. *International Journal of Aging and Human Development, 12*(1), 15–26.

Riley, J. W. (1905). *Songs o' cheer* (p. 55). Indianapolis, IN: Bobbs-Merrill.

Romaniuk, M. (1981). Review: Reminiscence and the second half of life. *Experimental Aging Research, 7,* 315–335.

Romaniuk, M., and Romaniuk, J. (1981). Looking back: An analysis of reminiscence function and triggers. *Experimental Aging Research, 7,* 477–489.

Rybarczyk, B., and Auerbach, S. (1990). Reminiscence interviews as stress management interventions for older patients undergoing surgery. *The Gerontologist, 39,* 522–528.

Sherman, E. (1985). A phenomenological approach to reminiscence and life review. *Clinical Gerontologist, 3*(4), 3–16.

Sherman, E., and Peak, T. (1991). Patterns of reminiscence and the assessment of late life adjustment. *Journal of Gerontological Social Work, 16*(1/2), 59–74.

Soltys, F., and Coats, L. (1995). The Sol Cos model: Facilitating reminiscence therapy. *Journal of Psychosocial Nursing and Mental Health Services, 33*(11), 21–26.

Stevens-Ratchford, R. (1992). The effect of life review reminiscence activities on depression and self-esteem in older adults. *American Journal of Occupational Therapy, 47,* 413–420.

Stevenson, G. (1959). Mental health hazards in later life. *The Canadian Nurse, 55*(5), 414–416.

Strack, F., Schwarz, N., and Gschneidinger, E. (1985). Happiness and reminiscing: The role of time perspective, affect, and mode of thinking. *Journal of Personality and Social Psychology, 49,* 1460–1469.

Taft, L., and Nehrke, M. (1990). Reminiscence, life review, and ego integrity in nursing home residents. *International Journal of Aging and Human Development 30,* 189–196.

Tekavec, C. (1982). *Self-actualization, reminiscence and life satisfaction in retired and employed older adults.* Unpublished doctoral dissertation, California School of Professional Psychology, Fresno.

Thornton, S., and Brotchie, J. (1987). Reminiscence: A critical review of the empirical literature. *British Journal of Clinical Psychology, 26,* 93–111.

Walker, L. S. (1984). *The relationships between reminiscing, health state, physical functioning, and depression in older adults.* Unpublished doctoral dissertation, The Catholic University of America, Washington, DC.

Weber, A., Harvey, J., and Stanley, M. (1987). The nature and motivation of accounts for failed relationships. In R. Burnett, P. McGhee, D. C. Clark (Eds.). *Accounting for relationships* (pp. 114–133). London: Methuen.

Webster, J. (1993). Construction and validation of the reminiscence functions scale. *Journal of Gerontology: Psychological Sciences, 48,* P256–P262.

Wong, P., and Watt, L. (1991). What types of reminiscence are associated with successful aging? *Psychology and Aging, 6,* 272–279.

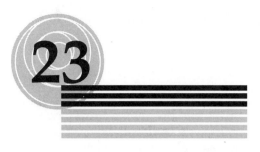

Patient Contracting

Margaret R. Simons

More than 50% of all Americans have chronic illnesses, many of which require the prescription of complex regimens. However, with chronic illness, there is no cure. These regimens can serve only to manage symptoms, reduce complications, and, it is hoped, stem the progression of the pathology. The regimens become part of individuals' daily activities, requiring permanent alterations in the way they live (Cameron & Gregor, 1987; Snyder, 1992). The ongoing ability or motivation of patients to carry out the recommended or prescribed behaviors that constitute these regimens is a continuing challenge, both for the patients themselves and for the health care providers who assist them. In 1979, Haynes, Taylor, and Sackett defined this challenge as compliance—"the extent to which a person's behavior (in terms of taking medications, following diets, or executing lifestyle changes) coincides with medical or health advice." Sackett and Snow (1979) noted a "distressingly wide gap" between the regimens recommended by clinicians and those adhered to by patients; the gap ranged from 10% to 94% in a comprehensive literature review of studies on compliance. Various studies since this landmark review have continued to confirm the disparity between prescribed treatments and actual patient behavior.

In addition to chronic illness, there is growing national concern regarding the behaviors and habits of many Americans that may contribute as risk factors to multiple health problems: obesity, smoking, and lack of exercise. Noncompliance with prescribed regimens as well as these unhealthy behaviors has many consequences. Baer (1986) identified multiple ramifications: increased medical costs because of the need for additional care for complications of disease, prolongation and exacerbation of disease, and increased incidence of usually preventable diseases. This, coupled with a marked increase in consumer consciousness of health care issues, points to the need for nursing interventions that will support patients in their self-care practices and behavior changes.

PATIENT CONTRACTING

Patient Contracting is a relatively new intervention, having gained attention only since the 1970s. Much of the early work was done in the fields of psychology and social work. Also known as contingency contracting, Patient Contracting has its basis in reinforcement as it is applied in behavior modification techniques. Reinforcement theory operates on the principle that the frequency of performance of a behavior can be increased when it is followed closely by a favorable consequence and, conversely, decreased when it is followed by an unfavorable or punishing consequence. Using Skinner's discoveries regarding human behavior (emphasizing consequences rather than causes of behavior) to change behavior through some form of operant conditioning is one of the cornerstones of the intervention of Patient Contracting. The principle that reward or reinforcement is contingent on the performance of a behavior is the other guiding premise (Steckel, 1982). There are basically two different types of contracting: the contingency contract and the therapeutic, or treatment, contract. The treatment contract differs from the contingency contract that will be discussed in this chapter, as it uses a more structured, legalistic approach to focus on the therapeutic work that is to be accomplished between the patient and the therapist (Rosen, 1978), and it does not use the principles of reinforcement.

Traditionally, health care providers have been accustomed to making decisions and implementing plans of care with little input from patients regarding their perception of how realistic or useful the treatment might be. One of the strengths of Patient Contracting is that it is based on the belief that all individuals have the right to self-determination, to make their own choices, and to become active in their own health care and an obligation to take some responsibility for their own well-being. In addition, health care providers have the opportunity to offer treatment that meets professional standards of care, while empowering patients to identify their own priorities, strengths, weaknesses, and methods of realistic goal-setting (Logan, 1984). Patient Contracting can help shift attention from disease processes themselves to the promotion of desired health behaviors, with patients taking responsibility for their own behavior changes. Janz, Becker, and Hartman (1984) cited multiple benefits from the use of Patient Contracting: clients become active participants in decision-making processes and make a commitment to behavior change; the contract fosters accountability and commitment between patients and their nurses; the written contract provides an instrument of communication for others involved in patients' care; and it facilitates the evaluation of progress.

Research Base

Patient Contracting as an intervention has been tested with multiple populations, although the majority of the research is in fields other than nursing. In 1989, Boehm conducted a review of research on Patient Contracting in the nursing literature for the period of 1965 to 1986. Compared to more than 300 research articles published in nonnursing literature, there were only 20 articles in the nursing literature, fewer than 8 of them being identified as research based. One of the most frequently cited nursing studies is that done by Swain and Steckel

(1981) in an experimental design with outpatients with hypertension. Patients who participated in contracts with reinforcers had higher knowledge levels about their hypertension, higher return visit rates, and decreases in diastolic blood pressure (Boehm, 1989; Snyder, 1992).

Two of the most common target outcomes of Patient Contracting are weight loss and smoking cessation. Janz et al. (1984) summarized multiple studies aimed at weight loss, using reinforcements such as money and personal items. Weight loss varied from 8.6 pounds to 32 pounds over a 12- to 16-week period. Target behaviors in the contracts included weight loss, self-monitoring, and attendance at group sessions. One of the conclusions drawn regarding these studies is that contracting can be very effective in the short term but that long-term effectiveness varies.

Several other studies have shown success with both children and adults. In 1993, Koch, Giardina, Ryan, MacQueen, and Hilgartner successfully used contingency contracting in a pediatric population with thalassemia: 76% of 23 patients were able to maintain improvement of adherence with their invasive medication regimen over a 6-month period. Solanto, Jacobson, Heller, Golden, and Hertz (1994) successfully used behavioral contracting to promote weight gain in adolescent inpatients with anorexia nervosa.

With adults, Leslie and Schuster (1991) demonstrated that contingency contracting significantly increased knowledge about safe exercise regimens in patients enrolled in outpatient cardiac rehabilitation. In 1991, Neale used behavioral contracting with patients classified as having high cholesterol. After contracting to adopt the American Heart Association (AHA) guidelines diet or engage in aerobic exercise or both, the contractors who fully met their contracts experienced the health benefits of lowered cholesterol or a decreased exercising heart rate.

The Process of Patient Contracting

The process of Patient Contracting is multistepped. A review of the literature provides seven recognized essential elements in the development of a good contract:

1. Behavioral analysis

2. Mutually agreed-upon goal(s)

3. Precise responsibilities of each person involved in the contract

4. Positive reinforcement and the timing of delivery of reinforcement

5. Potential consequences or sanctions for nonfulfillment of responsibilities

6. Specific dates for initiation, negotiation, and termination or renewal of the contract

7. A contract that is in written form and signed by all involved parties

Each step will be discussed in turn.

1. Behavioral analysis

The initial step in Patient Contracting is to assist the patient in assessing the presence or absence of a desired behavior, or behavioral analysis. This process is often the basis of the first visit or contact between the patient and nurse, and it is a way of establishing a baseline—a specific definition of the actual behavior as well as the number of times the behavior occurs in a day or week. Establishing a baseline is critical so that everyone has the same understanding of the behaviors to be measured, and it also provides a way to measure progress (Boehm, 1992; Snyder, 1992).

When analyzing behavior, it is also important to assess the effects of various environmental factors. These factors are commonly identified as antecedents and consequences. Antecedents are typically events that precede a behavior and are often strong enough to elicit the behavior. Examples of antecedents include places, thoughts or feelings, and other people. Consequences are generally events that follow a behavior, and they can be either positive (reinforcing) or negative. Examples of reinforcing consequences are praise from another person and feelings of pride. Examples of negative consequences are skeptical remarks from others and aligning oneself with those who have the same behavior one wants to change (Boehm, 1992; Snyder, 1992; Steckel, 1982).

The assessment or analysis of behavior is best accomplished by self-monitoring. Various self-monitoring techniques are available, including logs, diaries, counters, charts, and graphs. This gathering of data assists the patient (with the support of the nurse) in identifying occurrences of the behavior in question as well as influencing factors. This enables the patient to become more aware of his or her own perceptions of problems and potential solutions and to start the process of choosing behavioral strategies to learn, change, or maintain the desired behavior (Boehm, 1992).

2. Mutually agreed-upon goal(s)

Once the behavior analysis has been accomplished, the patient and nurse can together identify and prioritize desired goals. Even though the goals are mutually agreed-upon, they must initially be chosen by the patient and identified by the patient as significant. Both short- and long-term goals can be identified. Goals must be clearly and specifically described, realistic, measurable, preferably positive, and able to be accomplished in a reasonable amount of time. Often, goals should be broken down into small activities that are more specific and easily achieved, each smaller goal being reinforced as part of the process. This leads to a greater chance of success by building on successive accomplishments. It is often very rewarding to start with an easily accomplished behavior change, which leads the way for further progress toward larger goals. These smaller, very specific goals are also called contingent behaviors, as the delivery of the reinforcer is contingent on the performance of the behavior (Boehm, 1992; Janz et al., 1984; Snyder, 1992).

3. Precise responsibilities of each person involved in the contract

The precise responsibility or behavior required from each person in the contract to achieve the goal should be detailed. This may include setting time requirements for the performance of the behaviors, on the part of the patient as well as the nurse. Failure to define each party's level of accountability to the contract decreases the likelihood of success (Janz et al., 1984). The level of accountability and responsibility each party is willing to assume may well be a reflection of the quality of the relationship or the level of rapport between the patient and nurse. This step may also involve some exploration of a patient's own strengths and weaknesses as well as of available resources. Helping a patient identify ways to meet his or her own needs and solve problems fosters a sense of control and increases self-esteem and confidence (Kosnar, 1987). In addition, an important role of the nurse may be to assist in identifying other resources that the patient could use to achieve the agreed-upon goal(s).

4. Positive reinforcement and the timing of delivery of reinforcement

The selection of the reinforcement is almost as important as that of the positive behavior itself and, again, it is critical that it be the choice of the patient. A reinforcer is any consequence that strengthens a behavior (Snyder, 1992), and it is preferably positive when used in contingency contracting. Reinforcers are very individual—what is reinforcing for one person may not be for someone else. It should be noted that reinforcers are different from rewards. Reinforcers are directly tied to the performance of the target behavior and are used to help achieve the larger goal, whereas rewards are "pleasant consequences" that are not directly related to any behavior. A reward may be given after a goal is reached, but it is not a distinct part of the process of reinforcing and changing behavior (Snyder, 1992). Reinforcers may be intrinsic or extrinsic. A few highly motivated patients may find intrinsic reinforcers such as self-satisfaction and pride gratifying, but most people find extrinsic, more tangible reinforcers to be more effective when pursuing behavior change. Many potential reinforcers have been mentioned in the literature. In addition to material reinforcers such as lottery tickets, books, magazines, personal items, money, and tokens or points that can be cashed in for larger gifts as they are accumulated, many patients choose reinforcers that require the input of another person: uninterruped quiet time at home, a special time that is supported by a significant other, extra time with a health care provider, earlier appointment times, or assistance with undesirable tasks.

Planning the timing of the delivery of the reinforcement is also important. Typically, the closer in time the reinforcement occurs to the actual target behavior, the more likely it is to be effective in strengthening the behavior. The timing of the reinforcer can be modified over time as the behavior change is mastered and the focus is shifted from the reinforcement of behavior to maintaining the behavior change (Snyder, 1992). Again, the reinforcement has to be meaningful to the patient in order for it to foster goal attainment.

5. Potential consequences or sanctions for nonfulfillment of responsibilities

This component of the patient contract is not necessarily universally accepted. Janz et al. (1984) briefly discuss the use of "aversive consequences or sanctions" if any party fails to fulfill specified responsibilities. Although this could be interpreted as negative reinforcement, it is not used in place of the contingent positive reinforcer and may offer an additional motivation for some patients. Snyder (1992) offered an example in which a patient's reinforcer for not eating junk food was playing tennis with her roommate twice a week. In addition, a "penalty" was added, stating that if the patient did eat junk food, she had to clean their apartment. The penalty did not replace the reinforcer but provided an added incentive for complying with the terms of the contract.

6. Specific dates for initiation, negotiation, and termination or renewal of the contract

Once the goals, responsibilities, and reinforcers have been identified, time limits should be set to guide the process and facilitate evaluation. Like the goals, the time frame also must be realistic and measurable. Often, allotting extra time for goal achievement is wise in order to allow for sufficient progress to be made toward the goal. It can be frustrating and discouraging for both the patient and the nurse to see insufficient progress being made toward a goal (Snyder, 1992). A week is often a realistic time to set between appointments when dealing with outpatients who are trying to incorporate behavior change into their lives. When working in an inpatient or acute care setting, much shorter time frames may be needed in order to support smaller goals.

Time limits are used to guide evaluation, negotiation, and renewal or termination of a contract. Because goals often have to be broken down into smaller segments, multiple contracts may be required until the larger, overall goal is reached. Evaluation of progress toward specific goals allows for negotiation. The goals or time limits may not have been realistic, or external circumstances may have affected a party's ability to perform his or her part of the contract (Snyder, 1992). The process of patient contracting should be flexible, viewed as a working agreement that offers structure through a specific process and commitment to goal attainment while at the same time allowing for the human factor.

7. A contract that is in written form and signed by all involved parties

Although some literature alludes to verbal contracts, a written, signed contract creates a formal commitment between the parties involved in the contract. In addition, a written contract documents all the specifics that have been agreed upon, serves as a tangible history of progress toward desired goals, and can function as a form of communication with other health care providers and significant others who are involved. All involved parties should have a signed, dated copy of the contract, and it may be included in the patient's record (Boehm, 1992; Snyder, 1992).

Cautions

Several cautions should be observed when undertaking Patient Contracting. The first is that not all patients are appropriate candidates for contracting. Those who have minimal cognitive skills, those who are unwilling to become more active in their own health care and who place the authority and control of their own health outside themselves, and those who are unable to make their own decisions regarding their treatment because of the acuity of their illnesses or medical emergencies (Wilson, 1988) are probably not suitable participants. However, patients who are inappropriate for contracting at one point may have the capability or readiness at another time.

Another challenge is that Patient Contracting takes time to carry out. Because it is a process that must be gone through systematically and requires a certain level of commitment, contracting is an intervention that may require the scheduling of extra time or appointments with patients and perhaps their significant others (Snyder, 1992). In this era of cost-containment, it will become increasingly important that nurses be able to demonstrate that their interventions do facilitate behavior change, thus improving overall patient health by increasing healthy behavior, decreasing risk factors, and reducing disease complications.

Another consideration is that Patient Contracting should not be a substitute for other, more easily implemented and time-efficient interventions such as patient teaching and self-monitoring, which can and should be tried first when assisting patients with behavior change or enhancing compliance (Miller & Stark, 1994). Knowledge is not a guarantee of action, but behavior change cannot take place without the understanding of what activity is to be done, why it should be done, and how to actually do it. It cannot always be safely assumed that patients have the necessary understanding of their self-care behaviors to carry them out adequately.

Finally, the nurse should be careful when selecting outcome measures with which to evaluate long-term goal attainment. Only concrete, measurable outcomes that are directly related to the behavior change provide data for evaluation. These might include the keeping of appointments, weight loss, smoking cessation, or documentation of home monitoring. Koch et al. (1993) cite several studies that caution against the use of physiological outcome measures. Patients can sometimes improve despite low rates of adherence behavior or behavior change, and, alternatively, some do not improve despite high rates. For some disease states, the behavior change targeted may be only a part of the treatment regimen, so a physiological outcome does not necessarily measure the behavior change exclusively. Examples might include ferritin levels in thalassemia and glycosylated hemoglobin measurements in patients with diabetes whose treatment includes not only a targeted behavior of dietary changes but also a regimen of medication, exercise, and self-monitoring.

NIC INTERVENTION: PATIENT CONTRACTING

The above literature review, research base, and contracting process provide a foundation for the nursing intervention of Patient Contracting as contained in the Nursing Interventions Classification (NIC) (McCloskey & Bulechek, 1996). This intervention was originally developed as part of a master's thesis designed to identify and validate nursing interventions that are useful in enhancing compliance in patients with prescribed regimens. The intervention, its definition, and the nursing activities that operationalize the intervention were developed through a review of the literature and were empirically rated by nurse experts using the adapted Fehring method (Simons, 1992). The full intervention, including its definition and defining activities, is contained in Table 23–1.

McCloskey and Bulechek (1996) describe how choosing a nursing intervention for a particular patient is part of the clinical decision-making process of the nurse. For each patient, the nurse must identify a problem (or nursing diagnosis), consider the desired outcomes, and choose an intervention that will assist in meeting that outcome and in some way resolving the diagnosis. When determining whether or not to use an intervention, several factors should be considered: the desired patient outcome, the characteristics of the nursing diagnosis, the research base for the intervention, the feasibility of doing the intervention, the acceptability to the patient, and the capability of the nurse (McCloskey & Bulechek, 1996).

Once the intervention has been chosen, it is tailored to each individual patient by selecting the appropriate defining activities. The Patient Contracting intervention uses the process described earlier. Each of the discrete nursing activities in the intervention serves to break the process down into easily described and implemented steps. In order for the intervention to be most effective, activities should be selected that reflect each of the steps of the process described earlier (behavioral analysis, mutually agreed-upon goals, etc.), taking into consideration the patient and the nurse involved. The intervention, with selected, individualized activities, should provide guidance for the nurse in writing a patient contract. The complexity of the contract will vary, depending on the patient's needs, ability, and motivation as well as on the nurse's level of skill, comfort, and experience with the process.

Table 23–1 Patient Contracting

DEFINITION: Negotiating an agreement with a patient which reinforces a specific behavior change.

ACTIVITIES:

Encourage the patient to identify own strengths and abilities

Assist patient in identifying the health practices he/she wishes to change

Identify with patient the goals of care

Encourage patient to identify own goals, not those he/she believes the health care provider expects

Avoid focusing on diagnosis or disease process alone when assisting the patient in identifying goals

Assist the patient in identifying realistic, attainable goals

Assist the patient in identifying appropriate short- and long-term goals

Encourage the patient to write down own goals, if possible

State goals as easily-observed behaviors

State goals in positive terms

Assist the patient in breaking down complex goals into small, manageable steps

Clarify with the patient roles of the health care provider and the patient, respectively

Explore with the patient ways to best achieve the goals

Assist the patient in examining available resources to meet the goals

Assist the patient in developing a plan to meet the goals

Assist the patient in identifying present circumstances in the environment that may interfere with the achievement of goals

Assist the patient in identifying methods of overcoming environmental circumstances that may interfere with goal achievement

Explore with the patient methods for evaluating accomplishment of the goals

Foster an open, accepting environment for the creation of the contract

Facilitate involvement of significant others in the contracting process, if desired by the patient

Facilitate the making of a written contract, including all agreed-on elements

Assist the patient in setting time or frequency requirements for performance of behaviors/actions

Assist the patient in setting realistic time limits

Together with the patient, identify a target date for termination of the contract

Coordinate with the patient opportunities for review of the contract and goals

Facilitate renegotiation of contract terms, if necessary

Identify with the patient consequences or sanctions for not fulfilling the contract, if desired

Have the contract signed by all involved parties

Provide the patient with a copy of the signed and dated contract

Encourage the patient to identify appropriate, meaningful reinforcers/rewards

Encourage the patient to choose a reinforcer/reward that is significant enough to sustain the behavior

Specify with the patient timing of delivery of reinforcers/rewards

Identify additional rewards with the patient if original goals are exceeded, if desired

Instruct the patient on various methods of observing and recording behaviors

Assist the patient in developing some form of flow chart to assist in tracking the progress toward goals

Assist the patient in identifying even small successes

Explore with the patient reasons for success or lack of it

Source: McCloskey, J. C., and Bulechek, G. M. (1996). *Nursing interventions classification (NIC).* St. Louis: Mosby–Year Book.

NIC LINKAGE TO NANDA NURSING DIAGNOSES

The nursing intervention of Patient Contracting has been used with various patient groups in multiple settings. In general, the literature tends to point to the use of contracting in long-term chronic illnesses (Boehm, 1989), such as diabetes, hypertension, renal failure, and cardiovascular disease, and in behaviors and conditions that predispose patients to chronic illness (obesity, tobacco use, lack of exercise). More recently, contracting has also been used in assisting patients to increase adherence to their regimens (including medication compliance and self-monitoring), as well as with patients who are seeking to implement or increase more healthful behaviors in their lifestyles, such as healthful diets, increased exercise, and smoking cessation. The vast majority of these activities have taken place in outpatient and community settings. Boehm (1989) has suggested further exploration of contracting in short-term or acute care settings, citing potential areas of investigation such as weaning patients from ventilators, enhancing self-care of wounds and dressings, and assisting patients with postoperative behaviors such as deep breathing and coughing. In 1996, McCloskey and Bulechek reported on a survey that was done with practicing nurses to determine which nursing interventions from NIC were used most frequently, according to work setting and specialty area. Patient Contracting was noted to have high use by nonhospital nurses and high use by nonintensive care nurses.

In 1996, McCloskey and Bulechek provided a linkage list that linked all the NIC interventions with all the North American Nursing Diagnosis Association (NANDA) nursing diagnoses (as of 1994). In this linkage list, NANDA diagnoses are listed, and potentially useful NIC interventions are shown with each. It is suggested that the interventions be viewed at three levels: highlighted interventions, which are the treatments of choice for that diagnosis; suggested, or most essential interventions; and additional optional interventions that may also be considered for resolving the diagnosis. Patient Contracting is listed as a suggested intervention for the following diagnoses: Defensive Coping, Ineffective Individual Management of Therapeutic Regimen, and Noncompliance. As an additional optional intervention, Patient Contracting is listed under Body Image Disturbance, Decisional Conflict, Diversional Activity Deficit, Hopelessness, Ineffective Individual Coping, Altered Nutrition: More than Body Requirements, Altered Parenting, Powerlessness, Risk for Self-Mutilation, and the Self-Care Deficit diagnoses. Although Patient Contracting is not listed as an essential treatment of choice for any diagnoses, this author would add two diagnoses for which this intervention would also be useful: Knowledge Deficit and Health-Seeking Behaviors.

ASSOCIATED PATIENT OUTCOMES

As mentioned before, part of the clinical decision-making process of the nurse is selecting patient outcomes. Outcomes describe the behaviors and feelings of a patient in response to the nursing care provided. Serving as criteria against which to judge the success of a nursing intervention, outcomes are very individual, varying according to many factors—patient motivation, ability, and disease process; multiple environmental factors; and many aspects of the nurse and the interventions chosen. In addition to the NIC, another group has developed the Nursing Outcomes Classification (NOC). The NOC is a classification of patient outcomes that are sensitive to nursing treatments. Being able to make coherent associations among nursing diagnoses, nursing interventions, and nursing outcomes would meet at least three of the eight reasons put forth by the NIC team for a classification of nursing interventions: (1) To standardize nomenclature; (2) To expand nursing knowledge about the links among diagnoses, treatments, and outcomes; and (3) To establish language that communicates the unique function of nursing (McCloskey & Bulechek, 1996).

In an attempt to make some preliminary links based on a single nursing intervention, the identified nursing diagnoses have been linked with potential associated nursing outcomes based on utilization of the nursing intervention Patient Contracting (Table 23–2).

CASE STUDY

M is a 42-year-old woman who is married, works full-time as a secretary, and is the mother of two small children. During her annual physical approximately 6 months ago, M's primary care provider diagnosed her as having Type 2 diabetes mellitus. M has a significant family history of diabetes and is severely overweight, so the diagnosis was not a surprise to her. M and her provider agreed to attempt initially to control her diabetes with diet and activity alone. At the time of diagnosis, M attended an outpatient diabetes education program and received extensive instruction regarding her diabetes care regimen, including a personalized meal plan developed with the dietitian, an exercise plan, and home blood glucose monitoring. Upon completion of the education program, M scored 95% on a knowledge test.

During a return visit to the clinic with a diabetes nurse educator, M continued to verbalize good basic understanding of the concepts that were discussed in her education program. She felt that the meal plan was realistic for her and had been gradually losing weight. She had been performing home blood glucose monitoring daily at home, with fasting results running in the 150 to 220 mg/dL range consistently. M's greatest concern during the return visit was that she had been unable to consistently incorporate an exercise plan into her regimen. She understood that exercise would be beneficial because it would increase her rate of weight loss when used in conjunction with her dietary changes and would also help to improve diabetes control as reflected by her monitoring of her blood sugar at home, thus helping her to avoid diabetes medication.

In order to assist M in analyzing her behavior, the nurse asked that she perform self-monitoring at home for a week. M agreed to keep a diary about how much exercise she was currently doing, what kinds of thoughts or events helped or hindered her in performing exercise, and how she would like to see her current behavior changed or improved. On her return to the clinic the next week, M and the nurse noted that M's exercise was sporadic (less than twice a week). M said that it was difficult for her to exercise because of her work schedule and the necessity of taking care of her small children but that her husband had been very supportive of her weight loss and was interested in supporting her in her attempts to increase her exercise level.

After the behavioral analysis, M and the nurse were able to discuss her exercise goals. Initially, M set the very large goal for herself of exercising daily. On further discussion, she determined that this was probably not realistic for her, and she amended her goal to exercising 4 days per week. Because M found it difficult to find time to exercise at home, the two discussed alternatives, and M finally decided that because she had a 1-hour lunch break at work, it would be realistic for her to walk for 30 minutes at least 4 days per week during her lunch hour.

In discussing what might be a good reinforcer, M again stated that her husband was very interested in supporting her lifestyle changes. He had suggested that he give her some time alone on the weekends by taking the children out for several hours so that she could have time for reading and needlework, which she enjoyed but wasn't able to do often. It was decided that in return for M's successful completion of her weekly exercise objectives, her husband would take the children out of the house for 2 hours on Saturday morning, from 9 AM to 11 AM. Because M's husband wasn't able to attend her appointment, she contacted him by phone with her "proposal." He was very supportive and promised to sign the contract when he got home from work that day. In addition, the nurse agreed to continue weekly

Table 23–2 Nursing Diagnoses Linked with Nursing Outcomes Based on Use of the Patient Contracting Intervention

NANDA Nursing Diagnosis	NOC Outcome
Defensive Coping	Social Interaction Skills: An individual's use of effective interaction behaviors
Ineffective Individual Management of Therapeutic Regimen	Treatment Behavior: Illness or Injury: Personal actions to palliate or eliminate pathology
Noncompliance	Compliance Behavior: Actions taken on the basis of professional advice to promote wellness, recovery, and rehabilitation
Body Image Disturbance	Body Image: Positive perception of own appearance and body functions
Decisional Conflict	Decision Making: Ability to choose between two or more alternatives
Diversional Activity Deficit	Leisure Participation: Use of restful or relaxing activities as needed to promote well-being
Hopelessness	Hope: Presence of internal state of optimism that is personally satisfying and life-supporting
Ineffective Individual Coping	Coping: Actions to manage stressors that tax an individual's resources
Altered Nutrition: More Than Body Requirements	Nutritional Status: Body Mass: Congruence of body weight, muscle, and fat to height, frame, and gender
Altered Parenting, and Risk for Altered Parenting	Parenting: Provision of an environment that promotes optimum growth and development of dependent children
Powerlessness	Health Beliefs: Perceived Control: Personal conviction that one can influence a health outcome
Risk for Self-Mutilation	Self-Mutilation Restraint: Ability to refrain from intentional self-inflicted injury (non-lethal)
Self Care Deficit diagnoses (Bathing/Hygiene, Dressing/Grooming, and Feeding)	Self-Care: Activities of Daily Living (ADL): Ability to perform the most basic physical tasks and personal care activities
Knowledge Deficit	Knowledge: Health Behaviors: Extent of understanding conveyed about the promotion and protection of health Knowledge: Treatment Regimen: Extent of understanding conveyed about a specific treatment regimen
Health-Seeking Behaviors	Health-Promoting Behavior: Actions to sustain or increase wellness Adherence Behavior: Self-initiated action taken to promote wellness, recovery, and rehabilitation

Sources: North American Nursing Diagnosis Association (1996). *NANDA nursing diagnoses: Definitions and classification 1997–1998.* Philadelphia: Author; Johnson, M., and Maas, M. (Eds.) (1997). *Nursing outcomes classification* (NOC). St. Louis: Mosby–Year Book.

Table 23–3 Case Study Contract

CONTRACT

I, _____M_____, agree to exercise by walking for 30 minutes during my lunch hour, 4 days a week. I will keep a log of the days I exercise and share it with my husband weekly, as well as bring it to my appointments with the nurse educator. If I don't walk 4 times a week, I agree to take the children out for 2 hours on Saturday myself so my husband can play golf.

I, _____Husband_____, agree to take the children out every Saturday from 9 to 11 AM so M has time alone to read or do needlework or some other activity she enjoys.

I, _Nurse Educator_, agree to review M's log and contract with her weekly. I also agree to provide input regarding other parts of her regimen during the weekly ½-hour appointment time. At 1 month, if M has successfully met the contract each week for 4 weeks in a row, I will provide her with an additional reward of a free bottle of strips for her blood glucose meter.

Dates of contract: June 1, 1997, through July 1, 1997

_____ (Signature/date by patient)

_____ (Signature/date by husband)

_____ (Signature/date by nurse educator)

cc: M
    Husband
    Medical record
    Nurse educator

follow-ups of the contract, as well as provide input regarding other parts of M's diabetes regimen such as laboratory test interpretation, dietary feedback, and special recipes. M and the nurse formulated the contract in Table 23–3.

Over the course of several weeks, M and the nurse reviewed M's progress toward goals and renewed the contract on a weekly basis. Her husband continued to be supportive and met his obligation to supply the reinforcer every week. At the 1-month mark, the nurse gave M an additional reward of a free bottle of strips for her blood glucose meter. Over time, the interval between M's appointments with the nurse educator was lengthened, and M found that she was able to sustain her exercise behavior without the reinforcers and rewards. It had become habit, a part of her daily regimen. In addition, M continued to lose weight, and her blood sugars were better controlled, with fasting blood glucose levels in the 110 to 150 mg/dL range consistently.

CONCLUSION

Historically, Patient Contracting appears to be one of the most effective strategies available for enhancing patient compliance as well as for supporting patients in their self-care practices and behavior changes. Because of the formal nature of the contract, the documented effectiveness of reinforcement theory, and the collaborative relationship between the patients and their nurses, this process appears to enable nurses to more effectively and actively assist patients in being participants in their own plans of care, performing their own self-care, and implementing or changing desired health behaviors.

References

Baer, C. L. (1986). Compliance: The challenge for the future. *Topics in Clinical Nursing*, 7, 77–85.

Boehm, S. (1989). Patient contracting. In J. J. Fitzpatrick, R. L. Taunton, and J. Q. Benoliel (Eds.), *Annual review of nursing research* (Vol. 7, pp. 143–53). New York: Springer.

Boehm, S. (1992). Patient contracting. In G. M. Bulechek, and J. C. McCloskey (Eds.), *Nursing interventions: Essential nursing treatments* (pp. 425–433). Philadelphia: W.B. Saunders.

Cameron, K., and Gregor, F. (1987). Chronic illness and compliance. *Journal of Advanced Nursing, 12*, 671–676.

Haynes, R. B., Taylor, D. W., and Sackett, D. L. (1979). *Compliance in health care.* Baltimore: Johns Hopkins University Press.

Janz, N. K., Becker, M. H., and Hartman, P. E. (1984). Contingency contracting to enhance patient compliance: A review. *Patient Education and Counseling, 5*(4), 165–178.

Koch, D. A., Giardina, P. J., Ryan, M., MacQueen, M., and Hilgartner, M. W. (1993). Behavioral contracting to improve adherence in patients with thalassemia. *Journal of Pediatric Nursing, 8*(2), 106–111.

Kosnar, A. (1987). Contracting for care: A method to increase client compliance. *American Association of Occupational Health Nurses Journal, 35,* 493–495.

Leslie, M., and Schuster, P. A. (1991). The effect of contingency contracting on adherence and knowledge of exercise regimens. *Patient Education and Counseling, 18,* 231–241.

Logan, M. (1984). Health contracting: The client's perspective. *The Canadian Nurse, 80*(4), 27–29.

McCloskey, J. C., and Bulechek, G. M. (Eds.). (1996). *Nursing interventions classification (NIC)* (2nd ed.). St. Louis: Mosby–Year Book.

Miller, D. L., and Stark, L. J. (1994). Contingency contracting for improving adherence in pediatric populations. *Journal of the American Medical Association, 271*(1), 81–83.

Neale, A. V. (1991). Behavioral contracting as a tool to help patients achieve better health. *Family Practice, 8,* 336–342.

Rosen, B. (1978). Contract therapy. *Nursing Times, 74,* 119–121.

Sackett, D. L., and Snow, J. C. (1979). The magnitude of compliance and noncompliance in health care. In R. B. Haynes, D. W. Taylor, and D. C. Sackett (Eds.), *Compliance in health care.* Baltimore: Johns Hopkins University Press.

Simons, M. R. (1992). Interventions related to compliance. In G. M. Bulechek and J. C. McCloskey (Eds.), *The nursing clinics of North America, nursing interventions, 27*(2), 477–494.

Snyder, M. (1992). Contracting. In M. Snyder (Ed.), *Independent nursing interventions* (2nd ed., pp. 145–154). Albany, NY: Delman Publishers.

Solanto, M. V., Jacobson, M. S., Heller, L., Golden, N. H., and Hertz, S. (1994). Rate of weight gain of inpatients with anorexia nervosa under two behavioral contracts. *Pediatrics, 93*(Pt 1), 989–991.

Steckel, S. B. (1982). *Patient contracting.* Norwalk, CT: Appleton-Century-Crofts.

Swain, M. A., and Steckel, S. B. (1981). Influencing adherence among hypertensives. *Research in Nursing and Health, 4,* 213–222.

Wilson, M., and Boyer, C. (1988). A contract for change in diabetes self-management: Case report. *The Diabetes Educator, 14*(1), 37–40.

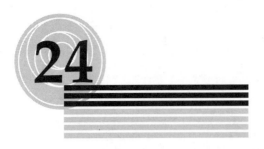

Preparatory Sensory Information

Norma J. Christman, Karin T. Kirchhoff,

and Marsha G. Oakley

Preparatory Sensory Information is the product of a program of research and theory development that spans approximately 25 years. It is based predominantly on the work of a nurse, Jean E. Johnson, and her colleagues in nursing, although investigators from other disciplines (Leventhal & Johnson, 1983; Wilson, 1981) have contributed to the empirical and theoretical base of this intervention. Preparatory Sensory Information, now frequently called Concrete Objective Information, describes the typical experiences associated with specific health care events (McHugh, Christman, & Johnson, 1982). The name of the intervention was modified to reflect research findings documenting the importance of using concrete and objective words to describe aspects of health care events that only patients experience, as well as to describe aspects that may be observed by health care providers or others (Johnson, Fieler, Jones, Wlasowicz, & Mitchell, 1997; Johnson & Lauver, 1989; Suls & Fletcher, 1985).

Experiences known only to the patient, or subjective experiences, are those sensations caused by a therapeutic or diagnostic procedure—that is, what will be felt, heard, tasted, seen, or smelled during the procedure. These sensory experiences are described in concrete, unambiguous terms. Also, they are described objectively; evaluative adjectives, such as *severe* or *excruciating*, are not attached to the descriptors of the sensory experiences. The cause of the sensation, when not self-evident, and its temporal features also are described. For example, Preparatory Sensory Information for a surgical patient includes not only the sensations associated with the surgical incision—tenderness, pressure, smarting, aching—but also the changes in these sensations that occur with movement (e.g., they may become sharp and seem to travel along the incision) and changes that occur over time (e.g., intensity declines with time).

Aspects of the experience that can be observed and verified by someone other than the patient include specific events associated with the procedure and their timing as well as the nature of the environment in which the procedure takes place (Johnson et al., 1997; McHugh et al., 1982). For example, for surgery description of these experiences may include information about the anesthesiology visit and when it will occur, the preoperative skin preparation and when it will be done, awakening in the recovery room, and when food and fluids will be permitted. The exact content of this part of the intervention necessarily varies with the specific practices, policies, and environment of the setting in which the procedure takes place. Whatever the exact content, these experiences also are described using concrete and objective terminology.

THEORETICAL-EMPIRICAL FOUNDATION

The self-regulation theory of coping guided the development and testing of Preparatory Sensory Information. Self-regulation theory also guides understanding the use of Preparatory Sensory Information and its effects on patients' ability to cope with health care procedures (Johnson, 1996; Johnson et al., 1997; Johnson & Lauver, 1989; Leventhal & Johnson, 1983). Self-regulation theory is concerned with the cognitive processing of information and its effects on human behavior. Schema formation is a concept central to self-regulation theory. A schema is a mental representation that structures and stores information from experience (Neisser, 1976). It directs the processing of incoming information, the retrieval of information stored from past experiences, the focus of attention, and the resulting behavior (Johnson & Lauver, 1989). Self-regulation theory posits two primary types of schema. A schema that draws attention to the emotionally arousing aspects of the experience focuses coping efforts on control of emotional responses. Alternatively, a schema that focuses attention on the concrete, objective features of an experience enhances problem-solving approaches to health care experiences (Johnson, 1996; Johnson et al., 1997; Johnson & Lauver, 1989; Leventhal & Johnson, 1983; Suls & Fletcher, 1985). Because Preparatory Sensory Information is composed of clear, unambiguous content related to specific aspects of an experience, it eases processing of incoming information, thereby enhancing interpretation and understanding of the experience (Johnson, Lauver, & Nail, 1989). When specific elements (e.g., the burning or tingling of an incision) of a more abstract experience (e.g., having surgery) are described, patients may more easily draw on past experiences similar to the specific element, which increases their confidence in their ability to cope with the new experience (Johnson & Lauver, 1989).

DEVELOPMENT OF SELF-REGULATION THEORY

Preparing patients for stressful health care procedures is a traditional part of nursing practice. For the most part, patients are given information or instruction thought to ease emotional distress, promote recovery, facilitate adherence to medical regimens, or in some way enhance health and well-being. Because many of these practices are based on tradition or beliefs inferred from educational theory, they provide little guidance for making clinical decisions about (1) which patients would benefit most from the information, (2) goals to be achieved by providing the information, and (3) criteria to use in evaluating patient responses to the information. Self-regulation theory provides guidance in making such clinical decisions because it goes beyond knowledge-based explanations of the effects of Preparatory Sensory Information on patient outcomes (Johnson et al., 1997).

As noted earlier, the specific aspects of Preparatory Sensory Information content were clarified through the research process. Initial research focused on determining the efficacy of describing typical procedure-related sensations. Because this type of information had not been used with patients, it was initially studied using healthy volunteers with whom a blood pressure cuff was used to induce ischemic pain as the stressful experience (Johnson, 1973). As expected, those who were given a description of the typical sensations reported less emotional distress during the experience than those who received only information about the procedure. With some evidence for the benefits of the sensation information, studies in patient populations were initiated.

The early clinical studies focused on the effects of sensation description, with patients undergoing relatively short-term stressful health care procedures such as gastroendoscopic examination, barium enema, cast removal, and nasogastric tube insertion. The effects of sensation description were tested against procedural information, or those experiences that are observable to others (Hartfield, Cason, & Cason, 1982; Johnson, Morrissey, & Leventhal, 1973), and in some cases also against usual care (Hartfield & Cason, 1981; Johnson, Kirchhoff, & Endress, 1975). These tests permitted comparison of the efficacy of sensation description with procedure information and, in turn, each of these with usual care. In other studies, the sensation description was combined with procedural information and tested against usual care, instruction in a coping strategy, or health education (Fuller, Endress, & Johnson, 1978; Johnson & Leventhal, 1974; Padilla et al., 1981; Rice, Sieggreen, Mullin, & Williams, 1988). In these short-term stressful health care situations, sensation description alone as well as when combined with procedural information reduced patients' emotional distress during or immediately following the stressful event.

A meta-analysis (Suls & Wan, 1989) also helped to clarify the effects of the different components of Preparatory Sensory Information. This statistical comparison of multiple studies done in a variety of clinical and laboratory situations indicated that, in contrast to description of the subjective sensations, description of the procedure yielded no benefits over that achieved in control groups. Yet the *combination* of describing both the sensations and the procedure yielded the greatest reduction of emotional distress. From both pragmatic and theoretical perspectives, these findings make sense. Pragmatically, separating sensory experiences from procedural elements of an experience may be difficult and artificial, especially for more complex or long-term health care events. From the theoretical perspective, combining both sensory and procedural information allows for more complete and accurate schema formation, thus easing interpretation and understanding of the event.

The more complex or long-term situations in which the effects of Preparatory Sensory Information were tested include surgery (Hill, 1982; Johnson, Christman, & Stitt, 1985; Johnson, Fuller, Endress, & Rice, 1978a; Johnson, Rice, Fuller, & Endress, 1978b; Wilson, 1981) and radiation therapy for cancer (Christman, 1997; Johnson, 1996; Johnson, Nail, Lauver, King, & Keys, 1988). From these studies, the importance of including information about the timing of elements in longer-lasting experiences was made explicit (Johnson et al., 1978a). A major contribution of these studies to the development of self-regulation theory was greater understanding of the link between schema-directed attentional focus and behavioral responses in short-term versus long-term health care events.

Compared with tests of the intervention with patients having short-term diagnostic or therapeutic procedures, Preparatory Sensory Information in longer and more complex stressful experiences affected primarily functional status outcomes, reflecting patients' positive problem-solving activities. There were few effects on emotional state. Providing Preparatory Sensory Information before abdominal surgery led to shorter hospital stays (Johnson et al., 1978a, 1978b; Wilson, 1981), earlier resumption of usual activities (Johnson et al., 1978a, 1978b), and reports of feeling more like one's normal self (Johnson et al., 1985). In patients having radiation therapy, Preparatory Sensory Information led to more involvement in usual recreation and pastime activities during and following treatment (Johnson, 1996; Johnson et al., 1988), and more social activities during treatment (Christman, 1997). Thus, in more complex long-term health care situations, the positive effects of focusing attention on the concrete, objective aspects of the event may become evident only over time (Suls & Fletcher, 1985).

Further understanding of how attentional focus on the concrete, objective elements of a stressful event enhances coping outcomes also was achieved in these long-term studies. Surgical patients given Preparatory Sensory Information reported perception of increased ability to deal with the experience and a belief that the experience would be less difficult for them (Johnson et al., 1985). Similarity between expectations and experience, understanding of experiences (Johnson et al., 1988), and lessened symptom uncertainty (Christman, 1997) explained the effects of Preparatory Sensory Information on patients having radiation therapy. These findings support the theoretical explanations concerning the means by which Preparatory Sensory Information produces its effects. With an understanding of the experience, the ability to find experiences similar to what is expected, and decreased symptom uncertainty (all evidence of schema formation), patients are able to effectively select coping strategies that enable them to regain or maintain usual functional activities (Johnson, 1996; Johnson et al., 1997).

In short-term situations, there are few problem-solving behaviors patients can use other than to cooperate with the procedure or to control their emotional response. Thus, studies of Preparatory Sensory Information in these situations reflect the outcomes of patients' behavioral attempts to cooperate and to control their emotions. In the more long-term stressful events, patients' behavioral options are less restricted. Here, the research findings suggest that over time, patients who receive Preparatory Sensory Information are better able to select coping strategies that lessen disruption in or speed resumption of usual daily activities. In summary, the research and theory indicate that schemata focusing attention on the concrete, objective elements of stressful health care experiences help patients know what to expect, thereby enhancing their ability to cope with the experience.

INDIVIDUAL DIFFERENCES

Some investigations of the effects of Preparatory Sensory Information have attempted to identify whether specific groups of patients may especially benefit from this intervention. Questions have been asked as to whether or not patients' coping styles or personal characteristics, such as a tendency to be anxious or optimistic, influence their response to Preparatory Sensory Information (Johnson, 1996; Miller & Mangan, 1983; Rainey, 1985; Sime & Libera, 1985; Watkins, Weaver, & Odegaard, 1986; Wilson, Moore, Randolph, & Hanson, 1982). Because the findings of these studies vary, it is not clear that personal characteristics such as these influence patient responses to Preparatory Sensory Information. More research and theory development are necessary to clarify the effects, if any, of such individual differences on the self-regulation of coping behaviors. It is important, however, to note that there is no clear evidence indicating that Preparatory Sensory Information produces negative effects in certain groups of patients.

COMBINING INSTRUCTIONS AND SENSORY INFORMATION

Another question important to nursing practice is whether or not Preparatory Sensory Information may be combined with instruction in specific coping strategies such as relaxation (Fuller et al., 1978; Wilson, 1981; Wilson et al., 1982), ambulation (Johnson et al., 1978a, 1978b, 1985), or distraction techniques (Johnson et al., 1985). Review of the studies investigating the effects of combining the information with instruction in a coping strategy suggests that such a combination was effective in those instances in which the instruction provided a behavior not already a part of the patient's repertoire of coping strategies (Hill, 1982; Johnson et al., 1978a, 1978b; Padilla et al., 1981). Further, the newly learned behavior was compatible with that supported by the Preparatory Sensory Information. For example, teaching ambulation techniques to preoperative patients is intended to increase ambulation and thereby speed recovery, the same type of behavioral outcome effected by Preparatory Sensory Information.

Explanations for lack of additive effects of Preparatory Sensory Information and instruction in a coping strategy (Fuller et al., 1978; Johnson et al., 1985; Wilson, 1981) may include incompatible behavioral responses, the presence of an existing effective strategy, or the need to use competing cognitive processes. For example, relaxation is intended to decrease activity, whereas other strategies such as ambulation and leg exercises increase activity that aids recovery. In other instances, such as pelvic examination (Fuller et al., 1978), the patient may have well-established behaviors that are used in preference to, or are incompatible with, the new technique. Finally, some combinations of information and instruction may not be effective because they require patients to use competing cognitive processes. The combination of Preparatory Sensory Information and distraction may be an example of such a situation (Johnson et al., 1985). Preparatory Sensory Information draws attention to event-related stimuli, whereas distraction requires blocking most of these stimuli from awareness.

When the findings concerning Preparatory Sensory Information are evaluated using the research utilization criteria identified by Haller, Reynolds, and Horsley (1979), the intervention is found to be useful for practice. The beneficial effects of Preparatory Sensory Information have been replicated in a wide variety of clinical settings, patient groups, and stressful health care events. Through conceptual replication, the research has contributed to the development of nursing knowledge; scientific merit is evident. The use of Preparatory Sensory Information involves little or no risk to patients, and its beneficial effects on coping with stressful health care procedures have been demonstrated. Nurses have clinical control in preparing patients for diagnostic and therapeutic procedures, and providing Preparatory Sensory Information is feasible. The cost-benefit ratio is more heavily weighed toward benefit than cost, as it provides a guide for selecting information that has a probability of being effective and replacing information that may not be effective.

Table 24–1   Sources of Typical Sensation Descriptors by Health Care Procedure

Procedure	Source
Abdominal surgery	Johnson, Rice, Fuller, & Endress, 1978b
	McHugh, Christman, & Johnson, 1982
Arteriography	Clark & Gregor, 1998
	Rice, Sieggreen, Mullin, & Williams, 1988
Barium enema	Hartfield & Cason, 1981
Breast biopsy, needle localization	Kelly & Winslow, 1996
Breast self-examination	Lauver & Keenan, 1991
Cardiac catheterization	Cason, Russell, & Fincher, 1992
Women's experiences	Cason & Landis, 1995
Cast removal	Johnson, Kirchhoff, & Endress, 1976
Chemotherapy	Greene, Nail, Fieler, Dudgeon, & Jones, 1994
	Rhodes, McDaniel, Hanson, Markway, & Johnson, 1994
Coronary artery bypass surgery	Moore, 1994
Gastroendoscopic examination	Johnson, Morrissey, & Leventhal, 1973
	Johnson & Leventhal, 1974
Mastectomy	
Mean 5.5 years postoperatively	Nail, Jones, Giuffre, & Johnson, 1984
1 to 12 months postoperatively	Lierman, 1988
Myelogram	Cason & Sample, 1995
Nasogastric tube insertion	Padilla et al., 1981
Radiation therapy	
Multiple sites	King, Nail, Kreamer, Strohl, & Johnson, 1985
Breast, prostate, lung, head and neck	Johnson, Fieler, Jones, Wlasowicz, & Mitchell, 1997
Tracheostomy	Oerman, McHugh, Dietrich, & Boyll, 1983

IMPLEMENTATION OF PREPARATORY SENSORY INFORMATION

The sensation descriptions of stressful health care events are listed by source in Table 24–1. Complete Preparatory Sensory Information messages for cast removal in children (Johnson, Kirchhoff, & Endress, 1976), needle-localization breast biopsy (Kelly & Winslow, 1996), cardiac catheterization (Cason, Russell, & Fincher, 1992), and myelogram (Cason & Sample, 1995) are currently published. These messages need only modification to incorporate setting-specific environmental and procedural variations. In addition to providing detailed Preparatory Sensory Information messages for use with patients having radiation therapy for breast, prostate, lung, and head and neck cancer, a book by Johnson et al. (1997) provides a more comprehensive explanation of self-regulation theory and its implementation in professional practice.

When information to guide development of Preparatory Sensory Information messages is not available in the literature, description of the sensory and procedural components of the message should be systematically obtained (McHugh et al., 1982). The procedural component of the message varies from setting to setting because of variation in practices, policies, and environment. Nursing staff observing the event can readily note the sequential elements and their timing and environmental changes as they occur. The typical sensations should be obtained by interviewing at least 15 patients who have undergone the experience for which the message is being prepared. During these interviews, patients may initially tend to describe their experience in general terms or in emotionally charged terms. It may be necessary to guide patients to use more specific and objective descriptors. It also is helpful if specific elements of the procedure are used to guide the interview about sensory experiences. Once these data are collected, they are reviewed for similarities, and those sensations reported by approximately 50% or more of the patients are incorporated into the message. Sensations should be described in objective terms; evaluative connotations such as *awful* or *intense* should not be used.

Combining the information gathered about the two components involves linking the sensory experiences to their causes and ensuring that the temporal qualities, such as frequency, duration, and change over time, are linked to appropriate sensations and procedural elements of the event. Once the message has been developed, it should be reviewed to make sure that it portrays a clear and objective picture of the event and the experiences a patient may anticipate. Specific activities for developing Preparatory Sensory Information messages (McCloskey & Bulechek, 1996) are summarized in Table 24–2.

Preparatory Sensory Information may be delivered verbally to individuals or groups of patients or by using printed or audiovisual techniques. One should not be concerned with omitting some of the sensory descriptors when providing the information verbally. Partial sensory description has been found to be as effective as a full sensory description (Johnson & Rice, 1974). Neither should one be concerned about the power of suggestion when using this intervention. Subjects given false sensory description did not report experiencing those sensations (Johnson & Rice, 1974); patients given Preparatory Sensory Information as well as those who were not given it reported experiencing similar sensations (McHugh et al., 1982).

When planning to use Preparatory Sensory Information with instruction in a coping strategy, it may be helpful to consider whether or not the two interventions are compatible in terms of their effects. As noted earlier, combining the informational intervention focusing attention on concrete, objective elements of

Table 24–2 Preparatory Sensory Information

DEFINITION: Describing both the subjective and objective physical sensations associated with an upcoming stressful health care procedure/treatment.

ACTIVITIES:

Identify the sensations surrounding the procedure/treatment

Describe the sensations in objective terms

Indicate the cause of a sensation

Present the sensations in the sequence that they are most likely to be experienced

Include information about the timing of events

Include information about the spatial characteristics of the environment in which the procedure/treatment takes place

Focus on the typical sensory experiences described by the majority of patients

Include typical sensations related to seeing, touching, smelling, tasting, and hearing, as appropriate to the procedure/treatment

Choose several words to describe each sensation, because one or the other of the descriptors should strike the patient as accurate

Use lay terms to describe the sensations

Use the word "pain" sparingly, but include it if it is typical

Personalize the information by using personal pronouns

Focus on the sensations to be experienced, but also include procedural information

Provide an opportunity for the patient to ask questions and clarify misunderstandings

Source: McCloskey, J. C., and Bulechek, G. M. (Eds.). (1996). *Nursing interventions classification (NIC)* (2nd ed.). St. Louis: Mosby–Year Book.

an experience with the teaching of a coping strategy such as distraction may not produce optimal patient outcomes.

APPROPRIATE CLIENT GROUPS AND ASSOCIATED NURSING DIAGNOSES AND OUTCOMES

Preparatory Sensory Information may be given to adults and to children 6 years of age or older who are able to understand verbal description of future events. Although younger children need to be prepared for stressful events, verbal description of the impending experience is not the most appropriate method for their level of cognitive development. Patients who have never experienced the anticipated procedure are most likely to benefit from Preparatory Sensory Information (McHugh et al., 1982), although patients who have had prior experience with the event also may benefit, because the information may be more accurate than their memories (Fuller et al., 1978). With health care events that occur frequently, such as daily or weekly venipuncture, patients' past experiences dominate the formation of expectations about the experience.

Because Preparatory Sensory Information is an intervention that facilitates coping or prevents disruption in coping, it is most useful for potential nursing diagnoses. At present, there are no appropriate potential diagnoses on the North American Nursing Diagnosis Association (NANDA)-approved listing (NANDA, 1994) for which this intervention may be used. We suggest Preparatory Sensory Information is most appropriately used for a diagnosis of Individual Coping, potential for enhanced. Risk factors (Bulechek & McCloskey, 1989) for such a diagnosis that may be modified by the use of Preparatory Sensory Information are indicative of possible inadequate schema formation and may include lack of prior experience with the stressful health care event, distant prior experience, anxiety due to the unknown, and tendency to focus on emotional aspects of experiences. Preparatory Sensory Information also may be useful as an intervention for the additional nursing diagnoses of Fear and Knowledge Deficit.

Overall, the major outcome affected by use of Preparatory Sensory Information is enhanced Coping (actions to manage stressors that tax an individual's resources [Johnson & Maas, p. 136]). Self-regulation theory and the research findings indicate other outcomes that may be affected. These include Fear Control (ability to eliminate or reduce disabling feelings of alarm aroused by an identifiable source [Johnson & Maas, p. 147]) and Knowledge: Treatment Procedure(s) (extent of understanding conveyed about procedure(s) required as part of a treatment regimen [Johnson & Maas, p. 196]). Use of Preparatory Sensory Information is more likely to enhance Fear Control for patients having relatively short diagnostic procedures and for those having a longer procedure who are especially fearful. Generally, for health care experiences of longer duration, Preparatory Sensory Information's effects will be reflected in indicators of functional status. Selection of specific indicators to be assessed should be based on consideration of those activities most likely to be threatened or interrupted by the particular health care event.

CASE STUDY

Mrs. O was a 62-year-old housewife who was scheduled to undergo external radiation therapy for early-stage endometrial cancer. She had been in good health up until her diagnosis. She was to receive daily treatments (excluding weekends) of 180 cGy over a period of 28 days, resulting in a total dose of 5,040 cGy of radiation. Her treatment was carried out on a linear accelerator in the oncology radiation center of a major university hospital.

Because of the recent diagnosis of cancer and undergoing an unfamiliar treatment experience, Mrs. O was facing a situation that could tax her resources for coping. Our goal was to enhance Mrs. O's potential for coping with radiation therapy and its side effects. The treatment was Preparatory Sensory Information delivered by audiocassette recording. The following are excerpts from the recording. The first excerpt is from the information provided before Mrs. O's first treatment, and the second is from that given on her third day of treatment.

Excerpt 1

"This recording describes the typical experiences that you can expect during your radiation treatments. The description is based on what patients similar to you have told us about what they saw, felt, and heard while having radiation treatment similar to yours.

"Before your treatment you will spend a few minutes in the waiting area of the radiation department. The technician will call you when it is time for your treatment. The treatment room is large. It contains a linear accelerator machine that houses the radiation source. The machine is big and has a table underneath it and an 'arm' that can be moved. The light in the room is dim; however, you may be aware of fluorescent lights along the wall, and you will see small beams of red light coming from the walls. These lights are used to help line up the area of your body to be treated. Below the arm of the accelerator is the table that you will lie on during your treatment. Once on the table you will be asked to slip your clothes down so that the marks placed on your body during simulation will be visible. The technician will then check your position on the table and will adjust the table itself. You may feel the table move up, down, backward, or forward. Once the machine, the table, and you are in the correct positions, the technician will leave the room and you will receive the first phase of the treatment. It is important that you lie perfectly still for your treatment. The technician will regulate the treatment from outside the room and will watch you on a television (TV) screen. You may notice the TV camera on the wall. You will

be able to talk to the technician through an intercom. .

"You will receive radiation doses from the linear accelerator when it is in four different positions: above you, below you, and on each side. The technician will come in and change the machine's position. When it is moving, it will make a clicking and humming sound like a motor. When it stops moving, the technician will leave the room, and you will hear a buzzing sound for a few seconds. This indicates that you are receiving the radiation. You will feel nothing during the treatment. The total time you will spend in the treatment room will be about 10 minutes. When it is finished, the technician will help you with your clothes and assist you down from the table."

Excerpt 2

"Women similar to you have told us about symptoms they've experienced while receiving radiation. While not all of the women experience them to the same degree, most tell us they experience diarrhea, fatigue, and nausea (Christman, Oakely, & Cornin, 1998).

"Diarrhea can begin in the second week of treatment and continue throughout your treatment. It is due to the effects of radiation on your bowels. It can occur at all times of the day; however, you may notice it more in the morning or during the evening hours. Your doctor will prescribe medications and give you information about foods to eat to help reduce the diarrhea.

"Fatigue, or being tired, can begin in the second week of treatment and will increase as your treatments continue. During your treatments you will notice the tiredness periodically during the day, .but particularly in the afternoon. Some women also experience periodic nausea or being 'sick to their stomach' during the first week of treatment or near the end of treatment. Any nausea you may have is not related to the effects of radiation on your body. More likely, it is due to changes in your routine, or it may be related to any feelings or concerns you may have about your treatment."

Evaluation

Mrs. O was an energetic and outgoing woman who had to curtail some of her activities due to her treatment schedule and side effects, but they did not change her daily routine entirely. She modified her social activities and planned more of them in her own home for the morning hours when she felt best. She wasn't able to keep up with all the housework but felt comfortable allowing her two daughters to take over the laundry and vacuuming. During the fourth week of treatment, Mrs. O stated that she was glad she had known what to expect during her treatments and that it had helped her plan her daily activities.

CONCLUSION

Clearly, Preparatory Sensory Information is an intervention that should be helpful to a wide variety of patients. Self-regulation theory enables nurses to link the use of Preparatory Sensory Information to appropriate nursing diagnoses and expected patient outcomes. Theory-guided practice involves the use of principles rather than step-by-step procedures and thereby promotes individualized, professional nursing care (Johnson et al., 1997).

References

Bulechek, G. M., and McCloskey, J. C. (1989). Nursing interventions: Treatments for potential nursing diagnoses. In R. M. Carroll-Johnson (Ed.), *Classification of nursing diagnoses*: *Proceedings of the eighth conference* (pp. 23–30). Philadelphia: J. B. Lippincott.

Cason, C. L., and Landis, N. (1995). Women's sensory experiences during cardiac catheterization. *Cardiovascular Nursing*, 31, 33–36.

Cason, C. L., Russell, D. G., and Fincher, S. B. (1992). Preparatory sensory information for cardiac catheterization. *Cardiovascular Nursing*, 28, 41–45.

Cason, C. L., and Sample, J. G. (1995). Preparatory information for myelogram. *Journal of Neuroscience Nursing*, 27, 182–187.

Christman, N. J. (1997). Enhancing functional outcomes during radiation therapy. Paper presented at the fourth national Conference on Cancer Nursing Research. Panama City Beach, FL, January 23–25.

Christman, N. J., Oakley, M. G., and Cronin, S. N. (1998). *Preparing women with cervical or uterine cancer for radiation therapy*. Manuscript submitted for publication.

Clark, C. R., and Gregor, F. M. (1998). Developing a sensation information message for femoral arteriography. *Journal of Advanced Nursing*, 13, 237–244.

Fuller, S. S., Endress, M. P., and Johnson, J. E. (1978). The effects of cognitive and behavioral control on coping with an aversive health examination. *Journal of Human Stress*, 4(4), 18–24.

Greene, D., Nail, L. M., Fieler, V. K., Dudgeon, D., and Jones, L. S. (1994). A comparison of patient-reported side-effects among three chemotherapy regimens for breast cancer. *Cancer Practice*, 2, 57–62.

Haller, K. B., Reynolds, M. A., and Horsley, J. A. (1979). Developing research-based innovation protocols: Process, criteria, and issues. *Research in Nursing and Health*, 2, 45–51.

Hartfield, M. J., and Cason, C. L. (1981). Effect of information on emotional responses during barium enema. *Nursing Research*, 30, 151–155.

Hartfield, M. J., Cason, C. L., and Cason, G. J. (1982). Effects of information about a threatening procedure on patients' expectations and emotional distress. *Nursing Research*, 31, 202–206.

Hill, B. J. (1982). Sensory information, behavioral instructions and coping with sensory alteration surgery. *Nursing Research*, 31, 17–21.

Johnson, J. E. (1973). Effects of accurate expectations about sensations on the sensory and distress components of pain. *Journal of Personality and Social Psychology*, 27, 261–275.

Johnson, J. E. (1996). Coping with radiation therapy: Optimism and the effect of preparatory interventions. *Research in Nursing and Health*, 19, 3–12.

Johnson, J. E., Christman, N. J., and Stitt, C. (1985). Personal control interventions: Short- and long-term effects on surgical patients. *Research in Nursing and Health*, 8, 131–145.

Johnson, J. E., Fieler, V. K., Jones, L. S., Wlasowicz, G. S., and Mitchell, M. L. (1997). *Self-regulation theory: Applying theory to your practice*. Pittsburgh, PA: Oncology Nursing Press.

Johnson, J. E., Fuller, S. S., Endress, M. P., and Rice, V. H. (1978a). Altering patients' responses to surgery: An extension and replication. *Research in Nursing and Health*, 1, 111–121.

Johnson, J. E., Kirchhoff, K. T., and Endress, M. P. (1975). Altering children's distress behavior during orthopedic cast removal. *Nursing Research*, 24, 404–410.

Johnson, J. E., Kirchhoff, K. T., and Endress, M. P. (1976). Easing children's fright during health care procedures. *MCN The American Journal of Maternal Child Nursing*, 1, 206–210.

Johnson, J. E., and Lauver, D. R. (1989). Alternative explanations of coping with stressful experiences associated with physical illness. *Advances in Nursing Science*, 11(2), 39–52.

Johnson, J. E., Lauver D. R., and Nail, L. M. (1989). Process of coping with radiation therapy. *Journal of Consulting and Clinical Psychology*, 57, 358–364.

Johnson, J. E., and Leventhal, H. (1974). Effects of accurate expectations and behavioral instructions on reactions during a noxious medical examination. *Journal of Personality and Social Psychology*, 29, 710–718.

Johnson, J. E., Morrissey, J. F., and Leventhal, H. (1973). Psychological preparation for an endoscopic examination. *Gastrointestinal Endoscopy*, 19, 180–182.

Johnson, J. E., Nail, L. M., Lauver, D., King, K., and Keys, H. (1988). Reducing the negative impact of radiation therapy on functional status. *Cancer*, 61, 46–51.

Johnson, J. E., and Rice, V. H. (1974). Sensory and distress components of pain: Implications for the study of clinical pain. *Nursing Research*, 23, 203–209.

Johnson, J. E., Rice, V. H., Fuller, S. S., and Endress,

M. P. (1978b). Sensory information, instruction in a coping strategy, and recovery from surgery. *Research in Nursing and Health, 1,* 4–17.

Johnson, M., and Maas, M. (Eds.). (1997). *Nursing outcomes classification (NOC).* St. Louis: Mosby–Year Book.

Kelly, P., and Winslow, E. H. (1996). Needle wire localization for nonpalpable breast lesions: Sensations, anxiety levels, and informational needs. *Oncology Nursing Forum, 23,* 639–644.

King, K. B., Nail, L. M., Kreamer, K., Strohl, R. A., and Johnson, J. E. (1985). Patients' descriptions of the experience of receiving radiation therapy. *Oncology Nursing Forum, 12*(4), 55–61.

Lauver, D., and Keenan, C. (1991). Identifying women's descriptions of breast tissue for the promotion of breast self-examination. *Health Care for Women International, 12,* 73–83.

Leventhal, H., and Johnson, J. E. (1983). Laboratory and field experimentation: Development of a theory of self-regulation. In P. J. Wooldridge, M. H. Schmitt, J. K. Skipper, and R. C. Leonard (Eds.), *Behavioral science and nursing theory* (pp. 189–262). St. Louis: Mosby.

Lierman, L. M. (1988). Sensory and physical alterations after mastectomy. *Health Care for Women International, 9,* 263–279.

McCloskey, J. C., and Bulechek, G. M. (Eds.). (1996). *Nursing interventions classification (NIC)* (2nd ed.). St. Louis: Mosby–Year Book.

McHugh, N. G., Christman, N. J., and Johnson, J. E. (1982). Preparatory information: What helps and why. *American Journal of Nursing, 82,* 780–782.

Miller, S. M., and Mangan, C. E. (1983). Interacting effects of information and coping style in adapting to gynecologic stress: Should the doctor tell all? *Journal of Personality and Social Psychology, 45,* 223–236.

Moore, S. M. (1994). Development of discharge information for recovery after coronary artery bypass surgery. *Applied Nursing Research, 7,* 170–177.

Nail, L., Jones, L. S., Giuffre, M., and Johnson, J. E. (1984). Sensations after mastectomy. *American Journal of Nursing, 84,* 1121–1124.

Neisser, U. (1976). *Cognition and reality.* San Francisco, CA: W. H. Freeman.

North American Nursing Diagnosis Association. (1994). *NANDA nursing diagnoses: Definition and classification 1995–1996.* Philadelphia: Author.

Oermann, M. H., McHugh, N. G., Dietrich, J., and Boyll, R. (1983). After a tracheostomy: Patients describe their sensations. *Cancer Nursing, 6,* 361–366.

Padilla, G. V., Grant, N. M., Rains, B. L., Hansen, B. C., Bergstrom, N., Wong, H. L., Hanson, R., and Kubo, W. (1981). Distress reduction and the effects of preparatory teaching films and patient control. *Research in Nursing and Health, 4,* 375–387.

Rainey, L. C. (1985). Effects of preparatory patient education for radiation oncology patients. *Cancer, 56,* 1056–1061.

Rhodes, V. A., McDaniel, R. W., Hanson, B., Markway, E., and Johnson M. (1994). Sensory perception of patients on selected antineoplastic chemotherapy protocols. *Cancer Nursing, 17,* 45–51.

Rice, V. H., Sieggreen, M., Mullin, M., and Williams, J. (1988). Development and testing of an arteriography intervention for stress reduction. *Heart and Lung, 17,* 23–28.

Sime, A. M., and Libera, M. B. (1985). Sensation information, self-instruction and responses to dental surgery. *Research in Nursing and Health, 8,* 41–47.

Suls, J., and Fletcher, B. (1985). The relative efficacy of avoidant and nonavoidant coping strategies: A meta-analysis. *Health Psychology, 4,* 249–288.

Suls, J., and Wan, C. K. (1989). Effects of sensory and procedural information on coping with stressful medical procedures and pain: A meta-analysis. *Journal of Consulting and Clinical Psychology, 57,* 372–379.

Watkins, L. O., Weaver, L., and Odegaard, V. (1986). Preparation for cardiac catheterization: Tailoring the content of instruction to coping style. *Heart and Lung, 15,* 382–389.

Wilson, J. F. (1981). Behavioral preparation for surgery: Benefit or harm? *Journal of Behavioral Medicine, 4*(1), 79–102.

Wilson, J. F., Moore, R. W., Randolph, S., and Hanson, B. J. (1982). Behavioral preparation of patients for gastrointestinal endoscopy: Information, relaxation, and coping style. *Journal of Human Stress, 8*(4), 13–23.

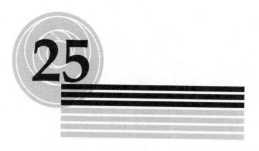

Communication Enhancement: Speech Deficit

Barbara J. Boss

Because communication is a form of social behavior (Hedge, 1995) and is far more than mere talk or speech, Communication Enhancement is a complex intervention designed to facilitate the rich social activity of communication. Hedge (1995) holds that communication may entail voice, articulation (phonology), language, fluency, and hearing. Boss and Lewis-Abney (1996) add pragmatics and cognitive abilities to that list. Facilitating communication competence (Holland, 1996), therefore, may involve enhancing (1) language (linguistic) competence, which includes voice, articulation, and fluency competence; (2) pragmatic competence; and (3) cognitive competence or hearing ability (Boss, 1984; 1991b; Boss & Lewis-Abney, 1996). Hearing is beyond the scope of this chapter and is not addressed.

Communication deficits frequently are (1) not adequately assessed, (2) misdiagnosed, or (3) mismanaged. Yet a communication deficit can be an extremely disabling problem for the person, family, friends, associates, and society in general as well as for health care providers.

Communication Enhancement often requires measures directed at (1) the creation of an external environment that facilitates attempts to communicate, (2) the promotion of behaviors by other persons that are experienced by the person with the communication deficit as positive and supportive, (3) the use of therapeutic techniques to improve the communication, and (4) the education of the person, family, and associates regarding Communication Enhancement techniques. Often a variety of health care professionals and assistive devices are helpful in enhancing communication.

REVIEW OF RELATED LITERATURE

A working knowledge of the types of communication deficits is essential for adequate assessment of the communication deficit(s) and the development of an appropriate Communication Enhancement strategy.

Language (Linguistic) and Speech Deficit

Language (linguistic) competence is the ability to form and use symbols and involves many processes—developing the thoughts to be communicated; selecting, formulating, and ordering the words; applying the rules of grammar; initiating the muscle, including vocal fold, movements to produce the speech or written words; controlling respiration to produce the required sounds and vocalization; and evaluating the output for correctness and need for corrective action (Boss & Lewis-Abney, 1996). Speech, the highly coordinated, sequential pattern of muscular contractions of the respiratory, larynx, pharynx, palate, tongue, and lip musculature (Adams & Victor, 1989), is considered part of language competence for the purposes of this chapter, because it results in verbal output.

Language acquisition, including speech development, is currently most often viewed as a multifactorial process involving innate maturational factors (Wexler, 1990) and experiential factors from within a cultural context (Harkness, 1990) or in a social-interaction context (Zukow, 1990), although a functionalist perspective is still argued by Dent (1990). Clearly, the intactness of the language neural network that mediates the comprehension and production of language is fundamental to language acquisition. What is still unclear is the exact locations of language centers and the degree of involvement of the right hemisphere in language comprehension and production (Feldman, Holland, Kemp, & Janosky, 1992; Locke, 1992). Functional brain imaging techniques such as positron-emission tomography (PET) and single photon emission computed tomography (SPECT) that are now available in research laboratories will end these debates. The resting brain and activation studies will greatly aid understanding of the language network within the brain (Demonet, Wise, & Frackowiak, 1993; Metter, 1995; Peterson, Fox, Posner, Mintun, & Raichle, 1988). For example, it has been established that there are unique networks for certain mental operations related to language. Passively viewing words activates most prominently an area along the inner surface of the left hemisphere (Posner & Raichle, 1994). Listening to words activates a group of areas in the temporal lobes of both hemispheres (Posner & Raichle, 1994). Speaking words aloud most prominently activates bilateral areas of the motor cortex and supplementary motor cortex, the insular cortex, and the middle cerebellum (Posner & Raichle, 1994). Generating verbs produces the most complex activity in the left frontal cortex, anterior cingulate, posterior temporal lobe, and right cerebellum (Posner & Raichle, 1994).

Wong (1994) and Hedge (1995) detail the stages of language development. The role of babbling in language development has been investigated (Hill & Singer, 1990; Locke & Pearson, 1990). Language competence appears to be unaffected by normal aging, although voice quality and loudness may change as the vocal folds age.

Language deficits are called language delays in infants and small children, developmental language disorders or developmental aphasias in older children, and acquired aphasia in children (Woods, 1995) and adults who have lost previously well-established language competence due to a brain injury. The clinical studies of adult aphasias are numerous and date back to Broca (1863,

1865) in the 1800s, but the study of developmental and acquired aphasias is just beginning (Klein, 1996; Paul, 1995; Tuchman, Rapin, & Shinnar, 1991). Some of the most pertinent new information in the field of aphasia is the documentation that metabolic changes occur in temporoparietal regions in all subjects with aphasia, regardless of the location of the structural lesion, which may be at a distant site (Metter, 1995). Cortical lesions are now known to be accompanied by metabolic changes in the ipsilateral basal ganglion and thalamus as well as in the contralateral cerebellum (Metter, 1995). Subcortical lesions have been documented to cause language deficits as well as cortical lesions (Metter, 1995). Prognosis for recovery has been found to correlate with regional cerebral blood flow (rCBF). Poor prognosis is associated with absence of increased blood flow in bilateral frontotemporal regions during certain activation tasks, whereas better recovery is correlated with blood flow to the area of the right hemisphere corresponding to Broca's on the left side (Metter, 1995). Benson and Arcadia (1996), Code & Muller (1995), and Kirschner (1995) provide a current discussion of the aphasias.

Speech difficulties may arise from articulation defects as experienced in Parkinson's disease, respiratory deficits as experienced in amyotrophic lateral sclerosis (ALS), voice (phonation) problems as follow a laryngectomy, resonation difficulties as experienced in myasthenia gravis, fluency problems as experienced with stuttering, and hearing loss. Loss of control of the vocal tract muscles, including the vocal folds, produces phonation deficits that cause consonant and vowel sound production to be disordered (Ackermann & Ziegler, 1991a). Clinical descriptions of classic patterns of speech problems exist in the literature (e.g., Adams & Victor, 1989), and some database descriptions can be found as well (Ackermann & Zeigler, 1991a, 1991b; Ansel & Kent, 1992; Darley, Aronson, & Brown, 1969a, 1969b; Kent et al., 1992; Kent et al., 1991; Murdock, Chenery, Strokes, & Hardcastle, 1991). Duffy (1995), Klein (1996), and McNeil (1997) address speech disorders and interventions.

Pragmatic Deficits

Pragmatic competence is "the use of language in terms of situational or social context" (Sohlberg & Mateer, 1989) and may be viewed as a distinct component of communication or as the overlying encompassing function of communication (Bates, 1979; Bloom & Lahey, 1970). Prosody (prosodia), gestures and pantomime, and facial expression are components of pragmatic competence. Ross (1985) defined prosodia as "the melody, pause, intonation, stresses, and accents applied to the articulatory line" and imparting affective tone, subtle gradation of meaning, and various emphases in spoken language (Bolton & Dashiell, 1984). Prosody generates dialects, conveys the speaker's emotional state and attitude, and places the language in its true context so that the full or real meaning is conveyed. Gestures (kinesics) are the use of limb, body, and facial movements associated with nonverbal communication to convey an emotional or attitudinal quality and are used to color, emphasize, and embellish speech (Ross, 1985). When kinesic activity is used for a semantic purpose—that is, to convey a specific meaning—it is referred to as pantomime (Critchley, 1970). Facial expression is the use of facial movements to convey mood and emotional state; it contributes to the dynamic nature of the communication.

Pragmatics is just developing as an area of speech and language pathology (Boss & Lewis-Abney, 1996), so the stages of development in childhood for prosody, gestures and pantomime, or facial expression have not been detailed in the literature. Clearly, children use pragmatics—specifically prosody, gestures, and facial expression—before they use language to express themselves, and they learn pragmatics in the social context of family, caregivers, and culture. Nor has pragmatic competence been examined specifically in aged persons, which is troubling in view of the known changes in retrieval of visual-spatial memories in elders, an ability that may well contribute to comprehension of gestures and facial expression.

Prosody is the most studied area of pragmatics, starting with Monrad-Krohn in 1947 (Monrad-Krohn, 1947a, 1947b, 1947c). The right brain's role in the emotional aspects of communication received more scientific attention in the 1970s (Blumstein & Cooper, 1974; Heilman, Scholes, & Watson, 1975; Ross & Mesulam, 1979; Tucker, Watson, & Heilman, 1977; Zuriff, 1974). Others (Borod, 1992; Cancelliere & Kertesz, 1990; Ross, 1981; Ross, Harney, deLaCoste-Utamsing, & Purdy, 1981; Ross, Holzapfel, & Freeman, 1983) have documented that right-hemisphere brain injury seriously impairs comprehension of the affective components of prosody and gestures. The more linguistic components, such as stress differences on segments of words, pause structure differences, and pitch changes, have been documented in both right- and left-hemisphere brain damage (Blumstein & Goodglass, 1972; Danly, Cooper, & Shapiro, 1983; Danly & Shapiro, 1982; Heilman, Bowers, Speedie, & Cosletter, 1983; Weintraub, Mesulam, & Kramer, 1981). Basal ganglia injury was the most common injury isolated by Cancelliere and Kertesz (1990), followed by anterior temporal and insular injury in aprosodia syndromes. Dent (1990), Gainotti and Lemmo (1976), and Goodglass and Kaplan (1963) found impairments in comprehension and performance of pantomime with left-hemisphere injury, and Ross and Mesulam (1979) found a relationship between loss of kinesic activity and right-sided brain injury; right inferior frontal injury resulted in loss of spontaneous gestural activity with apraxia. Developmental aprosodia has just recently begun to be explored (Basso, Farabola, Grassi, Laiacona, & Zanobio, 1990; Bell, Davis, Morgan-Fisher, & Ross, 1990).

High-Level Language Skills

Not only is the language network a cognitive network, but many cognitive activities carried out by the left hemisphere are language dependent. For example, memories are transferred and stored in the left hemisphere in a language format. Likewise, humans think in words (symbols). Left-hemisphere cognitive development closely parallels language development. Dysfunction in any cognitive network can significantly impair communication capabilities. In fact, a language impairment can be very difficult to distinguish from a cognitive impairment. Groher (1977) argued that disorientation to time and space, impaired recent memory, poor thinking, mistaken reasoning, poor understanding of the environment, and inappropriate behavior may produce confused language. Groher (1977) and Weinstein and Keller (1963) have documented that aphasia may resolve into a confused language pattern.

Related to attentional networks, dysfunction in the arousal network resulting in impaired consciousness (awakeness) eliminates language and restricts pragmatics to only inarticulate prosody such as groans, grimaces, or posturing. Impairment in the selective attention network prevents orienting to specific environmental stimuli, thus impairing the communication embedded in the auditory, visual, or tactile stimuli. Pragmatics can be markedly impaired when the right parietal lobe is affected.

With dysfunction in the recent memory network, the person appears forgetful and exhibits communication that appears confused and lacks meaningfulness, although syntax and semantics may be correct. Dysfunction in the remote memory network of the left hemisphere may produce a loss of comprehension of verbal or written language or both—that is, an aphasia—whereas dysfunction of the right hemisphere may result in aprosody, loss of facial expression, and loss of comprehension of gestures, pantomime, and facial expression. An individual unable to form and use concepts communicates as does a young child, with use of concrete and literal language as well as concrete and literal interpretations.

Impairment in the vigilance network mediated by the right frontal and parietal lobes (Posner & Raichle, 1994) produces an inability to remain alert and responsive to communicative stimuli. The person fails to notice, search for, or scan for relevant communication stimuli that should activate the selective attentional network. The person may not notice the gesture, the facial expression, the tone, or the voice calling his or her name.

Dysfunction in the detection networks, mediated in part by the cingulate gyrus, at its worst produces akinetic mutism (Posner & Raichle, 1994), a motionless individual who does not speak or exhibit any pragmatics. In less severe situations, the person appears apathetic and disinterested in communicating. Often he or she is unable to set a communication goal and plan how to achieve the communication. The person may not know what he or she wants to say or write or may not be able to put the language together to say or write it.

Impaired working memory (short-term representational memory) mediated by the dorsal-lateral frontal areas results in an inability to use internalized knowledge to guide behavior in the absence of informative external cues. Preestablished preferences (stay errors) cannot be inhibited, and the individual cannot use corrective feedback effectively.

Rehabilitation Approaches

The vast array of interventions for language deficits can be grouped into four approaches that are not mutually exclusive but derive from different psychological theories and often from different countries and cultures. Some interventions are grounded in a strong research base; others are derived from theory and have little empirical study to support the theory. The four approaches are as follows: (1) the classical or stimulation approach, which is based on the assumptions that aphasia is a central language deficit and that different language deficits are only quantitatively different; treating one aspect simultaneously treats all aspects, and the treatment is directed at improving access to language; (2) the Soviet approach based on Luria's theory (1970, 1973), which holds that aphasias are qualitatively different and that reorganization of the system to bypass the defect is necessary and is achieved through a highly individualized retraining program; (3) an operant conditioning approach based on Skinner's (1972) principles of operant conditioning; and (4) a psycholinguistic approach that focuses on linguistic criteria and substitute symbol systems.

In general, whatever approach is used, intervention strategies are individually tailored to the client. Improvement of spoken language is generally the goal of the intervention. Substitute skill models, such as lip reading; sign language; use of voice synthesizers; and use of written communications, including communication boards, spelling boards, cards, notebooks, picture boards, typewriters, computers, and other devices, are sometimes taught. Computer software programs to assist with communication are available. Listening interventions are generally used to treat auditory comprehension deficits. Wallace (1996) and White (1996) provide current suggestions for treatment programs.

Three additional approaches are used to address speech problems: (1) medical care for the underlying disorder to stabilize or improve the client's state, (2) surgical management or use of prosthetic devices, and (3) speech therapy based on behavioral methods and using communication aids (Boss & Lewis-Abney, 1996). With regard to pragmatic deficits, therapeutic interventions are in very early developmental stages, with only some trial remediation programs—predominantly for head-injured persons—currently existing, but published reports in the literature are lacking. Ehrlich and Spies (1985) and Sohlberg and Mateer (1989) have published material about their group approaches.

Cognitive intervention strategies are appropriate in addressing the cognitive network problems that generate communication deficits but are beyond the scope of this chapter. Sohlberg and Mateer (1989), Boss (1991a, 1993, 1994a, 1994b), and Chapey (1994) cover some cognitive strategies that would be appropriate.

Intervention Tools and Protocols

An appropriate Communication Enhancement strategy can be developed only from an assessment of the client's communication abilities and disabilities. This assessment includes information on the client's health history, developmental level, previous cognitive and communication abilities, and present communication abilities (Boss & Lewis-Abney, 1996). An adequate assessment of communication abilities includes assessment of language competence, including speech capabilities, pragmatic competence, and cognition. The assessment of language competence is well-established and includes evaluation of spontaneous speech, comprehension of verbal language, comprehension of written language, ability to name, ability to repeat, and ability to write (Boss & Lewis-Abney, 1996). Pragmatic assessment is less established and less known by health care providers. It includes evaluating comprehension and production of prosody, gestures and pantomime, and facial expression (Boss & Lewis-Abney, 1996). An adequate assessment of cognition as it relates to communication includes evaluation of the attentional networks of arousal and selective attention; the memory networks, including recent memory and remote memory; and executive attentional networks, including vigilance, detection, and working memory. Table 25–1 outlines clinical assessment parameters for language, pragmatics, and cognitive networks and provides examples of some standardized tests that are available for additional testing. The neuropsychologist and speech and language pathologist are resource professionals who assist with this assessment.

The goals of the intervention Communication Enhancement are to assist the client in achieving optimal communication, to assist the client in establishing a functional means of communication, to help establish an environment that is conducive to communication, to prevent injury, to help preserve the client's self-esteem, to promote social interaction, to assist the client in returning to social roles, to provide communication opportunities, to educate the client and family regarding the communication deficits, and to assist the client and family in establishing effective support networks (Boss & Lewis-Abney, 1996). When dysarthria or dysphonia are present, additional goals for the intervention Communication Enhancement include improving articulation and improving respiration, phonation, and resonance (Boss & Lewis-Abney, 1996). The Nursing Interventions Classification (NIC) intervention Communication Enhancement: Speech

Table 25–1 Language (Aphasia/Dysarthria), Pragmatic, and Cognitive Assessment and Standardized Tests

APHASIA ASSESSMENT

Spontaneous speech and reading
Comprehension of spoken words
Comprehension of written language
Ability to name
Ability to repeat
Ability to write

SPEECH ASSESSMENT

Spontaneous speech (assessed previously; see above)
Production of speech sounds
Movement of pharynx, tongue, face, and lips (Cranial Nerves VII, IX, X, and XII)

PRAGMATIC ASSESSMENT

Spontaneous affective prosody and gestures used in communicating
Ability to visually comprehend gestures
Ability to repeat, through imitation, linguistically neutral sentences with affective prosody
Ability to hear (auditorily comprehend) affective prosody
Internal emotional state

COGNITIVE ASSESSMENT

Arousability
Selective attention and orienting behaviors
Recent memory
Remote memory
Vigilance and ability to maintain alertness
Motivation, goal setting, and self-monitoring
Working memory (planning, initiating, and use of feedback)

EXAMPLES OF DYSPHASIA TESTS

Adults
  Bedside screening
    Aphasia Language Performance Scales
    Bedside Evaluation and Screening Scale
    Halstead-Wepman Aphasia Screening Test
  Comprehensive tests
    Boston Assessment of Severe Aphasia
    Boston Diagnostic Aphasia Examination
    Western Aphasia Battery
Children
  Denver Developmental Screening Test (DDST)
  Denver Prescreening Questionnaire (DPQ)

EXAMPLES OF SPEECH DISORDER TESTS

Adults
  Fisher-Logemann Test of Articulation Competence
  Frenchay Dysarthria Assessment
  Goldman-Fristoe Test of Articulation
Children
  Denver Articulation Screening Examination (DASE)

EXAMPLES OF PRAGMATIC DEFICIT TESTS

Adults
  Assessment of Nonverbal Communication/New England Pantomime Tests
  Communication Performance Scale
  Pragmatic Protocol

EXAMPLES OF RELATED COGNITIVE TESTS (not addressing language specifically)

Selective Attention
  Neglect in picture description tasks
Recent Memory
  Amnesia tests and ratings
  Immediate retention, retrieval, and recognition—verbal memory
  Immediate retention, retrieval, and recognition—visual memory
Remote Memory
  Abstract words, similarities, and differences
  Proverb interpretation
  Sorting tests
Detection
  Letter cancellation tasks
  Visual search tasks
Working memory
  Planning and purposeful behavior
  Motor impersistence and perseveration

Deficit (Table 25–2) can be used to work toward achievement of these goals. Each aspect of the intervention is discussed.

Environment

The first step in Communication Enhancement is to create an environment that encourages communication—that is, that makes the client's attempts to communicate easier and less stressful. No matter what type of communication deficit may exist, a calm, relaxed, and unhurried atmosphere is essential. Equipment should be placed so it is not distracting or intrusive. A schedule of activity should provide some degree of routine. Anxiety greatly compromises communication ability, so identifying and eliminating anxiety-provoking stimuli is critical, as is the use of anxiety-reducing measures discussed in other chapters of this book. Isolation does not help increase communication ability and should be avoided as well. Allow the patient to hear spoken language frequently, as appropriate, and carry on one-way conversations, as appropriate. Encourage participation in group activities.

However, if the primary communication deficit is in comprehending language or pragmatics, continuous, ongoing interaction is overwhelming and exhausting for the client. It is important to prevent undue fatigue and continuous exposure to stimuli and interactions. Even praise can be overwhelming and should be limited, as should the frequency and time length of communication stimulation and group activities. If the communication activity or interaction appears stressful or confusing at any point, it should be discontinued.

Table 25–2 Communication Enhancement: Speech Deficit

DEFINITION: Assistance in accepting and learning alternate methods for living with impaired speech.

ACTIVITIES:

Solicit family's assistance in understanding patient's speech, as appropriate

Allow patient to hear spoken language frequently, as appropriate

Provide verbal prompts/reminders

Give one simple direction at a time, as appropriate

Listen attentively

Use simple words and short sentences, as appropriate

Refrain from shouting at patient with communication disorders

Refrain from dropping your voice at the end of a sentence

Stand in front of patient when speaking

Use picture board, if appropriate

Use hand gestures, as appropriate

Perform prescriptive speech-language therapies during informal interactions with patient

Teach esophageal speech, as appropriate

Instruct patient and family on use of speech aids (e.g., tracheal-esophageal prosthesis and artificial larynx)

Encourage patient to repeat words

Provide positive reinforcement and praise, as appropriate

Carry on one-way conversations, as appropriate

Reinforce need for follow-up with speech pathologist after discharge

Use interpreter, as necessary

Source: McCloskey, J. C., and Bulechek, G. M. (Eds.). (1996). *Nursing interventions classification (NIC)* (2nd ed.). St. Louis: Mosby–Year Book: 180.

Support

Supportive behaviors from health care providers as well as family and friends are needed regardless of the type of communication deficit. Evidence of genuine concern is the cornerstone of supportive actions, accompanied by patience, acceptance, and a recognition of the frustration and difficulty the client is experiencing. Respect is evidenced when (1) the adult is always treated as an adult regardless of his or her current behavior and is involved in important decisions about his or her care and (2) the health care provider listens attentively and is observant and sensitive, which allows the provider to anticipate the client's needs and validate specific needs. The establishment of realistic short-term communication goals is fundamental, and excessive demands that cannot be met must be avoided. Then the client is encouraged in all his or her communication efforts and helped to develop a constructive and positive outlook by being given positive reinforcement and praise as appropriate even for the smallest gain, emphasizing what the client can do, working to build self-confidence, and reassuring the client that every person at times experiences difficulty, sometimes great difficulty, in expressing himself or herself. But in all cases, be honest about the prognosis for recovery and the difficulties entailed in reaching recovery. While protecting the client by not forcing communication or interactions he or she does not want, by changing the subject or activity if the client laughs or cries to excess, and by reminding the client how well he or she used to communicate, the client is at the same time encouraged to be as independent as he or she wishes to be and is provided with as many opportunities for self-care as possible. Being overly helpful and solicitous is to be avoided. Language and speech therapy or other interventions are initiated when the client is ready and interested. Reinforce the need for follow-up with the speech pathologist after discharge. Self-help organizations can be a valuable support system for both the client and the family. When comprehension and cognition are intact, it is critical that health care providers and family and friends not treat or permit others to treat the client as if he or she does not understand, is cognitively impaired, or is not present at all.

When language comprehension is impaired, use pragmatics—touch, tone of voice, gestures, facial expression, and pantomime—to communicate concern, caring, reassurance, and trustworthiness. A calm, unhurried manner is important. When pragmatic comprehension is impaired, all emotions and nonverbal intentions must be put into language. Say what you mean. Even if the client does not understand, do not talk about the client in front of him or her without attempting to involve the client as well. Nonjudgmentally accept paraphasia, "jargon language," cursing, and other behaviors, but attempt to clarify for the client that you do not understand.

Communication Facilitation

Some generally accepted principles of communication facilitation include the following: (1) distinguishing between a comprehension deficit and a production deficit and retraining each separately; (2) addressing comprehension deficits first because they are believed to be easier to achieve improvement in than are production deficits (Basso, 1987; Basso, Capitani, & Moraschini, 1982; Schuell, Jenkins, & Jimenez-Pabon, 1964); (3) using language in context, as it is a far better practice arena than are words and phrases used out of context; (4) being aware that improvement in one aspect of communication may be accompanied by improvement in other aspects; and (5) knowing that with practice, it is possible to improve functional communication efficiency or to develop an alternate pathway first at a voluntary level of control and then at an automatic level (Goodglass, 1987).

Some general principles for facilitating communication are to (1) use topics of interest or of current importance to the client to encourage spontaneous communication, (2) provide short but frequent interactions, (3) postpone communication when the client is fatigued or upset, and (4) encourage the client to use gestures and other forms of pragmatics when his or her language or speech is misunderstood (Boss & Lewis-Abney, 1996). Solicit the family's assistance in understanding the patient's speech, as appropriate, and use an interpreter when necessary. Perform prescriptive speech-language therapies during informal interactions with patients.

Whenever an aphasia or aprosodia is present, a slight comprehension deficit at the very least can be anticipated, so comprehension should be facilitated by (1) creating a quiet environment (e.g., turning off televisions and radios, removing unneeded equipment and items from view) so that communication can take place in a one-to-one interaction, at least early in the course of therapeutic intervention; (2) standing in front of the patient when speaking, securing the client's attention, including eye contact if possible, redirecting the client back to the communication partner if the client becomes distracted (Norman & Baratz, 1979), and refraining from dropping your voice at the end of a sentence; (3) speaking slowly and distinctly but maintaining natural pauses; (4) using simple words and short sentences, as appropriate; and (5) using short, simple instructions and explanations, giving one simple direction at a time, as appropriate, along with using gestures and pantomime as appropriate. Praise and reinforce appropriate responses, but tell the client when he or she is not understood, ask simple questions, and systematically point and gesture until the point is uncovered. If the the client does not comprehend or has misunderstood, signal that there was a miscommunication, refrain from shouting at the patient, including raising your voice or showing annoyance, and reword the communication using stronger gestures and facial expressions.

When comprehension is undisturbed and the communication deficit is in language or speech output, Communication Enhancement strategies include the following: (1) encourage all attempts to communicate, acknowledging the attempts and efforts; (2) allow the client to communicate for himself or herself, providing the person the opportunity to speak first and the time necessary to communicate; do not interrupt the client during attempts to communicate unless the client becomes frustrated (then interrupt or supply the word); (3) encourage automatic speech or imitation as well as singing, use self-talk (the client speaking about the activity being done by another person) and parallel talk (the client speaking aloud about what he or she is doing), and use expansion (the communication partner adding to the statement the client has made, expanding it); (4) request that statements be repeated or rephrased if they have not been understood, and assume some responsibility for misunderstanding the communication; (5) allow mistakes and do not insist that each word be pronounced perfectly; only occasionally correct the client if it is clearly necessary; (6) encourage the use of shorter statements if the client is distressed or fatigued or if the communication has been misunderstood (Piotrowski, 1978); and (7) if the client is having trouble, provide verbal prompts and reminders, also called cuing, by pronouncing the initial syllable of the word, encouraging the client to repeat the word after you, providing an open-ended sentence so the blank can be filled in, or writing down the word for the client to read (Norman & Baratz, 1979). Serve as a good communication model to imitate when the client is having difficulty. When there is a speech problem rather than a language problem, encourage the client to say one word at a time, with all the sounds in each word produced and the consonants emphasized. Also encourage the client to increase the volume of his or her voice. Specific exercise programs may improve articulation, resonance, and palatal, respiratory, and laryngeal muscle strength.

Education for Clients, Family Members, and Associates

The client should be helped to learn as much as possible, in the circumstance of a communication deficit, about the nature of the communication deficit, its causes, the prognosis for recovery, how to help himself or herself, and how to teach others how to help him or her communicate. A client is taught environmental strategies, support strategies, and communication facilitation strategies, including the use of speech aids such as a tracheal-esophageal prosthesis and esophageal speech or an artificial larynx, as appropriate. Realistic hope is to be supported, but unrealistic expectations are not to be encouraged.

Similarly, family members should be helped to learn about the nature of the communication deficit, its cause, the prognosis for recovery, how to create an environment that promotes communication, how to exhibit supportive behaviors, methods of facilitating communication, and the use of speech aids. Provide them with information about the behavioral changes in their loved one that often accompany a communication deficit. Help them learn to function as outside monitors of communication effectiveness for the client. Family members should be taught how to teach friends and associates Communication Enhancement techniques. Family and friends also should continue their normal activities and encourage the client to participate in appropriate activities, avoiding overprotectiveness as much as possible. Family and friends often need help to balance inclusion of the client in decision making with avoidance of overinvolvement in inconsequential decisions.

ASSOCIATED NURSING DIAGNOSES

A number of nursing diagnoses may be appropriate in the presence of a communication deficit, including the North American Nursing Diagnosis Association's (NANDA) diagnoses of Impaired Verbal Communication, Risk for Injury (related to impaired communication), Sensory/Perceptual Alterations, Self Care Deficit (related to impaired communication), Anxiety, Altered Family Processes, and Social Isolation. The diagnosis of impaired communication: written, emotional, gestural (Boss & Lewis-Abney, 1996) also applies.

ASSOCIATED PATIENT OUTCOMES

A number of nursing-sensitive patient outcomes from the Nursing Outcomes Classification (NOC) are appropriate for the intervention Communication Enhancement: Speech Deficit. They include the following:

1. Communication Ability—ability to receive, interpret, and express spoken, written, and non-verbal messages

2. Communication: Expressive Ability—ability to express and interpret verbal and/or non-verbal messages

3. Communication: Receptive Ability—ability to receive and interpret verbal and/or non-verbal messages

4. Compliance Behavior—actions taken on the basis of professional advice to promote wellness, recovery, and rehabilitation

5. Coping—actions to manage stressors that tax an individual's resources

6. Psychosocial Adjustment: Life Change—psychosocial adaptation of an individual to a life change

CASE STUDY

Mrs. EH was a 58-year-old woman who lived in a rural southeastern farming community. She had been in good health with no hospitalizations except for the birth of her children. She had no previously diagnosed chronic health problems and was on no medications at the time of her admission to the hospital. Her family history was positive for essential hypertension and cardiovascular disease. The day of admission and for several days prior, according to the family, Mrs. EH had complained of a bilateral throbbing headache and blurred vision and of generally not feeling well. In the early afternoon, Mrs. EH began "to act funny" and "seem confused," according to family members. It appeared to her husband and grown children that she had "lost her hearing." She was taken to the university medical center emergency room by family members by car, where her blood pressure was found to be 250/160, and, neurologically, she was found to have a dense Wernicke's (posterior, sensory, receptive) aphasia with no comprehension of verbal or written language. Motor, sensory, cerebellar, and cranial nerve findings were all within normal limits. Mrs. EH was admitted to neurology service with diagnoses of hypertension and left hemisphere stroke and was taken for a computed tomography (CT) scan, where an uncontrasted and then a contrasted brain CT scan were done. No evidence of a hypertensive bleed was found, and the CT scan was read as being consistent with cerebral ischemia, suggesting a left superior temporal lobe ischemic event.

During language testing, Mrs. EH was awake and alert. She was fluent, but her language output was jargon and jibberish. She could not read, and her writing made no sense. She gradually realized the communication problem was hers, not that of others. With this realization, she became more and more silent.

Mrs. EH smoked one to two packs of cigarettes a day, consumed a high-salt, high-fat diet (although she was not overweight), and was postmenopausal but receiving no estrogen therapy. She had health insurance that covered acute illness but had no provisions for rehabilitative services related to language-speech therapy.

The etiology of the ischemic stroke was investigated with carotid duplex, transcranial Doppler transthoracic echocardiogram, and clotting studies. No evidence of cardiac or aortic arch pathology was found. No large vessel carotid disease was present, and no hypercoagulable state was identified. Her final diagnosis was left superior temporal lobe ischemic stroke of small vessel origin. She was placed on enteric-coated aspirin 325 mg po qd. Her hypertension was worked up to rule out secondary hypertension, and a final diagnosis of essential hypertension was made, to be treated with smoking reduction leading to smoking cessation, a low-sodium (no added salt) diet, exercise, and medications—lisinopril 20 mg po qd and hydrochlorothiazide 12.5 mg po qd. She was also found to have some mild hypertrophic cardiomegaly and hyperlipidemia with very low high-density lipoprotein levels, which was further treated with a low-fat, low-cholesterol diet, because smoking cessation and exercise had already been described. Premarin 0.625 mg po qd was also initiated for its cardioprotective effects, because she had no contraindications.

Mrs. EH was provided with a calm, relaxed, and unhurried environment and as routine a schedule of activities as possible. She was encouraged to socialize with staff and other patients. Staff demonstrated concern, patience, acceptance, and recognition of her frustration. She was treated as a capable adult, and self-care was expected. Generally, effective communication was achieved using gestures, pantomime, pictures, drawings, touch, and tone of voice. The speech therapy department was consulted, but a therapist could see Mrs. EH on an inpatient basis for only two or three visits. While in the hospital, she worked well with pictures and drawings as a method of communication and was good at comprehending and using gestures and pantomime.

Education of the family regarding Mrs. EH focused on the nature of the communication problem, its cause, and ways to enhance communication using environmental manipulation, supportive behaviors, and facilitation techniques. The family members had great difficulty understanding what was wrong with Mrs. EH. She looked fine to them but acted strangely and different from usual, in their view. The nature of her communication loss escaped them. They had never heard of or seen a person with a stroke like this. Staff role-modeled the effective strategies and techniques that enhanced communication with Mrs. EH, but unfortunately, the family had much less success with Communication Enhancement than did the staff.

References

Ackermann, H., and Zeigler, W. (1991a). Articulatory deficits in Parkinsonian dysarthria: An acoustic analysis. *Journal of Neurology, Neurosurgery and Psychiatry, 54*, 1093–1098.

Ackermann, H., and Zeigler, W. (1991b). Cerebellar voice tremor: An acoustic analysis. *Journal of Neurology, Neurosurgery and Psychiatry, 54*, 74–76.

Adams, R., and Victor, M. (1989). *Principles of neurology* (4th ed.). New York: McGraw-Hill.

Ansel, B. M., and Kent, R. D. (1992). Acoustic-phonetic contrasts and intelligibility in the dysarthria associated with mixed cerebral palsy. *Journal of Speech and Hearing Research, 35*, 296–308.

Basso, A. (1987). Approaches to neuropsychological rehabilitation: Language disorders. In M. Meier, A. L. Benton, and L. Diller (Eds.), *Neuropsychological rehabilitation* (pp. 294–314). New York: Guilford Press.

Basso, A., Capitani, E., and Moraschini, S. (1982). Sex differences in recovery from aphasia. *Cortex, 18*, 469–475.

Basso, A., Farabola, M., Grassi, M. P., Laiacona, M., and Zanobio, M. E. (1990). Aphasia in left-handers: Comparison of aphasia profiles and language recovery in non–right-handed and matched right-handed patients. *Brain and Language, 38*, 233–252.

Bates, E. (1979). *The emergence of symbols: Cognition and communication in infancy.* New York: Academic Press.

Bell, W. F., Davis, D. L., Morgan-Fisher, A., and Ross, E. D. (1990). Acquired aprosodia in children. *Journal of Child Neurology, 5*(1), 19–26.

Benson, D. F., and Arcadia, A. (1996). *Aphasia: A clinical perspective.* New York: Oxford University Press.

Bloom, L., and Lahey, M. (1970). *Language development and language disorders.* New York: John Wiley.

Blumstein, S., and Cooper, W. (1974). Hemispheric processing of intonation contours. *Cortex, 10*, 146–158.

Blumstein, S., and Goodglass, H. (1972). The perception of stress as a semantic cue in aphasia. *Journal of Speech and Hearing Research, 15*, 800–806.

Bolton, S. O., and Dashiell, S. E. (1984). *Interaction checklist for augmentative communication: An observational tool to assess interactive behaviors.* Idyllwild, CA: Imaginart Communication Products.

Borod, J. C. (1992). Interhemispheric and intrahemispheric control of emotion: A focus on unilateral brain damage. *Journal of Consulting and Clinical Psychiatry, 60*, 339–348.

Boss, B. J. (1984). Dysphasia, dyspraxia, and dysarthria: Distinguishing features: II. *Journal of Neurosurgical Nursing, 16*, 211–216.

Boss, B. J. (1991a). Cognitive systems: Nursing assessment and management in the critical care environment. *AACN Clinical Issues in Critical Care Nursing, 2*, 685–698.

Boss, B. J. (1991b). Managing communication disorders in stroke. *Nursing Clinics of North America, 26*, 985–996.

Boss, B. J. (1993). The neurophysiological basis of learning: Attention and memory. Implications for SCI nurses. *SCI Nursing, 10*(4), 121–129.

Boss, B. J. (1994a). Coma and cognitive deficits. In E. Barker (Ed.), *Neuroscience nursing practice* (pp. 175–202). St. Louis: Mosby–Year Book.

Boss, B. J. (1994b). The neurophysiological basis of learning, Part 2: Concept formation and abstraction, reasoning and executive functions. Implications for SCI nurses. *SCI Nursing, 1*(1), 3–6.

Boss, B. J., and Lewis-Abney, K. (1996). Communication: Language and pragmatics. In S. P. Hoeman (Ed.), *Rehabilitation nursing process and application* (pp. 542–571). St. Louis: Mosby.

Broca, P. (1863). Localisation des functions cérébrales. Siège du langage articulé. *Bulletins-Société Anthropologies (Paris), 4*, 200.

Broca, P. (1865). Sur la faculté du langage articulé. *Bulletins-Société Anthropologies (Paris), 6*, 337–393.

Cancelliere, A. E., and Kertesz, A. (1990). Lesion localization in acquired deficits of emotional expression and comprehension. *Brain and Cognition, 13*, 133–147.

Chapey, R. (1994). *Language intervention strategies in adult aphasia* (3rd ed.). Baltimore: Williams & Wilkins.

Code, C., and Muller, D. J. (1995). *The treatment of aphasia.* San Diego: Singular Publishing Group.

Critchley, M. (1970). *Aphasiology and other aspects of language.* London: Edward Arnold.

Danly, M., Cooper, W. E., and Shapiro, B. (1983). Fundamental frequency, language processing, and linguistic structure in Wernicke's aphasia. *Brain and Language, 19*, 1–24.

Danly, M., and Shapiro, B. (1982). Speech prosody in Broca's aphasia. *Brain and Language, 16*, 171–190.

Darley, F. L., Aronson, A. E., and Brown, J. R. (1969a). Clusters of deviant speech dimensions in the dysarthrias. *Journal of Speech and Hearing Research, 12*, 462–496.

Darley, F. L., Aronson, A. E., and Brown, J. R. (1969b). Differential diagnostic patterns of dysarthria. *Journal of Speech and Hearing Research, 12*, 246–269.

Demonet, J. F., Wise, R., and Frackowiak, R. S. J. (1993). Language function explored in normal subjects by positron emission tomography: A critical review. *Human Brain Mapping, 1*, 39–47.

Dent, C. H. (1990). An ecological approach to language development: An alternative functionalism. *Developmental Psychobiology, 23*, 679–703.

Duffy, J. R. (1995). *Speech disorders substrates, differential diagnoses and management.* St. Louis: Mosby.

Ehrlich, J., and Spies, A. (1985). Group treatment of communication skills for head trauma patients. *Cognitive Rehabilitation, 3*, 32–37.

Feldman, H. M., Holland, A. L., Kemp, S. S., and Janosky, J. E. (1992). Language development after unilateral brain injury. *Brain and Language, 42*, 89–102.

Gainotti, G., and Lemmo, M. (1976). Comprehension of symbolic gestures in aphasia. *Brain and Language, 3*, 451–460.

Goodglass, H. (1987). Neurolinguistic principles and aphasia therapy. In M. Meier, A. Benton, and L. Diller (Eds.), *Neuropsychological rehabilitation* (pp. 315–326). New York: Guilford Press.

Goodglass, H., and Kaplan, E. (1963). Disturbance of gesture and pantomime in aphasia. *Brain, 86*, 703–720.

Groher, M. (1977). Language and memory disorders following closed head trauma. *Journal of Speech and Hearing Research, 20*, 212–223.

Harkness, S. (1990). A cultural model for the acquisition of language: Implications for the innateness debate. *Developmental Psychobiology, 23*, 727–740.

Hedge, M. H. (1995). *Introduction to communicative disorders* (2nd ed.). Austin, TX: PRO-ED.

Heilman, K. M., Bowers, D., Speedie, L., and Cosletter, H. B. (1983). The comprehension of emotional and nonemotional prosody. *Neurology, 33*(Suppl. 2), 241.

Heilman, K. M., Scholes, R., and Watson, R. T. (1975). Auditory affective agnosia: Disturbed comprehension of affective speech. *Journal of Neurology, Neurosurgery and Psychiatry, 38*, 69–72.

Hill, B. P., and Singer, L. T. (1990). Speech and language development after infant tracheostomy. *Journal of Speech and Hearing Disorders, 55*, 15–20.

Holland, A. L. (1996). Pragmatic assessment and treatment for aphasia. In G. L. Wallace (Ed.), *Adult aphasia rehabilitation* (pp. 161–173). Boston: Butterworth-Heinemann.

Kent, J. F., Kent, R. D., Rosenbeck, J. C., Weismer, G., Martin, R., Sufit, R., and Brooks, B. R. (1992). Quantitative description of the dysarthria in women with amyotrophic lateral sclerosis. *Journal of Speech and Hearing Research, 35*, 723–733.

Kent, R. D., Sufit, R., Rosenbeck, J. C., Kent, J. F., Weismer, G., Martin, R. E., and Brooks, B. R. (1991). Speech deterioration in amyotrophic lateral sclerosis: A case study. *Journal of Speech and Hearing Research, 34*, 1269–1275.

Kirschner, H. S. (1995). *Handbook of neurological speech and language disorders*. New York: Marcel Dekker.

Klein, E. (1996). *Clinical phonology. Assessment and treatment of articulation disorders in children and adults*. San Diego: Singular Publishing Group.

Locke, J. L. (1992). Thirty years of research on developmental neurolinguistics. *Pediatric Neurology, 8*, 245–250.

Locke, J. L., and Pearson, D. M. (1990). Linguistic significance of babbling: Evidence from a tracheostomized infant. *Journal of Child Language, 17*, 1–16.

Luria, A. R. (1970). *Traumatic aphasia: Its syndromes, psychology and treatment*. Le Hague: Mouton.

Luria, A. R. (1973). *The working brain, an introduction to neuropsychology*. Harmondsworth: Penguin.

McCloskey, J. C., and Bulechek, G. M. (Eds.). (1996). *Nursing interventions classification (NIC)* (2nd ed.). St. Louis: Mosby–Year Book.

McNeil, M. R. (1997). *Clinical management of sensorimotor speech disorders*. New York: Thieme.

Metter, E. J. (1995). In H. S. Kirschner (Ed.), *Handbook of neurological speech and language disorders* (pp. 187–212). New York: Marcel Dekker.

Monrad-Krohn, G. H. (1947a). Dysprosody or altered "melody of language." *Brain, 70*, 405–415.

Monrad-Krohn, G. H. (1947b). The prosodic quality of speech and its disorders. *Acta Psychiatrica Neurologica, 22*, 255–269.

Monrad-Krohn, G. H. (1947c). Altered melody of language ("dysprosody") as an element of aphasia. *Acta Psychiatrica Neurologica, 46* (Suppl.), 204–212.

Murdock, B. E., Chenery, J. H., Strokes, P. D., and Hardcastle, W. J. (1991). Respiratory kinematics in speakers with cerebellar disease. *Journal of Speech and Hearing Research, 34*, 768–780.

Norman, B., and Baratz, R. (1979). Understanding aphasia. *American Journal of Nursing, 79*, 2135–2138.

Paul, R. (1995). *Language disorders from infancy through adolescence: Assessment and treatment*. St. Louis: Mosby.

Peterson, S. E., Fox, P. T., Posner, M. I., Mintun, M., and Raichle, M. E. (1988). Positron emission tomographic studies of cortical anatomy of single word processing. *Journal of Cognitive Neuroscience, 1*(2), 153–170.

Piotrowski, M. (1978). Aphasia: Providing better nursing care. *Nursing Clinics of North America, 13*, 543–554.

Posner, M. I., and Raichle, M. E. (1994). *Images of mind*. New York: Scientific American Library.

Ross, E. D. (1981). The aprosodias: Functional-anatomic organization of the affective components of language in the right hemisphere. *Archives of Neurology, 38*, 561–569.

Ross, E. D. (1985). Modulation of affect and nonverbal communication by the right hemisphere. In M-M. Mesulam (Ed.), *Principles of behavioral neurology* (pp. 239–257). Philadelphia: F. A. Davis.

Ross, E. D., Harney, J. H., deLaCoste-Utamsing, C., and Purdy, P. (1981). How the brain integrates affective and propositional language into a unified brain function. Hypothesis based on clinicoanatomic evidence. *Archives of Neurology, 38*, 745–748.

Ross, E. D., Holzapfel, D., and Freeman, F. (1983). Assessment of affective behavior in brain damaged patients using quantitative acoustical-phonetic and gestural measurements. *Neurology, 33*(Suppl. 2), 219–220.

Ross, E. D., and Mesulam, M-M. (1979). Dominant language functions of the right hemisphere? Prosody and emotional gesturing. *Archives of Neurology, 36*, 144–148.

Schuell, H., Jenkins, J. J., and Jimenez-Pabon, E. (1964). *Aphasia in adults—diagnosis, prognosis and treatment*. New York: Harper & Row.

Skinner, B. F. (1972). *Cumulative records: A selection of papers*. New York: Appleton-Century-Crofts.

Sohlberg, M. M., and Mateer, C. A. (1989). *Introduction to cognitive rehabilitation: Theory and practice*. New York: Guilford Press.

Tuchman, R. F., Rapin, I., and Shinnar, S. (1991). Autistic and dysphasic children. I: Clinical characteristics. *Pediatrics, 88*, 1211–1218.

Tucker, D. M., Watson, R. T., and Heilman, K. M. (1977). Discrimination and evocation of affectively intoned speech in patients with right parietal disease. *Neurology, 27*, 947–958.

Wallace, G. L. (1996). *Adult aphasia rehabilitation*. Boston: Butterworth-Heinemann.

Weinstein, D., and Keller, W. (1963). Linguistic patterns of misnaming in brain injury. *Neuropsychologia, 1*, 79–90.

Weintraub, S., Mesulam, M-M., and Kramer, L. (1981). Disturbances in prosody. *Archives of Neurology, 38*, 742–744.

Wexler, K. (1990). Innateness and maturation in linguistic development. *Developmental Psychobiology, 23*, 645–660.

White, P. F. (1996). *Take time to talk* (2nd ed.). Boston: Butterworth-Heinemann.

Wong, D. L. (1994). *Whaley and Wong's nursing care of infants and children* (5th ed.). St Louis: Mosby–Year Book.

Woods, B. T. (1995). Acquired childhood aphasias. In H. S. Kirschner (Ed.), *Handbook of neurological speech and language disorders* (pp. 415–430). New York: Marcel Dekker.

Zukow, P. G. (1990). Socio-perceptual bases for the emergence of language: An alternative to innatist approaches. *Developmental Psychobiology, 23*, 705–726.

Zuriff, E. B. (1974). Auditory lateralization: Prosodic and syntactical factors. *Brain and Language, 1*, 391–404.

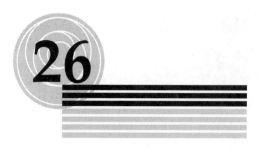

Genetic Counseling

Janet K. Williams and Debra L. Schutte

enetic Counseling has traditionally been provided to families of children with birth defects and genetic disorders. As genes for common chronic disorders are discovered, Genetic Counseling is becoming part of health care for individuals throughout the life span. Genetic Counseling is provided in primary care as well as specialty health care settings. When Genetic Counseling includes risk assessment and interpretation, it is provided by individuals with advanced education in genetics, including physicians, genetic counselors, social workers, and advanced practice nurses (APNs). The American Society of Human Genetics defines Genetic Counseling as a communication process that deals with the human problems associated with the occurrence, or the risk of occurrence, of a genetic disorder in a family (Ad Hoc Committee, 1975).

Genetic Counseling is an interactive helping process focusing on the identification and prioritization of strategies to promote a desirable outcome for an individual, family, or group manifesting or at risk for developing or transmitting a birth defect or genetic condition (Table 26–1). Professional nurses and APNs who are not genetic specialists incorporate aspects of Genetic Counseling into their practice when they assist individuals and families to learn about and cope with genetic information and to manage problems associated with genetic disorders. Knowledge of genetic principles and nursing concepts is essential for provision of Genetic Counseling interventions by nurses.

LITERATURE REVIEW

Genetics

The influence of inheritance on function and health has been recognized since early history. Present understanding of human genetics is based on Gregor

Table 26–1 Genetic Counseling

DEFINITION: Use of an interactive helping process focusing on the prevention of a genetic disorder or on the ability to cope with a family member who has a genetic disorder.

ACTIVITIES:

Establish a therapeutic relationship based on trust and respect

Provide privacy and ensure confidentiality

Discuss the purpose/goals of genetic counseling

Review life-style behaviors (e.g., use of alcohol, street drugs, and prescription medications) that place a fetus at risk, as appropriate

Review the genetic family history factors that place fetus at risk, as appropriate

Encourage appropriate diagnostic testing (e.g., DNA testing, amniocentesis, and chorionic villus sampling), which may predict the presence of a genetic disorder in patient or offspring

Discuss the advantages, risks, and costs of alternative diagnostic tests

Minimize any coercive action that could force the parents to intervene or to feel guilty because they choose not to act

Inform patient of specific treatments of genetic disorders, as appropriate (e.g., infant stimulation for children with Down syndrome and monitoring fever in sickle cell anemia)

Discuss the impact of the particular genetic disorder on the affected individual's general health status

Encourage expression of feelings

Monitor patients' response when they learn about own genetic risk factors

Assist patient to list and prioritize all possible alternatives to a problem

Institute crisis support skills with patient who is unable to determine a best course of action, such as in pregnancy termination

Assess family support for patient who undergoes a loss of a family member or pregnancy loss related to a genetic or birth defect condition

Support coping process in family members who are responsible for the ongoing care of an individual with a genetic disorder, such as Huntington disease

Provide referral to a member of a specialty genetic care team, as necessary

Provide referral to community resources, as needed

Source: McCloskey, J. C., and Bulechek, G. M. (1996). *Nursing interventions classification (NIC)* (p. 300). St. Louis: Mosby–Year Book.

Mendel's 1865 report of laws governing the transmission of units of heredity from parent to offspring (Mueller & Young, 1995). Approximately 40 years later, scientists suggested that units of heredity, later known as genes, are contained on chromosomes, which are threadlike structures in the cell nucleus. Renewed interest in Mendel's findings marked the beginning of the study of inherited diseases. In the 1950s, two achievements greatly enhanced scientists' understanding of disease inheritance. The first was the identification of the physical structure of deoxyribonucleic acid (DNA) by Watson and Crick, and the second was the correct specification of the 46 human chromosomes (Mueller & Young, 1995).

Hereditary information is transmitted from parent to offspring through DNA. However, all human diseases can be viewed as resulting from an interaction between a person's unique genetic makeup and the environment. In some diseases, the genetic component is so overwhelming that it expresses itself in a predictable manner. These diseases are termed genetic disorders (Goldstein & Brown, 1994). Some inherited disorders are due to the presence of an alteration in a gene, a sequence of DNA that directs the synthesis of a specific polypeptide chain. Research emerging from the Human Genome Project and other genetic research have identified mutations in specific genes for a number of single-gene inherited disorders, such as Huntington's disease (HD) and cystic fibrosis (CF). This project is a major international effort to map and sequence the entire human genome by the year 2005 as well as explore the ethical, legal, and social implications of human genome discoveries (Andrews, Fullarton, Holtzman, & Motulsky, 1994).

Understanding basic inheritance patterns and the implications of gene mutation discoveries underlies the professional nurse's ability to provide genetic counseling. When prepared with a background in genetics, the nurse may recognize the presence of a genetic disorder in an individual or a family when obtaining a comprehensive family health history. When several individuals in a family have the same condition, this may be due to one of the single-gene, or mendelian, patterns of inheritance (Table 26–2). In addition to recognizing the presence of an inherited disorder in a family, nurses can assist family members in understanding relationships between genes and the presence of an inherited disorder in themselves or other family members.

In addition to single-gene mutations and inheritance, genetic principles also include an understanding of chromosomes and the relationships between chromosome abnormalities and alterations in growth and development. Chromosomes are threadlike structures that contain numerous genes. People with chromosome disorders generally have alterations in growth and mental development and a higher incidence of congenital malformations (Thompson, McInnes, & Willard, 1991). Although many of these disorders are associated with a shortened life span, improvements in management have made it possible for some individuals with chromosome disorders to live into their adult years. In many cases, only one person with a chromosome disorder is found in a family. However, some chromosome rearrangements, known as translocations, can be passed on in families.

Another form of inheritance occurs when disease genes are found in the mitochondria, organelles in the cell cytoplasm involved in energy production. Disorders that affect both males and females but are passed through the mother

Table 26–2 Single-Gene Patterns of Inheritance

Autosomal Dominant (AD) Inheritance
  Usual recurrence risk—50%
  Disease phenotype seen in each generation
  Males and females equally likely to have condition
  Father-son transmission of disease gene is possible

Autosomal Recessive (AR) Inheritance
  Usual recurrence risk—25%
  Disease phenotype seen in siblings, but usually not in earlier generations
  Males and females equally likely to have condition
  Consanguinity sometimes seen, especially in rare disorders

X-Linked Recessive (XLR) Inheritance
  Sons have 50% risk to have gene and the disorder
  Daughters have 50% risk to have gene and be carriers
  Gene is passed from carrier mothers to offspring
  Gene is passed from males with the disorder to daughters, but not to sons

Source: Jorde, L., Carey, J., and White, R. (1995). *Medical genetics.* St. Louis: Mosby.

may be explained by the presence of disease genes in the mitochondria (Lewis, 1997).

In addition to conditions that have known patterns of inheritance, many traits are believed to be caused by a combination of numerous genes as well as by environmental factors. This is termed *multifactorial inheritance*. Examples of conditions with a multifactorial inheritance pattern include common congenital malformations as well as alcoholism, hypertension, and schizophrenia (Mueller & Young, 1995). Scientific understanding of genetic principles continues to evolve as new information emerges from genetic research. The challenge for nurses is to integrate new genetic knowledge into clinical practice in order to provide effective genetic services. Application of genetic counseling by nurses relies on maintenance of current knowledge of genetic principles.

Effectiveness of Genetic Counseling

Genetic Counseling is based on the identification and analysis of potential genetic risk factors in an individual, family, or group. The majority of clinical and research reports describing Genetic Counseling come from providers who offer Genetic Counseling to a specific population or in a specialty care setting. This literature provides some insight into the intervention and its effectiveness. However, variations in populations, methodology, and outcome measures limit generalizations.

KNOWLEDGE

Health teaching is a major component of Genetic Counseling. Examples of settings in which nurses provide information about genetic conditions include diagnostic and disease management programs such as those for phenylketonuria or sickle-cell disease. Oncology nurses may provide information to clients regarding genetic aspects of specific cancers in children and adults. Many studies of the effectiveness of Genetic Counseling include a measure of recall of information regarding risk of having a child with a genetic condition. For example, one of the early studies of individuals receiving Genetic Counseling in a general genetics clinic reported that only about half of the clients had a good understanding of the information received from Genetic Counseling (Leonard, Chase, & Childs, 1972). More recent studies of people receiving Genetic Counseling for CF carrier testing document a range of understanding of risk to have a child with CF from 46% to 89% (Clayton et al., 1995; Watson, Mayall, Lamb, Chapple, & Williamson, 1992).

Although recall of recurrence risk may appear relatively straightforward, numerous factors influence the ability of clients to understand and remember genetic information. These include the nature of the disorder, the client's reproductive intentions and familiarity with the condition, the length of time between the survey and when counseling was received, the counselor's style of presentation of information, the client's subjective perception of information, and the client's framework of existing ideas about health and disease (Hallowell & Richards, 1997; Michie, McDonald, & Marteau, 1997). Assessing recall of recurrence risks may not reflect important dimensions that influence understanding and reflect meaning of information to the Genetic Counseling client. In addition to how much information is retained, the interpretation of the information by the client and the client's evaluation of the information in light of his or her own expectations and interpretations are also important (Michie, McDonald, & Marteau, 1996).

Interactions between recall and time since receiving counseling and client education are factors that may also influence knowledge following Genetic Counseling. For example, 3 years after individuals had received Genetic Counseling as a part of CF carrier testing, 20% of carriers and more than 50% of those testing negative could not accurately recall their test results (Axworthy, Brock, Bobrow, & Marteau, 1996). Understanding of genetic information is also associated with the educational background of the client. Research groups pilot-testing carrier screening programs for CF in primary care settings report that knowledge of CF and carrier testing issues improved only for participants who had more than a high school education (Bernhardt et al., 1996; Clayton et al., 1995). Documentation of factors influencing understanding is important for nurses who incorporate genetic information in their nursing practice. Innovative strategies are needed to overcome obstacles limiting abilities of clients to understand and retain Genetic Counseling information.

DECISION MAKING AND HEALTH BEHAVIOR

Decision making is an integral component of Genetic Counseling when clients consider reproductive, diagnostic, and management options for genetic disorders. Decision making with regard to genetic information is especially difficult for many clients because of a lack of preparedness to consider new and different options for which no social guidelines exist (Shiloh, 1996). For example, the opportunity to have prenatal diagnosis or to learn whether one is a carrier of an inherited disease was not available to prior generations in the family. Many people are the first in their families to face such a decision. Many genetic-related decisions are based on probabilistic outcomes, and the desired outcome of a cure for or elimination of the disease is not an option in many situations. Relationships between Genetic Counseling, decision making, and health behavior are complex and poorly understood.

Decisions regarding reproduction have also been used as one measure of Genetic Counseling outcomes. However, reproductive decision making may be more strongly influenced by desire to have children than by perceived risk of a genetic condition (Marteau & Anionwu, 1995). Thus, attempts to link Genetic Counseling with reproductive decisions provide limited insight into relationships between Genetic Counseling, client variables, and subsequent reproductive behaviors.

Decisions regarding participation in predictive genetic testing programs are described in more recent studies. Predictive testing is possible when scientists have located or sequenced a gene for a disorder. Once a gene has been discovered, people who are at risk to have a mutation in the gene can have testing to identify whether the gene is present before the onset of symptoms of the disease. One example is genetic testing for the HD gene. Centers providing predictive testing for HD report that the proportion of clients entering these programs is smaller than what was expected from prior surveys to measure intent to use the test. Although initial studies of intention to participate in predictive HD testing reported a range of 32% to 65% of at-risk relatives indicating a desire for predictive testing, the proportion of people completing presymptomatic testing for HD is much smaller (Quaid, Brandt, Faden, & Folstein, 1989).

Other research describes factors that influence decisions to seek genetic testing. Desires to reduce uncertainty and to plan for the future are cited as reasons for having presymptomatic HD testing (Tibben, et al., 1993; Williams, Schutte, Forcucci, & Evers, 1997). Coping style and anxiety level are believed to influence decisions to seek genetic testing for familial cancers (Codori, 1997). Relationships of these variables to outcomes of genetic testing such as changes in health behaviors or psychological adjustment are as yet unknown.

PSYCHOLOGICAL WELL-BEING

Emotional well-being and psychological adjustment are of concern whenever individuals participate in Genetic Counseling. One body of knowledge describes coping with a diagnosis of mental retardation or a genetic disorder in one's child, characterized as chronic sorrow (Clubb, 1991; Olshanksky, 1962). Research describing the cyclic nature of this process and the differences in the process between mothers and fathers has increased understanding of this coping response (Damrosch & Perry, 1989; Wikler, Wasow, & Hatfield, 1981). The process of coping with a genetic condition is also described by nurse researchers who analyzed coping strategies used by school-age children and adolescents with CF and with hemophilia (Admi, 1995; Spitzer, 1992). Although not linked to Genetic Counseling interventions, these studies contribute to understanding of emotional responses to genetic information and provide data to guide implementation of emotional support aspects of the intervention.

More recent literature has included assessment of adjustment or coping in studies of individuals who participated in genetic testing programs to determine carrier status for the CF gene or in predictive testing programs for the HD gene. CF carrier testing programs have not reported adverse psychological consequences in individuals who participated in these programs. However, one 3-year follow-up study noted that some carriers (16%) reported feeling worried about their test results (Axworthy et al., 1996).

Programs providing predictive HD genetic testing include psychological assessments in their clinic protocols and program evaluations. A summary of studies of psychological effects of DNA testing for the HD gene notes that most tested individuals benefit psychologically from testing and feel relief from prior uncertainty. People with the HD gene who cope well have strong psychological defenses and satisfactory interpersonal relationships. Although most people who do not have the gene also have improved psychological functioning, a subgroup of gene-negative individuals experiences lack of relief, survivor guilt, and regret over prior decisions (Tibben, Timman, Bannink, & Duivenvoorden, 1997). Although the incidence of adverse events (e.g., psychiatric hospitalizations, depression, substance abuse, suicide) is small, these events have been documented in approximately 15% of individuals participating in the Canadian HD predictive program (Lawson et al., 1996). Data generated from clinical as well as formal research observations are needed to increase the body of knowledge regarding psychosocial aspects of genetic information and Genetic Counseling.

Nurse Providers of Genetic Counseling

Nurses' roles in Genetic Counseling have been identified in the nursing literature since the early 1960s. Initial descriptions focused on psychosocial support and case finding responsibilities of nurses in the community or in developmental disability programs (Forbes, 1966; Hillsman, 1966). The role of a clinical nurse specialist on a Genetic Counseling team was described by Fibison in 1983. This description formed the basis for subsequent distinction and delineation of the roles in Genetic Counseling of the nongenetic nurse and of the APN who specializes in Genetic Counseling.

These two levels of nursing practice have continued to be evident as genetic information has become part of nursing practice in a variety of settings. One of the most rapidly growing areas of nursing practice where Genetic Counseling is being provided by nurses is oncology nursing (MacDonald, 1997). Here, APNs in oncology are using genetic knowledge and Genetic Counseling as a part of their risk assessment and counseling practices. Genetic Counseling became a part of nursing's standardized language when it was included in the Nursing Interventions Classification (NIC) (McCloskey & Bulechek, 1992). Standards of genetics clinical nursing practice at the general and advanced practice levels are described by the International Society of Nurses in Genetics and the American Nurses Association (1998).

Genetic Counseling Intervention Protocols

The Genetic Counseling nursing intervention is composed of activities that are directed toward interactive discussions of genetic-related information and support of an individual's or family's coping abilities (see Table 26–1). Key components are described to illustrate the application of this intervention in nursing practice.

OBTAINING COMPREHENSIVE FAMILY HEALTH HISTORY

A core component of Genetic Counseling is reviewing a comprehensive family health history. A comprehensive family health history is used to identify individuals in the family who may be at risk to have an inherited condition or to pass a gene for the condition on to their children. Obtaining the history also offers the nurse the opportunity to observe family interactions and assess attitudes and understanding about a genetic disorder.

A comprehensive family health history includes the age and health status of children, parents, grandparents, and extended family members. The cause of death should be recorded for each deceased family member. The ethnic origins of family members should also be recorded, because some inherited conditions are more prevalent in specific ethnic groups. The family history should be recorded in a standardized format called a pedigree (Fig. 26–1) (Bennett et al., 1995).

Good interviewing skills are needed, and privacy and confidentiality of information obtained should be ensured. The process takes time, and the nurse will commonly speak with the individual or family on several occasions in order to complete the family history process. Information may not be known by younger family members, and family members may be reluctant to reveal information that is embarrassing to them. Genetic information is personal in nature, and people may be reluctant to reveal sensitive aspects of their family health history such as mental illness, mental retardation, pregnancy termination, or nonpaternity. A nonjudgmental approach with questions such as "Does your child or anyone in your family have a learning problem?" or "Is it possible that your partner is not the father of each of your children?" communicates respect for the individual and a desire to obtain accurate information (Williams, in press).

DISCUSSING DIAGNOSTIC TESTS

Genetic Counseling includes discussing advantages, risks, and costs of alternative diagnostic tests as well as minimizing any coercive actions that could force parents or other individuals to intervene or to feel guilty because they choose not to act. With the rapid pace of gene discoveries, many new genetic testing options, including DNA analysis, biochemical tests, and radiographs, are now available to people at any time during the life span. Genetic testing is currently

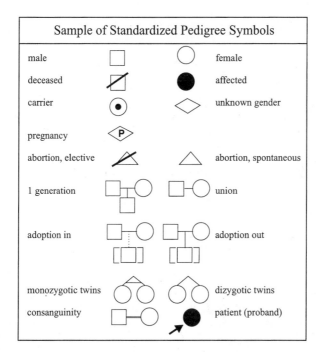

Sample of Standardized Pedigree Symbols

male □   ○ female

deceased   ● affected

carrier   ◇ unknown gender

pregnancy ⬦P

abortion, elective   △ abortion, spontaneous

1 generation   union

adoption in   adoption out

monozygotic twins   dizygotic twins

consanguinity   ● patient (proband)

Figure 26–1 Standardized pedigree symbols. (From Bennett, R., Steinhaus, K., Ulrich, S., Sullivan, C., Resta, R., Lochner-Doyle, D., Markel, D., Vincent, V., and Hamanish, J. [1995]. Recommendations for standardized human pedigree nomenclature. *American Journal of Human Genetics, 56*, 745–752, with permission of the University of Chicago Press.)

possible for the purposes of prenatal diagnosis of a fetus, diagnostic testing for an inherited condition in a child or adult, carrier detection of autosomal recessive or X-linked recessive genes, presymptomatic detection of autosomal dominant genes, and susceptibility testing of genes for familial disorders. All reveal information about the likelihood that a person has or will develop a genetic disorder. Although the estimated 50,000 to 80,000 genes in the human genome will likely be identified by the year 2003, understanding of potential adverse personal and social consequences of gene detection is developing at a much slower pace.

Genetic testing will be encountered by nurses in all areas of practice. One example is the opportunity for CF carrier testing during or before pregnancy. Elements of information that should be discussed with individuals and couples are the natural history of CF, its range of severity, survival rates, quality of life for the individual and the family, range of therapeutic options, and reproductive choices (Consensus Development Conference Statement, 1997).

Discussions of genetic screening and testing include additional components necessary to obtain informed consent (Table 26–3). Informed consent includes a discussion of potential risks and benefits of genetic testing. One risk is the potential for discrimination by employers or insurance providers. Loss of employment, rejection of applications for insurance, or increase in insurance rates are documented in case studies of people undergoing genetic testing for various conditions (Billings et al., 1992).

Genetic testing may also result in emotional distress, and some individuals experience difficulty communicating genetic information to family members who may benefit from it (Williams & Schutte, 1997). Genetic information is more personal than other medical information in that it divulges information about one's parents, siblings, and children; it can predict a person's likely medical future; and it has a history of being used to stigmatize and victimize individuals (Annas, 1995). Discussing potential benefits and risks as well as strategies to inform family members of test results is part of the nurse's intervention with

Table 26-3 Components of Informed Consent for Genetic Testing

Purpose of test
Nature of disorder
Reasons for participation
Benefits
Risks
Alternative procedures
Available interventions or treatment alternatives
Subsequent decisions that may be likely after receiving test results
Available counseling services
Disclosure to family members or third parties
Confidentiality standards
Rate of false-positive and false-negative results
Unexpected results

Source: Scanlon, C., and Fibison, W. (1995). *Managing genetic information: Implications for nursing practice.* Washington, DC: American Nurses Association.

clients considering genetic testing. Participation in the informed consent process requires that nurses be well informed regarding implications of genetic tests for the individual's well-being.

Genetic Counseling is rooted in a tradition of nondirective counseling. This is especially important when decisions regarding genetic testing or reproduction are being considered. Many situations in Genetic Counseling will raise ethical issues, and maintaining respect for persons and their autonomy is essential. When Genetic Counseling involves client education or a discussion of treatment options, a more directive approach is usually followed. Discussions of testing and treatment decisions may occur simultaneously and will require vigilance by the nurse to minimize any coercive actions by others with an interest in an individual's decisions.

ASSESSING FAMILY SUPPORT

Genetic conditions are a concern of the family, not only from a biological perspective, but also from a psychosocial perspective. Families share caregiving responsibilities for individuals with genetic conditions. For example, prompt recognition of early signs and symptoms of complications of sickle-cell disease by the family is an essential component of health maintenance for these children. In addition to knowledge of management of health problems, family members may desire counseling regarding the inheritance of this condition, family planning options, and support from organizations such as parent support groups (Selekman, 1993).

The family also is the transmitter of health information among its members. However, attitudes, family myths, and poor understanding of genetic inheritance may limit the ability of family members to share genetic information with each other. A study of women with a relative with hemophilia reported that the hereditary nature of hemophilia was never discussed in the parental home of approximately 20% of the women (Varekamp, Suurmeijer, Brocker-Vriends, & Rosendaal, 1992). Others report that decisions to have presymptomatic testing for HD may be made without discussions with or support from other family members (Williams et al., 1997). Awareness of knowledge, attitudes, and feelings of other family members is important when nurses provide Genetic Counseling activities to individuals and family members.

PROVIDING REFERRALS

Most people with genetic conditions need specific management and supportive services. Many genetic conditions are relatively rare, and locating providers with desired expertise may be difficult. Nurses who are knowledgeable about what services are available and how to access them can assist individuals in evaluating desired services. One example is the availability of health-related information on the Internet. However, clients may need assistance in assessing the quality of what they learn through this source.

Individuals may also wish to contact others with the same genetic disorder. This can occur through disease-specific organizations or through one-to-one contact. When the nurse arranges a contact, the selection of an experienced person or family is important; not all clients will be suitable. Individuals are most effective when they refrain from giving medical advice or from being judgmental about the newly diagnosed person's values or feelings. When a person with a genetic condition or his or her family indicates an interest in meeting others with this condition, the nurse should ensure that each person has given permission to share names and addresses with others (Williams, in press).

Some individuals want to contact disease-specific organizations. The Alliance of Genetic Support Groups (4301 Connecticut Avenue, NW, Suite 404, Washington, DC 20008) can provide information about specific groups or more general support organizations. Clients who have relatives with genetic conditions may need help in locating Genetic Counseling services. For example, some siblings of individuals with CF have not received genetic counseling and may have mistaken beliefs about their own carrier status (Fanos & Johnson, 1995). Likewise, spouses of individuals with genetic conditions may have received little information regarding the implications of the condition for their family or for their children's future health. Assessment of concerns of these family members and awareness of appropriate genetic service programs are important elements of the Genetic Counseling nursing intervention.

When nurses refer individuals to Genetic Counseling specialists for further assessment and counseling, explanation of the purpose of Genetic Counseling services is important. This can help individuals understand why they are being referred and what they can expect. People may be asked to bring medical records or family photographs of individuals with similar problems. Questions that the genetic specialist may answer include the following: What are the health implications of the disorder? What is the chance that it could occur in other family members? Can the disorder be detected prenatally, and what are the treatment options? (Williams, 1993).

POPULATIONS AND ASSOCIATED NURSING DIAGNOSES

Genetic Counseling may be indicated in a variety of situations. The most straightforward indication for Genetic Counseling is when a condition with a known or suspected genetic contribution is discovered. A more complete list of indications for Genetic Counseling includes the presence of a positive family history of a known or suspected genetic disorder, multifactorial disorder, progressive neurological disorder, mental retardation, or developmental delay. A personal or family history of multiple pregnancy loss is also appropriate for Genetic Counseling. Risk for inherited conditions, a nursing diagnosis under development, is based on these defining characteristics and related factors associated with genetic illness.

In addition, several existing North American Nursing Diagnosis Association (NANDA) (1996) diagnoses can be linked to the genetic counseling nursing intervention: Knowledge Deficit: disease process, Knowledge Deficit: health resources, Altered Growth and Development, Altered Family Processes, Decisional Conflict, and Social Isolation.

ASSOCIATED NURSING OUTCOMES

The identification of the desired outcomes of Genetic Counseling services is needed in order to evaluate their effectiveness. A nursing-sensitive outcome is defined as a measurable client or caregiver state, behavior, or perception that is influenced by and sensitive to nursing interventions (Johnson & Maas, 1997). Several Nursing Outcomes Classification (NOC) outcomes can be linked to the Genetic Counseling intervention. The use of NOC outcomes will enable standardized measurement of the effectiveness of Genetic Counseling in both practice and research. However, the ability to influence these outcomes will depend on the contributing factors and defining characteristics associated with the nursing diagnosis as well as the state of knowledge regarding the genetics of the associated disease process.

One outcome of Genetic Counseling, particularly explored in research, is enhanced knowledge. Specifically, client knowledge of the disease process can be monitored to determine the extent to which the client understands information conveyed about the disease, its pattern of inheritance, and the health implications for family members (Knowledge: Disease Process). Similarly, knowledge of health resources, including the plan for follow-up care and use of community resources, is particularly pertinent to the Genetic Counseling intervention (Knowledge: Health Resources).

Participation: Health Care Decisions is a nursing outcome central to the nondirective and participative nature of Genetic Counseling, defined as personal involvement in selecting and evaluating health care options. The essence of this outcome is the ability of the client to collaborate and negotiate with health care providers in determining and evaluating care options. Closely related to this outcome is Decision Making, which monitors the client's ability to actually choose between alternatives.

Individuals or families involved in Genetic Counseling, whether self- or provider-referred, are frequently concerned with their risk or another family member's risk of developing a disease or passing on a disease gene to offspring. The Risk Detection and Health Seeking Behavior outcomes may therefore be influenced by Genetic Counseling. The Risk Detection outcome monitors the client's ability to identify health threats, including family history and genetic background. The Health Seeking Behavior outcome monitors the client actions aimed at promoting wellness, recovery, and rehabilitation.

Several nursing-sensitive outcomes can be used to monitor the effectiveness of Genetic Counseling in meeting a client's psychosocial needs related to genetics and client health, such as Acceptance: Health Status, Anxiety Control, Coping, and Hope. Acceptance: Health Status concerns the client's ability to adjust to or reconcile his or her health circumstances. Relief from anxiety is frequently cited as an outcome of genetic testing in particular (Tibben et al., 1997; Williams & Schutte, 1997) and can be measured with the indicators of the Anxiety Control outcome. The Coping outcome monitors client actions directed at managing stressors. Finally, maintaining optimism and hope in the face of unexpected loss and uncertainty is an important outcome of Genetic Counseling that can be monitored through the indicators of the Hope outcome.

The nursing-sensitive outcomes described here provide an initial core set of concepts that can be influenced by the implementation of Genetic Counseling. It is likely that this list will expand as Genetic Counseling expands under the exponential growth of genetic knowledge and therapeutic options.

CASE STUDY

Jill is a 33-year-old woman who contacted her family nurse practitioner (FNP) following the diagnosis of her 32-year-old sister with unilateral breast cancer. Jill had read about breast cancer genes and genetic tests in the newspaper and expressed concern about her chances of developing breast cancer as well as the chances of her two young children. In addition to providing emotional support to Jill as she discussed her fears, the FNP obtained Jill's family health history, querying particularly about other family members with breast or ovarian cancer, age of onset, and whether the cancer was unilateral or bilateral (Fig. 26–2). Jill's mother and a maternal aunt had both been diagnosed with breast cancer in their late forties, both had unilateral disease, and both were still living following mastectomy. The FNP also determined Jill's current breast cancer screening practices. Jill stated she performed breast self-examinations periodically and had never had a mammogram. The FNP reviewed the breast self-examination technique with Jill as well as the current recommendations for mammograms. Given Jill's questions about genetic tests for breast cancer and her positive family history, the FNP discussed a referral to a regional Genet-

ics Counseling program so that Jill could obtain more detailed information about breast cancer genetics, the availability of genetic tests, the usefulness of genetic testing for Jill's family, and the potential risks and benefits of genetic tests. In addition, the FNP explored Jill's extended family dynamics and patterns of communication in anticipation of the genetic counselor's need to verify family member cancer diagnoses, requiring that Jill seek permission to obtain medical records from family members. Jill agreed to a genetics referral. Therefore, the FNP contacted the appropriate agency and with Jill's permission sent a copy of the family pedigree to the genetic specialist provider.

Shortly after the Genetic Counseling appointment, both Jill and her FNP received a summary letter from the genetics provider reviewing the information and options that were discussed at that meeting. At a follow-up appointment with the FNP, Jill reported that she had decided to obtain a baseline mammogram and continue with breast self-examination on a regular basis. In addition, she did not wish to pursue genetic testing for breast cancer genes at this time. During this discussion, the FNP explored Jill's understanding

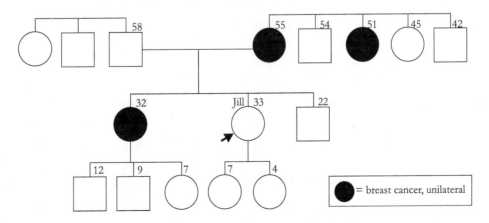

Figure 26–2   Case study of family pedigree.

of the information provided by the genetic specialists, provided emotional support, validated Jill's decisions, and facilitated Jill's chosen breast cancer surveillance strategies.

SUMMARY

Genetic information, once associated primarily with children and birth defects, is now pertinent across the life span as genetic research expands understanding of inheritance and its implications for health. Further research is needed to specify the outcomes associated with Genetic Counseling as well as the provider and client characteristics that maximize outcomes. However, skills in at least some aspects of the Genetic Counseling intervention will be increasingly necessary for nurses across all client populations and service settings.

References

Ad Hoc Committee on Genetic counseling of the American Society of Human Genetics. (1975). Genetic counseling. *American Journal of Human Genetics, 27*, 240–242.

Admi, H. (1995). Nothing to hide and nothing to advertise: Managing disease-related information. *Western Journal of Nursing Research, 17*(5), 484–501.

Andrews, L., Fullarton, J., Holtzman, N., and Motulsky, A. (1994). *Assessing genetic risks: Implications for health and social policy.* Washington, DC: National Academy Press.

Annas, G. (1995). Genetic prophecy and genetic privacy—Can we prevent the dream from becoming a nightmare? *American Journal of Public Health, 85*, 1196–1197.

Axworthy, D., Brock, D., Bobrow, M., and Marteau, T. (1996). Psychological impact of population-based carrier testing for cystic fibrosis: 3-year follow-up. *Lancet, 347*, 1443–1446.

Bennett, R., Steinhaus, K., Ulrich, S., Sullivan, C., Resta, R., Lochner-Doyle, D., Markel, D., Vincent, V., and Hamanish, J. (1995). Recommendations for standardized human pedigree nomenclature. *American Journal of Human Genetics, 56*, 745–752.

Bernhardt, B., Chase, G., Faden, R., Geller, G., Hofman, K., Tambor, E., and Holtzman, N. (1996). Educating patients about cystic fibrosis carrier screening in a primary care setting. *Archives of Family Medicine, 5*, 336–340.

Billings, P., Kohn, M., de Cuevas, M., Beckwith, J., Alper, J., and Natowicz, M. (1992). Discrimination as a consequence of genetic testing. *American Journal of Human Genetics, 50*, 476–482.

Clayton, E., Hannig, V., Pfotenhauer, J., Parker, R., Campbell, P., and Phillips, J. (1995). Teaching about cystic fibrosis carrier screening by using written and video information. *American Journal of Human Genetics, 57*, 171–181.

Clubb, R. (1991). Chronic sorrow: Adaptation patterns of parents with chronically ill children. *Pediatric Nursing, 17*, 461–466.

Codori, A., Slavney, P., Young, C., Miglioretti, D., and Brandt, J. (1997). Predictors of psychological adjustment to genetic testing for Huntington's disease. *Health Psychology, 16*(1), 36–50.

Consensus Development Conference Statement. (1997). *Genetic testing for cystic fibrosis.* Bethesda, MD: National Institutes of Health.

Damrosch, S., and Perry, L. (1989). Self-reported adjustment, chronic sorrow, and coping of parents of children with Down syndrome. *Nursing Research, 38*(1), 25–30.

Fanos, J., and Johnson, J. (1995). Perception of carrier status by cystic fibrosis siblings. *American Journal of Human Genetics, 57*, 431–438.

Fibison, W. (1983). The nursing role in the delivery of genetic services. *Issues in Health Care of Women, 4*, 1–15.

Forbes, N. (1966). The nurse and genetic counseling. *Nursing Clinics of North America, 1*, 679–688.

Goldstein J., and Brown, M. (1994). Genetic aspects of disease. In K. Isselbacher (Ed.), *Harrison's principles of internal medicine* (13th ed.). New York: McGraw-Hill.

Hallowell, N., and Richards, M. (1997). Understanding life's lottery. *Journal of Health Psychology, 2*(1), 31–43.

Hillsman, G. (1966). Genetics and the nurse. *Nursing Outlook, 14*, 34–39.

International Society of Nurses in Genetics and American Nurses Association. (1998). *Standards of genetics clinical practice.* Washington, DC: American Nurses Association.

Johnson, M., and Maas, M. (1997). *Nursing outcomes classification (NOC).* St. Louis: Mosby–Year Book.

Lawson, K., Wiggins, S., Green, T., Adam, S., Bloch, M., Hayden, M., & The Canadian Collaborative Study of Predictive Testing. (1996). Adverse psychological events occurring in the first year after predictive testing for Huntington's disease. *Journal of Medical Genetics, 33*, 856–862.

Leonard, C., Chase, G., and Childs, B. (1972). Genetic counseling: A consumers' view. *New England Journal of Medicine, 281*, 433–439.

Lewis, R. (1997). *Human genetics: Concepts and applications* (2nd ed.). Dubuque, IA: Wm. C. Brown.

MacDonald, D. (1997). The oncology nurse's role in cancer risk assessment and counseling. *Seminars in Oncology Nursing, 13*(2), 123–128.

Marteau, T., and Anionwu, E. (1995). Evaluating carrier testing: Objectives and outcomes. In T. Marteau and M. Richards (Eds.), *The troubled helix: Social and psychological implications of the new human genetics* (pp. 123–139). Cambridge, MA: Cambridge University Press.

Marteau, T., van Duijn, M., and Ellis, I. (1992). Effects of genetic screening on perceptions of health: A pilot study. *Journal of Medical Genetics, 29*, 24–26.

McCloskey, J., and Bulechek, G. (1992). *Nursing interventions classification (NIC)*. St. Louis: Mosby–Year Book.

Michie, S., McDonald, V., and Marteau, T. (1996). Understanding responses to predictive genetic testing: A grounded theory approach. *Psychology and Health, 11*, 455–470.

Michie, S., McDonald, V., and Marteau, T. (1997). Genetic counseling: Information given, recall and satisfaction. *Patient Education and Counseling, 32*(1–2), 101–106.

Mueller, R., and Young, I. (1995). *Emery's elements of medical genetics* (9th ed.). Edinburgh: Churchill Livingstone.

North American Nursing Diagnosis Association. (1996). *Nursing diagnoses: Definitions & classification 1997–1998*. Philadelphia: Author.

Olshansky, S. (1962). Chronic sorrow: A response to having a mentally defective child. *Social Casework, 43*, 190–193.

Quaid, K., Brandt, J., Faden, R., and Folstein, S. (1989). Knowledge, attitudes, and the decision to be tested for Huntington's disease. *Clinical Genetics, 36*, 431–438.

Selekman, J. (1993). Update: New guidelines for the treatment of infants with sickle cell disease. *Pediatric Nursing, 19*, 600–605.

Shiloh, S. (1996). Decision-making in the context of genetic risk. In T. Marteau and M. Richards (Eds.), *The troubled helix: Social and psychological implications of the new human genetics* (pp. 82–103). Cambridge, MA: Cambridge University Press.

Spitzer, A. (1992). Coping processes of school-age children with hemophilia. *Western Journal of Nursing Research, 14*(2), 157–169.

Thompson, M., McInnes, R., and Willard, H. (1991). *Genetics in medicine* (5th ed.). Philadelphia: W.B. Saunders.

Tibben, A., Frets, P., van de Kamp, J., Niermeijer, M., Vegter-van der Vlis, M., Roos, R., van Ommen, G., Duivenvoorden, H., and Verhage, F. (1993). Presymptomatic DNA-testing for Huntington disease; pretest attitudes and expectations of applicants and their partners in the Dutch program. *American Journal of Medical Genetics, 48*, 10–16.

Tibben, A., Timman, R., Bannink, E., and Duivenvoorden, H. (1997). Three-year follow-up after presymptomatic testing for Huntington's disease in tested individuals and partners. *Health Psychology, 16*(1), 20–35.

Varekamp, I., Suurmeijer, T., Brocker-Vriends, A., and Rosendaal, F. (1992). Hemophilia and the use of genetic counseling and carrier testing within family networks. In G. Evers-Kiebooms, J. Fryns, J. Cassiman, and H. Van den Berghe (Eds.), *Psychosocial aspects of genetic counseling. March of Dimes birth defects: Original article series, 28*(1) (pp. 139–148). New York: Wiley-Liss.

Watson, E., Mayall, E., Lamb, J., Chapple, J., and Williamson, R. (1992). Psychological and social consequences of community carrier screening programme for cystic fibrosis. *Lancet, 340*, 217–220.

Wikler, L., Wasow, M., and Hatfield, E. (1981). Chronic sorrow revisited: Parent vs. professional depiction of the adjustment of parents of mentally retarded children. *American Journal of Orthopsychiatry, 51*, 63–70.

Williams, J. (in press). Genetic counseling. In M. Craft-Rosenberg and J. Denehy (Eds.). *Nursing interventions for childbearing and childrearing families*. St. Louis Mosby-Year Book.

Williams, J. (1993). New genetic discoveries increase counseling opportunities. *American Journal of Maternal/Child Nursing, 18*(4), 218–222.

Williams, J., and Schutte, D. (1997). Benefits and burdens of genetic carrier information. *Western Journal of Nursing Research, 19*(1), 71–81.

Williams, J., Schutte, D., Forcucci, C., and Evers, C. (in press). *Decision making in adults seeking presymptomatic testing for Huntington disease*. Image: Journal of Nursing Scholarship.

Smoking Cessation Assistance

Kathleen A. O'Connell and Constance A. Koerin

Despite the scientific consensus and increased public awareness about the hazards of smoking to the health of smokers and those around them, 25% of the U.S. adult population continues to smoke. Rates among some low-income groups are as high as 34% (Centers for Disease Control and Prevention [CDC], 1996). In recent years, both the public health community and professional nurses have taken more active approaches to promoting smoking cessation and prevention. In 1996, new clinical practice guidelines for smoking cessation were widely disseminated (U.S. Department of Health and Human Services [USDHHS], 1996). Legal action by individuals and state agencies against tobacco companies and increasing indications that the U.S. Food and Drug Administration (FDA) will have more regulatory control over tobacco products are additional signs of the increased importance of smoking cessation to public health.

More than 46 million people in the United States have succeeded in quitting smoking (CDC, 1996). However, there is evidence that the decline in smoking rates among adults in the United States has reached a plateau. It may be that those who could easily quit smoking have already done so and that the adult smokers who remain are the "hard-core" smokers. Given its major health consequences, smoking itself has been called a chronic disease. Progress in smoking cessation treatment demands continuous assessment and monitoring by health care providers; smoking cessation requires a variety of behavioral and pharmacological interventions, and it is subject to frequent relapse.

Nursing interventions for smoking cessation are promising for several reasons. First, nurses are frequently in contact with groups most in need of help: those suffering from smoking-related diseases, pregnant women, and those in lower-income groups. Moreover, nurses in primary care and community health settings often follow up clients for much longer periods of time than do traditional smoking cessation counselors. This familiarity may make it possible to identify appropriate techniques and to help clients through several cessation attempts. In addition, nurses can use their expertise in pharmacology to give clients relevant information on the indications and contraindications for nicotine replacement and other drug therapies for smoking cessation.

The intervention described here is designed to help individual clients stop, rather than reduce, smoking. Abstinence is the generally accepted goal of smoking control programs, because approaches aimed at smoking reduction have not been shown to reduce disease risk. However, Hughes (1996) has suggested that increased restrictions on smoking and the continuation of a group of hard-core smokers will produce renewed interest in harm-reduction approaches, which allow for reduced nicotine use or alternative delivery systems to moderate the risk to those who are unable or unwilling to quit smoking altogether. The intervention described here is consistent with the Clinical Practice Guideline on smoking cessation (USDHHS, 1996).

RELATED LITERATURE

The nursing literature has shown increasing attention to the role of nurses in smoking cessation (Furlow & O'Quinn, 1996), and nurses have been involved in conducting intervention studies for smoking cessation among hospitalized patients (Miller, Smith, DeBusk, Sobel, & Taylor, 1997; Wewers, Bowen, Stanislaw, & Desimone, 1994) and minority populations (Ahijevych & Wewers, 1995). In addition, intervention studies abound in the psychological, medical, and pharmacological literature. Schwartz (1987) reviewed 416 intervention studies conducted between 1959 and 1985. Success rates appear low across all interventions (33% abstinence at 12 months is the best that can be expected, with much lower rates generally prevailing). Studies of interventions similar to the one described here are frequently termed *minimal interventions*. These studies are undertaken in outpatient facilities and involve physician's advice to quit smoking during a regularly scheduled office visit. This intervention may also include take-home reading materials for the clients and follow-up inquiry by the physician at subsequent appointments. Controlled studies indicate that such minimal interventions consisting of only advice by a physician yield about a 10.2% success rate at 6-month follow-up (USDHHS, 1996). When the advice is supplemented by problem solving and skill training, success rates increase to 13.7%. The use of social support increases success rates to about 15% (USDHHS, 1996). A study of a minimal intervention that involved both nurses and physicians in outpatient settings demonstrated a 6-month success rate of 15% when patients received advice from both physician and nurse and a 25% success rate when patients received advice and a self-quit manual (Janz et al., 1987). A meta-analysis on studies of the efficacy of nicotine replacement therapies showed 12-month success rates of about 18% for nicotine gum and 20.5% for the patch (Silagy, Mant, Fowler, & Lodge, 1994). Although these interventions have low success rates, when they are applied to large numbers of clients, they yield significant gains across the population. In addition, clients who fail can learn valuable information that may help them succeed on a subsequent attempt.

THE INTERVENTION

Table 27–1 lists the definition and activities involved in Smoking Cessation Assistance. The intervention described here is designed to be carried out by

Table 27–1 Smoking Cessation Assistance

DEFINITION: Helping a client to stop smoking.

ACTIVITIES:

Contact national and local resource organizations for resource materials

Record current smoking status and smoking history

Give smoker clear, consistent advice to quit smoking

Help choose best method for giving up cigarettes, when patient is ready to quit

Refer to group programs or individual therapists as appropriate

Assist patient with any self-help methods

Help patient plan specific coping strategies

Manage nicotine replacement therapy

Follow patient for 2 yr after quitting if possible, to provide encouragement

Help patient deal with any lapses

Support patient who begins smoking again by helping to identify what has been learned

Encourage relapsed patient to try again

Source: McCloskey, J. C., and Bulechek, G. M. (Eds.). (1996). *Nursing interventions classification (NIC)* (2nd ed.). St. Louis: Mosby–Year Book.

nurses who are practicing in outpatient clinics or community health settings where they have the opportunity to interact with clients directly over several weeks or months. Nurses interested in conducting smoking cessation interventions with hospitalized patients might consult articles by Wewers et al. (1994) or Miller et al. (1997).

Like many other health promotion activities, smoking cessation is largely a self-directed process. The nurse can encourage and inform, but the client ultimately decides whether to undertake smoking cessation. The type of encouragement and assistance offered should depend on the client's stage of change (Prochaska, 1996). Prochaska, DiClemente, and Norcross (1992) have identified five stages of self-change: precontemplation (unmotivated to quit smoking), contemplation (considering quitting in the next 6 months), preparation (intending to quit in the next 30 days), action (the first 6 months of quitting), and maintenance. Individuals sometimes get stuck in the contemplation stage, never proceeding to preparation or action. It is usually necessary to go through the entire cycle numerous times before maintenance is achieved.

Gather Resources

The first step is to prepare the practice setting by contacting national and local resource organizations to find out how they can help you. A variety of resources can be found on the World Wide Web. For instance, the Nursing Center for Tobacco Intervention (www.con.ohio-state.edu/tobacco/) is a Web site developed by nurse researchers Mary Ellen Wewers and Karen L. Ahijevych. The American Cancer Society (ACS) has sponsored a program called Tobacco-Free Young America, which enlists the aid of health care providers, including nurses. ACS provides a kit containing suggestions for methods that practitioners can use with their clients. ACS has also produced numerous written materials, booklets, and audiovisuals. The American Lung Association (ALA) has an excellent manual called *Freedom from Smoking* (1996), which can be given to smokers who are ready to quit, and the federal Office of Smoking and Health has a variety of materials. These and other organizations are constantly updating their selections. Some of the material is directed at specific client populations (pregnant women, Hispanic persons, teenagers). Community resources for quitting smoking might include smoking cessation referral services, group programs, and individual counseling.

Record Smoking Status and Smoking History

The next step is to set up a system to record the smoking status of all clients. The client records should contain a special section to record specific techniques tried and the outcomes of these. The section should include the smoking history information collected in the questionnaire discussed later. Assessments of smoking history and of quitting history are useful to guide smoking cessation. Questions can be administered by interview or questionnaire and should include the following:

1. How many cigarettes do you currently smoke per day?

2. How long have you been smoking regularly?

3. What brand and type of cigarette do you smoke? Filters? Menthol? Nicotine level? Tar level?

4. Do you use tobacco other than cigarettes (cigars, pipes, smokeless tobacco)?

5. How many times have you tried to quit smoking?

6. If you have tried to quit, what was the longest time you went without a cigarette?

7. How long ago was your most recent attempt to quit?

8. During that attempt, what kinds of problems did you have?

9. How many smokers do you live with? Work with?

10. How many of your friends are smokers?

11. How soon after awakening do you smoke your first cigarette of the day?

12. Have you ever tried nicotine replacement (gum, patch, spray, inhaler)? If so, what were your experiences with it?

Intercurrent and postintervention assessments are also necessary in order to determine how the clients are progressing. Such assessments should use interviews or questionnaires to determine self-reported cessation. The questions should include the following:

1. Have you smoked any tobacco at all, even a puff, since you quit smoking?

2. If so, when was the first time you smoked, and what were the circumstances?

3. How many cigarettes did you smoke at that time?

4. When was the next time you smoked?

5. How many cigarettes a day are you smoking now?

In addition to self-reported cessation, it is necessary to obtain an objective measure of smoking cessation. Numerous studies have shown that persons trying to quit smoking tend to underreport their smoking behavior. Objective indicators of cessation include expired air carbon monoxide levels and salivary, serum, or urinary cotinine (a metabolite of nicotine) levels. Expired air carbon monoxide levels can be determined with a portable instrument that costs $1,200 to $1,500. Nonsmoker values are usually less than 8 to 10 parts per million. Being outdoors in traffic, faulty car exhaust systems, and faulty furnace systems can raise carbon monoxide levels and may be responsible for some false positives. Salivary and serum cotinine levels are more expensive to measure but are also more specific indicators of smoking behavior. These assays are not easily performed, however, and usually require professional laboratory services. More economical urine dipstick methods of assessing nicotine and cotinine levels in practice settings are available (e.g., NicCheck I test kits from DynaGen, Inc., Cambridge, MA). However, if the client is using nicotine replacement therapy, cotinine levels are not a useful indicator of smoking cessation.

The nurse should institute plans to identify smokers in his or her caseload by asking all clients directly about their smoking history. Clients who have ever smoked should complete a smoking history questionnaire. Charts of those who have been abstinent for more than 2 years can be flagged with "Successful Ex-Smoker" stickers. "Recent Ex-Smoker" stickers should be used for those who have abstained for less than 2 years, and "Smoker" stickers should be used for those who are currently smoking (at any level). Recent ex-smokers should be given continued attention and encouragement. Records on successful ex-smokers and nonsmokers should be updated periodically in case their status changes.

Give Clear Advice to Quit Smoking

Current smokers must be given clear advice to quit smoking. Reviewing the client's smoking history, quitting history, and current smoking behavior is a good way to begin the interchange. Relating smoking to the client's current health problems or concerns is often effective in personalizing the message. In addition, the nurse needs to continue to demonstrate interest and concern about the client's smoking status at subsequent visits. It is common to hear smokers say that a health care provider told them to quit once (perhaps when they had a respiratory infection) but that the provider had not brought up the subject since. The health care provider might have concluded that advising the client to quit was useless, while the client simultaneously thought that the health care provider was not serious because the topic was mentioned only once. Continued interest provides a message to the client that smoking remains a concern.

Clients in the precontemplation phase are those who do not appear interested in quitting at present. They might be given a pamphlet about the benefits of quitting but should not be berated for smoking. Most smokers are aware of the general health effects of smoking. Many feel guilty or out of control where smoking is concerned. Others may behave defiantly in response to a nurse's concerns. Clients in the contemplation stage may be more amenable to discussing cessation. Exploring these clients' experiences with smoking and with trying to quit may help to illuminate specific concerns or problems. Let the client know that help is available when he or she is ready to quit smoking.

Help Choose the Best Method for Quitting

When the client has decided to quit smoking, the nurse can help him or her choose the best method for doing so. Such methods include group programs, individual therapy, and self-quit programs. Nicotine replacement therapy can usually be an adjunct to any of these and is highly recommended in the Clinical Practice Guideline on smoking cessation (USDHHS, 1996). However, the cost of nicotine replacement limits its practicality for many smokers.

Refer Clients to Group Programs or Individual Therapists

The ACS, the ALA, and many hospitals and health care agencies sponsor group programs. Group programs offer social support and structure to clients. Nurses interested in running group programs can take advantage of special training sessions offered by these organizations. However, group programs may be inappropriate for some clients. Clients with adequate resources may prefer individual therapy with a hypnotist, counselor, or behavioral therapist.

Assist Client with Self-Help Methods

Research indicates that most smokers prefer a self-quit method. Self-help materials are available from several sources. If the client wishes to embark on an individual self-help program, the nurse can facilitate the program by doing some or all of the following, depending on the client's needs and the nurse's availability.

1. Suggest or provide written self-help materials.

2. Offer to review the self-help materials with the client to identify specific aspects of the program with which the client may need help.

3. Help the client select a specific Quit Day and sign a "contract" stating that he or she will stop smoking on that day. The contract could include the nurse's promise to call the client on Quit Day (or the day before).

Help Plan Specific Coping Strategies

A coping strategy is a behavior or cognition that is helpful in preventing smoking behavior or in ameliorating, resisting, or preventing the urge to smoke. The best predictor of resisting the urge to smoke during a highly tempting situation is the enactment of either a behavioral or a cognitive coping strategy during the situation (Shiffman, Paty, Gnys, Kassel, & Hickcox, 1996). Types of coping strategies include anticipatory, immediate, and restorative (Shiffman, 1988). Anticipatory strategies are carried out before an actual urge and are used to prevent an urge or to prevent access to cigarettes. They include stimulus control strategies such as getting rid of cigarettes and ashtrays, as well as avoidance strategies such as sitting in the nonsmoking sections of restaurants. Immediate strategies are used in the presence of an urge and include distraction and substitution strategies and reminders of the reasons for quitting. Restorative strategies are those carried out after a lapse (a smoking occasion). They include getting rid of cigarettes and renewed commitment to refrain from smoking.

The nurse can also help the client identify sources of social support, plan specific coping strategies for a variety of situations in which abstinence may be threatened, and make a list of rewards for not smoking. Follow-up appointments at regular intervals to discuss progress and problems may be indicated. The exact nature of the nurse's involvement should depend on the needs of the client and on the setting where services are provided.

Manage Nicotine Replacement and Other Pharmacological Treatments

Several pharmacological therapies are available to assist with smoking cessation. These include nicotine replacement therapy and antidepressant medications. The recommendations in this section are based on the Clinical Practice Guideline on smoking cessation (USDHHS, 1996). However, new pharmacological therapies or therapy combinations may ultimately replace these formulations, and the nurse should keep informed about developments in this area.

Nicotine replacement therapy has been shown to increase the chances of successful quitting, especially when combined with behavioral counseling. The nicotine patch and gum delivery systems are available without prescription. Nicotine nasal spray (Hjalmarson, Franzon, Westin, & Wiklund, 1994) and inhalers (Schneider et al., 1996) have also been approved for use by the FDA.

Although both nicotine gum and the nicotine patch are effective, nicotine patch therapy is preferable to nicotine gum for most clients. Use of the patch is associated with fewer compliance problems, and it requires less time to train the client to use it effectively. The nicotine patch is marketed under several trade names. Recommended duration of treatment may vary from 8 to 10 weeks, and dosage per patch ranges from 21 mg/24 hr to 7 mg/24 hr. For specific usage, the package insert should be consulted.

The client should be cautioned not to smoke while using the nicotine patch. Instruct the client to remove the previous patch daily and to place a new patch in a relatively hairless area between the neck and waist. The most often reported side effect of nicotine patch use is a local skin reaction. These reactions are usually mild and self-limiting but may worsen over the course of therapy. Up to 50% of patients using the nicotine patch will have a local skin reaction, but discontinuation of nicotine patch treatment due to skin reaction occurs in less than 5% of clients. It is recommended that the patch site be rotated daily to minimize skin irritation.

Another reported side effect of patch usage in some clients is vivid, sometimes disturbing dreams due to continued nicotine intake during sleep. For this reason, the client may want to remove the patch at bedtime (16-hour use is recommended by one pharmaceutical manufacturer). The nurse should caution clients that their early morning withdrawal symptoms may be increased, in this case, until sufficient nicotine has been absorbed from the new patch.

Nicotine gum may be used based on client preference, previous failure with the nicotine patch, or problems with specific contraindications to the use of the patch (e.g., severe skin reactions). The gum is available in 2 mg and 4 mg (per piece) dosages. Often, clients do not use the nicotine gum frequently enough in the early stages of cessation to get the most benefit. In order to be effective in allaying withdrawal symptoms and smoking urges, at least 12 to 15 pieces of the gum (2 mg dose) should be chewed daily for the initial 1 to 3 months. Gum use should not exceed 30 pieces daily for the 2 mg dose (or 20 pieces daily for the 4 mg) and should be tapered off 3 to 6 months after cessation.

The nicotine in the gum must be absorbed through the oral mucous membranes and should be chewed slowly and intermittently over a 30-minute period. Correct technique involves chewing slowly until the client notices the peppery taste and tingling in the mouth. At that point, the client should hold or "park" the gum between the cheek and gums until the taste disappears and then resume this chewing cycle intermittently for 30 minutes. The client should avoid eating and drinking anything except water for 15 minutes before and after use of the gum. As mentioned with the patch, the client must be cautioned not to smoke while using nicotine gum. Persons with dental work who have trouble with regular gum may have difficulty with nicotine gum. Common side effects of nicotine gum include nausea, mouth soreness, hiccups, heartburn, sore throat, and jaw ache. These effects are usually mild and can often be relieved by correcting the client's chewing technique.

The nurse should consider individualizing treatment to fit the needs of the client. For light smokers (smoking 10 to 15 cigarettes per day or fewer), the starting dose of the nicotine patch or gum may be decreased. For clients who are highly dependent on nicotine (smoking more than 20 cigarettes per day and smoking within 30 minutes of awakening), the duration of use of higher patch doses may need to be adjusted. For those using nicotine gum, the 4 mg initial dose may be more appropriate.

When considering any nicotine replacement therapy, precautions should be taken with pregnant and lactating women. Clients in this group should first be encouraged to attempt cessation without nicotine replacement. The use of the patch or gum should be considered only if the increased likelihood of smoking cessation with its potential benefits outweighs the risk of nicotine replacement.

In clients with cardiovascular disease, nicotine replacement therapy should be used only after consideration of risks and benefits in particular groups. Therapy is particularly contraindicated in those in the immediate (within 4 weeks) post–myocardial infarction period, those with serious arrhythmias, and those with severe or worsening angina pectoris.

Most clients who choose to use nicotine replacement therapy report that it helps with their withdrawal symptoms but does not entirely eliminate craving for cigarettes. Clients often expect nicotine replacement therapy to be a "cure" for smoking. The nurse should stress that nicotine replacement therapy is a temporary aid in developing the habit of being a nonsmoker and that it must be supplemented with other coping strategies.

Evidence suggests that smoking is related to depressive symptoms and that cessation may initiate or exacerbate these symptoms (Anda et al., 1990). Antidepressants, especially those acting on dopamine pathways (e.g., Zyban), have been found to be useful in smoking cessation. Clients who have had problems with depression or negative affect in prior cessation attempts may benefit from the use of some types of antidepressant.

Follow Client for 2 Years after Quitting

The experience of smoking cessation changes as abstinence proceeds. Paul, one of the subjects in a study of smoking cessation (Cook, 1990), described the experience at several different points in the cessation process. "The first 3 weeks were kind of a steady level of discomfort that you could ignore, with sharp peaks of an alarm, your brain telling you to get that nicotine back into your system." During the fourth week, Paul reported, "The alarms have been going off a lot more frequently, but they are different. In the beginning, the urges were like a crushing weight that took minutes to go away. Now it's just quick little jabs in the chest." Eight weeks after cessation, Paul reported having "2 or 3 million desires to smoke"—mostly when seeing another person smoking. "Now," he said, "they are like cap gun explosions as you go through a day and they don't seem to be as severe as they were." Six months after cessation, Paul reported that his urges were not as strong as they used to be. "They're still somewhat frequent," he reported, "but certainly easier to ignore."

Reviewing the client's most tempting situations and assessing the frequency and strength of urges to smoke are excellent methods of determining the types of problems the client is currently having with the cessation attempt. It is important to congratulate the client for coping successfully and to help the client identify those circumstances that remain problematic or that might pose problems in the future, such as an upcoming deadline or a big party. The nurse should continue to follow up the client for at least 2 years, congratulating and encouraging at each visit. Many ex-smokers complain that they never get enough credit for quitting. While they are still struggling, their nonsmoking friends forget that they might still need encouragement. Follow-up should also include verifying abstinence with testing of carbon monoxide or urinary cotinine levels or other objective measures.

Help Client Deal with Any Lapses

A lapse is defined as a single smoking occasion after which abstinence is resumed. Several studies have shown that temptations to resume smoking often occur in negative affect situations, including situations involving anger, frustration, and feelings of deprivation (Cummings, Gordon, & Marlatt, 1980; O'Connell, Gerkovich, & Cook, 1995; O'Connell & Martin, 1987; Shiffman, 1982). Other research using concepts from the theory of psychological reversals shows that lapses in abstinence are also likely to occur when the ex-smoker is in a paratelic state (playful, sensation-oriented, and preferring high arousal levels) rather than a telic state (serious-minded, goal-oriented, preferring low arousal) (O'Connell, Cook, Gerkovich, Potocky, & Swan, 1990). Unfortunately, a single lapse after cessation is highly predictive of relapse. Several studies (Brandon, Tiffany, & Baker, 1986; O'Connell & Martin, 1987) indicate that 90% of those who smoke a single cigarette within the first 3 months of cessation will return to regular smoking within the year. The reasons for this are unclear. Marlatt and Gordon (1980) posited the abstinence violation effect, which occurs when an individual attributes a lapse to uncontrollable personal weakness. This attribution leads the individual to resume smoking. On the other hand, a single lapse might reinitiate withdrawal symptoms, which the individual may not be accustomed to dealing with, or the lapse might convince the ex-smoker that he or she can have a cigarette "now and then." An example from a study of highly tempting situations (Cook, 1990) illustrates the subject's experiences early in the cessation process.

Home alone 2 days after she quit smoking, Eileen was cleaning her family room when she found a cigarette left by her husband, who was a smoker. Apparently, it had fallen out of his pocket or pack and was lying on the sofa. Eileen recalled the incident: "When I saw it, then the hunger for a cigarette just got overwhelming at that point. I felt like there was no way I couldn't smoke it. I should have picked it up and run to the bathroom and thrown it into the [toilet] but I couldn't let myself do that, it was just a real addiction, a real need to smoke that cigarette. I don't think I would have smoked a cigarette if it hadn't just been there. It was just there. It was like being on a diet, walking into a room and a chocolate chip cookie is lying there, I mean, you know, you just can't resist. At the time, I didn't do anything I had been taught to do [to resist smoking]. As far as deep breathing or take time out, move from the situation, all that. It was just a total reaction of 'I've got to smoke this cigarette.'"

This example illustrates the importance (and the difficulty) of eliminating cigarettes from the environment, especially early in the cessation process. A cigarette is a strong stimulus to smoke, especially if there is no one else around to observe the behavior. The example also illustrates the role of strategies in preventing lapses. Eileen admitted that she used no strategies to resist smoking.

A client's report that he or she has lapsed (smoked, but resumed abstinence) or is smoking occasionally is considered a warning sign of impending relapse but also a sign that the client is still exercising considerable control over smoking. The initial lapse situation can be explored with the client to determine what factors contributed to the lapse. The client can be advised to institute (or reinstitute) rigorous stimulus control procedures, including disposing of all cigarettes and avoiding places where people are smoking or where cigarettes are available. The client should be informed that the lapses and occasional smoking tend to increase withdrawal symptoms and might make it harder to resist smoking. Other strategies for dealing with lapses include initiating or stepping up nicotine replacement therapy and helping the client find different ways of remembering to use strategies. Clients who have lapsed need support in understanding that the lapse is not a "sign" that the client is meant to return to smoking. Help the client review his or her reasons for quitting and the benefits. In addition, techniques that treat some of the nursing diagnoses caused by smoking cessation might be instituted. Any smoking during a cessation attempt is cause for concern, and the nurse should explain this to the client while being careful not to overreact to admissions of smoking, because such reactions may influence the client's tendency to give an accurate account of his or her smoking in the future.

Support the Client Who Begins Smoking Again

The relapse phase of the cessation process typically begins with a lapse. Thereafter, the individual engages in a period of struggle during which occasional smoking alternates with complete abstinence. Gradually, the smoking becomes more frequent, until regular smoking is resumed. Most lapses occur during the first 2 weeks after cessation, but the later phases of cessation also present problems. The nurse should be supportive, conveying that he or she knows how difficult it is to stop smoking and exploring with clients what they may have learned about themselves or about smoking during the attempt.

Encourage the Relapsed Client to Try Again

Dealing with the patient who has relapsed after attempting to quit smoking under the advice of his or her health care provider can be a difficult encounter. Both client and nurse may feel embarrassed about the failure. The client's self-efficacy for quitting and the nurse's self-efficacy for intervening may both be low. Nevertheless, the nurse should encourage the client to try again and remind both himself or herself and the client that most people who succeed at quitting must try numerous times before they succeed. The nurse may also consider suggesting alternative approaches: group support for the person who has tried self-quitting, or nicotine replacement therapy or antidepressants for those who did not use any pharmacological agents during their quit attempt.

ASSOCIATED NURSING DIAGNOSES

Smoking Cessation Assistance can be an appropriate intervention for several nursing diagnoses (North American Nursing Diagnosis Association [NANDA], 1994), including Activity Intolerance, Impaired Gas Exchange, Ineffective Airway

Clearance, Altered Health Maintenance, and Altered Cardiopulmonary Tissue Perfusion. Those who have independently decided that they need to quit smoking may be given the diagnosis of Health Seeking Behaviors, and those who refuse to quit or do not succeed may have diagnoses of Noncompliance or Ineffective Individual Management of Therapeutic Regimen.

Introducing a smoking cessation intervention may also *cause* some nursing diagnoses. These include Constipation, Diarrhea, Sleep Pattern Disturbance, Anxiety, and Altered Nutrition: Potential for More Than Body Requirements. These diagnoses are related to the withdrawal symptoms and to the finding that most recent ex-smokers gain weight in the process of smoking cessation. The average weight gain is less than 10 pounds, but about 10% of clients gain 30 or more pounds (Williamson et al., 1991). Most health care providers agree that the advantages of smoking cessation far outweigh the health disadvantage of weight gain. However, the psychological impact of the weight gain may predispose some clients to relapse or to refuse to attempt cessation (Klesges, Meyers, Klesges, & Lavasque, 1989). In addition, evidence suggests that smoking is related to depressive symptoms and that cessation may initiate or exacerbate these symptoms (Anda et al., 1990).

ASSOCIATED PATIENT OUTCOMES

The major outcome for all individuals who succeed with smoking cessation is the accomplishment of Risk Control: Tobacco Use, which can prevent many other untoward outcomes. At least short-term improvements in Self-Esteem and Well-Being are also common. Other likely outcomes are improved Respiratory Status: Gas Exchange, Respiratory Status: Ventilation, Tissue Perfusion: Cardiac, and Tissue Perfusion: Cerebral.

CASE STUDY

D was a 43-year-old professional woman who was going through a divorce at the start of her smoking cessation. Although she expected to be tempted to smoke when she was dealing with her estranged husband, these incidents were not associated with highly tempting situations. During the first 6 weeks of cessation, her only significant temptation occurred when she was bowling with friends who were smoking. Eleven weeks after quitting, D was at a bar for her birthday celebration. She described herself as euphoric, relaxed, and flirtatious. When she asked a member of the band with whom she was chatting for a cigarette, her girlfriend objected strenuously. "I think that I was trying to prove that I can have one and still stay smokeless," D said. "That I'm not addicted, or anything, I'm in control of the situation, and whatever it comes to I know that just one little cigarette is not going to put me back on that trodden path." She resumed abstinence after smoking a single cigarette.

About 2 months later (5 months after cessation),

D began to have problems with her daughter. These problems had been of concern to her for several weeks, but they were especially on her mind one evening when she was discussing the situation with friends. One of the friends was smoking, and D asked him for a cigarette. A few days later she was given some sample cigarettes at a convention she was attending, and thereafter she resumed smoking on a regular basis.

D's experience illustrates some of the perplexing aspects of smoking cessation. The stress of dealing with her husband, which occurred frequently during this period and which she expected, did not appear to induce an urge to smoke. However, D relapsed in a stressful situation that included a type of stress (problems with her daughter) she was not prepared to deal with. Although she had resisted temptation in situations where others were smoking and in stressful situations, the combination of a new stressor, smoking cues, and easy availability proved too much to control. It is unclear if her prior lapse at the bar influenced her subsequent relapse. Although D resumed abstinence after the lapse in the bar, during which she "proved" that she had control over her smoking habit, the feeling of control may have also given her a false sense of security. Control was demonstrated only for situations in which she was in a specific positive mood. Control in a negative mood is a different psychological experience. This example demonstrates that resisting smoking requires a variety of coping skills, because the skills that work in one situation may be ineffective or inappropriate in another.

CONCLUSION

Smoking Cessation Assistance can be carried out at different levels of intensity. The lowest level of intensity involves consistent tracking of the smoking status of clients, encouraging them to quit smoking, referring those who are ready to quit to smoking cessation programs, and following up on their progress. Higher-intensity interventions involve the nurse's involvement in the actual cessation process. The practitioner needs to have appropriate expectations about the success rates of such interventions, which are likely to be discouragingly low. More than 80% of clients who try to quit are likely to fail. It is therefore important for the nurse to remain motivated to continue the intervention program despite setbacks and to keep abreast of new techniques that might be helpful. In the final analysis, maintaining a smoking cessation intervention is quite similar to maintaining smoking cessation. A significant behavior change will be demanded, and overcoming disappointments and setbacks will be necessary. The rewards will be significant and compelling, but they are sometimes difficult to appreciate in the short term.

Acknowledgment

Case studies and examples were drawn from research project NR 10675 titled Reversal Theory and the Motivations for Health Behavior, funded by the National Center for Nursing Research, Mary Cook, Ph.D., Principal Investigator.

The authors acknowledge the assistance of Melba D. Small in the preparation of this chapter.

References

Ahijevych, K., and Wewers, M. E. (1995). Low-intensity smoking cessation intervention among African-American women cigarette smokers: A pilot study. *American Journal of Health Promotion, 9,* 337–339.

American Lung Association. (1996). *Freedom from smoking.* New York: Author.

Anda, R. F., Williamson, D. F., Escobedo, L. G., Mast E. E., Giovino, G. A., and Remington, P. L. (1990). Depression and the dynamics of smoking: A national perspective. *Journal of the American Medical Association, 264,* 1541–1545.

Brandon, T. H., Tiffany, S. T., and Baker, T. B. (1986). The process of smoking relapse. In F. M. Tims and C. G. Leukefeld (Eds.), *Relapse and recovery in drug abuse* (pp. 104–117). (NIDA Research Monograph No. 72). Rockville, MD: U.S. Public Health Service.

Centers for Disease Control and Prevention. (1996). Cigarette smoking among adults—United States, 1994. *Mortality and Morbidity Weekly Report, 45,* 588–590.

Cook, M. R. (1990). *Reversal theory and the motivations for health behavior* (Final Report: Grant NR10675). Kansas City, MO: Midwest Research Institute.

Cummings, C., Gordon, J. R., and Marlatt, G. A. (1980). Relapse: Strategies of prevention and prediction. In W. R. Miller (Ed.), *The addictive behaviors: Treatment of alcoholism, drug abuse, smoking and obesity* (pp. 291–321). New York: Pergamon Press.

Furlow, L., and O'Quinn, J. L. (1996). Research for practice: When the nurse says "stop," smokers listen. *American Journal of Nursing, 96* (3 Nurse Practitioner Extra Edition), 57.

Hjalmarson, A., Franzon, M., Westin, A., and Wiklund, O. (1994). Effect of nicotine spray on smoking cessation: A randomized, placebo-controlled, double-blind study. *Archives of Internal Medicine, 154,* 2567–2572.

Hughes, J. R. (1996). The future of smoking cessation therapy in the United States. *Addiction, 91,* 1797–1802.

Janz, N. K., Becker, M. H., Kirscht, J. P., Eraker, S. A., Billi, J. E., and Woolliscroft, J. O. (1987). Evaluation of a minimal-contact smoking cessation intervention in an outpatient setting. *American Journal of Public Health, 77,* 805–809.

Klesges, R. C., Meyers, A. W., Klesges, L. M., and Lavasque, M. E. (1989). Smoking and body weight and their effects on smoking behavior: A comprehensive review of the literature. *Psychological Bulletin, 106,* 204–230.

Marlatt, G. A., and Gordon, J. R. (1980). Determinants of relapse: Implications for the maintenance of behavior change. In P. O. Davidson and S. M. Davidson (Eds.), *Behavioral medicine: Changing health lifestyles* (pp. 410–452). New York: Brunner/Mazel.

Miller, N. H., Smith, P. M., DeBusk, R. F., Sobel,

D. S., and Taylor, C. B. (1997). Smoking cessation in hospitalized patients. *Archives of Internal Medicine, 157,* 409–415.

North American Nursing Diagnosis Association (NANDA). (1994). *NANDA nursing diagnoses: Definition and classification 1995–1996.* Philadelphia: Author.

O'Connell, K. A., Cook, M. R., Gerkovich, M. M., Potocky, M., and Swan, G. E. (1990). Reversal theory and smoking: A state-based approach to ex-smokers' highly tempting situations. *Journal of Consulting and Clinical Psychology, 58,* 489–494.

O'Connell, K. A., and Martin, E. J. (1987). Highly tempting situations associated with abstinence, temporary lapse, and relapse among participants in smoking cessation programs. *Journal of Consulting and Clinical Psychology, 55,* 367–371.

O'Connell, K. A., Gerkovich, M. M., and Cook, M. R. (1995). Reversal theory's mastery and sympathy states in smoking cessation. *Image: Journal of Nursing Scholarship, 27,* 311–316.

Prochaska, J. O. (1996). A stage paradigm for integrating clinical and public health approaches to smoking cessation. *Addictive Behaviors, 21,* 721–732.

Prochaska, J. O., DiClemente, C. C., and Norcross, J. C. (1992). In search of how people change: Applications to addictive behaviors. *American Psychologist, 47,* 1102–1114.

Schneider, N. G., Olmstead, R., Nilsson, F., Mody, F. V., Franzon, M., and Doan, K. (1996). Efficacy of a nicotine inhaler in smoking cessation: A double-blind, placebo-controlled trial. *Addiction, 91,* 1293–1306.

Schwartz, J. L. (1987). *Review and evaluation of smoking cessation methods: The United States and Canada 1978–1985* (NIH Publication No. 87-2940). Bethesda, MD: U. S. Department of Health and Human Services.

Shiffman, S. (1982). Relapse following smoking cessation: A situational analysis. *Journal of Consulting and Clinical Psychology, 50,* 71–86.

Shiffman, S. (1988). Behavioral assessment for smoking cessation. In D. M. Donovan and G. A. Marlatt (Eds.), *Assessment of addictive behaviors: Behavioral, cognitive, and physiological procedures* (pp. 139–181). New York: Guilford Press.

Shiffman, S., Paty, J. A., Gnys, M., Kassel, J. D., and Hickcox, M. (1996). First lapses to smoking: Within subjects analysis of real time reports. *Journal of Consulting and Clinical Psychology, 64,* 366–379.

Silagy, C., Mant, D., Fowler, G., and Lodge, M. (1994). Meta-analysis on efficacy of nicotine replacement therapies in smoking cessation. *Lancet, 343,* 139–142.

U.S. Department of Health and Human Services (USDHHS). (1996). *Smoking cessation: Clinical practice guideline, No. 18* (DHHS Publication No. [AHCPR] 96-0692). Washington, DC: USDHHS Public Health Service, Agency for Health Care Policy and Research.

Wewers, M. E., Bowen, J. M., Stanislaw, A. E., and Desimone, V. B. (1994). A nurse-delivered smoking cessation intervention among hospitalized postoperative patients—influence of a smoking-related diagnosis: A pilot study. *Heart and Lung, 23,* 151–156.

Williamson, D. F., Madans, J., Anda, R. F., Kleinman, J. C., Giovino, G. A., and Beyers, T. (1991). Smoking cessation and the severity of weight gain in a national cohort. *New England Journal of Medicine, 324,* 739–745.

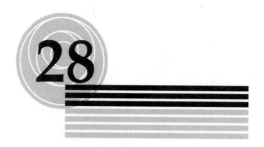

Music Therapy

Linda A. Gerdner and Kathleen C. Buckwalter

> There is a charm: a Power that sways the breast;
> Bids every Passion revel or be still;
> Inspires with Rage, or all your Cares dissolves;
> Can soothe Distraction, and almost Despair.
> That Power is Music.
>
> *John Armstrong (1744)*
> *(Schullian & Schoen, 1948, p. v)*

Since the advent of time, music has been used to ease the suffering of people; its influence on history, morals, and culture has long been noted. However, it was not until the 20th century that music as a form of treatment was investigated. In the 1990s, nursing has made a tremendous contribution to this ever-increasing base of knowledge.

Sears (1968) developed a theoretical framework encompassing three processes of Music Therapy: (1) experience within structure, (2) experience in self-organization, and (3) experience in relating to others. The content of Sears' framework can be individualized for a patient's own needs and abilities and is summarized later in this chapter. "Experience within structure refers to those behaviors of an individual that are required by and are inherent in musical experience" (Sears, 1968, p. 34). Music is an aural stimulant that evokes physical and psychological responses. Music provides for self-expression and allows individuals to communicate attitudes, feelings, and moods nonverbally, which can lead to an enhanced self-image. Musical activities often occur in groups and necessitate cooperation that fosters social interaction in addition to providing entertainment and recreation.

HISTORICAL PERSPECTIVES

Music has been used throughout history as a therapeutic influence. Early archaeological findings revealed crude musical instruments, although among primitive people music was primarily associated with dance and words. Altshuler (1948) stated that "the study of folk legends, fairy tales and myths . . . indicates that man has always attributed great power to music" (p. 269). Similarly, Herth

(1978) found that "accounts of the use of music in medicine date from the earliest times when music had a social function in every phase of life, civil and religious." When a primitive person became ill or injured, it was believed that a taboo had been broken or that a deity was angry. Music was then used to appease the gods (Radin, 1948).

The latter half of the 19th century and the early 20th century saw the beginnings of systematic study of music and its possible therapeutic benefits. Since the 1980s, nurses have made remarkable strides in testing the effects of music as an alternative or supplemental intervention in a wide variety of settings with diverse patient populations and conditions.

LITERATURE REVIEW

Music is one of the few interventions that can be considered truly holistic. Research and clinical findings support the use of music in a variety of physical and psychological conditions. It has also been shown to promote social interaction and spiritual well-being. A review of the literature that focuses on the holistic effects of music follows. The major studies are summarized in Table 28–1.

Physiological Effects

RESPIRATORY AND CARDIOVASCULAR SYSTEMS

The respiratory and cardiovascular systems are affected by music, with variations dependent on the pitch, intensity, and timber of sound (Diserens & Fine, 1939). As a physiological component of reduced anxiety, relaxing music was effective in reducing heart rate (Augustin & Hains, 1996; Barnason, Zimmerman, & Nieveen, 1995; Chlan, 1995; Davis-Rollans & Cunningham, 1987; White, 1992), respiratory rate (Chlan, 1995), and systolic blood pressure (Barnason et al., 1995; Updike, 1990; White, 1992). In addition, taped intrauterine sounds combined with synthesized female vocal singing resulted in a significant reduction in agitated behaviors and an improved oxygen saturation (as evidenced by pulse oximetry readings) in newborns (Collins & Kuck, 1991).

PAIN

Music alleviates both acute and chronic pain. With regard to acute pain, Herth (1978) found a 30% decrease in the use of pain medication with the use of therapeutic music. More recently, Whipple and Glynn (1992) noted that soothing music resulted in a significant increase in the pain thresholds of 10 healthy female volunteers. Music was effective in reducing the chronic pain associated with rheumatoid arthritis (Schorr, 1993) and cancer (Beck, 1991; Zimmerman, Pozehl, Duncan, & Schmitz, 1989).

Buckwalter (1976) evaluated the use of music in a variety of settings and with varied clinical populations while serving as a member of an "on-call" pain intervention team. Music was particularly effective when anxiety was a major component of the pain problem. For example, music positively influenced the course of treatment for patients with Crohn's disease and was also effective with adolescent trauma victims recuperating in Stryker frames. Because of the unusual and frequently awkward positioning associated with this latter treatment, these young patients were unable to watch television, read, or enjoy other diversionary activities for long periods of time. However, taped music (for this age group, usually rock music) provided distraction from the pain as well as

Table 28–1 Research on the Effects of Music Therapy

Condition	Subject Population	Author(s)
Physical		
Reduced heart rate	Mechanically ventilated patients	Chlan, 1995
	Preoperative patients	Augustin & Hains, 1996
	Post–coronary artery bypass grafting patients	Barnason, Zimmerman, & Nieveen, 1995
	Patients with myocardial infarction and other cardiac conditions	Davis-Rollans & Cunningham, 1987; White, 1992
Reduced respiratory rate	Mechanically ventilated patients	Chlan, 1995
	Acute myocardial infarction patients	White, 1992
Systolic blood pressure	Post–coronary artery bypass grafting patients; patients in coronary and surgical intensive care units	Barnason, Zimmerman, & Nieveen, 1995; Updike, 1990
Oxygen saturation levels	Premature infants	Standley & Moore, 1995
Acute pain/discomfort	Postoperative patients	Loesin, 1988; Mullooly, Levin, & Feldman, 1988
	Healthy female volunteers	Whipple & Glynn, 1992
	Patients receiving a bronchoscopy	Dubois, Bartter, & Pratter, 1995
Chronic pain	Patients with long-term and life-threatening illness	Magill-Levreault, 1993
	Women with rheumatoid arthritis	Schorr, 1993
	Cancer patients	Beck, 1991; Zimmerman, Pozehl, Duncan, & Schmitz, 1989
Mobility	Women (aged 65–99) possessing common characteristics of upper extremity osteoarthritis	Bernard, 1992
	Gait rehabilitation in persons with Parkinson's disease	McIntosh, Brown, Rice, & Thaut, 1997
Developmental delay	Children who are developmentally delayed in regard to hearing and speech, hand-eye coordination, personal-social interaction	Aldridge, Gustroff, & Neugebauer, 1995
Nausea and vomiting	Patients receiving chemotherapy	Frank, 1985
Food intake	Patients with severe dementia	Ragneskog, Brane, Karlsson, & Kihlgren, 1996
Sleep	Elderly patients	Mornhinweg & Voiginer, 1995
	Patients with dementia	Lindenmuth, Patel, & Chang, 1992
Psychological		
Anxiety	Intraoperative patients	Hinojosa & Steelman, 1995; Steelman, 1990; Stevens, 1990
	Preoperative ambulatory patients	Augustin & Hains, 1996
	Postoperative patients	Barnason, Zimmerman, & Nieveen, 1995; Mullooly, Levin, & Feldman, 1988
	Surgical patients	Kaempf & Amodei, 1989
	Patients in surgical holding area	Winter, Paskin, & Baker, 1994
	Post–myocardial infarction patients	Bolwerk, 1990; White, 1992
	Patients admitted to a cardiac care unit with a presumptive diagnosis of acute myocardial infarction	Guzzetta, 1989; Zimmerman, Pierson, & Marker, 1988
	Pediatric cancer patients undergoing bone marrow aspirations	Pfaff, Smith, & Gowan, 1989
	Chronically ill patients	Gross & Swartz, 1982
	College students with test anxiety	Mornhinweg, 1992; Stoudenmire, 1975; Stratton & Zalanowski, 1984; Summers, Hoffman, Neff, Hanson, & Pierce, 1990

Table continued on following page

Table 28–1 Research on the Effects of Music Therapy *(Continued)*

Condition	Subject Population	Author(s)
Psychological		
Agitation	Patients with severe dementia	Clair & Bernstein, 1994; Denney, 1997; Devereaux, 1997; Gerdner, 1992; Gerdner & Swanson, 1993; Goddaer & Abraham, 1994; Ragneskog, Kihlgren, Karlsson, & Norberg, 1996
Psychotic behavior	Psychiatric patients	Courtright, Johnson, & Baumgartner, 1990
Problematic behaviors	Restrained hospitalized patients	Janelli, Kanski, Jones, & Kennedy, 1995
High arousal behavior	Neonates	Kaminski & Hall, 1996
	Infants with bronchopulmonary dysplasia	Burke, Walsh, Oehler, & Gingras, 1995
Depression	Elderly patients	Hanser & Thompson, 1994
Mood	Mechanically ventilated patients; patients with myocardial infarction and other cardiac conditions; patients in coronary and intensive care units	Chlan, 1995; Davis-Rollans & Cunningham, 1987; Updike, 1990
Life review, ego integrity	Elderly patients	Bennette & Maas, 1988; McCloskey, 1990
Quality of life	Alzheimer's disease patients	Lipe, 1991; Lord & Garner, 1993
Social		
Social interaction	Patients with dementia	Clair & Bernstein, 1990
	Homeless patients	Peden, 1993
Spiritual		
Spiritual well-being	Patients with dementia	Gerdner, 1997
Cognition		
Cognitive functioning	Patients with dementia	Smith, 1986
	College students	Rauscher, Shaw, & Ky, 1993

diversionary activity regardless of the position of the bed frame, and when headphones were used, the music could be enjoyed around the clock.

Auditory stimulation, such as music, has a physiological effect on the body that may relate to the gate control theory of pain. Intense stimuli through the thalamus, midbrain, and brain stem produce modulating substances (e.g., endorphins, serotonin) that inhibit the release of neurotransmitters, therefore stimulating closure of the gate. Diversion of attention from the pain to a more pleasing stimulus (Zimmerman et al., 1989) decreases the adverse nature of the stimulus; thus, relaxation occurs that decreases muscle guarding at the painful site (Donovan, 1982).

MOBILITY

Early research conducted on musculoskeletal and neurological responses indicates that music affects muscular contraction and relaxation, muscle strength, and reflex action. Diserens and Fine (1939) found that muscular strength increased with the intensity and pitch of sound stimuli. Further studies concluded that the rhythm of the body responds to the rhythm of the music, which Van de Wall (1946) described as the kinesthetic response. This response is due to the interrelation and influence of sound vibration present in the body (McMahon, 1978). Other neurological effects appear to be due to the stimulation of the autonomic nervous system (Grunewald, 1953; Paul & Staudt, 1958).

A study conducted by Bernard (1992) compared the effects of music on exercise repetitions in 25 women ranging in age from 65 to 99 with upper extremity osteoarthritis. Subjects were able to perform an increased number of exercise repetitions during the presentation of fast-paced jazz than when no music was presented.

DEVELOPMENTAL DELAY

Music Therapy resulted in a clinically significant improvement in hearing, speech, hand-eye coordination, and social interaction in developmentally delayed children (Aldridge, Gustroff, & Neugebauer, 1995). The investigators attribute these results to the positive benefits of active listening and the eye-hand coordination required to play a musical instrument.

NAUSEA AND VOMITING

Many patients undergoing chemotherapy expect to experience nausea and vomiting. Frank (1985) hypothesized that this anticipatory anxiety potentiates the severity of nausea and vomiting and subsequently studied the effects of music and visual imagery on patients receiving chemotherapy. Findings indicated a decrease in the length of time patients experienced nausea and a perceived decrease in the degree of vomiting and the length of time that vomiting occurred.

Psychological Effects

In addition to physiological effects, music is believed to exert a powerful influence on the higher cerebral centers, as evidenced by its effects on attention, motivation, memory, and dreams (McMahon, 1978; Pickerell, Metzger, Wilde, Broadbent, & Edwards, 1954) as well as moods (Altshuler, 1948; Capurso, 1952).

Results of a pioneering study by Kerr as early as 1942 demonstrated an overwhelming confidence in music's psychological powers. Ninety-six percent of male subjects reported a favorable belief in the psychological effects of music; 77% thought it improved feelings toward associates; 90% felt it helped them when they were tired; 88% believed it soothed their nerves; 56% thought it helped their digestion; 90% thought it helped them in performing monotonous tasks; and 85% believed it helped them forget worries.

Altshuler (1948) maintained that in order to initiate psychotherapy, it is essential to remove states of inattention, anxiety, tension, and morbid moods, which is facilitated by the use of music. Subsequent research supported this view (Dickens & Sharpe, 1970). Herman (1954) identified the following therapeutic effects of music:

1. It has the property of attracting attention and prolonging its span. This is important in treating depression because it distracts the patient from depressive thought.

2. Music has the property of replacing one mood with another.

3. It has the ability to relieve inner tensions and conflicts.

4. The rhythmic stimuli produce physical motion, which draws attention of patients to things around them (p. 115).

Additional psychological effects of music include facilitating the ability to aid recall of past and present events; reinforcing identity, self-concept, and reality; and remitting the expression of fantasy (Diephouse, 1968; Munro & Mount, 1978; Van de Wall, 1946).

Music is thought to accomplish these effects in various ways. The musculoskeletal and neurological responses to music explain some of these effects (increased attention span, increased memory, increased physical motion, and decreased anxiety). Van de Wall (1946) suggested that music may initiate associational responses that connect ideas and emotions that are not directed cognitively or necessarily consciously. This type of mental response is highly subjective and is emotional rather than intellectual. The processes of association may explain music's ability to change moods and initiate recall of past and present events (Van de Wall, 1946). A third possible explanation for music's behavioral effects may be related to Altshuler's (1948) theory of thalamic response. The thalamus, being the seat of emotions, feelings, and sensations, is influenced by the pitch and rhythm of music, which in turn affects emotion and feelings.

These theories explain to some extent the effects of music on mental health, but the exact mechanism remains unknown. The responses to musical stimuli are rich in variation and subject to sociocultural influences. One's sociocultural background often determines choice of music and the pitch preferred. Music has a very personal and intimate meaning for each person, and this meaning is important when using music therapeutically (Maultsby, 1977).

ANXIETY

Music has also been used in an effort to decrease anxiety. Studies in brain hemisphere function provide some insight into why music may be considered a therapeutic intervention in alleviating anxiety. Bennett (1970), Dimond (1972), and Brydon and Nugent (1979) noted that the left hemisphere (which is usually dominant) has generally been considered rational, propositional, and analytical, whereas the right hemisphere has been considered more intuitive, appositional, gestalt-oriented, and symbolic. Similarly, Milner (1971) and King and Kimura (1972) reported that the right hemisphere is concerned with melodic patterns and imagery. In the words of Altshuler (1948),

> Music, even more than the spoken word, lends itself as a therapy because it meets with little or no intellectual resistance, and does not need to appeal to logic to initiate action . . . is more subtle and more primitive, and therefore its appeal is wider and greater (p. 267).

The effect of music on anxiety has been studied in a wide variety of conditions across the life span. Music was shown to reduce anxiety in preoperative patients (Augustin & Hains, 1996) and in patients waiting in a surgical holding area (Kaempf & Amodei, 1989; Winter, Paskin, & Baker, 1994).

Stoudenmire (1975) showed that brief anxiety-reduction techniques such as relaxing music and muscle relaxation training are effective methods of reducing anxiety. Updike (1990) found that music significantly reduced both the psychological and the physical components of anxiety in critically ill patients admitted to coronary and surgical intensive care units. Music also alleviated anxiety and promoted relaxation in patients suffering from acute cardiac conditions (Bolwerk, 1990; Davis-Rollans & Cunningham, 1987; White, 1992). Additional studies have reported that music decreases test anxiety (Mornhinweg, 1992; Peretti, 1975; Stanton, 1975; Stratton & Zalanowski, 1984; Summers, Hoffman, Neff, Hanson, & Pierce, 1990).

Studies have also evaluated the effects of music on infants. Burke, Walsh, Oehler, and Gingras (1995) used a case study approach to examine the effects of aural and vibrotactile music in reducing agitation and physiological instability following stress-producing interventions in infants with bronchopulmonary dysplasia. Results were as follows: (1) heart rate was not significantly affected by vibrotactile stimulation, but it was improved with the use of taped music; (2) oxygen saturation levels were improved during both of the music conditions; (3) both music conditions decreased the amount of time spent in a highly aroused state; (4) vibrotactile music increased the amount of time spent in a quiet alert state; (5) both music conditions increased the amount of time infants spent sleeping; and (6) infants displayed greater limb movement during the no-music condition. In addition, Kaminski and Hall (1996) found that newborns demonstrated fewer high arousal states during the presentation of soothing, lyrical music.

AGITATION

Goddaer and Abraham (1994) hypothesized that "relaxing" music would buffer the general noise level found in dining rooms in long-term care settings, thus exerting a calming effect that would reduce the frequency of agitated behaviors in persons with severe cognitive impairment. Significant reductions were observed in the cumulative incidence of total agitated behaviors (63.4%) as well as in the cumulative incidence of physically nonaggressive behaviors (56.3%) and verbally agitated behaviors (74.5%). These findings were supported when the study was replicated by Denney (1997). Similarly, a study conducted by Courtright, Johnson, and Baumgartner (1990) reported a decrease in disruptive behaviors exhibited by psychiatric patients when soothing background music was used in the cafeteria during meals.

Gerdner (1992) reported a reduction in agitated behaviors in subjects with Alzheimer's disease and related disorders (ADRD) during the immediate presentation of "individualized" music and during the following 30 minutes. Individualized music was defined as music that had special meaning to the person and had been integrated into the person's life (Gerdner, 1992). Because subjects suffered severe cognitive impairment, knowledgeable family members provided this information about their loved one's musical preference. These findings were supported when the study was replicated (Devereaux, 1997).

Music may be used as an alternative method of communication for persons in the advanced stages of ADRD. Anecdotal data indicate that receptive and expressive musical abilities are preserved in persons with advanced ADRD who have a decreased ability to understand verbal language. It is therefore believed that the cognitive processing of music and language are conducted independently. The exact means by which cognitive processing of music occurs is not known, and experts disagree on hypothesized theories (Aldridge, 1993; Petsche, Lindner, Rappelsberger, & Gruber, 1988). Gerdner (1997) theorizes that the presentation of carefully selected music that was meaningful to the person during the younger years will stimulate remote memory. The elicitation of memories associated with positive feelings (happiness, love, etc.) changes the focus of attention and provides an interpretable stimulus that overrides meaningless or confusing stimuli in the environment. This has a soothing effect on the person with ADRD, which in turn prevents or alleviates agitation. This theory is currently being tested more rigorously (Gerdner, 1995a).

DEPRESSION

The positive effects of music on persons diagnosed with major or minor depressive disorders have been well documented (Hanser, 1990; Hanser & Thompson, 1994). Hanser (1990) hypothesized that listening to music serves as a palliative strategy for coping with the stress and anxiety that underlie depression.

OTHER CLINICAL CONDITIONS

Preliminary studies reveal that music affects diverse populations in a variety of settings. For example, Scott (1970) found that productivity of minimally brain-damaged children was enhanced with background music. In addition, she noted a kinesthetic response of decreased lightheadedness with the application of Music Therapy. Munro and Mount (1978) demonstrated the usefulness of Music Therapy in palliative care, documenting the ability of music to bring comfort when words were inadequate and the facilitation of positive interactions and expression of feelings. Similarly, Salmon (1993) used music to assist terminally ill patients in experiencing, expressing, and working through their feelings, and McCloskey (1990) used music to facilitate reminiscence and life review in elderly persons. Clearly, more research into the varied applications of Music Therapy is warranted, and there is a need to replicate studies in given areas, so as to build a more systematic knowledge base.

Socialization

Research supports the use of music to enhance socialization across the life span. Hinds (1980) noted that music increased the number of social interactions of children in a group situation at a mental health unit. Peden (1993) implemented a program composed of live and recorded music for homeless adults in a nurse-managed clinic within a multiservice day shelter, and anecdotal evidence indicated an increase in socialization. In addition, homeless persons were more receptive to participating in a therapeutic relationship with psychiatric nursing staff following the music intervention. Despite their severely regressed condition, subjects with cognitive impairment have shown increased social interaction and increased participation during group singing sessions (Clair & Bernstein, 1990; Millard & Smith, 1989).

Spiritual Well-Being

There is much anecdotal evidence but limited empirical study to support the use of music to enhance spiritual well-being. Positive effects of music have been seen in persons in the advanced stages of dementia. Gerdner (1997) reports one such example in an elderly woman who was socially inaccessible. However, during the presentation of religious hymns per audiocassette, she frequently sang the lyrics in melody and occasionally in harmony. On one occasion, she even appeared to be praying. Gerdner (1991) reports another example of a woman residing in an adult day care center who was in the mild to moderate stages of dementia. This patient frequently appeared lethargic and rarely interacted with the other patients or staff, but when religious hymns were played, she would smile broadly and often sang along. During this time she would close her eyes tightly as if concentrating on the words. When asked how the music made her feel, she replied, "Good—I'm feeling lots of things—love for God!"

Cognition

A study by Rauscher, Shaw, and Ky (1993) garnered much attention regarding the cognitive effects of music. Thirty-six college students were each given three abstract reasoning tests taken from the Stanford-Binet intelligence scale. Each test was preceded by 10 minutes of (1) listening to Mozart's sonata for two pianos in D major; (2) listening to a relaxation tape; or (3) listening to silence. Students scored significantly better after listening to Mozart than after listening to the relaxation tape or to silence. Investigators excluded arousal as a cause for score differences on the basis of finding no interaction of main effect of pulse rate changes. They concluded that the "enhancing effect of the music condition is temporal, and does not extend beyond the 10-15 minute period during which subjects were engaged in each spacial task" (Rauscher et al., 1993, p. 611).

MUSIC AS A NURSING INTERVENTION

As suggested by the literature review, music has been used as an effective intervention in a variety of populations and by practitioners from a variety of disciplines, including nursing. Music Therapy as defined in the Nursing Interventions Classification (NIC) appears in Table 28–2. To achieve optimum results, the intervention must be tailored with the patient's specific condition(s) and desired outcome(s) in mind. For example, the use of music to facilitate communication in a patient with aphasia secondary to a cerebrovascular accident (CVA) (Taylor, 1989) is very different from that for an individual in the advanced stages of dementia (Gerdner, 1995a; Gerdner, 1997). Together, the nurse and patient can explore the option of using a musical intervention, taking into consideration the patient's background, musical interests, and abilities.

Personal Music Preference

Several of the activities prescribed by NIC focus on the patient's specific music preference. This preference appears to be influenced by emotional associations and learned response. Potential mediating variables in the selection of music

Table 28–2 Music Therapy

DEFINITION: Using music to help achieve a specific change in behavior or feeling.

ACTIVITIES:

Define the specific change in behavior that is desired (e.g., relaxation, stimulation, concentration, and pain reduction)

Determine the patient's interest in music

Identify the patient's musical preferences

Choose particular music selections representative of the patient's preferences, keeping in mind the behavior change desired

Make music tapes/compact discs and equipment available to patient

Ensure that tape/compact discs and equipment are in good working order

Provide earphones

Ensure that the volume is adequate but not too high

Avoid turning music on and leaving it on for long periods

Facilitate the patient's active participation (e.g., playing an instrument or singing), if this is desired and feasible within the setting

Avoid stimulating music after an acute head injury

Source: McCloskey, J. C., and Bulecheck, G. M. (Eds.). (1996). *Nursing interventions classification (NIC)* (2nd ed., p. 391). St. Louis: Mosby–Year Book.

include the patient's gender, previous experience and familiarity with music, musical interests and abilities, cultural background, and religious affiliation. To assess a patient's musical preference, nurses may use the Hartsock (1982) Music Preference Questionnaire (MPQ) (Table 28–3). The questionnaire was developed to determine patients' musical preferences by studying the effects of music on depression levels in immobilized patients. The MPQ requires approximately 15 minutes to complete (Hartsock, 1982). Information should be as specific as possible, to include song titles, performers, and preference for vocal or instrumental music (e.g., guitar, violin) (Gerdner, 1995b). If the patient is unable to provide this information (e.g., because of cognitive impairment), an adapted version of the questionnaire may be given to a family member who is knowledgeable with regard to the patient's music preferences (Gerdner, 1992). Following the acquisition of this information, the nurse will need to choose particular music selections representative of the preferences expressed.

Presentation of music must be tailored to the individual and the setting. The application of headphones may be discomforting to some patients, such as those with advanced dementia. In these cases, it may be more appropriate to play the music "free field." However, it is important to monitor the response of other patients in the immediate area if music is played free field. Music that is pleasing to one person may be disturbing to another. It is essential that the volume be

Table 28–3   Modified Hartsock Music Preference Questionnaire (MPQ)

The following questions are concerned with music likes. All information will be kept confidential.

1. The following is a list of different types of music. Please indicate your three (3) most favorite types with 1 being the most favorite, 2 the next, and 3 your third choice.

   _____ 1. Country and Western
   _____ 2. Classical
   _____ 3. Spiritual/Religious
   _____ 4. Rock
   _____ 5. Folk
   _____ 6. Blues
   _____ 7. Jazz
   _____ 8. Disco
   _____ 9. Other:

Please put a check (√) beside your choice in the following questions.

2. What form does your favorite music take?

   _____ 1. Vocal
   _____ 2. Nonvocal
   _____ 3. Both

3. What type of music makes you feel the most happy?

   _____ Country and Western
   _____ Classical
   _____ Spiritual/Religious
   _____ Rock
   _____ Folk
   _____ Blues
   _____ Jazz
   _____ Disco
   _____ Other:
   _____ None

4. Are there any specific songs/selections which make you feel happy?

5. When listening to music that makes you feel happy, is there any particular artist/performer you enjoy listening to most?

Table 28–3 Modified Hartsock Music Preference Questionnaire (MPQ) *(Continued)*

6. What type of music makes you feel the most sad?

_____ Country and Western
_____ Classical
_____ Spiritual/Religious
_____ Rock
_____ Folk
_____ Blues
_____ Jazz
_____ Disco
_____ Other:
_____ None

7. Before your hospitalization, how important a role did music play in your life?

_____ 1. Very important
_____ 2. Moderately important
_____ 3. Slightly important
_____ 4. Not important

8. Before your hospitalization, how often did you enjoy listening to music in a typical 24-hour period (day)?

_____ 1. Less than 1 hour
_____ 2. 1–3 hours
_____ 3. 4–6 hours
_____ 4. 7–9 hours
_____ 5. Over 10 hours

9. During your hospitalization, how often do you enjoy listening to music during a 24-hour period (day)?

_____ 1. Less than 1 hour
_____ 2. 1–3 hours
_____ 3. 4–6 hours
_____ 4. 7–9 hours
_____ 5. Over 10 hours

Source: Data from Hartsock, J. (1982). *The effects of music on levels of depression in orthopedic patients on prolonged bedrest.* Unpublished master's thesis, University of Iowa, Iowa City.

set at an appropriate level to ensure the patient's ability to hear the music. Music that is too loud or too soft may be annoying (Gerdner, 1995b). Also, impaired hearing may result in the distortion of sound, which itself may be a source of irritation. The length of time the music is presented should be determined on an individual basis according to the patient's tolerance and the evaluation of the desired effects.

Nurses should consider developing a portable patient listening library that houses tapes covering a broad spectrum of musical tastes. Philanthropic groups can be approached to purchase cassettes for the music library, and hospital volunteers can run the administrative and maintenance aspects of the library, thus freeing nurses for more professional activities, which include the identification of patients likely to benefit from Music Therapy.

Music is an auditory stimulus whose effects may be enhanced when used in combination with methods to stimulate other senses (taste, touch, visual, and olfactory). Thus, music can be used effectively in conjunction with other interventions. When used in combination with Reminiscence Therapy (see Chapter 22), it can enhance communication, socialization, and ventilation of feelings. Reminiscence Therapy can also be used to incorporate the past into the present, and dance and music can be used to increase mobility and socialization. In addition, singing or playing a musical instrument may provide a means to increase socialization and self-esteem.

Classifications of Music Used for Therapeutic Purposes

Music classifications such as classical, lullabies, and "new age" are reported to have therapeutic effects. Classical music has long been reported to have a relaxing effect on adults, whereas lullabies have been used for their soothing effects on infants. A commercial adaptation, the use of an audiotaped recording of lullabies superimposed over the sound of a human heart, is purported to promote sleep in newborns. In addition, O'Kelley (1996) describes the effective use of lullabies to induce relaxation and sleep in persons with ADRD.

New age is a contemporary classification of music that has been composed specifically to promote relaxation. Halpren has developed a subgroup of this music he calls "the anti-frantic alternative" (1989, p. 77). He describes the music as having "no recognizable melody, no insistent rhythmic pulse, and no recognizable harmonic progression," thereby providing an "effortless relaxation state." Halpren claims that because the music "does not stimulate the listener in a familiar conditioned pattern," it does not "unconsciously coerce" the listener into "responding in a prescribed fashion" (1989, p. 70). Halpren's music is not consistently effective, however. Gaffney (1982) studied the effects of one Halpren tape, "Spectrum Suite," on the anxiety level of immobilized patients and noted that the new age music chosen was not appreciated by older subjects. One participant commented that the music sounded "Oriental," and another stated that it was "strange music—sounds more like funeral music to me."

In addition, the tempo of music may also be adjusted to accommodate the patient's specific limitation. This method is commonly used in persons suffering from left hemisphere damage associated with a CVA. Despite the presence of aphasia, the person's ability to sing is usually retained. Consequently, singing (a sustained form of speech) may be used as an alternative method of communication in aphasic patients who have difficulty verbalizing or are unable to verbalize their needs. Tempos must be slower than normal to increase the available time to perceive and form syllables. Therefore, songs that have few words, with frequent repetition of fairly regular rhythmic patterns, are appropriate (Taylor, 1989, pp. 174–175). Patients are instructed to verbalize their needs using the melody of a specific song—for example, singing "I need a drink of water" to the melody of "Row, Row, Row Your Boat."

The "iso" principle is another method that focuses on the music's tempo to achieve a therapeutic effect. Music is selected to match the mood of the patient, focusing on the negative affect to be altered. For example, if the patient is sad, the music is matched to this mood. By stages, the content and quality of the music is changed toward a cheerful tone, thereby altering the mood of the patient in a more positive direction. A step-wise "vectoring" of music is used to facilitate the desired goal (Shatin, 1970).

NURSING DIAGNOSES ASSOCIATED WITH THE USE OF MUSIC THERAPY

Music Therapy is used in a wide variety of health care settings to alleviate a number of conditions (anxiety, agitation, and pain) and to enhance others (self-expression, self-esteem, and relaxation). Refer to Table 28–4 for a list of nursing diagnoses associated with the use of this intervention.

Table 28–4 Nursing Diagnoses and Associated Outcomes for Music Therapy

Nursing Diagnoses*	Nursing Outcomes†
Physical	
Pain	Comfort Level
Chronic Pain	Comfort Level
Impaired Physical Mobility	Ambulation: Walking
	Balance
	Joint Movement: Active
Altered Growth and Development	Child Development: 2 mo., 4 mo., 6 mo., 12 mo., 2 yr., 3 yr., 4 yr., 5 yr., 6–11 yr., 12–17 yr.
Altered Nutrition: Less Than Body Requirements	Nutritional Status: Food & Fluid Intake
Sleep Pattern Disturbance	Rest
	Sleep
Psychological	
Anxiety	Anxiety Control
	Concentration
Acute Confusion	Anxiety Control
	Memory
	Aggression Control
Chronic Confusion	Aggression Control
	Memory
	Anxiety Control
	Quality of Life
Impaired Memory	Memory
Altered Thought Processes	Memory
	Anxiety Control
	Aggression Control
	Quality of Life
Disorganized Infant Behavior	Anxiety Control
Risk For Disorganized Infant Behavior	Anxiety Control
Fear	Fear Control
Ineffective Individual Coping	Mood Equilibrium
Risk For Loneliness	Loneliness
Self Esteem Disturbance	Self-Esteem
Self-Concept Disturbance‡	Identity
Social	
Social Isolation	Social Involvement
Impaired Social Interaction	Social Involvement
Diversional Activity Deficit	Leisure Participation
Impaired Verbal Communication	Communication Ability
	Communication: Expressive Ability
	Communication: Receptive Ability
Spiritual	
Spiritual Distress	Spiritual Well-Being

*North American Nursing Diagnosis Association. (1994). *Nursing diagnosis: Definitions and classifications 1995–1996.* Philadelphia: Author.
†Johnson, M., and Maas, M. (Eds.). (1997). *Nursing outcomes classification (NOC).* St. Louis: Mosby–Year Book.
‡Not a NANDA diagnosis.

Table 28–5   Interview Questionnaire to Evaluate Effects of Music Therapy

May I tape this interview with you? All information will be kept strictly confidential.
How many minutes or hours did you listen to the music during a 24-hour period?
Did you listen more during the day or the night?
Was there any time when you felt like listening to music and were unable to?
Was there any time you would rather not have listened to your music?
Did you feel sad any time during the week?
Can you tell me about any event that occurred this week that has made you feel sad?
Did you feel like listening to music when you were sad? What type?
Did you feel happy any time during the past week?
Was there any event that occurred which made you feel happy?
Did you listen to music when you felt happy? What type?
Has there been any change in your music likes?
The type of music?
The songs?
Any other comments about the music?

Source: Hartsock, J. (1982). *The effects of music on levels of depression in orthopedic patients on prolonged bedrest.* Unpublished master's thesis, University of Iowa, Iowa City.

OUTCOMES ASSOCIATED WITH THE USE OF MUSIC THERAPY

The nursing outcomes associated with Music Therapy are listed in Table 28–4. Nurses should evaluate the impact of the music on the patient, as well as changes in musical preference. This can best be done using an interview schedule, such as the one developed by Hartsock (1982) (Table 28–5).

Glynn (1992) designed the Music Therapy Assessment Tool (MTAT) to specifically evaluate the effects of music on persons with ADRD. This instrument evaluates the effects during the presentation of music and following musical exposure. Categories of assessment include sensory-perceptual ability, verbal ability, nonverbal communication, affect, attention level, behavior, and rhythmic expression.

Nurses who introduce Music Therapy in an effort to change a particular aspect of patient care (e.g., pain, anxiety, depression) may wish to systematically measure the influence of the intervention on the variable of interest using standardized tools (e.g., Melzack-Wall's Pain Scales, Spielberger's State Trait Anxiety Inventory, Cohen-Mansfield Agitation Inventory, Beck Depression Inventory). These data may be supplemented with physiological measures (e.g., blood pressure, pulse) when appropriate.

CASE STUDIES

The following two case studies provide examples regarding assessment, implementation, and outcome measures associated with Music Therapy.

Case Study I

LR, a 42-year-old man, had suffered a massive abdominal wound from being shot at close range. The front and back dressings on LR's wound had to be changed and irrigated every 4 hours, a painful ordeal for both the patient and the nurse. LR was irritable and restless in anticipation of the dressing changes, which he dreaded. He was abusive to the staff throughout the experience and sullen and withdrawn at other times. His only other interaction with the nurses consisted of frequent and excessive demands for pain medications following the dressing changes. The second author was contacted by the nursing staff in an effort to help them deal with this "problem pain patient," and music was tested as an intervention. An initial interview with LR determined that his favorite type of music was rhythm and blues, and cassette tapes of this genre were recorded for his use. Approximately 30 minutes before each dressing change, LR began listening to the music with headphones attached to a bedside audiocassette player. He listened throughout the course of the dressing change (another 30 to 45 minutes) and for a short time afterward. Subjectively, LR reported being better able to cope with the experience of the dressing changes and feeling more relaxed and pain free because he could concentrate on the music rather than on the activity of the nurses. Objectively, a significant decrease was noted in the amount of pain medication LR requested, and significant increases were documented in terms of LR's hours of sleep per day, amount of food consumed, and positive interactions with the nursing staff. LR also requested that his family provide him with additional tapes to enable him to successfully cope with the painful and anxiety-laden experience of the dressing changes.

The individual in the second case study participated in a study to compare the effect of classical "relaxation" music to that of music preferred by a patient with ADRD (Gerdner, 1995a).

Case Study 2

Mrs. S was an 82-year-old woman diagnosed with ADRD who had severe cognitive impairment as indicated by a score of 6 on the Global Deterioration Scale (Reisberg, Ferris, deLeon, & Crook, 1982). She resided in a private room within a special care unit. On her bedside table was a photograph depicting her in a dance contest, which her daughter reported that she had attended weekly until the death of her husband. Mrs. S frequently wandered during baseline assessment. In addition, she exhibited general restlessness and performed repetitive mannerisms. She would frequently carry a towel close to her body and did not socially interact with the staff or other residents.

An audiotape of music performed by the Glen Miller Orchestra was played for 30 minutes two times a week for 6 weeks for Mrs. S. Her behavior was monitored and documented using a modi-

fied version of the Cohen-Mansfield Agitation Inventory (Cohen-Mansfield, 1986). The frequency of agitated behaviors decreased dramatically during the presentation of the individualized music and began increasing gradually during the 30 minutes following the presentation of music. However, it is important to note that it still remained lower than the frequency of agitated behaviors exhibited during baseline assessment. Anecdotal data indicated that Mrs. S would frequently smile broadly upon initiation of the preferred music. On one occasion she appeared to be "dancing with her feet and hands" while sitting in a chair. On other occasions she would sway to the rhythm of the music and clap her hands following the completion of selected songs. On one occasion she even stood up and danced with an imaginary partner. When a staff member entered the room and suggested that she sit down, Mrs. S replied, "I don't have time to sit down—there's music—I gotta dance." On another occasion she sang the words to "Gal from Kalamazoo" while swaying and snapping her fingers in rhythm to the music, then stated, "I just gotta dance." Upon completion of the music intervention on that day, she said, "My, my, I guess this dance is over." This was followed by a 2-week "washout" period in which Mrs. S's behaviors were monitored and documented during the same 60-minute interval of time without the presence of music. The frequency of agitated behaviors increased to a level comparable to baseline assessment. Next, an anthology of classical relaxation music was presented for 30 minutes two times a week for 6 weeks. There was a slight decrease in the frequency of agitated behaviors compared with that exhibited during baseline assessment. However, the frequency remained much higher than that exhibited during the presentation of individualized music. During this time Mrs. S frequently wandered, exhibited a "nervous laugh," performed repetitive mannerisms, and exhibited general restlessness. She did not overtly respond in any way to the classical relaxation music.

SUMMARY

Music has a long tradition of easing human suffering. Music is a holistic intervention that affects the physical, psychological, social, and spiritual aspects of patients. Nurses can use music as a diversionary or therapeutic intervention in a variety of health care settings and patient populations, limited only by their creativity. Musical preference should be incorporated into the initial assessment of each patient on admission. The patient's ethnic and religious background may influence this preference. The two most important variables governing the outcome of Music Therapy are the patient's personal music preference and his or her emotional status at the time of implementation. Music must be individualized based on both these factors. Flexibility is therefore an important aspect of implementation.

Music Therapy is relatively inexpensive and requires minimum time expenditure. Following instruction by nursing staff, music may be implemented by nursing assistants, activity staff, volunteers, and family members. An ongoing assessment should be conducted to determine the patient's response and the achievement of desired outcomes.

References

Aldridge, D. (1993). Music and Alzheimer's disease—assessment and therapy: Discussion paper. *Journal of the Royal Society of Medicine, 86*, 93–95.

Aldridge, D., Gustroff, G., and Neugebauer, L. (1995). A pilot study of music therapy in the treatment of children with developmental delay. *Complementary Therapeutic Medicine, 3*, 197–205.

Altshuler, I. A. (1948). Psychiatrist's experience with music as a therapeutic agent. In D. Schullian and M. Schoen (Eds.), *Music as medicine*. New York: Henry Schuman.

Augustin, P., and Hains, A. A. (1996). Effect of music on ambulatory surgery patients preoperative anxiety. *AORN Journal, 63*, 750, 753–756.

Barnason, S., Zimmerman, L., and Nieveen, J. (1995). The effects of music interventions on anxiety in the patient after coronary artery bypass grafting. *Heart and Lung, 24*(2), 124–132.

Beck, S. L. (1991). The therapeutic use of music for cancer-related pain . . . crossover study. *Oncology Nursing Forum, 18*, 1327–1337.

Bennett, J. (1970). The difference between right and left. *American Philosophical Quarterly, 1*, 175–191.

Bennette, S. L., and Maas, F. (1988). The effect of music-based life review on the life satisfaction and ego integrity of elderly people. *British Journal of Occupational Therapy, 51*, 433–436.

Bernard, A. (1992). The use of music as purposeful activity: A preliminary investigation. *Physical and Occupational Therapy in Geriatrics, 10*(3), 35–45.

Bolwerk, C. (1990). Effects of relaxing music on state anxiety in myocardial infarction patients. *Critical Care Nursing Quarterly, 13*(2), 63–72.

Brydon, K. A., and Nugent, W. R. (1979). Musical metaphor as a means of therapeutic communication. *Journal of Music Therapy, 16*(3), 149–153.

Buckwalter, K. C. (1976). *Use of music therapy in patients with pain*. Unpublished manuscript.

Burke, M., Walsh, J., Oehler, J., and Gingras, J. (1995). Music therapy following suctioning: Four case studies. *Neonatal Network, 14*(7), 41–49.

Capurso, A. (1952). The Capurso study. In E. Guthiel (Ed.), *Music and your emotions*. New York: Liveright Publishing Corporation.

Chlan, L. L. (1995). Psychophysiologic responses of mechanically ventilated patients to music: A pilot study. *American Journal of Critical Care, 4*, 233–238.

Clair, A. A., and Bernstein, B. (1990). A preliminary study of music therapy programming for severely regressed persons with Alzheimer's-type dementia. *Journal of Applied Gerontology, 9*, 299–311.

Clair, A. A., and Bernstein, B. (1994). The effect of no music, stimulative background music and sedative background music on agitated behaviors in persons with severe dementias. *Activities, Adaptation and Aging, 19*(1), 61–70.

Cohen-Mansfield, J. (1986). Agitated behaviors in the elderly II. Preliminary results in the cognitively deteriorated. *Journal of the American Geriatrics Society, 34*, 722–727.

Collins, S. K., and Kuck, K. (1991). Music therapy in the neonatal intensive care unit. *Neonatal Network, 9*(6), 23–26.

Courtright, P., Johnson, S., and Baumgartner, M. A. (1990). Dinner music: Does it affect the behavior of psychiatric inpatients? *Journal of Psychosocial Nursing and Mental Health Services, 28*(3), 37–42.

Davis-Rollans, C., and Cunningham, S. G. (1987). Physiologic responses of coronary care patients to selected music. *Heart and Lung, 16*, 370–378.

Denney, A. (1997). Quiet music an intervention for mealtime agitation? *Journal of Gerontological Nursing, 23*(7), 16–23.

Devereaux, M. A. (1997). *The effects of individualized music on cognitively impaired nursing home residents exhibiting agitation*. Unpublished master's thesis, College of St. Catherine, St. Paul, Minnesota.

Dickens, G., and Sharpe, M. (1970). Music therapy in the setting of a psychotherapeutic center. *British Journal of Medical Psychology, 43*, 83–94.

Diephouse, J. (1968). Music therapy: A valuable adjunct to psychotherapy with children. *Psychiatric Quarterly Supplement, 42*, 75–85.

Dimond, S. (1972). *The double brain*. Baltimore: Williams & Wilkins.

Diserens, C., and Fine, H. (1939). *A psychology of music*. Cincinnati, OH: College of Music.

Donovan, M. (1982). Cancer pain: You can help. *Nursing Clinics of North America, 17*, 713–728.

Dubois, J. M., Bartter, T., and Pratter, M. R. (1995). Music improves patient comfort level during outpatient bronchoscopy. *Chest, 108*(1), 129–130.

Frank, J. M. (1985). The effects of music therapy and guided visual imagery on chemotherapy induced nausea and vomiting. *Oncology Nursing Forum, 12*(5), 47–52.

Gaffney, J. M. (1982). *The use of music therapy to decrease* state anxiety in immobilized patients. Unpublished master's thesis, University of Iowa, Iowa City.

Gerdner, L. A. (1991). *Therapeutic use of music in persons with Alzheimer's disease and related disorders.* Unpublished manuscript.

Gerdner, L. A. (1992). *The effects of individualized music on elderly clients who are confused and agitated.* Unpublished master's thesis, University of Iowa, Iowa City.

Gerdner, L. A. (1995a). *Individualized vs. classical music on agitation in ADRD* (NIH F31 NR07090-01A1). Bethesda, MD: National Institute of Nursing Research.

Gerdner, L. A. (1995b). *Practice protocol: Individualized music intervention.* Iowa City, IA: Research Development and Dissemination Core, Geriatric Nursing Research Intervention Center, University of Iowa.

Gerdner, L. A. (1997). An individualized music intervention for agitation. *Journal of the American Psychiatric Nurses Association, 3*(6), 177–184.

Gerdner, L. A., and Swanson, E. A. (1993). Effects of individualized music on elderly patients who are confused and agitated. *Archives of Psychiatric Nursing, 7*(5), 282–291.

Glynn, N. J. (1992). The music therapy assessment tool in Alzheimer's patients. *Journal of Gerontological Nursing, 18*(1), 3–9.

Goddaer, J., and Abraham, I. L. (1994). Effects of relaxing music on agitation during meals among nursing home residents with severe cognitive impairment. *Archives of Psychiatric Nursing, 8*(3), 150–158.

Gross, J. L., and Swartz, R. (1982). The effects of music therapy on anxiety in chronically ill patients. *Music Therapy, 2*(1), 43–51.

Grunewald, M. (1953). A physiological aspect of experiencing music. *American Journal of Psychotherapy, 7*, 59–67.

Guzzetta, C. E. (1989). Effects of relaxation and music therapy on patients in a coronary care unit with presumptive acute myocardial infarction. *Heart and Lung, 18*, 609–615.

Halpren, S. (1989). A new age of music in medicine. In M. H. M. Lee (Ed.), *Rehabilitation, music and human well-being* (pp. 76–97). St. Louis: MMB Music.

Hanser, S. B. (1990). A music therapy strategy for depressed older adults in the community. *Journal of Applied Gerontology, 9*, 283–297.

Hanser, S. B., and Thompson, L. W. (1994). Effects of a music therapy strategy on depressed older adults. *Journal of Gerontology, 49*, P265–P269.

Hartsock, J. (1982). *The effects of music on levels of depression in orthopedic patients on prolonged bedrest.* Unpublished master's thesis, University of Iowa, Iowa City.

Herman, E. P. (1954). Music therapy in depression. In E. Padolsky (Ed.), *Music therapy.* New York: Philosophical Library.

Herth, K. (1978, October). The therapeutic use of music. *Supervisor Nurse*, 22–23.

Hinds, P. S. (1980). Music: A milieu factor with implications for the nurse therapist. *Journal of Psychiatric Nursing, 18*, 28–33.

Hinojosa, R., and Steelman, V. (1995). A research critique. Intraoperative music therapy: Effects on anxiety, blood pressure. *Plastic Surgery Nursing, 15*(4), 228–231.

Janelli, L. M., Kanski, G. W., Jones, H. M., and Kennedy, M. C. (1995). Exploring music interventions with restrained patients. *Nursing Forum, 30*(4), 12–18.

Johnson, M., and Maas, M. (Eds.). (1997). *Nursing outcomes classification (NOC).* St. Louis: Mosby-Year Book.

Kaempf, G., and Amodei, M. E. (1989). The effect of music on anxiety: A research study. *AORN Journal, 50*(1), 114–118.

Kaminski, J., and Hall, W. (1996). The effect of soothing music on neonatal behavioral states in the hospital newborn nursery. *Neonatal Network, 15*(1), 45–54.

Kerr, W. A. (1942). Psychological effects of music as reported by 162 defense trainers. *Psychological Record, 5*, 205–210.

King, G., and Kimura, D. (1972). Left-ear superiority in dichotic perception in vocal nonverbal sounds. *Canadian Journal of Psychology/Review of Canadian Psychology, 26*(2), 111–117.

Lindenmuth, G. F., Patel, M., and Chang, P. K. (1992, March-April). Effects of music on sleep in healthy elderly subjects with senile dementia of the Alzheimer's type. *American Journal of Alzheimer's Care and Related Disorders and Research*, 13–20.

Lipe, A. W. (1991). Using music therapy to enhance the quality of life in a client with Alzheimer's dementia: A case study. *Music Therapy Perspectives, 9*, 102–105.

Loesin, R. G. R. (1988). Effects of preferred music and guided imagery music on the pain of selected postoperative patients. *ANPHI Papers, 23*(1), 2–4.

Lord, T. R., and Garner, J. E. (1993). Effects of music on Alzheimer patients. *Perceptual and Motor Skills, 76*, 451–455.

Magill-Levreault, L. (1993). Music therapy in pain and symptom management. *Journal of Palliative Care, 9*(4), 42–49.

Maultsby, M. (1977). Combining music therapy with rational behavior therapy. *Journal of Music Therapy, 14*(2), 89–96.

McCloskey, J. C., and Bulechek, G. M. (Eds.). (1996). *Nursing interventions classification (NIC)* (2nd ed.). St. Louis: Mosby-Year Book.

McCloskey, L. J. (1990, Winter). The silent heart sings. *Generations*, 63–65.

McIntosh, G. C., Brown, S. H., Rice, R. R., and Thaut, M. H. (1997). Rhythmic auditory-motor facilitation of gait patterns in patients with Parkinson's disease. *Journal of Neurology, Neurosurgery, and Psychiatry, 62*(1), 22–26.

McMahon, T. (1978). Music therapy for training and growth. *Australian Nurses Journal, 7*(11), 5–6.

Millard, K. A., and Smith, J. M. (1989). The influence of group singing therapy on the behavior of Alzheimer's disease patients. *Journal of Music Therapy, 16*(2), 58–70.

Milner, B. (1971). Interhemispheric differences in the localization of psychological processes in man. *British Medical Bulletin, 27*, 1172–1277.

Mornhinweg, G. C. (1992). Effects of music preference and selection on stress reduction. *Journal of Holistic Nursing, 10*(2), 101–109.

Mornhinweg, G. C., and Voiginer, R. R. (1995). Music for sleep disturbances in the elderly. *Journal of Holistic Nursing, 13*, 248–254.

Mullooly, V. M., Levin, R. F., and Feldman, H. R. (1988). Music for postoperative pain and anxiety. *Journal of the New York State Nurses Association, 19*(3), 4–7.

Munro, S., and Mount, B. (1978). Music therapy in palliative care. *CMA Journal, 119*, 1029–1034.

O'Kelley, S. (1996, February 8–9). Oral presentation at the Tenth Annual Joseph & Kathleen Bryan Alzheimer's Disease Research Center Conference, Duke University Medical Center, Durham, NC.

Paul, R., and Staudt, V. M. (1958). Music therapy for the mentally ill: 1. A historical sketch and a brief review of the literature on the physiological effects and an analysis of the elements of music. *Journal of General Psychology, 59,* 167–176.

Peden, A. R. (1993). Music: Making the connection with persons who are homeless. *Journal of Psychosocial Nursing and Mental Health Services, 31,* 17–31.

Peretti, P. (1975). Changes in galvanic skin response as affected by musical selection, sex, and academic discipline. *Journal of Psychosocial Nursing and Mental Health Services, 89,* 183–187.

Petsche, H., Lindner, K., Rappelsberger, P., and Gruber, G. (1988). The EEG—an adequate method to concretize brain processes elicited by music. *Music Perceptions, 6*(2), 133–159.

Pfaff, V. K., Smith, K. E., and Gowan, D. (1989). The effects of music-assisted relaxation on the distress of pediatric cancer patients undergoing bone marrow aspirations. *Child Health Care, 18*(4), 232–236.

Pickerell, K. L., Metzger, J. T., Wilde, N. J., Broadbent, T.R., and Edwards, B. F. (1954). The use and therapeutic value of music in the hospital and operating room. In E. Podolsky (Ed.), *Music therapy.* New York: Philosophical Library.

Radin, P. (1948). Music and medicine among primitive peoples. In D. Schullian and M. Schoen (Eds.), *Music as medicine.* New York: Henry Schuman.

Ragneskog, H., Brane, S., Karlsson, I., and Kihlgren, M. (1996). Influence of dinner music on food intake and symptoms common in dementia. *Scandinavian Journal of Caring Science, 10*(1), 11–7.

Ragneskog, H., Kihlgren, M., Karlsson, I., and Norberg, A. (1996). Dinner music for demented patients: Analysis of video-recorded observations. *Clinical Nursing Research, 5,* 262–282.

Rauscher, F. H., Shaw, G. L., and Ky, K. N. (1993). Music and spatial task performance. *Nature, 6447,* 611.

Reisberg, B., Ferris, S. H., deLeon, M. J., and Crook, T. (1982). The global deterioration scale for assessment of primary degenerative dementia. *American Journal of Psychiatry, 139,* 1136–1139.

Salmon, D. (1993). Music and emotion in palliative care. *Journal of Palliative Care, 9*(4), 42–48.

Schorr, J. A. (1993). Music and pattern change in chronic pain. *Advanced Nursing Science, 15*(4), 27–36.

Schullian, D., and Schoen, M. (Eds.). (1948). *Music as medicine.* New York: Henry Schuman.

Scott, T. J. (1970). The use of music to reduce hyperactivity in children. *American Journal of Orthopsychiatry, 40,* 677–680.

Sears, W. W. (1968). Process in music therapy. In E. T. Gaston (Ed.), *Music in therapy* (pp. 30–44). New York: Macmillan Company.

Shatin, L. (1970). Alteration of mood via music: A study of the vectoring effect. *Journal of Psychology, 75,* 81–86.

Smith, G. H. (1986). A comparison of the effects of three treatment interventions on cognitive functioning of Alzheimer's patients. *Music Therapy, 6A*(1), 41–56.

Standley, J. M., and Moore, R. S. (1995). Therapeutic effects of music and mother's voice on premature infants. *Pediatric Nursing, 21,* 509–512.

Stanton, H. E. (1975). Music and test anxiety: Further evidence for an interaction. *British Journal of Educational Psychology, 45,* 80–82.

Steelman, V. M. (1990). Intraoperative music therapy: Effects on anxiety, blood pressure. *AORN Journal, 52,* 1026–1028.

Stevens, K. (1990). Patients' perceptions of music during surgery. *Journal of Advanced Nursing, 15,* 1045–1051.

Stoudenmire, J. (1975). A comparison of muscle relaxation training and music in the reduction of state and trait anxiety. *Journal of Clinical Psychology, 31,* 490–492.

Stratton, V. N., and Zalanowski, A. H. (1984). The relationship between music, degree of liking, and self-reported relaxation. *Journal of Music Therapy, 21*(4), 184–192.

Summers, S., Hoffman, J., Neff, E. J. A., Hanson, S., and Pierce, K. (1990). The effects of 60 beats per minute music on test taking anxiety among nursing students. *Journal of Nursing Education, 29*(2), 66–70.

Taylor, D. B. (1989). A neuroanatomical model for the use of music in the remediation of aphasic disorders. In M. H. M. Lee (Ed.), *Rehabilitation, music and human well-being* (pp. 168–178). St. Louis: MMB Music.

Updike, P. (1990). Music therapy results for ICU patients. *Dimensions of Critical Care Nursing, 9*(1), 39–45.

Van de Wall, W. (1946). *Music in hospitals.* New York: Russell Sage Foundation.

Whipple, B., and Glynn, N. J. (1992). Quantification of the effects of listening to music as a noninvasive method of pain control. *Scholarly Inquiry for Nursing Practice, 6*(1), 43–62.

White, J. M. (1992). Music therapy: An intervention to reduce anxiety in the myocardial infarction patient. *Clinical Nurse Specialist, 6*(2), 58–63.

Winter, M. J., Paskin, S., and Baker, T. (1994). Music reduces stress and anxiety of patients in the surgical holding area. *Journal of Post Anesthesia Nursing, 9,* 340–343.

Zimmerman, L. M., Pierson, M. A., and Marker, J. (1988). Effects of music on patients in coronary care units. *Heart and Lung, 17,* 560–566.

Zimmerman, L., Pozehl, B., Duncan, K., and Schmitz, R. (1989). Effects of music in patients who had chronic cancer pain. *Western Journal of Nursing Research, 11,* 298–309.

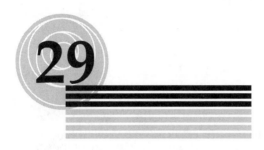

Health Education

Mary Lober Aquilino

The ends of health education are achieved best where they are harnessed to the felt needs and motivations of the community itself.

Guy W. Steuart

Health Education, an essential component of comprehensive health care, is a strategy aimed at reducing morbidity and mortality and enhancing wellness by influencing lifestyle choices. The Nursing Interventions Classification (NIC) defines Health Education as "developing and providing instruction and learning experiences to facilitate voluntary adaptation of behavior conducive to health in individuals, families, groups, or communities" (McCloskey & Bulechek, 1996). This includes making appropriate health-related decisions regarding personal behavior, use of health resources, and involvement in societal health efforts such as influencing health policy and contributing to health-related causes (Clark, 1996).

Health Education differs from patient teaching in that, although it ultimately affects the individual, it is designed for delivery to groups and focuses on health promotion and disease prevention, not disease treatment. It is primarily concerned with enabling decision making by elucidating motivation, attitudes, values, and beliefs rather than merely dispensing information. In addition, Health Education emphasizes client responsibility for health and involves an ongoing process, not a one-time encounter (Smith & Maurer, 1995; Whitman, Graham, Gleit, & Boyd, 1992).

Health Education is an integral part of professional nursing practice. In the role of health educator, nurses serve as consultants or advocates ensuring that clients are knowledgeable of the facts, are motivated and mobilized to act, and are supported in their efforts to change behavior. The nurse guides individuals or groups in examining their own health values and suggests means for achievement of client-desired outcomes (Whitman et al., 1992).

RELATED RESEARCH

Theoretical Underpinnings

Health Education is both a field of study and a health intervention. The concepts and theories of many disciplines, including sociology, psychology, education, and the health sciences, support Health Education. Related concepts include health, health promotion, disease prevention, learning, health behavior, health beliefs, health values, self-care, self-efficacy, and empowerment (Abrams, Emmons, & Linnan, 1997; Glanz, Lewis, & Rimer, 1997; Nutbeam, 1996).

Many of these concepts and theories have been incorporated into models useful for planning and delivering Health Education programs, including the health belief model, the health promotion model, and the PRECEDE/PROCEED model. A very brief description of each of these models follows.

The health belief model was developed more than 30 years ago as a framework for examining the reasons some individuals take actions to avoid illness or to minimize health risks, whereas others fail to do so. It is based on three factors: (1) the individual's readiness to consider behavioral change, (2) the existence and power of environmental forces that influence behavior change, and (3) the actual behaviors (Dignan & Carr, 1992). According to this model, individual perceptions of susceptibility to disease and severity of disease affect the perceived threat of disease, which in turn influences the likelihood that an individual will heed a recommended preventive health action. It also takes into account modifying variables such as age, gender, social class, and cues to action that influence these individual perceptions (Dignan & Carr, 1992).

The health promotion model, introduced 20 years later, is a representation of the complex biopsychosocial processes that motivate individuals to engage in behaviors directed toward the enhancement of health. It integrates constructs from expectancy-value theory and social cognitive theory and is based on assumptions that emphasize the active role of the client in shaping and maintaining health behaviors and in modifying the environmental context for health behaviors. Unlike the health belief model, it is approach oriented (Pender, 1996).

The PRECEDE/PROCEED model is an intervention model that provides a structure for identifying variables related to health problems, health behaviors, and program implementation. The model depicts the steps involved in designing, implementing, and evaluating a Health Education program, in addition to describing the interrelatedness of the variables. This model was designed specifically for program development (Dignan & Carr, 1992).

Health Education Programs

Examples of Health Education programs are prevalent not only in the nursing literature but also in literature pertaining to medicine, public health, and the social sciences. The topics of Health Education programs are frequently dictated by the actual, leading, or suspected causes of disability and death and the evidence that changes in lifestyle behavior can affect the occurrence or course of disease. Currently, the actual causes of morbidity and mortality include tobacco use, diet and activity patterns, alcohol use, microbial agents, toxic agents, firearms, sexual behavior, motor vehicles, and illicit drug use (McGinnis & Foege, 1993).

Table 29–1 presents examples of Health Education topics related to these causes of disability or death, with suggested groups to target for intervention.

Table 29–1 Examples of Health Education Topics and Related Target Groups

Topics	Target Group
Nutrition	Preschoolers
Smoking	School-age children
Sexual behavior	Adolescents
Workplace safety	Young adults
Exercise	Adults
Home safety	Older adults
Infection control	Child care workers
Heart-healthy behaviors	Community—all ages

Ethical Considerations

As health educators, nurses have certain ethical responsibilities. The first is possession of current, accurate, and unbiased health information. Is the health behavior change that is being promoted supported by rigorous ongoing research or merely by one greatly publicized study? Premature recommendations to adopt health-related behaviors have previously met with lack of success, frequent reversals of advice, and unfulfilled promises concerning what the behaviors would achieve for the adopters (Becker, 1993).

Responsible health educators not only ensure that presentations are evidence based and unexaggerated, but also ensure that the meaning and significance of the information provided is well understood by the recipient. Temptation to be self-righteous or paternalistic must be resisted when helping people comprehend the implications of their health decisions and choices. It is preferable to use values clarification instead of indoctrination and to guide decision making rather than advance personal positions. In short, health educators must avoid coercion, persuasion, or manipulation in an effort to promote client responsibility and empowerment (Becker, 1993; Sharkey, Graham-Kresge, & White, 1995).

Health educators must also be aware of the social, cultural, and political environment of the individuals or groups to be educated. Becker (1993) argues that because health habits are acquired within social groups such as families or communities, personal behavior is not usually the primary determinant of health status. He blames the individual-responsibility approach for establishing "health as a New Morality by which character and personal worth are judged." Lowenberg (1995) supports this argument in her warning concerning "the ideology of choice," which reflects predominant views that individuals are "responsible for" and "choose" their disease. These arguments give credence to group and community approaches to Health Education that address the contextual determinants of morbidity and mortality.

Finally, health educators are responsible for protecting individual rights, treating people equally, ensuring privacy and confidentiality, and obtaining informed consent (Breckon, Harvey, & Lancaster, 1994). Health Education should be available to all people regardless of race, geography, or socioeconomic situation. These ethical considerations are consistent with the NIC definition that charges the health educator "to facilitate the *voluntary* adaptation of behavior conducive to health in individuals, families, groups, or communities [emphasis added]."

Future Directions

Renewed interest in prevention of disease and disability through lifestyle change has drawn attention to the need for quality Health Education programs. Current changes in the health care system are providing additional supports and opportunities for such programs. At the same time, emphasis is shifting from individual behaviors bearing the full responsibility for health to broader social and economic determinants. Moving Health Education toward social action is foreseeable and consistent with its historical roots (Glanz et al., 1997; McKinley, 1996).

Other future challenges for health educators include the need to develop culturally sensitive educational materials and media messages as well as new strategies for dissemination of information and delivery of interventions. There is a continuing need to rectify the disparity in death and disability rates faced by low-income and minority groups. This can be achieved only through special emphasis on the health needs of these groups and increased efforts in reaching the disenfranchised. Because technology such as computers and even telephones does not reach a sizable portion of the population, other strategies must be used. In addition, the relevance of topics continually changes. There will be a need to focus more attention on the health of the elderly as the population ages. Futurists predict that lifestyles will become more isolated, leading to increased need for mental health interventions. Anticipating the Health Education needs of various segments of the population is critical to successful intervention.

Health Education has already experienced an increased use of technology. Computers are now being used to analyze nutrients in the diet, design and monitor weight-loss programs, and perform health risk appraisals. Fiberoptic networks and the Internet allow exchange of ideas over great distances and in remote locations. Mass media are bursting with health messages and opportunities for interaction through radio and television talk shows. As the use of technology increases, the challenge for the health educator is to help the client filter the available health information, because the integrity and the quality of the message are sometimes lost (Abrams et al., 1997; Breckon et al., 1994; Gott, 1995).

USING NIC ACTIVITIES

Table 29–2 presents the NIC intervention Health Education. To facilitate discussion of the Health Education activities, they have been categorized into targeting, program development, program implementation, program evaluation, and gaining external support. Each NIC activity is discussed within this framework.

Targeting

Targeting, a salient feature of Health Education, requires the nurse to examine data regarding the leading causes of morbidity and mortality for a given segment of the population defined by such characteristics as age, gender, ethnicity, occupation, or lifestyle. These data are derived from aggregate and population assessments at the community, state, national, and global levels. There is a plethora of health data available through local and state governments, departments of public health, national organizations such as the Centers for Disease Control and Prevention (CDC), and international organizations such as the World Health Organization (WHO).

During the 1990s, the U.S. Department of Health and Human Services (USDHHS) facilitated the development of national health promotion and disease prevention guidelines that are delineated in *Healthy People 2000: National Health Promotion and Disease Prevention Objectives*. The hope is that use of these guide-

Table 29-2 Health Education

DEFINITION: Developing and providing instruction and learning experiences to facilitate voluntary adaptation of behavior conducive to health in individuals, families, groups, or communities.

ACTIVITIES:

Target high-risk groups and age ranges that would benefit most from health education

Target needs identified in *Healthy People 2000—National Health Promotion and Disease Prevention Objectives* or other local, state, and national needs

Identify internal or external factors that may enhance or reduce motivation for healthful behavior

Determine personal context and sociocultural history of individual, family, or community health behavior

Determine current health knowledge and life-style behaviors of individual, family, or target group

Assist individuals, families, and communities in clarifying health beliefs and values

Identify characteristics of target population that affect selection of learning strategies

Prioritize identified learner needs based on client preference, skills of nurse, resources available, and likelihood of successful goal attainment

Formulate objectives for health education program

Identify resources (e.g., personnel, space, equipment, and money) needed to conduct program

Consider accessibility, consumer preference, and cost in program planning

Strategically place attractive advertising to capture attention of target audience

Avoid use of fear or scare techniques as strategy to motivate people to change health or life-style behaviors

Emphasize immediate or short-term positive health benefits to be received by positive life-style behaviors, rather than long-term benefits or negative effects of noncompliance

Incorporate strategies to enhance the self-esteem of target audience

Develop educational materials written at a readability level appropriate to target audience

Teach strategies that can be used to resist unhealthful behavior or risk taking, rather than give advice to avoid or change behavior

Keep presentation focused, short, and beginning and ending on main point

Use group presentations to provide support, and lessen threat to learners experiencing similar problems or concerns, as appropriate

Use peer leaders, teachers, and support groups in implementing programs to groups less likely to listen to health professionals or adults (i.e., adolescents), as appropriate

Use lectures to convey the maximal amount of information, when appropriate

Use group discussions and role playing to influence health beliefs, attitudes, and values

Use demonstrations/return demonstrations, learner participation, and manipulation of materials when teaching psychomotor skills

Use computer-assisted instruction, television, interactive video, and other technologies to convey information

Use teleconferencing, telecommunications, and computer technologies for distance learning

Involve individuals, families, and groups in planning and implementing plans for life-style or health behavior modification

Determine family, peer, and community support for behavior conducive to health

Use social and family support systems to enhance effectiveness of life-style or health behavior modification

Emphasize importance of healthful patterns of eating, sleeping, exercising, and so on, to individuals, families, and groups who model these values and behaviors to others, particularly children

Use variety of strategies and intervention points in educational program

Plan long-term follow-up to reinforce health behavior or life-style adaptations

Design and implement strategies to measure client outcomes at regular intervals during and after completion of program

Design and implement strategies to measure program and cost-effectiveness of education, using this data to improve the effectiveness of subsequent programs

Influence development of policy that guarantees health education as an employee benefit

Encourage policy whereby insurance companies give consideration for premium reductions or benefits for healthful life-style practices

Source: McCloskey, J. C., and Bulechek, G. M. (Eds). (1996). *Nursing interventions classification (NIC)* (2nd ed.). St. Louis: Mosby–Year Book.

lines will "reduce preventable disease and disability, enhance quality of life, and reduce disparities in the health status of populations within our society" (USDHHS, 1991, p. 1). Individual states and communities have used these guidelines to develop similar objectives based on their needs.

The broad national goals cited in *Healthy People 2000* are to increase the span of healthy life for Americans, reduce health disparities among Americans, and achieve access to preventive services for all Americans. Objectives are grouped into the three broad categories of health promotion, health protection, and preventive services. Health Education is an integral part of efforts in all three areas. In particular, health promotion is concerned with lifestyle choices and the social context in which such decisions are made. Priority areas include physical activity and fitness, nutrition, tobacco, alcohol and drugs, family planning, mental health and mental disorders, and violent and abusive behavior. Health protection encompasses environmental and regulatory measures that confer protection on large population groups. Areas addressed include unintentional injuries, occupational safety and health, food and drug safety, and oral health. Objectives in this area focus on community approaches to protecting health. The third category of preventive services includes counseling, screening, immunization, and chemoprophylactic interventions for individuals in clinical settings. Priority areas include maternal and infant health, heart disease and stroke, diabetes and chronic disabling conditions, human immunodeficiency virus (HIV) infection, sexually transmitted diseases, and infectious diseases. The health needs of all age groups are represented. These objectives provide guidance in selecting worthy targets for health education and guidelines for measuring outcomes. The following are examples of *Healthy People 2000* objectives potentially related to Health Education:

1. Increase to at least 30% the proportion of people aged 6 and older who engage regularly, preferably daily, in light to moderate physical activity for at least 30 minutes per day.
2. Reduce cigarette smoking to a prevalence of no more than 15% among people aged 20 and older.
3. Reduce by 20% the proportion of people who possess weapons that are inappropriately stored and therefore dangerously available (USDHHS, 1991).

Program Development

CONSIDERING TARGET GROUP CHARACTERISTICS

Identification of factors that will affect both participation in Health Education activities and the outcome of that participation is essential to program success. Individual, family, and community factors include beliefs, values, knowledge, skills, positive and negative incentives, lifestyle, and socioeconomic status. Identification and prioritization of beliefs and values are critical to Health Education outcomes. The nurse must recognize that deep-seated beliefs and values are not easily changed and that attempts to encourage behavior that is in conflict with these beliefs and values may lead to superficial versus intrinsic behavior change.

In addition to beliefs and values, the knowledge and skills that an individual, group, or community possesses will influence the nature of the Health Education program. Health educators need to assess how much is already known about a given topic and whether or not misinformation exists. The cognitive and physical developmental levels of the target group must also be determined in order to design instruction that can be understood and acted on. For example, the elderly tend to learn more slowly, and children are sometimes more comfortable with computer-aided instruction than are adults. Most learners benefit from visual cues and hands-on experience, yet modifications may need to be made for physically or mentally challenged individuals.

Receptivity to the information presented depends on relevance to the learner. Learners must feel both a need for information and a desire to change behavior in order for the intervention to be successful. Receptivity may depend on the individual's current state or perception of health and emotional readiness. This sometimes demands capturing the "teachable moment." It is likely that an individual will take a closer look at exercise, diet, and smoking immediately after a cardiac arrest. Similarly, communities are more likely to initiate and attend to education regarding proper handling of food after an outbreak of *Escherichia coli* infection or hepatitis.

Health educators need to recognize sociocultural influences on individuals, families, and communities. Educational programs need to be sensitive to primary language, literacy, and cultural or religious beliefs and values. Use of educational materials that are uninterpretable or in conflict with personal beliefs will fail to achieve the desired outcome (Murray & Zentner, 1997; Smith & Maurer, 1995).

ELICITING SUPPORT

One of the first steps in the development of a Health Education program is to recruit planning group members. An important consideration in selecting a planning group is inclusion of representatives of the target population. Participation of target group members in the planning process ensures that the ideas and desires of the target group will be represented and increases the likelihood that the target group will ultimately support the program (Dignan & Carr, 1992).

INSTRUCTIONAL DESIGN

In designing a Health Education program, the needs of the learners should be prioritized in collaboration with the target group. This will increase the likelihood of participation and support for the program. In addition to health educator skills, available resources, and potential for success, prioritization can be based on the urgency of the problem or the potential for certain interventions to address multiple needs. For example, a contaminated water supply is generally a more urgent problem than motor vehicle safety.

Educational objectives should clearly state what the target audience of the educational program should know or in what way they should behave differently following the intervention. The objectives serve as the framework for the Health Education program. In developing and stating learning objectives, it is important to identify the type of learning expected. There are three types or domains of learning objectives—cognitive, psychomotor, and affective—and each domain can be further delineated into subcategories. Objectives should be stated precisely and in measurable terms. The *Healthy People 2000* objectives stated previously are good examples of usable objectives.

Using the program objectives as a guide, materials and personnel required for developing, maintaining, and evaluating the Health Education objectives must be identified. Personnel include administrative support and technical assistance staff, as well as those who will implement the intervention. It is necessary to be very specific regarding the number and types of people, the equipment, the physical space, and the supplies needed. Coordinating efforts with other related activities can sometimes minimize resource needs. Numerous local, state, and national organizations and agencies, both private and public, offer materials for Health Education that have been developed for both the educator and the learner. Included are pamphlets, videos, posters, models, and computer software that are frequently available for free or for a nominal cost.

Health Education is more than presentation of information. It includes continuing clarification of values and reinforcement of efforts to reduce risk and maintain health. Adoption of healthy behaviors such as smoking cessation, weight reduction, and regular exercise does not usually occur without great effort and encouragement over an extended period of time. The role of the health educator is to guide the individuals or groups undertaking health behavior changes by providing accurate and useful information and ongoing support. It takes the average smoker several attempts before actually quitting smoking. Similarly, although most dieters are able to shed extra pounds, few are able to maintain a healthy weight for more than a year after the initial weight loss. Thus, providing realistic goals and regular follow-up for such Health Education efforts is critical to success.

Program Implementation

PUBLIC RELATIONS AND MARKETING

Public relations and marketing are not usually part of the repertoire of the nurse. However, the success of Health Education programs is largely dependent on reaching and engaging the intended audience. Programs that are not known cannot be used. Marketing lets people know what services are available and how to use them. In addition, decision makers need to know about the benefits of programs to be encouraged to provide financial support (Breckon et al., 1994).

Public relations is a management tool designed to improve people's opinions of programs or agencies. Because a press agent or public relations director is not always available or affordable, a staff member can be trained for this task. An effective public relations program (1) involves the entire organization, (2) is consistently supported by the program administrator, (3) demands that a single person be responsible for coordination, and (4) relies heavily on personal contact and a positive working relationship with members of the media (Breckon et al., 1994).

Marketing involves determining the orientation of consumer groups toward programs or products in order to select those most likely to succeed. With little concern about opinions, marketing works to determine what people want or need. It requires assessing the environment in which the program under consideration will be introduced, determining competing influences, and developing a strategic plan for implementation (Breckon et al., 1994). Marketing questions that the planner of a Health Education program might ask include the following: Where do teenagers hang out? What magazines do people older than 65 read? Who reads bulletin boards at the library? What time of day do children watch television? Is there a local event scheduled at the same time as a Health Education offering that will either enhance or diminish attendance?

MOTIVATION AND SUPPORT IN BEHAVIOR CHANGE

Fear of an event that is perceived as distant or unlikely does not usually increase healthy behavior. In fact, intense fear can actually immobilize an individual, limiting the ability to even attend to the unhealthy behavior. However, likely and immediate negative consequences do result in more favorable health practices. For example, increased seat belt use has more to do with concern about fines than with avoiding injury or death. In addition, it is preferable to state the consequences of health-related behaviors in the positive. Certain individuals are more likely to refrain from smoking because of a desire to breathe more efficiently or to have whiter teeth now than because of a fear of future disability (Job, 1988).

Changing attitudes regarding health behaviors is often the most difficult challenge. Because individuals tend to adopt the attitudes of family and friends, it is important to include significant others in the Health Education process. This includes not only assessing the values and beliefs of the family and community of which the target individuals are a part, but also eliciting the help of these support systems in implementing and sustaining health behavior changes. Changing the contents of the home refrigerator or adding reduced-fat items to the local restaurant menu are as important to healthy eating behaviors as is patient education regarding dietary fat.

EDUCATIONAL/TEACHING STRATEGIES

Strategies for providing Health Education are limited only by the creativity of the program designer. However, as mentioned previously, it is critical to match the strategy to the target group, considering such factors as group size, age, and gender. The medium for delivery is often as critical as the message. Television is appropriate for relaying certain information to certain groups, whereas personal contact is preferable for others. In this age of technology and information explosion, getting people to attend to and have confidence in the health information presented is often a challenge. A 30-second public service announcement may gain attention, but reinforcement strategies might be required to convince people of the validity of the message. Mass media—newspapers, radios, television, the World Wide Web—generally work best when (1) the message is simple and factual, (2) the change is close to present practice or directed to those already motivated to change, (3) the target group is highly educated, and (4) the desired decisions are short term. Examples of media messages include news releases, press conferences, public service announcements, and short advertisements through the radio, newspapers, billboards, posters, brochures, or newsletters.

The latest technologies used in health promotion and disease prevention efforts are those that involve the use of computers and modems that allow global communication and instant access to health information and consultation. An example is E ZOOT, a multiline electronic bulletin board system developed in Canada aimed at promoting adolescent health. This system allows users to exchange health-related information with volunteer moderators or other participants and view or download health-related files that are collected and transcribed by a systems operator. This medium allows not only the distribution of health information but also personal interaction through moderated discussion and counseling. Preliminary evaluations of this new technology are promising (Gott, 1995).

Program Evaluation

Evaluation continues to present an enormous challenge to health educators. "The quality of evaluation in health education has been an important obstacle to better interventions and wider acknowledgment of the importance of health education in improving public health" (Nutbeam, Smith, & Catford, 1996). There seem to be more questions than answers. Should process or product, direct or indirect indicators, knowledge, attitudes, or behaviors be measured? Should evaluation occur during or following the intervention, how many times, and at what intervals? Finally, with the number of extraneous factors that are difficult to control, how can change be attributed to the program itself? (Abrams et al., 1997; Dignan & Carr, 1992).

Recently, attention has been focused on economic indicators of success, such as cost-benefit and cost-effectiveness. This increases the challenge from merely demonstrating that the program produced the desired effect to showing that the benefits derived from the intervention were worth the expenditure and that there is no other intervention that can achieve similar results at a lower cost (Dignan, 1995; Macdonald, Veen, & Tones, 1996; Phillips & Holtgrave, 1997).

Gaining External Support for Health Education

In the role of the health educator, the nurse must continue to be an advocate for health-related initiatives. Staying informed concerning policy issues related to Health Education, campaigning, and contacting lawmakers or other decision makers are essential to supporting the changes necessary for improving Health Education. This includes rallying for Health Education funding as well as work-site and community policies that enhance or support Health Education efforts. It may be as simple as convincing an employer to increase the number of breaks for pregnant employees or as complex as developing legislation regarding water quality.

ASSOCIATED NURSING DIAGNOSES AND APPROPRIATE CLIENT GROUPS

Health Education is an intervention that can be carried out almost anywhere with any group of individuals that is willing and cognitively able to comprehend and respond to a given message or program. This includes the majority of the population from preschool to late adulthood who live and work in a variety of settings including homes, schools, communities, work sites, health care sites, and the consumer marketplace (Glanz et al., 1997). Audiences include not only

Table 29–3 NANDA Nursing Diagnoses Associated with Health Education

Ineffective Community Coping
Potential for Enhanced Community Coping
Ineffective Management of Therapeutic Regimen, Community
Altered Health Maintenance
Health Seeking Behaviors (Specify)
Effective Management of Therapeutic Regimen, Individual
Risk for Injury
Knowledge Deficit (Specify)
Noncompliance (Specify)
Risk for Trauma
Risk for Infection
Nutrition
Risk for Altered Parenting
Ineffective Management of Therapeutic Regimen, Family
Ineffective Management of Therapeutic Regimen, Individual

Source: North American Nursing Diagnosis Association (NANDA). (1994). *Nursing diagnosis: Definitions and classification, 1995–1996.* Philadelphia: Author.

segments of the population at risk for disease or in search of healthier lifestyles but also people who influence the health of others, such as parents, teachers, health care providers, and politicians.

A list of current North American Nursing Diagnosis Association (NANDA) nursing diagnoses that are related to Health Education appears in Table 29–3. Although this list includes many of the potential diagnoses, others will undoubtedly be added as nurses focus on the aggregate as the unit of nursing care.

ASSOCIATED OUTCOMES

Most of the direct outcomes of Health Education fall in the "health knowledge and behavior" domain of the nursing outcomes taxonomy (Iowa Outcomes Project, 1997). Included in this domain are the classes of health behavior, health beliefs, health knowledge, and risk control and safety. In addition, outcomes from the functional health domain in the classes of growth and development, those in the physiological domain in the classes of immune response and nutrition, those in the psychosocial health domain in the classes of psychological well-being and social interaction, those in the perceived health domain in the classes of health and life quality, and those in the family health domain in the classes of family caregiver status and maltreatment resolution are also related to Health Education. Table 29–4 presents the outcome labels from these domains. Indirectly, Health Education can be linked to most health outcomes.

Table 29–4 NOC Outcomes Associated with Health Education

Abuse Protection	Immunization Behavior
Adherence Behavior	Knowledge: Breastfeeding
Child Development: 2 months	Knowledge: Child Safety
Child Development: 4 months	Knowledge: Diet
Child Development: 6 months	Knowledge: Disease Process
Child Development: 12 months	Knowledge: Energy Conservation
Child Development: 2 years	Knowledge: Health Behaviors
Child Development: 3 years	Knowledge: Health Resources
Child Development: 4 years	Knowledge: Infection Control
Child Development: 5 years	Knowledge: Medication
Child Development: Middle Childhood (6–11 years)	Knowledge: Personal Safety
	Knowledge: Prescribed Activity
Child Development: Adolescence (12–17 years)	Knowledge: Substance Use Control
	Knowledge: Treatment Procedure(s)
Compliance Behavior	Knowledge: Treatment Regimen
Decision Making	Leisure Participation
Health Beliefs	Parenting
Health Beliefs: Perceived Ability to Perform	Risk Control
	Risk Control: Alcohol Use
Health Beliefs: Perceived Control	Risk Control: Drug Use
Health Beliefs: Perceived Resources	Risk Control: Sexually Transmitted Diseases (STD)
Health Beliefs: Perceived Threat	Risk Control: Tobacco Use
Health Orientation	Risk Control: Unintended Pregnancy
Health Promoting Behavior	Risk Detection
Health Seeking Behavior	Well-Being

Source: Johnson, M., and Maas, M. (Eds.). (1997). *Nursing outcomes classification (NOC).* St. Louis: Mosby–Year Book.

CASE STUDIES

There are numerous examples of Health Education interventions that have been developed and implemented by nurses and other health educators. The following examples have been chosen as case studies because the reports include outcome evaluations. Although it is not always feasible to design rigorously controlled studies of each Health Education program delivered, it is difficult to demonstrate the effectiveness of the intervention without such a design.

Case Study 1—Sun Safety

Program Design

Twelve classes of 4- to 5-year-olds were recruited from local preschools, and each class was randomly assigned to an intervention or control group. The intervention group received a sun safety curriculum, and the control group did not. All children were pretested at the onset of the study and tested again at 2 and 7 weeks after the intervention.

Health Education Intervention: Sun Safety Curriculum

Sun safety was defined as the development and practice of positive health habits aimed at protecting skin and staying healthy. Three units, each addressing a simple sun safety concept—cover up, find shade, and ask for sun-safe things (e.g., sunscreen, sunglasses)—were presented to the intervention groups. Presenters of the units received special training. Units were team taught using two teachers per session, and one session (unit) was presented on each of 3 consecutive days. Activities included puppet shows, games, art activities, and songs and storybooks on sun safety, and key characters "Sunny the Bear" and "Shadow the Frog" conveyed and reinforced sun-safe messages in all activities. Units were developmentally based and age appropriate, with objectives focusing on children's cognition and attitudes concerning sun safety. Parents received parallel educational material.

Rationale

Research evidence supported both the intervention and the curriculum content. First, excessive exposure to solar radiation is known to play a role in the etiology of skin cancers, and a link may exist between severe sunburn in childhood and greatly increased risk of skin cancers later in life. Second, behaviors adopted during childhood are likely to carry over to later life. In addition, many skin cancers can be prevented by practicing such behaviors as reducing sun exposure during peak hours of intensity, wearing protective apparel, and regularly applying sunscreen.

Evaluation

Children were questioned by trained interviewers using pictures to which children would point or make limited responses. This format was chosen based on the developmental level of the children. There was no attempt to measure behavior, just knowledge.

Results

The curriculum had a significant effect on the knowledge and comprehension components of cognition. The application component of cognition was not significantly changed by the curriculum, possibly because of the preoperational developmental stage of the participants (Loescher, Emerson, Taylor, Christensen, & McKinney, 1995, pp. 939–943).

Case Study 2—Cardiovascular Risk Reduction

Program Design

Forty-six work sites were randomly assigned to one of the following two interventions:

1. A "usual" intervention of 5 minutes of counseling
2. 2 hours of behaviorally based education on dietary changes to lower serum cholesterol

Health Education Intervention

Workers were recruited to participate in the program by flyers, posters, and word-of-mouth within work sites. Workers with cholesterol levels of 200 mg or higher were invited to participate. The "usual" intervention consisted of 5 minutes of counseling immediately followed by cholesterol testing. It included American Heart Association (AHA) Step 1 diet education counseling and brochures describing the importance of reducing blood cholesterol by reducing fat in the diet. The education intervention was the same as the comparison program but included 2 hours of nutrition education delivered in multiple sessions over the next month, mostly at work during work times, and conducted in small groups by health professionals. The teaching was based on behavioral, skill-based principles and was designed to increase both knowledge and skills, including how to choose and prepare low-fat foods and the cholesterol-lowering effects of reduced fat in the diet.

Rationale

Research suggests that reducing blood cholesterol level can reduce the risk of coronary heart disease. In addition, providing work-site testing and education may attract a greater cross-section of adults in the community and provide better access to screening and education services.

Evaluation

Participant cholesterol levels were measured.

Results

Cholesterol levels differed little between the two intervention groups 6 months after screening, but after 12 months, those with the education intervention showed a 6.5% drop in cholesterol as compared with a 3% drop for the others. Nutritional education in work sites may be a useful way to lower the risk of heart disease (Byers et al., 1995).

References

Abrams, D., Emmons, K., and Linnan, L. (1997). Health behavior and health education: The past, present, and future. In K. Glanz, F. Lewis, and B. Rimer (Eds.), *Health behavior and health education: Theory, research and practice* (2nd ed., pp. 453–478). San Francisco: Jossey-Boss Publishers.

Becker, M. (1993). A medical sociologist looks at health behavior. *Journal of Health and Social Behavior, 34,* 1–6.

Breckon, D., Harvey, J., and Lancaster, R. (1994). *Community health education: Settings, roles, and skills for the 21st century* (3rd ed.). Gaithersburg, MD: Aspen Publishers.

Byers, T., Millis, R., Anderson, J., Dusenbury, L., Gorsky, R., Kimber, C., Krueger, S., Mokdad, A., and Perry, G. (1995). The costs and effects of a nutritional education program following work-site cholesterol screening. *American Journal of Public Health, 85,* 650–655.

Clark, M. (1996). *Nursing in the community* (2nd ed.). Stamford, CT: Appleton & Lange.

Dignan, M. (1995). *Measurement and evaluation of health education* (3rd ed.). Springfield, IL: Charles C Thomas.

Dignan, M., and Carr, P. (1992). *Program planning for health education and promotion* (2nd ed.). Philadelphia: Lea & Febiger.

Glanz, K., Lewis, F., and Rimer, B. (1997). The scope of health promotion and health education. In K. Glanz, F. Lewis, and B. Rimer (Eds.), *Health behavior and health education: Theory, research and practice* (2nd ed., pp. 3–18). San Francisco: Jossey-Boss Publishers.

Gott, M. (1995). *Telematics for health.* New York: Radcliff Medical Press.

Iowa Outcomes Project. (1997). *Taxonomy of nursing outcomes classification (NOC).* Iowa City, IA: University of Iowa College of Nursing.

Job, R. (1988). Effective and ineffective use of fear in health promotion campaigns. *American Journal of Health Promotion, 78*(2), 163–167.

Loescher, L., Emerson, J., Taylor, A., Christensen, D., and McKinney, M. (1995). Educating preschoolers about sun safety. *American Journal of Public Health, 85,* 939–943.

Lowenberg, J. (1995). Health promotion and the "ideology of choice." *Public Health Nursing, 12,* 319–323.

Macdonald, G., Veen, C., and Tones, K. (1996). Evidence for success in health promotion: Suggestions for improvement. *Health Education Research, 11,* 367–376.

McCloskey, J. C., and Bulechek, G. M. (Eds). (1996). *Nursing interventions classification (NIC)* (2nd ed.). St. Louis: Mosby–Year Book.

McGinnis, J., and Foege, W. (1993). Actual causes of death in the United States. *Journal of the American Medical Association, 270,* 2207–2212.

McKinley, J. (1996). Health promotion through health public policy: The contribution of complementary research methods. In Pan American Health Organization, *Health promotion: An anthology* (Scientific Publication No. 557). Washington, DC: World Health Organization.

Murray, R., and Zentner, J. (1997). *Health assessment and promotion strategies throughout the lifespan* (6th ed.). Stamford, CT: Appleton & Lange.

Nutbeam, D. (1996). Health promotion glossary. In Pan American Health Organization, *Health promotion: An anthology* (Scientific Publication No. 557). Washington, DC: World Health Organization.

Nutbeam, D., Smith, C., and Catford, J. (1996). Evaluation in health education: A review of progress, possibilities and problems. In Pan American Health Organization, *Health promotion: An anthology* (Scientific Publication No. 557). Washington, DC: World Health Organization.

Pender, N. (1996). *Health promotion in nursing practice* (3rd ed.). Stamford, CT: Appleton & Lange.

Phillips, K., and Holtgrave, D. (1997). Using cost-effectiveness/cost-benefit analysis to allocate health resources: A level playing field for prevention? *American Journal of Preventive Medicine, 13*(1), 18–25.

Sharkey, P., Graham-Kresge, S., and White, G. (1995). Defining health education: Health, values, and responsibility. *Health Values, 19*(6), 23–29.

Smith, C., and Maurer, F. (Eds.). (1995). *Community health nursing: Theory and practice.* Philadelphia: W.B. Saunders.

U.S. Department of Health and Human Services (USDHHS). (1991). *Healthy people 2000: National health promotion and disease prevention objectives* (USDHHS Publication No. (PHS) 91-50012). Washington, DC: Author.

Whitman, N., Graham, B., Gleit, C., and Boyd, M. (1992). *Teaching in nursing practice: A professional model* (2nd ed.). Norwalk, CT: Appleton & Lange.

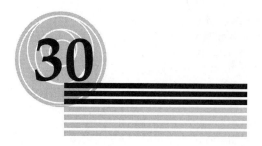

Substance Use Prevention

Julia Hagemaster

Substance abuse is acknowledged as the number-one health problem in this country, placing a tremendous burden on the nation's health care system and causing health care costs to spiral (Horgan, 1993). More than $150 billion is spent each year on alcohol and drugs, and more than $120 billion is paid by society in health care expenses and decreased work productivity (National Nurses Society on Addictions [NNSA], 1994). All aspects of public and private life are affected in terms of harm to family, economy, public safety, the workplace, disadvantaged groups, and the future of young people. Substance abuse accounts for more deaths, illnesses, and disabilities than any other preventable condition. In fact, one in four of the 2 million U.S. deaths each year are related to alcohol, illicit drug, or tobacco use (Horgan, 1993).

Although the use and misuse of substances can be traced back thousands of years, alcohol, tobacco, and other drug abuse (ATODA) has fluctuated throughout this century in response to changes in public tolerance and political activities (Horgan, 1993; Sullivan, 1995). Alcohol consumption reached its peaks during war years (the Civil War, World War I, World War II) and its lowest points during Prohibition and the Depression. During the 1990s, its use declined because of the raising of the minimum drinking age to 21 and the shift from consumption of distilled spirits to consumption of beer and wine, which have lower ethanol content. The latest indices, however, are pointing toward a new rise in use of alcohol. The history of illicit drug use is also marked by shifts in public attitudes and policies; illicit drug use peaked in the late 1970s for most drugs and declined in most segments of the population during the 1980s and 1990s. There is continued concern over the use of marijuana and cocaine and its derivative, "crack," especially considering the fact that declines in frequency of use since

1985 are not statistically significant (National Institute on Alcohol Abuse and Alcoholism [NIAAA], 1992). Regardless, trends show that frequent heavy use is unchanged; mortality related to ATODA remains high, especially for drug-related acquired immunodeficiency syndrome (AIDS) and drug-related crime (Horgan, 1993). This country has the highest rate of teenage alcohol and drug use of any industrialized nation in the world (NNSA, 1994).

There are some positive indicators. Much harm associated with substance abuse has been prevented through the combined efforts of federal, state, and local governments and private citizen groups, but there is still much to be done. The U.S. Department of Health and Human Services' (USDHHS) Public Health Service has addressed the need for decreasing ATODA through the government's *Healthy People 2000: National Health Promotion and Disease Prevention Objectives* (1991b). This set of objectives is aimed at decreasing the use of alcohol, illicit drugs, and tobacco in order to increase the span of healthy life for all Americans, to reduce health disparities among diverse population groups, and to achieve access to prevention services for everyone. Achieving these objectives depends on widespread support of prevention programs from health care professionals, community groups, businesses, and private citizens.

LITERATURE REVIEW

In 1995, former Surgeon General C. Everett Koop wrote that the most important gains in prolonging life have come from community prevention successes. "Diseases are of two types: those we develop inadvertently and those we bring upon ourselves by failure to practice preventive measures" (Koop, 1995). The concept of prevention is defined by the National Nurses Society on Addictions (NNSA) (1994) as a "proactive process which empowers individuals and systems to meet the challenges of life events and transitions by creating and reinforcing conditions that promote healthy behaviors and lifestyles."

The comprehensiveness of substance abuse prevention programs in this country continues to improve. Unimodal interventions such as drug education, self-esteem building, and peer resistance are being replaced by more multimodal approaches that involve children, families, schools, and entire communities (USDHHS, 1991a). A longitudinal assessment project measuring drug and alcohol use by adolescents, high school seniors, and young adults has been ongoing since 1976 at the University of Michigan Institute for Social Research (Johnston, O'Malley, & Bachman, 1986). Commonly referred to as the Monitoring the Future Study, this project is a rigorously designed annual survey of the attitudes and behaviors of randomly selected samples of students in the 12th grade, high school graduates, and college students in the 19 to 30 age range. It is conducted each year in order to monitor trends in substance abuse and drug-related attitudes of adolescents and young adults at significant transitional points in their lives.

These kinds of epidemiological studies are critical to understanding the drug use patterns in segments of the population most at risk for substance involvement and the factors that contribute to that risk. The important question for researchers is not simply how substance abuse can be prevented but how and under what circumstances it can be prevented among each of the subpopulations in our society (USDHHS, 1991a). It has become evident that no single factor triggers substance abuse but rather that multiple determinants of individual and environmental factors combine to cause susceptibility (Jones & Battjes, 1985; Orford, 1985; Sameroff & Fiese, 1988).

Treatment strategies applied to adolescents often attempt to change undesirable behaviors related to substance abuse, delinquency, violence, school dropout, and pregnancy after problems have already surfaced. Catalano and Hawkins (1986) and Haggerty, Hawkins, and Muir (1989) are researching a more proactive approach to identifying risk factors that increase the chances of adolescent health and behavior problems as well as protective factors that can help buffer young people from these problems. Their risk-focused prevention strategy is based on the simple premise that to prevent problems from occurring, one must identify factors that increase the risk of problem development and use strategies to reduce risks and enhance protective factors. In conjunction with this work, the state of Kansas joined five other states for a Federal Prevention Needs Assessment Study funded by the Center for Substance Abuse Prevention (CSAP). With direction from the Social Development Research Group of the University of Washington, the Catalano and Hawkins risk and protective factor framework was used to create a standardized set of indicators to aid in the identification of high-risk behaviors (Southeast Kansas Education Service Center [SKESC], 1994). An archival indicator study (the systematic tracking and monitoring of risk and protective indicators) has just been completed in which each state in the six-state consortium collected data at the state, regional, and county levels. Trends occurring throughout these sectors of the country indicate that there is an overall increase in the percentage of adolescents who are trying the more common drugs, including alcohol. There is, however, a decrease in the percentage of adolescents who are trying cocaine and steroids and a decrease in daily use of all drugs. Community risk levels appear to be increasing in terms of juvenile arrests, social welfare programs, and health-related issues. The effect of these increased community risk levels may be buffered by an increase in the average per capita income and in immunization rates. Family risk levels seem to be rising in areas of adult drug-related disease, deaths, arrests, and imprisonment. One family risk indicator, that of divorce, appears to be on the decline. Unlike the community domain, the family domain demonstrates no buffers. The school environment shows two positive trends. There is an increase in average daily attendance and an increase in American College Test (ACT) scores. Unfortunately, the individual and peer domain indicates an increase in vandalism and ATODA-related arrests for 10- to 14-year-olds and shows no increase in positive variables (SKESC, 1994).

In looking at biological risk factors in the population, there is mounting evidence of genetic predisposition to addictions. Children of alcoholics and other drug users are more likely to demonstrate substance abuse and dependence at younger ages and to increase use more quickly. Pollock, Schneider, Gabrielli, and Goodwin (1987) used a meta-analysis to evaluate 32 familial alcoholic studies to examine parent-offspring alcoholism rates. The task was to determine whether alcoholism rates of fathers of alcoholics are greater than those of mothers and to evaluate the patterns of alcoholism (father to son versus daughter and mother to son versus daughter). Data collected on the parents of 8,071 alcoholics in these 32 studies indicate that male and female alcoholics are more likely to come from families in which the biological father is an alcoholic. In contrast, only female alcoholics are more likely to come from homes in which the biological mother is an alcoholic. These findings suggest that sons and daughters of male alcoholics and daughters of female alcoholics may be at higher risk for alcoholism.

Discovering markers of alcoholism risk is useful in determining the contribution of genetic factors to vulnerability. These markers provide the initial step in prevention intervention by revealing susceptibility (Hill & Steinhauer, 1993). Previous studies of alcoholic men demonstrated deficits in the P300 component of event-related brain potentials (ERPs). Hill and Steinhauer (1993) examined ERPs in a sample of 25 alcoholic women, 31 nonalcoholic sisters of these women, and 30 control women. Results demonstrate a significant difference in the magnitude of the P300 component between women selected on the basis of their familial risk for developing alcoholism. In the visual modality, there is almost a 50% decrement in voltage between alcoholic women and controls. The P300 amplitude reduction among alcoholic women might be irreversible brain dysfunction caused by chronic alcoholism, or the lower amplitude of the P300 wave may be a marker for the possible development of alcoholism within high-risk families. These results hold promise for screening young girls to determine possible risk status.

In addition to adolescent, young adult, and middle-aged groups, another high-risk population is the elderly. Prevention efforts are severely compromised because many older people live alone and drink secretly, self-reporting may be unreliable, retirement and fewer social outings reduce the opportunity for detection by employers and others, and family members often choose to protect them from the embarrassment of being labeled with a drinking problem (Gupta, 1993; Hesse & Savitsky, 1987; Thibault & Maly, 1993). Another problem associated with this age group is not substance abuse but substance misuse. With so many age-related illnesses and different specialist physicians for each ailment, the number of medications used can be forgotten by the patient who goes from one office to another. Synergistic effects of prescription medications can be alarming. Many elderly also have a tendency to save and share medications.

Although Substance Use Prevention research is receiving increased attention, there are several gaps that need to be addressed (NNSA, 1990): (1) most studies have been done on white, middle-aged males and have been generalized to other groups without consideration for differences; (2) more research needs to be done with minorities, the elderly, women, homosexuals, and adolescents; (3) more controlled evaluations of primary prevention are needed because most studies have been retrospective; (4) variables of tertiary prevention involving rehabilitation should be done in terms of outcome measures; (5) terminology needs to be operationally defined; and (6) nurses need to increase the complexity of their research by advancing to levels three and four of Dickhoff and James' (1968) levels of research. This is not a comprehensive listing of all the areas needed in future research but rather a starting place for action.

NURSING INTERVENTION AND PATIENT OUTCOME

Nurses play important roles in the success and effectiveness of programs that ensure the health of individuals, families, and communities. Traditional roles include serving as (1) educators for individual, family, workplace, and community health concerns; (2) providers of health care, including assessment and early identification of risk factors for substance abuse problems, counseling, intervening, and referring; and (3) coordinators or collaborators functioning as members of multidisciplinary teams to strengthen the overall health of the community (NNSA, 1994).

There are many practice settings for nurses involved in Substance Use Prevention. These involve places where information about addiction can be taught to groups or individuals, such as schools, community groups, organizations, and health care agencies. Table 30–1 provides a succinct listing of nursing activities

Table 30–1   Substance Use Prevention

DEFINITION: Prevention of an alcoholic or drug use lifestyle.

ACTIVITIES:

Assist patient to tolerate increased levels of stress, as appropriate

Prepare patient for difficult or painful events

Reduce irritating or frustrating environmental stress

Reduce social isolation, as appropriate

Support measures to regulate the sale and distribution of alcohol to minors

Lobby for increased drinking age

Recommend responsible changes in the alcohol and drug curricula for primary grades

Conduct programs in schools on the avoidance of drugs and alcohol as recreational activities

Encourage responsible decision making about lifestyle choices

Recommend media campaigns on substance use issues in the community

Instruct parents and teachers in the identification of signs and symptoms of addiction

Assist patient to identify substitute tension-reducing strategies

Support or organize community groups to reduce injuries associated with alcohol, such as SADD and MADD

Survey students in grades 1 to 12 on the use of alcohol and drugs and alcohol-related behaviors

Instruct parents to support school policy that prohibits drug and alcohol consumption at extracurricular activities

Assist in the organization of post-activities for teenagers for such functions as prom and homecoming

Facilitate coordination of efforts between various community groups concerned with substance use

Source: McCloskey, J., and Bulechek, G. (1996). *Nursing interventions classification (NIC)* (2nd ed.). St. Louis: Mosby–Year Book.

for the intervention Substance Use Prevention identified in the Nursing Interventions Classification (NIC) system (McCloskey & Bulechek, 1996). In order to examine appropriate actions, it is necessary to distinguish among primary, secondary, and tertiary prevention efforts.

Primary Prevention

Primary prevention involves action taken to prevent disease or disability. Specific nursing interventions relate to (1) educating clients about drugs and addictive behaviors; (2) recognizing individuals at high risk for substance abuse; (3) identifying early signs and symptoms of drug use and misuse; (4) assisting clients in developing effective plans to limit and monitor the use of alcohol or other drugs; (5) incorporating ATODA content into health teaching of clients; (6) using peer counseling to cultivate positive, nonjudgmental attitudes toward abusers; (7) increasing public awareness of use of alcohol or other drugs with prescription medications; (8) presenting information to expectant mothers in prenatal clinics on the effects of substance use on the fetus; (9) alerting psychiatric nurses and other health care workers about the fact that substance abuse can hide or exaggerate symptoms during treatment; and (10) helping clients understand the importance of developing lifestyles that foster holistic health (Burns, Thompson, & Ciccone, 1993; NNSA, 1990). Another important action for nurses involves effecting social change through legislation and policy making. In this way, community norms can be changed in relation to drug use, violence, and crime. Taxation on alcohol and cigarettes is just one illustration of a community law that affects consumption. Higher rates of taxation serve to decrease rates of alcohol and nicotine use. Resources for referral in primary prevention include school programs, community workshops, self-help groups, and legislative activities.

Secondary Prevention

Secondary Substance Use Prevention occurs during the acute phase of addiction treatment. Nursing roles are focused on stopping the addictive process and preventing disability. Interventions include (1) early case finding to prevent more serious effects of misuse, (2) holistic assessments to identify early problems, (3) self-help with an emphasis on self-management, (4) recognizing psychosocial effects, and (5) encouraging individual and group counseling (Burns et al., 1993; NNSA, 1990). Referral sources for secondary Substance Use Prevention involve ATODA outpatient services (e.g., assessments, counseling, workshops), mental health outpatient services, and self-help groups.

Tertiary Prevention

This level of prevention refers to the recovery phase of addiction, which is often a lifelong process. Nurses working with clients at this stage need to understand the difference between lapse and relapse and to assist clients in their efforts to function in drug-free environments that support their health and well-being. *Lapse* is defined as a single drinking incident during a period of sobriety, which may or may not result in relapse. *Relapse,* on the other hand, is a return to frequent use after a period of abstinence—a return to addiction (Einstein, 1994). Interventions focus on aftercare in a variety of settings, such as outpatient treatment facilities, partial hospitalization programs, halfway houses, and other residential care programs (Burns et al., 1993; NNSA, 1990). Referral sources include both outpatient and inpatient substance abuse service groups.

Regardless of whether interventions are geared toward primary, secondary, or tertiary levels of prevention, nurses would expect to influence a number of patient outcomes. There are currently 190 identified patient outcomes listed in the Nursing Outcomes Classification (NOC) (Johnson & Maas, 1997). Five of these relate to Substance Use Prevention efforts. The first is Knowledge: Substance Use Control and is defined as the extent of understanding conveyed about managing substance use safely. The second, third, and fourth are similar in that each relates to Risk Control (Alcohol Use, Drug Use, and Tobacco Use) and are defined as any action to eliminate or reduce alcohol, drug, or tobacco use that poses a threat to health. The final patient outcome that applies to Substance Use Prevention is Substance Addiction Consequences, a compromise in health status and social functioning as a result of addiction (Johnson & Maas, 1997).

Cultural Implications

Nurses need to be aware of the fact that patterns of substance use and abuse are affected by the client's culture. Effective community prevention programs require mutual respect for racial and ethnic differences while also acknowledging relatedness. It is not enough simply to be "culturally aware." Nurses need to take the next step toward cultural competence, whereby they increase their understanding and appreciation of cultural differences and similarities within, among, and between groups. This requires a willingness to incorporate community-based values, traditions, and customs in order to develop focused programs (Gordon & Freeman, 1996).

An interesting tool to help the nurse explore a culture and understand how it affects personal behaviors and thoughts is the "Circle of Culture" developed by the National Institute on Drug Abuse (1980). This worksheet contains a 10-

Table 30–2 Nursing Diagnoses Common to Addictions

Nursing Diagnosis	Defining Characteristics
I. Biological Responses	
A. Risk for Injury	A. Ataxia; history of flashbacks; history of seizure
B. Self Care Deficit	B. Intolerance to activity; diminished self-esteem; discomfort
C. Risk for Infection	C. Homeless lifestyle; practice of unsafe sex; severe withdrawal syndrome
D. Sleep Pattern Disturbance	D. Sleep pattern reversal; mild, fleeting nystagmus
E. Altered Nutrition; Less Than Body Requirements	E. Report of inadequate dietary intake; change in appetite; dental caries
F. Altered Growth and Development: biological	F. Infants of chemically dependent mothers; newborn exhibiting drug-induced sedation; retardation of brain growth
II. Cognitive Responses	
A. Knowledge Deficit	A. Verbalization of knowledge deficit
B. Noncompliance	B. Continuing pattern of addiction; verbalization of noncompliance; inability to set goals
III. Psychosocial Responses	
A. Impaired Verbal Communication	A. Inability to express feelings; slurring of speech; inappropriate speech patterns
B. Ineffective Individual Coping	B. Ineffective coping with feelings of defeat; replacing one chemical with another; ineffective choices and actions
C. Self-Esteem Disturbance	C. Body image disturbance; low self-esteem; social withdrawal; role performance; role conflict
D. Social Isolation	D. Nonverbal behaviors; staying in room; refusing to join group
E. Altered Family Processes	E. Disturbed social communication; dependency; loss of family support system
F. Altered Parenting	F. Continued substance abuse while breast-feeding; verbalization of role frustration; lack of parental attachment behavior
G. Altered Growth and Development: psychosocial	G. Lack of trust in adults; fear of losing control; harsh self-criticism
IV. Spiritual Responses	
A. Spiritual Distress	A. Distress in human spirit caused by guilt, shame, grief, self-blame; lack of meaning in life
B. Powerlessness	B. Passivity; a perceptual experience of loss of control; inappropriate efforts to assert control over self
C. Hopelessness	C. Diminished trust; frequent crying spells; flat affect, sadness
D. Grieving	D. Potential, perceived, or actual loss of a significant object or person

Source: Modified from American Nurses Association. (1988). *Standards of addictions nursing practices with selected diagnoses and criteria.* Kansas City, MO: Author.

section pie chart that allows one to write out ideas that apply to each category for the selected cultural group. It can be surprising to learn how little or how much is known about another racial or ethnic group and where stereotypes are hidden.

NURSING DIAGNOSES

The nurse formulates nursing diagnoses based on information that has been collected through client assessment. Nursing theory and knowledge of addictions is combined with these data in a decision-making process to determine appropriate diagnoses. Clarity and conciseness are accomplished by using nursing diagnoses that already have been developed by the North American Nursing Diagnosis Association (NANDA). To date, more than 100 nursing diagnoses have been identified and approved in its Taxonomy I. Table 30–2 contains 19 diagnoses with defining characteristics that pertain specifically to addiction (American Nurses Association [ANA] & NNSA, 1988; Thomas & Handley, 1995). Other nursing diagnoses also may be used and related to the addicted client (whether individual, family, or group) through defining characteristics and level of prevention. Substance Use Prevention will be the intervention of choice for some of these diagnoses.

CASE STUDY

JD is a 13-year-old, sixth-grade boy who was sent to the school nurse's office in a large midwestern inner-city school. His art teacher sent him there after discovering that he had cut his own arm intentionally with scissors. JD stated that he had injured himself in art class because of boredom and displayed little concern for the behavior. After treating the superficial wound, the nurse continued her nursing assessment with questions related to his classes, lifestyle, and goals for the future.

JD stated that his eating and sleeping habits were centered around late-night "hanging out" with friends who belonged to a gang. The gang provided him with transportation, entertainment, food, and clothing. It was not uncommon for him to be out until one or two o'clock in the morning and then try to sleep for a few hours, if at all. JD stated that he had no curfew and that his father was a marijuana user. He recalled having his own first marijuana joint as a very young boy and stated that he continued to use occasionally. He claimed that he did not use alcohol.

In looking at a decisional balance grid, JD was asked to describe the pros and cons involved in maintaining his present behavior and those involved in changing to healthier behaviors. Throughout the motivational interviewing, he

identified no reason to change because more of his needs were being met in his present situation than would be met if he altered his behavior. He stated that he had more material and emotional support from gang members who were not in school. He denied the health risks of marijuana except for a noticeable decrease in concentration. His major health concerns were insomnia and worry for his sick mother. JD stated that he was still able to attend school but that he did little schoolwork at home. On leaving the office, he agreed to think more about the decisional balance grid and to meet again to discuss further concerns.

The school nurse arranged a meeting with the school principal and counselor. She learned that JD had been seeing the counselor regularly and that the principal and teachers were concerned with his failing grades and absenteeism. There had been a report that he had marijuana in the school building 1 month ago, but no evidence was found when he and his locker were searched. JD and his sixth-grade classmates were near the completion of a 6-month DARE (Drug Awareness, Resistance, and Education) program conducted by an officer with the city police department. General response to the program had been positive. The nurse, who was assigned to the school as part of a university faculty practice plan, suggested that some of her nursing students provide a three-session program on refusal skills and goal setting. An inservice session also could be provided to teachers to learn (1) how to recognize signs and symptoms of substance abuse, (2) risk assessment, (3) current school policy and procedures related to student possession of illegal substances, (4) use of school substance abuse surveillance surveys, and (5) available community resources, including the district Drug-Free Schools Center and the Regional Prevention Center. The nurse then arranged a meeting with JD's parents, the principal, and the school counselor. The parents were supportive of the plan and agreed to seek counseling for their son and to work on their own parenting skills and discipline (Hicks, 1997).

References

American Nurses Association (ANA) and National Nurses Society on Addictions. (1988). *Standards of addictions nursing practice*. Kansas City, MO: ANA.

Burns, E., Thompson, A., and Ciccone, J. (1993). *Springer series on the teaching of nursing: An addictions curriculum for nurses and other helping professionals* (Vol. 1). New York: Springer Publishing.

Catalano, R., and Hawkins, J. (1986). *Preventing relapse among former substance abusers: A model for developmental research*. Seattle, WA: University of Washington Center for Social Welfare Research.

Dickhoff, J., and James, P. (1968, May-June). A theory of theories: A position paper. *Nursing Research, 17*(3), 197–203.

Einstein, S. (1994). Relapse revisited: Failure by whom and what? *International Journal of Addictions, 29*, 409–413.

Gordon, J., and Freeman, E. (1996). *Multicultural training in alcohol, tobacco and other drug abuse: Multicultural community development*. Lawrence, KS: University of Kansas Press.

Gupta, K. (1993). Alcoholism in the elderly. *Postgraduate Medicine, 93*, 203–206.

Haggerty, K., Hawkins, J., and Muir, G. (1989). *Together! Planning guide, communities in action to prevent youth drug abuse*. Seattle, WA: University of Washington Social Development Research Group.

Hesse, K., and Savitsky, J. (1987). The elderly. In H. Barnes, M. Aronson, and T. Delbanco (Eds.), *Alcoholism: A guide for the primary care physician*. New York: Springer-Verlag.

Hicks, V. (1997). *Case study interview*. Kansas City, KS: University of Kansas School of Nursing.

Hill, S., and Steinhauer, S. (1993). Event-related potentials in women at risk for alcoholism. *Alcohol, 10*, 349–354.

Horgan, C. (1993). *Substance abuse: The nation's number one health problem*. NJ: Institute for Health Policy, Brandeis University.

Johnson, M., and Maas, M. (Eds.). (1997). *Nursing outcomes classification (NOC)*. St. Louis: Mosby–Year Book.

Johnston, L., O'Malley, P., and Bachman, J. (1986). *Drug use among American high school students, college students and other young adults: National trends through 1985* (DHEW Pub. No. 87-1535). Rockville, MD: National Institute on Drug Abuse.

Jones, C., and Battjes, R. (1985). *Etiology of drug abuse: Implications for prevention* (Research Monograph No. 56). Rockville, MD: National Institute on Drug Abuse.

Koop, C. E. (1995). Editorial: A personal role in health care reform. In M. Stoil and G. Hill (Eds.), *Preventing substance abuse: Interventions that work* (p. 1). New York: Plenum Press.

McCloskey, J., and Bulechek, G. (Eds.). (1996). *Nursing interventions classification (NIC)* (2nd ed.). St. Louis: Mosby-Year Book.

National Institute on Alcohol Abuse and Alcoholism (NIAAA). (1992). *Surveillance report #23. Apparent per capita alcohol consumption: National, state, and regional trends, 1977–1990*. Rockville, MD: NIAAA, Division of Biometry and Epidemiology.

National Institute on Drug Abuse. (1980). *Training of trainers: Cultural identity*. Rockville, MD: Author.

National Nurses Society on Addictions. (1990). *Core curriculum of addictions nursing* (L. Jack, Ed.). Stokie, IL: Midwest Education Association, Inc.

National Nurses Society on Addictions. (1994). *Prevention of alcohol, tobacco, & other drug problems: An independent study for nurses*. Pittsburgh, PA: Center for Substance Abuse Prevention.

Orford, J. (1985). *Excessive appetites: A psychological view of addictions*. New York: John Wiley & Sons.

Pollock, V., Schneider, L., Gabrielli, W., and Goodwin, D. (1987). Sex of parent and offspring in the transmission of alcoholism: A meta-analysis. *Journal of Nervous and Mental Disease, 175*, 668–673.

Sameroff, A., and Fiese, B. (1988). Conceptual issues in prevention. In D. Shaffer and I. Phillips (Eds.), *Project prevention*. Washington, DC: American Academy of Child and Adolescent Psychiatry.

Southeast Kansas Education Service Center (SKESC). (1994). *Kansas communities that care archival indicators: 1988–1993*. Topeka, KS: Kansas Alcohol and Drug Abuse Services.

Sullivan, E. (Ed.). (1995). *Nursing care of clients with substance abuse*. St. Louis: Mosby.

Thibault, J., and Maly, R. (1993). Recognition and treatment of substance abuse in the elderly. *Primary Care, 20*, 155–165.

Thomas, M., and Handley, S. (1995). Substance abuse diagnosis. In E. Sullivan (Ed.), *Nursing care of clients with substance abuse*. St. Louis: Mosby.

U.S. Department of Health and Human Services, Public Health Service. (1991a). *Drug abuse and drug abuse research* (DHHS Pub. No. [ADM] 91-1704). Rockville, MD: Author.

U.S. Department of Health and Human Services, Public Health Service. (1991b). *Healthy people 2000: National health promotion and disease prevention objectives* (DHHS Pub. No. 91-50212). Washington, DC: Author.

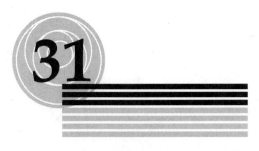

Mood Management

Mary Kanak

In the Nursing Interventions Classification (NIC) (McCloskey & Bulechek, 1996), the intervention of Mood Management is defined as "providing for safety and stabilization of a patient who is experiencing dysfunctional mood." This NIC intervention is intended for use in treating patients who have mood disorders as they are defined by the fourth edition of *Diagnostic and Statistical Manual of Mental Disorders* of the American Psychiatric Association (APA), also known as the DSM-IV (APA, 1994). The DSM-IV divides mood disorders into five categories: (1) depressive disorders (also known as "unipolar depressions"), (2) bipolar disorders, (3) mood disorders due to a general medical condition, (4) substance-induced mood disorders, and (5) mood disorders not otherwise specified. These disorders are characterized by disturbances in the regulation of emotion, ranging from intense elation or irritability (mania) to severe depression. Although mood fluctuation is a normal phenomenon for all of us as we respond to the circumstances of daily living, individuals with mood disorders experience moods or mood changes that are extreme and persist to the point where they impair the ability to function effectively, safely, and comfortably.

The importance of effective treatment of mood disorders, and thus the need for the Mood Management intervention in a classification of nursing interventions, becomes evident given the widespread prevalence of these psychiatric disorders and the toll they exact from the afflicted individual, his or her loved ones, and society at large. The lifetime prevalence of developing any mood disorder is 19.3%—14.7% for men, 23.9% for women (Kessler et al., 1994). Mood disorders account for more than 565,000 hospital admissions, 7.4 million hospital days, and 13 million physicians' visits annually (Depression Guideline Panel,

1993a). It is estimated that the direct and indirect costs of mood disorders total $16 billion per year (Depression Guideline Panel, 1993a).

The NIC intervention Mood Management is composed of those nursing activities that address the issues of safety and the recovery of a healthier level of mental and physical functioning in patients who are experiencing or recovering from a mood disorder. Although the manic and depressive episodes of mood disorders have what initially appear to be very different clinical presentations, a closer look reminds us that they sit on the same mood continuum (although at opposite ends), and thus the needs for nursing care are very similar. For example, the nurse may need to assist both the depressed and the manic patient with grooming; the former because he or she lacks energy and motivation to do this task independently, the latter because he or she is so overenergized that he or she is unable to focus and complete even the simplest of tasks. The NIC intervention Mood Management consolidates the nursing activities for mania and depression under a single nursing intervention label.

LITERATURE REVIEW

The nursing intervention label of Mood Management is new and not yet well represented as a term in the health care literature. However, with the publication of the second edition of the NIC (McCloskey & Bulechek, 1996), the term is now included in the Cumulative Index for Nursing and Allied Health Literature (CINAHL). Although, as of yet, there is little referenced in the health care literature under the term Mood Management, there has been much written about the treatment and management of depression and mania. This literature is reflected in the NIC intervention Mood Management and is reviewed here.

The literature shows that treatment focuses on (1) alleviating the dysfunctional mood (depression or mania) and (2) compensating for the functional deficits that result from the dysfunctional mood. The treatments for dysfunctional mood are pharmacotherapy (medications), psychotherapy, electroconvulsive therapy, and light therapy. Nurses are involved in the delivery of all these treatments to varying degrees, often in collaboration with professionals from other health care disciplines.

In terms of the functional deficits seen in mood-disordered patients, nurses assume the primary role in planning and providing care that compensates for these deficits. Depressed or manic moods are often accompanied by a constellation of symptoms pertaining to changes in appetite, weight, sleep, psychomotor activity, energy level, and possibly thoughts of self-harm or death. Psychotic features (e.g., hallucinations, delusions, bizarre behavior and speech) may also be present. These symptoms result in safety risks, self-care deficits, cognitive deficits, social deficits, and knowledge deficits. Nursing care addresses these deficits, ensuring that the patient maintains a healthy and safe level of functioning while awaiting the therapeutic benefit of the somatic treatments or psychotherapy that targets the dysfunctional mood. This literature review first discusses the nursing role in the treatments of pharmacotherapy, psychotherapy, electroconvulsive therapy, and light therapy, and then the review addresses nursing care of the functional deficits seen during depressed and manic episodes.

Treatment of Dysfunctional Mood: Nursing Care

In the early 1990s, a multidisciplinary group of health care providers was organized by the Agency for Health Care Policy and Research (AHCPR). The purpose of this group was to study the current literature on the treatment of depression and to make recommendations for treatment. This group, named the Depression Guideline Panel, published its findings and recommendations in a three-part series. Although all three volumes are recommended reading for any health care provider caring for depressed patients, it is the second volume that is particularly relevant to this literature review. The second volume is titled *Depression in Primary Care: Volume 2. Treatment of Major Depression. Clinical Practice Guideline, Number 5* (Depression Guideline Panel, 1993b). It focuses on the treatment of depression, making specific recommendations for treatments with a review of the research base supporting each treatment.

Volume 2 of the guidelines (Depression Guideline Panel, 1993b) divides treatment into two phases: acute and continuation. The goals of acute treatment are "to reduce and ultimately to remove all signs and symptoms of the depressive syndrome, and to restore occupational and psychosocial function to that of the asymptomatic state" (p. 1). When the patient responds to acute treatment with a remission of symptoms, continuation therapy is used to reduce the likelihood of relapse and recurrence. The recommended treatments for depression include pharmacotherapy (medications), psychotherapy, pharmacotherapy combined with psychotherapy, electroconvulsive therapy, and light therapy. These treatments can be appropriately used in both the acute and the continuation phases of treatment. The Depression Guideline Panel was careful to avoid labeling treatment activities as belonging to any one discipline, because many of the treatments can now be provided by a variety of disciplines. For example, psychotherapy can be provided by a variety of health care providers ranging from a psychiatrist to a psychiatric nurse to a counselor. Another example is pharmacotherapy, which can be provided by a physician as well as by appropriately licensed physician assistants and advanced practice nurses. Although the Depression Guideline Panel (1993b) did not specifically delineate the role of the nurse in the aforementioned treatments, the nursing literature is explicit and is reviewed here.

PHARMACOTHERAPY: NURSING ACTIVITIES

Medications have been shown to be effective in treating all forms of mood disorder, with the therapeutic mode of action being at the level of the neurotransmitter disturbance within the central nervous system (Depression Guideline Panel, 1993b). Several classes of antidepressants exist for the treatment of depressive symptoms. Antimanic drugs such as lithium and certain anticonvulsants are used to treat mania or hypomania. Psychotic symptoms that may accompany depressive or manic episodes are usually treated with antipsychotic medications. Anxiolytic or anti-anxiety drugs are often helpful in treating anxiety that may be present with a mood disorder.

The literature states that nursing activities in pharmacotherapy include collaborating with the prescribing clinician to assess and plan for the patient's medication needs, teaching patients and their families about the medications, administering the medications, monitoring the patient for intended and unintended effects of the medications, documenting and communicating these observations to other team members, treating adverse drug effects, and drawing blood or monitoring blood levels of particular medications, such as lithium, to determine appropriateness of medication dose and patient compliance (Chitty, 1996; Depression Guideline Panel, 1993b; Hagerty, 1996; Laraia, 1995; McFarland, Wasli, & Gerety, 1997; Pennebaker & Riley, 1995; Sherr, 1996). Nurses also play an important role in monitoring and promoting the patient's medication compliance through medication teaching and by developing a rapport that allows the patient to discuss feelings and concerns about the medications (Hagerty, 1996; Pennebaker & Riley, 1995). Advanced practice nurses have been granted prescriptive privileges in many states and now assume the additional responsibility of prescribing and managing the medications of patients with mood disorders (Hagerty, 1996; Laraia, 1995; Pennebaker & Riley, 1995).

PSYCHOTHERAPY: NURSING ACTIVITIES

Psychotherapy has been shown to be an effective modality in treating patients with mood disorders (Depression Guideline Panel, 1993b). Psychotherapy is a broad term that includes a variety of different approaches. Parloff (1982) has identified at least 250 subtypes of psychotherapy. The AHCPR Depression Guideline Panel (1993b) recommends five types of psychotherapy for the treatment of the depressive episodes: interpersonal therapy, cognitive therapy, behavioral therapy, brief dynamic therapy, and marital therapy. In addition, psychoanalytical therapy, family therapy, and group therapy have also been identified as useful psychotherapies to treat depression (Buffum & Madrid, 1995; Fortinash & Holoday-Worret, 1995; Hagerty, 1996; McFarland et al., 1997; Stuart, 1995; Tommasini, 1995).

Hagerty (1996) points out that despite differences in terms of theoretical framework and approach, the various psychotherapies all share a common formula for success. Successful therapy results from establishment of a therapeutic relationship between the patient and the therapist, understanding and support, instillation of hope, provision of a framework that the patient can use to understand and examine his or her problems, and opportunities to develop new coping skills. The goals of any psychotherapy approach with mood-disordered patients are similar: a remission of symptoms, improved level of functioning, and prevention of a relapse or a recurrence (Depression Guideline Panel, 1993b).

It is recommended that psychotherapy be conducted by professionals who have received specific training in this discipline. The nursing literature clearly indicates that psychotherapy is within the realm of the psychiatric nurse (Buffum & Madrid, 1995; Chitty, 1996; Fortinash & Holoday-Worret, 1995; Hagerty, 1996; McFarland et al., 1997; Stuart, 1995; Tommasini, 1995). The American Nurses Association (ANA) (1994), in its practice standards for psychiatric–mental health nursing practice, identifies the certified clinical specialist in psychiatric–mental health nursing as the appropriate provider of psychotherapies. These psychotherapies include individual, group, family, and child psychotherapy. Generally, there is agreement with this standard in the current psychiatric–mental health nursing literature, but authors do differ in terms of the roles of the psychiatric–mental health generalist in psychotherapeutic interventions. Buffum and Madrid (1995) state that the generalist may be a group therapist or cotherapist as well as lead groups that promote patient activity and socialization, provide psychoeducation, teach tasks such as social skills, or provide a support system for group members. Antai-Otong (1995a) states that the generalist may provide other types of counseling, such as crisis intervention or grief counseling. These types of counseling provide support, help the patient marshal available resources, and facilitate coping and problem solving by the patient. Hagerty (1996) designates the generalist role in family or marital therapy as one of collaboration with the advanced practice nurse to assess the need for such therapy and then make referrals to appropriate therapists. Hagerty (1996) sees the role of the generalist in group therapy as assessing the suitability of patients for participation in groups, encouraging patients to attend, conducting groups (if trained to do so), listening, allowing ventilation of feelings, and reinforcing patients' insights. Other nursing authors discuss the various applications of group therapy in patients with mood disorders but do not differentiate between the roles of the generalist and the advanced practitioner in these groups (Fortinash & Holoday-Worret, 1995; McFarland et al., 1997; Stuart, 1995).

ELECTROCONVULSIVE THERAPY: NURSING ACTIVITIES

Electroconvulsive therapy (ECT) is typically used to treat those patients with a severe or psychotic form of depression. It may also be used for less severe depressions that have failed to respond to other therapies or for patients at high risk for suicide or for whom the antidepressant medications are contraindicated because of medical conditions (Depression Panel Guideline, 1993b). ECT is provided by a specialist, usually a psychiatrist, with nurses providing adjunctive care before, during, and after the treatment. Several organizations have delineated the nursing role in the provision of ECT. The ANA (1994) states that the role of the nurse in ECT is to provide education and support to the patient and family, to assess and determine the patient's pretreatment level of functioning, to prepare the patient for the actual treatment, and to monitor the patient's response to the treatment. The APA Task Force on Electroconvulsive Therapy (1990) concurred with the ANA that the role of the nurse is to educate the patient and family about ECT, as well as to organize the care (including setup of the treatment area, medications, and equipment) and to promote patient safety and knowledge about the treatment. Anesthesia during ECT may be provided by a certified nurse anesthetist.

LIGHT THERAPY: NURSING ACTIVITIES

Light therapy, also known as phototherapy, is a treatment option for mild to moderate seasonal nonpsychotic depressive episodes (Avery et al., 1991; Depression Guideline Panel, 1993b; Lam, Buchanan, Mador, & Corral, 1992). The patient is exposed to light that is brighter than usual indoor light for specified time periods in the morning or evening on a daily basis. This decreases the mood symptoms seen in seasonal depressive episodes (Lewy, Sack, & Singer, 1990; Rao et al., 1992; Wehr, Skwerer, Jacobsen, Sack, & Rosenthal, 1987). Dawn simulation is another form of light therapy that involves more gradual exposure to dimmer light earlier in the sleep cycle (Terman & Schlager, 1990). Nursing activities with light therapy include engaging the client in the informed-consent process, teaching the patient and family about the treatment, and assessing the patient for treatment side effects (Antai-Otong, 1995b). Nurses may also set up the equipment and assist the patient with the treatment.

Treatment of Functional Deficits: Nursing Care

As mentioned previously, the mood-disordered patient often experiences a variety of functional deficits, especially during the acute phase of the illness, that require skilled nursing care. The following is a literature-based discussion of those nursing activities that target (1) safety risks to the patient and others, (2) self-care deficits, (3) cognitive deficits, (4) social deficits, and (5) knowledge deficits.

SAFETY: NURSING ACTIVITIES

Because of the nature of the mood disorders, safety is a priority in the provision of nursing care. The emotional symptoms of a mood disorder may place the individual at high risk to harm self or others. Such symptoms in the depressed patient include depressed mood, irritability or anger, or feelings of hopelessness. The emotional symptoms during a manic or hypomanic episode consist of an abnormally and persistently elevated, expansive, or irritable mood. The manic patient may lack insight as to what is rational or safe behavior and may thus behave in ways that endanger himself or herself as well as others. If irritable, he or she may be easily provoked to have a temper outburst. Thus, the nurse must determine whether the patient presents a safety risk and initiate the necessary precautions to safeguard the patient or others who are at risk for physical harm (Chitty, 1996; Fortinash & Holoday-Worret, 1995; Hagerty, 1996; McFarland et al., 1997; Schultz & Videbeck, 1994; Stuart, 1995; Tommasini, 1995). These precautions may take a variety of forms depending on the condition of the particular patient and the resources available to manage the safety risk. Hospitalization in a protected environment is recommended if the patient is at serious risk for self-harm or violence (Fortinash & Holoday-Worret, 1995; McFarland et al., 1997). Suicide or violence precautions include increased surveillance of the patient in a protective environment as well as behavior management strategies (e.g., limit setting, patient contracting). If the patient requires more protection than such precautions provide, interventions such as the use of anxiolytic or sedating medications, physical restraint, or seclusion may be necessary (Chitty, 1996; Fortinash & Holoday-Worret, 1995; Hagerty, 1996; McFarland et al., 1997; Schultz & Videbeck, 1994; Stuart, 1995; Tommasini, 1995).

SELF-CARE DEFICITS: NURSING ACTIVITIES

As a result of the illness, the mood-disordered patient may experience an increased or decreased appetite with corresponding body weight changes, hyposomnia or hypersomnia, psychomotor retardation or agitation, fatigue, and poor grooming. An appropriate level of physiological and behavioral functioning may be maintained by the nurse monitoring the patient's self-care ability and assisting as needed if the patient is unable to adequately care for himself or herself (Fortinash & Holoday-Worret, 1995; Hagerty, 1996; Schultz & Videbeck, 1994; Stuart, 1995; Tommasini, 1995). Such assistance may pertain to fluid and nutritional intake, elimination of body wastes, level of physical activity and environmental stimulation, and the sleep-wakefulness cycle (Chitty, 1996; Hagerty, 1996; Schultz & Videbeck, 1994; Stuart, 1995; Tommasini, 1995). Fortinash and Holoday-Worret (1995) as well as McFarland et al. (1997) caution that if the deficits are severe, it may be necessary to arrange for hospitalization or supervised care. These authors also emphasize the importance of communicating to the patient that he or she will be expected to assume increasing responsibility for self-care as he or she is able.

COGNITIVE DEFICITS: NURSING ACTIVITIES

Depression affects cognitive functioning by diminishing memory and the ability to think, concentrate, or make decisions. The cognitive symptoms seen in mania, and to a lesser degree in hypomania, include racing thoughts, flight of ideas, limited insight into seriousness of the condition, and poor judgment in the areas of personal, social, and occupational needs and activities. The nurse may intervene with activities that compensate for the patient's cognitive deficits while awaiting restoration of more normal functioning in this area.

Hagerty (1996) and Schultz and Videbeck (1994) recommend that the nurse constantly monitor the cognitive functioning of the patient (e.g., ability to process information, memory, concentration, attention, decision-making ability) to determine which deficits are present and to what degree. The acutely ill patient may be incapable of efficiently processing incoming verbal stimuli, so he or she may need to be approached with simple, concrete, here-and-now language during interactions (Hagerty, 1996; Schultz & Videbeck, 1994). Memory problems can be addressed with written or pictorial aid, such as a written daily schedule to assist the patient in moving more smoothly through the routine of the day (Chitty, 1996; Fortinash & Holoday-Worret, 1995; Schultz & Videbeck, 1994; Stuart, 1995). The patient may be cognitively impaired to a degree where he or she is unable to make decisions and, in this case, the nurse or a significant other may need to make decisions for the patient. However, as the patient recovers cognitive abilities, it is appropriate for the nurse to encourage simple decision making as a means of promoting a sense of control and competence in the patient (Hagerty, 1996; McFarland et al., 1997). The ability to make decisions is a life skill necessary for successful coping. Some patients may have lacked decision-making skills before their illness, and this may have been a contributing factor to the onset of the depressed or manic episode. McFarland et al. (1997) recommend that the nurse teach the client decision-making skills as necessary.

Both depressed and manic patients may experience changes in perceptual functioning, such as hallucinations or delusions (e.g., paranoid, grandiose). A variety of nursing authors (Chitty, 1996; Fortinash & Holoday-Worret, 1995; Schultz & Videbeck, 1994) suggest that these symptoms may be effectively managed by establishing a trusting relationship in which the patient feels emotionally safe and therefore comfortable in seeking validation of his or her perceptions from the trusted caregiver. One means of accomplishing this goal is by providing a limited number of consistent caregivers. Hagerty (1996) emphasizes the need for the nurse to reflect on the themes, feelings, and meanings behind the patient's words or perceptions rather than challenge the actual content of the delusion or hallucination. Fortinash and Holoday-Worret (1995) advocate that the nurse gently assist the patient to correct misinterpretations about the environment, self, and experiences through recall of events and problem solving. Additionally, the patient needs positive reinforcement for differentiating between reality-based and non-reality-based thinking (Chitty, 1996; Fortinash & Holoday-Worret, 1995; Hagerty, 1996). If the patient is too psychotic for these techniques, it may be necessary to use distraction, by directing the patient's attention to here-and-now activities and topics (Fortinash & Holoday-Worret, 1995; Hagerty, 1996; Schultz & Videbeck, 1994).

SOCIAL DEFICITS: NURSING ACTIVITIES

Withdrawal from friends, family, and social activities is a social symptom of depression. The nurse intervenes with activities targeting increased socialization. Initially, this may consist of the nurse arranging to spend time with the patient at regular, prearranged times for interaction (Chitty, 1996; Fortinash & Holoday-Worret, 1995; Hagerty, 1996; Schultz & Videbeck, 1994; Stuart, 1995). As the patient is able to tolerate more social stimulation, the nurse may encourage the patient to gradually engage in one-to-one interactions with others and attend groups, meetings, and social activities (Chitty, 1996; Hagerty, 1996; Schultz & Videbeck, 1994; Tommasini, 1995). Social skills training and assertiveness training may be appropriate for the depressed patient who lacks skills or confidence in his or her ability to deal effectively with people.

Social difficulties seen in mania and hypomania consist of intrusiveness, disruptiveness, and difficulty with social boundaries. In the case of the manic patient, the nurse provides feedback on the appropriateness of social behaviors, as well as limit-setting and behavioral management strategies to ensure that the patient's behavior does not infringe on the rights of others in the environment (Chitty, 1996; Fortinash & Holoday-Worret, 1995; McFarland et al., 1997; Schultz & Videbeck, 1994; Tommasini, 1995). If these nursing activities are unsuccessful in promoting appropriate behavior, the manic patient may need to be removed to a less stimulating environment where opportunities for social interaction are limited in number and more closely supervised.

KNOWLEDGE DEFICITS: NURSING ACTIVITIES

Nurses typically assume the responsibility for educating the depressed or manic patient and significant others about the illness and the corresponding treatment (Chitty, 1996; Fortinash & Holoday-Worret, 1995; Hagerty, 1996; McFarland et al., 1997; Schultz & Videbeck, 1994; Stuart, 1995; Tommasini, 1995). Nurses educate patients and their significant others about treatment in terms of medications, preprocedural teaching, and coping skills and resources. Patient and family knowledge in these areas is key to compliance with treatment and ultimately to recovery and prevention of relapse.

THE NIC INTERVENTION OF MOOD MANAGEMENT

The intervention of Mood Management was developed for the second edition of the NIC (McCloskey & Bulechek, 1996). Practicing nurses who were familiar with the first edition of the NIC (McCloskey & Bulechek, 1992) suggested the development of this intervention for inclusion in the second edition of NIC. Further impetus was provided by the 1993 publication of the AHCPR clinical guidelines for depression (Depression Guideline Panel, 1993a, 1993b, 1993c). As a result, the intervention of Mood Management was developed by a group of psychiatric and mental health nurses who, in doing so, used a review of the literature as well as clinical experience gained from working with mood-disordered patients. The intervention was then submitted to the larger NIC research team, which included representation from a large number of clinical nursing specialties besides mental health, for review. Suggestions from the group were incorporated into the current version of Mood Management. An overview of the intervention follows.

The NIC intervention of Mood Management (Table 31–1) is defined as "providing for safety and stabilization of a patient who is experiencing dysfunctional mood" (McCloskey & Bulechek, 1996). The intervention begins with a cluster of nursing activities that target safety and proceeds to clusters of nursing activities that pertain to self-care deficits, cognitive deficits, psychotherapy, pharmacotherapy, ECT, phototherapy, knowledge deficit (patient and family education), and social deficits. Although the intervention is already lengthy and comprehensive, the literature review for this chapter reveals some additional nursing activities that will enhance the intervention. These activities are included in the following discussion of the intervention, as well as submitted to the NIC research team for inclusion in Mood Management in the third edition of NIC that is planned.

Nursing activities within the safety cluster of Mood Management include monitoring for safety risks and then instituting appropriate precautions to safeguard the patient and others who may be at risk because of contact with the patient. Typically, the safety risks are suicide, self-mutilation, or violent behavior directed toward others. The various safety precautions and protective activities are of a level of sophistication and detail sufficient to merit recognition as discrete interventions within NIC. The author refers the user to the following NIC safety interventions: Anger Control Assistance, Area Restriction, Behavior

Table 31–1 Mood Management

DEFINITION: Providing for safety and stabilization of a patient who is experiencing dysfunctional mood.

ACTIVITIES:

Determine whether patient presents safety risk to self or others

Initiate necessary precautions to safeguard the patient or others at risk for physical harm

Monitor self-care ability

Assist with self-care, as needed

Monitor fluid and nutritional intake

Assist patient to maintain adequate hydration and nutritional status

Monitor physical status of patient (e.g., body weight and hydration)

Monitor and regulate level of activity and stimulation in environment in accord with patient's needs

Assist patient to maintain a normal cycle of sleep/wakefulness (e.g., scheduled rest times, relaxation techniques, and limit caffeine and medications)

Provide opportunity for physical activity (e.g., walking, or riding the exercise bike)

Monitor cognitive functioning (e.g., concentration, attention, and decision-making ability)

Assist patient to consciously monitor mood (e.g., 1 to 10 rating scale and journaling)

Encourage patient, as appropriate, to take an active role in treatment and rehabilitation

Assist patient to identify precipitants of dysfunctional mood (e.g., chemical imbalances, situational stressors, and physical problems)

Assist patient to identify feelings underlying the dysfunctional mood

Assist patient to ventilate feelings in an appropriate manner (e.g., punching bag, art therapy, and vigorous physical activity)

Assist patient to identify aspects of precipitants that can/cannot be changed

Assist in identification of available resources and personal strengths/abilities that can be used in modifying the precipitants of dysfunctional mood

Teach new coping and problem-solving skills

Provide cognitive restructuring, as appropriate

Administer mood-stabilizing medications (e.g., antidepressants, lithium, hormones, and vitamins)

Monitor patient for medication side effects and impact on mood

Assist physician with the provision of electroconvulsive therapy (ECT) treatments, when they are indicated

Monitor the physiological and mental status of the patient immediately after ECT

Assist with the provision of "phototherapy" to elevate mood

Provide procedural teaching to patient who is receiving ECT or phototherapy

Monitor patient's mood for response to ECT or phototherapy

Provide medication teaching to patient/significant others

Provide illness teaching to patient/significant others, if dysfunctional mood is illness based (e.g., depression, mania and premenstrual syndrome)

Provide guidance about development and maintenance of support systems (e.g., support groups and counseling)

Source: McCloskey, J. C., and Bulechek, G. M. (1996). *Nursing interventions classification (NIC)* (2nd ed., pp. 388–389). St. Louis: Mosby–Year Book.

Management: Self-Harm, Elopement Precautions, Environmental Management: Safety, Environmental Management: Violence Prevention, Fire Setting Precautions, Limit Setting, Physical Restraint, Seclusion, and Surveillance: Safety (McCloskey & Bulechek, 1996).

The second cluster of activities within Mood Management targets the patient's self-care deficit. The intervention of Mood Management recommends that the nurse assist the patient to meet these self-care deficits by monitoring the patient's self-care ability and physical status (e.g., body weight, hydration) and assisting, as needed, to maintain appropriate food and fluid intake, elimination patterns, rest and sleep, and personal grooming and hygiene. For more detailed guidance in these areas, the nurse can refer to related NIC interventions, which include Energy Management, Exercise Promotion, Electrolyte Management, Fluid Management, Nutrition Therapy, Self-Care Assistance: Bathing/Hygiene, Self-Care Assistance: Dressing/Grooming, Self-Care Assistance: Feeding, and Self-Care Assistance: Toileting.

Mood Management contains a third cluster of activities that target cognitive deficits; these consist of monitoring cognitive functioning and regulating the level of activity and stimulation in the patient's environment. This latter activity includes incoming stimuli (e.g., verbal communications, television, general activity of other individuals in the patient's vicinity) that may exceed the patient's cognitive processing abilities. This portion of the intervention could be expanded to include additional cognitive activities found in the literature review. These include (1) using simple, concrete, here-and-now language; (2) using written or pictorial memory aids (e.g., a written daily schedule); (3) limiting decision-making situations until cognitive abilities improve; and (4) teaching decision-making skills as needed. Additionally, an activity referring the nurse to the NIC interventions Hallucination Management and Delusion Management could be added to the cognitive cluster.

The next cluster of activities in Mood Management pertains to psychotherapy. These activities include assisting or encouraging the patient to (1) monitor his or her mood by rating it on a 1 to 10 rating scale or by journaling, (2) identify precipitants of dysfunctional mood, (3) ventilate feeling in an appropriate manner (e.g., by using a punching bag or engaging in art therapy or vigorous physical activity), (4) identify precipitants that can or cannot be changed, (5) identify resources for modifying precipitants that can be changed, (6) learn new coping and problem-solving skills, and (7) engage in cognitive restructuring. In the future, for the convenience of the nurse who is not qualified to provide psychotherapy, an additional activity may be added with regard to referring the patient to an appropriate provider for psychotherapy.

The nurse's role in pharmacotherapy is reflected in a cluster of activities that concern the administration of medications, monitoring for therapeutic effects and side effects, and educating the patient and family about medications. The medication prescription and management role of the advanced practice nurse, although not reflected in the current version of Mood Management, will be recommended for inclusion in future versions of this intervention.

Another cluster of Mood Management activities deals with nursing roles in the provision of ECT and phototherapy. These consist of providing preprocedural teaching, assisting with delivery of the treatment, and monitoring the patient for therapeutic effects and side effects of the treatment.

The knowledge deficit cluster includes several education activities that address potential knowledge deficits of the patient and his or her family regarding the illness and its treatment (medications, procedures).

The last cluster addresses the social deficits of the mood-disordered patient by assisting the patient to develop and maintain support systems. Additional social activities from the literature would greatly enhance this aspect of care. These activities include the nurse (1) arranging to interact with the patient at regular, prearranged times; (2) encouraging the patient, as he or she can tolerate, to engage in one-to-one interactions with others and attend groups, meetings, and social activities; (3) providing feedback on the appropriateness of social behaviors; (4) developing limit-setting and behavioral modification strategies to promote desired social behaviors; and (5) relocating the patient who is overstimulated by the surrounding environment to a low-stimulus environment. Additionally, an activity could be added that refers the nurse to the NIC interventions of Behavior Modification: Social Skills and Assertiveness Training for those depressed patients who lack skills or confidence in their ability to deal effectively with people.

MOOD MANAGEMENT: INTENDED USERS

It is evident from earlier discussions in this chapter that patients afflicted with mood disorders are the intended patient population for this intervention. However, the "intended users" of this intervention need to be identified. Mood Management was developed for use by both nonpsychiatric and psychiatric nurses. Because of the widespread prevalence of mood disorders and the current health care climate, it is likely that nurses from all clinical specialties will encounter patients with depression and mania in their practice. For example, in today's era of managed care and limited access to inpatient hospitalization, a community health nurse may be responsible for managing the care of a moderately depressed patient in the home. Similarly, a staff nurse on an inpatient orthopedic unit may find himself or herself caring for a patient with a fractured limb in traction who is also experiencing a manic episode. Nonpsychiatric nurses often feel inexperienced and apprehensive about caring for these patients and appreciate some guidance as to how to treat the mood disorder. The NIC intervention Mood Management was developed to provide guidance to nurses caring for mood-disordered patients in both psychiatric and nonpsychiatric settings. It encompasses nursing activities that are used in inpatient, outpatient, and community settings and that are appropriate when dealing with the continuum of illness from acute episodes through the recovery and maintenance stages of treatment. These activities are appropriate for use with both children and adults who have mood disorders.

TIPS FOR USING THE INTERVENTION MOOD MANAGEMENT

In the course of initiating the Mood Management intervention with a particular patient, nurses may have questions about the selection of appropriate Mood Management activities for that patient. Does every mood-disordered patient need every nursing activity? If not, how does one decide which activities are necessary? The Iowa Intervention Project (McCloskey & Bulechek, 1996) recommends that six factors be considered when choosing an intervention: (1) the desired patient outcomes, (2) the active nursing diagnoses, (3) the adequacy of the research or literature base for the activities, (4) the feasibility of carrying out the activity, (5) the acceptability to the patient, and (6) the capability of the nurse. These six factors can also be applied to the process of selecting activities, especially with an intervention such as Mood Management that has linkages with numerous nursing diagnoses and outcomes (Table 31–2). Identification of the relevant nursing diagnoses and the desired patient outcomes is the first step in selecting the activities. A diagnosis reflects a specific need for care, whereas the outcome describes the patient's response to care. If the nurse has these two pieces of information, it becomes evident by perusing the intervention of Mood Management which activity(ies) will provide the appropriate linkage between the diagnosis and the desired outcome(s). Thereafter, the final decision of whether to use these activities requires screening with the remaining four factors mentioned: adequacy of the literature base, feasibility (e.g., time, cost, interaction with other activities), acceptability to the patient, and capability of the nurse (e.g., knowledge, psychomotor and interpersonal skills, ability to effectively access needed resources within the health care setting).

The nurse may want to refer the patient to other providers if the appropriate nursing activities are not feasible in his or her practice settings or if the patient care needs exceed his or her capabilities. An example of this would be the community health nurse who is caring for a depressed patient in the home. If the patient becomes actively suicidal, it is unlikely that the community health nurse can provide the level of observation and protective environment in the patient's home that is necessary to safeguard the patient against suicide. In this instance, it would be appropriate to hospitalize the patient on a unit where psychiatric nurses can provide suicide precautions.

NURSING DIAGNOSES AND PATIENT OUTCOMES ASSOCIATED WITH MOOD MANAGEMENT

The North American Nursing Diagnosis Association (NANDA) (1996) states that nursing diagnoses "provide a basis for selection of nursing interventions to achieve outcomes for which the nurse is accountable" (p. 8). This definition emphasizes the conceptual flow and linkages that exist between nursing diagnoses, nursing interventions, and patient outcomes. The purpose of this section is to identify those nursing diagnoses and patient outcomes that are linked with the intervention of Mood Management. The NANDA nomenclature is used in the discussion of nursing diagnoses. The Nursing Outcomes Classification (NOC) (Johnson & Maas, 1997) provides an excellent framework and the necessary standardized nomenclature to discuss patient outcomes. Table 31–2 illustrates the NANDA nursing diagnoses and NOC patient outcomes that are associated with the intervention of Mood Management. Diagnoses and accompanying outcomes are arranged in clusters that reflect areas of patient need: dysfunctional mood, safety, self-care deficits, cognitive deficits, social deficits, and knowledge deficits.

Nursing diagnoses triggered by the dysfunctional mood are Self Esteem Disturbance, Ineffective Individual Coping, Defensive Coping, and Hopelessness. These problems may be contributing factors to the development of, as well as symptoms of, the depressive and manic episodes. The Mood Management activities that target dysfunctional mood have already been thoroughly discussed and are not reiterated here except to state that these activities attempt to effect positive change in the NOC outcomes of Self-Esteem, Coping, Impulse Control, Anxiety Control, Mood Equilibrium, and Hope.

The safety needs generated by depression or mania necessitate the nursing diagnoses of Risk for Violence: Self-Directed or Directed at Others; Self Mutilation, Risk for; and Injury, Risk for. The safety activities within Mood Management

Table 31–2 Nursing Diagnoses and Patient Outcomes Associated with the NIC Intervention of Mood Management

NANDA Nursing Diagnoses	NOC Patient Outcomes
MOOD	
Self Esteem Disturbance	Self-Esteem: Personal judgment of self-worth.
Ineffective Individual Coping	Coping: Actions to manage stressors that tax an individual's resources.
	Impulse Control: Ability to self-restrain compulsive or impulsive behaviors.
	Anxiety Control: Ability to eliminate or reduce feelings of apprehension and tension from an unidentifiable source.
Defensive Coping	Mood Equilibrium: Appropriate adjustment of prevailing emotional tone in response to circumstances.
Hopelessness	Hope: Presence of internal state of optimism that is personally satisfying and life-supporting.
SAFETY	
Violence, Risk for, Self-Directed or Directed at Others	Aggression Control: Ability to restrain assaultive, combative or destructive behavior toward others.
	Suicide Self-Restraint: Ability to refrain from gestures and attempts at killing self.
Self Mutilation, Risk for	Self-Mutilation Restraint: Ability to refrain from intentional self-inflicted injury (non-lethal).
Injury, Risk for	Safety Behavior: Personal: Individual or caregiver efforts to control behaviors that might cause physical injury.
SELF-CARE	
Self Care Deficit	Self-Care: Activities of Daily Living (ADL): Ability to perform the most basic physical tasks and personal care activities.
Constipation	Bowel Elimination: Ability of the gastrointestinal tract to form and evacuate stool effectively.
Fatigue	Rest: Extent and pattern of diminished activity for mental and physical rejuvenation.
Altered Nutrition, More or Less Than Body Requirements	Nutritional Status: Extent to which nutrients are available to meet metabolic needs.
	Hydration: Amount of water in the intracellular and extracellular compartments of the body.
Sleep Pattern Disturbance	Sleep: Extent and pattern of sleep for mental or physical rejuvenation.
COGNITIVE	
Sensory/Perceptual Alterations	Distorted Thought Control: Ability to self-restrain disruption in perception, thought processes, and thought content.
	Cognitive Orientation: Ability to identify person, place, and time.
	Identity: Ability to distinguish between self and non-self and to characterize one's essence.
Thought Processes, Altered	Distorted Thought Control: Ability to self-restrain disruption in perception, thought processes, and thought content.
	Cognitive Ability: Ability to execute complex mental processes.
	Concentration: Ability to focus on a specific stimulus.
	Decision Making: Ability to choose between two or more alternatives.
	Information Processing: Ability to acquire, organize, and use information.
	Memory: Ability to cognitively retrieve and report previously stored information.
Communication, Impaired Verbal	Communication Ability: Ability to receive, interpret, and express spoken, written and non-verbal messages.
SOCIAL	
Social Interaction, Impaired	Social Interaction Skills: An individual's use of effective interaction behaviors.
	Impulse control: Ability to self-restrain compulsive or impulsive behaviors.

Table continued on following page

Table 31-2 Nursing Diagnoses and Patient Outcomes Associated with the NIC Intervention of Mood Management *(Continued)*

NANDA Nursing Diagnoses	NOC Patient Outcomes
SOCIAL	
Social Isolation	Social Involvement: Frequency of an individual's social interactions with persons, groups, or organizations.
	Loneliness: The extent of emotional, social, or existential isolation response.
	Social Support: Perceived availability and actual provision of reliable assistance from other persons.
KNOWLEDGE	
Knowledge Deficit	Knowledge: Disease Process: Extent of understanding conveyed about a specific disease process.
	Knowledge: Medication: Extent of understanding conveyed about the safe use of medication.
	Knowledge: Treatment Procedure(s): Extent of understanding and skills conveyed about procedure(s) required as part of a treatment regimen.
	Knowledge: Treatment Regimen: Extent of understanding and skills conveyed about a specific treatment regimen.
	Compliance Behavior: Actions taken on the basis of professional advice to promote wellness, recovery, and rehabilitation.

Sources: Johnson, M., and Maas, M. (1997). *Nursing outcomes classification (NOC).* St. Louis: Mosby–Year Book; North American Nursing Diagnosis Association. (1996). *Nursing diagnoses: Definitions and classification 1997–1998.* Philadelphia: Author.

attempt to promote Aggression Control, Suicide Self-Restraint, Self-Mutilation Restraint, and Safety Behavior in the mood-disordered patient.

The self-care needs that often accompany acute depression or mania drive the nursing diagnoses of Self Care Deficit; Constipation; Fatigue; Nutrition, Altered (More or Less Than Body Requirement); and Sleep Pattern Disturbance. The self-care activities within Mood Management promote a healthy level of functioning with regard to the NOC outcomes of Self-Care: Activities of Daily Living (ADL), Bowel Elimination, Rest, Nutritional Status, Hydration, and Sleep.

The cognitive deficits of these patients result in the nursing diagnoses of Sensory/Perceptual Alterations; Thought Processes, Altered; and Communication, Impaired Verbal. Nursing activities promote the outcomes of Distorted Thought Control, Cognitive Orientation, Identity, Cognitive Ability, Concentration, Decision Making, Information Processing, and Memory.

The social impairments of depression or mania result in the diagnoses of Social Interaction, Impaired and Social Isolation. The expected outcomes of Mood Management include increases in Social Involvement, Social Interaction Skills, Impulse Control, Role Performance, and Social Support, as well as decreased feelings of loneliness.

The needs of the patient for knowledge regarding the illness and its treatment necessitate the diagnosis of Knowledge Deficit. Mood Management activities that target the knowledge deficits of the patient and his or her family have the expected NOC outcomes of Knowledge: Disease Process, Knowledge: Medication, Knowledge: Treatment Procedure(s), Knowledge: Treatment Regimen, and Compliance Behavior.

CASE STUDY—MAJOR DEPRESSIVE DISORDER

The following is a typical scenario in which the intervention of Mood Management would be instituted. It illustrates how Mood Management can be applied from the onset of an acute mood disorder through the continuation phase of treatment.

D was a 45-year-old married man who presented with a 1-month history of depressed mood, loss of pleasure from life, social withdrawal, and a more recent onset of suicidal ideation with a plan to shoot himself. His verbalizations were limited, his rate of speech was slowed, and he had some difficulty comprehending when people spoke to him. Because of decreased ability to concentrate and a diminished energy level, D had been unable to function at work and so had been staying home in bed most of the time. Other depressive symptoms experienced were a decreased appetite, with a recent 15-pound weight loss, diminished personal grooming, and difficulty sleeping. The nursing diagnoses made were Violence, Risk for (self directed); Self Care Deficit; Altered Nutrition, Less Than Body Requirements; Sleep Pattern Disturbance; Thought Processes, Altered; Impaired Verbal Communication; Social Isolation; Ineffective Individual Coping; Hopelessness; and Knowledge Deficit. The nursing staff instituted the intervention of Mood Management to deal with the many problems D was experiencing as a result of his severely depressed mood. Targeted NOC outcomes included Suicide Self-Restraint, increased ability to engage in Self Care: Activities of Daily Living (ADL), improved Nutritional Status, adequate Sleep, increased Cognitive Ability and Information Processing, improved Communication Ability and Social Involvement, improved Coping, increased Hope, and increased Knowledge of the Disease Process, Medication, and Treatment Procedures.

The admitting psychiatrist placed D on a locked psychiatric nursing unit where the environment had been designed to accommodate the safety needs of suicidal patients. Because of the intensity of D's suicidal ideation, the nursing staff placed him on suicide precautions that included round-the-clock one-to-one observation. D needed assistance from the nursing staff to eat food, drink fluids, and engage in personal grooming tasks. He did not sleep well, and the nursing staff intervened with behavioral strategies to promote

sleep that included a regular sleep schedule and, eventually, administration of an antidepressant medication that had a sedating effect. The nursing staff administered D's medications, monitoring him for side effects and treatment response. The nursing staff provided and reviewed printed medication education materials to D and his family to familiarize them with the antidepressant. Written and verbal communication that was directed toward D was simplified and provided at a slowed rate so that he was able to cognitively process it.

Because of the severity of his suicidal ideation and his depressive symptoms (as well as a past history of depression and a serious suicide attempt), it was decided to treat D with a course of ECT in addition to the antidepressant medication. The nursing staff provided education to D and his family about the ECT treatments. Additionally, the nursing staff prepared D for each of his six ECT treatments, assisted with the actual treatment procedure, monitored D in the recovery area after each treatment, and provided feedback to other treatment team members about D's response to treatment.

After 2 weeks of treatment, D began to respond positively to the ECT treatments and medications. His mood improved, the suicidal ideation disappeared, and his affect brightened. D's speech increased to a more conversant level and appropriate rate, and he seemed better able to process speech that others directed toward him. D's appetite returned, and he began to restore the weight previously lost. Personal grooming improved without any prompting from the nursing staff. With daily encouragement from the nursing staff, he attended recreational activities and interacted with other patients, as well as his family when they visited. His concentration improved, as evidenced by his ability to follow television coverage of his favorite sports team.

With the return of more normal cognitive functioning, D, during his daily meeting with his primary nurse, began to verbalize his feelings and reflect on stressors that had contributed to his depression. The primary nurse worked with D to identify more adaptive coping strategies for dealing with stress and emotions. These included developing more assertive interpersonal skills, using progressive muscle relaxation, engaging in regular physical exercise, and using a four-step problem-solving strategy for evaluating and generating solutions to problem situations that he encountered in his daily life. In consultation with the multidisciplinary treatment team, the primary nurse referred D to an inpatient cognitive therapy group led by a psychiatric–mental health clinical nurse specialist.

D continued to show improvement in his mood and functioning level, verbalizing hope for the future. He indicated that he was ready to resume full-time employment at his previous job. The discharge plan included continued treatment with the antidepressant medication and regular outpatient follow-up of his illness and medications. D was referred to a psychiatric–mental health clini-

cal nurse specialist in the community who was licensed to prescribe and manage psychiatric medications and was also a member of the provider panel sanctioned by D's insurance company. This provider was also certified in individual psychotherapy and continued to work with D on cognitive therapy, assertiveness training, relaxation, and application of problem-solving strategies. At 12 months after discharge, D remained relatively symptom free with continued antidepressant treatment and individual psychotherapy. He reported satisfaction with his marriage and home life and was reported to be performing well on the job. He was regularly attending sporting events with enjoyment and expressed happy anticipation about the upcoming birth of his first grandchild.

SUMMARY

The care and treatment of the mood-disordered patient has always been a challenge, given the broad scope and severity of impairment imposed by these disorders. However, in today's health care environment, this challenge has been magnified by the emphasis on cost-efficient care with predictable patient outcomes. Mood Management comprehensively addresses this broad scope of impairment and the corresponding nursing treatment activities. Thus, when combined with relevant NANDA diagnoses and NOC outcomes, Mood Management becomes a very useful clinical tool, greatly increasing the probability that desired patient outcomes are attained within a reasonable time and at a reasonable cost.

References

American Nurses Association. (1994). *A statement on psychiatric–mental health clinical nursing practice and standards of psychiatric–mental health clinical nursing practice.* Washington, DC: American Nurses Publishing.

American Psychiatric Association. (1994). *Diagnostic and statistical manual of mental disorders* (4th ed.). Washington, DC: Author.

American Psychiatric Association Task Force on Electroconvulsive Therapy. (1990). *The practice of electroconvulsive therapy: Recommendations for psychiatric training and privileging.* Washington, DC: American Psychiatric Association.

Antai-Otong, D. (1995a). Individual psychotherapy. In D. Antai-Otong and G. Kongable (Eds.), *Psychiatric nursing. Biological and behavioral concepts* (pp. 453–467). Philadelphia: W.B. Saunders.

Antai-Otong, D. (1995b). Electroconvulsive therapy and other biological therapies. In D. Antai-Otong and G. Kongable (Eds.), *Psychiatric nursing. Biological and behavioral concepts* (pp. 577–594). Philadelphia: W.B. Saunders.

Avery, D. H., Khan, A., Dager, S. R., Cohen, S., Cox, G. B., and Dunner, D. L. (1991). Morning or evening bright light treatment of winter depression? The sig-

nificance of hypersomnia. *Biological Psychiatry, 29,* 126.

Buffum, M., and Madrid, E. (1995). Group psychotherapy. In D. Antai-Otong and G. Kongable (Eds.), *Psychiatric nursing. Biological and behavioral concepts* (pp. 486–506). Philadelphia: W.B. Saunders.

Chitty, K. K. (1996). Clients with mood disorders. In H. S. Wilson and C. R. Kneisel (Eds.), *Psychiatric nursing* (pp. 323–359). Menlo Park, CA: Addison-Wesley.

Depression Guideline Panel. (1993a). *Depression in primary care: Volume 1. Detection and diagnosis. Clinical practice guideline, number 5.* Rockville, MD: U.S. Department of Health and Human Services, Public Health Service, Agency for Health Care Policy and Research.

Depression Guideline Panel. (1993b). *Depression in primary care: Volume 2. Treatment of major depression. Clinical practice guideline, number 5.* Rockville, MD: U.S. Department of Health and Human Services, Public Health Service, Agency for Healthcare Policy and Research.

Depression Guideline Panel. (1993c). *Depression in primary care: Detection, diagnosis and treatment. Quick reference guide for clinicians, number 5.* Rockville, MD:

U.S. Department of Health and Human Services, Public Health Service, Agency for Health Care Policy and Research.

Fortinash, K. M., and Holoday-Worret, P. A. (1995). Mood disorders. In K. M. Fortinash and P. A. Holoday-Worret (Eds.), *Psychiatric nursing care plans* (pp. 48–73). St. Louis: Mosby.

Hagerty, B. (1996). Mood disorders: Depression and mania. In K. M. Fortinash and P. A. Holoday-Worret (Eds.), *Psychiatric mental health nursing* (pp. 251–283). St. Louis: Mosby.

Johnson, M., and Maas, M. (Eds.). (1997). *Nursing outcomes classification* (*NOC*). St. Louis: Mosby.

Kessler, R. C., McGonagle, K. A., Zhao, S., Nelson, C. E., Hughes, M., Eshleman, S., Wittchen, H. U., and Kendler, K. S. (1994). Lifetime and 12-month prevalence of DSM-IIIR psychiatric disorders in the U.S. *Archives of General Psychiatry, 51,* 8–19.

Lam, R. W., Buchanan, A., Mador, J. A., and Corral, M. R. (1992). Hypersomnia and morning light therapy for winter depression. *Biological Psychiatry, 31,* 1062–1064.

Laraia, M. T. (1995). Psychopharmacology. In G. W. Stuart and S. J. Sundeen (Eds.), *Principles and practice of psychiatric nursing* (pp. 663–702). St. Louis: Mosby.

Lewy, A. J., Sack, R. L., and Singer, C. M. (1990). Bright light, melatonin, and biological rhythms in humans. In J. Montplaisir and R. Godbout (Eds.), *Sleep and biological rhythms* (pp. 99–112). New York: Oxford University Press.

McCloskey, J. C., and Bulechek, G. M. (Eds.). (1992). *Nursing interventions classification* (*NIC*). St. Louis: Mosby–Year Book.

McCloskey, J. C., and Bulechek, G. M. (Eds.). (1996). *Nursing interventions classification* (*NIC*) (2nd ed.). St. Louis: Mosby–Year Book.

McFarland, G. K., Wasli, E., and Gerety, E. K. (1997). Mood disorders. In G. K. McFarland, E. Wasli, and E. K. Gerety (Eds.), *Nursing diagnoses and process in psychiatric mental health nursing* (pp. 243–262). Philadelphia: J.B. Lippincott.

North American Nursing Diagnosis Association. (1996). *Nursing diagnoses: Definitions and classification 1997–1998.* Philadelphia: Author.

Parloff, M. B. (1982). Psychotherapy research evidence and reimbursement decisions: Bambi meets Godzilla. *American Journal of Psychiatry, 138,* 718–727.

Pennebaker, D. F., and Riley, J. (1995). Psychopharmacological therapy. In D. Antai-Otong and G. Kongable (Eds.), *Psychiatric nursing. Biological and behavioral concepts* (pp. 543–576). Philadelphia: W.B. Saunders.

Rao, M. L., Muller-Oerlinghausen, B., Mackert, A., Strebel, B., Stieglitz, R. D., and Volz, H. P. (1992). Blood serotonin, serum melatonin and light therapy in healthy subjects and inpatients with nonseasonal depression. *Acta Psychiatrica Scandinavica, 86,* 127–132.

Schultz, J. M., and Videbeck, S. D. (1994). *Manual of psychiatric nursing care plans.* Philadelphia: J.B. Lippincott.

Sherr, J. D. (1996). Psychopharmacology and other biologic therapies. In K. M. Fortinash and P. A. Holoday-Worret (Eds.), *Psychiatric mental health nursing* (pp. 531–564). St. Louis: Mosby.

Stuart, G. (1995). Emotional responses and mood disorders. In G. W. Stuart and S. J. Sundeen (Eds.), *Principles and practice of psychiatric nursing* (pp. 413–451). St. Louis: Mosby.

Terman, M., and Schlager, D. S. (1990). Twilight therapeutics, winter depression, melatonin and sleep. In J. Montplaisir and R. Godbout (Eds.), *Sleep and biological rhythms: Basic mechanisms and applications to psychiatry* (pp. 113–128). New York: Oxford University Press.

Tommasini, N. R. (1995). The client with a mood disorder (depression). In D. Antai-Otong and G. Kongable (Eds.), *Psychiatric nursing. Biological and behavioral concepts* (pp. 157–189). Philadelphia: W.B. Saunders.

Wehr, T. A., Skwerer, R. G., Jacobsen, F. M., Sack, D. A., and Rosenthal, N. E. (1987). Eye versus skin phototherapy of seasonal affective disorder. *American Journal of Psychiatry, 144,* 753–757.

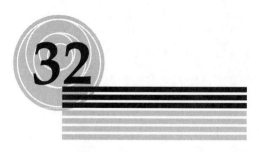

Animal-Assisted Therapy

Kathie M. Cole

The application of Animal-Assisted Therapy in the health service field has become increasingly popular. Animal-Assisted Therapy is acknowledged and used as an adjunctive therapy for nurses (Barba, 1995; Baun, Bergstrom, Langston, & Thoma, 1984; Carmack, 1991; Carmack & Fila, 1989; Cole & Gawlinski, 1995; Duncan, 1995a; Gammonley, 1995) and other health care professionals to maintain and promote optimal well-being. Animal-Assisted Therapy as a nursing intervention can be used to promote cognitive, physical, psychosocial, and spiritual benefits to patients in a variety of settings. Animal-Assisted Therapy has been demonstrated as beneficial to patients in nursing homes (Yates, 1987), hospitals (Kale, 1992b), hospices (Chinner & Dalziel, 1991), outpatient programs (Cawley, Cawley, & Retter, 1994), rehabilitation programs (Allen & Blaskovich, 1996), psychiatric facilities (Holcomb & Meacham, 1989), schools (Nebbe, 1995; Weatherill, 1993), and prisons (Walsh & Mertin, 1994), within the guidelines and policy of each facility.

Organized efforts to train guide dogs for people with visual impairments began approximately 80 years ago (Stuckey, 1982). Since the 1960s, the role of the service animal has expanded (Duncan, 1998), and service dogs are now used to alert the hearing impaired, warn a person of an oncoming seizure, and assist with physical or emotional impairments. Levinson (1962) presented case study results that showed successful psychotherapeutic treatment, together with his "cotherapist" dog, Jingles, in severely withdrawn children. Levinson (1964) believed pets were valuable adjuncts to therapy in facilitating and expediting healthy communication in both the home and the office therapy setting. He coined the term *pet therapy*, despite the skepticism of his audience. Other colleagues (Corson & Corson, 1973; Corson, Corson, Gwynne, & Arnold, 1977) supported his research in the technique of what we now call Animal-Assisted Therapy.

Today, the most progressive nonprofit organization advocating the use of animals to help people promote their health, increase independence, and improve quality of life is the Delta Society. The Delta Society was developed in 1977 by a group of health professionals under the leadership of physician Michael McCullough (Bustad, 1996). The Delta Society's first president was veterinarian Leo K. Bustad, dean of a veterinary college and a pioneer in human-animal bond theory and application. The founders of the Delta Society were interested in the relationship between pet owners, pets, and caregivers; thus the triangle symbol or "Delta" name was used.

LITERATURE REVIEW

The application of Animal-Assisted Therapy in the health service field has become increasingly popular based on scientific research studies showing physiological, cognitive, physical, psychosocial, and spiritual benefits.

Physiological Benefits

Several Animal-Assisted Therapy studies have elicited physiological signs of the relaxation response such as decreased blood pressure and heart rate (Friedman, Katcher, Thomas, Lynch, & Messent, 1983; Wilson, 1987), decreased blood pressure and skin conductance (Allen, Blascovich, Tomaka, & Kelsey, 1991), and decreased heart rate and respiratory rate (Baun, et al., 1984). Baun et al. (1984) conducted a study of the change in blood pressure, heart rate, and respiratory rate in three groups: group 1 (subject reading quietly), group 2 (subject petting own dog, or "bonded"), and group 3 (subject petting strange dog). Results showed group 2 (subject with bonded dog) experienced the same physiological effects (decrease in heart rate and respiratory rate over time) as did group 1 (subject reading quietly). The investigators reported an initial increase in blood pressure, heart rate, and respiratory rate when the dog first came into the room, which was referred to as "the greeting response." It seems the later decrease in heart rate and respiratory rate shows a relaxation response from the dog's presence over time. A research study that described Animal-Assisted Therapy as relaxing was the study of contemplation of a fish tank (Katcher, Segal, & Beck, 1984), in which the investigator also suggested to his subjects that it would be a relaxing experience. Because the blood carries oxygen, nutrition, and regulating hormones to every cell in the body, it would appear that an improvement in circulation from relaxation or beneficial effects of animal interaction can provide a positive physiological counterbalance to stress.

Anderson, Reid, and Jennings (1992) looked at pet ownership and risk factors for cardiovascular disease and found male pet owners across the age continuum to have significantly lower plasma triglyceride levels and systolic blood pressures than did men who did not own pets. Results of Friedmann, Katcher, Lynch, and Thomas's (1980) well-known study of 1-year survival rates among patients who had experienced myocardial infarction showed a significant increase in survival rate in pet owners regardless of the type of pet. One might suggest that personality may have an influence on beneficial effects of pet ownership; however, Friedman and Thomas (1985) looked at a sample of 300 college students exposed to a battery of tests, and results showed that pet owners and non–pet owners do not differ in personality. In the Cardiac Arrhythmia

Suppression Trial (CAST), 1-year survival data were obtained showing that both "pet ownership and social support are significant predictors of survival, independent of the effects of other psychosocial factors and physiologic status" (Friedman & Thomas, 1995).

Cognitive Benefits

Thirty elderly nursing home residents were given birds to care for and showed an improvement of self-concept and attitude toward others compared with a control group (Mugford & M'Comisky, 1975). In one study, 20 people were tested in a laboratory setting and a home environment with or without a dog present. An overall decrease in anxiety was measured in both settings with the dog, with more attention given to the dog in the laboratory setting (Sebkova, 1977). Increased memory recall may be tested with Animal-Assisted Therapy as patients learn about the therapy dog's age, breed, color, and size and are later asked to reverbalize information about the therapy dog (10 minutes later or next day) (Delta Society, 1996b). Adolescents identified with special education needs showed an increase in self-concept after an 8-week therapeutic horseback riding program (Cawley et al., 1994). Animal-Assisted Therapy has been shown to provide an excellent vehicle for clinical assessment and diagnosis for all patients and an added opportunity for social interaction among isolated patients (Holcomb & Meacham, 1989). Supervising therapists at the University of California–Los Angeles (UCLA) Medical Center in the geriatric neuropsychiatric area report an increase in focusing of attention and a decrease in agitation among this population when in an Animal-Assisted Therapy group session. To improve patient consciousness, an animal is placed next to a patient in bed, and the patient is assisted in stroking the animal to arouse neurological status. An increased acceptance of health status may occur as the dog lies in bed with the patient, snuggled to one side as the patient talks to the dog and reminisces toward acceptance of health circumstances. Nursing staff of a geriatric hospital reported an increase in patient responsiveness, pleasure, and reality therapy as a result of resident cats (Brickel, 1979). A therapy cat is introduced to the client, and the Animal-Assisted Therapy therapist assists the patient in stroking the animal and placing the cat on the patient's lap to be stroked independently. Topics about this pet, such as his or her name, activities, care, and characteristics, can be discussed.

Physical Benefits

Increased upper extremity muscle function can occur with Animal-Assisted Therapy in quadriplegia patients, demonstrated by placing a dog on a raised table and having the patient groom the dog, with resultant increase in muscle function (McLaughlin, 1996). Increased joint mobility or improved hand coordination can occur with collar and leash manipulation. With the dog in a closed area, the patient manipulates buckles from on to off to on again. Encourage the patient to stroke the animal's ears during times of frustration or fatigue. Improve shoulder movement by having the patient throw a ball to be retrieved by the dog. The patient will improve ambulatory skills by walking to the dog at the end of parallel bars or a hallway. Natural mobilization of the pelvis, lumbar spine, and hip joints based on the transfer of movement from a horse to a patient occurs with hippotherapy (use of horse in physiotherapy) (Baker, 1994; Cohen, 1992; Copeland, 1992) and results in increased strength, mobility, and balance. This form of therapeutic riding is highly recommended for multiple sclerosis and cerebral palsy patients (Yasikoff & Kunzle, 1995). Increased physical or psychological comfort can occur with Animal-Assisted Therapy by placing a fish aquarium in a patient's room and instructing the patient to contemplate the fish aquarium for 20 minutes and telling him or her that this will increase comfort level or relaxation (Katcher et al., 1984). Speech may be elicited from the patient by asking the patient to give commands to a dog (e.g., sit, lie down, stay, come, retrieve).

Psychosocial Benefits

The literature on children's attachment to companion animals suggests that many of the functions of social support may be served by pets (Melson & Schwartz, 1994). "Children's attachment to companion animals has been shown to be positively related to their sense of self-esteem either directly or indirectly according to stage of development and type of pet" (Triebenbacher, 1998). Children in the home reported pets as those they turn to for psychological or emotional support when they are happy, sad, or angry (Bryant, 1985). Classroom lessons learned by children in animal-based projects include the fragility of life and the importance of respect for living things. To promote child adaptation to hospitalization with Animal-Assisted Therapy, a visiting therapy dog is used to assist in diversion of a child from physical examination. Start by offering the patient a stuffed toy. Slowly introduce a small, friendly, well-trained, low-reactive dog into the session (Woolverton, 1993). Increased self-esteem may occur with Animal-Assisted Therapy by allowing the child to take the dog down the corridor for a walk (Kale, 1992a). With parental permission for a child or adult patient permission, a Polaroid picture may be taken for the patient to keep. In one adult psychiatric group at UCLA Medical Center, patients are encouraged to sketch the Animal-Assisted Therapy dog. The canine model provides a paw print signature to add to the sharing experience. One study shows a decrease in depression when an elderly day care population of men were introduced to an aviary in their physical environment (Holcomb, Jendro, Weber, & Nahan, 1997). The effect of interacting with an unknown pet dog was a decrease in anxiety among college students (Wilson, 1991). Encourage the patient to watch the visiting therapy dog, promote proximity, and stroke the dog for comfortable intervals of 10 to 15 minutes. In another study, fish aquariums placed in patients' rooms resulted in an increase in caregiver-patient socialization demonstrated by lengthened medical visits (Hart, 1992). The Alzheimer's disease patient population shows positive social effects from Animal-Assisted Therapy (Kongable, Stolley, & Buckwalter, 1990). In the presence of an Animal-Assisted Therapy dog, a group of Alzheimer's disease patients showed increased smiles, tactile contacts, and leans toward and looks at the dog (Batson et al., 1995). The term *therapeutic riding* is used to describe all rehabilitative uses of the horse (Engel, 1992; North American Riding for the Handicapped Association, 1993), including equine-assisted psychotherapy (Klüwer, 1988, 1994; Scheidhacker, 1994), where goals such as ego strengthening, self-confidence, and social competence may be obtained (Fitzpatrick & Tebay, 1995). A study of hospitalized patients showed that this population opened up lines of communication to people caring for their pets at home (Friedman, Katcher, & Meislich, 1983). Introduction of nonpoison-ous snakes into group activities of children with disabilities, adolescents with behavior problems, and the elderly in nursing homes has been shown to be successful (Shalev, 1996).

Spiritual Benefits

Fila (1991) describes a case study in which implementation of Animal-Assisted Therapy with a guinea pig and a dog for a long-term hospitalized vascular patient renewed the patient's positive outlook, decreased his stress, and improved his well-being from a state of withdrawal and expressed hopelessness. One nurse described a case study of a young girl who was visited by her pet Labrador Blackie in the hospital during her last week of life and the positive impact it had on her (MacInnis, 1991). Nursing home residents reminisce about positive interactions with a once-owned pet to renew their spirituality or meaningful connections. One meaningful connection described by Bustad (1996) was that of an 11-year-old boy who was severely affected by Duchenne's muscular dystrophy. Weakness and depression in both body and spirit had taken over this young boy until a horse named Dancer entered his life. Together they developed a special relationship and competed in the National Association of Sports for Cerebral Palsy, where they won three gold medals. Before Michael's condition deteriorated, he was asked to attend a banquet to be the recipient of the Delta Society's President's Award (in honor of impressive animal-person relationships). Michael accepted the award with the following words:

> Every hour of every day
> Three hundred sixty-five days a year,
> I ride.
> I ride in a blue and silver wheelchair.
> It bothers me when people stare,
> But maybe they really do care.
> There are many things I can't do.
> Wouldn't this upset you, too?
> One and a half hours a day,
> About fifty-two days a year,
> I ride.
> I ride a dark brown Connemara.
> Dancer is my very best friend.
> Upon her I often depend.
> Without wheels, she makes me feel free!
> That's all I really want to be.
> (Bustad, 1996, p. 32)

IMPLEMENTING THE INTERVENTION

The Nursing Interventions Classification (NIC) intervention Animal-Assisted Therapy appears in Table 32–1. Before implementing Animal-Assisted Therapy, it is important to have a solid foundation including, at a minimum, facility assessment, patient population assessment, staff responsibility determination, animal screening criteria, and clearly written policies and procedures (Arkow, 1982; Delta Society, 1992, 1996a). Experts for each population or setting must develop their own inclusion and exclusion criteria at each facility. Animal selection is an important consideration in regard to the specific patient population and the nature of the injury. For instance, dogs and cats are more interactive companions than turtles, fish, and hamsters; this quality is displayed by proximity-seeking behavior such as tail wagging, purring, and initiation to be petted (Melson, 1988). Consultation from a Delta-certified animal evaluator is highly recommended. Written policies should address the overall philosophy and rationale for the Animal-Assisted Therapy program for that facility. An example

Table 32–1   Animal-Assisted Therapy

DEFINITION: Purposeful use of animals to provide affection, attention, diversion, and relaxation.

ACTIVITIES:

Determine patient's acceptance of animals as therapeutic agents

Teach patient/family purpose and rationale for having animals in a care environment

Enforce rigid screening and training of animals in therapy program

Fulfill health inspectors' rules concerning animals in an institution

Provide therapy animals for patient, such as dogs, cats, horses, snakes, turtles, gerbils, guinea pigs, and birds

Facilitate patient's holding and petting therapy animals

Encourage repeated stroking of the therapy animal

Facilitate patient's watching therapy animals

Encourage patient's expression of emotions to animals

Arrange for patient to exercise with therapy animals

Encourage patient to play with therapy animals

Encourage patient to feed/groom animals

Source: McCloskey, J. C., and Bulechek, G. M. (1996). *Nursing interventions classification (NIC)* (2nd ed.). St. Louis: Mosby–Year Book.

of steps to conduct a volunteer or owner dog visit for hospital inpatients is illustrated in Table 32–2.

Suggested therapeutic activities or techniques that address cognitive, physical, psychosocial, and spiritual needs can be incorporated into the standard visit. An activity care plan should be developed to identify goals, select Animal-Assisted Therapy activity, and target desired outcomes. Examples of goals, activities, and outcomes taken from literature examples appear in Table 32–3.

Table 32–2   Example of Protocol for Hospital Volunteer/Owner Dog Visit

1. Primary nurse rules out exclusion criteria.
2. Patients are asked by RN [registered nurse] if they would like a dog visit.
3. After verbal consent, physician's order is obtained.
4. Verbal consent is obtained from roommate if present.
5. Order is transcribed to unit's Animal-Assisted Therapy log book by name sticker.
6. Volunteer handler/dog team arrives and refers to log book.
7. Volunteer handler/dog team identifies themselves to patient.
8. Patient washes hands with no rinse antiseptic gel before and after visit.
9. Patient dictates visit (dog on bed, chair, or floor).
10. A sheet is placed over bed linen as a barrier.
11. One visit may take 15 to 20 minutes.
12. Number of visits depends on volunteer handler/dog team stamina.
13. Volunteer handler/dog team disposes of linen and washes hands.
14. Volunteer handler/dog team document patient visit or AAT [Animal-Assisted Therapy] patient outcome.
15. Volunteer handler/dog team reports off to charge nurse.

Source: Cole, K., and Gawlinski, A. (1995). Animal-assisted therapy in the intensive care unit. *Nursing Clinics of North America, 30,* 529–537.

Table 32–3 Examples of Goals, Activities, and Outcomes

Goal	Animal-Assisted Therapy Activity/Technique	Nursing Outcomes Classification
Cognitive		
1. Increase patient attention and knowledge, and provide diversion from facility environment demonstrated by reverbalization of information taught	1. Bring animal to individual or group for show and tell. Teach patient/client about history of animal, foods eaten, sleep habits, play, and overall care	1. Concentration: Ability to focus on a specific stimulus
2. Increase memory recall with Animal-Assisted Therapy (AAT) demonstrated by patient reverbalization of dog's name, breed, color, and size (Delta Society, 1996b)	2. Patients learn about therapy dog's age, breed, color, and size and later are asked to reverbalize information about therapy dog (10 minutes later or next day)	2. Memory: Ability to cognitively retrieve and report previously stored information
3. Decrease feelings of guilt at a chemical dependency treatment facility with AAT demonstrated by verbalization of past drug behavior and goals for the future (Delta Society, 1996b)	3. Interact with small farm animals, using animals as a bridge between staff and patient to communicate	3. Adherence Behavior: Self-initiated action taken to promote wellness, recovery, and rehabilitation
4. Improved consciousness demonstrated by patient movement or verbalization while in proximity to dog	4. Place animal next to patient in bed and assist patient in stroking animal	4. Neurological Status: Consciousness: Extent to which an individual arouses, orients, and attends to the environment
Physical		
1. Increase relaxation with AAT demonstrated by the contemplation of a fish aquarium (Katcher, Segal, & Beck, 1984)	1. Provide actual fish aquarium and instruct patients to contemplate a fish or fish aquarium for 20 minutes and tell them this will increase feelings of relaxation (hands are kept out of water)	1. Comfort Level: Feelings of physical and psychological ease
2. Increase muscle function with AAT demonstrated by increased strength, mobility, and balance during hippotherapy (Yasikoff & Kunzle, 1995)	2. Hippotherapy via natural mobilization of pelvis, lumbar spine, and hip joints (highly recommended for patients with multiple sclerosis and cerebral palsy)	2. Joint Movement: Active: Range of motion of joints with self-initiated movement
3. Increase upper extremity muscle function with AAT in quadriplegia patient with upper extremity weakness, demonstrated by patient grooming dog (McLaughlin, 1996)	3. Visiting therapy dog is supervised by physical therapist and supported by animal owner to place dog on raised table and have patient groom dog	3. Muscle Function: Adequacy of muscle contraction needed for movement
4. Patient will improve ambulatory skills, demonstrated by walking to animal	4. Dog is stationed at end of parallel bars or end of 40-foot hallway, and patient ambulates to greet dog	4. Ambulation: Walking: Ability to walk from place to place

Table continued on opposite page

Table 32–3 Examples of Goals, Activities, and Outcomes *Continued*

Goal	Animal-Assisted Therapy Activity/Technique	Nursing Outcomes Classification
Psychosocial		
1. Decrease anxiety with AAT demonstrated by an increase in relaxed body posture and facial expression (Wilson, 1991)	1. Facilitate patient's watching visiting/resident therapy dog and promote proximity and stroking animal at comfortable intervals of 10–15 minutes	1. Anxiety Control: Ability to eliminate or reduce feelings of apprehension and tension from an unidentifiable source
2. Decreased loneliness with AAT, demonstrated by interaction with a pet animal (Duncan, 1995b)	2. Provide AAT animal visits to patients at home, nursing homes, hospitals, hospice, rehabilitation facilities, psychiatric facilities, and prisons, within guidelines and policy of each facility	2. Loneliness: The extent of emotional, social, or existential isolation response
3. Initiate verbal communication with AAT, demonstrated by patient giving dog commands or describing animal's coat	3. Introduce AAT dog and explain to patient dog's ability and level of understanding to commands (i.e., sit, lie down, stay, come)	3. Communication: Expressive Ability: Ability to express and interpret verbal and/or nonverbal messages
4. Increase social involvement with AAT in Alzheimer's disease patients, demonstrated by presence of AAT dog to decrease agitation	4. Schedule regular visits to facility geared toward Alzheimer's disease patients. Questions and answers about dog care and reminiscence are common	4. Social Support: Perceived availability and actual provision of reliable assistance from other persons
Spiritual		
1. Increase acceptance of health status, demonstrated by increased reminiscence in maintaining spirit	1. Dog's position is dictated by patient (may snuggle to one side in bed), and patient strokes the dog and reminisces	1. Acceptance: Health Status: Reconciliation to health circumstances
2. Health promoting behavior, demonstrated by pet acquisition and care (Serpell, 1991)	2. Support pet ownership (desire and provision of animal care needs are met); utilize community resources in the prevention of pet separation from owners	2. Health Promoting Behavior: Actions to sustain or increase wellness
3. Increase quality of life, demonstrated by increased smiles and cheerfulness during dog interaction (Kongable, Stolley, & Buckwalter, 1990)	3. AAT dog visitation to a unit for Alzheimer's disease patients three times a week for 1 hour or as tolerated: Assist patient in gently petting the dog	3. Quality of Life: An individual's expressed satisfaction with current life circumstances
4. Increase spiritual well-being (provide meaningful connection for patient) with AAT, demonstrated by reminiscence	4. Patient talks about past experiences with previous animals and their past, present, or future in general	4. Spiritual Well-Being: Personal expressions of connectedness with self, others, higher power, all life, nature, and the universe that transcend and empower the self

North American Nursing Diagnosis Association (NANDA) (1996) diagnoses suggested for Animal-Assisted Therapy include the following:

Anxiety
Communication, Impaired Verbal
Confusion, Chronic
Diversional Activity Deficit
Hopelessness
Individual Coping, Ineffective
Loneliness, Risk for
Pain

Physical Mobility, Impaired
Powerlessness
Relocation Stress Syndrome
Self Esteem Disturbance
Social Interaction, Impaired
Social Isolation
Spiritual Distress

Nursing Outcomes Classification (NOC) outcomes suggested for Animal-Assisted Therapy include the following:

Acceptance: Health Status
Adherence Behavior
Ambulation: Walking
Anxiety Control
Caregiver-Patient Relationship
Child Development: Middle
    Childhood (6–11 years)
Circulation Status
Comfort Level
Communication Ability
Compliance Behavior

Concentration
Hope
Joint Movement: Active
Leisure Participation
Loneliness
Memory
Muscle Function
Self-Esteem
Social Involvement
Spiritual Well-Being
Well-Being

CASE STUDIES

Case Study 1

Assessment and History

Mr. P was becoming increasingly withdrawn and hopeless during the long waiting period for a heart transplant. Mr. P was a very pleasant 45-year-old, seemingly happy man, who was admitted January 10, 1997 with idiopathic cardiomyopathy, precipitated by flulike symptoms 6 months before admission. Mr. P had three loving and supportive children and a wife and owned a small yet lucrative construction company. Mr. P's blood type was O positive. This was significant, because large hearts with type O blood are the most uncommon. Mr. P's cardiac output was low, and he was categorized as status one, meaning he would stay in the confines of the cardiac care unit on intravenous inotropes of dobutamine and renal dose dopamine in addition to frequent intravenous diuretics until transplant. After 6 weeks of hospitalization, the nursing staff had acknowledged his difficulty coping with the hospitalization; he showed signs of anxiety, depression, and hostility, demonstrated by frequently requesting anxiolytics, staying in bed all day, refusing company other than his immediate family, refusing to eat foods

that contained any nutrition, and drinking more water than he was supposed to despite his already fluid-overloaded state. Most distressing to the staff was that, after 3 months of hospitalization, Mr. P was found bent over in a chair with his head in his hands, crying uncontrollably.

SOAP Note

S: I'm feeling worse every day. I'm thirsty all the time and scared for my family."

O: Three months after being hospitalized in the same room, the patient was found in his chair with his face in his hands, crying uncontrollably.

A: Appears patient is accustomed to being a support person for family and friends and is having difficulty coping with current health status.

P: Place a saltwater fish tank in Mr. P's room with colorful fish for him to name, feed, and care for until he receives a heart transplant. The patient was instructed not to put his hands in the fish tank water.

Nursing Diagnosis/Problem

Ineffective Individual Coping related to situational crisis.

Goals and Evaluation

Improve coping, as demonstrated by the patient's ability to identify needs and solve problems with staff and family, increased frequency of smiles and relaxed facial expression when focusing on fish aquarium, diversion from health status, getting out of bed to feed fish, increased frequency of conversation, fewer requests for anxiolytics, and verbalization that the fish aquarium is relaxing to him.

Patient Response

The fish aquarium in Mr. P's room became a bridge for socialization between staff, patient, and family. Mr. P verbalized that the aquarium was peaceful and soothing and kept him company at night when he felt especially alone. Mr. P was able to demonstrate his responsible nature by making sure the fish were fed daily.

Case Study 2

Assessment and History

AM was a 29-year-old woman from Kansas City, Missouri, who worked as an archivist and lived on a large farm, where she spent much of her leisure time outdoors. AM had been diagnosed in her hometown with breast cancer. She had a modified mastectomy and all the lymph nodes removed on her right side, in addition to chemotherapy treatments. It was recommended that AM undergo a bone marrow transplant (stem cell) for immune defense purposes. AM received her transplant at a facility 2,000 miles away from home in February; however, her course was complicated by a rare problem called veno-occlusive disease, which caused severe liver impairment that prolonged her hospitalization by 4 months. AM had one picture at her bedside of her three dogs, Gwen, Kate, and Duncan. AM's parents were deceased, and her family support consisted of a close friend and a boyfriend who commuted back and forth from Kansas City. By March 20, AM was, by inspection, severely jaundiced, withdrawn, and listless; her cachectic silhouette was weak, and she remained motionless in the bed. AM seemed depressed, and her eyes remained

closed most of the time. Although AM was neutropenic, the staff, including the primary attending physician, believed that Animal-Assisted Therapy visits, which historically were perceived by AM to be a strong support and resource, would carry more benefit than risk in this very sick, withdrawn woman.

SOAP Note

S: "I miss my dogs very much. I hope they are okay. There is nothing I can do about it."

O: AM was severely jaundiced, withdrawn, and listless; her cachectic silhouette was weak; and she remained motionless in bed, frequently with her eyes closed, and only responded if necessary.

A: AM appeared to be depressed and hopeless.

P: Start Animal-Assisted Therapy visits twice a week for 30 minutes or as tolerated as one nursing intervention as an adjunct to AM's excellent medical care.

Nursing Diagnosis/Problem

Hopelessness related to situational crisis.

Goal and Evaluation

Improved mood, demonstrated by the patient's opening her eyes when the dog team arrived, increased frequency of smiles, eye contact, increased conversation, increased mobility, stroking and cuddling with the dog, relaxed facial expression of reverie, cognitive interest, and patient verbalization of improved well-being.

Patient Response

At her weakest, AM would open her eyes with interest and softly dictate where she would like the dog placed in the bed. AM would snuggle and look at the dog in reverie as she talked to the volunteer owner about her own dogs and home. AM reported, "The dogs were a healing force that lifted my spirits and ability to get well. I looked forward to my visits. They helped me breathe." On AM's last Animal-Assisted Therapy visit, with a warm and grateful "thank you" and a tear of joy, it was now her turn to say "goodbye" and head home to her own furry friends.

CONCLUSION

Animal-Assisted Therapy is being recognized as a nursing intervention that focuses on optimizing wellness and the healing process. Refined medical knowledge of the brain and discoveries in physics about what stimuli affect, neutralize, or protect us from the ill effects of stress and how they accomplish this will help guide us to a better understanding, utilization, and respect for our relationship with animals. Convincing case studies and scientific research tell us that animals can have beneficial effects for many people from all age groups, from the residential to the tertiary setting. It is the responsibility of the people to take good stewardship over their pets, assist them in good health, teach them polite public behavior, and learn about their needs and means of communication or language as we teach them ours.

References

Allen, K. M., and Blaskovich, J. (1996). The value of service dogs for people with severe ambulatory disabilities. *Journal of the American Medical Association, 275,* 1001–1006.

Allen, K. M., Blascovich, J., Tomaka, J., and Kelsey, R. M. (1991). Presence of human friends and pet dogs as moderators of autonomic responses to stress in women. *Journal of Personality and Social Psychology, 61,* 582–589.

Anderson, W. P., Reid, C. M., and Jennings, G. L. (1992). Pet ownership and risk factors for cardiovascular disease. *Medical Journal of Australia, 157,* 298–301.

Arkow, P. (1982). *How to start a pet therapy program.* Alameda, CA: The Latham Foundation.

Baker, E. (1994). Precautions and contraindications to therapeutic riding: A framework for decision-making. In *Proceedings of the 8th International Therapeutic Riding Congress* (pp. 70–72). Levin, New Zealand: National Training Resource Center.

Barba, B. E. (1995). The positive influence of animals: Animal-assisted therapy in acute care. *Clinical Nurse Specialist, 9*(4), 199–202.

Batson, K., McCabe, W., Baun, M. M., Mara, M., and Wilson, C. (1995, September 6). The effect of a therapy dog on socialization and physiologic indicators of stress in persons diagnosed with Alzheimer's disease. C. C. Wilson and D. C. Turner (Eds.), *Companion animals in human health* (pp. 203–215). Thousand Oaks, CA: Sage Publishing.

Baun, M. M., Bergstrom, N., Langston, N. F., and Thoma, L. (1984). Physiological effects of human/companion animal bonding. *Nursing Research, 33*(3), 126–129.

Brickel, C. N. (1979). The therapeutic roles of cat mascots with a hospital based population: A staff survey. *Gerontologist, 19,* 368–372.

Bryant, B. K. (1985). The neighborhood walk: A study of sources of support in middle childhood from the child's perspective. *Monographs of the Society for Research and Childhood Development, 50* (Serial 210).

Bustad, L. K. (1996). The importance of animals to the well-being of people. In *Compassion: Our last great hope* (2nd ed., pp. 39–44). Renton, WA: Delta Society.

Carmack, B. J. (1991). The role of companion animals for persons with AIDS/HIV. *Holistic Nursing Practice, 5,* 24–31.

Carmack, B. J., and Fila, D. (1989). Animal-assisted therapy: A nursing intervention. *Nursing Management, 20*(5), 96–101.

Cawley, R., Cawley, M. S., and Retter, M. (1994). Therapeutic horseback riding and self-concept in adolescents with special educational needs. *Anthrozoös, 7*(2), 129–134.

Chinner, T. L., and Dalziel, F. R. (1991). An exploratory study on the viability and efficacy of a pet-facilitated therapy project within a hospice. *Journal of Palliative Care, 7*(4), 13–20.

Cohen, B. (1992). Therapy is a key word in equine treatment. *Advance: The Physical Therapy Weekly, 8,* 48.

Cole, K., and Gawlinski, A. (1995). Animal-assisted therapy in the intensive care unit: A staff nurse's dream comes true. *Nursing Clinics of North America, 30,* 529–537.

Copeland, J. (1992). Three therapeutic aspects of riding for the disabled. In B. Engel (Ed.), *Therapeutic riding programs: Instruction and rehabilitation* (pp. 19–20). Durango, CO: B. Engel Therapy Services.

Corson, I. S., and Corson, E. O. (1973). *Proposal for research project designed to facilitate therapy of adults and adolescent psychiatric and psychosomatic patients and shorten hospital stay.* Columbus: Ohio State University.

Corson, S. A., Corson, E. O., Gwynne, P., and Arnold, L. E. (1977). Pet dogs as nonverbal communication links in hospital psychiatry. *Comprehensive Psychiatry, 18,* 61–72.

Delta Society. (1992, May). *Pet partners: Clinical applications of animal-assisted therapy workshop.* Renton, WA: Author.

Delta Society. (1996a, November). *Standards of practice for animal-assisted activities and animal-assisted therapy.* Renton, WA: Author.

Delta Society. (1996b, November). *Animal-assisted therapy in the healthcare professions.* Renton, WA: Author.

Duncan, S. L. (1995a, September 6). Service dogs: The evolving role of dogs in the lives of people with disabilities. In *Animals, health and quality of life.* Geneva, Switzerland: International Association of Human–Animal Interaction Organizations.

Duncan, S. L. (1995b). Loneliness: A health hazard of modern times. *InterActions, 13*(1), 5–9.

Duncan, S. L. (1998). The importance of training standards and policy for service animals. In C. Wilson and D. C. Turner (Eds.), *Companion animals in human health* (pp. 251–266). Thousand Oaks, CA: Sage Publishing.

Engel, B. T. (Ed.). (1992). *Therapeutic riding programs: Instruction and rehabilitation.* Durango, CO: B. Engel Therapy Services.

Fila, D. (1991). The significance of companion animals to a geriatric vascular case study. *Holistic Nursing Practice, 5,* 2.

Fitzpatrick, J. C., and Tebay, J. M. (1995). Hippotherapy and therapeutic riding. In C. C. Wilson and D. C. Turner (Eds.), *Companion animals in human health* (pp. 41–58). Thousand Oaks, CA: Sage Publications.

Friedmann, E., Katcher, A., Lynch, J., and Thomas, S. (1980). Animal companions and one-year survival of patients after discharge from a coronary care unit. *Public Health Reports, 95,* 307–312.

Friedmann, E., Katcher, A., Thomas, S., Lynch, J., Messent, P. (1983). Social interaction and blood pressure. Influence of animal companions. *Journal of Nervous and Mental Disease, 171,* 461–465.

Friedmann, E., Katcher, A., and Meislich, D. (1983). When pet owners are hospitalized: Significance of companion animals during hospitalization. In A. H. Katcher and A. M. Beck (Eds.), *New perspectives on our lives with animal companions* (pp. 346–350). Philadelphia: University of Pennsylvania Press.

Friedmann, E., and Thomas, S. (1985). Health benefits of pets for families. In M. B. Sussman (Ed.), *Pets in the family* (pp. 191–203). New York: Haworth Press.

Friedmann, E., and Thomas, S. A. (1995). Pet ownership, social support, and one-year survival after acute myocardial infarction in the cardiac arrhythmia suppression trial (CAST). *American Journal of Cardiology, 76,* 1213–1217.

Gammonley, J. (1995, September 6–9). *A role delineation study for certification in animal assisted therapy.* Paper presented at the 7th International Conference on Human–Animal Interactions. Animals, Health and Quality of Life (Selected abstract). Geneva, Switzerland.

Hart, L. A. (1992). *Aquarium fish for recovery of coronary patients in intensive care.* Paper presented at the 6th International Conference on Human–Animal Interactions, Montreal, Canada.

Holcomb, R., Jendro, C., Weber, B., and Nahan, U. (1997). Use of an aviary to relieve depression in elderly males. *Anthrozoös, 10*(1), 32–36.

Holcomb, R., and Meacham, M. (1989). Effectiveness of an animal-assisted therapy program in an inpatient psychiatric unit. *Anthrozoös, 2*(4), 259–264.

Kale, M. (1992a). How some kids gain success, self-esteem with animals. *InterActions, 10,* 1317.

Kale, M. (1992b). Kids & animals: A comforting hospital combination. *Interactions, 10*(3), 17–21.

Katcher, A. H., Segal, H., and Beck, A. (1984). Comparison of contemplation and hypnosis for the reduction of anxiety and discomfort during dental surgery. *American Journal of Clinical Hypnosis, 27,* 14–21.

Klüwer, B. (1994). Psychomotoric movement: Observation in hippotherapy. In *Proceedings of the 8th International Therapeutic Riding Congress* (pp. 79–87). Levin, New Zealand: National Training Resource Center.

Klüwer, C. (1988). The specific contribution of the horse in different branches of therapeutic riding for the disabled. In *Proceedings of the 6th International Therapeutic Riding Conference* (pp. 268–294). (Information available through H. Brcko, 19 Alcaine Court, Thornhill, Ontario, Canada L3T 2G8).

Kongable, L. G., Stolley, J. M., and Buckwalter, K. C. (1990, Fall). Pet therapy for Alzheimer's patients: A survey. *Journal of Long-Term Care Administration,* 17–21.

Levinson, B. (1962). The dog as "Co-therapist." *Mental Hygiene, 46,* 59–65.

Levinson, B. (1964). Pets: A special technique in child psychotherapy. *Mental Hygiene, 48,* 243–248.

MacInnis, K. (1991). Blackie. *American Journal of Nursing, 84.*

McLaughlin, C. (1996, January 29). Bow-wow: What a difference animal assistance can make. *ADVANCE for Physical Therapists,* 10.

Melson, G. F. (1988). Availability of and involvement with pets by children: Determinants and correlates. *Anthrozoös, 2,* 265–273.

Melson, G. F., and Schwartz, R. (1994, October). *Pets as social supports for families with young children* (pp. 1–16). Paper presented to Delta Society, New York.

Mugford, R., & M'Comisky, J. (1975). Some recent work on the psychotherapeutic value of caged birds with old people. In R. Anderson (Ed.), *Pet animals and society.* London: Bailiere Tindall.

Nebbe, L. (1995). *Nature as a guide.* Minneapolis, MN: Educational Media Corp.

North American Nursing Diagnosis Association. (1987). *Classifications of nursing diagnosis: Proceedings of the seventh national conference.* St. Louis: C.V. Mosby.

North American Riding for the Handicapped Association. (1993). *NARHA guide.* Denver, CO: Author.

Scheidhacker, M. (1994). *Die arbeit mit dem pferd in psychiatrie und psychotherapie* [Working with the horse in psychiatry and psychotherapy]. Warendorf, Germany: Schnell, Buch and Druck.

Sebkova, J. (1977). *Anxiety levels as affected by the presence of a dog.* Unpublished master's thesis, University of Lancaster, Bailrigg, Lancaster, England. Cited in M. B. Sussman (Ed.). (1985). *Pets and the family.* New York: Haworth Press.

Serpell, J. (1991). Beneficial effects of pet ownership on some aspects of human health and behaviour. *Journal of the Royal Society of Medicine, 84,* 717–720.

Shalev, A. (1996). Snakes: Interactions with children with disabilities and the elderly—some psychological considerations. *Anthrozoös, 9*(4), 182–187.

Stuckey, K. (Ed.). (1982). *The world book encyclopedia* (Vol. 8). Chicago: World Book-Childcraft International.

Triebenbacher, S. L. (1998). The relationship between attachment to companion animals and self-esteem: A developmental perspective. In C. C. Wilson and D. C. Turner (Eds.), *Companion animals in human health* (pp. 135–148). Thousand Oaks, CA: Sage Publications.

Walsh, P. G., and Mertin, P. G. (1994). The training of pets as therapy dogs in a women's prison: A pilot study. *Anthrozoös, 7*(2), 124–128.

Weatherill, A. (1993). Pets at school: Child-animal bond sparks learning and caring. *InterActions, 11*(1), 7–9.

Wilson, C. C. (1987). Physiological responses of college students to a pet. *Journal of Nervous and Mental Disease,* 606–612.

Wilson, C. C. (1991). The pet as an anxiolytic intervention. *Journal of Nervous and Mental Disease, 179,* 482–489.

Woolverton, M. C. (1991, October). *Reducing children's stress during physical examination by having them play with animals during the procedure.* Paper presented at the 10th Annual Conference of the Delta Society. Portland, Oregon.

Woolverton, M. (1993, February). An observation study on the responses of children to the presence of animal during neuromuscular examination. In *First international congress: Mexico 1993 human-animal companionship: Health benefits.*

Yasikoff, N., and Kunzle, U. (1995, September 7). Hippotherapy-K. In *Animals, health, and quality of life.* Geneva, Switzerland: International Association of Human-Animal Interaction Organizations.

Yates, J. (1987). Project pup: The perceived benefits to nursing home residents. *Anthrozoös, 1*(3), 188–192.

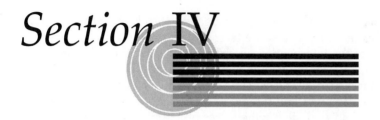

Section IV

Safety Interventions
Overview: Care That Supports Protection against Harm

Gloria M. Bulechek

Joanne C. McCloskey

One of the primary concerns of nurses is the safety of the patient and the provision of a safe environment for care delivery. Many of the monitoring and assessment functions of nurses are directed at detecting risks. In this section, we cover six safety interventions.

In Chapter 33, Cynthia M. Dougherty discusses the intervention of **Surveillance**, which can be used with a variety of patient populations, although it is a key intervention in critical care settings. According to Dougherty, Surveillance is similar to observation but goes beyond observation by emphasizing a greater variety of methods to gather data and, most importantly, including an evaluation component that then directs further data-gathering activities. Dougherty reviews the literature related to the field of intelligence, from which the concept was abstracted, and then discusses the limited research on use of Surveillance as a nursing intervention. Two elements are essential to the implementation of the intervention: time and the parameters of interest, such as vital signs or blood gas levels. Some of the associated nursing diagnoses and outcomes are identified, and a case study of a patient with the diagnosis of Decreased Cardiac Output illustrates the use of Surveillance in a critical care patient.

Safety is also a major concern in persons who are chronically confused. The intervention of **Dementia Management** is discussed in Chapter 34 by Jacqueline M. Stolley, Linda A. Gerdner, and Kathleen C. Buckwalter as the treatment for those with dementia or chronic confusion. Although many conditions can cause a chronic state of confusion, the most common is Alzheimer's disease. The authors first delineate the stages of Alzheimer's disease and the associated behavioral states and losses. They explain the Progressively Lowered Stress Threshold (PLST) model of care, which helps a caregiver modify the chronically confused patient's environment to provide less stress. The authors review some screening tools that help assess the level of cognitive functioning and then discuss details of the intervention according to the six principles of the PLST model: maximizing safe functioning, giving unconditional positive regard, determining limits of activity, listening, modifying the environment, and giving support to the caregiver and family. The intervention is aimed at maximizing the strengths and minimizing the losses of chronically confused patients, who have multiple needs and present a major challenge to caregivers. The intervention is used for the nursing diagnosis of Chronic Confusion and has several possible appropriate outcomes. A case study of a patient with advanced Alzheimer's disease is included to illustrate some of the intervention principles and activities discussed in the chapter.

Chapter 35, by Perle Slavik Cowen, addresses the other end of the age spectrum with a focus on the intervention of **Abuse Protection: Child.** According to Cowen, there are five types of child maltreatment: physical abuse, neglect, sexual abuse, emotional abuse, and emotional neglect. Eighty-two percent of maltreatment fatalities involve children younger than the age of 5. The literature on child maltreatment is extensive, and Cowen reviews and summarizes the risk factors (sociocultural, family, parental-caretaker, and child) and the signs and symptoms. She discusses both physical and environmental indicators and the child behavioral indicators that should be monitored in order to determine maltreatment. She reviews the classification of the North American Nursing Diagnosis Association (NANDA), the Nursing Interventions Classification (NIC), and the Nursing Outcomes Classification (NOC) and makes recommendations that each of these, while helpful now, should be further developed to include more specificity related to the population and type of maltreatment. Several tools are described that assist in evaluating at-risk families. A case study of a single homeless mother with an 11-month-old daughter is used to illustrate the application of the intervention Abuse Protection: Child and the usefulness of specified activities.

Another important safety intervention is **Suicide Prevention,** because suicides are the ninth leading cause of death in the United States. In Chapter 36, Rosemary Ferdinand reviews the risk factors for suicide within the categories of demographic factors, psychosocial factors, and chronic illness. Most completed suicides are by persons who are psychiatrically ill at the time of suicide, and the chapter offers an orientation to related psychiatric illnesses. The second half of the chapter elaborates on the research base for each of the NIC activities related to the intervention, providing specific directions to the provider for carrying out the activity. The chapter includes identification of the related nursing and psychiatric diagnoses and related patient outcomes. Ferdinand points out that positive orientation or the accomplishment of some intermediate outcomes (such as Coping, Impulse Control, or Grief Resolution) can indicate that the risk for suicide is lessening. The chapter concludes with a case study that demonstrates the application of the intervention at the specific activity level.

The risk of falling with the resultant injuries is a concern for many, with the highest incidence of falls occurring in the toddler and elderly years. Virginia Kilpack and Mary E. Godin begin Chapter 37, on **Fall Prevention,** with some interesting statistics on who falls and what happens to them. The old view that falls occur by chance or are a normal result of growing old has now changed to the view that falls are predictable and can be prevented. The authors review the research on falls in acute care settings, long-term care settings, and community settings. They provide an overview of the variety of screening tools that identify risk factors and probability of falling. Common variables placed on a risk assessment tool are history of falls, age, medical condition, medications, physical status, mental status, ambulatory devices, and protective restraining devices. Deciding on the specific intervention strategies or activities is challenging because of the variety of reasons that people fall. The chapter concludes with the identification of associated nursing diagnoses and patient outcomes and a case study.

A growing percentage of the population suffers from adverse reactions to products containing latex. This is associated with increased use of latex gloves by health care workers but is also caused by use of other latex products. In Chapter 38, Victoria M. Steelman reviews the literature as to types of reactions, routes of exposure, allergenicity of products, groups at increased risk, and changes for clinical practice. The intervention **Latex Precautions** includes screening of patients, communication, latex avoidance, monitoring, and patient education. The intervention is used with the nursing diagnoses of Risk for Injury and Knowledge Deficit related to latex allergy. The overall effectiveness of the intervention can be determined by the outcome Immune Hypersensitivity Control. A case study in which the intervention is used with a surgical patient is presented.

Surveillance

Cynthia M. Dougherty

Monitoring the health status of patients is an integral part of nursing practice and central to the nurse's role. During the 1990s, the number of illnesses increased, and the types of interventions dramatically increased in technological complexity, requiring the development of highly specialized monitoring skills in nursing. If monitoring of a particular parameter of interest is unnecessary, then nursing care is usually not required. Acute care hospitalization is needed when the patient or his or her family are not able to carry out therapeutic regimens at home or require the expert monitoring capability of nurses. Monitoring functions often go unrecognized as important nursing interventions, but close attention to health parameters is often the patient's first defense against injury or complications.

DEFINITION

Surveillance is defined as the application of behavioral and cognitive processes in the systematic collection of information used to make judgments and predictions about a person's health status. The intervention Surveillance is defined in the Nursing Interventions Classification (NIC) (McCloskey & Bulechek, 1996) as the "purposeful and ongoing acquisition, interpretation, and synthesis of patient data for clinical decision-making" (see Table 33–1). Surveillance is similar to observation, in that the gathering of information through watching, feeling, or touching is part of this intervention. However, Surveillance extends beyond observation in two ways: it emphasizes a greater variety of methods to gather data, and, more importantly, it includes an evaluation component. Surveillance is similar to nursing assessment, with assessment occurring at a single point in time. An initial assessment of health status is made at the time of first contact with a health care provider or institution, such as at hospital admission or at an annual physical examination. Surveillance becomes a nursing intervention when it involves the ongoing collection of information in order to identify and subvert potential problems. After the initial assessment is complete, a decision is made about Surveillance of future signs or symptoms in order to identify a problem, observe the progress of a current problem, or determine that no problem exists.

In nursing, Surveillance is the same as monitoring. In the quality assurance paradigm, monitoring is defined as "the systematic and ongoing collection and organization of data related to the indicators of quality and appropriateness of important aspects of care, and the comparison of cumulative data with thresholds for evaluation related to each indicator" (Joint Commission on Accreditation of Healthcare Organizations [JCAHO], 1988, p. 148). Monitoring is the measurement of small but important parts of care, practice, or staff performance. In the NIC, the word *monitor* is used at the activity level to indicate the surveillance of specific activities; the terms *surveillance* and *monitoring* are used at the intervention label level. The resulting data are reviewed, and judgments are made as to whether a problem exists. If problems are identified, either more extensive measurement is necessary or actions are taken to resolve them (Duquette, 1991).

Benner (1984) has identified seven domains of nursing practice, of which three domains describe essential elements of nursing monitoring and Surveillance. These include (1) the diagnostic and monitoring function, (2) effective management of rapidly changing situations, and (3) administering and monitoring therapeutic interventions and regimens. Within the category of diagnostic and monitoring functions of nursing, Benner (1984) has identified the competencies of detection and documentation of significant changes in a patient's condition, providing an early warning signal, and anticipating problems: future think, understanding the particular demands and experiences of an illness, and assessing the patient's potential for wellness and for responding to various treatment strategies (p. 97). She emphasized that the diagnostic and patient monitoring functions are central to the nurse's role yet are not fully recognized or legitimized. In discussing this domain, nurses described the importance of recognizing subtle patient changes within narrow margins of safety and knowing how to react appropriately. Nurses with experience in caring for similar patients develop specialized skills and knowledge that help them become experts.

Within the domain of effective management of rapidly changing situations, the nursing competencies of skilled performance in extreme life-threatening emergencies, contingency management (rapid matching of demands and resources in emergencies), and identifying and managing crises were identified. This domain encompasses the ability to rapidly detect a problem and to institute the help necessary to solve it. Determining accurate Surveillance parameters will enhance the nurse's ability to pick up early warning signs that a serious problem could develop (Benner, 1984).

Finally, Surveillance is needed to determine the therapeutic effects of interventions and regimens on treatments instituted to resolve health problems. Within this domain, essential nursing competencies include starting and maintaining intravenous (IV) therapy, administering medications accurately and safely, preventing and intervening in skin breakdown, and creating wound management strategies (Benner, 1984). Descriptions of competencies in this domain are well outlined in procedure books throughout varying health care situations. The nurse's role in determining the effectiveness of a given therapy involves collecting the necessary information about indicators expected to change as a result of therapy and conveying information to others when change has not occurred. Many of the interventions in the NIC include monitoring activities as an important component of the intervention.

Surveillance involves both a behavioral and a cognitive process. The behavioral component of Surveillance concerns the collection of information from both primary and secondary sources. Direct data collection includes inspection, palpation, percussion, and auscultation (Timerding, 1989; Yacone, 1987). Secondary sources of information may involve the use of several types of highly technical equipment. New monitoring parameters and devices used in health care are always becoming available, with nurses being primarily responsible for using the devices correctly in order to produce reliable and valid data. The cognitive component of Surveillance includes studying, interpreting, analyzing, and evaluating data to indicate a range of possibilities and to isolate those factors influencing a situation (Dulles, 1963). This process involves knowing where to look for information, remembering how frequently certain observations are required, and knowing when to expect a change in response to treatment (Carrieri, Stotts, Levinson, Murdaugh, & Holzemer, 1982; Reyes, 1987). A basic understanding of normal and abnormal findings is essential (Chan, 1989; Thompson, 1989). Perception and the ability to relate sensory stimuli to a knowledge base or to previous experience are two important elements of Surveillance. Nurses are responsible for interpreting signs and symptoms with a high degree of accuracy and reporting abnormalities to those responsible for changing treatment (Yacone, 1987).

RELATED LITERATURE AND RESEARCH

The concept of Surveillance has been abstracted from literature primarily in the field of intelligence related to espionage. In this field, Surveillance suggests that a judgment has been made by some governmental unit that the behavior being monitored is outside the range of legitimate political activities. In the case of the person being watched, the class of events under Surveillance is categorized as potentially threatening, and the individual functions appropriately in terms of avoiding or minimizing possible negative consequences. *Intelligence*, a synonym of *surveillance*, involves the process of information gathering followed by evaluation, judgment, or prediction, and then reporting the findings to an organization or group participating in the policymaking process (Blum, 1972).

The process of Surveillance involves an ongoing development of information about events, persons, groups, and even attitudes of large segments of the public (Blum, 1972). Surveillance must have planning and structure. Objectives are outlined, priorities established, and obstacles examined. Information that is gathered is of little value unless it reaches the hands of decision makers. In priority cases, someone has to decide what constitutes important information. Special watch is kept to scan incoming data for anything of critical nature, clues are sorted, and ideas are exchanged as to the development of an impending crisis. Because there is not time to submit every item for detailed analysis, raw intelligence can be dangerous without an understanding of the circumstances from which it was gathered. Therefore, information must be interpreted within a context (Dulles, 1963).

Because the concept of Surveillance has emerged in the field of intelligence, implications of deviance and secrecy have been associated with it. When viewed in the light of police operations, criminal investigations, and political or intelligence activities, Surveillance stigmatizes or labels those behaviors under close watch as deviant. When applied to a hospital situation, where patients have voluntarily placed themselves in the care of professionals for the purpose of remedying a health problem, the act of Surveillance is legitimate and appropriate. In this instance, the information that is gathered forms the basis for monitoring a diagnosis and instituting prompt intervention. Therefore, in health care situations, Surveillance is both legitimate and necessary for optimizing health status.

Critical care units in hospitals were established for the purpose of monitoring signs and symptoms in order to intervene quickly in life-threatening situations (Timerding, 1989). Patients in critical care units receive more frequent and detailed Surveillance activities than any other population of ill people. This type of Surveillance activity requires the nurse to possess highly specialized knowledge and skills in order to practice safely. Without Surveillance in the critical care situation, important information is likely to be overlooked, and problems of life-threatening proportion may be either missed altogether or misidentified. The essence of successful Surveillance, then, involves the piecing together of minute amounts of information that, when evaluated separately, may appear unrelated and insignificant.

Very little research has been reported in which Surveillance has been tested as an appropriate nursing intervention for specific nursing diagnoses. Most descriptions of Surveillance as a nursing intervention are embedded within the nursing assessment section of physical assessment textbooks. Within the last decade, the American Association of Critical-Care Nurses (AACN) published a manual of outcome standards for nursing care of the critically ill that included Surveillance as a nursing intervention for every nursing diagnosis listed (AACN, 1990).

Three related studies (Dougherty, 1985; Hubalik, 1981; Wessel, 1981) have demonstrated that Surveillance activities are legitimate and important in critical care situations involving patients with severe cardiovascular disorders. Nurses used both medical and nursing diagnoses to determine the parameters of interest for Surveillance activities. Examples are taking vital signs, evaluating laboratory values, monitoring electrocardiogram changes, and regulating fluid intake (Wessel, 1981). Several other authors have reported the importance of implementing Surveillance in pediatric populations (Curry & Duby, 1994; Kang, Barnard, & Oshio, 1994), those in life-threatening situations (Hebra, 1994), those with diabetes mellitus (Tilly, Belton, & McLachlan, 1995), those with acute respiratory conditions (Graybeal, 1994), and those requiring home care (McNeal, 1996).

The NIC research program has identified nursing activities related to the nursing intervention Surveillance (Table 33–1). The activities were validated and reported by Titler (1992), who also validated nine additional specific interventions related to the concept of Surveillance. These included Invasive Hemodynamic Monitoring, Intracranial Pressure (ICP) Monitoring, Neurologic Monitoring, Shock Prevention, Vital Signs Monitoring, Fluid Monitoring, Electrolyte Monitoring, and Acid-Base Monitoring. Specific behaviors of the nurse in implementing the interventions were specified and validated using Fehring's (1986) methodology. Further testing of the use of each intervention is needed in order to determine the practice settings where these interventions are most used and how they are related to patient care outcomes.

INTERVENTION TOOLS AND PROTOCOL

Two elements are essential to any Surveillance tool: *time*, measured in seconds, minutes, hours, or days, and *parameters of interest*, such as vital signs or blood

Table 33–1 Surveillance

DEFINITION: Purposeful and ongoing acquisition, interpretation, and synthesis of patient data for clinical decision-making.

ACTIVITIES:

Determine patient's health risk(s), as appropriate

Obtain information about normal behavior and routines

Select appropriate patient indices for ongoing monitoring, based on patient's condition

Establish the frequency of data collection and interpretation, as indicated by status of the patient

Facilitate acquisition of diagnostic tests, as appropriate

Interpret results of diagnostic tests, as appropriate

Retrieve and interpret laboratory data; contact physician, as appropriate

Explain diagnostic test results to patient and families

Monitor patient's ability to do self-care activities

Monitor neurological status

Monitor behavior patterns

Monitor vital signs, as appropriate

Collaborate with physician to institute invasive hemodynamic monitoring, as appropriate

Collaborate with physician to institute ICP monitoring, as appropriate

Monitor comfort level, and take appropriate action

Monitor coping strategies used by patient and family

Monitor changes in sleep patterns

Monitor oxygenation and initiate measures to promote adequate oxygenation of vital organs

Initiate routine skin surveillance in high-risk patient

Monitor for signs and symptoms of fluid and electrolyte imbalance

Monitor tissue perfusion, as appropriate

Monitor for infection, as appropriate

Monitor nutritional status, as appropriate

Monitor gastrointestinal function, as appropriate

Monitor elimination patterns, as appropriate

Monitor for bleeding tendencies in high-risk patient

Note type and amount of drainage from tubes and orifices and notify the physician of significant changes

Troubleshoot equipment and systems to enhance acquisition of reliable patient data

Compare current status with previous status to detect improvements and deterioration in patient's condition

Initiate and/or change medical treatment to maintain patient parameters within the limits ordered by the physician, using established protocols

Facilitate acquisition of interdisciplinary services (e.g., pastoral services or audiology), as appropriate

Obtain a physician consult when patient data indicates a needed change in medical therapy

Institute appropriate treatment, using standing protocols

Prioritize actions, based on patient status

Analyze physician orders in conjunction with patient status to ensure safety of the patient

Obtain consultation from the appropriate health care worker to initiate new treatment or change existing treatments

Source: McCloskey, J. C., and Bulechek, G. M. (Eds.). (1996). *Nursing interventions classification (NIC)* (2nd ed., pp. 536–537). St. Louis: Mosby–Year Book.

gas levels. Several examples of tools exist in the form of flow sheets used in acute care areas. Standard monitoring procedures for patients are sometimes established by clinical protocols in each institution. These protocols provide clues as to the appropriate parameters of interest to monitor for various types of problems. The medical and nursing diagnoses help determine the frequency of data collection, as well as the types of information needed in the Surveillance effort. In general, the more critical or life-threatening the situation is, the more frequently the parameters of interest should be monitored and evaluated. Successful implementation of the nursing intervention Surveillance will result in the prevention of complications and the stabilization of health problems. This depends on the nurse's ability to diagnose the problem requiring the intervention of Surveillance, the ability to choose the appropriate parameters of interest, and the appropriate use of information that is gathered.

After an initial assessment of health concerns has taken place, or it is determined that the patient has one of the at-risk nursing diagnoses, appropriate nursing interventions to target these problems are identified. Prioritized nursing diagnoses that require further Surveillance are determined. The exact parameters of interest that will be subsequently monitored are sometimes determined by the types of monitoring devices that are placed on the patient or by those body systems that require close watching. The only other decision to be made about the parameters of interest is the frequency of monitoring. This is determined by the patient acuity and the potential for harm if important information is not available in a timely manner.

Once baseline determinations of the parameters of interest are made, the frequency of subsequent monitoring is determined. The time of the parameters may change as further information is collected or a pattern in the data becomes apparent. New parameters may be selected for monitoring, and the time interval may be changed to increase or decrease the frequency of monitoring as is warranted. When greater stability is achieved in a parameter, the frequency of the monitoring interval can be safely decreased. The decision to change a parameter of interest or the frequency of monitoring interval is made by both nurses and physicians.

ASSOCIATED NURSING DIAGNOSES AND OUTCOMES

The target populations for Surveillance are those in life-threatening situations, those who are not able to care for themselves independently, those who exhibit self-destructive behaviors, those who are members of at-risk groups, and those who because of physical or mental impairments are not able to care for themselves safely. As identified by the NIC (McCloskey & Bulechek, 1996), the following primary diagnoses often require this intervention: Infant Behavior: Risk for Disorganized, Injury: Risk for, Positioning: Risk for, Sensory/Perceptual Alterations: Tactile, Skin Integrity: Impaired, and Trauma: Risk for, with monitoring interventions being identified for several other nursing diagnoses. The degree to which the potential or actual problem is life-threatening or poses a problem of safety will determine whether Surveillance, alone or in combination with other interventions, is indicated.

Outcomes of the intervention Surveillance are the amelioration of the defining characteristics identified in each specific nursing diagnosis for which Surveillance would be instituted. For example, the nursing diagnosis Infant Behavior: Risk for Disorganized would be treated with the nursing intervention of Surveillance over developmental progress of the infant across the life span from birth

Table 33–2 Nursing Diagnoses and Patient Outcomes Associated with the Nursing Intervention Surveillance

Diagnosis	Intervention	Outcome
Decreased Cardiac Output	Surveillance Invasive Hemodynamic Monitoring Shock Prevention Fluid Monitoring	Cardiac Pump Effectiveness Cardiac Pump Effectiveness Vital Signs Status Fluid Balance
Risk for Disorganized Infant Behavior	Surveillance	Child Development: 12 months
Risk for Injury	Surveillance: Safety	Safety Behavior: Personal Risk Control Safety Status: Falls Occurrence
Risk for Positioning	Surveillance: Safety	Risk Control Body Positioning: Self-Initiated
Sensory/Perceptual Alterations: Tactile	Surveillance: Safety	Neurological Status
Impaired Skin Integrity	Skin Surveillance	Tissue Integrity: Skin & Mucous Membranes
Risk for Trauma	Skin Surveillance	Tissue Integrity: Skin & Mucous Membranes

to 5 years. The patient outcome for this diagnosis is Child Development within normal limits for a particular age category through age 5 years (Johnson & Maas, 1997). Using the nursing diagnosis Impaired Skin Integrity and instituting the nursing intervention Skin Surveillance, the patient outcome would be Tissue Integrity: Skin & Mucous Membranes (Johnson & Maas, 1997) (Table 33–2).

CASE STUDY

B was a 27-year-old male construction worker who developed congestive cardiomyopathy following a viral infection. He contracted a subsequent respiratory infection, which exacerbated his congestive heart failure, placing him in a life-threatening condition. In order to save his life, he was hospitalized in the coronary care unit, and intra-aortic balloon pumping (IABP) was instituted in order to resolve cardiogenic shock. The primary nursing diagnosis for B was Decreased Cardiac Output, defined as a decrease in volume of blood ejected from the heart due to factors influencing stroke volume or heart rate. The antecedent condition leading to B's Decreased Cardiac Output was a decreased ventricular contractility resulting from the cardiomyopathy.

This episode of Decreased Cardiac Output was not the first for B, but this time it was complicated by continued enlargement and dilation of the heart. The compensatory mechanisms that normally increase cardiac output when a decrease in stroke volume has occurred were ineffective in maintaining a steady state, because B's cardiac reserve had been depleted. Because his cardiac output could not be maintained on the medical regimen, B was being considered for a heart transplant as the only remaining medical treatment that could improve his condition.

After B returned from the cardiac catheterization laboratory, where right and left catheterization was completed and an intra-aortic balloon pump was inserted, he was reattached to all monitoring capabilities in the coronary care unit. Equipment used for monitoring included a left femoral Swan-Ganz catheter, a left femoral arterial line, a right femoral intra-aortic balloon pump, two right femoral intravenous lines, a urinary catheter, a cardiac monitor, a ventilator, a nasogastric tube, and left subclavian intravenous lines. At the time the primary nurse first came in contact with B, he was experiencing a further decrease in his cardiac output, indicating that cardiogenic shock and death were imminent if prompt action was not instituted.

A number of factors led to the selection of the nursing intervention of Surveillance for B. Desired outcomes included early detection of an impending cardiopulmonary disaster, early detection of complications, successful resolution of the decreased cardiac output, detection of minor changes in hemodynamic state, establishment of priorities of care so that important areas would not be overlooked, development of a plan to deal with future developments in care, and resolution of the instability in cardiac function long enough for B to receive a cardiac transplant. These goals have been found to be of primary importance for critically ill cardiac patients (Chan, 1989; Timerding, 1989; Yacone, 1987).

The behavioral aspect of Surveillance included inspecting, palpating, percussing, and auscultating B's body, equipment, and environment. This encompassed vital signs, pulmonary artery pressure, cardiac output, urine output, oxygen status, medication titration, heart and lung sounds, peripheral circulation, skin color and temperature, secretions, hygienic care, intravenous titration, and laboratory values. The cognitive components of Surveillance for B included looking, seeing, estimating, understanding, interpreting, analyzing, and evaluating the parameters identified. These cognitive aspects may not always be readily apparent to someone observing the nurse who performs Surveillance, particularly if the nurse is merely standing at the patient's bedside and thinking. But because the frequency of recording and reporting is common to nurses in critical care, this cognitive component is reflected in the nurse's notes that imply that judgments are made. The cognitive component is also observable when the nurse notes an abnormality and either reports it to the physician or takes action by titrating medications, changing the position of the patient, increasing the rate of intravenous fluids, giving emergency drugs, implementing protocols, collecting subsequent laboratory samples, or making a conscious effort to continue to watch a particular parameter.

In this case study, Surveillance was implemented as a nursing intervention for the purpose of preventing cardiopulmonary disaster. The final step of the process involves an evaluation of the success of the intervention in reducing B's problem of Decreased Cardiac Output and in rapidly detecting changes in stability. It would be unrealistic to think that Bill's cardiomyopathy could be resolved by Surveillance; however, rapid detection and evaluation of changes in the cardiovascular system prompted immediate action. From the time the nursing intervention was instituted, B remained alive and reasonably stable for 4 days. By close monitoring and early action, it was hoped that the cardiogenic shock would be stabilized so that B could be transferred for a heart transplant. Surveillance of hemodynamics, urine, laboratory values, and medications prevented major cardiopulmonary complications until approximately 1 hour before his death. Surveillance prompted prioritizing needs, quick intervention, and detection of minor changes and most likely extended the life span of B beyond what would have been expected. This intervention allowed time for family members to begin the grief process in coping with this crisis. In Nursing Outcomes Classification (NOC) terms, one of the outcomes achieved by the intervention was Grief Resolution for family members.

SUMMARY

■

The nursing intervention Surveillance is described as an intervention important for individuals facing life-threatening conditions, those who are unable to independently care for themselves, and those exhibiting self-destructive behaviors. The application of both cognitive and behavioral processes is used to make judgments about a person's health status. Perception and the ability to relate sensory stimuli to a knowledge base or previous experience are important elements of Surveillance. Nurses are responsible for interpreting signs and symptoms as accurately as possible and reporting abnormalities. Future research should address the essential elements of various types of monitoring interventions with specific patient populations and relate these interventions to patient care outcomes.

References

American Association of Critical-Care Nurses. (1990). *Outcome standards for nursing of the critically ill.* Laguna Nigel, CA: Author.

Benner, P. (1984). *From novice to expert.* Menlo Park, CA: Addison-Wesley.

Blum, R. H. (1972). *Surveillance and espionage in a free society.* New York: Praeger.

Carrieri, V., Stotts, N., Levinson, J., Murdaugh, C., and Holzemer, W. L. (1982). The use of cardiopulmonary assessment skills in the clinical setting. *Western Journal of Nursing Research, 4*(1), 5–17.

Chan, E. S. (1989). Nursing assessment following cardiac resuscitation. *Nursing, 3*(36), 30–31.

Curry, D. M., and Duby, J. C. (1994). Developmental surveillance by pediatric nurses. *Pediatric Nursing, 20*(1), 40–44.

Dougherty, C. M. (1985). Decreased cardiac output. *Nursing Clinics of North America, 20,* 787–799.

Dulles, A. (1963). *The craft of intelligence.* New York: Harper & Row.

Duquette, A. M. (1991). Approaches to monitoring practice: Getting started. In P. Schroeder (Ed.), *Monitoring and evaluation in nursing* (pp. 7–25). Gaithersburg, MD: Aspen Publishers.

Fehring, R. J. (1986). Validating diagnostic labels: Standardized methodology. In M. E. Hurley (Ed.), *Classification of nursing diagnoses: Proceedings of the sixth conference* (p. 183). St. Louis: C.V. Mosby.

Graybeal, J. M. (1994). Advances in respiratory monitoring. *RT: The Journal of Respiratory Care Practitioners, 7*(4), 31–34.

Hebra, J. D. (1994). The nurse's role in continuous dysrhythmia monitoring. *AACN Clinical Issues for Critical Care Nursing, 5*(2), 178–185.

Hubalik, K. T. (1981). *Nursing diagnosis associated with heart failure in critical care nursing.* Unpublished master's thesis, University of Illinois, Chicago.

Johnson, M., and Maas, M. (1997). *Nursing outcomes classification (NOC).* St. Louis: Mosby–Year Book.

Joint Commission on Accreditation of Healthcare Organizations. (1988). Guide to clinical indicators. In *Accreditation manual for hospitals.* Chicago: Author.

Kang, R., Barnard, K., and Oshio, S. (1994). Description of the clinical practice of advanced practice nurses in family-centered early intervention in two rural settings. *Public Health Nursing, 11,* 376–384.

McCloskey, J. C., and Bulechek, G. M. (Eds.). (1996). *Nursing interventions classification (NIC)* (2nd ed.). St. Louis: Mosby–Year Book.

McNeal, G. J. (1996). High-tech home care: An expanding critical care frontier. *Critical Care Nurse, 16*(5), 51–58.

Reyes, A. V. (1987). Monitoring and treating life-threatening ventricular dysrhythmias. *Nursing Clinics of North America, 22*(1), 61–76.

Thompson, C. (1989). The nursing assessment of the patient with cardiac pain on the coronary care unit. *Intensive Care Nursing, 5*(4), 147–154.

Tilly, K. E., Belton, A. B., and McLachlan, J. F. C. (1995). Continuous monitoring of health status outcomes: Experience with a diabetes program. *Diabetes Education, 21,* 413–419.

Timerding, B. L. (1989). Cardiopulmonary monitoring and sudden cardiac death. *Topics in Emergency Medicine, 11*(2), 12–22.

Titler, M. G. (1992). Interventions related to surveillance. *Nursing Clinics of North America, 27,* 495–516.

Wessel, S. L. (1981). *Nursing functions related to the nursing diagnosis decreased cardiac output.* Unpublished master's thesis, University of Illinois, Chicago.

Yacone, L. A. (1987). Cardiac assessment. *RN, 50*(5), 42–48.

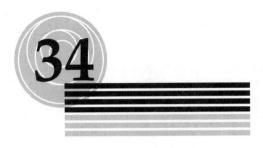

Dementia Management

Jacqueline M. Stolley, Linda A. Gerdner, and

Kathleen C. Buckwalter

ementia is a chronic, progressively deteriorating disease that is socially disabling and makes unusually high demands on medical, nursing, social, and economic resources. Dementia Management incorporates the provision of symptomatic and supportive measures that include such diverse actions as modification of the environment to prevent under- and overstimulation or correction of physiological stressors to prevent excess disability.

Dementia, or chronic confusion, is different from delirium, or acute confusion. Dementia is irreversible and a result of actual brain damage, whereas delirium is reversible and unrelated to permanent brain damage. Therefore, it is important for nurses to distinguish between delirium and dementia and to understand that a person with dementia can also experience an acute episode of delirium, exhibiting exacerbated symptoms related to physical or environmental causes. Anything that interrupts or violates the dynamic equilibrium of person, body, self, and the environment can result in delirium. Aged persons are particularly vulnerable to disequilibrium due to losses associated with the aging process and various sociocultural factors that increase the perception of stress (Hall & Buckwalter, 1987). This chapter focuses on the nursing intervention for persons with dementia, which results in progressive, deteriorating declines in cognitive and functional abilities.

DEMENTIA

Although there are 70 different conditions that can cause dementia in the middle and late years (Blass, 1982; Katzman, 1986), Alzheimer's disease (AD) is the most common, affecting 60% to 75% of the elderly who have dementia (Hull,

1996; Jellinger, Danielczyk, Fischer, & Gabriel, 1990). AD is a progressive disorder characterized by losses of memory, intellectual and language ability, and general competency over a period from 8 to 10 years after diagnosis, and ending in death. AD affects approximately 10% of individuals between ages 65 and 75 and 25% of individuals older than age 85 (Evans et al., 1989). Because of the costs of long-term care and the duration of dementia, 80% to 90% of persons with the condition are cared for in the home by family members (Office of Technology Assessment [OTA], 1987). The remainder are cared for in institutions, but only after several years, when family members are no longer able to provide adequate care. It is estimated that at least 50%, and perhaps as many as 70%, of all nursing home residents have some type of dementia. Institutionalization may be inevitable as the disease progresses (Berger, 1985).

The diagnosis of AD is made by exclusion of other possible causes of dementia (Weiner, Tintner, & Bonte, 1996). Several other degenerative brain diseases present with behaviors similar to those found in AD, although their etiologies are quite different. Multi-infarct dementia (MID), or vascular dementia, accounts for about 15% to 20% of all dementing illnesses (Malone, 1994; Mirsen & Hachinski, 1988). When infarcts occur, cognitive and functional abilities diminish in abrupt, steplike fashion rather than in the gradual, almost imperceptible decline noted in AD. MID and AD coexist in another 7% to 18% of the cases of dementia (Malone, 1994; Mirsen & Hachinski, 1988). Other rare conditions account for around 13% of the dementias, including Pick's disease, Creutzfeldt-Jakob disease, Parkinson's disease, Huntington's disease, normal-pressure hydrocephalus, and acquired immunodeficiency syndrome (AIDS). AIDS is among the fastest-growing cause of dementia, especially in young adults.

Symptoms of AD typically progress in stages or phases. Reisberg, Ferris, DeLeon, and Crook (1982) defined the stages of AD using the Global Deterioration Scale (GDS). The GDS measures deterioration in seven stages, with stage 1 being normal (indicating no cognitive decline) and stage 7 being late dementia (indicating very severe cognitive decline). A simpler method delineates disease progression into four states: forgetfulness, confusion, ambulatory dementia, and the terminal or end stage (Hall & Buckwalter, 1987). In the forgetful stage, a loss of short-term memory is seen, and the client may use memory aids but also become depressed because he or she is aware that something is wrong with his or her memory. AD is usually not diagnosable at this stage.

In the second stage, confusion and memory declines are more pronounced, and the client becomes disoriented to time, place, person, and things, usually in that order. Decline in instrumental activities of daily living (IADLs) becomes apparent, although denial of the memory loss is common. Because clients may fear they are "losing their mind," they are at increased risk for depression. The client may confabulate to cover for memory loss and may seem to have more problems with memory, judgment, and temper when fatigued. In this stage, the client may need assistance in the home and may also need day care.

In the ambulatory dementia stage, functional losses in activities of daily living (ADLs) become much more apparent, and these losses progress with time and the amount and location of brain damage. The client in this third stage of AD loses the ability to reason, communicate verbally, and plan for safety. With disease progression, the client may become more withdrawn and self-absorbed, but depression lifts as the client become less aware of his or her disabilities. Evidence of a decreased ability to tolerate stress is seen in episodes of night awakening, wandering, pacing, increased confusion, belligerence, agitation, withdrawal, and combative behavior. At this point, institutional care is usually needed.

In the final, end stage of the disease, the client no longer recognizes family members or even his or her own reflection in the mirror. The client is often mute or may yell spontaneously and loses purposeful activity ability, including walking. Weight loss is common because of changes in glucose metabolism, and the client often forgets how to eat, swallow, and chew. As a result, problems associated with immobility occur, and incontinence is common. Seizure activity may emerge in this stage. At this stage, institutionalization is most certain.

Progressively Lowered Stress Threshold

Because of ego-sensory impairments and diminished perceptual and cognitive processes that interfere with the AD client's ability to interact successfully with the environment, control of the environment is essential for care management. Repetitive behaviors, catastrophic reactions, and inappropriate behaviors are symptoms of this impairment (Gerdner, Hall, & Buckwalter, 1996; Hall & Buckwalter, 1987). The Progressively Lowered Stress Threshold (PLST) model of care asserts that persons with AD require a modified environment because of declining functional and cognitive abilities. According to the PLST model, persons with AD have a decreasing ability to cope with stress as the disease progresses (Hall & Buckwalter, 1987).

Hall (1991) has described three types of behavior that may be present throughout the course of the disease: baseline or normative behavior, where the client is still cognitively and socially accessible; anxious behavior, which is a response to stress; and dysfunctional behavior, when excess stress is not reduced and the client with dementia cannot process the amount, complexity, or intensity of stimuli. These behaviors correspond to the amount of brain damage and the progression of the disease (Table 34–1).

According to the PLST model, the losses associated with AD and other

---

Table 34–1 Behavioral States Associated with Alzheimer's Disease

BASELINE	The client remains cognitively accessible. The client possesses a basic awareness of the environment and is able to interact and function, limited only by the amount of neurological deficits. The client also remains socially accessible. The client is able to communicate wants and needs and respond to the communication of others in an appropriate manner.
ANXIOUS	The client becomes anxious when feeling stress. Symptoms of anxious behavior may be complaints of a feeling of uneasiness. Eye contact is poor or absent, and psychomotor activity may increase in response to the avoidance of the noxious stimuli. Communication abilities usually remain intact.
DYSFUNCTIONAL	The client becomes dysfunctional if stress levels continue or increase. The client becomes catastrophic and cognitively and socially inaccessible. Communication is impaired, and the client is unable to interpret the environment appropriately (Wolanin & Phillips, 1981). The client may be fearful and panic-stricken and actively avoid noxious stimuli (Hall, 1991). Increased confusion, purposeful wandering, night awakening, "sundowner's syndrome," agitation, fearfulness, panic, combativeness, and sudden withdrawal are exhibited with catastrophic, dysfunctional behavior. The client may experience these symptoms infrequently early in the disease, but with disease progression they increase in frequency and intensity (Hall, 1991).

Source: Adapted from Hall, G. R. (1991). Altered thought processes: SDAT. In M. Maas and K. C. Buckwalter (Eds.), *Nursing diagnoses and interventions for the elderly.* Menlo Park, CA: Addison-Wesley.

Table 34–2 Symptom Clusters Associated with Progressive Dementing Illness

Cognitive (Intellectual)	• Memory loss, initially for recent events • Loss of time sense • Inability to abstract • Inability to make choices and decisions • Inability to reason and problem solve • Poor judgment • Altered perceptions and ability to identify visual and auditory stimuli • Less expressive and receptive language abilities
Affective Response to Perceptions of Loss (Personality)	• Loss of affect • Diminished inhibitions, emotional lability, spontaneous conversation with loss of tact, loss of control of temper, and inability to delay gratification • Decreased attention span • Social withdrawal and avoidance of complex or overwhelming stimuli • Increasing self-preoccupation • Antisocial behavior • Confabulation, perseveration • Psychotic features, such as paranoia, delusions, and hallucinations
Conative (Planning)	• Loss of general ability to plan activities • Inability to carry out voluntary activities or activities requiring thought to set goals, organize, and complete task • Functional loss, starting with IADL's; these progress to losses in ADLs • Motor apraxia • Increased fatigue with exertion or cognition, loss of energy reserve • Frustration, refusal to participate, or expressions of helplessness when losses are challenged • Increased thought about function tends to worsen performance
Progressively Lowered Stress Threshold (PLST)	• Catastrophic behaviors • Confused or agitated night awakening • Purposeful wandering • Violent, agitated, or anxious behavior • Withdrawal or avoidance behavior, such as belligerency • Noisy behavior • Purposeless behavior • Compulsive behavior • Other cognitively and socially inaccessible behaviors

Source: Adapted from Hall, G. R. (1988). Care of the patient with Alzheimer's disease living at home. *Nursing Clinics of North America, 23*(1), 31–46.

irreversible dementias fall into four symptom clusters: cognitive or intellectual losses, affective or personality losses, conative or planning losses, and PLST (Hall & Buckwalter, 1987) (Table 34–2). Dementia Management is directed largely toward providing supportive care to compensate for these losses and flows logically from the PLST framework. In planning interventions for persons with AD or other diseases manifested by chronic confusion, the following assumptions are made:

1. All humans require some control over their person and their environment and need some degree of unconditional positive regard.

2. All behavior is rooted and has meaning; therefore, all catastrophic and stress-related behaviors have a cause.

3. The confused or agitated client is not comfortable and should be regarded as frightened. All clients have the right to be comfortable.

4. The client exists in a 24-hour continuum. Care cannot be planned or evaluated on an 8-hour-shift basis (Hall, 1991; Hall & Buckwalter, 1987, p. 401).

Intervention activities for the client with dementia include the provision of symptomatic and supportive measures and are based on these four assumptions. Using this framework and the following principles, nurses can provide effective intervention and care for clients with dementia and their families:

1. Maximize the level of safe function by supporting all areas of loss in a prosthetic manner.

2. Provide the client with unconditional positive regard.

3. Use behaviors indicating anxiety and avoidance to determine limits of levels of activity and stimuli.

4. Teach caregivers to listen to the client, evaluating verbal and nonverbal responses.

5. Modify the environment to support losses and enhance safety.

6. Provide ongoing support, care, and problem solving for caregivers (Gerdner et al., 1996, p. 243; Hall & Buckwalter, 1987, p. 401; McCloskey & Bulechek, 1996, pp. 201–202).

INTERVENTION TOOLS

An appropriate intervention must take into account the degree of loss of the individual suffering from dementia. Thus, it is important to obtain accurate physical, social, and psychological histories of the client to determine premorbid personality and strategies used by the in-home caregiver to provide comfort.

The Mini Mental Status Examination (MMSE) is a useful screening tool for ascertaining the current cognitive level of the client and assessing cognitive loss on an ongoing basis (Folstein, Folstein, & McHugh, 1975). This test contains 10 items that measure recent and past memory, temporal orientation, language, quick recall, and ability to abstract and calculate, as well as assess affective and conative losses (Hall, 1991). The MMSE is a quick and easy method for nurses to obtain baseline measures of cognitive status and to determine changes over time. However, this instrument requires that the person be able to respond verbally and in writing, and it is not sensitive to changes in the last stage of the disease (Reisberg et al., 1984). The Global Deterioration Scale (GDS) measures function in seven clinically identifiable stages (Reisberg et al., 1982). However, neither the MMSE nor the GDS measures cognitive and functional ability with any precision at the time before death (Gerdner & Hall, in press).

The Functional Assessment Staging (FAST) was created to mirror the seven stages measured in the GDS and designed to characterize aspects of the patient's daily functioning in stages ranging from normal to severe dementia (Reisberg et al., 1984). The FAST is particularly useful because it is sensitive to functional changes related to the severity of the disease and provides more detail on the functional status than do the MMSE and GDS in the late stage of AD (Gerdner & Hall, in press).

Other parameters that must be assessed in order to determine appropriate intervention strategies are sleep patterns; medication use (especially psychoactive drugs); food intake and weight; socialization before and after institutionalization; episodes of anxious, confused, agitated, or purposeful wandering; combative or otherwise dysfunctional behavior; functional level; and family's satisfaction with care. Another area of paramount importance in assessment is the cultural aspects of the person with dementia.

Dementia Management

The intervention of Dementia Management can be associated with the six principles identified earlier and is specified in more detail in this section. The definition of Dementia Management is the "provision of a modified environment for the patient who is experiencing a chronic confusional state" (McCloskey & Bulechek, 1996) (Table 34–3).

Maximizing Safe Functioning

Nurses must prevent and treat the occurrence of excess disability, a condition that exists when the disturbance of functioning is greater than might be accounted for by basic physical illness or cerebral pathology (Dawson, Kline, Wianko, & Wells, 1986). Excess disability is thought to be caused by five factors: fatigue; change in routine (caregiver or environment); multiple competing stimuli; frustration and affective responses resulting from unrealistic expectations to perform; and physiological causes such as illness, discomfort, pain, or medication reactions (Gerdner et al., 1996; Hall & Buckwalter, 1987). Catastrophic reactions or dysfunctional behavior can result from any of these factors, causing excess disability.

Manifestations of dysfunctional behavior include wandering, night awakening, agitation, fearfulness, panic, combativeness, and sudden withdrawal. Nurses can be alert to anxious behavior that often leads to dysfunctional behavior by observing the client for loss of eye contact and attempts to avoid offending stimuli. Prevention or containment of the five factors listed is a key element of Dementia Management.

FATIGUE

Persons with AD and other chronic confusional states tend to react to stress or frustration by becoming more active, not knowing their levels of fatigue tolerance. In addition, sleep patterns tend to be altered, with an upset in diurnal rhythms. Nurses must be alert to this and provide for structured rest periods or quiet times at mid-morning and mid-afternoon. These rest periods prevent fatigue, allowing for a reduction in stress levels and promoting effective sleep patterns. In addition, rest periods provide the client with time to recover from stressful activities such as morning care and mealtimes.

CHANGE IN ROUTINE

It is important to provide a structured routine for persons with dementia. Because of memory loss and diminished intellectual functioning, the demented client has an increased need for security. Security is enhanced by providing a structured routine, familiar caregivers, and a secure environment. Because the client does not need to rely on planning skills for most activities, the use of a consistent routine is effective (Hall, 1991; Schwab, Rader, & Doan, 1985). For example, bath times, mealtimes, rest periods, and activities should be at approximately the same time every day. If possible, caregivers should be consistent, providing the client with the security of a familiar face. Room changes and

Table 34–3 Dementia Management

DEFINITION: Provision of a modified environment for the patient who is experiencing a chronic confusional state.

ACTIVITIES:

Include family members in planning, providing, and evaluating care, to the extent desired

Identify usual patterns of behavior for such activities as sleep, medication use, elimination, food intake, and self-care

Determine physical, social, and psychological history of patient, usual habits, and routines

Determine type and extent of cognitive deficit(s), using standardized assessment tool

Monitor cognitive functioning, using a standardized assessment tool

Determine behavioral expectations appropriate for patient's cognitive status

Provide a low-stimulation environment (e.g., quiet, soothing music; nonvivid and simple, familiar patterns in decor; performance expectations that do not exceed cognitive processing ability; and dining in small groups)

Provide adequate but nonglare lighting

Identify and remove potential dangers in environment for patient

Place identification bracelet on patient

Provide a consistent physical environment and daily routine

Prepare for interaction with eye contact and touch, as appropriate

Introduce self when initiating contact

Address the patient distinctly by name when initiating interaction, and speak slowly

Give one simple direction at a time

Speak in a clear, low, warm, respectful tone of voice

Use distraction, rather than confrontation, to manage behavior

Provide unconditional positive regard

Avoid touch and proximity, if this causes stress or anxiety

Provide caregivers that are familiar to the patient (e.g., avoid frequent rotations of assignments)

Avoid unfamiliar situations, when possible (e.g., room changes and appointments without familiar people)

Provide rest periods to prevent fatigue and reduce stress

Monitor nutrition and weight

Provide space for safe pacing and wandering

Avoid frustrating patient by quizzing with orientation questions that cannot be answered

Provide cues—such as current events, seasons, location, and names—to assist orientation

Seat patient at small table in groups of three to five for meals, as appropriate

Allow to eat alone, if appropriate

Provide finger foods to maintain nutrition for patient who will not sit and eat

Provide patient a general orientation to the season of the year by using appropriate cues (e.g., holiday decorations, seasonal decorations and activities, and access to contained, out-of-doors area)

Decrease noise levels by avoiding paging systems and call lights that ring or buzz

Select television or radio activities based on cognitive processing abilities and interests

Select one-to-one and group activities geared to the patient's cognitive abilities and interests

Label familiar photos with names of the individuals in photos

Select artwork for patient rooms featuring landscapes, scenery, or other familiar images

Ask family members and friends to see the patient one or two at a time, if needed, to reduce stimulation

Discuss with family members and friends how best to interact with the patient

Assist family to understand it may be impossible for patient to learn new material

Limit number of choices patient has to make, so not to cause anxiety

Provide boundaries, such as red or yellow tape on the floor, when low stimulus units are not available

Place patient's name in large block letters in room and on clothing, as needed

Use symbols, other than written signs, to assist patient to locate room, bathroom, or other equipment

Avoid use of physical restraints

Monitor carefully for physiological causes of increased confusion that may be acute and reversible

Remove or cover mirrors, if patient is frightened or agitated by them

Source: McCloskey, J. C., and Bulechek, G. M. (1996). *Nursing interventions classification (NIC)* (2nd ed., p. 201). St. Louis: Mosby–Year Book.

redecorating are discouraged, as is changing the location of activities. The client should not be exposed to changes in the environment unless he or she has experienced no dysfunctional behavior in the past associated with these activities.

MULTIPLE COMPETING STIMULI

Because demented clients are frequently deficient in cognitive and social accessibility, it is important to modify stimuli and simplify the environment. Persons with dementia have more difficulty interpreting the environment because of brain damage and sensoriperceptual deficits. For example, many demented persons become distracted and confused when eating in a large group, resulting in inability to consume appropriate nutrients. Thus, mealtimes should be modified as small-group or solitary activities.

Noise levels on a unit for persons with dementia should be decreased. Paging systems, ringing phones, yelling, banging, and even the noise of a disruptive client can be disturbing and become a source of agitation for the client with dementia. Television and radio use should be carefully monitored.

Pictures and photographs should be simple, because persons with dementia frequently misinterpret them as real. Therefore, artwork featuring landscapes and scenery is preferable. Photographs should be of familiar persons and labeled with their name to enable the demented client to identify the person in the photograph. Holiday and seasonal decorations provide cues to the client about the time of year. However, these decorations must be more subtle than those for clients who are not cognitively impaired to prevent overstimulation and dysfunctional behaviors.

Visits should occur at regular times if possible, and only one or two persons should visit at a time. Large-group activities, such as a family reunion, may need to be avoided unless the client has shown comfort and pleasure with these activities or they can be modified so that the demented client is with only one or two familiar persons at a time. Visitors should be instructed on appropriate topics to address, especially past events, and be reminded not to "test" the client or expect him or her to have memories or abilities that no longer are there.

UNREALISTIC EXPECTATIONS AND AFFECTIVE RESPONSE TO LOSS

Stress and frustration are frequently the result of expectations of others that go beyond the client's capabilities. This deals with diminished moods (e.g., depression) when the client is told he or she cannot do something or is not allowed to participate—for example, being told, "You can't drive the car," or "You are not allowed to come to bingo because you are disruptive." Unrealistic expectations of others and subsequent depression of the client with AD have been part of the impetus for the development of dedicated Special Care Units (SCUs) for demented persons in nursing facilities.

Persons with dementia have short-term memory deficits. Research involving reality orientation (RO) has shown that this technique is not beneficial and may, in fact, cause agitation and distress to clients with AD, reminding them of their deficits (Dietch, Hewett, & Jones, 1989; Hogstel, 1979; Nodhturft & Sweeney, 1982; Parker & Somers, 1983). The caregiver, however, may use an informal RO approach that will help the client with general orientation. For example, stating, "It's a very warm day for October" provides cues to the general time of year without the expectation of the client's remembering the exact date or season.

Routines should be simplified and choices limited. A demented person may not be able to understand the concept of getting dressed, but if the nurse simplifies the process with step-by-step directions, the client may function well. For example, the nurse might present a shirt while explaining exactly what behavior is expected: "Put your right arm in this sleeve; put your left arm in the other sleeve. Now button the shirt." In selecting clothing, it is important to give minimal choices while preserving the dignity of choice, because with dementia the decision-making process is impaired. Thus, the caregiver may present only two items of clothing for the client to choose from rather than opening the closet and asking the client the more general question, "What do you want to wear?"

Demented clients frequently become catastrophic and combative because of negative feedback from others. The client may behave inappropriately and be told, "Don't do that," or "You're out of your mind." This negative feedback is confusing to the demented client who has difficulty defining his or her own space and property. Because of disinhibition, the client may not eat properly, failing to use utensils. Rather than correcting the client, the caregiver should provide foods that are easily eaten with fingers. Caregivers may place red or yellow tape on floors to provide visual boundaries for the demented client. Yellow cloth drapes fastened with Velcro have been known to keep demented clients in their own rooms or out of others' rooms without using restraints. Identifying a demented client's room with his or her name in large block letters or a photograph easily visible outside the door helps the person identify his or her own space. Red or yellow are universal colors that say "Stop" or "Caution"; they are also the wavelength of light on the color spectrum most visible to aging eyes. It is important to identify all items of clothing and other property with the client's name and have the person with dementia wear identification in case of wandering. The Alzheimer's Association has a client identification program called "Safe Return" that is available through most local chapters.

The use of physical restraints must be avoided for demented persons. They cause dysfunctional, catastrophic behaviors; loss of self-image; dependency; and increased confusion and may precipitate regressive behavior and withdrawal or angry, belligerent behavior (Mion, Frengley, Jakovcic, & Makino, 1989; Strumpf & Evans, 1991). The use of restraints has little or no safety value and may actually be hazardous, resulting in iatrogenic illnesses, falls, and prolonged hospitalization (Creditor, 1993; Tinetti, Liu, Marottoli, & Ginter, 1991). Alternatives to restraints should be used and include the red and yellow tape and drapes, which can be effective in delineating boundaries and discouraging wandering. Nurses should look for the meaning of the behavior if the client wanders or is combative and direct their activities toward that underlying cause. Other alternatives to restraints are providing comfort measures, manipulating the environment with lighting or functional furniture, and planning appropriate activities. Restraints should be used only if they enable a client to function at the highest level possible, not for the convenience of the staff.

PHYSICAL STRESSORS

Normal aged individuals do not present with physiological disorders in the same manner as younger persons. Because of changes in pain tolerance, temperature regulation, baroreceptors, and so forth, symptoms may not clearly point to a disease process until it has become well progressed. Persons with dementia experience diminished perception, interpretation, and communication. Excess disability and catastrophic reactions are often the result of deviations in their physiological condition. When a demented person becomes more acutely confused or agitated, the caregiver should first check for physiological causes, such as pain or the need to urinate or defecate. After ruling out this need, the presence of an infectious process should be investigated. Treatment of pneumonia or a urinary tract infection can result in dramatic improvement, yet the only presenting symptom may be an acute increase in confusion. Similarly, constipation and dehydration can cause an acute episode of confusion, and caregivers should prevent these conditions by establishing regular bowel programs and providing adequate fluids. Adequate fluid intake is especially important because the demented person does not always interpret thirst and request fluids.

Other common physiological causes of acute confusion are medications and electrolyte imbalances. When a demented client experiences an acute episode of confusion, the nurse must first rule out physiological and treatable causes through thorough assessment, consultations with the physician, and observation.

Unconditional Positive Regard

The inability of persons with chronic dementia to interpret the environment and the disinhibition experiences make it important for nurses to use unconditional positive regard. Caregivers must accept the demented client and avoid giving negative feedback for inappropriate behaviors. Verbal and nonverbal messages can be used to communicate acceptance and affection. Touch is an especially important form of communication and conveys unconditional acceptance. Studies have shown positive effects of touch for demented clients, such as an increase in facial expression, eye contact, and body movements relative to being touched (Burnside, 1979; Langland & Panicucci, 1982). Touch should be natural and unhurried and convey respect (Ryden, 1992). Feil (1992, 1993) reported that certain types of touching, such as stroking the face from earlobe to chin, can elicit pleasant memories and have a calming effect. Relaxation and decreased agitation have resulted from hand massage and therapeutic touch (Snyder, Egan, & Burns, 1992). The caregiver, however, must be cautious to use touch appropriately and congruently with his or her own personality and that of the demented client.

Bartol (1979) emphasizes the use of nonverbal communication in the AD client and states that nonverbal communication may be sharpened as other abilities decline. The person with AD is responsive to emotional undertones in the environment, touch, facial expression, eye contact, tone of voice, and posture (Bartol, 1979; Ryden, 1992). Principles of communication with the client with dementia include the following:

- Use short words, simple sentences, and no pronouns (only nouns), and begin each conversation by identifying yourself and calling the person by name.
- Speak slowly and clearly, lowering voice tone, not volume, unless the patient is deaf.
- If you ask a question, wait for a response, and ask only one question at a time.
- If you repeat a question, repeat it exactly.
- Use humor whenever possible, but this humor should not be directed toward the client (Bartol, 1979).

Using these principles, caregivers convey unconditional positive regard and act to preserve the demented client's dignity, helping to save face. Unless clients request otherwise, formal caregivers should address them by their surname, rather than by first name or by nicknames such as "Granny," to convey respect.

Levels of Activity and Stimuli

Caregivers must assess behavior indicating anxiety and avoidance to determine appropriate levels of activity and stimuli. In so doing, dysfunctional, catastrophic episodes can be diminished or prevented. Table 34–1 describes anxious and dysfunctional behaviors that nurses can use as a guide in determining activity and stimulation levels for clients with AD. Anxiety can often be relieved by providing the appropriate amount and kind of stimuli according to the client's response, along with periodic rest periods.

Exposure to television and radio should be minimal and carefully monitored. Persons with dementia may have difficulty interpreting the media appropriately and may misinterpret television and radio, sensing people on television as "little people in the room" or a radio voice as an auditory hallucination. If television is used, it is important to evaluate the programs watched. Old movies may be comforting to the aged in general and especially to persons with dementia, because their long-term memory is frequently intact. Nature shows or movies with beautiful scenery can provide positive diversional activity. Radios should be tuned to stations that play classical music or music of the 1930s and 1940s. However, it is important to obtain a thorough history when planning activities centered around music. The client may dislike classical music and enjoy country music, in which case the caregiver should provide the appropriate programming. Other activities should be simple and geared toward the client's capabilities. High stimulation activities should be carefully evaluated, be followed by periods of rest, and include only a small group of clients. One-on-one activities are most effective if geared to the client's cognitive ability and interests.

Because of the progressive deterioration associated with most forms of dementia, it is important for all caregivers to remember that it may be impossible for the demented person to learn new material. Short-term memory abilities are greatly diminished or absent, and the inability to comprehend or relearn can result in frustration. All tasks must be geared toward the client's level of intellectual functioning, consist of short and simple directions, and be rewarding for the client at some level. Demented clients have good days and bad days, and what was performed proficiently on one day may be an impossible task the next. To plan tasks and activities that maximize strengths while minimizing weaknesses, caregivers need a thorough history of the client's likes and dislikes, premorbid abilities, education, capabilities, and occupation.

Listening and Evaluating

Caregivers must listen to demented clients, evaluating verbal and nonverbal responses in order to prevent anxiety and assess for physiological discomfort. For example, a demented client who continually asks for "Mama" may be expressing a need for nurturing and affection, as well as the unconditional positive regard that is generally encompassed by the concept of mother. By validating the client's underlying need, the caregiver can provide an effective and affirming intervention. Validation is an alternative to reality orientation and has shown some effectiveness in caring for the person with AD (Feil, 1993). Validation requires that the caregiver enter the demented client's reality, rather than bring the client into the "here and now." Although validation has potential and certainly seems to increase client comfort, research has not yet conclusively established the value of this activity (Day, 1997).

Modifying the Environment

More than two decades ago, Lawton (1977) identified the need for environmental modification that coincides with decreasing competence, in order to maintain and enhance the well-being of demented clients. Similarly, Kruzich (1986) found that environmental factors influence social integration as much as the client's level of physical and psychological functioning.

The low-stimulus SCU ideally offers opportunities to encourage patient control, to modify but not eliminate stimulation, to individualize the schedule, and to modify the internal environment and provide successful, client-appropriate activities and programming. There are no hard and fast rules for creating and maintaining an SCU for demented clients, but general guidelines may be followed to ensure optimum functioning (Ronch, 1987). These guidelines continue to be relevant today. They include the following:

- Provide a coherent, thematically consistent program of environmental stimulation that promotes and predisposes toward prosocialization and adaptive behavior.
- Encourage the client's independent social interaction with peers, family, and staff.
- Provide a personalized, dignified, safe, and secure environment with maximum predictability.
- Employ trained, supervised staff.
- Manage wandering, agitation, and so forth as responses to cognitive overload.
- Use chemical or physical restraints only for the betterment of the client, not the staff.
- Provide family support.
- Prevent and reduce staff burnout through proper interviewing, orientation, training, ventilation, and relaxation.
- Make evaluation of the client a preadmission requirement using current screening techniques.
- Provide for continued evaluation of the client.
- Be nonjudgmental in analyzing problem behavior and in evaluating the effect of programming on staff, families, and clients.
- Encourage the highest degree of client adaptation by meeting a wide range of needs and being responsive to other individuals and groups.

Individualized, consistent, safe, and supportive care is the hallmark of effective SCUs for demented clients, which provide for management of symptoms, environmental adaptation, and caregiver support (Gwyther, 1985). Expected outcomes of following these general guidelines are restoration of self-worth, stress reduction, acceptance of cognitive impairment, establishment of a calm, secure community, and focus on client strengths. Investigations of SCUs have reported mixed results with regard to improvement in cognitive and functional abilities (Maas, Swanson, and Buckwalter, 1994; Sloane & Mathew, 1991). However, research has shown positive effects of SCUs in areas of resident interactions and activities, catastrophic reactions, and decreased use of chemical and physical restraints (Cleary, Clamon, Price, & Shullaw, 1987; Hall, Kirshling, & Todd, 1986; Maas et al., 1994; Sloane & Mathew, 1991). Further outcome research in this area is currently under way through the SCU cooperative initiative, funding 10 major SCU studies of cost, family, staff, and patient outcomes.

Caregiver and Family Support

Caregivers of persons with dementia can become exhausted in view of the inexorably progressive nature of the disease. Demented clients rarely give positive feedback for care. Education for family and staff caregivers should incorporate the principles outlined, as well as stress management techniques to prevent burnout. Family members must be supported through support groups and education about the stages of the disease. Involving the family in planning and implementing care provides for good family–staff–client relations and helps facilitate a feeling of usefulness for family members and of comfort for the client. Information, support, and education are the primary strategies to assist caregivers in caring for the person with dementia.

Physical Care

Because of the progressive nature of AD and other dementias, the ability to care for self diminishes until the client is totally dependent by the end stage. Interventions to prevent emaciation, prevent pressure areas, control incontinence, enhance mobility, and meet self-care needs are essential. Nurses are referred to other chapters (e.g., Chapters 1–7) focusing on these problems. The subject of this chapter, however, is those problems unique to the demented client.

ASSOCIATED NURSING DIAGNOSES

A number of nursing diagnoses are associated with dementia. In the past, one of the most common nursing diagnoses used was Altered Thought Processes, which described a state in which the person had difficulty interpreting the environment, cognitive dissonance, distractibility, memory deficit problems, egocentricity, and hyper- or hypovigilance. However, the most recent diagnosis, and perhaps the most germane, was added to the North American Nursing Diagnosis Association (NANDA) taxonomy in 1994 (Carroll–Johnson & Paquette, 1994). This diagnosis, Chronic Confusion, is designed particularly for persons with AD. The definition of Chronic Confusion is "an irreversible, long-standing and/or progressive deterioration of intellect and personality characterized by decreased ability to interpret environmental stimuli and decreased capacity for intellectual thought processes and manifested by disturbances of memory, orientation, and behavior" (Carroll–Johnson & Paquette, 1994; Gordon, 1995, p. 281). Other NANDA diagnoses that could be suitable for persons with AD are Impaired Verbal Communication, Risk for Injury, High Risk for Violence, and Sensory/Perceptual Alterations. Some nursing diagnoses are more appropriate for the caregiver, including such NANDA diagnoses as Caregiver Role Strain or Ineffective Individual Coping.

NURSING-SENSITIVE OUTCOMES

Several nursing-sensitive outcomes (Johnson & Maas, 1997) are expected and can be achieved with the intervention of Dementia Management. These outcomes include, but are not limited to, Safety Behavior: Personal: individual or caregiver efforts to control behaviors that might cause physical injury; Comfort Level: feelings of physical and psychological ease; Symptom Severity: extent of perceived adverse changes in physical, emotional, and social functioning; and Caregiver Well-Being: primary care provider's satisfaction with health and life circumstances. Outcomes must be individualized depending on the nursing assessment, driving interventions that result in quality of life for the person with dementia and his or her caregiver(s).

CASE STUDY

M is a 77-year-old woman who was admitted to the SCU of a local nursing facility 2 years ago with AD diagnosed 5 years previously. She is in the third stage of AD, moving quickly to the fourth. M was living in her home in Michigan with live-in help until her admission, but her mental condition has deteriorated to such a degree that the visiting nurse and her paid caregiver agreed that it was unwise to keep her at home. She became increasingly dependent in her ADLs, began wandering, and experienced night awakening. Her caretaker was unable to cope. It was felt that M should be placed in a nursing facility near her younger son in Iowa. M's only other diagnosis is emphysema with no presenting symptoms, for which she is not treated. M takes only a multivitamin daily and medication as needed for constipation.

M is dependent in all ADLs. Her son visits infrequently because M no longer recognizes him, and it is distressing for him to see her with such cognitive decline. Most of the day, M wanders around her room, chattering and tearing the sheets off the beds. She does respond to her name and seems to recognize her frequent caregivers, whom she wants to touch and hug.

M's speech is jargon, with many words meaningless to others. When focused by staff, she will follow simple directions, dance with staff, and even hum along to old songs when staff are singing to her. M dislikes being alone and will eat only if she can sit on someone's lap or at least very near the person. She will not nap unless someone lies in bed with her to get her to sleep.

M's communication is limited. At times her speech is spontaneous—"Leave me alone," when someone is doing something she does not like, such as combing her hair—and profanity comes easily, illustrating the lowered inhibitions frequently observed in persons with AD. Sometimes she cries for no apparent reason but accepts the comfort offered by the staff. M detests bathing or showering, and this is one of the most difficult aspects of her care. Staff members are very affectionate with M, and she seems appreciative of the acceptance.

M responds well to touch, her main form of communication. Her attention is focused only on certain cues: touch, imitation of her chattering, and singing. She listens briefly when her name is called, and when in distress, M is able to make appropriate sounds. Her language and reality base have been altered because of her cognitive deficits, but she is able to interpret affection and caring, with an appropriate response. According to her family, M has never wanted to be alone, and this social response remains intact. She frequently reaches out for caregivers as they pass her by. Her attention span is poor, but hugging, dancing, or singing will maintain her focus for several minutes. She is unable to participate actively in communication unless directed by staff. Her major strength is her love of human contact and the warm manner in which she responds to touch. When using the intervention of Dementia Management for M, her primary mode of communication must be considered. Touch and affection are used to get her attention and to comfort her when she is distressed. The staff members of the nursing facility were able to use several of the activities that flow from the PLST model and are consistent with the Nursing Interventions Classification (NIC) intervention Dementia Management:

- Always call M by name when communicating with her (she prefers her first name). Identify yourself. In this way, M's attention can be focused, even if only for moments, and her social role can be preserved.

- Use touch and hugs whenever possible except when M is not receptive (when she is angry). M is particularly dependent on nonverbal language and is able to participate actively in physical touch and communication.

- Use exaggerated facial expressions and gestures when communicating. This will enhance verbal communication with nonverbal cues.

- Mimic M's jargon to get her attention, and then proceed with the task at hand.

- Sing with M, and perhaps dance with her too, in order to have an effective quiet time together, especially if M has been upset.

- Make sure M is an active participant in communication and other interactions.

- Redirect inappropriate behavior. If she is angry or hostile, leave and return in 5 minutes, or have another caregiver take over. Because of M's impairments in communication, it is fruitless for staff to explain or reason with her. Use whatever communication abilities M possesses at the time, and do not expect more than what she is capable of.

- Provide for rest periods. It is frequently necessary for a caregiver to lie in bed with M in order to get her to rest.

- Provide for safety. Keep all toxic materials, such as cleaning fluids, perfumes, and even some plants, out of reach. Assess M's walking ability and provide for rest if she seems unsteady.

- Provide support and education, especially about communication techniques and the plan of care, for the family so that they may accept M as she is, deal with her appropriately, and become involved in her care.

SUMMARY

Clients with dementia experience losses in both the cognitive and the physical domains. By maximizing strengths and minimizing losses, the nurse can intervene to promote an optimum level of functioning for these individuals. Clients must be viewed holistically, and activities that focus on diversion, self-care, anxiety, communication, planning losses, memory losses, and the provision of unconditional positive regard must be emphasized.

Acknowledgment

The authors gratefully acknowledge the conceptual contribution and ongoing support of Geri Hall.

References

Bartol, M. A. (1979). Nonverbal communication in patients with Alzheimer's disease. *Journal of Gerontological Nursing, 5*(4); 21–31.

Berger, E. Y. (1985, November–December). The institutionalization of patients with Alzheimer's disease. *Nursing Homes,* 22–28.

Blass, J. P. (1982). Dementia. *Medical Clinics of North America, 66,* 1143–1160.

Burnside, I. M. (1979). Alzheimer's disease: An overview. *Journal of Gerontological Nursing, 3*(4), 14–20.

Carroll-Johnson, R. M., and Paquette, M. (1994). *Classification of nursing diagnoses: Proceedings of the tenth conference.* Philadelphia: J. B. Lippincott.

Cleary, T. A., Clamon, C., Price, M., and Shullaw, G. (1987). A reduced stimulus unit: Effects on patients with Alzheimer's disease and related disorders. *Gerontologist, 28*(4), 511–514.

Creditor, M. C. (1993). Hazards of hospitalization of the elderly. *Annals of Internal Medicine, 118,* 219–223.

Dawson, P., Kline, K., Wianko, D., and Wells, D. (1986). Preventing excess disability in patients with Alzheimer's disease. *Geriatric Nursing, 1,* 298–330.

Day, C. R. (1997). Validation therapy: A review of the literature. *Journal of Gerontological Nursing, 24*(4), 29–34.

Dietch, J. T., Hewett, L. J., and Jones, S. (1989). Adverse effects of reality orientation. *Journal of the American Geriatrics Society, 37,* 974–976.

Evans, D. A., Funkenstein, H. H., Albert, M. S., Scherr, P. A., Cook, N. R., Chown, M. J., Hebert, L. E.,

Hennekens, C. H., and Taylor, J. O. (1989). Prevalence of Alzheimer's disease in a community population of older persons. *Journal of the American Medical Association, 262,* 2551–2557.

Feil, N. (1992, May–June). Validation therapy. *Geriatric Nursing,* 129–133.

Feil, N. (1993). *The validation breakthrough.* Baltimore: Health Professions Press.

Folstein, M., Folstein, S., and McHugh, P. (1975). Minimental state: A practical method for grading the cognitive state of patients for the clinician. *Journal of Psychiatric Research, 12,* 189–198.

Gerdner, L. A., and Hall, G. R. (In press). Historical development of nursing diagnosis from altered thought to chronic confusion. In M. Maas, T. Reimer, M. Hardy, M. Titler, and K. Buckwalter (Eds.), *Nursing diagnoses and interventions and outcomes for the elderly.* Thousand Oaks, CA: Sage Publications.

Gerdner, L. A., Hall, G. R., and Buckwalter, K. C. (1996). Caregiver training. *Image, 28,* 241–246.

Gordon, M. (1995). *Manual of nursing diagnosis, 1995–96.* St. Louis: Mosby.

Gwyther, L. P. (1985). *Care of the Alzheimer's patient: A manual for nursing home staff.* Chicago: Alzheimer's Disease and Related Disorders Association, and Washington, DC: American Health Care Association.

Hall, G. R. (1991). Altered thought processes: SDAT. In M. Maas and K. Buckwalter (Eds.), *Nursing diagnoses and interventions of the elderly.* Menlo Park, CA: Addison-Wesley.

Hall, G. R., and Buckwalter, K. C. (1987). Progressively lowered stress threshold: A conceptual model for care of adults with Alzheimer's disease. *Archives of Psychiatric Nursing, 1,* 309–406.

Hall, G., Kirshling, M., and Todd, S. (1986). Sheltered freedom: The creation of a special Alzheimer's unit in an intermediate level facility. *Geriatric Nursing, 7*(3), 132–136.

Hogstel, M. (1979). Use of reality orientation with aging confused patients. *Nursing Research, 28*(3), 161–165.

Hull, M. (1996). Oral presentation. Alzheimer's Conference, Friday Center at Duke University, Chapel Hill, NC.

Jellinger, K., Danielczyk, W., Fischer, P., and Gabriel, E. (1990). Clinicopathological analysis of dementia disorders in the elderly. *Journal of Neurological Science, 95,* 239–258.

Johnson, M., and Maas, M. (Eds.). (1997). *Nursing outcomes classification (NOC).* St. Louis: Mosby–Year Book.

Katzman, R. (1986). Alzheimer's disease. *New England Journal of Medicine, 314,* 964–973.

Kruzich, J. M. (1986). The chronically mentally ill in nursing homes: Issues in policy and practice. *Health and Social Work, 11*(1), 5–14.

Langland, R. M., and Panicucci, C. (1982). Effects of touch on communication with elderly confused clients. *Journal of Gerontological Nursing, 8,* 152–155.

Lawton, M. P. (1977). The impact of the environment on aging and behavior. In J. E. Birren and K. W. Schaie (Eds.), *Handbook of psychology and aging.* New York: Van Nostrand Reinhold.

Maas, M., Swanson, E., and Buckwalter, K. C. (1994). Alzheimer's special care units. *Nursing Clinics of North America, 29,* 173–194.

Malone, M. J. (1994). Multi-infarct dementia (MID). *The Journal of the South Carolina Medical Association, 90,* 539–542.

McCloskey, J. C., and Bulechek, G. M. (1996). *Nursing interventions classification (NIC)* (2nd ed., pp. 201–202). St. Louis: Mosby–Year Book.

Mion, L. C., Frengley, J. D., Jakovcic, C. A., and Makino, J. A. (1989). A further exploration of the use of physical restraints in hospitalized patients. *Journal of the American Geriatrics Society, 37,* 949–956.

Mirsen, T., and Hachinski, V. (1988). Epidemiology and classification of vascular and multi-infarct dementia. In J. S. Meyer, H. Lechner, J. Marshall, and J. F. Toole (Eds.), *Vascular and multi-infarct dementia* (pp. 61–76). Mount Kisco, NY: Futura.

Nodhturft, B. L., and Sweeney, N. M. (1982). Reality orientation therapy for the institutionalized elderly. *Journal of Gerontological Nursing, 8,* 396–401.

Office of Technology Assessment. (1987). *Losing a million minds: Confronting the tragedy of Alzheimer's disease and other dementias.* Washington, DC: U.S. Congress.

Parker, C., and Somers, C. (1983, May–June). Reality orientation on a geropsychiatric unit. *Geriatric Nursing,* 163–165.

Reisberg, B., Ferris, S. H., Arnand, R., DeLeon, M. J., Schneck, M. K., Buttinger, C., and Borenstein, J. (1984). Functional staging of dementia of the Alzheimer's type. *Annals of the New York Academy of Science, 435,* 481–483.

Reisberg, B., Ferris, S. H., DeLeon, M. J., and Crook, T. (1982). The Global Deterioration Scale (GDS): An instrument for the assessment of primary degenerative dementia. *American Journal of Psychiatry, 139,* 1136–1139.

Ronch, J. L. (1987). Special Alzheimer's units in nursing homes: Pros and cons. *American Journal of Alzheimer's Care and Research, 2*(4), 10–19.

Ryden, M. B. (1992). Alternatives to restraints and psychotropics in the care of aggressive, cognitively impaired elderly persons. In K. C. Buckwalter (Ed.) *Geriatric mental health nursing: Current and future challenges* (pp. 84–93). Thorofare, NJ: Slack.

Schwab, M., Rader, J., and Doan, J. (1985). Relieving the fear and anxiety in dementia. *Journal of Gerontological Nursing, 11*(6), 8–15.

Sloane, P., and Mathew, L. (1991). *Specialized dementia units in nursing homes.* Baltimore: Johns Hopkins University Press.

Snyder, M., Egan, E., and Burns, K. (1992). Efficacy of hand massage and therapeutic touch in decreasing agitated behaviors in dementia. *Gerontologist, 32,* 303.

Strumpf, N. E., and Evans, L. K. (1991). The ethical problems of prolonged physical restraint. *Journal of Gerontological Nursing, 17*(2), 27–33.

Tinetti, M. E., Liu, W., Marottoli, R. A., and Ginter, S. F. (1991). Mechanical restraint use among residents of skilled nursing facilities. *JAMA, 265,* 468–471.

Weiner, M. F., Tintner, R., and Bonte, F. J. (1996). The dementia workup. In M. F. Weiner (Ed.), *The dementias, diagnosis, management, and research* (2nd ed., pp. 65–99). Washington, DC. American Psychiatric Press.

Wolanin, M., and Phillips, L. (1981). *Confusion: Prevention and care.* St. Louis: C.V. Mosby.

Abuse Protection: Child

Perle Slavik Cowen

Nursing interventions in child maltreatment cover a broad spectrum of roles and approaches throughout the family life span. Different levels of family functioning require adaptations in the nursing role, therapeutic approach, and helping activities. Primary preventive interventions are directed at the general population in order to prevent or reduce the occurrence of child maltreatment, whereas secondary preventive interventions are targeted at high-risk groups, and tertiary interventions are focused on preventing further injury or harm to children who have been maltreated. The Abuse Protection: Child intervention in the Nursing Interventions Classification (NIC) is associated with Domain 4–Safety (care that supports protection against harm), and it is within Class V–Risk Management (interventions to initiate risk reduction activities and continue monitoring risks over time) (McCloskey & Bulechek, 1996). This NIC intervention subsumes all types of child maltreatment, includes activities directed at all three preventive levels, and is defined as "identification of high-risk, dependent-child relationships and actions to prevent possible or further infliction of physical, sexual, or emotional harm or neglect of basic necessities of life" (McCloskey & Bulechek, 1996).

Despite increasing scholarly publications, health care professionals still lack integrated knowledge regarding assessment, diagnosis, preventive interventions, outcomes, and reporting criteria of child maltreatment. Standardized nursing care classification systems, including that of the North American Nursing Diagnosis Association (NANDA) (1990), the NIC (McCloskey & Bulechek, 1996), and the Nursing Outcomes Classification (NOC) (Johnson & Maas, 1997), offer the potential for a more effective approach to the prevention and treatment of child maltreatment. However, because these systems were developed independently, their categorizations, definitions, variables, criteria, and prioritization for concept development differ. A more seamless linkage between these classification systems could provide guidance to both practitioners and researchers in addressing this multidimensional problem. The purpose of this chapter is to review the research basis for the Abuse Protection: Child NIC intervention and to shed new light on the nursing care of victims and potential victims of child maltreatment through integration of current research and the previously mentioned classification systems.

DEFINITION

Child maltreatment was first described as *battered child syndrome* in 1962 (Kempe, Silverman, Steele, Drogmeuller, & Silver, 1962) and was further delineated in 1974 when Congress passed PL 93-247, which defines child abuse and neglect as "the physical or mental injury, sexual abuse, negligent treatment or maltreatment of a child under the age of eighteen by a person who is responsible for the child's welfare under the circumstances which indicate that the child's health or welfare is harmed or threatened thereby" (Child Abuse Prevention and Treatment Act of 1974, 1974). Criminal, dependency, and reporting statutes define child maltreatment for enforcement purposes in all 50 states; however, there are differences in the encompassing nature of both their specificity and their boundaries (Cicchetti & Carlson, 1989). Generally, child maltreatment is addressed in terms of acts of commission (intentional infliction of harm) or acts of omission (harm occurring through neglect). Researchers typically use conceptual definitions that delineate five distinct types of child maltreatment: physical abuse, neglect, sexual abuse, emotional abuse, and emotional neglect (Table 35–1). Individual cases may present with multiple types of maltreatment,

Table 35–1 Types of Child Maltreatment

Type	Definition
PHYSICAL ABUSE	Intentional acts resulting in bodily harm, anguish, and pain to a child; acts that are typically at variance with the history given of them; unreasonable confinement, punishment, or assault; repeated patterns of physical punishment with short- or long-term effects.
PHYSICAL NEGLECT	Willful or negligent acts or omissions that deprive the child of minimum food, shelter, clothing, supervision, physical or mental health care, or other care necessary to maintain life or health; failure to provide for a care need despite having the resources or being aware of available resources that could fulfill the need.
SEXUAL ABUSE	Any form of sexual contact including incest, rape, molestation, prostitution, or participation in sexual acts; acts that are typically perpetrated through threats of force, coercion, or misrepresentation.
PSYCHOLOGICAL ABUSE	Verbal assault that dehumanizes and damages immediately or ultimately the behavioral, cognitive, affective, or physical functioning of the child; acts include name calling, ridiculing, humiliating, threatening, terrorizing, inducing fear of isolation or removal, exploiting, and missocializing.
PSYCHOLOGICAL NEGLECT	Failure to satisfy the emotional or psychological needs of a child, which damages immediately or ultimately the behavioral, cognitive, affective, or physical functioning of the child through isolation and failure to provide minimum social or cognitive stimulation.

in varying degrees of severity, with resultant physical, psychological, and developmental harm to the child.

Physical abuse includes the intentional use of physical force resulting in bodily harm, anguish, or pain and includes such acts of violence as striking (with or without an object), hitting, beating, pushing, shaking, kicking, pinching, burning, inappropriately administering medications, and using age-inappropriate physical restraints. Although many people accept the notion that spanking is harmful, it remains a common practice, and many states explicitly exclude corporal punishment from child abuse statutes (Barnett, Miller-Perrin, & Perrin, 1997).

Generally, child neglect is defined as the failure of the child's parents or caretakers to provide the child with the basic necessities of life when financially able to do so or when offered reasonable means to do so, including minimally adequate care in the areas of shelter, nutrition, health, supervision, education, affection, and protection. State statutes often classify specific subpopulations of neglect by the type of action that the parent or caretaker fails to take (Crittenden, 1992), and researchers have identified the existence of child neglect in many forms, including abandonment, educational, emotional, health care, household sanitation, nutritional, personal sanitation, physical, shelter, supervision, fostering delinquency, and prenatal neglect (Barnett et al., 1997; Dubowitz & Black, 1994; McHugh, 1992).

Although there is basic agreement as to what constitutes severe child neglect, specific types and individual cases of neglect often have different underlying causes (see "Risk Factor Identification") that create ethical dilemmas. Because many parents engage in some kind of neglectful behavior, at least occasionally, the issue of severity is critical in assessing the future risk to the child and in designing realistic interventions. Several factors are considered in assessing the severity of neglect, including the frequency, duration, and type of neglect; age of the child; potential consequences to the child's development; and the degree of danger to the child. Fatal neglect has been associated both with chronic deprivation of the basic necessities of life (Rosenberg, 1994; Wilkey, Pearn, Petrie, & Nixon, 1982) and with situational failures to supervise the activities of young children (Margolin, 1990; Rosenberg, 1994).

Sexual abuse is any form of sexual contact with a child, who by nature is incapable of giving consent, and includes rape, sodomy, coerced nudity, molestation, prostitution, and taking of sexually explicit photographs. Psychological or emotional abuse is defined as the infliction of mental anguish through verbal acts, including name calling, ridicule, humiliation, intimidation, threats, or harassment, whereas psychological neglect is the nonverbal infliction of mental anguish through use of the "silent treatment" or social isolation. The often intangible aspects of psychological abuse and neglect are typically assessed by the degree of deviance that a child displays in order to be considered in need of protection (Wolfe, 1991).

PREVALENCE

Results of the Annual Fifty State Survey (46 states actually provided data) indicate that 3.1 million cases of child maltreatment were reported in 1996, up 0.2% from 1995 (Wang & Daro, 1997). The average substantiation rate was 31%, with 14 of every 1,000 U.S. children found to be victims of child maltreatment following investigation. The distribution of substantiated cases included neglect–60%, physical abuse–23%, sexual abuse–9%, emotional maltreatment–4%, and other–5%. During 1996, an estimated 1,046 children died from maltreatment (30 states reporting), with the rate of fatalities for children younger than 5 years at 5.4 per 100,000 children. Data from annual surveys between 1994 and 1996 indicated that 43% of the child victims died as a result of neglect, 54% died from abuse, and 4% died as a result of both forms of maltreatment. Younger children were the most at risk for loss of life, with the 3-year data indicating that 82% of maltreatment fatalities involved children who were younger than 5 years, and 43% involved infants younger than 1 year. These figures represent the lowest estimate of the problem, because they depend on the level of involvement of Child Protective Services and the varying levels of comprehensive investigation into child mortality cases by local authorities as well as classification variances among the states in reporting deaths due to child maltreatment (Wang & Daro, 1997).

LITERATURE REVIEW

Theoretical perspectives on the causes and correlates of child maltreatment are many and varied (Cicchetti & Carlson, 1989). The inability of the single-dimensional models to adequately address the known characteristics of child maltreatment has resulted in multidimensional models including the ecological model of child maltreatment (Garbarino, 1977). This model is derived from the ecological model of human development (Bronfenbrenner, 1977) and is a paradigm for examining the complex interactions between parental and child characteristics, intra- and extrafamilial stressors, and the social and cultural systems that affect families. The model offers a framework for considering available supports and resources in relation to a topology of four levels that have been adapted to include individual, familial, social, and cultural factors (Howze & Kotch, 1987). Additionally, the model provides a framework for understanding the relationships between stress, social support systems, and child maltreatment and is further adapted to provide guidance to child maltreatment preventive intervention efforts (Fig. 35–1).

Risk Factor Identification

The importance of early identification and intervention lies in its potential for reducing or preventing the occurrence of child maltreatment. Those variables that have been associated with child maltreatment can be classified into four separate domains: sociocultural, family, parental–caretaker, and individual characteristics of the child (Table 35–2). Stress arising from these domains may be situational, acute, or chronic in nature. However, it should be noted that research to date has not indicated that there are any factors present in all child maltreatment circumstances that are absent in all nonmaltreatment circumstances. Thus, there is no litmus test for child maltreatment, only related risk factors whose identification provides the opportunity for preventive interventions to be directed at stressful environments, interpersonal relationships, and parental psychosocial problems, with securing the child's safety and optimal growth and development as the desired outcomes.

SOCIOCULTURAL FACTORS

Although child maltreatment is reported among all socioeconomic groups, it is disproportionately reported among poor families (Council, 1993). Physical child abuse and child neglect have been highly correlated with poverty, whereas

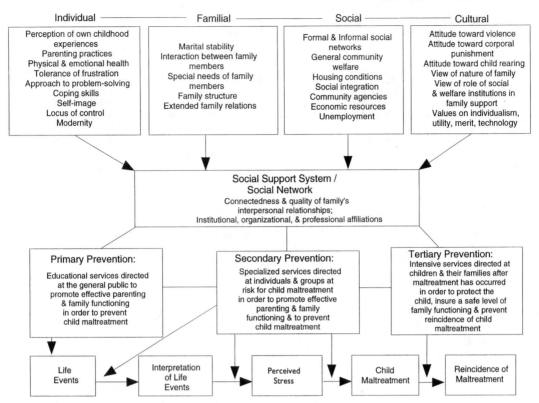

Figure 35–1 The ecological model of child maltreatment: implications for prevention. (Adapted from *Child Abuse & Neglect*, 8[4], Howze, D.C. and Kotch, J.B., Implications for the primary prevention of child abuse and neglect, 401–9, Copyright [1984], with permission from Elsevier Science Ltd, The Boulevard, Langford Lane, Kidlington OX5 16B, UK.)

neglect has been found to be concentrated among the poorest of the poor who typically reside in inadequate housing (Pelton, 1985; Wolock & Horowitz, 1979, 1984). Income level has also been associated with the severity level of neglect, with higher-income families generally associated with less severe forms of neglect, presumably because they have more resources at their disposal (Claussen & Crittenden, 1991). National Incidence Study data showed strong income-related differences for all forms of child maltreatment, including an incidence of physical abuse three and a half times greater among children from families with annual incomes less than $15,000 than from families with incomes greater than $15,000. Physical neglect was nine times greater, emotional neglect was almost five times greater, and sexual abuse was six times greater (Sedlak, 1991). Self-reports on the Conflict Tactics Scales indicate that lower socioeconomic status is a risk factor for violent behaviors toward children, particularly severe violence (Gelles & Straus, 1988; Straus, 1980), and mothers with young children living below the poverty line have been found to be at greatest risk of violent behavior toward children (Connelley & Straus, 1992; Gelles, 1992).

According to the 1995 official poverty measure, 20.8% of all U.S. children were poor (more than 14 million children, including more than 5 million preschoolers younger than 6 years), compared with a child poverty rate of approximately 15% in the early 1970s (Baugher & Lamison-White, 1996). Poverty is not represented equally across different demographic groups; African-American and His-

Table 35–2 Risk Factors Associated with Child Maltreatment

Sociocultural	Family	Parent/Caretaker	Child
Acceptance of corporal punishment of children	Geographical or social isolation from family and friends	Anxiety and/or depression	A child engaged in protracted crying
Depletion of economic resources in the community	Harsh discipline strategies and lack of positive parenting behavior	Fears, disturbances of affect, poor peer relationships, and other symptoms associated with victimization as a child	Children 5 years of age or younger, particularly children younger than 1 year of age
Economic stress, poverty, underemployment	Headed by young parents with lower educational levels and larger number of closely spaced children	Inappropriate expectations of child, inconsistent parenting practices	Children with significantly more major and minor health problems in the first year of life
Glorification of violence	Life stress and distress	Limited or dysfunctional coping skills	Children with subtle developmental abnormalities, such as attention deficits
Homelessness	Low rate of positive interaction among family members	Limited financial and household management skills	Female children age 7 to 12 whose mothers are unavailable (child sexual abuse)
Inadequate support and educational services	Negative family interactions and family problems	Low self-esteem, poor motivation, poor impulse control, or limited social competencies	Infants or children with feeding problems
Lack of or restricted access to health care	Poor problem-solving abilities	Poor physical health	Multiple-birth children (twins, triplets, etc.)
Lack of respite and crisis child care	Previous child removed from family or placed with relatives	Psychological problems associated with being abused or rejected as a child (excessive hostility, anger, unhappiness, rigidity, distress, flattened affect)	Preterm, low-birthweight, handicapped infants
Limited or unavailable prevention services in the community	Unequal burden on one parent for child-rearing, typically mother	Role reversal—expectations that the child will meet the caretaker's needs	Seriously ill newborns
Low priority for culturally competent parenthood education and training programs	Violent interactions, with marital conflict, domestic abuse, and sibling violence	Stress-related symptoms that affect emotional or physical health	Teenagers 15 to 17 years old, particularly boys (physical abuse)
	Violent, antisocial behavior with a history of aggressive or criminal behavior outside of the family	Substance abuse	
		Unrealistically high expectations of the child	
		Violent, antisocial behavior	

panic children and children in mother-only families are disproportionately poor, and although most poor children are white, almost 90% of children who experience poverty for at least 5 years are African-American (Corcoran & Chaudry, 1997). Factors associated with poverty include family structure, labor market, changes in employment (job termination), and changes in family composition (Corcoran & Chaudry, 1997). Given the strong relationship between low income and child maltreatment, some researchers posit that we should fully expect the incidence of child maltreatment to increase as the poverty rate for children continues to rise (Pelton, 1994). The term *societal neglect* has been suggested to characterize American tolerance for childhood poverty (Fund, 1991).

The relationship between unemployment and child maltreatment has been

reported in several studies (Gabinet, 1983; Krugman, Lenherr, Betz, & Fryer, 1986; Whipple & Webster-Stratton, 1991), with violent behavior toward children strongest for fathers who are employed part-time, possibly as a result of their higher frustration levels than those of fathers who are unemployed (Straus, 1980). The association between unemployment and maltreatment has been reported in studies of individuals (Gabinet, 1983; Whipple & Webster-Stratton, 1991) and communities, where longitudinal studies demonstrated that increased rates of child maltreatment are preceded by periods of high job loss (Steinberg, Catalano, & Dooley, 1981). The exact mechanism for this increase, which is presumed to be the result of increased stress, was not directly measured. However, other studies have found unemployment to be related to increased anxiety, depression, and hostility among men, with increased somatic complaints, hostility, depression, and anxiety found among their wives (Liem & Liem, 1988).

Child maltreatment rates have also been found to be higher in poor neighborhoods with fewer social resources than in equally deprived neighborhoods where social resources (such as respite and crisis child care) were perceived to be higher (Garbarino & Sherman, 1980). The relationship between poverty and child maltreatment is complex; most poor parents are not abusive, and poverty alone is not a sufficient or necessary antecedent for child maltreatment (Council, 1993). The ecological perspective argues that as the environment in which a family lives becomes more stressful, or is perceived as such, the parents may rely more and more on coercion and violence to control irritating daily events, including interactions with their children (Bronfenbrenner, 1977; Garbarino, 1977; Garbarino, Sebes, & Schellenbach, 1984; Howze & Kotch, 1987). As well as the indirect manner (stress) in which poverty may lead to child maltreatment, there is little doubt that poverty is directly hazardous to children, requiring parental hypervigilance of the environment (deteriorated housing, fires, lead poisoning, crime), management of scarce financial resources, and provision of constant supervision of children with little or no margin for error (Pelton, 1994).

Health disparities between low-income and high-income groups are almost universal for all dimensions of health care, and, as a result, low-income groups have been targeted as a special population for health promotion interventions in the *Healthy People 2000* national health goals (U.S. Department of Health and Human Services [USDHHS], 1990). Neglect in particular has been related to the inaccessibility or unaffordability of health care (Barnett et al., 1997). Studies of health care utilization suggest that nonfinancial barriers also make it difficult for individuals, especially poor rural children, adolescents, and women, to obtain both health care and health promotion services (Klerman, 1992). Nonfinancial barriers may hinder care-seeking among these groups even when they have adequate resources to purchase care. For the uninsured or inadequately insured, these nonfinancial barriers increase the risk of inadequate health care and often result in nonexistent preventive care (Klerman, 1992). The lack of public transportation often prohibits poor, rural families from completing public support program recertification at their countywide or districtwide office as well as limits their access to preventive or illness-related health care. According to federal surveys, children in nonmetropolitan areas are less likely to see a physician or dentist or to have access to nurse-managed preventive care than are those in metropolitan areas as a result of such access barriers (Hughes & Rosenbaum, 1989; Larson, 1991). The higher rates of mortality and morbidity among rural children as compared with urban children in areas such as postneonatal mortality, injuries, and acute conditions may be related to the resultant delays in securing medical care quickly and the lack of health promotion educational services (Klerman, 1991, 1992).

It is also postulated that societal acceptance and glorification of violence and the presence of domestic abuse and child maltreatment contribute to the level of violence in society (Eron, Huesmann, Lefkowitz, & Walder, 1984), resulting in what the popular press has termed a "culture of violence" in the western world. Children who grow up in a climate of violence, either as maltreated children or as observers of domestic abuse, are more likely to commit acts of violence compared with children who have not grown up in a climate of violence (Spaccarelli, Coatsworth, & Bowden, 1995; Spaccarelli, Sandler, & Roosa, 1994). The exposure of children and young adults to violent television has been shown to result in behavior more aggressive than that of children in control groups (Eron et al., 1984). Physical discipline (corporal punishment) has been viewed by many as one end of a continuum of abusive behavior (Council, 1993); however, survey data have shown that many people consider such acts to be an acceptable part of punishment (Graziano & Namaste, 1990; Wauchope & Straus, 1990). Straus (1991, 1994) contends that spanking is harmful because it both legitimizes violence and gives the implicit message of acceptance, which contributes to violence in other aspects of society. His research has shown that the more children are spanked, the more likely they are to be violent toward siblings, commit juvenile delinquency and serious crimes, and be abusive spouses or abusive parents (Straus, 1991).

Cultural practices have not been linked to differential rates or types of maltreatment (Council, 1993); however, individual cases of child harm related to cultural practices have been reported in the literature. Divergent health and child care practices and beliefs have been the primary sources of cultural conflict in identifying child maltreatment (Korbin, 1994). For example, the Vietnamese curing practice of "coin rubbing" occasionally leaves bruises that have been mistaken for intentional harm instead of the nurturing practice they represent (Yeatman, Shaw, Barlow, & Bartlett, 1976). However, practitioners and child protective workers must also acknowledge that some cultural practices may cause injury or be harmful to children, particularly if they are used exclusively to treat a condition for which more effective therapy is indicated (e.g., coin rubbing for meningitis instead of antibiotics and coin rubbing). Some cultural practices have been found by health practitioners to be very dangerous, such as the use of "azarcon" and "greta," indigenous medications used to cure empacho (an illness some Hispanic persons define as a bolus in the stomach that must be purged) that were found to be almost pure lead (Trotter, Ackerman, Rodman, Martinez, & Sorvillo, 1983). Culturally competent parent education programs have been successful in diminishing such harmful practices (Korbin, 1994). Other cases have been reported where parents claimed their actions, which were found to be maltreatment, represented cultural practices that were either not associated with their cultural heritage or were family subversions of a cultural heritage (Korbin, 1994). Researchers have noted that although an extreme position on ethnocentrism (belief that one's cultural beliefs and practices are superior) can result in false-positive misidentification, an extreme relativist runs the risk of false negatives or missed cases (Korbin, 1994). It has been suggested that culturally informed assessment and treatment of child maltreatment should include determination of whether the cultural practices are viewed as maltreating by other cultures, but not the one in question; the situation represents an idiosyncratic departure from one's cultural practices; or the situation represents societally induced harm to children beyond the control of parents or caretakers (Council, 1993; Korbin, 1994).

FAMILY FACTORS

Maltreatment is a family problem, with the majority of instances involving either the direct actions of parents or their failure to protect the child. Disruptions in all aspects of family relations, not just parent–child, are often present in the families of maltreated children, with anger and conflict pervasive in abusive families and social isolation more prevalent in neglectful families (Council, 1993; Crittenden, 1985b). Family structure has been associated with sexual abuse, with stepfathers more likely to abuse children than biological fathers, and it has been postulated that exposure of children to unrelated men (single mothers' dating relationships) also increases this risk (Conte, 1990; Faller, 1990; Finkelhor, 1984a; Finkelhor & Baron, 1986).

Additional family factors that have been linked to child maltreatment include geographical or social isolation from family and friends (Crittenden, 1985b; Polansky, Gaudin, & Kilpatrick, 1992; Straus, 1980; Wauchope & Straus, 1990; Wolock & Horowitz, 1984); harsh discipline strategies and lack of positive parenting behavior (Oldershaw, Walters, & Hall, 1986; Trickett & Kuczynski, 1986); younger parents with lower education levels and a larger number of closely spaced children (Cicchetti & Carlson, 1989; Council, 1993; National Center on Child Abuse and Neglect, 1988; Zuravin, 1991); interaction among family members that is characterized by a low rate of positive interaction, a higher rate of negative interaction, and family problems (Bousha & Twentyman, 1984; Crittenden, 1985a, 1985b; Oldershaw et al., 1986); life stress and distress (Oldershaw et al., 1986; Pelton, 1985, 1994; Trickett & Kuczynski, 1986; Whipple & Webster-Stratton, 1991; Wolock & Horowitz, 1984); violent family interactions characterized by marital discord, domestic violence, and sibling violence (Bolton & Bolton, 1987; Cicchetti & Carlson, 1989; Garbarino et al., 1984; Gelles & Straus, 1988; Hutchings, 1988; Jean-Giles & Crittenden, 1990; Straus, Gelles, & Steinmetz, 1980; Wauchope & Straus, 1990), with wife assault believed to occur in approximately 40% of cases of physical child abuse in which both partners are living in the home (Jaffe, Wolfe, & Wilson, 1990); and violent, antisocial families with a history of aggressive or criminal behavior outside the family (Abel, Becker, Cunningham-Rathner, Mittleman, & Rouleau, 1988; Pagelow, 1989; Patterson, 1982).

Physically abusing families are characterized by negative daily interactions—anxious relationships between some family members and other family members who respond more negatively to aversive communication or interactions (Crittenden, Partridge, & Claussen, 1991; Lynch & Cicchetti, 1991). Research findings indicate that hostility and aggression often underlie abusers' smiles and affectionate behavior, which may explain the process whereby children (and the adults they become) are more likely to distrust and misuse ordinary communication signals (Crittenden, 1995). Although a wide range of family functioning has been reported in neglectful families, observations of family interactions have shown neglectful families to be more chaotic, less able to resolve conflict, less cohesive, less verbally expressive, and less warm and empathetic than a matched comparison group (Gaudin, Polansky, Kilpatrick, & Shilton, 1996), and researchers have noted that the needs of everyone in the family tend to be neglected (Crittenden, 1992; Dubowitz & Black, 1994; Gaudin et al., 1996; Pelton, 1994).

Familial sexual abuse is not randomly distributed among all possible adult–

child dyads (Hoagwood, 1990); instead, the most likely (in descending order) is male relative–daughter incest, father–daughter, father–son, mother–son, and mother–daughter (Finkelhor, 1986). Although the mean age of the offender is 32½ years (American Humane Association, 1988), evidence suggests that a substantial proportion of offenders are adolescents (Gomes-Schwartz, Horowitz, & Cardarelli, 1990). Family factors related to child sexual abuse include an estranged family; a mother who is absent, ill, or otherwise not protective of the child; unusual sleeping or rooming conditions; the erosion of social networks; and the lack of social support for the mother (Finkelhor, 1984a, 1984b; Finkelhor & Hotaling, 1984; Gomes-Schwartz et al., 1990).

There is a paucity of literature related to the family characteristics of emotionally abusive or neglectful families; however, studies have characterized such families as having more psychosocial problems, poor coping skills, and greater levels of perceived stress (Hickox & Furnell, 1989). Researchers have postulated that vulnerable families may also include those in situational crisis related to such life stressors as death, divorce, relocation, and unemployment (Crittenden, 1996).

PARENTAL AND CARETAKER FACTORS

Very dissimilar approaches to childrearing can emerge from the interaction of two fundamental dimensions of parenting, which include the degree of parental "authority" and the degree of parental "sensitivity" (Baumrind, 1971; Maccoby & Martin, 1983). Parents who are very demanding while failing to recognize their child's limitations and needs typify the pattern of physically and emotionally abusive parents, whereas parents who place few demands and little or no structure on their children typify a neglectful, uninvolved style of parenting (Wolfe, 1991). Specific characteristics of parental personality have been extensively reported to increase the likelihood of abusive or neglectful behavior (Azar & Rohrbeck, 1986; Belsky & Vondra, 1989; Cicchetti & Carlson, 1989; Council, 1993; Cowen, 1997; Crittenden, 1996; Dubowitz & Black, 1994; Garbarino et al., 1984; Gaudin et al., 1996; Hoagwood, 1990; Mehl, Coble, & Johnson, 1990; Polansky et al., 1992; Spaccarelli et al., 1995; Wauchope & Straus, 1990; Wolfe, 1987, 1991) and are only briefly reviewed in this section (see Table 35–2).

Identified parental and caregiver risks for child maltreatment include a history of depression, anxiety, and antisocial relations that are associated with subsequent disruption in social relations and social support and an inability to cope with stress (Council, 1993; Whipple & Webster-Stratton, 1991; Wolfe, 1985, 1991); excessive hostility, anger, harsh parenting, disturbances of affect, and other psychological characteristics associated with a history of maltreatment during childhood (Cappell & Heiner, 1990; Gelles & Straus, 1987; Milner, Robertson, & Rogers, 1990; Simons, Whitbeck, Conger, & Chyi-In, 1991; Whipple & Webster-Stratton, 1991); substance abuse, which has been implicated both in rendering parents less able or willing to interact with their children and in aggressive acts toward children (Famularo, Kinscherff, & Fenton, 1992; Famularo, Stone, Barnum, & Wharton, 1986; Murphy et al., 1991; Whipple & Webster-Stratton, 1991), as well as in impeding children's development related to maternal ingestion during pregnancy (Kelly, 1992); and a history of violent or antisocial behavior (Abel et al., 1988; Pagelow, 1989; Patterson, 1982), with research indicating that 49% of incestuous fathers and stepfathers sexually abuse children outside the family at the same time as they are abusing their own children (Abel et al., 1988).

Additional characteristics that have been associated with neglecting parents include an immature, childlike personality related to low self-esteem; poor impulse control; limited financial and household management skills; and limited social competencies (Pianta, Egeland, & Erickson, 1989; Polansky et al., 1992). Abusive parents have been found to demonstrate inappropriate expectations of the child, disregard for the child's needs and abilities, role reversal with expectations that the child will meet their needs, beliefs that the child intentionally annoys them, and inconsistent childrearing practices (Azar, Robinson, Hekimian, & Twentyman, 1984; Azar & Rohrbeck, 1986; Bauer & Twentyman, 1985; Cicchetti, 1990; Crittenden, 1996; Daro, 1988; Whipple & Webster-Stratton, 1991).

Poor parental physical health and stress-related symptoms have been related to child physical and emotional neglect (when the parent is physically or psychologically immobilized and unable to provide care) and child physical and emotional abuse (Brayden, Altemeier, Tucker, Dietrich, & Vietze, 1992; Crittenden, 1996; Hoagwood, 1990; Lahey, Conger, Atkeson, & Treiber, 1984; Whipple & Webster-Stratton, 1991). Violent behavior has also been associated with the following underlying health conditions: (1) illnesses including hypoglycemia, seizure disorders, central nervous system vasculitis, hyperthyroidism, infections, cardiopulmonary insufficiency, dehydration with resulting electrolyte imbalances, severe pain, and brain lesions such as tumors, abscesses, and trauma-related conditions; (2) exposure to toxins including carbon monoxide, hydrocarbons, inorganic mercury, and boric acid; (3) ingestion, overdose, or withdrawal from psychoactive drugs including alcohol, benzodiazepines, amphetamines, phencyclidine (PCP), corticosteroids, digitalis, lidocaine, pentazocine, narcotic analgesics, and those drugs with anticholinergic effects that can produce atropinism (atropine, scopolamine, neuroleptics, and tricyclic antidepressants); and (4) major mental disorders including schizophrenia and bipolar affective disorders (Barry, 1984).

CHILD FACTORS

Child health, intellectual, or developmental characteristics have been reported to contribute to the emergence of abusive or neglectful parent–child interactions (Belsky & Vondra, 1989). Some researchers contend that the "goodness of fit" between child and parent characteristics influences the child's vulnerability to maltreatment (Dubowitz & Black, 1994). Others have postulated that additional care burdens placed on an already stressed or incapable family system result in a breakdown of parental coping abilities (Pianta et al., 1989). Professional reporting dilemmas related to the excessive demands of technology-dependent children on their parents or caretakers have also been reported (Johnson, 1993).

As previously noted, children 5 years of age or younger, particularly children younger than 1 year of age, are the most frequently reported victims of maltreatment (particularly physical abuse and neglect) (Wang & Daro, 1997), with adolescents (particularly boys) also at risk (American Humane Association, 1988). Other vulnerable child characteristics include difficult temperament (impulsivity, protracted crying) (Belsky & Vondra, 1989), conduct disorders (Whipple & Webster-Stratton, 1991), factors related to increased care demands such as prematurity and low birth weight (Herrenkohl, Herrenkohl, & Egolf, 1983), feeding problems that may lead to maternal detachment (Powell, Low, & Spears, 1987), chronic disabilities and physical impairments (USDHHS, 1993), developmental disabilities (Ammerman, 1991; Ammerman, Hasselt, Hersen, McGonigle, & Lubetsky, 1989), and a large number of closely spaced children within the family (Holden, Willis, & Corcoran, 1992). Child characteristics that result from maltreatment (aggressive, provocative, and approach-avoidant behaviors) may be important factors in reabuse or revictimization (Dodge, Bates, & Pettit, 1990; Wolfe, 1985).

The majority of child sexual victims are female, with 7 to 12 years of age as the most vulnerable age for onset (Finkelhor, 1993). Other characteristics of children vulnerable to sexual abuse include having a mother who is ill or disabled, living with parents whose relationship is conflicted, living with a stepfather or without one's natural parents for extended periods of time, living with parents who have substance abuse problems, and having few close friends (Finkelhor, 1993; Finkelhor & Baron, 1986; Finkelhor & Hotaling, 1984).

SIGNS AND SYMPTOMS

Physical and behavioral indicators of child maltreatment have been widely reported and are summarized in Table 35-3 (Abel et al., 1988; Alter-Reid, Gibbs, Sigal, Lachenmeyer, & Massoth, 1986; Ambrose, 1989; Azar & Rohrbeck, 1986; Barnett et al., 1997; Briere & Runtz, 1988; Burgdorff, 1980; Burgess, Hartman, & Kelley, 1990; Cantwell, 1987; Casey, 1991; Deblinger, McLeer, Atkins, Ralphe, & Foa, 1989; Dykes, 1986; Finkelhor, 1993; Finkelhor & Baron, 1986; Fordham, 1992; Garbarino, Stott, & Faculty of Erikson Institute, 1989; Gaudin et al., 1996; Heindl, Krall, Salus, & Broadhurst, 1979; Margolin, 1990; McHugh, 1992; Mehl et al., 1990; Polansky et al., 1992; Reece, 1994; Rosenberg, 1987, 1994; Tharinger, Horton, & Millea, 1990; Williams, 1991; Wolfe, 1987, 1991; Young, 1981). Although a single indicator does not necessarily prove that child maltreatment is occurring, the repeated occurrence of an indicator, the presence of several indicators, or the appearance of serious injury or a critical marker should alert the nurse to the possibility of child maltreatment. The physical indicators of child maltreatment may be mild to severe, and although dramatic cases of physical abuse or neglect are readily diagnosed by the experienced practitioner, cases involving psychological abuse or neglect can be more difficult to identify (Barnett et al., 1997; Crittenden, 1996; Wolfe, 1991). Behavioral indicators of maltreatment may exist alone or may accompany physical indicators. They may appear as subtle clues that something is amiss, or they may raise questions that leave one with the "something is not right here" mindset.

The role of the informed inquisitor is absolutely fundamental to the assessment of child maltreatment. The reporting of suspected child maltreatment to state authorities enlists the assistance of Child Protective Services, whose professional staff have expertise and resources in this area. Diagnosis, management, and prevention of child maltreatment should never occur in isolation but rather should involve a multidisciplinary team of well-coordinated professionals from nursing, medicine, social work, clinical psychology, and other disciplines when indicated (speech pathology, audiology, and so forth). In the acute setting, several aspects of the presentation should alert the clinician to the possibility of mistreatment, including long delays between injuries and treatment (lacerations healing through secondary intention); unexplained, discrepant, or implausible explanations of illnesses or injuries; alleged self-inflicted injuries or claims that the child is "accident prone"; repeated emergency visits or admissions due to dehydration; noncompliance with medication or care prescriptions; and the rapid departure of parents or caretakers following the admission of a child with a critical illness in tandem with infrequent visitation during the hospitalization. Initial contact in the community or home setting allows assessment of environmental clues such as inadequate hygiene or physical safety precautions; unused or grossly contaminated assistive equipment for technology-dependent children;

Table 35-3 Physical and Behavioral Indicators of Child Maltreatment

Physical/Environmental Indicators	Child Behavioral Indicators
Neglect	

Abandonment

Emotional Neglect

Inadequate age-appropriate emotional support; parents emotionally distant/unavailable; bald patches on infant's scalp; physical delays.

Nutritional Neglect

Inadequate age-appropriate food and fluids; inadequate growth, failure to thrive; dehydration, starvation; wasting of subcutaneous tissue.

Health Care Neglect

Inadequate basic preventive care, care during illnesses, timely visits to health professional, and/or maintenance of professionally prescribed health care routines for acute and chronic illnesses. Indicators include the following:

- Lack of immunization documentation; contraction of a preventable disease
- Failure to seek dental treatment for visually untreated caries, oral infections, and pain
- Failure to seek vision, hearing, or speech assessment when indicators of problems are present
- Repeated failure to keep appointments for routine and follow-up care
- Advanced stage of acute illness related to failure to seek initial treatment
- Persistence or worsening of a symptom that should improve with treatment or medication
- Failure to administer medications or infrequent administration, as evidenced by laboratory testing, lack of a known side effect of medication, delay or failure to fill prescription at pharmacy, lack of request for medication refills, and unused medications
- Incomplete dietary records and/or medication journals for children with chronic diseases such as diabetes and phenylketonuria
- Frequent exacerbations in chronic illness that are not consistent with severity of disease pathology
- Worn-out or unworn special shoes or braces
- Reports from home visitors of children who are technology dependent that needed equipment is dirty, frequently contaminated, not used, or used infrequently
- Reports from siblings that caretakers either refuse to provide or inconsistently provide prescribed treatment such as chest physical therapy, dietary regimens, medications, or dressing changes
- Mortality related to a failure to seek treatment or provide care for acute or chronic health conditions

Physical Neglect

Chaotic family lifestyle; deterioration in most areas of family functioning.

- Substandard housing is common; homelessness
- Housekeeping is practically nonexistent; living areas may be littered with rotting food, garbage, and animal feces; environmental hazards are present and accessible
- No routine for activities of daily living; emotional indifference to child's well-being
- Children may sleep on floor mattresses without sheets or blankets

Child Behavioral Indicators:

- Apathy, watchful wariness
- Assuming adult roles/responsibilities
- Begging, stealing food
- Cognitive and social developmental delays
- Constant fatigue/listlessness
- Extended stays at school in young children (early arrival/late departure)
- Inappropriate affection seeking; needy personality
- Infants with stiff body position; resist being held
- Truancy in older children
- States there is no caretaker
- Substance abuse; delinquency; criminal activity

Table continued on following page

Table 35–3 Physical and Behavioral Indicators of Child Maltreatment *(Continued)*

Physical/Environmental Indicators	Child Behavioral Indicators

Physical Neglect
- Children are bathed on an irregular basis; They may be encrusted with dirt and have foul odors
- Children's clothes are dirty, ragged, ill-fitting, and inappropriate for extreme weather conditions
- Children are left unattended; supervision is often inadequate even when caretakers are present
- Injuries and fatalities related to falls; corrosive, hydrocarbon, and lead poisonings; prescription or illegal drug/alcohol ingestions; burns related to playing with matches. Deaths due to drowning, electrocution, poisonings; burns and smoke inhalations associated with house fires; strangulation; choking; falls from windows; and gun accidents

Supervision Neglect
Inadequate protection and guidance of children, including protection from environmental hazards. Parents may be in the home but impaired as a result of substance abuse, physical or mental illness, low intelligence, or immaturity, or may delegate their children's care to an inadequate caretaker or leave young children alone

Physical Abuse

Unexplained Bruises and Welts
Located on eyes, mouth, lips, torso, buttocks, genitalia, thighs, and calves
Injuries might be in shape of object used to produce them (e.g., sticks, belts, hairbrushes, buckles)
Regularly appear after absence, weekend, or vacation

Unexplained Lacerations or Abrasions
To mouth, lips, gums, eyes, genitals
In various stages of healing
Human bite marks of adult size

Burns
Pattern burns: suggest object used (e.g., iron, stove grate, electric burner)
Circular burns: on feet, face, hands, chest, or buttocks; suggest cigar/cigarette
Immersion burns: "socklike, glovelike, or donutlike" appearance from area being immersed in very hot water or oil; typically arms, legs, buttocks
Friction burns: result from rope friction on legs, arms, neck, or torso

Unexplained Fractures
Of skull, face, nose, long bones
Multiple or spiral fractures caused by twisting motion
Shaft fractures from direct blows
Fractures in various stages of healing

Head Injuries
Blows to head typically cause intracranial, subdural, and intraventricular hemorrhaging
Whiplash shaken infant syndrome typically causes intracranial, subdural, and intraocular hemorrhaging
Child presented nonresponsive or apneic

Münchausen's Syndrome by Proxy
Illness is simulated or produced by parent or someone in parental role
Acute symptoms abate when child is separated from perpetrator
Disease that is resistant to treatment and signs and symptoms are changing

Child Behavioral Indicators:
- Afraid to go home
- Apprehensive when other children cry
- Behavioral extremes: aggressiveness/withdrawal
- Capable of only superficial relationships
- Feels deserving of punishment
- Frightened of parents
- Inappropriate or precocious maturity
- Indiscriminately seeks affection; needy personality
- Lies very still while surveying surroundings
- Manipulative behavior to get attention
- No age-appropriate separation anxiety
- Nonreactive to painful procedures
- Poor self concept
- Reports injury by parents
- Responds to questions in monosyllables
- Vacant or frozen stare
- Wary of adult contacts

Table continued on opposite page

Table 35–3 Physical and Behavioral Indicators of Child Maltreatment *(Continued)*

Physical/Environmental Indicators	Child Behavioral Indicators
Sexual Abuse	
Acquired sexually transmitted diseases Difficulty in walking or sitting Dramatic change in previously well-managed chronic illness Genital or anal injuries or lacerations Masked complaints—genital symptoms, straddle injuries, constipation Poor sphincter tone Pregnancy Recurrent urinary tract infections Reddened or traumatized genitals Psychosomatic complaints Torn, stained, or bloody underclothing	• Betrayal feelings: anger, grief, depression, dependency, impaired ability to trust others • Poor peer relationships • Sense of powerlessness / hopelessness: anxiety, fear, phobias, nightmares, insomnia, hypervigilance, aggressive behavior; change in school performance; delinquency or running away • Sophisticated sexual knowledge; sexualization; prostitution • Stigmatization: feelings of guilt, shame, isolation, low self-esteem, suicidal idealization; self-injurious behaviors; substance abuse • Sudden massive weight loss or gain • Withdrawal and fantasy
Emotional Abuse	
Failure to thrive Lags in physical development Speech disorders	• Attempted suicide • Behavior extremes • Cognitive developmental lags • Conduct / learning disorders • Habit disorders • Neurotic traits / psychoneurotic reactions

inadequate provision for shelter, food, clothing, or care needs; and the absence of nurturing behaviors on the part of the parent or caregiver as observed or reported by neighbors or other relatives. In all settings, observation of parent–child interactions is important, with indicators of maltreatment including the child's being fearful, agitated, or overly quiet in the presence of the parent; parental behavior that includes repeated interruptions of the nurse's and child's conversation, use of a harsh tone, demeaning statements, lack of concern, or treating the child as if he or she were invisible; and hostile or negative nonverbal interactions (Crittenden, 1995, 1996; Crittenden & Ainsworth, 1990; Crittenden et al., 1991; Pianta et al., 1989).

Accurate documentation in cases of suspected maltreatment is crucial and should include verbatim information obtained from interviews of the child, parents, alleged perpetrator, and witnesses; the stated provocation for treatment or request for services; health history, including any "accidental injuries"; a detailed description of the physical examination including the child's functional, cognitive, nutritional, and hygiene status; precise descriptions and photographs of injuries including parental or caregiver explanations as to how and when they occurred; parent–child interaction; parental behavior during the interview process; and an environmental assessment either during the initial interview (if occurring in the community setting) or through follow-up. The tone of the discussion should be professional, nonjudgmental, and supportive.

Nurses who work with children and their families have a unique role in detecting child maltreatment, particularly with regard to the physical and developmental manifestations of the child and the interaction patterns between the parents and the child. Nurses can often identify maltreatment during their initial physical examination of the child or during their history interview with the child and the parents. Their background in child growth and development is superior to that of most social workers, and thus it is their expertise that often forms the basis for questions that arise related to the child's behavior or the parent–child interaction patterns.

The involvement of the nurse is typically initiated because of the child's need for acute or preventive health care services. When it is necessary to interview the child concerning possible maltreatment, nurses must keep in mind that the child may be hurt, in pain, fearful, or confused and may have been threatened not to say anything. Because children vary in their linguistic and interactive competence, it cannot be assumed that interviewing methods suitable for adults will work with children (Garbarino et al., 1989). Additional factors that must be considered include the child's cognitive development, psychological competence, language development, level of socialization, and cultural background.

NURSING CLASSIFICATION SYSTEMS AND CHILD MALTREATMENT

Nursing classifications that are specific to the type of maltreatment, victim population, parent or caregiver risks or inabilities, and preventive level (prevention versus protection) offer the most guidance to both practitioners and researchers. The defining characteristics of physical abuse, physical neglect, sexual abuse, psychological abuse, and psychological neglect differ substantially, indicating the need to address each as a unique problem. There are too many pathophysiological, developmental, and behavioral differences among infant-toddler, adolescent, young adult, and elder populations to merit broad generalizations about the effect of maltreatment. The value of distinguishing between individuals who are at risk for maltreatment and those who have been maltreated lies within the specificity it accords all aspects of nursing practice and research.

Nursing diagnoses (NANDA, 1990), NIC nursing interventions (McCloskey & Bulechek, 1996), and NOC nursing outcomes (Johnson & Maas, 1997) each demonstrate strengths in some of these areas. However, nursing diagnoses are not population specific and are generally not type specific, outcomes are not population specific, and interventions are not type specific at the category level but are specific in identification areas within the intervention. The continued development of these classification systems will result in categories that provide exacting descriptors of child maltreatment phenomena such as child maltreatment: physical neglect (NANDA); physical neglect protection: child (NIC); and child neglect recovery: physical (NOC). The following discussion of the current nursing classification systems' approach to child maltreatment demonstrates that the major barrier to linkage of these systems lies in the lack of nursing diagnoses that specifically address the child maltreatment victim.

Within nursing diagnoses, child maltreatment is primarily addressed through parental or caregiver risks and inabilities, including Altered Family Processes; Altered Role Performance; Caregiver Role Strain; Risk for Caregiver Role Strain; Family Coping: Compromised, Ineffective; Family Coping: Disabling, Ineffective;

Growth and Development, Altered; Ineffective Management of Therapeutic Regimen: Family; Parental Role Conflict; Parenting, Altered; Parenting, Risk for Altered; Self Esteem Disturbance; Social Isolation; and High Risk for Violence: Self-Directed or Directed at Others. Although victim symptomatology may be addressed through a variety of physical and psychological states that result from maltreatment (e.g., Altered Nutrition, Less Than Body Requirements; Pain; Anxiety; Fear), this is not a comprehensive or succinct method of clustering the defining characteristics related to the types of child maltreatment. The only type of child maltreatment that is specifically addressed is sexual abuse (Rape-Trauma Syndrome, Rape-Trauma Syndrome: Compound Reaction, and Rape-Trauma Syndrome: Silent Reaction); however, the defining characteristics are not population (child) specific. Nursing diagnoses are available for primary preventive concepts (Potential for Enhanced Community Coping) and secondary and tertiary preventive concepts (Ineffective Management of Therapeutic Regimen: Community); however, they are not specific to the concept of maltreatment or to child and childrearing populations.

Nursing diagnoses are needed that incorporate the known risk factors and signs and symptoms of child maltreatment in order to provide guidance and direct linkages for primary, secondary, and tertiary preventive interventions and outcome indicators. As well as improving both practice and research, this would greatly facilitate the identification of child maltreatment within nursing minimum data sets, which could further assist local and state public health departments to benchmark progress toward patient and community health goals.

NURSING INTERVENTION

The NIC intervention Abuse Protection: Child includes identifiers for all types of mistreatment, is restricted to a unique population, identifies caregiver risks and inabilities, and provides a variety of primary, secondary, and tertiary preventive activities (Table 35–4) (McCloskey & Bulechek, 1996). The further delineation of this intervention by maltreatment type could provide the opportunity for clustering type-specific activities as well as afford the clinician a more user-friendly format.

The health professional's role in comprehensive assessment, intervention, and prevention of child maltreatment has been well described (Allen & Hollowell, 1990; Barnard & Bee, 1984; Browne, 1989; Campbell & Humphreys, 1984, 1993; Cowen, 1997; Craft & Staudt, 1991; Dubowitz & Black, 1994; Heindl et al., 1979; Herbert, 1987; Mehl et al., 1990; Melton & Barry, 1994; Polansky et al., 1992; Reece, 1994; Rhodes, 1987). Key components of effective nursing intervention include the nurse's ability to adequately identify indicators of mistreatment, describe the nature of the maltreatment in a detailed and comprehensive manner, identify necessary case management components as a key member or leader of a multidisciplinary team, promote maximum independence and self-care of the family through innovative teaching strategies, coordinate activities between acute and community settings to ensure continuity of care, provide direct care and serve as the child's advocate, provide counseling to the family to help them identify coping strategies for stressful situations, identify social support resources and assist the family in accessing needed services, determine the effectiveness of the parents in their ability to meet the child's safety and care needs, coordinate efforts with Child Protective Services to ensure that the safety needs of the child are met, serve as an expert witness in cases involving legal

Table 35–4   Abuse Protection: Child

DEFINITION: Identification of high-risk, dependent-child relationships and actions to prevent possible or further infliction of physical, sexual, or emotional harm or neglect of basic necessities of life.

ACTIVITIES:

Identify mothers who have a history of late (4 months or later) or no prenatal care

Identify parents who have had another child removed from the home or have placed previous children with relatives for extended periods

Identify parents who have a history of substance abuse, depression, or major psychiatric illness

Identify parents who demonstrate an increased need for parent education (e.g., parents with learning problems, parents who verbalize feelings of inadequacy, parents of a first child, teen parents)

Identify parents with a history of domestic violence or a mother who has a history of numerous "accidental" injuries

Identify parents with a history of unhappy childhoods associated with abuse, rejection, excessive criticism, or feelings of being worthless and unloved

Identify crisis situations that may trigger abuse (e.g., poverty, unemployment, divorce, homelessness, and domestic violence)

Determine whether the family has an intact social support network to assist with family problems, respite child care, and crisis child care

Identify infants / children with high-care needs (e.g., prematurity, low birth weight, colic, feeding intolerances, major health problems in the first year of life, developmental disabilities, hyperactivity, and attention deficit disorders)

Identify caretaker explanations of child's injuries that are improbable or inconsistent, allege self-injury, blame other children, or demonstrate a delay in seeking treatment

Determine whether a child demonstrates signs of physical abuse, including numerous injuries in various stages of healing; unexplained bruises and welts; unexplained pattern, immersion, and friction burns; facial, spiral, shaft or multiple fractures; unexplained facial lacerations and abrasions; human bite marks; intracranial, subdural, intraventricular, and intraocular hemorrhaging; whiplash shaken infant syndrome; and diseases that are resistant to treatment and / or have changing signs and symptoms

Determine whether the child demonstrates signs of neglect, including poor or inconsistent growth patterns, failure to thrive, wasting of subcutaneous tissue, consistent hunger, poor hygiene, constant fatigue and listlessness, bald patches on scalp or other skin afflictions, apathy, unyielding body posture, and inappropriate dress for weather conditions

Determine whether the child demonstrates signs of sexual abuse, including difficulty walking or sitting; torn, stained, or bloody underclothing; reddened or traumatized genitals; vaginal or anal lacerations; recurrent urinary tract infections; poor sphincter tone; acquired sexually transmitted diseases; pregnancy; promiscuous behavior or prostitution; a history of running away, sudden massive weight loss or weight gain, aggression against self, or dramatic behavioral or health changes of undetermined etiology

Determine whether the child demonstrates signs of emotional abuse, including lags in physical development, habit disorders, conduct learning disorders, neurotic traits / psychoneurotic reactions, behavioral extremes, cognitive developmental lags, and attempted suicide

Encourage admission of child for further observation and investigation as appropriate

Record times and durations of visits during hospitalizations

Monitor parent-child interactions and record observations

Determine whether acute symptoms in child abate when child is separated from family

Determine whether parents have unrealistic expectations for child's behavior or whether they have negative attributions for their child's behavior

Monitor child for extreme compliance, such as passive submission to invasive procedures

Monitor child for role reversal, such as comforting the parent, or overactive or aggressive behavior

Listen to pregnant woman's feelings about pregnancy and expectations about the unborn child

Monitor new parents' reactions to their infant, observing for feelings of disgust, fear, or disappointment in gender

Monitor for a parent who holds newborn at arm's length, handles newborn awkwardly, asks for excessive assistance, and verbalizes or demonstrates discomfort in caring for the child

Monitor for repeated visits to clinics, emergency rooms, or physicians' offices for minor problems

Establish a system to flag the records of children who are suspected victims of child abuse or neglect

Monitor for a progressive deterioration in the physical and emotional state of the infant / child

Determine parent's knowledge of infant / child basic care needs and provide appropriate child care information as indicated

Instruct parents on problem solving, decision making, and childrearing and parenting skills, or refer parents to programs where these skills can be learned

Table continued on opposite page

Table 35–4   Abuse Protection: Child *(Continued)*

DEFINITION: Identification of high-risk, dependent-child relationships and actions to prevent possible or further infliction of physical, sexual, or emotional harm or neglect of basic necessities of life.

ACTIVITIES:

Help families identify coping strategies for stressful situations

Provide parents with information on how to cope with protracted infant crying, emphasizing that they should not shake the baby

Provide the parents with noncorporal punishment methods for disciplining children

Provide pregnant women and their families with information on the effects of smoking, poor nutrition, and substance abuse on the baby's and their health

Engage parents and child in attachment-building exercises

Provide parents and their adolescents with information on decision-making and communication skills and refer to youth services counseling as appropriate

Provide older children with concrete information on how to provide for the basic care needs of their younger siblings

Provide children with positive affirmations of their worth, nurturing care, therapeutic communication and developmental stimulation

Provide children who have been sexually abused with reassurance that the abuse was not their fault and allow them to express their concerns through play therapy appropriate for age

Refer at-risk pregnant women and parents of newborns to nurse home visitation services

Refer at-risk families with a Public Health Nurse referral to ensure that the home environment is monitored, that siblings are assessed, and that families receive continued assistance

Refer families to human services and counseling professionals as needed

Provide parents with community resource information that includes addresses and phone numbers of agencies that provide respite care, emergency child care, housing assistance, substance abuse treatment, sliding-fee counseling services, food pantries, clothing distribution centers, health care, human services, hot lines, and domestic abuse shelters

Inform physician of observations indicative of abuse or neglect

Report suspected abuse or neglect to proper authorities

Refer a parent who is being battered and at-risk children to a domestic violence shelter

Refer parents to Parents Anonymous for group support as appropriate

Source: McCloskey, J. C., and Bulechek, G. M. (1996). *Nursing interventions classification (NIC)* (2nd ed.). St. Louis: Mosby–Year Book.

intervention, and, most importantly, provide guidance for the prevention of child maltreatment.

Since the 1970s, increasing public concern about child maltreatment has resulted in the development of a diverse base of primary, secondary, and tertiary preventive interventions. Several actions have been identified as increasing the probability of reducing child maltreatment within diverse populations, including those that (1) initiate parenting support programs prior to or as close to the birth of their first child as possible; (2) provide parent enhancement services that are tied to a child's specific development and that recognize the unique challenges in caring for and disciplining children of various ages; (3) provide opportunities for parents to model the interactions or discipline methods being promoted through intervention; (4) provide an adequate dosage (i.e., more than 6 months) of interventions focused on changing parental attitudes and strengthening parenting and personal skills; (5) provide parents with community resource information in order to ensure the safety of children beyond the immediate intervention period; (6) provide a balance of home-based and group-based alternatives for both parents who are not comfortable in group settings and those who desire such interaction; and (7) provide program activities that recognize the cultural differences in family functioning and parent–child interactions (Daro, 1996).

Both home-based and center-based child maltreatment prevention programs have demonstrated a wide range of positive client outcomes. Studies have identified gains that included (1) improved mother–infant bonding and maternal capacity to respond to the child's emotional needs (Affholter, Connell, & Nauta, 1983; Dickie & Gerber, 1980; Field, Widmayer, Greenberg, & Stoller, 1985; O'Connor, Vietze, Sherrod, Sandler, & Altemeier, 1980); (2) demonstrated ability to care for the child's physical and developmental needs (Field et al., 1985; Gabinet, 1979; Gutelius, Kirsch, MacDonald, Brooks, & McErlean, 1977; Larson, 1980; Love, Nauta, Coelen, Hewett, & Ruopp, 1976; Olds & Henderson, 1990; Olds, Henderson, Chamberlin, & Tatelbaum, 1986; Olds & Kitzman, 1990; Travers, Nauta, & Irwin, 1982); (3) fewer subsequent unintended pregnancies (Badger, 1981; McAnarney et al., 1978; Olds & Henderson, 1990; Olds et al., 1986); (4) more consistent use of health care services and job training opportunities (Olds & Kitzman, 1990; Powell, 1986); and (5) lower welfare use, higher school completion rates, and higher employment rates (Badger, 1981; Gutelius et al., 1977; Olds & Kitzman, 1990; Pelton, 1994; Powell, 1986).

A study that reviewed randomized trials of prenatal and infancy home-visitation programs for socially disadvantaged women and children indicated that some home-visitation programs were effective in (1) improving women's health-related behaviors during pregnancy, the birth weight and length of gestation of babies born to smokers and young adolescents, parents' interaction with their children, and children's developmental status; (2) reducing the incidence of child abuse and neglect, childhood behavioral problems, emergency department visits and hospitalizations for injury, and unintended subsequent pregnancies; and (3) increasing mothers' participation in the work force (Olds & Kitzman, 1990). The authors noted that home-visit programs with the greatest chances of success have the following three characteristics: (1) they are based either explicitly or implicitly on ecological models, (2) they are designed to address the ecology of the family during pregnancy and the early childrearing years with nurse home visitors who establish a therapeutic alliance with the families, and (3) they are targeted to families at greater risk for maternal and child health problems by virtue of their poverty and lack of personal and social resources (Olds & Kitzman, 1990). Additionally, a variety of home-visitor programs emphasizing different topics (e.g., health, education, child development, social supports) have proved successful in reducing the likelihood for child maltreatment (Olds & Kitzman, 1993). Home-visiting services have been identified as the best documented preventive effort and as the intervention holding the most promise (U.S. Advisory Board on Child Abuse and Neglect, 1991).

A review of the effects of maltreatment on child development posits that many of the effects that maltreated children exhibit (poor self-esteem and self-regulation, aggressive and rejecting or withdrawn and isolated relations with peers, lags in cognitive and academic competence, and elevated levels of behavioral symptomatology) appear to be based on insecurity issues reflecting an expectation of unresponsive, unavailable, or rejecting adults (Aber, Allen, Carlson, & Cicchetti, 1990). In a study of a home-based parent–infant stimulation program for premature offspring of teenage mothers, a number of positive effects were reported, including (1) at 4 months, the intervention infants showed more optimal growth, developmental test performance, and face-to-face interactions; (2) their mothers rated their infants' temperament more optimally, expressed more realistic developmental milestones and childrearing attitudes, and received higher ratings on face-to-face interactions; and (3) at 8 months, the intervention group received more optimal home stimulation and infant temperament scores (Field et al., 1985).

The programs that have succeeded in changing outcomes for high-risk children and their families differ in fundamental ways from prevailing services. Successful intervention programs see the child in the context of the family and the family in the context of its surroundings. They offer (1) support to parents who need help with their lives before they can make use of services for their children; (2) a broad spectrum of services including concrete help with basic necessities such as food, transportation, clothing, and respite child care; (3) services that are coherent and integrated, with staff crossing traditional professional and bureaucratic boundaries; (4) staff members who are fundamentally flexible and render services ungrudgingly and at a high level of intensity; (5) professionals who are perceived by clients as people they can trust who care about and respect them; and (6) professionals who are able to redefine their roles and venture into nontraditional settings and provide services at nontraditional hours (Connell, Kubisch, Schorr, & Weiss, 1995).

Domestic violence prevention training is clearly indicated for pregnant and parenting mothers and their husbands or partners as an intervention to prevent child maltreatment. A research study of the effectiveness of cognitive-behavioral skill training for male spouse abusers reported dramatic decreases in occurrences of violent behaviors after treatment and up to 1 year following participation in the program (Hamberger & Hastings, 1988). The major components of the therapeutic interventions included cognitive restructuring (learning to monitor, identify, and modify self-talk associated with negative emotional arousal), self-imposed time-outs, communication and assertiveness, and active coping. An additional study that assessed anger control group therapy interventions for battering couples reported that following participation in the program, 85% of the families were free of further violence and remained so for 6 months following interventions (Deschner & McNeil, 1986).

The continuity of nursing care between and among care settings is essential for effective nursing intervention with at-risk families. Many care mapping and case management models of care have been developed in response to cost-containment measures. If they functioned to organize and integrate available services on behalf of at-risk families, they could provide structure to continuity efforts. However, some delivery systems are precipitously moving families between acute and community settings without regard for the continuity of nursing care needed between these modalities. Advanced nurse practitioners who coordinate their clients' care have the ability to follow their clients' progress across settings. In order to link knowledge about diagnoses, treatments, and outcomes and to facilitate the ability of nurses to articulate their professional activities, nurses must become adept at contributing to and using the NIC system (McCloskey & Bulechek, 1996). The continued evolution of this system offers hope to nurses working with at-risk families in all practice settings that their care activities can be communicated, linked, mandated, and reimbursed.

Child abuse legislation in each state mandates the reporting of suspected child maltreatment and broadly sets forth the process through which reporting occurs. In general, these processes describe the conditions for reporting, who reports, and where reports are filed, as well as the legal protection afforded the reporter. Currently, all states mandate that nurses report child maltreatment (Fraser, 1986). However, because of the diversity in laws, particularly in regard to definitions, nurses should obtain a copy of their particular state's reporting statute and study its provisions carefully.

Protocols and Tools for Intervention

Record keeping or the documentation of evidence is vital, because it substantiates the basis for "reasonable belief" and provides the legal basis for state intervention on behalf of the child. Nursing history, assessments, interventions, and referrals are considered "germane to the diagnosis and treatment of the child" and therefore qualify as admissible during a court hearing. Entries should be recorded immediately following contact with the family because they are admissible evidence only if they are recorded at or near the time of the event (Krietzer, 1981). Documentation should reflect accuracy, timeliness, and objectivity and be devoid of "feelings" or conclusions that are made without documented evidence.

Several tools are available to assist the nurse in assessing and evaluating at-risk families. However, it should be noted that, to date, research has not indicated that there are any factors that are present in all abusing parents and absent in all nonabusing parents (Wolfe, 1987). The Child Abuse Potential Inventory is a 160-item, client-administered screening device that was determined to correctly classify 82.7% of known abusive parents in a retrospective study (Milner, Gold, & Wimberley, 1986). The Parenting Stress Index consists of 101 items that measure the amount of stress experienced by the parent as a result of the parenting role, and it also includes a life stress scale (Abidin, 1990). A Nursing Child Assessment by Satellite Training (NCAST) assessment tool consists of 73 items that were developed to evaluate critical features in parent–infant interaction (Barnard & Bee, 1984). The Checklist for Child Abuse Evaluation (Petty, 1995) is a 264-item tool used for investigation and evaluation of children and adolescents who may have been maltreated. Clinicians may use the entire checklist or only applicable sections, including those on emotional abuse, sexual abuse, physical abuse, neglect, and treatment recommendations and issues. McCoy's (1995) Sexual Abuse Screening Inventory is a 61-item checklist, within eight behavior categories, that can be very helpful in routine screening of children entering day camp, group homes, or emergency shelters.

Browne (1989) developed a 13-item checklist based on known risk factors and conducted a retrospective study involving a matched sample of 62 known abusing families and 124 nonabusing families. Nurse health visitors in conjunction with professional colleagues completed the checklist for both groups. Interestingly, although the tool could correctly classify 86% of the cases, the best predictor of child maltreatment was the health visitor's perception of whether the parent was indifferent, intolerant, or overanxious. The author concludes that perinatal screening for child maltreatment should have at least three stages: (1) perinatal screening for stressful social and demographic characteristics, resulting in identification of a target group for further screening; (2) screening of the target group at 3 to 6 months after birth for their perception of the newborn and their perceived parenting and life stress; and (3) assessment of the infant's attachment to the primary caregiver and parental sensitivity to the infant's behavior at 9 to 12 months after birth.

Because children vary in their linguistic and interactive competence, it cannot be assumed that interviewing methods suitable for adults will work with children (Garbarino et al., 1989). Additional factors that must be considered include the child's cognitive development, psychological competence, language development, level of socialization, and cultural background. In general, it is important to start with openness, a good basis in child development, and an empathetic approach. Basic techniques include the following: (1) use sentences with only three to five more words than the number of words in the child's average sentence, (2) use names rather than pronouns, (3) use the child's terms, (4) ask the child to repeat what you have said, (5) rephrase questions the child does not understand, (6) avoid asking young children questions involving a time sequence, (7) do not respond to every answer with another question, and (8) be careful in interpreting responses to very specific questions because children are apt to be very literal (Garbarino et al., 1989). A variety of age-appropriate early intervention strategies that address the developmental needs of children are available (Brown, Thurman, & Pearl, 1993).

ASSOCIATED PATIENT OUTCOMES
■

NOC outcomes are comprehensive in provision of type-specific outcome indicators for the preventive and treatment concerns of both the child and the parent or caregiver (Johnson & Maas, 1997). The addition of population-specific indicators would greatly increase the outcomes' utility in addressing the differing issues of these groups. Patient outcomes are usually selected by the patient or family members in consultation with the nurse because the outcomes must be important to the patient (Johnson & Maas, 1997). This contrasts with the situation for children, who under the law are unable to protect themselves or make decisions in their own best interests, including those involving medical treatment or social services. Recognition of these considerations, as well as those related to the significant developmental differences between adults and children, lends support for the notion of population-based outcome indicators. Outcomes associated with child maltreatment include Abuse Protection; Abuse Cessation; Abuse Recovery: Physical; Abuse Recovery: Sexual; Abuse Recovery: Emotional; Caregiver Stressors; Caregiver Performance: Direct Care; Caregiver Performance: Indirect Care; Caregiver Emotional Health; Caregiver Home Care Readiness; and Abusive Behavior Self-Control (Johnson & Maas, 1997).

CASE STUDY

S, a 21-year-old single mother of an 11-month-old daughter named April, became homeless when her brother and his family moved from the area and declined to take her and April with them. Previously, S's sister-in-law had cared for April while S worked as a waitress at a local restaurant, and S had given most of her salary to her brother to pay for the housing and child care. S had lived only 3 months in this small town (population: 5,000) located in a rural midwest county, which did not have any designated low-income housing, apartment complexes, or public transportation. She subsequently rented a rural farmhouse that had been used to store grain and moved in with April and her few belongings. She had just enough money to pay the electricity deposit and to purchase $50.00 worth of fuel oil for heat, which was a necessity during the cold November weather. Two days after moving in, S's car broke down, and she was unable to travel the 2 miles to town and thus could not go to work, buy food for herself or her daughter, or seek any agency help. She did not have a telephone and could not contact anyone for assistance. After 3

days, she stood in the road and flagged down a farmer, and she and April were able to obtain a ride into town. She presented at the local community support agency and asked for the home visiting nurse to examine April, because she was "sick and feels real hot."

Abuse Protection: Child

The home visiting nurse initiated the intervention Abuse Protection: Child and implemented the following activities to further identify S's and April's needs and to provide preventive action:

1. *Determine whether the child demonstrates signs of neglect.* In assessing April, the nurse found her to have adequate growth and development, good hygiene, a left otitis media and cold symptoms, and adequate hydration (although she appeared to be hungry and immediately took crackers that were offered to her); the nurse found S to be comforting to April during the examination and observed S holding April close to her body, hugging her, and talking to her in a soothing manner that quieted April.

Although S's stomach was rumbling with hunger the entire time, her full attention was on April's needs.

2. *Identify crisis situations that may trigger abuse.* In this case S did not have adequate resources such as transportation to her job or money to obtain basic necessities, including food and supplies, medication for April's otitis media, and diapers.

3. *Determine whether the family has an intact social support network to assist with family problems, respite child care, and crisis care.* Because S had no identifiable support system, the home health nurse obtained medication for April from an emergency fund and assisted S in placing April in the crisis child care program for the day while they worked on other resource issues. Both S and April were provided with breakfast through emergency funds, and April received meals throughout the day and a bath at the local crisis child program.

4. *Provide parents with community resource information that includes addresses and telephone numbers of agencies that provide (only appropriate areas selected) respite care, emergency child care, housing assistance, food pantries, clothing distribution centers, health care, and human services.* A home health aide was assigned to assist S in traveling to the appropriate agencies and obtaining assistance. She was able to obtain some emergency funds from the Department of Human Services and was assigned a case worker, she was able to have her car towed to town and to have a new battery installed, and she was able to obtain food and extra clothing for herself and April. Her case worker assisted her in applying for emergency fuel oil support and filed papers to begin collecting child support payments from April's father (a high school sweetheart who had joined the army and wanted nothing to do with them). S was also able to sign April up for sliding-scale respite care services that would allow S to keep her job.

5. *Help families identify coping strategies for stressful situations.* That afternoon, the home visiting nurse drove S home to examine the "bugs" that S said were everywhere and to assess the home environment. The nurse found that the farmhouse was "crawling with cockroaches" as a result of its being used for grain storage. She was able to help S identify another waitress at work with whom she could spend the night while they "bug bombed the farmhouse," and April would be able to spend the night in crisis care. It required 3 days of bug bombing to rid the house of cockroaches, and the community agency staff and S literally used snow shovels to collect the cockroaches from the floor. S was provided with supplies and did a thorough job of cleaning the house. Mr. Piper, the local farmer who had given S the ride during the height of her crisis, stopped by with his wife during this process and asked if they could be of assistance. The visiting nurse suggested that S might be able to obtain some furniture from the Goodwill agency in a city located 30 miles away. The next day Mr. and Mrs. Piper took S to the Goodwill store, and she was able to obtain $200 worth of used furniture, including a bed for herself, a kitchen table and chairs, a davenport, an area rug for the living room, and a playpen for April. The Pipers said that they would stop by daily to check on S and April.

6. *Determine parents' knowledge of infant and child basic care needs and provide appropriate child care information as indicated.* The visiting nurse assessed S's knowledge of April's nutritional, developmental, and safety needs. She provided S with a home safety checklist, and they went through the house and childproofed all areas. The nurse also provided S with some developmental stimulation cards and toys for April, noncorporal punishment discipline methods, and methods for coping with a crying child, while emphasizing that S should never shake April when she cries. The nurse also monitored their parent–child interactions on a biweekly basis.

7. *Identify parents who demonstrate an increased need for parent education.* S had verbalized to the nurse that she did not know whether she could be an adequate parent; she had been abused and neglected as a child, and she wanted to do "a good job with April." The nurse helped S enroll in a Bavolek Nurturing parent education program at the local community agency. S attended this

program weekly for 15 weeks, enjoyed meeting several other young parents in her classes, and made several friends. She stated that she felt much more capable of being "a real parent" to April.

8. *Instruct parents on problem solving, decision making, and childrearing and parenting skills.* Three months after S's original crisis, her nurse and social worker convinced her that

she should return to school at the local community college to obtain her general equivalency diploma. S accomplished this within 9 months and is now enrolled in a paralegal program at the college. April is flourishing in the respite care program and seems to have adopted the Pipers as her grandparents, and they have been very supportive of both S and April.

References

Abel, G., Becker, J., Cunningham-Rathner, J., Mittleman, M., and Rouleau, J. (1988). Multiple paraphiliac diagnosis among sex offenders. *Academy of Psychiatry and the Law, 16*(2), 153–168.

Aber, J. L., Allen, J. P., Carlson, V., and Cicchetti, D. (1990). The effects of maltreatment on development during early childhood: Recent studies and their theoretical, clinical and policy implications. In D. Cicchetti and V. Carlson (Eds.), *Child maltreatment: Theory and research on the causes and consequences of child abuse and neglect* (pp. 579–619). New York: Cambridge University Press.

Abidin, R. R. (1990). *Parenting stress index.* Charlottesville, VA: Pediatric Psychology Press.

Affholter, D., Connell, D., and Nauta, M. (1983). Evaluation of the child and family resource program: Early evidence of parent-child interaction effects. *Evaluation Review, 7*(1), 65–79.

Allen, J. M., and Hollowell, E. E. (1990). Nurses and child abuse/neglect reporting: Duties, responsibilities, and issues. *Journal of Practical Nursing, 40*(2), 56–59.

Alter-Reid, K., Gibbs, M. S., Sigal, H., Lachenmeyer, J. R., and Massoth, N. A. (1986). Sexual abuse of children: A review of the empirical findings. *Clinical Psychology Review, 6,* 249–266.

Ambrose, J. B. (1989). Orofacial signs of child abuse and neglect: A dental perspective. *Pediatrician, 16*(3–4), 188–192.

American Humane Association. (1988). *Highlights of official child abuse and neglect reporting–1986.* Denver, CO: Author.

Ammerman, R. T. (1991). The role of the child in physical abuse: A reappraisal. *Violence and Victims, 6,* 87–101.

Ammerman, R. T., Hasselt, V. D., Hersen, M., McGonigle, J. J., and Lubetsky, M. J. (1989). Abuse and neglect in psychiatrically hospitalized multihandicapped children. *Child Abuse and Neglect, 13,* 335–343.

Azar, S. T., Robinson, D. R., Hekimian, E., and Twentyman, C. T. (1984). Unrealistic expectations and problem-solving ability in maltreating and comparison mothers. *Journal of Consulting and Clinical Psychology, 52,* 687–691.

Azar, S. T., and Rohrbeck, C. A. (1986). Child abuse and unrealistic expectations: Further validation of the Parent Opinion Questionnaire. *Journal of Consulting and Clinical Psychology, 54,* 867–868.

Badger, E. (1981). Effect of a parent education program on teenage mothers and their offspring. In K. G. Scott, T. Field, and E. Robertson (Eds.), *Teenage parents and their offspring.* New York: Grune & Stratton.

Barnard, K. E., and Bee, H. L. (1984). The assesment of parent-infant interaction by observation of feeding and teaching. In T. B. Braselton and H. Als (Eds.), *Behavioral assessment of newborn infants* (pp. 199–128). Hillsdale, NJ: Lawrence Erlbaum Associates.

Barnett, K., Miller-Perrin, C., and Perrin, R. (1997). *Family violence across the lifespan.* Thousand Oaks, CA: Sage Publications.

Barry, D. (1984). Pharmacotherapy in violent behavior. In S. Saunders, A. Anderson, C. Hart, and G. Rubenstein (Eds.), *Violent individuals and families: A handbook for practitioners.* Springfield, IL: Charles C Thomas.

Bauer, W. D., and Twentyman, C. T. (1985). Abusing, neglectful, and comparison mothers' responses to child-related and non-child-related stressors. *Journal of Consulting and Clinical Psychology, 53,* 335–343.

Baugher, E., and Lamison-White, L. (1996). *Poverty in the United States, 1995* (Current Population Reports, P-60, no. 194). Washington, DC: U.S. Government Printing Office, U.S. Bureau of the Census.

Baumrind, D. (1971). Current patterns of parental authority. *Developmental Psychology, 4*(1 Pt 2), 1–103 (monograph).

Belsky, J., and Vondra, J. (1989). Lessons from child abuse. The determinants of parenting. In D. Cicchetti and V. Carlson (Eds.), *Child maltreatment: Theory and research on the causes and consequences of child abuse and neglect* (pp. 153–202). New York: Cambridge University Press.

Bolton, F. G., and Bolton, S. R. (1987). *Working with violent families.* Newbury Park, CA: Sage Publications.

Bousha, D., and Twentyman, C. (1984). Mother-child interactional style in abuse, neglect and control groups: Naturalistic observations in the home. *Journal of Abnormal Psychology, 93,* 106–114.

Brayden, R. M., Altemeier, W. A., Tucker, D. D., Dietrich, M. S., and Vietze, P. (1992). Antecedents of child neglect in the first two years of life. *The Journal of Pediatrics, 120,* 426–429.

Briere, J., and Runtz, M. (1988). Symptomatology associated with childhood sexual victimization in a nonclinical adult sample. *Child Abuse and Neglect, 12*(1), 51–59.

Bronfenbrenner, U. (1977). Toward an experimental ecology of human development. *American Psychologist, 32,* 513–531.

Brown, W., Thurman, S. K., and Pearl, L. F. (Eds.). (1993). *Family-centered early intervention with infants and toddlers: Innovative cross-disciplinary approaches.* Baltimore: Paul Bookes Publishing.

Browne, K. (1989). The health visitor's role in screening for child abuse. *Health Visitor, 62,* 275–277.

Bulechek, G., and McCloskey, J. (1992). Nursing diagnoses, interventions and outcomes. In G. Bulechek and J. McCloskey (Eds.), *Nursing interventions: Essential nursing treatments.* Philadelphia: W.B. Saunders.

Burgdorff, K. (1980). *Recognition and reporting of child maltreatment: Findings from the national incidence and severity of child abuse and neglect.* Washington, DC: National Center on Child Abuse and Neglect.

Burgess, A., Hartman, C., and Kelley, S. (1990). Assessing child abuse: The TRIADS checklist. *Journal of Psychosocial Nursing and Mental Health Services, 28*(4), 6–8, 10–14.

Campbell, J., and Humphreys, J. (1984). *Nursing care of victims of family violence.* Reston, VA: Reston Publishing.

Campbell, J., and Humphreys, J. (1993). *Nursing care of survivors of family violence* (2nd ed.). St. Louis: Mosby.

Cantwell, H. (1987). *Physical neglect.* Chicago: National Committee for the Prevention of Child Abuse.

Cappell, C., and Heiner, R. B. (1990). The intergenerational transmission of family aggression. *Journal of Family Violence, 5,* 135–151.

Casey, N. (1991). Willful neglect. *Nursing Standards, 5*(49), 3.

Child Abuse Prevention and Treatment Act of 1974. (1974). Public Law 93-247. *U.S. Statutes at Large, 88,* 4–8.

Children's Defense Fund. (1991). *The state of America's children.* Washington, DC: Author.

Cicchetti, D. (1990). How research on child maltreatment has informed the study of child development: Perspectives from developmental psychopathology. In D. Cicchetti and V. Carlson (Eds.), *Child maltreatment: Theory and research on the causes and consequences of child abuse and neglect* (pp. 377–431). New York: Cambridge University Press.

Cicchetti, D., and Carlson, V. (Eds.). (1989). *Child maltreatment: Theory and research on the causes and consequences of child abuse and neglect.* Cambridge: Cambridge University Press.

Claussen, A. H., and Crittenden, P. M. (1991). Physical and psychological maltreatment: Relations among types of maltreatment. *Child Abuse and Neglect, 15,* 5–18.

Connell, J. P., Kubisch, A. C., Schorr, L. B., and Weiss, C. H. (Eds.). (1995). *New approaches to evaluating community initiatives: Concepts, methods, and contexts.* Washington, DC: Apen Institute.

Connelley, C. D., and Straus, M. A. (1992). Mother's age and risk for physical abuse. *Child Abuse and Neglect, 16,* 703–712.

Conte, J. R. (1990). *A look at child sexual abuse.* Chicago: National Committee for Prevention of Child Abuse.

Corcoran, M. E., and Chaudry, A. (1997). The dynamics of childhood poverty. In R. Behrman (Ed.), *The future of children* (Vol. 7, pp. 40–54). Los Altos, CA: Center for the Future of Children, The David and Lucile Packard Foundation.

Council, N. R. (1993). *Understanding child abuse and neglect.* Washington, DC: National Academy Press.

Cowen, P. S. (1997). Child maltreatment: Nursing's changing role. In J. McCloskey and H. K. Grace (Eds.), *Current issues in nursing* (pp. 731–741). St. Louis: Mosby.

Craft, J. L., and Staudt, M. M. (1991). Reporting and founding of child neglect in urban and rural communities. *Child Welfare, 70,* 359–370.

Crittenden, P. (1992). *Preventing child neglect.* Chicago: NCPCA Publications.

Crittenden, P., Partridge, M., and Claussen, A. (1991). Family patterns of relationship in normative and dysfunctional families. *Development and Psychology, 3,* 491–512.

Crittenden, P. M. (1985a). Maltreated infants: Vulnerability and resilience. *Journal of Child Psychology and Psychiatry, 26,* 85–96.

Crittenden, P. M. (1985b). Social networks, quality of childrearing and child development. *Child Development, 56,* 1299–1313.

Crittenden, P. M. (1995). Attachment and psychopathology. In S. Goldberg, R. Muir, and J. Kerr (Eds.), *Attachment theory: Social, developmental, and clinical perspectives.* Hillsdale, NJ: Analytic Press.

Crittenden, P. M. (1996). Research on maltreating families. In J. Briere, L. Berliner, J. Bulkley, C. Jenny, and T. Reid (Eds.), *The APSAC handbook on child maltreatment.* Thousand Oaks, CA: Sage Publications.

Crittenden, P. M., and Ainsworth, M. D. S. (1990). Child maltreatment and attachment theory. In D. Cicchetti and V. Carlson (Eds.), *Child maltreatment: Theory and research on the causes and consequences of child abuse and neglect* (pp. 432–463). New York: Cambridge University Press.

Daro, D. (1988). *Confronting child abuse: Research for effective program design.* New York: The Free Press.

Daro, D. (1996). Preventing child abuse and neglect. In J. Briere, L. Berliner, J. Bulkley, C. Jenny, and T. Reid (Eds.), *The APSAC handbook on child maltreatment* (pp. 343–358). Thousand Oaks, CA: Sage Publications.

Deblinger, E., McLeer, S. V., Atkins, M. S., Ralphe, D., and Foa, E. (1989). Post-traumatic stress in sexually abused, physically abused, and nonabused children. *Child Abuse and Neglect, 13,* 403–408.

Deschner, J., and McNeil, J. (1986). Results of anger control training for battering couples. *Journal of Family Violence 1*(2), 111–121.

Dickie, J., and Gerber, S. (1980). Training in social competence: The effects on mothers, fathers, and infants. *Child Development, 51,* 1248–1251.

Dodge, K. A., Bates, J. E., and Pettit, G. S. (1990, December). Mechanisms in the cycle of violence. *Science, 250,* 1678–1683.

Dubowitz, H., and Black, M. (1994). Child neglect. In R. M. Reece (Ed.), *Child abuse: Medical diagnosis and management* (pp. 279–297). Malvern, PA: Lea & Febiger.

Dykes, L. J. (1986). The whiplash shaken infant syndrome: What has been learned? *Child Abuse and Neglect, 10,* 211–221.

Eron, L. L., Huesmann, L. R., Lefkowitz, M. M., and Walder, L. O. (1984). How learning conditions in early childhood—including mass media—relate to aggression in later adolescence. *Psychological Reports, 9,* 291–334.

Faller, K. (1990). *Understanding child sexual maltreatment.* Newbury Park, CA: Sage Publications.

Famularo, R. A., Kinscherff, R., and Fenton, T. (1992). Parental substance abuse and the nature of child maltreatment. *Child Abuse and Neglect, 14,* 439–444.

Famularo, R. A., Stone, K., Barnum, R., and Wharton, R. (1986). Alcoholism and severe child maltreatment. *American Journal of Orthopsychiatry, 56,* 481–485.

Field, T., Widmayer, S., Greenberg, R., and Stoller, S. (1985). Home- and center-based intervention for teenage mothers and their offspring. In S. Harel and N. J. Anastasiow (Eds.), *The at-risk infant: Psycho/social/medical aspects* (pp. 29–38). Baltimore, MD: Paul H. Brooks Publishing.

Finkelhor, D. (1984a). *Child sexual abuse: New theory and research*. New York: The Free Press.

Finkelhor, D. (1984b). How widespread is child sexual abuse? *Children Today, 13,* 18–20.

Finkelhor, D. (Ed.). (1986). *A sourcebook on child sexual abuse*. Newbury Park, CA: Sage Publications.

Finkelhor, D. (1993). Epidemiological factors in the clinical identification of child sexual abuse. *Child Abuse and Neglect, 17,* 67–70.

Finkelhor, D., and Baron, L. (1986). High risk children. In D. Finkelhor (Ed.), *A sourcebook on child sexual abuse*. Beverly Hills, CA: Sage Publications.

Finkelhor, D., and Hotaling, G. T. (1984). Sexual abuse in the National Incidence Study of child abuse and neglect: An appraisal. *Child Abuse and Neglect, 8,* 23–32.

Fordham, H. (1992). Child abuse: Physical neglect the most common form. *Michigan Medicine, 91*(9), 28.

Fraser, B. (1986). A glance at the past, a gaze at the present, a glimpse of the future: A critical analysis of the development of child abuse reporting statues. *Journal of Juvenile Law, 10,* 641–686.

Fund, C. S. D. (1991). *The state of America's children*. Washington, DC: Children's Defense Fund.

Gabinet, L. (1979). Prevention of child abuse and neglect in an inner-city population: II. The program and the results. *Child Abuse and Neglect, 3,* 809–817.

Gabinet, L. (1983). Child abuse treatment failures reveal need for redefinition of the problem. *Child Abuse and Neglect, 7,* 395–402.

Garbarino, J. (1977). The human ecology of child maltreatment. *Journal of Marriage and the Family, 39,* 721–735.

Garbarino, J., Sebes, J., and Schellenbach, C. (1984). Families at-risk for destructive parent-child relations in adolescence. *Child Development, 55,* 174–183.

Garbarino, J., and Sherman, D. (1980). High-risk neighborhoods and high-risk families. *Child Development, 51,* 188–198.

Garbarino, J., Stott, F., and Faculty of Erikson Institute. (1989). *What children can tell us*. San Francisco: Jossey-Bass, Inc.

Gaudin, J. M., Polansky, N. A., Kilpatrick, A. C., and Shilton, P. (1996). Family functioning in neglectful families. *Child Abuse and Neglect, 20,* 363–377.

Gelles, R. J. (1992). Poverty and violence toward children. *American Behavioral Scientist, 35,* 258–274.

Gelles, R. J., and Straus, M. A. (1987). Is violence toward children increasing? *Journal of Interpersonal Violence, 2,* 212–222.

Gelles, R. J., and Straus, M. A. (1988). *Intimate violence*. New York: Simon and Schuster.

Gomes-Schwartz, B., Horowitz, J. M., and Cardarelli, A. P. (1990). *Child sexual abuse: The initial effects*. Newbury Park, CA: Sage Publications.

Graziano, A. M., and Namaste, K. A. (1990). Parental use of physical force in child discipline: A survey of 679 college students. *Journal of Interpersonal Violence, 5,* 449–463.

Gutelius, M., Kirsch, A., MacDonald, S., Brooks, M., and McErlean, T. (1977). Controlled study of child health supervision: Behavioral results. *Pediatrics, 60,* 294–304.

Hamberger, K., and Hastings, J. (1988). Skills training for treatment of spouse abusers: An outcome study. *Journal of Family Violence, 8,* 121–131.

Heindl, C., Krall, C., Salus, M., and Broadhurst, D. (1979). *The nurse's role in the prevention and treatment of child abuse and neglect*. Washington, DC: U.S. Department of Health, Education, and Welfare.

Herbert, C. P. (1987). Expert medical assessment in determining probability of alleged child sexual abuse. *Child Abuse and Neglect, 11,* 213–221.

Herrenkohl, R. C., Herrenkohl, E. C., and Egolf, B. P. (1983). Circumstances surrounding the occurrence of child maltreatment. *Journal of Consulting and Clinical Psychology, 51,* 424–431.

Hickox, A., and Furnell, J. (1989). Psychosocial and background factors in emotional abuse of children. *Child: Care, Health and Development, 15,* 227–240.

Hoagwood, K. (1990). Parental functioning and child sexual abuse. *Child and Adolescent Social Work, 7,* 377–387.

Holden, K. W., Willis, D. J., and Corcoran, M. (1992). Chapter 2. In D. J. Willis, E. W. Holden, and M. Rosenber (Eds.), *Prevention of child maltreatment: Developmental and ecological perspectives*. New York: John Wiley.

Howze, D. C., and Kotch, J. B. (1987). Disentangling life events, stress, and social support: Implications for primary prevention of child abuse and neglect. *Child Abuse and Neglect, 8,* 401–409.

Hughes, D., and Rosenbaum, S. (1989). An overview of maternal and infant health services in rural America. *Journal of Rural Health, 5,* 299–319.

Hutchings, N. (1988). *The violent family: Victimization of women, children and elders*. New York: Human Sciences Press.

Jaffe, P., Wolfe, D., and Wilson, S. (1990). *Children of battered women*. Newbury Park, CA: Sage Publications.

Jean-Giles, M., and Crittenden, P. (1990). Maltreating families: A look at siblings. *Family Relations 39*(3), 323–329.

Johnson, C. (1993). Physicians and medical neglect: Variables that affect reporting. *Child Abuse and Neglect, 17,* 605–612.

Johnson, M., and Maas, M. (1997). *Nursing outcomes classification (NOC)*. St. Louis: Mosby.

Kelly, S. J. (1992). Parenting stress and child maltreatment in drug-exposed children. *Child Abuse and Neglect, 16,* 317–328.

Kempe, H., Silverman, F., Steele, B., Drogmeuller, W., and Silver, H. (1962). The battered-child syndrome. *Journal of the American Medical Association, 181,* 17–24.

Klerman, L. V. (1991). The health of poor children. In A. Huston (Ed.), *Children in poverty* (pp. 79–105). New York: Cambridge University Press.

Klerman, L. V. (1992). Nonfinancial barriers to the receipt of medical care. In *The future of children* 2(1) (pp. 171–185). Los Altos, CA: Center for the Future of Children.

Korbin, J. E. (1994). Sociocultural factors in child maltreatment. In G. Melton and F. Barry (Eds.), *Protecting children from abuse and neglect* (pp. 182–223). New York: Guilford Press.

Krietzer, M. (1981). Legal aspects of child abuse. *Nursing Clinics of North America, 16,* 149–160.

Krugman, R. D., Lenherr, M., Betz, L., and Fryer, G. E. (1986). The relationship between unemployment and physical abuse of children. *Child Abuse and Neglect, 10,* 415–418.

Lahey, B. B., Conger, R. D., Atkeson, B. M., and Treiber, F. A. (1984). Parenting behavior and emotional status of physically abusive mothers. *Journal of Consulting and Clinical Psychology, 52,* 1062–1071.

Larson, C. (1980). Efficacy of perinatal and postpartum home visits on child health and development. *Pediatrics, 66,* 191–197.

Larson, C. S. (1991). Overview of state legislative and judicial responses. In R. E. Behrman (Ed.), *The future of children* (Vol. 1, pp. 72–84). Los Altos, CA: Center for the Future of Children, The David and Lucile Packard Foundation.

Liem, R., and Liem, J. H. (1988). Psychological effects of unemployment on workers and their families. *Journal of Social Issues, 44*(4), 87–105.

Love, J., Nauta, M., Coelen, C., Hewett, K., and Ruopp, R. (1976). *National home start evaluation: Final report, findings and implications.* Ypsilanti, MI: High Scope Educational Research Foundation.

Lynch, M., and Cicchetti, D. (1991). Patterns of relatedness in maltreated and non-maltreated children: Connections among multiple representational models. *Development and Psychopathology, 3,* 207–226.

Maccoby, E., and Martin, J. (1983). Socialization in the context of the family: Parent-child interaction. In E. M. Hetherington (Ed.), *Handbook of child psychology: Vol. 4. Socialization, personality, and social development* (Vol. 4, pp. 1–101). New York: Wiley.

Margolin, L. (1990). Fatal child neglect. *Child Welfare, 69,* 309–319.

McAnarney, E., Roghmann, K., Adams, B., Tatlebaum, R., Kash, C., Coulter, M., Plume, M., and Charney, E. (1978). Obstetric, neonatal, and psychosocial outcome of pregnant adolescents. *Pediatrics, 61*(2), 199–205.

McCloskey, J. C., and Bulechek, G. M. (1996). *Nursing interventions classification (NIC).* St. Louis: Mosby-Year Book.

McCoy, D. (1995). *Sexual abuse screening inventory (SASI).* Odessa, FL: Psychological Assessment Resources.

McHugh, M. (1992). Child abuse in a sea of neglect: The inner-city child. *Pediatric Annals, 21,* 504–507.

Mehl, A. L., Coble, L., and Johnson, S. (1990). Munchausen syndrome by proxy: A family affair. *Child Abuse and Neglect, 14,* 577–585.

Melton, G. B., and Barry, F. D. (1994). *Protecting children from abuse and neglect: Foundations for a new national strategy.* New York: Guilford Press.

Milner, J., Gold, R., and Wimberley, R. (1986). Prediction and explanation of child abuse: Cross-validation of the Child Abuse Potential Inventory. *Journal of Consulting and Clinical Psychology, 54,* 865–866.

Milner, J. S., Robertson, K. R., and Rogers, D. L. (1990). Childhood history of abuse and adult child abuse potential. *Journal of Family Violence, 5,* 15–34.

Murphy, J. M., Jellinek, M., Quinn, D., Smith, G., Poitrast, F. G., and Gkoshko, M. (1991). Substance abuse and serious child maltreatment: Prevalence, risk, and outcome in a court sample. *Child Abuse and Neglect, 15,* 197–211.

National Center on Child Abuse and Neglect. (1988). *Study findings: Study of national incidence and prevalence of child abuse and neglect: 1988.* Washington, DC: U.S. Department of Health and Human Services.

North American Nursing Diagnosis Association. (1990). *Taxonomy I revised.* St. Louis: Author.

O'Connor, S., Vietze, P., Sherrod, K., Sandler, H., and Altemeier, W. (1980). Reduced incidence of parenting inadequacy following rooming-in. *Pediatrics, 66,* 176–182.

Oldershaw, L., Walters, G., and Hall, D. (1986). Control strategies and noncompliance in abusive mother-child dyads: An observational study. *Child Development, 57,* 722–732.

Olds, D., and Kitzman, H. (1993). Review of research on home visitation for pregnant women and parents of young children. In R. Behrman (Ed.), *The future of children* (Vol. 3). Los Altos, CA: The David and Lucile Packard Foundation.

Olds, D. L., and Henderson, C. R. (1990). The prevention of maltreatment. In D. Cicchetti and V. Carlson (Eds.), *Child maltreatment: Theory and research on the causes and consequences of child abuse and neglect* (pp. 722–763). New York: Cambridge University Press.

Olds, D. L., and Kitzman, H. (1990). Can home visitation improve the health of women and children at environmental risk? *Pediatrics, 86*(1), 108–116.

Olds, D. S., Henderson, C. R., Chamberlin, R., and Tatelbaum, R. (1986). Preventing child abuse and neglect: A randomized trial of nurse home visitation. *Pediatrics, 78,* 65–78.

Pagelow, M. D. (1989). The incidence and prevalance of criminal abuse of other family members. In L. Ohlin and M. Tonry (Eds.), *Family violence Vol. II* (pp. 263–313). Chicago: University of Chicago Press.

Patterson, G. (1982). *Coercive family processess.* Eugene, OR: Castalia Publishing.

Pelton, L. (1985). *The social context of child abuse and neglect.* New York: Human Science Press.

Pelton, L. H. (1994). The role of material factors in child abuse and neglect. In G. Melton and F. Barry (Eds.), *Protecting children from abuse and neglect* (pp. 131–181). New York: Guilford Press.

Petty, J. (1995). *Checklist for child abuse evaluation.* Odessa, FL: Psychological Assessment Resources.

Pianta, R., Egeland, B., and Erickson, M. F. (1989). The antecedents of maltreatment: Results of the mother-child interaction research project. In D. Cicchetti and V. Carlson (Eds.), *Child maltreatment: Theory and research on the causes and consequences of child abuse and neglect* (pp. 203–253). New York: Cambridge University Press.

Polansky, N. A., Gaudin, J. M., and Kilpatrick, A. C. (1992). Family radicals. *Children and Youth Services Review, 14,* 19–26.

Powell, D. (1986). Parent education and support programs. *Young Children 41*(3), 47–53.

Powell, G. F., Low, J. L., and Spears, M. A. (1987). Behavior as a diagnostic aid in failure to thrive. *Journal of Development and Behavioral Pediatrics, 8,* 18–24.

Reece, R. M. (Ed.). (1994). *Child abuse: Medical diagnosis and management.* Philadelphia: Waverly.

Rhodes, A. M. (1987). The nurse's legal obligations for reporting child abuse. *The American Journal of Maternal Child Nursing, 12,* 313.

Rosenberg, D. (1994). Fatal neglect. *APSAC Advisor, 7*(4), 38–40.

Rosenberg, D. A. (1987). Web of deceit: A literature review of Munchausen syndrome by proxy. *Child Abuse and Neglect, 11,* 547–563.

Sedlak, A. J. (1991). *National incidence and prevalence of child abuse and neglect: 1988. Revised report.* Rockville, MD: Westat.

Simons, R. L., Whitbeck, L. B., Conger, R. D., and Chyi-In, W. (1991). Intergenerational transmission of harsh parenting. *Developmental Psychology, 27,* 159–171.

Spaccarelli, S., Coatsworth, J. D., and Bowden, B. S. (1995). Exposure to serious family violence among incarcerated boys: Its association with violent offending and potential mediating variable. *Violence and Victims, 10,* 163–182.

Spaccarelli, S., Sandler, L. N., and Roosa, M. (1994). History of spouse violence against mother: Correlated risks and unique effects in child mental health. *Journal of Family Violence, 9,* 79–88.

Steinberg, L., Catalano, R., and Dooley, D. (1981). Economic antecedents of child abuse and neglect. *Child Development, 52*, 975–985.

Straus, M., Gelles, R., and Steinmetz, S. (1980). *Behind closed doors: Violence in the American family.* Garden City, NJ: Anchor/Doubleday.

Straus, M. A. (1980). Stress and physical child abuse. *Child Abuse and Neglect, 4*, 75–88.

Straus, M. A. (1991). Discipline and deviance: Physical punishment of children and violence and other crimes in adulthood. *Social Problems, 38*, 133–154.

Straus, M. A. (1994). *Beating the devil out of them: Corporal punishment in American families.* New York: Lexington Books.

Tharinger, D., Horton, C. B., and Millea, S. (1990). Sexual abuse and exploitation of children and adults with mental retardation and other handicaps. *Child Abuse and Neglect, 14*, 301–312.

Travers, J., Nauta, M., and Irwin, N. (1982). *The effects of a social program: Final report of the child and family resource program's infant and toddler component.* Cambridge, MA: ABT Associates.

Trickett, P., and Kuczynski, L. (1986). Children's misbehaviors and parental discipline strategies in abusive and nonabusive families. *Developmental Psychology, 22*, 115–123.

Trotter, R., Ackerman, A., Rodman, D., Martinez, A., and Sorvillo, F. (1983). "Azarcon" and "greta": Ethnomedical solutions to epidemiological mystery. *Medical Anthropology Quarterly, 14*(3), 3, 18.

U.S. Advisory Board on Child Abuse and Neglect. (1991). *Creating caring communities: Blueprint for an effective federal policy on child abuse and neglect.* Washington, DC: U.S. Department of Health and Human Services.

U.S. Department of Health and Human Services. (1990). *Healthy people 2000: National health promotion and disease prevention guidelines* (DHHS Publication No. [PHS] 91-50213). Washington, DC: U.S. Government Printing Office.

U.S. Department of Health and Human Services. (1993). *A report on the maltreatment of children with disabilities* (Vol. Publication No. 105-89-1630). Washington, DC: Author.

Wang, C. T., and Daro, D. (1997). *Current trends in child abuse reporting and fatalities: Results of the 1996 annual fifty state survey* (Working paper number 808). Chicago: National Committee to Prevent Child Abuse.

Wauchope, B. A., and Straus, M. A. (Eds.). (1990). *Physical violence in American families: Risk factors and adaptations to violence in 8,145 families.* New Brunswick, NJ: Transaction Books.

Whipple, E. E., and Webster-Stratton, C. (1991). The role of parental stress in physically abusive families. *Child Abuse and Neglect, 15*, 279–291.

Wilkey, I., Pearn, J., Petrie, G., and Nixon, J. (1982). The ecology of adolescent maltreatment: A multilevel examination of adolescent physical abuse, sexual abuse, and neglect. *Journal of Consulting and Clinical Psychology, 59*, 449–457.

Williams, J. (1991, January 6). The real tragedy of crack babies isn't drugs. *The Des Moines Sunday Register.* Section C, p. 3.

Wolfe, D. A. (1985). Child-abusive parents: An empirical review and analysis. *Psychological Bulletin, 97*, 462–482.

Wolfe, D. A. (1987). *Child abuse: Implications for child development and psychopathology.* Newbury Park, CA: Sage Publications.

Wolfe, D. A. (1991). *Preventing physical and emotional abuse of children.* New York: Guilford Press.

Wolock, I., and Horowitz, B. (1979, June). Child maltreatment and maternal deprivation among AFDC-recipient families. *Social Service Review, 53*, 175–194.

Wolock, I., and Horowitz, B. (1984). Child maltreatment as a social problem: The neglect of neglect. *American Journal of Orthopsychiatry, 54*, 530–543.

Yeatman, G. W., Shaw, C., Barlow, M. J., and Bartlett, G. (1976). Pseudobattering in Vietnamese children. *Pediatrics, 58*, 616.

Young, L. (1981). *Physical child neglect.* Chicago: The National Committee for the Prevention of Child Abuse.

Zuravin, S. J. (1991). Unplanned child bearing and family size: Their relationship to child neglect and abuse. *Family Planning Perspectives, 23*(4), 155–161.

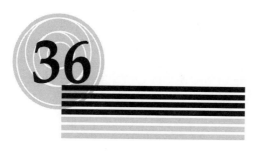

Suicide Prevention

Rosemary Ferdinand

Approximately 25,000 people die by suicide per year; as a result, suicide is the ninth leading cause of death in the United States. One of every 8 to 10 attempts is successful. The average rate is 12.7 suicides per 100,000 deaths, increasing to 19.2 per 100,000 deaths in persons older than 65 years. Adolescent suicide has increased threefold over the last 25 years to 10 per 100,000 deaths per year (Stern, 1995). The overwhelming majority of completed suicides (more than 90%) are in individuals who are psychiatrically ill at the time of suicide (Ghosh & Victor, 1994).

Relevant definitions of suicide in the literature include the following (Ghosh & Victor, 1994; Lego, 1996):

- Suicide: Self-inflicted death.
- Suicidal thoughts: Thoughts of self-annihilation. Active suicidal thoughts involve a fantasy or plan of killing oneself. Passive suicidal thoughts involve a wish to die without taking action—for example, "I wish I were dead."
- Parasuicide: Self-destructive behavior and nonfatal suicide attempts.

The Suicide Prevention intervention in the taxonomy structure for the Nursing Interventions Classification (NIC) (McCloskey & Bulechek, 1996) is associated with Domain 4—Safety: Care that supports protection against harm. The intervention is further associated with two level 2 classes: Class U—Crisis Management: Interventions to provide immediate short-term help in both psychological and physiological crisis, and Class V—Risk Management: Interventions to initiate risk-reduction activities and continue monitoring risks over time. According to the numeric code assigned to the intervention, Suicide Prevention belongs primarily to the Crisis Management class.

REVIEW OF THE RELATED LITERATURE

The activities associated with the Suicide Prevention intervention in the NIC address management of an acute suicidal crisis as well as management of risk for suicide. Knowledge of the risk factors associated with suicide is critical to these activities and is explored in this section.

Demographic Profiles (Ghosh & Victor, 1994; Stern, 1995)

- Age: Rates of suicide rise steadily with age, and suicide is associated with fears of social alienation and physical debilitation. Suicide among teenagers is on the rise.
- Sex: Men and boys complete suicide two to three times more often than women and girls and use more violent means; women and girls attempt suicide three to four times more frequently than men and boys.
- Marital status: Those who are married are at highest risk, followed by those who are widowed, separated, divorced, or single.
- Race: White people have the highest risk for suicide, followed by Native Americans, African Americans, Hispanic Americans, and Asian Americans. The rates for both white and African-American females are low compared with those for men. The rate for African-American men peaks between ages of 20 and 40, declines, and then increases again after 75. White male rates for completed suicides initially peak between ages 20 and 40, level off between ages 40 and 65, and rapidly increase after age 65. The suicide rate for white males aged 85 and older is 50 per 100,000 deaths.
- History of attempts or threats: Nearly 50% of those with successful suicides have made an earlier attempt. In some studies, more than 50% of near-lethal overdoses have been preceded by another attempt. The risk increases if previous efforts to obtain help met with negative or variable results.
- Family history: A history of successful suicide of a family member is a risk factor.
- Occupation: Rates for suicide are highest for executives, followed by administrators, owners of businesses, professionals, and semiskilled workers.
- Finances: Suicide risk increases with financial resources and the presence of threatened financial loss.
- Sexual orientation: Higher risk is associated with active bisexual and inactive homosexual orientations.
- Sleep: Risk increases with the number of hours of sleep per night.
- Weight change: Risk increases with weight gain or 1% to 9% loss.

General Risk Profiles (Ghosh & Victor, 1994)

- High risk: Older than age 45, male, white, living alone, in poor health
- Low risk: Younger than age 45, female, nonwhite, living with others, in good health

Psychosocial Risk Factors (Ghosh & Victor, 1994; Stern, 1995)

Risk for suicide increases with a history of psychiatric disorders or coexisting psychiatric disorders, especially affective illness (mood disorders), substance abuse, eating disorders, and posttraumatic stress disorder (Ghosh & Victor, 1994). Features associated with specific mental conditions are as follows.

DEPRESSION

The presence of a major depressive disorder accounts for 50% of completed suicides. The risk of suicide increases if psychosis coexists and is 5 times greater for patients with delusional depressive features. Approximately 15% of patients with a major affective disorder will eventually die by suicide. Any of the following are symptoms of depression (American Psychiatric Association, 1994):

Suicidal Ideation and Hopelessness.

Thoughts of suicide are in themselves a diagnostic symptom of depression.

Recurrent Thoughts of Death.

Depressed patients will report that they "see" themselves as dead or that they "feel" dead inside. This ideation is different from the normal fear of death seen at the beginning of anticipatory grief.

Depressed Mood.

This may be indicated by your patient's report, "I feel sad," or it may be observed by others.

Anhedonia.

This refers to diminished interest or pleasure in daily activities. Assess this characteristic by asking if your patient's enthusiasm or level of participation in his or her daily activities has changed or decreased. Family members or others may also describe this to you.

Significant Weight Loss or Weight Gain.

Although weight loss may be associated with many illnesses, it should still be evaluated as an indicator of depression.

Insomnia or Hypersomnia.

Evaluate any alterations in patterns of sleep, including deficits or increases.

Psychomotor Agitation or Retardation.

Observe your patient for evidence of physical restlessness or slowed movement. This may also be reported by others.

Fatigue or Loss of Energy.

Again, fatigue is associated with many chronic physical illnesses; its presence should alert you to the possibility of depression.

Feelings of Worthlessness, Excessive or Inappropriate Guilt.

Your patient may say to you, "I don't deserve to live. . . I shouldn't be doing this to my family. . . I deserve to die."

Difficulty Concentrating or Thinking.

You may observe that your patient is indecisive or has difficulty following you in conversation.

BIPOLAR DISORDER

Bipolar disorder is characterized by episodes of mania as well as depression. Features of mania include exaggerated, expansive, or elevated mood; inflated self-esteem; grandiosity; decreased need for sleep; and pressured or excessive speech (Paquette, 1991).

The suicide rate in untreated bipolar disorder patients is as high as 20%. The predisposing factor is not the manic state, but the presence of depression that accompanies a mixed bipolar state. The mixed bipolar state is associated with a particularly high risk of suicide because of the combination of a highly dysphoric mood and a high level of energy and perturbation.

SCHIZOPHRENIA AND OTHER THOUGHT DISORDERS

Diagnoses of thought disorders, including schizophrenia, account for 10% of completed suicides. Thought disorders are a deadly combination with coexistent depression; depressed patients with delusions are at highest risk. The risk for suicide increases when paranoia or command hallucinations urging self-destruction are present. The risk is greatest in young men with high premorbid achievement and high self-expectations. In the first few years of the illness, this population may be in remission and enter a depressive recovery phase of the illness. Although not psychotic, they may recognize the loss of functioning and that their lives have been fundamentally changed by schizophrenia.

ALCOHOLISM AND DRUG DEPENDENCE

Alcoholism and drug dependence account for 25% of completed suicides, making this combination the second most common diagnosis among victims of suicide. Substance use or intoxication may disinhibit depressed patients and facilitate a suicide attempt as well as result in high-risk behaviors leading to automobile accidents and drug overdoses. Chemical dependency increases the suicide risk in a patient fivefold. Although alcohol is the single most prevalent substance, the majority of suicides occur in those patients with multiple-substance abuse.

Characteristics of substance abusers who commit suicide include the following: 20 to 39 years old; male; concurrent alcohol abuser and user of multiple substances (especially opiates, sedatives, amphetamines, and cocaine); mean age of onset 15 years; mean duration of disorder 9 years; chronic use; history of drug overdoses; comorbid psychiatric syndrome (especially depression, borderline personality disorder, and psychosis); recent (<6 weeks) interpersonal loss; childhood history of hyperactivity, incorrigibility, family financial difficulties, family suicidal behaviors, parental abuse, or living in foster homes; and family history of psychiatric syndromes (depression, suicide, or alcoholism) (Ghosh & Victor, 1994).

PERSONALITY DISORDERS

Histrionic, antisocial, and borderline personality disorders account for 5% of completed suicides. Histrionic personality disorder is characterized by pervasive and excessive emotionality and attention-seeking behaviors. Antisocial personality disorder involves a pervasive pattern of disregard for, and violation of, the rights of others. Borderline personality disorder is characterized by a pervasive pattern of instability of personal relationships, self-image, and affect as well as marked impulsivity (American Psychiatric Association, 1994).

Impulsivity may predispose a patient to suicide, and dysphoric patients frequently attempt suicide. Addressing suicidal behavior in the patient with borderline personality disorder is especially challenging with respect to making the distinction between a potentially lethal attempt and chronic self-mutilation or suicide attempts as a way of life. Characterisitcs of borderline psychopathology that have been associated with high risk for suicide include impulsivity, hopelessness, despair, antisocial features, and interpersonal aloofness (Kernberg, 1984).

Chronic Illness, Pain, or Terminal Illness

Many people who complete suicide are physically ill. These illnesses are frequently chronic medical conditions such as cancer, chronic obstructive pulmonary disease, and chronic pain. The diagnosis of acquired immunodeficiency syndrome (AIDS) has been established as a special suicide risk factor. Male persons with AIDS are 7.4 times more likely than demographically similar men and 66 times more likely than the general population to complete suicide (Marzurk, 1988). Related risk factors of the chronically ill for suicide include delirium, dementia, suffering, and hopelessness.

Delirium describes alterations in the level of consciousness. Awareness of the environment is less clear, with decreased ability to focus or to maintain attention. You may observe cognitive changes, including memory deficits and language disturbances. Disorientation and perceptual disturbances may also present and fluctuate over the course of the day.

Cognitive disturbances are frightening to patients. They will fear they are "losing their minds." Fear of living their last days out of touch with reality is also frequently cited by patients considering suicide as an option.

Dementia refers to alterations in cognition and is associated with the advanced stages of many physical illnesses. Symptoms include memory impairments, difficulty executing physical tasks (apraxia), failure to recognize or name familiar objects despite intact sensory function (agnosia), and impaired organizational skills, demonstrated by difficulties in planning and sequencing tasks. Impairments in judgment related to disinhibition are particularly associated with suicide risk. A patient's normal controls may be altered, resulting in high-risk behavior (e.g., driving a car while taking large doses of pain medication). As with delirium, these symptoms can be frustrating and distressing to the patient. The plan of care should address supporting the cognitive deficits, organizing the environment, and facilitating control by the patient.

Fear of prolonged suffering and a painful death are the most frequently cited reasons in surveys of patients considering suicide as an option. Adequate pain control must be given the highest priority in the plan of care. To assess a patient's pain, an objective rating scale, such as a visual analogue or descriptive scale, should be used. Suffering is a subjective experience, and each patient will assign unique meanings to his or her symptoms. Ask how the patient feels about his or her current condition to assess his or her evaluation of quality of life.

Hopelessness has been identified as a significant clinical risk factor for suicide (Beck, Brown, Berchick, Stewart, & Steer, 1990). To have hope means to anticipate a future that is good. Hope also involves a view to the future, and so you must also be interested in the patient's expectations and plans for the future.

Summary

Thorough familiarity with the risks associated with suicide is essential in preventing completion; however, it is not a guarantee that a patient's future behavior can be accurately predicted. The activities associated with this intervention are consistent with the literature and can be implemented to reduce the risk of completion.

Table 36–1 Suicide Prevention

DEFINITION: Reducing the risk of self-inflicted harm for a patient in crisis or severe depression.

ACTIVITIES:

Determine whether the patient has specific suicide plan identified
Encourage the person to make a verbal no-suicide contract
Determine history of suicide attempts
Protect patient from harming self
Place patient in least restrictive environment that allows for necessary level of observation
Demonstrate concern about patient's welfare
Refrain from negatively criticizing
Remove dangerous items from the patient's environment
Place patient in room with protective window coverings, as appropriate
Observe closely during suicidal crisis
Instruct patient and significant other in signs, symptoms and basic physiology of depression
Instruct family that suicidal risk increases for severely depressed patients as they begin to feel better
Facilitate discussion of factors or events that precipitated the suicidal thoughts
Escort patient during off-ward activities, as appropriate
Provide psychiatric counseling, as appropriate
Facilitate support of patient by family and friends
Instruct family on possible warning signs or pleas for help patient may use
Refer patient to psychiatrist, as needed

Source: McCloskey, J. C., and Bulechek, G. M. (1996). *Nursing interventions classification* (NIC) (2nd ed.). St. Louis: Mosby–Year Book.

SUICIDE PREVENTION INTERVENTION AND RELATED ACTIVITIES

The activities associated with Suicide Prevention are shown in Table 36–1. They are as follows.

Determine whether the patient has specific suicide plan identified.

Be prepared to be direct; talking about suicide will not "cause" the person to become suicidal. Not asking the questions only serves to further isolate the suicidal individual. A direct approach will give the patient permission to discuss any suicidal thoughts she or he may be having. One way to start is by asking, "Has it gotten to the point that you are thinking of killing yourself?" (Ferdinand, 1995). Ask the patient about suicide plans. Is there a definite plan? Are the means available? Are the means lethal? Is there a chance for rescue? (Stern, 1995).

Encourage the person to make a verbal no-suicide contract.

According to Ghosh and Victor (1994), the establishment of a therapeutic alliance with the suicidal patient is the single most important task in preventing suicide. Making a no-suicide contract can be a powerful first step toward gaining control in a suicidal crisis. Be empathetic, demonstrate concern, and ask the patient to state that he or she will not commit suicide.

Determine history of suicide attempts.

Ask the patient, "Have you ever tried to kill yourself before?" If a previous suicide attempt was made, what was the risk? Was the method dangerous? What were the chances for rescue—was the attempt in a place where the patient could be discovered or in a setting where there was a very low chance for rescue? Did the patient believe the method would work? Is the patient disappointed that he or she survived? Was the attempt impulsive? Had the patient gotten his or her affairs in order or made changes to a will? (Stern, 1995).

Protect patient from harming self.

Separate the patient from any means of self-destruction (Beeber, 1996). Patients in an acute suicidal crisis may need to be restrained when other, less restrictive means of protection are ineffective.

Place patient in least restrictive environment that allows for necessary level of observation.

Appropriate environments can include a community setting with others in attendance or a crisis intervention setting (Beeber, 1996). Patients who are at high risk for suicide should be hospitalized and prevented from fleeing the hospital. These include patients who are psychotic and suicidal, are older than 45 years, have made a violent attempt for which they took precautions to avoid rescue, are refusing help, or have no social supports (Stern, 1995).

Demonstrate concern about patient's welfare.

Be empathetic and listen actively in addition to telling the patient that you are there to maintain his or her safety. The patient may reject your help, which can be evidence of the patient's efforts to maintain control. Taking a slow and patient approach allows the patient to align with the nurse and with efforts to control the urge of self-destruction (Beeber, 1996).

Refrain from negatively criticizing.

The nurse's communication should be directed toward establishing a therapeutic alliance with the patient. Judgmental or negative critical messages will only serve to further isolate the patient. The risk for suicide has been noted to increase with the negativity of the health care provider's reaction (Ghosh & Victor, 1994).

Remove dangerous items from the patient's environment.

If the patient is being counseled over the telephone, as in a crisis intervention setting, ask the patient to throw the means of self-destruction (e.g., knife, gun) out the window, flush pills down the toilet, or drop car keys down a drain or heat register (Beeber, 1996). In a hospital setting, remove all sharp objects such as scissors, razors, and eating utensils; long objects such as belts and ties; and other dangerous objects such as glass bottles and metal cans.

Place patient in room with protective window coverings, as appropriate.

Protective devices may include nonshattering glass reinforced with wire, locks, and metal guards on windows.

Observe closely during suicidal crisis.

During the acute suicidal crisis, self-destructive impulses are strong and have overwhelmed the patient's ability to control them. The patient must be closely monitored to ensure adequate safety.

Instruct patient and significant other in signs, symptoms and basic physiology of depression.

Depression is a frequent precursor to suicidal ideation. Educating the patient and significant others in the signs and symptoms of depression, including supplying written resources, can enhance recognition and coping with a potential crisis (Beeber, 1996).

Instruct family that suicidal risk increases for severely depressed patients as they begin to feel better.

This phenomenon is related to the abatement of the vegetative symptoms of depression. As the patient recovers, he or she may have the energy required to act on suicidal ideation.

Facilitate discussion of factors or events that precipitated the suicidal thoughts.

Once the acute crisis has been stabilized and a therapeutic alliance established, the nurse can assist the patient to identify the events that precipitated the suicidal ideation. The patient can begin to identify alternative coping strategies.

Escort patient during off-ward activities, as appropriate.

During the acute suicidal crisis, this activity can help protect the patient from suicidal impulses. After the acute crisis, the activity supports the development of the nurse–patient relationship.

Provide psychiatric counseling, as appropriate.

The nurse can provide counseling to address feelings of hopelessness and helplessness and sources of pain, to help develop problem solving and social skills, and to help cope with mental illnesses such as depression and schizophrenia. Advance practice nurses can provide psychotherapy as indicated.

Facilitate support of patient by family and friends.

Social isolation is a critical risk factor for suicide. The nurse can provide education and resources, such as a referral to support groups or family or group therapy, to assist the development of meaningful relationships.

Instruct family on possible warning signs or pleas for help patient may use.

The nurse can provide information on symptoms associated with the exacerbation of specific diseases, such as depression or schizophrenia. Crisis resources should also be identified.

Refer patient to psychiatrist, as needed.

In outpatient settings, all suicidal ideation must be taken seriously and referred for psychiatric follow-up. In inpatient settings, suicidal behavior and ideation must be documented and communicated to all members of the treatment team. As previously stated, the overwhelming majority of completed suicides (more than 90%) are in individuals who are psychiatrically ill at the time of suicide (Ghosh & Victor, 1994).

ASSOCIATED NURSING DIAGNOSES AND APPROPRIATE CLIENT GROUPS

■

The following nursing diagnoses have been linked to the Suicide Prevention intervention in the NIC (McCloskey & Bulechek, 1996):

- Body Image Disturbance
- Grieving, Dysfunctional
- Hopelessness
- Post-Trauma Response
- Self Mutilation, Risk for
- Social Interaction, Impaired
- Violence, Risk for: Self-Directed or Directed at Others

Table 36–2 lists each nursing diagnosis, its definition, and whether the intervention of Suicide Prevention is suggested or optional.

Three of the nursing diagnoses identified in Table 36–2—Hopelessness; Social Interaction, Impaired; and Violence, Risk for: Self-Directed or Directed at Others—have been linked in the literature (Paquette, 1991) to the following diagnoses from the *Diagnostic and Statistical Manual of Mental Disorders*, fourth edition (DSM-IV) (American Psychiatric Association, 1994):

- Major Depressive Episode
  According to the DSM-IV, five or more of the following symptoms must

Table 36–2   Related Nursing Diagnoses for Suicide Intervention

Nursing Diagnosis	Definition	Suicide Prevention
Body Image Disturbance	Disruption in the way one perceives one's body image	S
Grieving, Dysfunctional	Extended, unsuccessful use of intellectual and emotional responses by which individuals attempt to work through the process of modifying self-concept based on the perception of loss	O
Hopelessness	A subjective state in which an individual sees limited or no alternatives or personal choices available and is unable to mobilize energy on own behalf	O
Post-Trauma Response	The state of an individual experiencing a sustained painful response to an overwhelming traumatic event(s)	O
Self Mutilation, Risk for	A state in which an individual is at risk to perform an act on the self to injure, not kill, which produces tissue damage and tension relief	S
Social Interaction, Impaired	The state in which an individual participates in an insufficient or excessive quantity or ineffective quality of social exchange	O
Violence, Risk for: Self-Directed or Directed at Others	A state in which an individual experiences behaviors that can be physically harmful either to the self or others	S

O = Optional
S = Suggested
Source: North American Nursing Diagnosis Association. (1996). *Nursing diagnoses: Definitions and classification 1997–1998.* Philadelphia: Author; McCloskey, J. C., and Bulechek, G. M. (1996). *Nursing interventions classification (NIC)* (2nd ed.). St. Louis: Mosby–Year Book.

have been present during the same two-week period: depressed mood, diminished interest or pleasure, significant weight loss or weight gain, insomnia or excessive sleep, psychomotor agitation or retardation, fatigue or energy loss, feelings of worthlessness or excessive and inappropriate guilt, diminished ability to think or concentrate, and recurrent thoughts of death or suicidal ideation. In order for the diagnosis of major depressive disorder to be made, one of the symptoms must be depressed mood or loss of interest or pleasure.

- Major Depression, Single Episode
This diagnosis indicates a single episode of major depression.
- Major Depression, Recurrent Episode
This diagnosis indicates the presence of two or more major depressive episodes, separated by an interval of at least 2 months.
- Dysthymia
Dysthymia is characterized by a chronically depressed mood with at least two of the following: poor appetite or overeating, insomnia or excessive sleep, low energy or fatigue, low self-esteem, poor concentration or difficulty making decisions, and feelings of hopelessness.
- Bipolar Disorder, Manic
This diagnosis indicates the presence of at least one or more manic episodes. To make the diagnosis of mania, an abnormally and persistently elevated mood must be present and last at least one week. Additionally, three or more of the following should be present: inflated self-esteem, decreased need for sleep, patient more talkative than usual, flight of ideas or the subjective feeling that thoughts are racing, distractibility, psychomotor agitation, and excessive involvement with pleasurable activities that are associated with a high potential for negative consequences (buying sprees, sexual indiscretions).
- Bipolar Disorder, Mixed
A mixed bipolar episode is characterized by a period of at least one month in which the criteria for both major depressive episode and mania are met nearly every day.
- Cyclothymia
This diagnosis is characterized by chronic fluctuations in mood between hypomanic and depressive states. Hypomania can be viewed as an attenuated form of mania, in which the features of mania may be present, but to a lesser degree. Additionally, no psychosis or delusions may be present.

Clients associated with the following categories of comorbid conditions that increase the risk of suicide (Beeber, 1996) should also be considered for the Suicide Prevention intervention: Substance Use Disorder, Schizophrenia, Mood Disorders (Bipolar Disorders, Major Depressive Episode, Organic Mental Disorders, Personality Disorders [Histrionic, Antisocial, Borderline], Anxiety Disorders [Post-Traumatic Stress Disorder]).

ASSOCIATED PATIENT OUTCOMES
■

The Suicide Prevention intervention can be expected to achieve the following patient outcomes from the Nursing Outcomes Classification (NOC) (Johnson & Maas, 1997).

- Suicide Self-Restraint—Ability to refrain from gestures and attempts at killing self
- Coping—Actions to manage stressors that tax an individual's resources
- Safety Behavior: Personal—Individual or caregiver efforts to control behaviors that might cause physical injury
- Will to Live—Desire, determination, and effort to survive

A positive orientation on the following outcomes can reduce the risk for completion of suicide:

- Acceptance: Health Status—Reconciliation of health circumstances
- Anxiety Control—Ability to eliminate or reduce feelings of apprehension and tension from an unidentifiable source
- Cognitive Orientation—Ability to identify person, place, and time
- Dignified Dying—Maintaining personal control and comfort with the approaching end of life
- Distorted Thought Control—Ability to self-restrain disruption in perception, thought processes, and thought content
- Fear Control—Ability to eliminate or reduce disabling feeling of alarm aroused by an identifiable source
- Grief Resolution—Adjustment to actual or impending loss
- Hope—Presence of internal state of optimism that is personally satisfying and life-supporting
- Impulse Control—Ability to self-restrain compulsive or impulsive behaviors
- Loneliness—The extent of emotional, social, or existential isolation response
- Mood Equilibrium—Appropriate adjustment of prevailing emotional tone in response to circumstances
- Pain Control Behavior—Personal actions to control pain
- Pain: Disruptive Effects—Observed or reported disruptive effects of pain on emotions and behavior
- Pain Level—Amount of reported or demonstrated pain
- Psychosocial Adjustment: Life Change—Psychosocial adaptation of an individual to a life change
- Quality of Life—An individual's expressed satisfaction with current life circumstances
- Risk Control: Alcohol Use—Actions to eliminate or reduce alcohol use that poses a threat to health
- Risk Control: Drug Use—Actions to eliminate or reduce drug use that poses a threat to health
- Self-Esteem—Personal judgment of self-worth
- Social Interaction Skills—An individual's use of effective interaction behaviors
- Social Involvement—Frequency of an individual's social interactions with persons, groups, or organizations
- Social Support—Perceived availability and actual provision of reliable assistance from other persons
- Spiritual Well-Being—Personal expression of connectedness with self, others, higher power, all life, nature, and the universe that transcend and empower the self
- Symptom Control Behavior—Personal actions to minimize perceived adverse changes in physical and emotional functioning
- Symptom Severity—Extent of perceived adverse changes in physical, emotional, and social functioning
- Well-Being—An individual's expressed satisfaction with health status

CASE STUDY

M, a 21-year-old man who was diagnosed six months earlier as having schizophrenia following a psychotic episode at college, was hospitalized for 10 days and discharged on psychotropic medication. He returned to college, where he was living before the hospitalization. Since his return, he has not been attending classes and has increasingly withdrawn from his friends. He has been admitted to an inpatient unit after attempting to kill himself with a rifle on the previous night. Admitting blood work indicates that alcohol was present. M's parents have flown in to see him. They report that his communications with them have decreased considerably in the past 4 weeks.

Applying the Suicide Prevention Intervention

- Protect patient from harming self. Admission to the hospital's psychiatric ward is a first step to separate M from any means of self-destruction. M should be monitored closely to determine the need for restraints if other, less restrictive, means of protection are ineffective.

- Place patient in least restrictive environment that allows for necessary level of observation. M meets the high risk for suicide criteria and has been appropriately hospitalized. He should be prevented from fleeing the hospital.

- Demonstrate concern about patient's welfare. Communicate to M that you are there to maintain his safety. M may reject your help. Be prepared to take a slow approach to allow him to align with you to work toward controlling his urges for self-destruction.

- Refrain from negatively criticizing. Focus your communication on establishing a therapeutic alliance with M. Judgmental or negative critical messages will only serve to further isolate him.

- Remove dangerous items from the patient's environment. Remove all sharp objects such as scissors, razors, and eating utensils; long objects such as belts and ties; and other dangerous objects such as glass bottles and metal cans.

- Place patient in room with protective window coverings, as appropriate. Ensure that the environment provides nonshattering glass reinforced with wire, locks, and metal guards on windows.

- Observe closely during suicidal crisis. M should be closely monitored, because he is still in the acute suicidal crisis where self-destructive impulses are strong and have recently overwhelmed his ability to control them.

- Instruct patient and significant others in signs, symptoms, and basic physiology of depression. M is most likely in the depressive recovery stage of schizophrenia. His family reports that he is attending college on an academic scholarship and was the valedictorian of his high school class. With the acute psychosis under control, M may be realizing the implications of the disease and may be prone to depression. Educate both M and his family in the signs and symptoms of depression and provide written resources to enhance recognition and coping with a potential crisis.

- Instruct family that suicidal risk increases for severely depressed patients as they begin to feel better. Although M may not be formally diagnosed with depression, this phenomenon may still occur, and providing education to M and his family is appropriate.

- Facilitate discussion of factors or events that precipitated the suicidal thoughts. Encourage M to discuss the losses he perceives related to the disease and any other events that may have precipitated the crisis, and assist him to identify alternative coping strategies.

- Escort patient during off-ward activities, as appropriate. During the acute suicidal crisis, this activity can help protect M from suicidal impulses, and, after the acute crisis, this activity supports the development of your relationship with M.

- Provide psychiatric counseling, as appropriate. Provide counseling to address feelings of hopelessness and helplessness and develop problem-solving and social skills as well as skills for coping with schizophrenia.

- Facilitate support of patient by family and friends. M has isolated himself from family and friends. Refer M to support groups or family or group therapy to assist the development of meaningful relationships.

- Instruct family on possible warning signs or pleas for help patient may use. Provide information on symptoms associated with the exacerbation of schizophrenia and identify crisis resources.

- Refer patient to psychiatrist, as needed. mented and communicated suicidal behavi and ideation must be reported to all members of the treatment team. Reinforce compliance with follow-up care.

References

American Psychiatric Association. (1994). *Diagnostic and statistical manual of mental disorders* (4th ed.). Washington, DC: Author.

Beck, A., Brown, G., Berchick, R., Stewart, B. L., and Steer, R. A. (1990). Relationship between hopelessness and ultimate suicide: A replication with psychiatric outpatients. *American Journal of Psychiatry, 147*, 190–195.

Beeber, L. S. (1996). The client who is suicidal. In S. Lego (Ed.), *Psychiatric nursing: A comprehensive reference* (pp. 208–212). Philadelphia: Lippincott-Raven.

Ferdinand, R. (1995, December). I'd rather die than live this way. *American Journal of Nursing, 95* (12), 42–47.

Ghosh, T., and Victor, B. S. (1994). Suicide. In R. E. Hales, S. C. Yudofsky, and J. A. Talbott (Eds.), *American psychiatric press textbook of psychiatry* (pp. 1251–1271). Washington, DC: American Psychiatric Press.

Johnson, M., and Maas, M. (1997). *Nursing Outcomes Classification (NOC).* St. Louis: Mosby–Year Book.

Kernberg, O. (1984). *Severe personality disorders: Psychotherapeutic strategies.* New Haven, CT: Yale University Press.

Lego, S. (1996). Glossary. In S. Lego (Ed.), *Psychiatric nursing: A comprehensive reference* (p. 632). Philadelphia: Lippincott-Raven.

Marzurk, P. M. (1988). Increased risk of suicide in persons with AIDS. *JAMA, 259*, 1333–1337.

McCloskey, J. C., and Bulechek, G. M. (1996). *Nursing interventions classifications (NIC)* (2nd ed.). St. Louis: Mosby–Year Book.

Paquette, M. (1991). *Psychiatric nursing diagnosis care plans for DSM-III-R.* Boston: Jones and Bartlett.

Stern, T. A. (1995, October 20–22). Evaluation of suicide risk. In *Psychopharmacology.* Boston: Harvard Medical School and Massachusetts General Hospital.

37

Fall Prevention

Virginia Kilpack and Mary E. Godin

awrence and Maher define a fall as "an unplanned slip to the floor, whether or not injury was sustained" (1992, p. 23). Falls and avoiding a fall are complex phenomena that result from the interaction of a multitude of intrinsic and extrinsic risk factors (Benson & Luscardi, 1995; Mitchell & Jones, 1996; Tideiksaar, 1997). Individuals of all ages fall, with the highest incidence occurring in early childhood and old age (Garrettson & Gallagher, 1985; Hogue, 1982; Mosenthal, Livingston, Elcavage, Merritt & Stucker, 1995).

Falls have been identified as the most common cause of injury and the most frequent reason for emergency department visits among all age groups (Garrettson & Gallagher, 1985; Hogue, 1982; Province et al., 1995). An analysis of death certificates done by the National Safety Council (1995) revealed falls in all age groups ranked second as cause of death behind motor vehicle trauma. Unintentional injuries, which most often are the result of a fall, have been cited as the sixth leading cause of death in people older than 65, especially those age 85 and older (Runge, 1993; Sattin, 1992). Unlike in toddlers, elder falls tend to become more, rather than less, of a hazard with advancing age (Berryman, Gaskin, Jones, Tolley & MacMullen, 1989).

Once viewed as a normal consequence of aging or as accidents that occurred randomly or "by chance," falls are beginning to be regarded as predictable events that can often be prevented (Hogue, 1992; Tideiksaar, 1997). Therefore, the goal of any Fall Prevention program should be the identification of at-risk individuals in order to facilitate the development and implementation of effective strategies that minimize or prevent the likelihood of a fall (Wood & Cunningham, 1992). When designing Fall Prevention activities, it is critical to remember that most Fall Prevention activities need to be executed by health care providers or caregivers rather than by the individual at risk to fall (Hogue, 1982).

LITERATURE REVIEW

Epidemiology of Falls

Falls continue to be a common and potentially preventable cause of morbidity and mortality among young children and the elderly (Mosenthal et al., 1995; Sattin, 1992). Lambert and Sattin (1988) showed a 100-fold rise in death rates among individuals age 5 to 85 years who experienced a fall. Similar findings were documented by Mosenthal et al. (1995), who conducted a study to determine the epidemiology and risk factors of patients following a fall event. Results showed that falls constituted 9% of total trauma admissions and carried an 11% mortality rate. Of the 356 patients, children younger than 13 accounted for 61 falls, with only one death. The elderly, 64 years and older, accounted for only 44 falls but more than 50% of deaths. When compared with children, the elderly who fall have a risk of hospitalization that is 10 times higher and a risk of death that is 8 times higher than these same risks in children who fall (Runge, 1993).

Regardless of clinical setting, approximately 10% to 15% of all falls result in serious injuries. About 1% of the elderly who fall suffer a hip fracture, 5% suffer a bone fracture at other sites, and 5% suffer a soft-tissue injury (Sattin, 1992; Tinetti & Speechley, 1989; Tinetti, Speechley, & Ginter, 1988). Twenty-five percent of elderly persons who suffer a fractured hip have been found to die within one year of injury, compared with a 15% mortality rate in the general population of the same age (Hendrich, 1988; Magaziner, Simonsick, Kashner, Hebel, & Kenzora, 1989).

Financially, the cost of caring for falls in the elderly exceeds $15 billion each year (Runge, 1993). Upon discharge, the majority of these individuals are transferred to nursing homes (Tinetti, Lui, & Claus, 1993). Even in the absence of physical injuries, a fall may lead to anxiety and fear of falling, decreased mobility, restriction of activities, social isolation, depression, loss of self-confidence, and loss of independence (Tideiksaar, 1997; Tinetti, Rickman, & Powell, 1990).

Acute Care Settings

Acute and long-term care facilities have been found to have the highest incidence rates for patient falls (Rubenstein et al., 1988). In the acute care setting, falls account for 40% to 90% of all hospital incidents (Foreman, 1989; Jones & Smith, 1989; Raz & Baretich, 1987). Among all age groups that are hospitalized, the elderly are recognized to be at the greatest risk for falling (Rymes & Jaeger, 1988). Studies have demonstrated that falls in the elderly can be an indication of the onset of acute illness or exacerbation of chronic illness (Rubenstein, Robbins, Josephson, Schulman, & Osterweil, 1990).

Estimates show that one of every five elderly persons will fall a minimum of once during a hospital stay, and at least 50% of these fallers will suffer multiple falls (Caley & Pinchoff, 1994; Hendrich, Nyhuis, Kippenbrock, & Soja, 1995). Most falls tend to happen during the first week of hospitalization and again after week 3 of hospitalization (Tack, Ulrich, & Kehr, 1987). The majority of older persons admitted to the hospital after a fall generally do not return to their previous level of independence (Oreskovich, Howard, Copass, & Carrico, 1984).

Various researchers have attempted to establish a profile of characteristics that describe patients most at risk for falls in an acute care setting (Foster & Kohlenberg, 1996; Hendrich, 1988; Hendrich et al., 1995; Janken, Reynolds, & Swiech, 1986; Jones & Smith, 1989; Kippenbrock & Soja, 1993; Nevitt, Cummings, & Hudes, 1991; Spellbring, 1992; Tinetti et al., 1988). To date, no studies have been able to identify a consistent set of risk factors that are applicable to all patients across every health care setting (Janken et al., 1986; Raz & Baretich, 1987). In a review of risk profiles, Whedon and Shedd (1989) concluded that none of the high-risk profiles were sensitive enough or specific enough to warrant their use as predictive instruments for falls in any patient population.

Most patient fall studies have focused on retrospective chart reviews. In contrast, Kippenbrock and Soja (1993) conducted a descriptive study in a large midwestern acute care hospital to identify risk factors for falling from the patient's perspective. For the study, interviews were conducted with elderly patients (age 60 to 85 years) within 48 hours of each patient's fall. Open-ended questions were asked to gain information about the patient's perceptions of the fall, factors related to the fall, patient outcomes, and suggestions for preventing falls. Study results showed that the most frequent risk factors, in order of their most common occurrence, were confusion, a cardiovascular medical diagnosis, decreased lower extremity mobility, generalized weakness, elimination needs, and an orthopedic medical diagnosis. The risk factors identified in this study support the high-risk factors previously described in the literature on falls.

Long-Term Care Settings

Each year, at least 40% to 50% of patients in nursing homes fall, with more than 40% of these individuals experiencing multiple falls (Gurwitz, Sanchez-Cross, Eckler, & Matulis, 1994; Howe, 1994; Rubenstein et al., 1988), In a review describing the epidemiology of falls in long-term care facilities, Rubenstein et al. (1988) reported a mean annual incidence rate of 165 falls per 100 beds.

Although fall-related injuries, especially fractures, are a source of considerable morbidity and mortality among elderly nursing home residents, few studies have been done in this area. Cali and Kiel (1995) conducted a five-year retrospective study in a long-term rehabilitation center in Boston. The purpose of the study was to assess the incidence of fall-related fractures and the circumstances surrounding the fall events. Subjects consisted of residents age 65 to 104 years with a radiologically documented fracture that was the direct result of a fall. Study results showed that 313 fractures occurred during the study period. Of these fractures, 296 (95%) were fall related, with hip fractures constituting 50% of the total number of fractures. The majority of these fall-associated fractures (89%) were found in residents without a history of recurrent falls and with moderate functional impairment. A review of the incident reports found that 42% of falls occurred during the day shift, 55% of falls took place in the resident's bedroom or adjoining bathroom, and 67% of falls occurred during ambulation. An unexpected finding of the study was that 16% of fractures occurred in the presence of a wet floor.

In many health care facilities, especially long-term care settings, physical restraints are often used as a safety measure against patient falls (Watson & Mayhew, 1994). Although there is scant evidence to support the use of restraints as a method to prevent falls (Evans & Strumpf, 1989), there is a plethora of data demonstrating that fall-related injuries are more numerous and serious in restrained patients (Rubenstein, Miller, Postel, & Evans, 1983). Tinetti, Lui, and

Ginter (1992) conducted a study that assessed restraint use and fall-related injuries among a group of twelve nursing homes. Results revealed that an increased use of restraints was accompanied by an increase in the number of falls and fall-associated injuries. Specifically, 5% of unrestrained residents versus 17% of restrained residents suffered a serious fall-related injury.

An eight-site clinical intervention study, called Frailty and Injuries: Cooperative Studies of Intervention Techniques (FICSIT) (Province et al., 1995), was jointly funded by the National Institute on Aging and the National Center for Nursing Research for the purpose of preventing falls and frailty in older persons. Two of the clinical trial sites involved nursing home settings (Fiatarone et al., 1993; Mulrow, Gerety, Kanten, DeNino, & Cornell, 1993). The Boston FICSIT site (Fiatarone et al., 1993) was a nursing home and involved 100 residents, age 70 to 100 years, who were ambulatory and at high risk to fall and did not have severe dementia. Each patient was randomly assigned to one of four treatment groups for a ten-week period. The goal of the study was to improve muscle strength through progressive resistance training of lower extremities and/or multinutrient supplementation. In the San Antonio FICSIT site, Mulrow et al. (1993) recruited 194 nursing home residents age 60 and older who were functionally dependent in two or more activities of daily living but were not severely cognitively impaired. Subjects were randomized to either the intervention group, which received one-on-one physical therapy sessions three times per week for 16 weeks, or the control group, which received structured social visits for 16 weeks. A preplanned meta-analysis of the FICSIT trials (Province et al., 1995) showed that none of the exercise interventions had a significant effect on the incidence of *injurious* falls but that treatment, including the use of exercises for elderly adults, reduced the *risk* of falls.

Community Settings

The lowest incidence rates for falls have been found among elderly persons living in the community (Luukinen, Koski, Honkanen, & Kivela, 1995; Rubenstein et al., 1988). Each year, approximately one quarter of community dwellers age 65 to 74 years and one third or more elderly persons age 75 years and older suffer a fall. About 20% of all elderly persons who fall will fall again within six months (Vellas et al., 1992). Because many of the falls experienced by elderly community residents are unreported, the incidence of falls in this population may be much higher (Tideikaar, 1997).

Many researchers (Hale, Delaney, & McGaghie, 1992; Rodriquez et al., 1991; Sattin, 1992; Shepherd, Lutz, Miller, & Main, 1992) have found that the majority of falls experienced by older adults occur inside the home. The most common locations of falls in the home environment, in order of frequency, include the bedroom, bathroom, living room, and stairways (Campbell, Borrie, & Spears, 1989). Some of the more commonly identified environmental hazards in the home setting are transferring from excessively low or high bed or chair heights, using low toilet seats without support grab bars, walking in poorly lighted rooms, and wearing improper footwear (Fleming & Pendergast, 1993; Hornbrook et al., 1991; Sattin, 1992).

It is well known that the causes of falls are multifactorial. Several investigators (Galindo-Ciocon, Ciocon, & Galindo, 1995; Maki, Holliday, & Topper, 1991; Woolley, Czaja, & Drury, 1997) have demonstrated gait and balance disorders to be the second most frequent cause of falls in the elderly, after environmental factors. One research team (Galindo-Ciocin et al., 1995) conducted a study to ascertain the effects of gait training on the incidence of falls and on the improvement of gait and balance among elderly (age 65 and older) community residents. These subjects had difficulty walking and suffered at least one fall within three months of the initiation of the study. Each subject received Fall Prevention education and was referred to a physical therapist for gait training three times a week for one month. Results showed that physical therapy–guided gait training improved gait and balance as well as decreased the number of falls.

Researchers have also studied the effects of exercise in reducing falls and fall-related injuries in the elderly (Province et al., 1995; Reinsch, MacRae, Lachenbruch, & Tobis, 1992). Five of the eight sites for the FICSIT clinical intervention trials (Buchner et al., 1993; Hornbrook, Stevens, & Wingfield, 1993; Tinnetti et al., 1993; Wallace, Ross, Huston, Kundel, & Woodworth, 1993; Wolf, Kutner, Green, & McNeely, 1993) were community sites. The Yale FICSIT trial (Tinetti et al., 1993) recruited 300 ambulatory community residents age 70 and older who were health maintenance organization (HMO) members. Investigators compared a targeted fall-reduction strategy with social visits and usual care. Interventions included medication adjustments, behavioral changes, patient education, and home-based exercise for a three-month period, with a 12-month follow-up. Results showed that the Yale FICSIT interventions for decreasing falls were feasible and effective.

IDENTIFICATION OF INTERVENTION PROTOCOLS

Fall Prevention is a complex intervention that must take into account numerous patient-related and environment-related factors. Many studies identify a myriad of fall risk factors and describe how to determine patients at high risk for falling (Janken et al., 1986; Myers, Baker, Van Natta, Abbey, & Robinson, 1991; Nevitt et al., 1991; Rapport et al., 1993; Spellbring, 1992; Tinetti et al., 1988). On the basis of such reports, preventive strategies have been advised. The diverse measurement methodologies, in addition to inconsistencies in the multiple risk factors investigated and discrepancies among the interventions chosen, can make applying study findings to clinical practice perplexing. Uncontrolled intervention studies often show positive outcomes in reducing the incidence of falls (Croft & Foraker, 1992; Kilpack, Boehm, Smith, & Mudge, 1991; Mitchell & Jones, 1996; Ruckstuhl, Marchionda, Salmons, & Larrabbee, 1991; Tack et al., 1987), but the few controlled studies have not always demonstrated this effect (Hornbrook et al., 1994; Lauritzen, Petersen, & Lund, 1993; Reinsch et al., 1992; Rubenstein et al., 1990; Wagner et al., 1994). Fall Prevention protocols and tools in current references are divided into two major categories: (1) risk assessment screening tools to determine patient probability of falling and (2) intervention checklists or programs.

Risk Assessment

A variety of screening tools for identifying risk factors and probability of falling are used by nurses to determine when the intervention Fall Prevention (Table 37–1) is appropriate. Hendrich et al. (1995) have made a contribution to risk factor assessment that incorporates a nursing standard for interventions. At a large tertiary care hospital, over an interval of one month, they conducted a retrospective case-control study that included a sample of 102 falls as found on incident reports and 236 nonfall charts. A risk factor instrument developed by Hendrich (1988) was modified for this study, and logistic regression was used

Table 37–1   Fall Prevention

DEFINITION: Instituting special precautions with patient at risk for injury from falling.

ACTIVITIES:

Identify cognitive or physical deficits of the patient that may increase potential of falling in a particular environment

Identify characteristics of environment that may increase potential for falls (e.g., slippery floors and open stairways)

Monitor gait, balance, and fatigue level with ambulation

Assist unsteady individual with ambulation

Provide assistive devices (e.g., cane and walker) to steady gait

Maintain assistive devices in good working order

Lock wheels of wheelchair, bed, or gurney during transfer of patient

Place articles within easy reach of the patient

Instruct patient to call for assistance with movement, as appropriate

Teach patient how to fall as to minimize injury

Post signs to remind patient to call for help when getting out of bed, as appropriate

Use proper technique to transfer patient to and from wheelchair, bed, toilet, and so on

Provide elevated toilet seat for easy transfer

Provide chairs of proper height, with backrests and armrests for easy transfer

Provide bed mattress with firm edges for easy transfer

Use physical restraints to limit potentially unsafe movement, as appropriate

Use side rails of appropriate length and height to prevent falls from bed, as needed

Place a mechanical bed in lowest position

Provide a sleeping surface close to the floor, as needed

Provide seating on bean bag chair to limit mobility, as appropriate

Place a foam wedge in seat of chair to prevent patient from arising, as appropriate

Use partially-filled water mattress on bed to limit mobility, as appropriate

Provide the dependent patient with a means of summoning help (e.g., bell or call light) when caregiver is not present

Answer call light immediately

Assist with toileting at frequent, scheduled intervals

Use a bed alarm to alert caretaker that individual is getting out of bed, as appropriate

Mark doorway thresholds and edges of steps, as needed

Remove low-lying furniture (e.g., footstools and tables) that presents a tripping hazard

Avoid clutter on floor surface

Provide adequate lighting for increased visibility

Provide night light at bedside

Provide visible handrails and grab bars

Place gates in open doorways leading to stairways

Provide nonslip, nontrip floor surfaces

Provide a nonslip surface in bathtub or shower

Provide sturdy, nonslip step stools to facilitate easy reaches

Provide storage areas that are within easy reach

Provide heavy furniture that will not tip if used for support

Orient patient to physical "setup" of room

Avoid unnecessary rearrangement of physical environment

Ensure that patient wears shoes that fit properly, fasten securely, and have nonskid soles

Instruct patient to wear prescription glasses, as appropriate, when out of bed

Educate family members about risk factors that contribute to falls and how they can decrease these risks

Instruct family on importance of handrails for stairs, bathrooms and walkways

Assist family in identifying hazards in the home and modifying them

Instruct patient to avoid ice and other slippery outdoor surfaces

Institute a routine physical exercise program that includes walking

Post signs to alert staff that patient is at high risk for falls

Collaborate with other health care team members to minimize side effects of medications that contribute to falling (e.g., orthostatic hypotension and unsteady gait)

Provide close supervision and/or a restraining device (e.g., infant seat with seat belt) when placing infants/young children on elevated surfaces (e.g., table and highchair)

Table continued on following page

Table 37–1 Fall Prevention *Continued*

DEFINITION: Instituting special precautions with patient at risk for injury from falling.

ACTIVITIES:

Remove objects that provide young child with climbing access to elevated surfaces

Maintain crib side rails in elevated position when caregiver is not present, as appropriate

Provide a "bubble top" on hospital cribs of pediatric patients who may climb over elevated side rails, as appropriate

Fasten the latches securely on access panel of incubator when leaving bedside of infant in incubator, as appropriate

Source: McCloskey, J. C., and Bulechek, G. M. (Eds.). (1996). *Nursing interventions classification (NIC)* (2nd ed., p. 272). St. Louis: Mosby–Year Book.

to develop a multivariate risk factor model showing seven risk factors: recent history of falls (the most significant factor), depression, altered elimination pattern, dizziness or vertigo, primary cancer diagnosis, confusion, and altered mobility. Relative risk values converted to risk points were used to assess the patient's level of fall risk. A sensitivity of 77% (79 of 102) and a specificity of 72% (169 of 236) were calculated for this model. The risk factor assessment tool includes a Fall Prevention intervention based on the seven intrinsic conditions associated with a fall event. The categories of intervention include promoting patient independence, teaching patient and family about fall risk, increasing the nurse's awareness of the patient's risk to fall, meeting elimination needs, and providing ambulatory assistance to high-risk patients; these were formulated from extensive literature review and fall reports at multiple institutions. The risk score determines the level of intervention to initiate. The tool is streamlined and takes less than one minute to complete on each shift. Further research is needed to test the value of this risk factor model for specialized patient care groups such as pediatrics, critical care, and rehabilitation.

McCollam (1995), at a Veterans Affairs Medical Center (VAMC), describes the use of the Morse Fall Scale (MFS) (Morse, Morse, & Tylko, 1989), a falls identification instrument that is research based. This scale consists of six scored variables: history of falling, secondary diagnosis, intravenous therapy, use of ambulatory aids, gait, and mental status. Statistical analysis showed that a score of 45 or greater identified 70% of fallers. Over a three-month period, 458 patients on a cardiology–general medicine unit at VAMC were assessed for fall risk, yielding a total of 30 falls or near falls for 23 patients. The VAMC results of sensitivity and specificity compared favorably with the original MFS research and with the interrater reliablity coefficient. Because this instrument takes only one minute to complete, McCollam added the MFS to nursing admission assessment forms, encouraging its use to reassess patients whenever a change in condition occurred. Nursing inservice sessions stressed the need to initiate interventions on patients assessed at risk to fall, but only 50% to 58% of high-risk patients had care plans or nursing orders prescribing interventions. The interventions used were not described. Although the reported number of falls increased by 24%, this research-based innovation reduced the number of serious injuries from 11 in the year before implementation to four in the year after implementation. Adopting the MFS for general use requires adjustment of the cutoff scores for different patient groups. McCollam recommends that a falls assessment instrument be accompanied by a strong Fall Prevention program.

The critical variables in predicting fall-prone status have not yet been identified, but the literature contains a range of contributing risk factors (Foster & Kohlenberg, 1996; Llewellyn, Martin, Schekleton, & Firlit, 1988; Mitchell & Jones, 1996; Soja et al., 1992; Spellbring, 1992; Wood & Cunningham, 1992). Common variables placed on a risk assessment tool are history of falls; age; medical condition; current medications; physical status (with attention to mobility, sensory deficits, and elimination pattern); mental status; ambulatory devices; and protective restraining devices. The first activity listed under Fall Prevention (see Table 37–1) recommends the identification of cognitive or physical deficits of patients that may increase potential for falling. The use of risk assessment instruments exemplifies implementation of this activity. Risk factors can be used to describe or predict individuals who are more likely to fall, thus cuing the nurse or caregiver to initiate intervention activities to reduce that risk.

Intervention Strategies

Deciding on the activities to administer to prevent falls can be challenging because the ample literature has no standardized strategy, but certain themes are beginning to emerge (Table 37–2). A frequently used approach in health care institutions is to educate nurses, multidisciplinary groups, and nonprofessional staff about the causes of patient falls, demonstrate safety precautions to take, provide a risk assessment tool, and, over a set interval, give periodic feedback on the fall and fall injury rates. In addition, colored bracelets or dots are used to identify the fall-prone patient, and, depending on the agency setting, a

Table 37–2 Common Components of a Fall Prevention Program

Component	Content
Education Sessions	Includes nursing department, multidisciplinary groups, and nonprofessional staff; causes of patient falls and safety precautions are presented.
Definition of a Fall	Describes what is included in the identification of a fall incident for that institution; a definition might include near falls.
Risk Assessment Tool	Usually designed for a specific patient population after a retrospective audit is completed; patients are assessed at admission and at every shift or when status changes occur.
Intervention Strategy	Suggests (in list form) Fall Prevention activities to choose and individualize; a standard care plan may be written; risk score may direct the activities to initiate.
Color Coding	Visually identifies at-risk patients for all persons serving them; yellow, red, green, or orange bracelets or dots for care plan, call system, and doorway are used.
Program Pamphlet	Presents the Fall Prevention program to patient and family and explains how they can participate; generic pamphlet for all staff may be created to announce the program.
Safety Equipment	Provides an automatic concurrent evaluation of protective equipment available on site.
Multidisciplinary Approach	Uses the experts to analyze the multifaceted aspects of a fall and to make recommendations.
Feedback	Reports of fall and fall injury rate are periodically posted and discussed.
Compliance Measurement	Completion of a modified risk management form may be used to evaluate the appropriateness of nursing care before the fall event.

combination of activities from the intervention Fall Prevention (see Table 37–1) will be part of a standard care plan or program guideline that can be individualized (Brady et al., 1993; Foster & Kohlenberg, 1996; Mitchell & Jones, 1996; Sweeting, 1994; Trummer et al., 1996; Wood & Cunningham, 1992).

Patients who have been identified as fall prone must have immediate intervention, and several authors have illustrated the successful components of their programs. A nursing quality assessment committee in a large medical center developed a Fall Prevention protocol that identified three levels of risk and the intervention activities to be taken at each level (Ruckstuhl et al., 1991). Level 1 is for all patients and includes intervention activities such as eliminating environmental hazards, orienting the patient to surroundings, keeping assistive devices within reach, and maintaining the bed in the lowest position. Level 2 includes both toddlers and adults and describes patients who understand their need for help but have poor balance or are taking medications affecting blood pressure, conciousness, or elimination. The activities for level 2 add instructing the patient to ask for assistance, keeping side rails up, and keeping items of use close to the patient. Level 3 includes infants as well as adults and represents patients at highest risk due to disorientation, behavioral changes, or sensory or balance problems. The activities at this level require increased patient observation and assistance, additional night lighting, reorientation, and, if necessary, restraints or patient sitters. Patients are reassessed with this tool at the beginning of each shift to accommodate any changes in condition. This Fall Prevention protocol heightened staff's awareness of factors associated with falls, and the number of falls and serious injuries was dramatically reduced.

A large rehabilitation center within a medical center designed a Fall Prevention program that was the result of a quality improvement activity on a geriatric unit (Brady et al., 1993). Two levels of safety were identified, and emphasis was placed on patient reassessment every eight hours, plus offering assistance with toileting, fluids, and nutrition and with any other request every four hours. An easy-to-read handout was developed to explain and reinforce the Fall Prevention program to patients and families. The safety levels indicated the planned interventions that should occur at each shift. This had implications for time management because it promoted scheduled interventions to alleviate the multiple patient calls for assistance in the midst of other important aspects of care. This program, which gave nurses a sense of increased control over both patient safety and time management, resulted in a decrease in patient falls of more than 80%.

Croft and Foraker (1992), at a community hospital, used a green-dot system for alerting staff to a patient's high-risk status, but it was not sufficient to reduce the number of falls. Falls were noted to increase after visiting hours, when side rails were left down and call bells were moved out of patient's reach. A pamphlet was created that instructed families about specific approaches to take for a safe bedside environment: patient's call bell is always within reach, side rails are up when the family leaves, light is on in the bathroom at all times, bed wheels are locked, slippers or nonskid socks are on patient when walking, and family stops at the nurses' station when a visit ends. Special attention was given to an explanation of why patients can become confused when admitted to a hospital. This consistently applied approach provided a considerable drop in fall rate.

Knowing elderly patients can fail to seek preventive help for falls, Tibbitts (1996) designed a one-page educational handout for office patients. The handout cites a fall statistic of people older than 65 and then lists common risk factors of the elderly, with brief statements about what to do if they have any of these factors. The closing section of the handout guides the family in what they can do to help, such as looking for environmental hazards in the home, noticing the patient's stability when walking, and responding to complaints of dizziness or weakness. The content is of the most salient type and is based on evidence that education and therapy aimed at modifying multiple risk factors have been shown to reduce falls in elderly outpatients by about 12% (Tinetti et al., 1994).

ASSOCIATED NURSING DIAGNOSES AND CLIENT GROUPS

Research demonstrates that fall risk can be modified and that falls should not be considered an inevitable happening. Although the nursing diagnosis Risk for Injury is appropriate for clients along the entire continuum of life, it is most applicable for fall-prone individuals, such as infants and toddlers, adults in health care institutions, and the elderly. It is well established that many falls occur during walking or when an activity requires a change in the body position (Wolter & Studenski, 1996). Balance control is based on the integration of our sensory input system, a central processing system, and an effector system that acts in response to the sensory input (Patla, Frank, & Winter, 1992); thus the nursing diagnoses Auditory Sensory/Perceptual Alterations, Visual Sensory/Perceptual Alterations, and Risk of Trauma can reflect issues of balance control and the need for protection through Fall Prevention. Another important linkage is with the nursing diagnosis Acute Confusion. When compared to young persons, adults are likely to have a greater incidence of mental status change as an intrinsic risk factor (Lach et al., 1991); therefore most adult fall risk assessment instruments include measurement of cognitive function.

Three other diagnoses—Chronic Confusion, Impaired Physical Mobility, and Bathing/Hygiene Self Care Deficit—consider Fall Prevention an optional intervention, with clinical decision making determining the appropriateness. It may seem unusual that the nursing diagnosis Impaired Physical Mobility does not regard Fall Prevention as a primary intervention; however, this diagnosis clearly directs first-choice interventions toward exercise therapy and positioning (McCloskey & Bulechek, 1996).

ASSOCIATED PATIENT OUTCOMES

Outcome statements serve nurses as a means for measuring the success of implementing selected nursing interventions. Using a fall incidence report as the only outcome measurement for Fall Prevention intervention could be misleading, because patients who become stronger and more active may take more risks to avoid deconditioning. This type of patient may fall but avoid injury and continue to be active; thus, the nurse would probably choose several outcomes sensitive to the Fall Prevention intervention. Patient outcomes most likely to be considered for adults and children are as follows (Johnson & Maas, 1997):

Caregiver Performance: Direct Care

Provision by family care provider of appropriate personal and health care for a family member or significant other

Caregiver Performance: Indirect Care

Arrangement and oversight of appropriate care for a family member or significant other by family care provider

Child Safety Knowledge

Extent of understanding conveyed about safely caring for a child

Knowledge: Personal Safety

Extent of understanding conveyed about preventing unintentional injuries

Risk Control

Actions to eliminate or reduce actual, personal, and modifiable health threats

Risk Detection

Actions taken to identify personal health threats

Safety Behavior: Fall Prevention

Individual or caregiver actions to minimize risk factors that might precipitate falls

Safety Behavior: Home Physical Environment

Individual or caregiver actions to minimize environmental factors that might cause physical harm or injury in the home

Safety Status: Falls Occurrence:

Number of falls in the past week

CASE STUDY

Mrs. B is a 68-year-old widow with a 10-year history of arthritis in both knees and a recent cataract in her left eye. For the last two years, she has been living in the home of her married daughter, and this has been of mutual benefit because Mrs. B enjoys helping the family with meal preparation and supervising the grandchildren. Early one morning, Mrs. B had sudden dizziness and weakness on her left side and complained of a headache. She was taken quickly to the community hospital, where she was diagnosed with a right-sided cerebrovascular accident (CVA). Basic support measures included frequent neurological checks, vital sign measurement, oxygen and drug therapy, intravenous fluids, and physical therapy. While in the hospital, she developed some muscle atrophy as a result of bed rest and the painful arthritis in her knees. She was placed on a nonsteroidal anti-inflammatory drug and was able to bear weight with a quad cane four days before discharge. During her acute CVA illness, she exhibited spatial perceptual deficits and denial of her left side and showed impulsive behavior with some lack of awareness of her deficits.

At admission, Mrs. B was assessed to be at high risk for falling, and her care plan, call system, and doorway were labeled with a yellow dot. During the third day of hospitalization, as the nurse was helping Mrs. B bathe, the nurse was interrupted by a brief telephone call. Before leaving the room, the nurse placed the bed in the lowest position and pulled up the upper side rails. When the nurse returned, Mrs. B's bed alarm was sounding, and Mrs. B was on the floor, sitting in urine. Although the only injury was a small elbow bruise, the nurse reviewed the care plan and wrote additional Fall Prevention activities under the nursing diagnosis Risk for Injury. The following actions were carried out:

1. Mrs. B was moved to a room closer to the nurses' station.
2. The bed was made more visible from the doorway and Mrs. B's right side faced toward the doorway.
3. A large paddle call light was installed on the right side of the bed.
4. Use of the call light was reviewed with Mrs. B on each shift.
5. Staff were requested to remind Mrs. B to ask or call for assistance.

6. A toileting schedule was posted, and the female urinal was kept in easy reach from the bed.
7. The physical exercise program was reassessed but could not be increased because of the pain of Mrs. B's arthritis.
8. A meeting was held with Mrs. B and her daughter regarding the possible need for a soft vest restraint.

On day 6 of hospitalization, Mrs. B began to ambulate with a quad cane. At this time, the physical therapy and nursing departments reassessed her environment and added an elevated toilet seat, a brightly colored call chain by the toilet, and a wedged seat cushion for her lounge chair. Night lights were kept on at all times, Mrs. B's shoes were brought in, and all wastebaskets were moved to the edge of the room. Mrs. B

continued to have impulsive behavior and, while in the bathroom, suffered a second fall resulting in a lacerated eyebrow. The daughter believed her mother would be better at home in familiar surroundings and requested no further rehabilitation. The nurse, physical therapist, and case manager met with Mrs. B's daughter to arrange for a home assessment and to continue teaching her about the environmental hazards unique to her mother's care.

Mrs. B's second fall was analyzed by a multidisciplinary team to determine whether appropriate care was in place before the fall event occurred. The Fall Prevention program had been carried out as planned, but considerable discussion focused on the safety of allowing a patient with a right-sided CVA to toilet without direct supervision; standing outside the bathroom door was the standard in place when Mrs. B fell.

CONCLUSION

Falling is one of the most serious and common problems faced by the elderly. Falls and fall-related injuries create additional health care costs by prolonging length of hospitalization, creating the need for additional diagnostic tests or surgeries, and placing the elderly at risk for disability and loss of function. Falls are also a frequent reason that health professionals are sued for medical negligence. Given the magnitude of problems associated with falls, Fall Prevention must become a priority for all clinicians, researchers, and health policymakers. As the number of elderly persons age 65 and older continues to grow (U.S. Department of Commerce, 1995), it will become even more critical to develop effective and feasible fall prevention strategies.

References

Benson, C., and Luscardi, P. (1995). Neurologic antecedents to patient falls. *Journal of Neuroscience Nursing, 27,* 331–337.

Berryman, E., Gaskin, D., Jones, A., Tolley, F., and MacMullen, J. (1989). Point by point: Predicting elders' fall. *Geriatric Nursing, 10,* 199–201.

Brady, R., Chester, E., Pierce, L., Salter, J., Schreck, S., and Radziewicz, R. (1993). Geriatric falls: Prevention strategies for the staff. *Journal of Gerontological Nursing, 19*(9), 26–32.

Buchner, D., Cress, M., Wagner, W., de Lateur, B., Price, P., and Abrass, I. (1993). The Seattle FICSIT/Move it study: The effect of exercise on gait and balance in old adults. *Journal of the American Geriatrics Society, 41,* 321–325.

Caley, L., and Pinchoff, D. (1994). A comparison study of patient falls in a psychiatric setting. *Hospital and Community Psychiatry, 45,* 823–825.

Cali, C., and Kiel, D. (1995). An epidemiologic study of falls-related fractures among institutionalized older people. *Journal of the American Geriatrics Society, 43,* 1336–1342.

Campbell, A., Borrie, M., and Spears, G. (1989). Risk factors for falls in a community-based prospective study of people 70 years and older. *Journal of Gerontology, 44,* 112–117.

Croft, W., and Foraker, S. (1992). Working together to prevent falls. *RN, 55*(11), 17–19.

Evans, L. K., and Strumpf, N. E. (1989). Tying down the elderly: A review of the literature on physical restraint. *Journal of the American Geriatrics Society, 2,* 65–74.

Fiatarone, M., O'Neill, E., Doyle, N., Clements, K., Roberts, S., Kehayias, J., Lipsitz, L., and Evans, W. (1993). The Boston FICSIT study: The effects of resistance training and nutritional supplementation on physical frailty in the oldest old. *Journal of the American Geriatrics Society, 41,* 333–337.

Fleming, B., and Pendergast, D. (1993). Physical conditions, activity pattern, and environment as factors in falls by adult care facilities. *Archives of Physical Medicine and Rehabilitation, 75,* 454–456.

Foreman, M. (1989). Confusion in the hospitalized elderly: Incidence, onset, and associated factors. *Research in Nursing and Health, 12,* 21–29.

Foster, K., and Kohlenberg, E. (1996). Patient falls in a tertiary rehabilitation setting. *Rehabilitation Nursing Research, 5*(1), 23–29.

Galindo-Ciocon, D., Ciocon, J., and Galindo, D. (1995). Gait training and falls in the elderly. *Journal of Gerontological Nursing, 21*(6), 11–17.

Garrettson, L., and Gallagher, S. (1985). Falls in children and youth. *Pediatric Clinics of North America, 32*, 153–162.

Gurwitz, J. H., Sanchez-Cross, M. T., Eckler, M. A., and Matulis, J. (1994). The epidemiology of adverse and unexpected events in the long-term care setting. *Journal of the American Geriatrics Society, 42*(11), 33–38.

Hale, W., Delaney, M., and McGaghie, W. (1992). Characteristics and predictors of falls in elderly patients. *Journal of Family Practice, 34*, 577–581.

Hendrich, A. (1988). An effective unit-based fall prevention plan. *Journal of Nursing Quality Assurance, 3*(1), 28–36.

Hendrich, A., Nyhuis, A., Kippenbrock, T., and Soja, M. E. (1995). Hospital falls: Development of a predictive model for clinical practice. *Applied Nursing Research, 8*(3), 129–139.

Hogue, C. (1982). Injury in later life. Part 2. Prevention. *Journal of the American Geriatrics Society, 30*, 276–278.

Hogue, C. (1992). Managing falls: The current basis for practice. In S. G. Funk, E. M. Tourquist, M. T. Champagne, and R. A. Weise (Eds.), *Key aspects of elder care—Managing falls, incontinence, and cognitive impairment* (pp. 41–55). New York: Springer Publishing.

Hornbrook, M. C., Wingfield, D., Stevens, V., Hollis, J., and Greenlick, M. (1991). Falls among older persons: Antecedents and consequences. In R. Weindruch, E. Hadley, and M. Ory (Eds.), *Reducing frailty and falls in older persons* (pp. 106–125). Springfield, IL: Charles C Thomas.

Hornbrook, M. C., Stevens, V. J., Wingfield, D. J. (1993). Seniors' program for injury control and education. *Journal of the American Geriatrics Society, 41*, 309–314.

Hornbrook. M. C., Stevens, V. J., Wingfield, D. J., Hollis, J., Greenlick, M., and Ory, M. (1994). Preventing falls among community-dwelling older persons: Results from a randomized trial. *Gerontologist, 34*, 16–23.

Howe, J. S. (1994). Preventing falls through environmental assessment. *Nursing Homes, 43*(5), 10–11, 16–19.

Janken, J., Reynolds, B., and Swiech, K. (1986). Patient falls in the acute care setting: Identifying risk factors. *Nursing Research, 35*, 215–219.

Johnson, M., and Maas, M. (1997). *Nursing outcomes classification (NOC)*. St. Louis: Mosby–Year Book.

Jones, W., and Smith, A. (1989). Preventing hospital incidents: What we can do. *Nursing Management, 20*(9), 58–60.

Kilpack, V., Boehm, J., Smith, N., and Mudge, B. (1991). Using research-based interventions to decrease patient falls. *Applied Nursing Research, 4*(2), 50–56.

Kippenbrock, T., and Soja, M. (1993). Preventing falls in the elderly: Interviewing patients who have fallen. *Geriatric Nursing, 14*, 205–209.

Lach, H., Reed, A., Arfken, C., Miller, J., Paige, G., Birge, S., and Peck, W. (1991). Falls in the elderly: Reliability of a classification system. *Journal of the American Geriatrics Society, 39*(2), 197–202.

Lambert, D., and Sattin, R. (1988). Death from falls, 1978–1984. *Morbidity and Mortality Weekly Report, 37*(1), 21–26.

Lauritzen, J., Petersen, M., and Lund, B. (1993). Effect of external hip protectors on hip fractures. *Lancet, 341*, 11–13.

Lawrence, J., and Maher, P. (1992). An interdisciplinary falls consult team: A collaborative approach to patient falls. *Journal of Nursing Care Quality, 6*(3), 21–29.

Llewellyn, J., Martin, B., Shekleton, M., and Firlit, S. (1988). Analysis of falls in the acute surgical and cardiovascular surgical patient. *Applied Nursing Research, 1*, 116–121.

Luukinen, H., Koski, K., Honkanen, R., and Kivela, S. (1995). Incidence of injury-causing falls among older adults by place of residence: A population-based study. *Journal of the American Geriatrics Society, 43*, 872–876.

Magaziner, J., Simonsick, E., Kashner, T., Hebel, J., and Kenzora, J. (1989). Survival experience of aged hip fracture patients. *American Journal of Public Health, 79*, 274–278.

Maki, B., Holliday, P. and Topper, A. (1991). Fear of falling and postural performance in the elderly. *Journal of Gerontology: Medicine and Science, 46*(4), M123–M131.

McCloskey, J. C., and Bulechek, G. M. (Eds.). (1996). *Nursing interventions classification (NIC)* (2nd ed., p. 272). St. Louis: Mosby-Year Book.

McCollam, M. (1995). Evaluation and implementation of a research-based falls assessment innovation. *Nursing Clinics of North America, 30*(3), 507–515.

Mitchell, A., and Jones, N. (1996). Striving to prevent falls in an acute care setting—Action to enhance quality. *Journal of Clinical Nursing, 5*, 213–220.

Morse, J., Morse, R., and Tylko, S. (1989). Development of a scale to identify the fall-prone patient. *Canadian Journal of Aging, 8*, 366–377.

Mosenthal, A., Livingston, D., Elcavage, J., Merritt, S., and Stucker, S. (1995). Falls: Epidemiology and strategies for prevention. *Journal of Trauma: Injury, Infection, and Critical Care, 38*, 753–756.

Mulrow, C., Gerety, M., Kanten, D., DeNino, L., and Cornell, J. (1993). Effects of physical therapy on functional status of nursing home residents. *Journal of the American Geriatrics Society, 41*, 326–328.

Myers, A. H., Baker, S. P., Van Natta, M. L., Abbey, H., and Robinson, E. (1991). Risk factors associated with falls and injuries among elderly institutionalized persons. *American Journal of Epidemiology, 133*, 1179–1190.

National Safety Council. (1995). *Accident facts*. Chicago: Author.

Nevitt, M. C., Cummings, S. R., and Hudes, E. S. (1991). Risk factors for injurious falls: A prospective study. *Journal of Gerontology, 46*, M164–M170.

Oreskovich, M., Howard, J., Copass, M., and Carrico, C. J. (1984). Geriatric trauma: Injury patterns and outcomes. *Trauma, 24*, 565–572.

Patla, A., Frank, J. S., and Winter, D. A. (1992). Balance control in the elderly: Implications for clinical assessment and rehabilitation. *Canadian Journal of Public Health, 83*, 529–533.

Province, M., Hadley, E., Hornbrook, M., Lipsitz, L., Miller, J., Mulrow, C., Ory, M., Sattin, R., Tinetti, M., and Wolf, S. (1995). The effects of exercise on falls in elderly patients. *Journal of the American Medical Association, 273*, 1341–1347.

Rapport, L. J., Webster, J. S., Flemming, K. L., Lindberg, J., Godlewski, M., Brees, J., and Abadee, P. (1993). Predictors of falls among right-hemisphere stroke patterns in the rehabilitation setting. *Archives of Physical Medicine and Rehabilitation, 74*, 621–626.

Raz, T., and Baretich, M. (1987). Factors affecting the incidence of patient falls in hospitals. *Medical Care, 25*(3), 185–195.

Reinsch, S., MacRae, P., Lachenbruch, P., and Tobis, J. (1992). Attempts to prevent falls and injury: A prospective community study. *Gerontologist, 32,* 450–456.

Rodriquez, J., Sattin, R., DeVito, C., Wingo, P., and the Study to Assess Falls Among the Elderly Group. (1991). Developing an environmental hazards assessment instrument for falls among the elderly. In R. Weindruch, E. Hadley and M. Ory (Eds.), *Reducing frailty in older persons* (pp. 263–276). Springfield, IL: Charles C Thomas.

Rubenstein, H., Miller, F., Postel, S., and Evans, H. B. (1983). Standards of medical care based on consensus rather than evidence: The case of routine bedrail use for the elderly. *Law, Medicine, and Health Care, 11,* 271–276.

Rubenstein, L., Robbins, A., Schulman, B., Rosado, J., Osterweil, D., and Josephson, K. (1988). Falls and instability in the elderly. *Journal of American Geriatrics Society, 36,* 278–288.

Rubenstein, L. Z., Robbins, A. S., Josephson, K. R., Schulman, B., and Osterweil, D. (1990). The value of assessing falls in an elderly population: A randomized clinical trial. *Annals of Internal Medicine, 113,* 308–316.

Ruckstuhl, M., Marchionda, E., Salmons, J., and Larrabee, J. H. (1991). Patient falls: An outcome indicator. *Journal of Nursing Care Quality, 6*(1), 25–29.

Runge, J. (1993). The cost of injury. *Emergency Medical Clinics of North America, 11,* 241–253.

Rymes, J., and Jaeger, R. (1988). Falls: Prevention and management in the institutional setting. *Clinics in Geriatric Medicine, 4,* 613–622.

Sattin, R. (1992). Falls among older people: A public health perspective. *Annual Review of Public Health, 13,* 489–508.

Shepherd, J., Lutz, L., Miller, R., and Main, D. S. (1992). Patients presenting to family physicians after a fall: A report from the ambulatory sentinel practice network. *Journal of Family Practice, 35*(1), 43–48.

Soja, M. E., Kippenbrock, T. A., Hendrich, A. L., and Nyhuis, A. (1992). A risk model for patient fall prevention. In S. G. Funk, E. M. Tornquist, M. T. Champagne, and R. A. Wiese (Eds.), *Key aspects of elder care—Managing falls, incontinence, and cognitive impairment* (pp. 65–70). New York: Springer Publishing.

Spellbring, A. (1992). Assessing elderly patients at high risk for falls. A reliability study. *Journal of Nursing Care Quality, 6*(3), 30–35.

Sweeting, H. (1994). Patient fall prevention—A structured approach. *Journal of Nursing Management, 2,* 187–192.

Tack, K., Ulrich, B., and Kehr, C. (1987). Patient falls: Profile for prevention. *Journal of Neuroscience Nursing, 19*(2), 83–89.

Tibbitts, G. (1996). Patients who fall: How to predict and prevent injuries. *Geriatrics, 51*(9), 24–31.

Tideiksaar, R. (1997). *Falling in old age—Prevention and management,* (2nd ed., pp. 6–7, 10, 29–51, 52–167). New York: Springer Publishing Company.

Tinetti, M., Baker, D., Garrett, P., Gottschalk, M., Koch, M., and Horwitz, R. (1993). Yale FICSIT: Risk factor abatement strategy for fall prevention. *Journal of the American Geriatrics Society, 41,* 315–320.

Tinetti, M. E., Baker, D., McAvay, G., Claus, E., Garrett, P., Gottschalk, M., Koch, M., Trainor, K., and Horwitz, R. (1994). A multifactorial intervention to reduce the risk of falling among elderly people living in the community. *New England Journal of Medicine, 331,* 821–827.

Tinetti, M., Lui, W., and Claus, E. (1993). Predictors and prognosis of inability to get up after falls among older persons. *Journal of the American Medical Association, 116,* 369–374.

Tinetti, M., Lui, W., and Ginter, S. (1992). Mechanical restraint use and fall-related injuries among residents of skilled nursing facilities. *Annals of Internal Medicine 116,* 369–374.

Tinetti, M., Rickman, D., and Powell, L. (1990). Falls efficacy as a measure of fear of falling. *Journal of Gerontology, 45,* 239–243.

Tinetti, M., and Speechley, M. Prevention of falls among the elderly. *New England Journal of Medicine, 320,* 1055–1059.

Tinetti, M. E., Speechley, M., and Ginter, S. F. (1988). Risk factors for falls among elderly persons living in the community. *New England Journal of Medicine, 319,* 1701–1707.

Trummer, K., Foster, B., Hartman, L., Lewis-Vais, C., and Sullivan, H. (1996). Protecting confused patients from falls. *American Journal of Nursing, 96*(7), 16R–16X.

U.S. Department of Commerce, Economics and Statistics Administration, Bureau of the Census. (1995). Statistical brief: Sixty-five plus in the United States. Washington, DC: Author.

Vellas, B., Garry, P., Wayne, S., Baumgartner, R., and Albarede, J. (1992). A comparative study of falls, gait and balance in elderly persons living in North America (Albuquerque, NM, USA) and Europe (Toulouse, France): Methodology and preliminary results. In B. Vellas, M. Toupet, L. Rubinstein, and Y. Christian (Eds.), *Falls, balance and gait disturbances in the elderly* (pp. 93–116). Paris: Elsevier.

Wagner, E. H., LaCroix, A. Z., Grothaus, L., LeVielle, S., Hecht, J., Artz, K., Odle, K., Bucher, D. (1994). Preventing disability and falls in older adults: A population-based randomized trial. *American Journal of Public Health, 84,* 1800–1806.

Wallace, R., Ross, J., Huston, J., Kundel, C., and Woodworth, G. (1993). Iowa FICSIT trial: The feasibility of elderly wearing a hip joint protective garment to reduce hip fractures. *Journal of the American Geriatrics Society, 41,* 338–340.

Watson, M., and Mayhew, P. (1994). Identifying fall risk factors in preparation for reducing the use of restraints. *Medical Surgical Nurse, 3*(1), 25–35.

Whedon, M., and Shedd, P. (1989). Prediction and prevention of patient falls. *Image, 21*(2), 106–114.

Wolf, S., Kutner, M., Green, R., and McNeely, E. (1993). The Atlanta FICSIT study with two exercise interventions to reduce frailty in elders. *Journal of the American Geriatrics Society, 41,* 329–332.

Wolter, L., and Studenski, S. (1996). A clinical synthesis of falls intervention trials. *Topics in Geriatric Nursing, 11*(3), 9–12.

Wood, L., and Cunningham, G. (1992). Fall risk protocol and nursing care plan. *Geriatric Nursing, 13,* 205–206.

Woolley, S., Czaja, S., and Drury, C. (1997). An assessment of falls in elderly men and women. *Journal of Gerontology: Medicine and Science, 52A*(2), M80–M87.

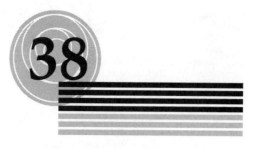

Latex Precautions

Victoria M. Steelman

Numerous case reports have been reviewed describing adverse reactions to products containing natural rubber latex (hereafter referred to as *latex*) (Steelman, 1995). These reactions range in severity and include contact dermatitis, urticaria, edema, rhinoconjunctivitis, wheezing, bronchospasm, and death. The increased numbers of these reports are associated with the increased use of latex examination gloves in health care. In 1987, with the implementation of universal precautions, health care workers began routinely wearing latex gloves when contacting blood and body fluids. Consequently, these frequent exposures have led to sensitization and reactions in patients with chronic health conditions and in health care workers. The sensitization rates have increased dramatically, creating a challenge to nurses in hospitals, clinics, long-term care facilities, and the community.

Providing safe care for sensitized patients is problematic for a number of reasons. First, health care providers often do not know what a latex allergy is, which patients have the allergy, and what modifications in care should be made. The preponderance of latex in the environment and the difficulty in identifying it compound this problem. Furthermore, exposures to the allergen are not always predictable. Patients encounter different health care providers, ancillary staff, visitors, and other patients. Any of these individuals could cause an inadvertent exposure to latex. A patient may be treated in different areas of a facility (e.g., operating room, radiology department, inpatient unit) or may transfer between agencies. With each change, plans of care need to be modified before the patient arrives. Poor communication creates confusion. Lastly, sensitized patients need comprehensive education to prevent life-threatening reactions. Unfortunately, nurses are often ill prepared to provide the needed information.

REVIEW OF THE LITERATURE

A review of the literature provides valuable insight into latex, types of reactions, routes of exposure, allergenicity of products, groups at increased risk, and changes that have been recommended for clinical practice. This knowledge provides a foundation for a nursing intervention outlining care of patients at high risk for a latex allergy.

Natural Rubber Latex

Natural rubber latex is the milky, white sap of the *Hevea brasiliensis* plant, more commonly known as the rubber tree. During the manufacturing process, a variety of chemicals (e.g., stabilizers, accelerators, vulcanizers) are compounded with the latex to give the product specific physical properties (Subramaniam, 1995; Truscott, 1995). Either plant proteins in the latex or chemical additives can trigger reactions to products containing latex. However, the reactions that occur are quite different.

Types of Reactions

Hypersensitivity to latex products manifests clinically as either a type IV (delayed hypersensitivity) or a type I (immediate hypersensitivity) reaction (Table 38–1). Type IV reactions are by far the more common (84%) (Heese, von Hintzenstern, Peters, Koch, & Hornstein, 1991; von Hintzenstern, Koch, Peters, & Hornstein, 1991). Multiple exposures over weeks and months lead to sensitization (Ownby, 1995). Re-exposure of the skin triggers sensitized T lymphocytes to stimulate proliferation of other lymphocytes and mononuclear cells, resulting in tissue inflammation and allergic contact dermatitis. Therefore, symptoms are always localized to the area of skin contacting the latex product (Hamann, 1993; Kelly, Kurup, Reijula, & Fink, 1994; Ownby, 1995). Symptoms appear after 6 to 48 hours of contact and include erythema, itching, and vesicles; symptoms may

Table 38–1 Reactions to Natural Rubber Latex Products

	Delayed Hypersensitivity (Type IV)	Immediate Hypersensitivity (Type I)
PHYSIOLOGICAL MECHANISM	T lymphocyte	Immunoglobulin E
RESPONSE	Localized	Generalized
ONSET OF SYMPTOMS	6–48 hr	<30 min
SYMPTOMS	Erythema, itching, vesicles, fissures, eczema	Urticaria, edema, rhinoconjunctivitis, wheezing, respiratory distress, cardiovascular collapse
USUAL EXPOSURE	Long-term skin contact (e.g., wearing gloves, rubber boots, or elastic clothing)	Skin and mucous membrane contacts, invasive procedures, parenteral administration, inhaled (e.g., on glove powder)
TRIGGERING AGENT	Chemical accelerators used in manufacturing process	Natural rubber latex plant proteins
SERIOUSNESS	Discomfort	Can be life-threatening

progress to fissures and eczema (Ownby, 1995). Because these symptoms are associated with prolonged contact, the exposure usually results from wearing a latex product (e.g., gloves, condom catheter). Type IV reactions are triggered by chemical accelerators used in the manufacturing process, primarily thiurams (Conde-Salazar, del-Rio, Guimaraens, & Gonzalez, 1993; Heese et al., 1991; von Hintzenstern et al., 1991).

Immediate hypersensitivity (type I) reactions are far less common. In sensitized individuals, an antilatex IgE antibody stimulates mast cell proliferation and basophil histamine release, leading to anaphylaxis (Alenius, Turjanmaa, Makinen-Kiljunen, Reunala, & Palosuo, 1994; Alenius et al., 1995; Kelly et al., 1994). Therefore, symptoms may be generalized and distant to the area contacting latex. These hypersensitivity reactions are immediate, taking only minutes to manifest. Symptoms are more severe, ranging from urticaria or rhinoconjunctivitis to wheezing and bronchospasm (Alenius et al., 1994; Ownby, 1995). This type of a reaction may result from transient exposure to a latex product (e.g., examination with gloves, blood pressure cuff, or balloon). Unlike the less serious type IV reaction, type I reactions are triggered by the latex proteins themselves and constitute a *latex allergy* (Alenius et al., 1995; Kurup, Murali, & Kelly, 1995; Ownby, 1995). Because these reactions are systemic, individuals developing this allergy, regardless of past symptoms, are at risk for life-threatening anaphylaxis.

Exposures

Five routes of exposure to latex proteins have resulted in serious, type I reactions: (1) cutaneous, (2) mucous membrane, (3) inhalation, (4) internal tissue, and (5) parenteral (Steelman, 1995). Although most cutaneous exposures have been to surgical and examination gloves, other health care products (e.g., anesthesia masks, tourniquets, blood pressure cuffs) and nonmedical products (e.g., balloons, koosh balls, sporting goods) have also triggered reactions (Dillard & MacCollum, 1992; Steelman, 1995). More severe reactions have occurred when the skin was moist from handwashing or perspiration and readily absorbed the water-soluble proteins.

Many systemic reactions have resulted from latex proteins contacting mucous membranes (Steelman, 1995). These exposures have occurred in dentistry (e.g., gloves, dams, prophylaxis cups), in health care (e.g., gloves, catheters), and at home (e.g., balloons, koosh balls, enema kits, gloves, contraceptives) (Hamann, 1993; Steelman, 1995). The most severe reactions, including 16 reported deaths, have resulted from latex contacting rectal mucosa during enema administration (Dillard & MacCollum, 1992).

Systemic reactions also occur when the proteins are inhaled. This type of exposure usually occurs when latex proteins, bound to glove powder, are aerosolized (Tarlo, Sussman, Contala, & Swanson, 1994; Vandenplas, Delwiche, Evrard et al., 1995). This results in exposure to the conjunctival, nasal, and respiratory tract mucosa, as well as cutaneous contact when powder settles (Alenius et al., 1994; Beezhold, Kostyal, & Wiseman, 1994).

Internal tissues readily absorb latex proteins during surgery and other invasive procedures. Although reports of intraoperative anaphylaxis associate these reactions with surgical gloves, many other latex products are used during surgery (e.g., syringes, instruments, catheters) (Steelman, 1995).

Intravascular administration of very small amounts of latex proteins can be life-threatening. Disposable syringes, medication vial stoppers, and intravenous tubing have all triggered serious reactions (Dillard & MacCollum, 1992; Kwitten, Sweinberg, Campbell, & Pawlowski, 1995; Setlock, Cotter, & Rosner, 1993; Yassin et al., 1992). Disposable syringes have been shown to leech latex proteins into contrast dye, causing anaphylactic reactions in a series of patients (Hamilton, 1984). In another study, saline stored in syringes triggered reactions in some sensitized subjects (Melton, 1992).

Allergenicity of Products

Systemic reactions are triggered when water-soluble proteins on the surface of latex products are absorbed by sensitized individuals. The amount of extractable latex proteins on products varies greatly, with the largest amount found on gloves and balloons (Yunginger et al., 1994). Using a inhibition immunoassay, a greater than 3,000-fold variability in allergenicity was found among different brands of gloves (Yunginger et al., 1994). The highest amounts were found on powdered examination gloves (<5–16,300 AU [allergenic units]/mL), followed by powdered surgical gloves (<5–12,100 AU/mL). Significantly lower levels were found on powderless examination gloves (<5–151 AU/mL) and powderless surgical gloves (<5–61 AU/mL). Of all other products tested, balloons were found to contain the highest amount of extractable latex proteins (4,700 AU/mL). Condoms and anesthesia bags contained 50 AU/mL, and intravenous tubing, nasopharyngeal airways, and nipples contained less than 5 AU/mL (Yunginger et al., 1994).

The Role of Glove Powder

Research has demonstrated that glove powder binds to latex proteins (Beezhold & Beck, 1992). The bound proteins are then aerosolized when gloves are dispensed from the box, donned, or removed from hands (Beezhold et al., 1994). As much as 974 ng of latex per cubic meter of air was found in the breathing zone of the anesthetist in an operating room, a greater amount than is found on most medical products (Swanson et al., 1994). Very high levels of latex (300–2,536 ng/m^3) in the air have also been found in clinics, inpatient units, and intensive care units where powdered exam gloves are being used (Steelman, 1997a). This demonstrates the magnitude of an exposure from even using powdered latex gloves in the same room as a sensitized individual. A study showed that use of powdered gloves is a major contributor to the amount of latex in the air (Heilman, Jones, Swanson, & Yunginger, 1996). As little as 0.6 ng of latex in the air triggers respiratory symptoms in sensitized individuals and has led to occupational asthma in health care workers (Baur, Chen, & Allmers, 1998; Brugnami, Marabini, Siracusa, & Abbritti, 1995; Vandenplas, Delwiche, Evrard et al., 1995). This health condition is chronic and does not resolve if the individual leaves the setting. However, symptoms can be minimized. Conversion to powder-free examination gloves has resulted in a reduction in levels of latex in the air (39–311 ng/m^3 to <0.02 ng/m^3) (Tarlo et al., 1994). A study of health care workers with latex-induced asthma found that using gloves with lower protein concentrations reduced the risk of exhibiting asthmatic reactions (Vandenplas, Delwiche, Depelchin et al., 1995). The appropriateness of using vinyl goves for standard (universal) precautions has also been studied. Vinyl goves have much higher failure rates in use (43% to 85%) than do latex examination gloves (4% to 18.4%) (Korniwiecz et al., 1990; Korniwiecz et al., 1993; Korniwiecz et al., 1994; Olsen et al., 1993). Because of this high failure rate, the hands of health care workers are more likely to become contaminated with pathogens when wearing vinyl gloves than when wearing latex gloves.

Prevalence and High-Risk Groups

In 1987, a Finnish study found 0.8% of the general population to be allergic to latex (Turjanmaa, 1987). Studies since then have evaluated the prevalence of latex allergies in individuals with frequent exposures, particularly in patients with congenital anomalies and in individuals who are occupationally exposed. Up to 72% of patients with spina bifida are allergic to latex (Ellsworth, Merguerian, Klein, & Rozycki, 1993; Konz et al., 1995; Pearson, Cole, & Jarvis, 1994; Porri et al., 1997; Tosi, Slater, Shaer, & Mostello, 1993; Yassin et al., 1992). Numerous case reports indicate that patients with exstrophy of the bladder are also at high risk for a latex allergy (Steelman, 1995). This group has multiple surgeries, frequent catheterizations, and other exposures similar to those of patients with neural tube defects. A study of pediatric subjects compared (1) subjects with neural tube defects, (2) subjects with other conditions also requiring multiple surgeries during the first years of life, and (3) a control group (Porri et al., 1997). Fifty-nine percent of the spina bifida patients, 55% of the multiple-surgery group, and none of the control group were allergic to latex. Therefore, the condition of spina bifida itself is not a predisposing factor. Rather, the risk factor is frequent exposures to latex during the first years of life.

Individuals with frequent occupational exposure to latex (e.g., health care workers) are also at increased risk of sensitization. In 1987, in Finland, 4.5% of hospital workers tested positive to a glove-use test for latex allergy (Turjanmaa, 1987). In Europe, the highest prevalence has been found among surgeons (7.4% to 9.9%) and operating room nurses (5.6% to 10.7%) (Arellano, Bradley, & Sussman, 1992; Lagier, Vervloet, Lhermet, Poyen, & Charpin, 1992; Turjanmaa, 1987). Prevalence in American health care workers has been reported to range from 5% to 17% (Kaczmarek et al., 1996; Kibby & Akl, 1997; Konrad, Fieber, Gerber, Schuepfer, & Muellner, 1997; Yassin et al., 1994). The severity of symptoms from latex contact appears to be worsening in health care workers, in response to continued frequent exposures. In 1988, 98% of sensitized subjects reported only cutaneous symptoms (Turjanmaa, Laurila, Makinen-Kiljunen, & Reunala, 1988). More recent studies have found asthma and severe anaphylactic reactions to be associated with latex exposure (Turjanmaa, Makinen-Kiljunen, Reunala, Alenius, & Palosuo, 1995; Yassin et al., 1994).

Individuals allergic to latex are more likely to have other allergies. Up to 80% are atopic, as opposed to 20% of the general population (Bubak et al., 1992; Wrangsjo, Osterman, & van Hage-Hamsten, 1994). Latex-allergic individuals frequently report allergies to foods (fruits, vegetables, nuts); this is at least partially explained by a cross-reactivity between these plant proteins (Ahlroth et al., 1995; Blanco et al., 1994; Lavaud et al., 1995). Yet it is unclear if these other food allergies predispose individuals to latex allergy, or if the food allergies develop after sensitization to latex. Up to 60% of latex-allergic persons have a history of hand eczema, but a recent study found that eczema was not a risk factor for development of an allergy to latex in health care workers (Charous, Hamilton, & Yunginger, 1994; Yassin et al., 1994). Indeed, sensitization may be the result of respiratory, rather than cutaneous, exposures in some individuals.

Recommendations

Climbing sensitization rates are the result of frequent exposures to products containing high levels of extractable latex proteins. It is clear from the research that powdered, high-allergen gloves are unsafe for patients and health care workers. Yet, to date, these gloves remain in use in many health care settings. Primary prevention of sensitization and prevention of reactions to aerosolized latex require elimination of these products from all health care settings (Steelman, 1996, 1997). The American Academy of Allergy, Asthma and Immunology (AAAI), the American College of Allergy and Immunology (ACAI), and the National Institute for Occupational Safety and Health (NIOSH) (1997) endorse this recommendation (Latex Hypersensitivity Committee, 1995; Task Force on Allergic Reactions to Latex, 1993). Because of the high allergen content in balloons, which can also trigger respiratory exposures in sensitized patients and health care workers, no rubber balloons should be used in health care facilities. Because in-use failure rates of vinyl gloves are very high, the gloves routinely used for standard precautions should be low-allergen, powder-free latex gloves.

Because of the high rates of latex allergies among patients with spina bifida, and their frequent anaphylaxis to latex, the AAAI, the ACAI, and Steelman (1995) recommend latex avoidance for patients with neural defects undergoing procedures (Latex Hypersensitivity Committee, 1995; Task Force on Allergic Reactions to Latex, 1993). Because patients with exstrophy of the bladder are also at high risk, the AAAI and Steelman (1995) recommend that these patients be treated with latex avoidance as well (Task Force on Allergic Reactions to Latex, 1993). Because most patients have not been tested for an allergy to latex, the AAAI and Steelman (1995) also recommend that any patient with a history consistent with a latex allergy be treated with latex avoidance (Task Force on Allergic Reactions to Latex, 1993). Because exposures to latex occur throughout health care settings and the community, latex avoidance should be used wherever care is being provided.

A NURSING INTERVENTION

Specific protocols for operating rooms and gerontological nursing departments and recommendations for nurse anesthetists have been published elsewhere (Steelman, 1995, 1996, 1997b). A more generalizable, research-based intervention, which can be used in any setting, is included in the Nursing Interventions Classification (NIC) (McCloskey & Bulechek, 1996) (Table 38–2). The purpose of the intervention Latex Precautions is twofold: primary prevention of sensitization of high-risk patients and prevention of reactions in sensitized individuals. This nursing treatment includes screening of patients, communication, latex avoidance, monitoring, and patient education. *The effectiveness of this intervention relies on the total absence of powdered latex gloves in the setting.*

Patient Screening

It is essential to screen all patients for high risk for an allergy to latex. This step is taken to identify patients who should be treated with latex avoidance. High-risk patients include (1) any patient with a neural tube defect (e.g., spina bifida) or exstrophy of the bladder, (2) any patient with a positive latex allergy test, and (3) any patient with a history of systemic symptoms from latex contact (Steelman, 1995).

The nurse should review the patient's medical history to identify whether the patient has had a neural tube defect or exstrophy of the bladder. This activity can be undertaken by either interviewing the patient or reviewing the medical record. Identified patients should be treated with latex avoidance, regardless of their allergy status.

Table 38–2 Latex Precautions

DEFINITION: Reducing the risk of a systemic reaction to latex.

ACTIVITIES:
Question patient or appropriate other about history of neural tube defect (e.g., spina bifida) or congenital urological condition (e.g., exstrophy of the bladder)
Question patient or appropriate other about history of systemic reactions to natural rubber latex (e.g., facial or scleral edema, tearing eyes, urticaria, rhinitis, and wheezing)
Refer patient to allergist for allergy testing, as appropriate
Record allergy or risk in patient's medical record
Place allergy band on patient
Post sign indicating latex precautions
Survey environment and remove latex products
Monitor latex-free environment
Monitor patient for signs and symptoms of a systemic reaction
Report information to physician, pharmacist, and other care providers, as indicated
Administer medications, as appropriate
Instruct patient and family about risk factors for developing a latex allergy
Instruct patient and family about potential for reaction
Instruct patient and family about latex content in products and substitution with nonlatex products, as appropriate; wearing a medical alert tag; and notifying care providers
Instruct patient and family about signs of a reaction
Instruct patient and family about emergency treatment
Instruct patient and family about administration of epinephrine, as appropriate
Instruct visitors about latex-free environment

Source: McCloskey, J. C., and Bulechek, G. M. (1996). *Nursing interventions classification (NIC)* (2nd ed.). St. Louis: Mosby–Year Book.

If the patient's history is negative, the nurse should continue screening to determine whether the patient has a history of systemic reactions to latex. Many sensitized individuals are unaware of the cause of symptoms or consider them minor and unimportant. When asked about allergies, the patient may report only allergies to medications. Therefore, it is important to ask specific questions about contacts with latex to elicit this information. Because many patients do not know that latex, in this context, means natural rubber, the words *latex* and *rubber* should both be used. Because the research has shown that gloves and balloons have the highest allergen content, these examples are the best. A simple question such as "Have you ever had any problems with or reactions to latex or rubber, such as balloons and gloves?" solicits valuable information. If the answer is "no," it is unlikely that the patient has an allergy to latex, and no latex avoidance is necessary. If the answer is "yes," further questioning is done to determine whether the patient is reporting a type I reaction or a type IV reaction. A list of systemic symptoms indicative a type I reaction is helpful for this purpose (Table 38–3). If the patient denies any systemic symptoms, standard care is provided. However, if the patient reports systemic symptoms, latex avoidance should be used.

Referral to an allergist for testing is sometimes necessary to weigh the costs and benefits of a specific treatment. Even if postponed until a later date, this referral provides valuable information for the patient and for health care providers planning future care. The nurse should facilitate this referral.

Communication

The need for latex avoidance should be communicated to other health care providers. The patient's medical record should be flagged to indicate this re-

Table 38–3 Signs and Symptoms of a Systemic Reaction to Natural Rubber Latex

Skin: Hives

Face: Erythema, edema, itching

Eyes: Erythema around eyes; tearing; edema of eyelids, sclera

Nose: Erythema, itching, rhinorrhea, congestion

Mouth, throat: Edema of the lips, tongue, and throat; perioral itching

Chest: Tightness of chest, shortness of breath, wheezing, bronchospasm

Cardiovascular system: Hypotension, shock, cardiovascular collapse, cardiac arrest

Other: Abdominal pain, nausea, vomiting, diarrhea

quirement. This can be done by use of a traditional allergy label stating "latex precautions" on the front of the chart or by a computerized flag. The intervention should be recorded in the plan of care and medication order form. It is important to notify all persons who might inadvertently expose the patient to latex. A sign should be placed on the door to the patient's room and on the patient's transport cart or wheelchair. Placing a sign over the patient's bed is insufficient, because latex products might continue to be used in close proximity. An allergy or "latex precautions" band is also a helpful reminder. If the patient will be treated in another area, notification should be made well in advance, preferably at least 1 day earlier, to allow time for preparation before patient arrival. The pharmacist should also be notified in advance to ensure the availability of latex-free medications.

Latex Avoidance

Latex avoidance should not be implemented indiscriminately, for several reasons. First, a great deal of extra work may be required in procedural areas (e.g., operating room) to verify that supplies are latex free. Second, medications need to be latex free, and substitutions may be suboptimal (e.g., patient-controlled analgesia may not be an option). Lastly, indiscriminate use diminishes compliance with latex avoidance.

The environment should be surveyed to identify and remove products containing latex. Ideally, this should be done before patient arrival and regularly thereafter (e.g., once per shift). Although it is impossible to remove all latex from the environment (e.g., wheels on bed), it is important to remove the items that may pose a risk to the patient. This includes items that come in contact with the patient or those that may release latex proteins into the air (Table 38–4). Special attention should be placed on bandages, catheters, clothing that stretches, medications and medication administration supplies, and respiratory therapy equipment. The content of these products varies among manufacturers. Therefore, the development of an institution-specific list of latex products and alternatives is valuable. A basket of latex-free supplies is also helpful. Whenever additional supplies are going to be used, it is important to verify that they are also latex free.

Monitoring the Patient

The patient should be routinely monitored for symptoms of a systemic reaction. The level of monitoring depends on the patient's treatment and condition. For

Table 38–4 Medical Products Containing Natural Rubber Latex*

Bandages/tape: Ace wrap, Band-Aids, Coban, Eshmarch, cloth adhesive tape, waterproof tape

Bedding: Rubber sheets, reusable underpads

Blood pressure cuffs: Bladder and tubing

Catheters/tubes: Nasogastric, nephrostomy, rectal, red rubber

Clothing: Antiembolism stockings, support garments, elastic

Gloves: Chemotherapy, examination, surgical, utility†

Medications/intravenous: Buretrols, intravenous tubing, medication vial stoppers

Respiratory therapy: Ambu bags, anesthesia bags, nasopharyngeal airways

Stethoscopes

Tourniquets

*Products by some manufacturers contain natural rubber latex. This list is not all inclusive and is subject to change.
†The term *hypoallergenic* does not mean *latex-free*.

minor symptoms, the physician should be notified and medication administered as per order (e.g., antihistamine). The environment should be surveyed to locate the cause of the reaction, and the item should be removed. If the reaction is severe, the nurse should administer emergency medications as per institutional protocol (e.g., epinephrine). Care must be taken to avoid exposures to latex when managing this emergency.

Patient Education

Education of the patient and family is a critical, often overlooked, component of Latex Precautions. Unlike instructions regarding medication allergies, patients sensitized to latex need to understand much more than to avoid the allergen (Table 38–5). The family or caregiver plays a key role in prevention of exposures and should participate in this interaction. First, patients need to understand that latex, in this context, means natural rubber latex. An explanation of how this differs from synthetic rubber and latex paint (which does not contain latex) should be made clear. Second, patients need to understand what an allergy is and what range of symptoms could occur. Routes of exposure should be reviewed, along with how to avoid products that contain latex. The latter should be patient specific, focusing on the lifestyle of the individual. For example, a young mother needs to know more about infant and toddler supplies and toys. Someone athletically inclined may need to know more about sporting goods and exercise equipment. Most teenagers and adults need information about alternatives for protected sexual intercourse.

Patients need to be given recommendations on how to communicate the allergy, including the importance of a medical alert tag and how to obtain one.

Table 38–5 Key Elements of Patient Education

Natural rubber latex	Communication
Latex allergy	Signs and symptoms of a reaction
Routes of exposure	Emergency treatment of a reaction
Latex avoidance	

They also need to be instructed about the importance of notifying a number of key individuals, such as teachers, babysitters, dentists, and other health care providers. Recommending that the patient or care provider notify these individuals in advance of the need for care may eliminate unnecessary confusion and inadvertent exposures.

The patient needs to be instructed about signs and symptoms indicating a need for treatment and the importance of using prescribed medications when symptoms appear. For example, an antihistamine may resolve less serious symptoms. A bronchodilator may be prescribed for asthmatic reactions. Many sensitized patients have received a prescription for an epinephrine pen. The nurse should emphasize the importance of carrying the pen at all times and explain when to use it and how to administer the medication. All patients and care providers need to know how to activate the emergency medical system. All visitors need to know the importance of latex avoidance. A sign asking visitors to stop at the nurses' station before entering the patient's room prevents delivery of balloons or other avoidable exposures.

RELATED NURSING DIAGNOSES

The intervention Latex Precautions may be used to treat two existing nursing diagnoses approved through the North American Nursing Diagnosis Association (NANDA) (1992). One diagnosis, which addresses the overall patient need, is Risk for Injury. The definition of this diagnosis is, "A state in which an individual is at risk of injury as a result of environmental conditions interacting with the individual's adaptive and defensive resources." Sensitized individuals have a maladaptive physiological response to an environmental condition—the presence of a latex protein. This diagnosis addresses the potential for a range of reactions, from urticaria, rhinoconjunctivitis, and scleral edema to life-threatening airway compromise.

Patients often lack the knowledge needed to prevent exposures and treat reactions. In these cases, Knowledge Deficit related to latex allergy is an appropriate nursing diagnosis. This diagnosis is treated with the seven teaching activities within the intervention Latex Precautions including those related to (1) risk factors; (2) potential for reaction; (3) latex content and substitution; (4) wearing a medical alert tag and notifying care providers; (5) signs of a reaction, (6) emergency treatment; and (7) administration of epinephrine.

RELATED NURSING-SENSITIVE OUTCOMES

The Nursing Outcomes Classification (NOC) (Johnson & Maas, 1997) contains a number of patient outcomes that may be used to evaluate the effectiveness of Latex Precautions. The overall effectiveness of the intervention may be determined by the outcome Immune Hypersensitivity Control. This outcome is defined as the "extent to which inappropriate immune responses are suppressed." Long-term effectiveness of the intervention may also be determined by the outcome Quality of Life, defined as "an individual's expressed satisfaction with current life circumstances." Respiratory Status: Ventilation is an alternate outcome, defined as "movement of air in and out of the lungs." This outcome may be valuable for evaluating the management of a patient with latex-induced asthma.

Five different outcomes may be used to describe the effect of patient teaching activities within Latex Precautions. Knowledge: Disease Process is defined as the "extent of understanding and skills conveyed about a specific disease process." This outcome evaluates two activities: (1) "Instruct patient and family about risk factors for developing a latex allergy" and (2) "Instruct patient and family about potential for a reaction." Knowledge: Health Behaviors is defined as the "extent of understanding conveyed about the promotion and protection of health." This outcome measures the effectiveness of the activity, "Instruct patient and family about latex content in products and substitutions with nonlatex products, as appropriate; wearing a medical alert tag; and notifying care providers." An alternate outcome for this purpose is Knowledge: Treatment Procedure(s), defined as the "extent of understanding conveyed about procedure(s) required as part of a treatment regimen." The outcome Knowledge: Health Resources is defined as the "extent of understanding conveyed about healthcare resources." This outcome evaluates the effectiveness of the activity, "Instruct patient and family about emergency treatment." The activity, "Instruct patient and family about administration of epinephrine, as appropriate" may be measured by the outcome Knowledge: Medication. This outcome is defined as the "extent of understanding conveyed about the safe use of medication."

CASE STUDY

Ms. H is a 34-year-old woman being seen for preoperative screening in an ambulatory surgery center. A laparoscopy and tubal ligation are planned for the following day. Ms. H has worked as a nursing assistant in a long-term care facility for the past 15 years. She has had two previous surgeries, a dilatation and curettage and an adenotonsillectomy. She has no history of congenital anomaly. Nurse Akre questions her about allergies, and Ms. H reports that she is allergic to penicillin, chestnuts, and tape. Nurse Akre asks whether she has any other allergies, to which Ms. H responds, "Just hay fever." Nurse Akre asks, "Have you ever had any problems or reactions to latex or rubber, such as balloons or gloves?" Ms. H pauses and then says, "Yes. I can't wear the gloves at work." When questioned further, she reports a history of hives on her arms and swelling of her eyes when she wears the gloves.

Based on this information, Nurse Akre determines that Ms. H it at high risk for a latex allergy and records the nursing diagnosis Risk for Injury in the nurses' notes. She continues implementation of the intervention Latex Precautions. She places a "latex precautions" sign on the door and surveys the room for latex products. She removes a box of examination gloves and obtains a cart of latex-free supplies. She continues questioning Ms. H, who reports two episodes of scleral edema and wheezing after contact with bal-

loons and wheezing and hives during a dental examination. Nurse Akre writes "latex precautions" on the front of the medical record and on the documentation form. She directs the unit clerk to contact Dr. Smith. After conferring with Dr. Smith, the decision is made to proceed with surgery using latex avoidance. Nurse Akre directs the clerk to notify the operating room charge nurse, the anesthesiologist, the postanesthesia nurse, the radiology department, and the pharmacy. Nurse Akre instructs Ms. H about risk factors for a latex allergy and explains the use of latex avoidance. Phlebotomy is performed using nitrile examination gloves and a nonlatex tourniquet. Gauze and silk tape are used instead of a Band-Aid. A preoperative chest X-ray film is taken using latex avoidance. Nurse Akre monitors the patient for signs and symptoms of a reaction. None occur. The operating room nurse reviews the surgical supplies needed for completion of the intended surgery and orders latex-free alternatives (e.g., gloves, drapes, dressing, tape, syringes, intravenous tubing, medications).

The morning of surgery, Nurse Akre prepares Ms. H with latex avoidance. She places a "latex precautions" bracelet on Ms. H's wrist and applies nonlatex antiembolism stockings. The intravenous line is inserted using nitrile gloves and nonlatex tubing and is secured with silk tape. The operating room nurse surveys the operating room and verifies that the products used are latex free. She places a "latex precautions" sign on the door and on the postoperative transport cart. Ms. H is transferred to the operating room, where she is continuously monitored for a reaction to latex. While surgery is under way, the postanesthesia care nurse surveys the environment and replaces latex supplies with latex-free alternatives (e.g., blood pressure cuff, stethoscope, oximeter probe). She assists the nurse in the second-stage recovery area to prepare that area as well.

Surgery proceeds as planned, and Ms. H is subsequently transferred to the postanesthesia care unit. Her plan of care is implemented in that area as well as in the second-stage recovery area. She is continuously monitored for signs of a reaction to latex. None occur. Before discharge, the second-stage recovery nurse discusses a possible referral to an allergist with Dr. Smith, who concurs that this is advisable. The referral is discussed with Ms. H, and an appointment is made for her. The nurse evaluates the outcome of the intervention, determines that no hypersensitivity reaction has occurred during this hospitalization, and records this information under Immune Hypersensitivity Control. Ms. H is discharged.

One week later, Ms. H is seen in the allergy clinic. Nurse Zelensky implements Latex Precautions. The allergist administers a skin prick test and diagnoses an allergy to natural rubber latex. Nurse Zelensky records the nursing diagnosis Knowledge Deficit related to latex allergy in the medical record and prepares to provide the patient education needed. Nurse Zelensky instructs Ms. H and her significant other about the allergy, risk factors, and potential for a systemic reaction. She reviews common products that contain latex, as well as alternative nonlatex products. She provides Ms. H with a list of latex products and alternatives, a latex-free condom, and an order form for a medical alert tag. She instructs the patient about the importance of wearing the tag at all times and notifying care providers. She gives Ms. H a letter from the allergist diagnosing the allergy, along with a list of care providers to notify (e.g., pharmacist, dentist, family practitioner, gynecologist, hospital). Nurse Zelensky reviews signs and symptoms of a reaction to latex and appropriate treatment for minor as well as serious reactions. She provides Ms. H with a prescription for an epinephrine pen and assists her in practicing using the device. Nurse Zelensky provides Ms. H with telephone numbers to use if she has questions at a later time.

Ms. H indicates that she understands the instructions. This is recorded under the following outcomes: (1) Knowledge: Disease Process; (2) Knowledge: Health Behaviors; (3) Knowledge: Health Resources; and (4) Knowledge: Treatment Procedure(s). Under Knowledge: Medication, Nurse Zelensky records the return demonstration of use of an epinephrine pen.

SUMMARY

With the increasing rates of sensitization of latex, Latex Precautions has become an important part of nursing care. The purpose of the intervention is to prevent sensitization of high-risk patients as well as prevent systemic reactions in sensitized individuals. This intervention is based on research, case reports, and expert opinion, which have been reviewed here. Latex Precautions is comprehensive, providing guidance for screening and identification of high-risk patients, latex avoidance, communication, and patient education. Inclusion of this treatment within the NIC provides clear linkages with NANDA diagnoses and NOC outcomes. These linkages provide a mechanism to determine frequency of use, associated costs, and effectiveness of the intervention. Application of the intervention in a clinical setting can be complex, requiring specific activities to be repeated as the patient moves through the health care system. This type of application has been depicted through a case study using Latex Precautions in a surgical patient. However, the intervention can be used in any nursing specialty and in any setting.

References

Ahlroth, M., Alenius, H., Turjanmaa, K., Makinen-Kijunen, S., Reunala, T., and Palosuo, T. (1995). Cross-reacting allergens in natural rubber latex and avocado. *Journal of Allergy and Clinical Immunology, 96*(2), 167–173.

Alenius, H., Kalkkinen, N., Lukka, M., Turjanmaa, K., Reunala, T., Makinen-Kiljunen, S., and Palosuo, T. (1995). Purification and partial amino acid sequencing of a 27-kD natural rubber allergen recognized by latex-allergic children with spina bifida. *International Archives of Allergy and Immunology, 106*, 258–262.

Alenius, H., Turjanmaa, K., Makinen-Kiljunen, S., Reunala, T., and Palosuo, T. (1994). IgE immune response to rubber proteins in adult patients with latex allergy. *Journal of Allergy and Clinical Immunology, 93*, 859–863.

Arellano, R., Bradley, J., and Sussman, G. (1992). Prevalence of latex sensitization among hospital physicians occupationally exposed to latex gloves. *Anesthesiology, 77*, 905–908.

Baur, X., Chen, Z., and Allmers, H. (1998). Can a threshold limit value for natural rubber latex airborne allergens be defined? *Journal of Allergy and Clinical Immunology, 101*(1Pt. 1), 24–27.

Beezhold, D., and Beck, W. C. (1992). Surgical glove powders bind latex antigens. *Archives of Surgery, 127*, 1354–1357.

Beezhold, D. H., Kostyal, D. A., and Wiseman, J. (1994). The transfer of protein allergens from latex gloves. A study of influencing factors. *AORN Journal, 59*, 605–613.

Blanco, C., Carrillo, T., Castillo, R., Castillo, R., Quiralte, J., and Cuevas, M. (1994). Latex allergy: Clinical features and cross-reactivity with fruits. *Annals of Allergy, 73*, 309–314.

Brugnami, G., Marabini, A., Siracusa, A., and Abbritti, G. (1995). Work-related late asthmatic response induced by latex allergy. *Journal of Allergy and Clinical Immunology, 96*, 457–464.

Bubak, M. E., Reed, C. E., Fransway, A. F., Yunginger, J. W., Jones, R. T., and Hunt, L. W. (1992). Allergic reactions to latex among health-care workers. *Mayo Clinic Proceedings, 67*, 1075–1079.

Charous, B. L., Hamilton, R. G., and Yunginger, J. W. (1994). Occupational latex exposure: Characteristics of contact and systemic reactions in 47 workers. *Journal of Allergy and Clinical Immunology, 94*(1), 12–18.

Conde-Salazar, L., del-Rio, E., Guimaraens, D., and Gonzalez, D. A. (1993). Type IV allergy to rubber additives: A 10-year study of 686 cases. *Journal of the American Academy of Dermatology, 29* (2 Pt. 1), 176.

Dillard, S. F., and MacCollum, M. A. (1992). Reports to FDA: Allergic reactions to latex containing medical devices. In *Program and proceedings of the International Latex Conference: Sensitivity to latex in medical devices*, Baltimore, MD.

Ellsworth, P. I., Merguerian, P. A., Klein, R. B., and Rozycki, A. (1993). Evaluation and risk factors of latex allergy in spina bifida patients: Is it preventable? *Journal of Urology, 150* (2 Pt. 2), 691–693.

Hamann, C. P. (1993). Natural rubber latex protein sensitivity in review. *American Journal of Contact Dermatitis, 4*(1), 4–21.

Hamilton, C. (1984). Contamination of contrast agents by rubber components of 50-ml disposable syringes. *Radiology, 152*, 539–540.

Heese, A., von Hintzenstern, J. V., Peters, K.-P., Koch, H. U., and Hornstein, O. P. (1991). Allergic and irritant reactions to rubber gloves in medical health services: Spectrum, diagnostic approach, and therapy. *Journal of American Academy of Dermatology, 25* (5 Pt. 1), 831–839.

Heilman, D., Jones, R., Swanson, M., and Yunginger, J. W. (1996). A prospective, controlled study showing that rubber gloves are the major contributor to latex aeroallergen levels in the operating room. *Journal of Allergy and Clinical Immunology, 98*, 325–330.

Johnson, M., and Maas, M. *Nursing outcomes classification (NOC).* (1997). St. Louis: Mosby-Year Book.

Kaczmarek, R. G., Silverman, B. G., Gross, T. P., Hamilton, R. G., Kessler, R., Arrowsmith-Lowe, J. T., and Moore, R. M. (1996). Prevalence of latex specific IgE antibodies in hospital personnel. *Annals of Allergy, Asthma, and Immunology, 76*(1), 51–56.

Kelly, K. J., Kurup, V. P., Reijula, K. E., and Fink, J. N. (1994). The diagnosis of natural rubber latex allergy. *Journal of Allergy and Clinical Immunology, 93*, 813–816.

Kibby, T., and Akl, M. (1997). Prevalence of latex sensitization in a hospital employee population. *Annals of Allergy, Asthma, and Immunology, 78*(1), 41–44.

Konrad, C., Fieber, T., Gerber, H., Schuepfer, G., and Muellner, G. (1997). The prevalence of latex sensitivity among anesthesiology staff. *Anesthesia and Analgesia, 84*, 629–633.

Konz, K. R., Chia, J. K., Kurup, V. P., Resnick, A., Kelly, K., and Fink, J. N. (1995). Comparison of latex hypersensitivity among patients with neurologic defects. *Journal of Allergy and Clinical Immunology, 95* (5 Pt. 1), 950–954.

Korniwiecz, D., Kirwin, M., Cresci, K., and Larsen, E. (1993). Leakage of latex and vinyl exam gloves in high and low risk clinical settings. *American Industrial Hygiene Association Journal, 54*(1), 22–26.

Korniwiecz, D., Kirwin, M., Cresci, K., Sing, T., Choo, T., Wool, M., and Larsen, E. (1994). Barrier protection with examination gloves: Double versus single. *American Journal of Infection Control, 22*(1), 12–15.

Korniwiecz, D., Laughton, B., Cyr, W., Lytle, C., and Larsen, E. (1990). Leakage of virus through used vinyl and latex examination gloves. *Journal of Clinical Microbiology, 28*(4), 787–788.

Kurup, V., Murali, P., and Kelly, K. J. (1995). Latex antigens. *Immunology and Allergy Clinics of North America, 15*(1), 45–59.

Kwitten, P. L., Sweinberg, S. K., Campbell, D. E., and Pawlowski, N. A. (1995). Latex hypersensitivity in children: Clinical presentation and detection of latex-specific immunoglobulin E. *Pediatrics, 95*, 693–699.

Lagier, F., Vervloet, D., Lhermet, I., Poyen, D., and Charpin, D. (1992). Prevalence of latex allergy in operating room nurses. *Journal of Allergy and Clinical Immunology, 90* (3 Pt. 1), 319–322.

Latex Hypersensitivity Committee. (1995). Latex allergy—an emerging healthcare problem. *Annals of Allergy, Asthma, and Immunology, 75*(1), 19–21.

Lavaud, F., Prevost, A., Cossart, C., Guerin, L., Bernard, J., and Kochman, S. (1995). Allergy to latex, avocado pear, and banana: Evidence of a 30 kd antigen in immunoblotting. *Journal of Allergy and Clinical Immunology, 95*, 557–564.

McCloskey, J. C., and Bulechek, G. M. (Eds). (1996). *Nursing interventions classification (NIC)* (2nd ed.) St. Louis: Mosby–Year Book.

Melton, A. L. (1992). Allergenicity of latex syringe components. In *Program and proceedings of the International*

Latex Conference: Sensitivity to latex in medical devices, Baltimore, MD.

National Institute for Occupational Safety and Health. (1997). *Preventing allergic reactions to natural rubber latex in the workplace* (DHHS [NIOSH] Publication No. 97–135). Cincinnati, OH.

North American Nursing Diagnosis Association. (1992). *NANDA nursing diagnoses: Definition and classification.* St. Louis: Author.

Olsen, R., Lynch, P., Coyle, M., Cummings, J., Bokete, T., and Stamm, W. (1993). Examination gloves as barriers to hand contamination in clinical practice. *JAMA, 270*(3), 350–353.

Ownby, D. R. (1995). Manifestations of latex allergy. *Immunology and Allergy Clinics of North America, 15*(1), 31–43.

Pearson, M. L., Cole, J. S., and Jarvis, W. R. (1994). How common is latex allergy? A survey of children with myelodysplasia. *Developmental Medicine and Child Neurology, 36*(1), 64–69.

Porri, F., Pradal, M., Lerniere, C., Birnbaum, J., Mege, J. L., Lanteaume, A., Charpin, D., Vervloet, D., and Camboulives, J. (1997). Association between latex sensitization and repeated latex exposure in children. *Anesthesiology, 86*, 599–602.

Setlock, M. A., Cotter, T. P., and Rosner, D. (1993). Latex allergy: Failure of prophylaxis to prevent severe reaction. *Anesthesia and Analgesia, 76*, 650–652.

Steelman, V. M. (1995). Latex allergy precautions: A research-based protocol. *Nursing Clinics of North America, 30*, 475–493.

Steelman, V. M. (1996). Latex allergy: Implications for the nurse anesthetist. *Current Reviews for Nurse Anesthetists, 19*, 26–31.

Steelman, V. (1997a). Prevalence and risk factors of adverse reactions to natural rubber latex among nursing personnel. Doctoral dissertation, University of Iowa, Iowa City.

Steelman, V. M. (1997b). *Research-based protocol: Latex precautions.* Iowa City, IA: The University of Iowa Gerontological Nursing Interventions Research Center.

Subramaniam, A. (1995). The chemistry of natural rubber latex. *Immunology and Allergy Clinics of North America, 15*(1), 1–20.

Swanson, M. C., Bubak, M. E., Hunt, L. W., Yunginger, J. W., Warner, M. A., and Reed, C. E. (1994). Quantification of occupational latex aeroallergens in a medical center. *Journal of Allergy and Clinical Immunology, 94* (3 Pt. 1), 445–451.

Tarlo, S. M., Sussman, G., Contala, A., and Swanson, M. C. (1994). Control of airborne latex by use of powder-free gloves. *Journal of Allergy and Clinical Immunology, 93*, 985–989.

Task Force on Allergic Reactions to Latex. (1993). American Academy of Allergy and Immunology. Committee report. *Journal of Allergy and Clinical Immunology, 92* (1 Pt. 1), 16–18.

Tosi, L. L. Slater, J. E., Shaer, C., and Mostello, L. A. (1993). Latex allergy in spina bifida patients: Prevalence and surgical implications. *Journal of Pediatric Orthopedics, 13*, 709–712.

Truscott, W. (1995). The industry perspective on latex. *Immunology and Allergy Clinics of North America, 15*(1), 89–121.

Turjanmaa, K. (1987). Incidence of immediate allergy to latex gloves in hospital personnel. *Contact Dermatitis, 17*, 270–275.

Turjanmaa, K., Laurila, K., Makinen-Kiljunen, S., and Reunala, T. (1988). Rubber contact urticaria: Allergenic properties of 19 brands of latex gloves. *Contact Dermatitis, 19*, 362–367.

Turjanmaa, K., Makinen-Kiljunen, S., Reunala, T., Alenius, H., and Palosuo, T. (1995). Natural rubber latex allergy: The European experience. *Immunology and Allergy Clinics of North America, 15*(1), 71–88.

Vandenplas, O., Delwiche, J. P., Depelchin, S., Sibille, Y., Vande Weyer, R., and Delaunois, L. (1995). Latex gloves with a lower protein content reduce bronchial reactions in subjects with occupational asthma caused by latex. *American Journal of Respiratory Care Medicine, 151* (3 Pt. 1), 887–891.

Vandenplas, O., Delwiche, J. P., Evrard, G., Aimont, P., van der Brempt, X., Jamart, J., and Delaunois, L. (1995). Prevalence of occupational asthma due to latex among hospital personnel. *American Journal of Respiratory Care Medicine, 151*(1), 54–60.

von Hintzenstern, J., Koch, H. U., Peters, K.-P., and Hornstein, O. P. (1991). Frequency, spectrum and occupational relevance of type IV allergies to rubber chemicals. *Contact Dermatitis, 24*, 244–252.

Wrangsjo, K., Osterman, K., and van Hage-Hamsten, M. (1994). Glove-related skin symptoms among operating theatre and dental care unit personnel (II). Clinical examination, tests and laboratory findings indicating latex allergy. *Contact Dermatitis, 30*(3), 139–143.

Yassin, M. S., Lierl, M. B., Fischer, T. J., O'Brien, K., Cross, J., and Steinmetz, C. (1994). Latex allergy in hospital employees. *Annals of Allergy, 72*, 245–249.

Yassin, M. S., Sanyurah, S., Lierl, M. B. Fischer, T. J., Oppenheimer, S., Cross, J., O'Brien, K., Steinmetz, C., and Khoury, J. (1992). Evaluation of latex allergy in patients with meningomyelocele. *Annals of Allergy, 69*, 207–211.

Yunginger, J. W., Jones, R. T., Fransway, A. F., Kelso, J. M., Warner, M., and Hunt, L. W. (1994). Extractable latex allergens and proteins in disposable medical gloves and other rubber products. *Journal of Allergy and Clinical Immunology, 93*, 836–842.

Section V

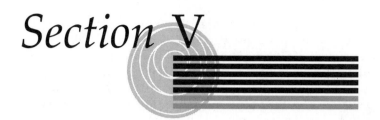

Health System Interventions

Overview: Care That Supports Effective Use of the Health Care Delivery System

Gloria M. Bulechek

Joanne C. McCloskey

A ll nurses have two roles: a provider of direct care and a manager of the environment where care takes place. As the health care system changes and becomes more complex, interventions related to the management of the environment become more important to the success of more clinically oriented interventions. An important aspect of this care is the nurse's role as mediator between the health system and the patient and family.

The first intervention in the section, **Patient Rights Protection**, discusses the nurse's legal role in protection of the health care rights of patients. Kay Weiler and Sue Moorhead begin Chapter 39 by overviewing the constitutional rights to privacy and free exercise of religion and the common law right to self-determination. The activities in the intervention are reviewed in these three sections, and the legal basis for each activity is discussed. Many of the intervention's activities are in the area of self-determination, which has had extensive litigation. The authors discuss the Patient Self-Determination Act of 1990, do-not-resuscitate orders, and the advance directives of living will and durable power of attorney. Because the North American Nursing Diagnosis Association (NANDA) has no diagnosis in this area, they propose the nursing diagnosis of potential loss of self-determination. Vulnerable populations include frail adults, institutionalized adults, educationally limited adults, isolated adults without a spokesperson, and adults who have not given verbal or written advance directives to anyone. Six appropriate outcomes are identified. A case study discussing the Nancy Cruzan/Missouri Supreme Court decision of 1983 is used to illustrate many of the activities of the intervention. The chapter is basic reading for all nurses and illustrates the legal foundation for this important nursing intervention.

The second intervention in this section further illustrates the nurse's mediator role. In Chapter 40, Toni Tripp-Reimer, Pamela J. Brink, and Carol S. Pinkham discuss the intervention of **Culture Brokerage**, whereby the nurse bridges and links the orthodox health care system with the patient of a different culture. The focus may target the patient, the practitioners, or both. The authors say that in order to effectively deliver the intervention, the nurse must have cultural competence, which they define as more than awareness and sensitivity to cultural differences. A review of the literature includes the history and present-day use of the intervention. The authors point out that Culture Brokerage is of particular use today when the nurse is confronted with a situation involving ethical issues. The authors discuss several strategies to implement the intervention including cultural assessment, negotiation, use of time, and use of a translator. The intervention is useful for many diagnoses but is usually triggered by the diagnosis of Noncompliance. Two case studies illustrate the use of this intervention. As the world's population becomes increasingly mobile, nurses in all countries will encounter patients from other parts of the globe. This intervention will assist them in delivering care for anyone who comes from a different culture.

The intervention **Visitation Facilitation** is discussed in Chapter 41 by Jeanette M. Daly. This intervention of promoting beneficial visits from family members and friends is relevant to patients in all settings. Daly reviews the literature related to visitation in the categories of patients' opinions, families' needs, nurses' opinions, policies, and ethical and legal considerations. Visiting policies vary by institution and specialty area. Nurses' perceptions of family visits differ from those of patients and family members; nurses favor a restriction of visits, whereas family members desire no or few restrictions. Daly argues for a flexible policy that is adjusted for the situation and the patient's condition. Appropriate related diagnoses and outcomes are included, as are two short case studies.

The intervention **Sustenance Support** is addressed in Chapter 42 by Juanita K. Hunter. The definition of the intervention is "helping a needy individual/family to locate food, clothing, or shelter." This intervention is frequently used by community health nurses, often with people who are homeless, but it is also used by other types of nurses and is appropriate for other populations. Hunter first discusses the origins of the intervention in religious traditions of charity. She reviews nursing's emphasis on providing for patients' basic needs from the theory of Maslow and the writings of nursing theorists. She addresses how the nurse helps an individual or family find food, clothing, and shelter and includes addresses and telephone numbers of helping organizations. Two case studies illustrate the complex and challenging patient situations nurses may encounter for which this intervention is appropriate.

The last chapter in this section, and in the book, is on **Telephone Consultation**. The practice of nursing over the telephone is rapidly growing as demands of time increase and in response to concerns about cost. Sheila A. Haas and Ida A. Androwich first discuss the reasons for the growth of practice over the telephone and then cover three issues related to telephone consultation: cost-effectiveness, workload, and standardized language. They argue that, despite trends to use nonprofessionals for telephone calls, only professional nurses have the necessary preparation and skills for telephone interventions. Currently, the Nursing Interventions Classification (NIC) has only one telephone intervention. Haas and Androwich, with the help of 11 colleagues, have developed and proposed a revision to this intervention and the addition of three others. Two case studies illustrate the use of two of the newly proposed interventions—Surveillance: Telephone and Triage: Telephone. The chapter illustrates how the changes and evolving nursing roles in practice should inform and change the standardized languages used for documentation and communication.

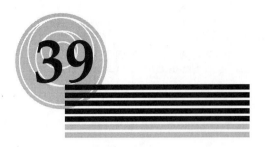

Patient Rights Protection

Kay Weiler and Sue Moorhead

It is important to note at the outset that this intervention is based on patients' rights. "Statements of rights provide vital protections of life, liberty, expression, and property. They protect against oppression, unequal treatment, intolerance, arbitrary invasion of privacy, and the like" (Beauchamp & Childress, 1994, pp. 69–70).

> Rights are justified claims that individuals and groups can make upon others or upon society. To have a right is to be in a position to determine, by one's choices, what others are to do or need not do. Rights give us a claim based on a system of rules that authorize us to affirm, demand, or insist upon what is due. If a person possesses a right, others are validly constrained from interfering with the exercise of that right. Claiming will hereafter be understood as a rule-governed activity. The rules may be legal rules, moral rules, institutional rules, or rules of games, but all rights exist or fail to exist because the relevant rules either allow or disallow the claim or entitlement in question. These rules distinguish valid claims from invalid claims (Beauchamp & Childress, 1994, p. 71).

The intervention of Patient Rights Protection is based on legal rules that grant a competent American adult the right to accept or to reject health care treatment. Patient rights are derived from the constitutional rights to privacy and free exercise of religion and the common law right to self-determination. All these legal rights provide the structure and backbone for the activities identified by this nursing intervention (McCloskey & Bulechek, 1996).

The right to privacy is not explicitly stated in the Constitution; this right has been found within the penumbra or zone of rights in the 9th (*Griswold v. Connecticut*, 1965) and 14th amendments (*Roe v. Wade*, 1973). Although the Constitution does not definitively state the right to privacy, the Supreme Court has determined that this fundamental right is implied in the intent and wording of the Constitution (*Griswold v. Connecticut*, 1965). This right recognizes the individual's interest in preserving "the inviolability of his person" (*Superintendent of Belchertown v. Saikewicz*, 1977, p. 424; *quoting Pratt v. Davis*, 1905, p. 166). The New Jersey Supreme Court established that the constitutional right to privacy is "broad enough to encompass a patient's decision to decline medical treatment under certain circumstances" even if that personal decision would foreseeably result in death (*Matter of Quinlan*, 1976, p. 663).

The constitutional right to freedom of religion is in the first amendment of the Constitution, which states, "Congress shall make no law respecting an establishment of religion, or prohibiting the free exercise thereof" (Constitution of the United States, Amendment 1, 1791). The amendment has two distinct aspects. The first phrase prohibits Congress from establishing a religion; this is referred to as the establishment clause. After prohibiting Congress from establishing a mandatory religion, the second phrase protects the individual's right to the free exercise of his or her own religion. The establishment clause has not been applicable to cases involving health care treatment decisions. The free exercise clause has, however, been examined in relation to the individual's right to refuse life-sustaining treatment based on the religious conviction that the treatment is in opposition to the individual's right to the free exercise of his or her religious beliefs.

The common law right of self-determination has been described as follows: "No right is held more sacred, or is more carefully guarded by the common law, than the right of every individual to the possession and control of his own person, free from all restraint or interference of others, unless by clear and unquestionable authority of law" (*Matter of Conroy*, 1985, p. 1221, citing *Union Pacific Railroad Co. v. Botsford*, 1891, p. 251). Another description of this right is, "Every human being of adult years and sound mind has a right to determine what shall be done with his own body" (*Schloendorff v. Society of New York Hospital*, 1914, p. 93).

THE NURSING INTERVENTION PATIENT RIGHTS PROTECTION

The intervention Patient Rights Protection was published in the first edition of the Nursing Interventions Classification (NIC) (McCloskey & Bulechek, 1992) and was one of the very first interventions developed to serve as a template for intervention development (Table 39–1). As the intervention was discussed by the research team, its relationship with the role of the nurse as an advocate was clearly identified. The decision was made to keep this intervention focused on the rights of patients interacting with the health care system in general, regardless of setting. As the taxonomy for the NIC classification was developed, Patient Rights Protection was placed in the domain called Health System, defined as "care that supports effective use of the health care delivery system" (McCloskey & Bulechek, 1996, p. 68), and in the class called Health System Mediation, defined as "interventions to facilitate the interface between patient/family and the health care system" (McCloskey & Bulechek, 1996, p. 68). From its inception, this intervention identified the important links between the patient, the family and significant others connected to the patient, and the health care system. Specifically, this intervention described a variety of factors that could infringe on a patient's rights.

Table 39–1 Patient Rights Protection

DEFINITION: Protection of health care rights of a patient, especially a minor, incapacitated, or incompetent patient unable to make decisions.

ACTIVITIES:

Provide patient with "Patient's Bill of Rights"

Provide environment conducive for private conversations between patient, family, and health care professionals

Protect patient's privacy during activities of hygiene, elimination, and grooming

Determine whether patient's wishes about health care are known

Determine who is legally empowered to give consent for treatment or research

Work with physician and hospital administration to honor patient and family wishes

Refrain from forcing the treatment

Note religious preference

Know the legal status of living wills in the state

Honor a patient's wishes expressed in a living will or durable power of attorney for health care, as appropriate

Honor written "Do Not Resuscitate" orders

Assist the dying person with unfinished business

Note on medical record any observable facts bearing on the testator's mental competency to make a will

Intervene in situations involving unsafe or inadequate care

Be aware of mandatory reporting requirements in the state

Limit viewing of the patient's record to immediate health care providers

Maintain confidentiality of patient data

Source: McCloskey, J. C., and Bulechek, G. M. (Eds.). (1996). *Nursing interventions classification (NIC)* (2nd ed.). St. Louis: Mosby–Year Book.

Patients at Risk

Most patients, merely by having been admitted to an inpatient facility (e.g., acute care facility, rehabilitation or long-term care facility) perceive that they have lost some autonomy and decision-making ability. Efforts to meet all the patients' care needs may necessitate organization of daily care routines, medication administration, and the integration of numerous other diagnostic and therapeutic activities. Therefore, individual preferences for awakening, personal hygiene, and other personal lifestyle preferences may need to be altered to fit the organizational needs of the clinical unit or even the needs of the entire health care facility (Annas, 1992; Kelly, 1976). The intervention Patient Rights Protection must also be vigorously applied to vulnerable patients who have limited abilities to protect themselves in the health care environment (e.g., children, cognitively compromised or debilitated patients, terminally ill patients, patients with very limited physical capacity to protect themselves from bodily assault) (Annas, 1992; Dew, 1992; Kelly, 1976).

NURSING ACTIVITIES INCLUDED IN PATIENT RIGHTS PROTECTION

The activities identified for the intervention are derived from the legal obligations that nurses have to their patients. Specifically, patients retain the legal rights to privacy, religion, and self-determination, even if they are admitted to inpatient care settings. Historically, nurses have advocated for patients' legal rights in the health care system. A closer examination of this intervention allows the activities in this intervention to be clustered under the constitutional rights to privacy and free exercise of religion and the common law right to self-determination.

Privacy

Nursing activities that are derived from the patient's right to privacy include (1) the protection of the patient's privacy during activities of hygiene, elimination, and grooming; (2) provision of an environment conducive to private conversations between patient, family, and health care professionals; (3) limiting viewing of the patient's record to immediate health care providers; and (4) maintaining confidentiality of patient data. The protection of bodily privacy is one of the most fundamental nursing activities and may be implemented by the use of drawn curtains, closed doors, and bathrobes or blankets used for draping. The protection of conversations may be more difficult to achieve, because many patients share rooms with other patients. However, providing the patient and others with a quiet room located on the clinical unit or indicating to the patient that the other patient in the room will be absent for a specified period of time allows the patient and visitors to have private discussions. Sensitive information, such as progress reports during surgery, should be delivered in a private setting whenever possible.

Protection of the right to privacy is also demonstrated in the nursing activities related to patient's records. Nurses should always keep patient's records and data in an area that is not readily accessible to the public. This has traditionally meant that the records for each unit were kept in a central location at the nurses' station. With the increased use of computerized record keeping and computerized charting, additional measures need to be implemented to protect patients' privacy. Specifically, the nurse should position the computer screen so that people walking past the computer are not able to read patient data. If patient data are printed from the computer, the printouts should not be thrown into the regular trash or recycling containers; the printouts should be shredded. Access to computer passwords should be protected so that unauthorized personnel cannot access the patient data. In addition, the nurse should not access patient records unless there is a legitimate need for information that will assist in providing patient care (Bialorucki & Blaine, 1992).

In addition to the protection of written or computerized patient data, the patient's privacy must also be protected by not verbally disclosing confidential information to the patient's friends or family members unless the patient has clearly authorized the disclosure. Nurses should not make verbal disclosures either in face-to-face interactions or through telephone contacts (Bialorucki & Blaine, 1992).

Free Exercise of Religion

The nursing activity "note religious preference" is based on the individual's right to the free exercise of religion. This activity assumes that the notation of religious preference will assist health care providers in respecting the individual's religious preference and in seeking religious resources as appropriate. This nursing activity is important when the patient's decision to refuse life-sustaining treatment has been based on personal religious convictions (Ferdinand, 1996). In legal cases involving a minor or an adult with diminished decision-making skills, the courts have been reluctant to honor the right of free exercise of religion when the right has been asserted by a surrogate decision maker.

Self-Determination

Protecting the patient's right to self-determination is becoming increasingly more complex because many patients have sought judicial review. Three categories of nursing activities for Patient Rights Protection are (1) the patient's right to make decisions for himself or herself regarding personal health care, (2) the patient's right to extend his or her right to make personal decisions to a surrogate or substitute decision maker, and (3) the patient's right to make decisions regarding his or her own personal bodily integrity.

The judicial review of multiple cases involving controversies regarding patient rights and health care facilities' obligations precipitated extensive attention to a patient's right to self-determination. These cases initially arose with the issue of whether the patient had a right to self-determination in health care treatment decisions (*Jacobson v. Massachusetts*, 1905; *Schloendorff v. Society of New York Hospital*, 1914). After the legal right was established, the breadth of the right and specific aspects of the right were questioned and litigated (*Brophy v. New England Sinai Hosp., Inc.*, 1986; *Cruzan v. Director, Missouri Department of Health*, 1990; *Griswold v. Connecticut*, 1965; *Matter of Conroy*, 1985; *Matter of Quinlan*, 1976; *Roe v. Wade*, 1973; *Superintendent of Belchertown v. Saikewicz*, 1977).

The extensive litigation exploring the patient's right to self-determination prompted federal legislation, the Patient Self-Determination Act (PSDA), to enhance the patient's role in health care treatment decisions (PSDA, 1990). The PSDA requires that all adults admitted to inpatient, nursing home, home health, and hospice care receive information about the legal options available in that state for documenting present or future health care treatment decisions. The legislation was enacted "to provide written information to each such individual concerning . . . an individual's rights under State law . . . to make decisions concerning such medical care, including the right to accept or refuse medical or surgical treatment and the right to formulate advance directives. . . ." The legislation also required the health care facility to "provide the written policies of the provider or organization respecting the implementation of such rights" and "to document in the individual's medical record whether or not the individual has executed an advance directive" (PSDA, 1990).

The purpose of the PSDA is not to require patients to have such a document, but to make people aware of the alternatives available to them. With increased patient knowledge and awareness, it is expected that the number of patients with advance directives will increase. It is also expected that nurses will have increased encounters with these documents (Johns, 1996; Weiler, Eland, & Buckwalter, 1996).

PERSONAL SELF-CARE

Seven of the activities involved in Patient Rights Protection evolve from the patient's right to make decisions for himself or herself regarding personal self-care. These activities are (1) determine whether patient's wishes about health care are known, (2) work with physician and hospital administration to honor patient and family wishes, (3) know the legal status of living wills in the state, (4) determine who is legally empowered to give consent for treatment or research, (5) honor written do-not-resuscitate orders, (6) assist the dying person with unfinished business, and (7) note on medical record any observable facts bearing on the testator's mental competency to make a will.

With the passage of the PSDA, the first four activities listed under personal self-care should have become essential components of every admission to an acute care, long-term care, hospice, or home health agency (PSDA, 1990; Teno, Sabatino, Parisier, Rouse, & Lynn, 1993). The PSDA requires that a representative of the health care institution ask the patient whether he or she has an advance directive. If the patient has an advance directive, the institution is directed to include a copy of the document, if available, in the health care record. After documentation of the patient's wishes about health care, the next logical activity is to honor the patient's wishes. If the patient has questions about advance directives, the institution should have a policy regarding how the patient will be directed to obtain information about those questions (PSDA, 1990). The ability to recognize whether the patient has expressed his or her wishes for health care treatment in a legal advance directive is based on the premise that the nurse has gained accurate knowledge of the legal advance directives available in the specific state in which care is being delivered.

The nursing activity "honor written 'Do Not Resuscitate' orders" is focused on the patient's right to exercise self-determination by requesting or concurring with a physician's determination that resuscitation after the cessation of respiration or cardiac function is futile. The order must be a physician's order; however, the physician's decision should be made in consultation with the patient if he or she is capable of participating in the decision-making process (Aiken & Catalano, 1994; *Payne v. Marion General Hospital*, 1990). This activity allows the patient the ultimate opportunity to determine when or if life has become more burdensome than beneficial or more degrading or painful than tolerable. The decision regarding a do-not-resuscitate order should be clearly documented in the health care record and routinely reviewed (Aiken & Catalano, 1994). It is essential for nurses to recognize that a do-not-resuscitate order is not synonymous with the lack of supportive care, pain relief, respect, or caring (Fowler, 1989).

The nursing activities "assist the dying person with unfinished business" and "note on medical record any observable facts bearing on the testator's mental competency to make a will" are not directly related to protection of the patient's right to self-care regarding health care treatment decisions. However, these activities recognize the importance of other significant aspects of the patient's life and death. The dying patient may need to have a last conversation with a significant loved one or to plan for and document whom he or she has chosen to care for any minor or incapacitated children. Additionally, the patient may have unfinished business related to his or her profession or employment situation, such as communicating information about where important files are kept or about important scheduled meetings. The documentation regarding the patient's mental ability to write a will is not directly related to the physical health care of the patient. However, the documentation may have a critical impact on later questions concerning the cognitive ability of the patient to have recognized the extent of his or her estate and the range of options available for distribution of assets. Both of these activities will certainly assist the patient with organizing and planning for some important aspects of his or her life and approaching death.

SELF-DETERMINATION BY A SURROGATE DECISION MAKER

The second category of activities is derived from the patient's right to self-determination as exercised by a surrogate decision maker and is described in the activity "honor a patient's wishes expressed in a living will or durable power of attorney for health care, as appropriate." The litigation surrounding the patient's right to self-determination in health care treatment decisions has also prompted state legislative action regarding authorizing the creation of advance directives for future health care treatment decisions.

Decisions to provide advance directives for future health care treatment decisions may be formalized in one of the two forms of written advance directives: living will and durable power of attorney. The living will authorizes an adult to document personal decisions regarding the administration of life-sustaining treatment. By putting health care treatment preferences in writing, the individual provides directions to be followed in the event that the person is in a terminal condition *and* unable to participate in medical treatment decisions. The living will does not name a specific surrogate decision maker for future health care treatment decisions. The living will does, however, identify to the health care provider, at the time that a life-sustaining procedure needs to be made, the patient's previously expressed wishes for care (Uniform Rights of the Terminally Ill Act, 1989). The second form of written advance directive is the durable power of attorney for health care. Specific characteristics of a durable power of attorney for health care are (1) the person writing the document must be mentally competent at the time that the document is created, (2) it is a private agreement, and (3) the document must contain words demonstrating that the relationship was intended to continue even if the person who wrote it became incapacitated or disabled (Uniform Durable Power of Attorney Act, 1984, 1987).

The durable power of attorney for health care does specify the person who is responsible for making future health care treatment decisions. In addition to naming a specific person, the durable power of attorney for health care offers greater flexibility; because it is not limited to life-sustaining measures, it may apply to nursing home placement or other forms of nonemergency treatment. However, durable power of attorney for health care does require that the person writing the document have someone who is willing to serve in the role of substitute decision maker. Unfortunately, many individuals do not have a close relative or friend who is able and willing to serve as the substitute decision maker, so those individuals are limited to using the living will for future health care treatment decisions.

PROTECTION OF BODILY INTEGRITY

The third category of activities associated with the person's right to self-determination concerns the right to protection of bodily integrity. These activities include (1) refrain from forcing treatment, (2) be aware of mandatory reporting requirements in the state, and (3) intervene in situations involving unsafe or inadequate care.

An adult may give informed consent for direct personal health care. The patient must receive specific information in order to make an informed decision: the nature of the treatment or intervention, benefits of the proposed treatment or procedure, risks involved in accepting the proposed care, desired outcomes, reasonably available alternatives, and consequences to the patient if no care is given (Guido, 1997). Informed consent may be received from the patient or from a substitute decision maker, such as the attorney-in-fact named in a durable power of attorney for health care or a court-appointed guardian.

The logical corollary of the informed consent doctrine is the patient's right to not have treatment forced upon him or her. If the nurse does proceed with care, even after the patient has indicated that he or she does not want the treatment or procedure, the nurse and other health care providers may be liable for assault and battery upon the patient (*Schloendorff v. Society of New York Hospital*, 1914). Assault, in the health care environment, may be characterized as a patient's being threatened with potential harm, believing that the threatening person is capable of creating the harm, and being fearful that the harm will occur (Brent, 1997). Assault may or may not be accompanied by battery. Battery occurs if the patient has refused physical contact or care and the health care provider continues the treatment and actually touches the patient (*Anderson v. St. Francis–St. George Hospital*, 1992; *Foflygen v. R. Zemel*, 1992; *Lounsbury v. Capel*, 1992; *Schloendorff v. Society of New York Hospitals*, 1914).

Additional nursing activities associated with the protection of bodily integrity include an awareness of mandatory reporting laws. Most states have legislation that protects vulnerable populations from direct or indirect physical or psychological harm. Nurses must recognize that physical or psychological harm may be initiated by friends, family, or caregivers in the home or institutional setting. In addition to direct harm, nurses must also recognize their responsibility to protect patients who are in violent, abusive, or negligent care settings. Protection from harm must be provided in the home, respite, or institutional care settings (Weiler & Slavik Cowen, in press).

Provision of Information

The final activity for the Patient Rights Protection intervention, "provide patient with 'Patient's Bill of Rights,' " is based on the American Hospital Association's (AHA) publication, "Patient's Bill of Rights" (American Hospital Association [AHA], 1978). In 1969, the Joint Commission on Accreditation of Hospitals (JCAH) issued a statement that scarcely mentioned the problems that patients encountered within the health care system. In response to the JCAH statement, the National Welfare Rights Organization presented a statement in 1970 that offered 26 proposals for identifying and protecting patients' rights. The proposals were then examined, debated, and finalized into the AHA's Patient's Bill of Rights (Beauchamp & Childress, 1989).

When the American Association of Homes for the Aging and the American Nursing Home Association joined the JCAH in 1988, the commission became the Joint Commission on Accreditation of Healthcare Organizations (JCAHO) (Annas, 1992). The current goal of the JCAHO is respecting patient rights to improve patient outcomes (JCAHO, 1997). One of the standards that association hospitals are expected to meet is, "Each patient receives a written statement of his or her rights" (JCAHO, 1997, pp. R1–5). The intent of the standard is to assist patients, who are likely to be frightened and confused by the necessity for a hospital admission, to understand and exercise their patient rights (JCAHO, 1997, pp. R1–5). This standard and intent indicate that the patient should receive a written statement of rights. The standard does not stipulate that the statement must be the AHA's Patient's Bill of Rights; however, a written copy of the health care provider's patient bill of rights should be provided to the patient.

The AHA's Patient's Bill of Rights is not a statement of the patient's legal rights but is a combination of moral and legal rights (Trandel-Korenchuk, 1982). Only the legal rights, such as the right to privacy and the right to make personal decisions regarding health care treatment, are legally enforceable (Trandel-Korenchuk, 1982). The rights that are not based on legal precedent are not enforceable in the courts, such as "patient has the right to know what hospital rules and regulations apply to his conduct as a patient," and are dependent on the good will of the facility (AHA, 1978; Trandel-Korenchuk, 1982). The lack of clarification regarding which rights are legally enforceable and which are moral, but not legal, rights is a significant limitation of the document.

Since the establishment of the Patient's Bill of Rights, interest in protecting patients has been increasing, as documented in the literature. Many publications focus on describing the document and its implications for nurses (Brent, 1994; Cahill, 1994; Fiesta, 1988; Klop, van Wijmen & Philipsen, 1991; Ramsey, 1990; Scanlon, 1993). Others have focused on the intent and outcomes of the PSDA (Davis, 1992; Greve, 1994; Teno et al., 1993). In addition, the role of the nurse as an advocate and a protector of patient rights to autonomy, confidentiality, and dignity is also documented in the nursing literature that supports this intervention (Nelson, 1988; Prins, 1992; Trandel-Korenchuk, 1982).

ASSOCIATED NURSING DIAGNOSES

Since the development of the intervention Patient Rights Protection, little literature in terms of nursing diagnoses has been developed or refined through the North American Nursing Diagnosis Association (NANDA). As linkage work between NIC and NANDA has been attempted, the absence of this type of diagnosis is more obvious, but nursing as a profession has not addressed this issue. Work on identifying a diagnosis using the NANDA patient problem classification was developed for a book dealing with the elderly (Weiler & Moorhead, in press). The result of this work was a suggested diagnosis of Potential Loss of Self-Determination.

The nursing diagnosis Potential Loss of Self-Determination has been proposed as a problem that could be resolved by the nurse using the intervention Patient Rights Protection. The defining characteristics include (1) mental capacity, (2) the presence of an advance directive for health care, and (3) the availability of a substitute decision maker. The proposed signs and symptoms are (1) the potential or actual loss of decision-making capacity, (2) a change in physical capacity, (3) a change in mental capacity, (4) a change in health status, (5) a change in the caregiver's usual pattern of responsibility regarding the patient, (6) family members' or caregivers' uncertainty regarding patient's wishes concerning treatment, and (7) incongruence between one's stated wishes regarding treatment and the treatment provided by caregivers (Weiler & Moorhead, in press). Related factors include (1) a change in the level of personal independence, (2) institutionalization, (3) lack of an advocate, (4) change in others' perception of patient's decision-making capacity, (5) lack of knowledge of advance directive, and (6) lack of an advance directive (Weiler & Moorhead, in press).

The diagnosis of Potential Loss of Self-Determination may be appropriate for a variety of vulnerable groups. The defining characteristics, signs and symptoms, and related factors identify situations or qualities that describe a variety of vulnerable populations. Specifically, the loss of self-determination may be experienced by physically or cognitively frail adults, institutionalized adults, educationally limited adults, isolated adults without a spokesperson or an advocate, and adults who have not given verbal or written advance directives for their family, friends, or caregivers (Weiler & Moorhead, in press).

ASSOCIATED NURSING OUTCOMES

Linkages between the NANDA patient problems and the NIC interventions have been established (McCloskey & Bulechek, 1996); also, linkages between

NANDA diagnoses and Nursing Outcomes Classification (NOC) outcomes have been identified (Johnson & Maas, 1997). However, because there is no accepted NANDA diagnosis for this patient problem, the literature does not provide clear linkages between this intervention, NANDA, and the NOC outcomes (Johnson & Maas, 1997). The authors suggest that outcomes that may be important for this intervention are Caregiver Stressors, Dignified Dying, Grief Resolution, Participation: Health Care Decisions, Well-Being, and Will to Live (Johnson & Maas, 1997).

CASE STUDY

This case study identifies six activities associated with Patient Rights Protection. The applicable nursing activities include all three categories of activities related to the patient's right to self-determination: (1) the patient's right to make decisions for himself or herself regarding personal health care, (2) the patient's right to extend his or her right to make personal decisions to a surrogate or substitute decision maker, and (3) the patient's right to make decisions regarding his or her own personal bodily integrity.

On the night of January 11, 1983, Nancy Cruzan lost control of her car. . . . The vehicle overturned, and Cruzan was discovered lying face down in a ditch without detectable respiratory or cardiac function. Paramedics were able to restore her breathing and heartbeat at the accident site, and she was transported to a hospital in an unconscious state. . . . She [was in] what is commonly referred to as a persistent vegetative state. . . . After it had become apparent that Nancy Cruzan had virtually no chance of regaining her mental faculties, her parents asked hospital employees to terminate the artificial nutrition and hydration procedures. All agree that such removal would cause her death. The employees refused. . . . The parents then sought and received authorization from the state trial court for termination.

The Supreme Court of Missouri reversed on a divided vote. . . . We granted certiorari to consider the question whether Cruzan has a right under the United States Constitution which would require the hospital to withdraw life-sustaining treatment from her. . . .

The logical corollary of the doctrine of informed consent is that the patient generally possesses the right not to consent, that is, to refuse treatment. . . . The issue is not whether, but when, for how long, and at what cost to the individual [a] life may be briefly extended. . . .

The choice between life and death is a deeply personal decision of obvious and overwhelming finality. We believe Missouri may legitimately seek to safeguard the personal element of this choice through the imposition of heightened evidentiary requirements.

In our view, Missouri has permissibly sought to advance these interests through the adoption of a "clear and convincing" standard of proof. . . . The Supreme Court of Missouri held that . . . the testimony adduced at trial did not amount to clear and convincing proof of the patient's desire to have hydration and nutrition withdrawn.

The judgment of the Supreme Court of Missouri is Affirmed (*Cruzan v. Director*, 1990).

Discussion

Nancy Cruzan was injured in an automobile accident on January 11, 1983, and the next month a gastrostomy feeding tube was placed. At the time of her accident, Nancy Cruzan had never written any advance directive regarding her potential health care treatment. Nancy had, however, had serious discussions with a housemate about her beliefs regarding the quality of life that she would find intolerable and not worth living. In October 1987, her parents, as her guardians, petitioned the county court judge to remove the feeding tube; the request was approved. The Missouri Attorney General appealed the case to the Missouri Supreme Court, which overturned the lower court ruling because there was no clear and convincing evidence of what Nancy would have wanted if she could have chosen her own course of treatment (*Cruzan v. Harmon*, 1988).

The Missouri Supreme Court decision was appealed to the U.S. Supreme Court, and the state Supreme Court decision was upheld. Therefore, under the U.S. Supreme Court ruling, the gastrostomy feeding tube could not be removed from Nancy (*Cruzan v. Director*, 1990).

As identified in Table 39–1, a person has a legal right to self-determination and a right to privacy. The critical question in the U.S. Supreme Court decision was whether the state of Missouri could require clear and convincing evidence of the individual's previously stated or written preferences for health care treatment before authorizing the withdrawal of treatment. This question was particularly important because the removal of the gastrostomy tube would hasten Nancy's death.

The U.S. Supreme Court held that Missouri could require clear and convincing evidence of the individual's preferences before removing life-sustaining treatment. For Nancy, this indicated that either more information was needed to clearly and convincingly establish her preferences before her accident or Nancy would have to continue to live with a gastrostomy tube. In August 1990, Nancy's parents brought a second petition with additional testimony regarding Nancy's comments made before her accident. The state of Missouri did not object. The Cruzan's second request for removal of the feeding tube was granted on December 14, 1990. Nancy Cruzan died on December 26, 1990.

Suggested Interventions and Outcomes

Nancy Cruzan was unable to make her own decisions about health care treatment because she was in a persistent vegetative state and was not able to participate in the decision-making process. However, her parents were convinced that Nancy had made her wishes known during conversations with her housemate. Her parents, as her guardians, assumed the role of her substitute decision makers and hoped for a dignified death.

The Cruzan case vividly demonstrated six nursing activities of Patient Rights Protection. The activities focused on the patient's right to self-determi-nation and included all three of the subcategories of self-determination previously discussed: (1) the patient's right to make decisions for himself or herself regarding personal health care, (2) the patient's right to extend his or her right to make personal decisions to a surrogate or substitute decision maker, and (3) the patient's right to make decisions regarding his or her own personal bodily integrity. Specifically, the activities included were as follows: (1) determine whether patient's wishes about health care are known, (2) work with physician and hospital administration to honor patient and family wishes, (3) know the legal status of living wills in the state, (4) honor a patient's wishes expressed in a living will or durable power of attorney for health care, as appropriate, (5) refrain from forcing the treatment, and (6) determine who is legally empowered to give consent for treatment or research.

Nancy Cruzan's parents exerted extensive time and energy to convince the Missouri courts that Nancy had made her wishes for health care known and that their request for removal of the gastrostomy tube was an expression of her previously determined decision. The Cruzans did not have the support of the physician and hospital administration in carrying out Nancy's wishes. In fact, the hospital was assisted by the state attorney general's office in objecting to removal of the life-sustaining treatment. Nancy's parents asserted that Nancy, if she could participate in the discussion, would want to have the gastrostomy tube removed. Nancy had not written a living will but had given verbal instructions regarding her future wishes. Nancy's parents believed that the gastrostomy tube was being forced on Nancy against her wishes and against their wishes as Nancy's legally authorized substitute decision makers.

FUTURE DIRECTIONS

The intervention of Patient Rights Protection is not a new concept. Legal cases from the early 1900s indicate that the relationship between patients and health care providers has been the subject of legal controversies for almost a century. The current concerns regarding Patient Rights Protection are as follows: How do patients exert their legal rights? Is it the patient or the health care facility who has the responsibility to insure patient rights? What recourse do patients have if they feel a moral or legal right has been violated?

All the activities identified in this intervention are based on legal theory and precedent and are enforceable under established law except one: to provide each patient with a copy of a patient bill of rights. This activity is based on ethical and moral considerations and is not enforceable under the law. It is important to note that the breadth of many of the legal rights has expanded as multiple cases have been explored. It is also important to recognize that new rights have been established in the 1990s (PSDA, 1990). It is essential that nurses be aware of the legal precedents and statutes that provide the framework for this intervention and follow legal cases that support this right.

New interventions such as Self-Determination Enhancement should be developed to assist patients and families with issues such as participation in health care treatment decision making and the patient's right to refuse treatment. Finally, an outcome such as Self-Determination Control or Patient Rights Protection needs to be developed for the NOC (Johnson & Maas, 1997).

SUMMARY

This chapter summarizes the challenges that nurses face as they attempt to assist patients to explore and exercise their patient rights. In order for nurses to serve as facilitators and advocates for patient rights, nurses must understand the legal rights to privacy, free exercise of religion, and self-determination. Nurses must continue to recognize the importance of the patients' legal rights within the health care system and must continue to develop nursing diagnoses, interventions, and outcomes that address this issue.

The American Nurses Association Code for Nurses explicitly identifies the nurse's role of patient autonomy. The code states, "The nurse provides services with respect for human dignity and the uniqueness of the client unrestricted by considerations of social or economic status, personal attributes, or the nature of health problems" (American Nurses Association, 1985). The accompanying interpretive statements clarify that clients have a moral right to determine what will be done to their own person and that "truth-telling and the process of reaching informed choice underlie the exercise of self-determination" (American Nurses Association, 1985). Nurses also need to recognize and support the patient's legal rights. The complexity of health care and the impact of technology on treatment options dictate the continued emphasis on the role of nurses as patient advocates into the next century. Protecting the rights of patients is one intervention that supports this role in a complex health care system.

References

Aiken, T. D., and Catalano, J. T. (1994). *Legal, ethical, and political issues in nursing.* Philadelphia: F. A. Davis.

American Hospital Association. (1978). A Patient's Bill of Rights. *Hospitals, 52*(22), 112.

American Nurses Association. (1985). *Code for nurses with interpretive statements.* Kansas City: Author.

Anderson v. St. Francis–St. George Hospital, 614 N.E. 2d 841 (Ohio 1992).

Annas, G. J. (1992). *The rights of patients.* Totowa, NJ: Humana Press.

Beauchamp, T. L., and Childress, J. F. (1989). *Principles of biomedical ethics* (3rd ed.). New York: Oxford University Press.

Beauchamp, T. L., and Childress, J. F. (1994). *Principles of biomedical ethics* (4th ed.). New York: Oxford University Press.

Bialorucki, T., and Blaine, M. J. (1992). Protecting patient confidentiality in the pursuit of the ultimate computerized information system. *Journal of Nursing Care Quality, 7*(1), 53–56.

Brent, N. J. (1994). Protecting the AIDS patient's right to make treatment decisions. *Home Healthcare Nurse, 12*(2), 10–11.

Brent, N. J. (1997). *Nurses and the law: A guide to principles and applications.* Philadelphia: W. B. Saunders.

Brophy v. New England Sinai Hospital., Inc., 497 N.E.2d 626 (Mass. 1986).

Cahill, J. (1994). Are you prepared to be their advocate? Issues in patient advocacy. *Professional Nurse, 9,* 371–372, 374–375.

Constitution of the United States. (1791). Amendment 1.

Constitution of the United States. (1791). Amendment 9.

Constitution of the United States. (1868). Amendment 14.

Cruzan v. Director, Missouri Department of Health, 110 S. Ct. 2841 (1990).

Cruzan v. Harmon, 760 SW 2d. 408 (Mo. 1988).

Davis, M. C. (1992). The client's right to self-determination. *Caring, 11*(6), 26–32.

Dew, B. (1992). Do those who cannot speak really have a voice? *Law, Medicine and Health Care, 20*, 316–319.

Ferdinand, R. (1996). Ethical dilemmas. Jehovah's Witnesses and advance directives. *American Journal of Nursing, 96* (3 Nurse Practice Extra Edition), 64.

Fiesta, J. (1988). Nurses' duty to disclose. *Nursing Management, 19*(1), 30–32.

Foflygen v. R. Zemel, 615 A.2d 1345 (Pennsylvania 1992).

Fowler, M. D. M. (1989). When did "do not resuscitate" mean "do not care"? *Heart and Lung, 18*, 424–425.

Greve, P. (1994). Has the PSDA made a difference? *RN, 57*(2), 59, 61, 63–64.

Griswold v. Connecticut, 381 U.S. 479 (1965).

Guido G. W. (1997). *Legal issues in nursing* (2nd ed.). Stamford, CT: Appleton & Lange.

Jacobson v. Massachusetts, 197 U.S. 11 (1905).

Johns, J. L. (1996). Advance directives and opportunities for nurses. *Image: The Journal of Nursing Scholarship, 28*(2), 149–153.

Johnson, M., and Maas, M. (Eds.). (1997). *Nursing outcomes classification (NOC)*. St. Louis: Mosby–Year Book.

Joint Commission on Accreditation of Healthcare Organizations. (1997). *Comprehensive accreditation manual for hospitals: The official handbook*. Oakbrook Terrace, IL: Author.

Kelly, L. Y. (1976). The patient's right to know. *Nursing Outlook, 24*(1), 26–32.

Klop, R., van Wijmen, F. C. B., and Philipsen, J. (1991). Patients' rights and the admission and discharge process. *Journal of Advanced Nursing, 16*(4), 408–412.

Lounsbury v. Capel, 836 P.2d 188 (Utah 1992).

Matter of Conroy, 486 A.2d 1209 (1985).

Matter of Quinlan, 355 A.2d 647 (1976).

McCloskey, J. C., and Bulechek, G. M. (1992). *Nursing interventions classification (NIC)*. St. Louis: Mosby–Year Book.

McCloskey, J. C., and Bulechek, G. M. (1996). *Nursing interventions classification (NIC)*. (2nd ed.). St. Louis: Mosby–Year Book.

Nelson, M. L. (1988). Advocacy in nursing: How has it evolved and what are its implications for practice? *Nursing Outlook, 36*(3), 136–141.

Patient-Self Determination Act, Pub. L. No. 101–508. (1990).

Payne v. Marion General Hospital, 549 N.E.2d 1043 (1990).

Pratt v. Davis, 118 Ill. App. 161, 166 (1905), *aff'd* 224 Ill. 300, 79 N.E.562 (1906).

Prins, M. M. (1992). Patient advocacy: The role of nursing leadership. *Nursing Management, 23*(7 Long Term Care Edition), 78–80.

Ramsey, M. K. (1990). Patient rights and obligations. *Advancing Clinical Care, 5*(1), 29–30.

Roe v. Wade, 410 U.S. 113 (1973).

Scanlon, C. (1993). Safeguarding a patient's right to self-determination. *American Nurse, 5*(10), 20–21.

Schloendorff v. Society of New York Hospital, 105 N.E. 92 (1914).

Superintendent of Belchertown v. Saikewicz, 370 N.E.2d 417 (Mass. 1977).

Teno, J. M., Sabatino, C., Parisier, L., Rouse, F., and Lynn, J. (1993). The impact of the Patient Self-Determination Act's requirement that states describe law concerning patients' rights. *Journal of Law, Medicine and Ethics, 21*(1), 102–108.

Trandel-Korenchuk, D. M. (1982). Patients' rights and the preservation of human dignity. *Nursing Administration Quarterly, 6*, 83–86.

Uniform Durable Power of Attorney Act (U.L.A.). (1984). § 1 and comments.

Uniform Durable Power of Attorney Act (U.L.A.). (1987). § 2.

Uniform Rights of the Terminally Ill Act (U.L.A.). (1989). §2.

Union Pacific Railroad Co. v. Botsford, 141 U.S. 250 (1891).

Weiler, K., Eland, J., and Buckwalter, K. C. (1996). Iowa nurses' knowledge of living wills and perceptions of patient autonomy. *Journal of Professional Nursing, 12*, 245–252.

Weiler, K., and Moorhead, S. (In press). Self determination. In M. Maas, K. C. Buckwalter, M. Hardy, T. Tripp-Reimer, and M. Titler (Eds.), *Nursing diagnoses, interventions and outcomes for the elderly* (2nd ed.). Thousand Oaks, CA: Sage Publications.

Weiler, K., and Slavik Cowen, P. (In press). Legal and ethical issues for elders in transition. In E. Swanson and T. Tripp-Reimer (Eds.), *Advances in gerontological nursing: Working with the elderly in transition*. New York: Springer Publishing.

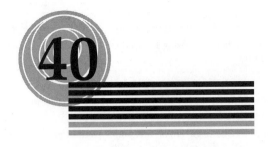

Culture Brokerage

Toni Tripp-Reimer, Pamela J. Brink,
and Carol S. Pinkham

Culture Brokerage is an act of mediation in which messages, instructions, and belief systems are manipulated and processed from one group to another. As a nursing intervention, Culture Brokerage primarily involves the nurse's acting as a mediator between clients and members of the biomedical health professions. Culture Brokerage may be used whenever there are separate culture groups and a need to establish links between them. As a nursing intervention, Culture Brokerage occurs most obviously between minority clients and orthodox health professionals. Brokerage, however, is sometimes necessary between the popular culture of the lay client and the scientific culture of the health professional. Culture Brokerage is defined in the Nursing Interventions Classification (NIC) (McCloskey & Bulechek, 1996) as "bridging, negotiating, or linking the orthodox health care system with a patient and family of a different culture" (Table 40–1).

Brokers are individuals who occupy linkage roles between sectors of a society. Sussex and Weidman (1975) identified nursing personnel as the bearers and transmitters of a professional health culture in which patients and staff are interlocked in processes of learning, supporting, and changing behavior in mutually beneficial ways. Culture Brokerage is a nursing intervention more than an intervention for other health professionals because nursing education emphasizes the social as well as the biological sciences, and nurses generally have the closest relationships with the client's family and significant others.

Weidman (1982) states, "In the context of clinical activities, culture brokerage encourages behavior by health professionals which theoretically should lead to greater success for the clinician and a better outcome for the patient. In order for the health practitioner to negotiate between divergent health beliefs and

Table 40–1   Culture Brokerage

DEFINITION: Bridging, negotiating, or linking the orthodox health care system with a patient and family of a different culture.

ACTIVITIES:

Determine the nature of the conceptual differences that the patient and nurse have of the illness

Discuss discrepancies openly and clarify conflicts

Negotiate, when conflicts cannot be resolved, an acceptable compromise of treatment based on biomedical knowledge, knowledge of the patient's point of view, and ethical standards

Allow the patient more than the usual time to process the information and work through a decision

Appear relaxed and unhurried in interactions with the patient

Allow more time for translation, discussion, and explanation

Use nontechnical language

Determine the "belief variability ratio"—the degree of distance the patient sees between self and cultural group

Use a language translator, if necessary (e.g., signing, or Spanish)

Include the family, when appropriate, in the plan for adherence with the prescribed regimen

Translate the patient's symptom terminology into health care language that other professionals can more easily understand

Provide information to the patient about the orthodox health care system

Provide information to the health care providers about the patient's culture

Source: McCloskey, J. C., and Bulechek, G. M. (1996). *Nursing interventions classification (NIC)* (2nd ed.). St. Louis: Mosby–Year Book.

practices, it is necessary to determine the nature of the beliefs and concerns that guide the patient's behavior. Only then can areas of difference or incompatibility be determined. And only after these are identified can mediation be attempted" (p. 211).

If used properly, the intervention of Culture Brokerage can result in the following benefits in clinical situations:

1. A more comprehensive understanding of the client by the practitioner and a more realistic treatment plan
2. Greater congruence between the patient's perception of illness and the practitioner's perception of the patient's pathology
3. Increased compatibility between the client's notions of desired treatments and the scientific therapeutic regimen
4. Increased client satisfaction and adherence and decreased practitioner frustration.

Culture Brokerage has a broader scope than that of most nursing interventions, which are directed primarily toward altering aspects of the client's system. Culture Brokerage may focus on the client, on the health professional, or on mediation between both. Thus, Culture Brokerage may take three basic forms:

1. Culture Brokerage may target the client to facilitate management of the illness and its consequences. This presumes the nurse broker understands what is important to the client and how the illness is interpreted. Cultures have differing values and beliefs pertaining to role expectations, family lifestyles, child-rearing activities, patterns of authority, occupational patterns, religious prescriptions, educational achievements, political affiliation,

and dietary practices. Nurses who understand the client's specific orientation in these areas can anticipate illness-oriented problems that derive from the particular culture base.

2. Culture Brokerage may assist practitioners in adapting biomedical methods, communications, or intervention strategies into culturally appropriate ones. DeSantis (1994) suggested an additional component of this form: Culture Brokerage as mediating between nurses or other professional colleagues from different cultural groups or health care delivery systems.

3. Culture Brokerage may simultaneously target the client and the health practitioner, as when the client and the practitioner have different views about the cause, meaning, or treatment of an illness. In this case, each person's perspective needs to be translated to the other.

Basic to Culture Brokerage is cultural competence. Cultural competence has been defined as a "set of congruent behaviors, attitudes, and policies that come together in a system, agency or amongst professionals and enables that system, agency, or those professionals to work effectively in cross-cultural situations" (Cross, Bazron, Dennis, & Isaacs, 1989, p. iv). The term *cultural competence* has come to widely reflect the need to extend beyond awareness and sensitivity (which often lose power after the assessment phase) and to plan, implement, and evaluate interventions on the basis of cultural factors. The mandate in nursing is evident in publications by the American Academy of Nursing (Lenburg et al., 1995; Meleis, Isenberg, Loerner, Lacey, & Stern, 1995). The components of cultural competence include awareness of and sensitivity to cultural differences; knowledge of cultural values, beliefs, and behaviors; and skill in working with culturally diverse populations. These characteristics, however, reside in the practitioner and are prerequisite to using Culture Brokerage as an intervention.

An important component of Culture Brokerage is an understanding of the distinction between the concepts of disease and illness (Eisenberg, 1977; Kleinman, Eisenberg, & Good, 1978; Tripp-Reimer, 1984). Diseases are abnormalities in the structure and function of body organs and systems; they are problems of biological malfunctioning. Illness, on the other hand, encompasses the subjective experiences of the individual who is sick and includes the way this sickness is perceived and experienced by the individual and the social group. In other words, or more simply, illness involves *perceived symptoms*, whereas disease involves the *underlying pathology*. The client is predominantly concerned with illness. Medicine is primarily concerned with disease: its etiology, pathology, and treatment. Nursing uses both the model of illness and the model of disease and mediates between the two.

In order to use Culture Brokerage successfully, the nurse needs knowledge of the client's culture and its influence on health beliefs and behaviors. The nurse also must have insight into the culture of scientific health professionals to ascertain which elements are crucial to clinical effectiveness and which are superfluous. Finally, the nurse needs skills in communication and negotiation for mediating between the two systems.

RELATED LITERATURE ON CULTURE BROKERAGE

The concept of the culture broker emerged from the discipline of anthropology. The earliest work on culture brokers by Wolf (1956) and Geertz (1960) looked at individuals who served as middlemen between groups at local and national levels. These local men usually lived in small villages and served as the economic or political intermediaries between their own group at the local level and a group at the national level. Brokers tend to emerge in situations involving culture change or culture conflict. Consequently, the broker role has been apparent particularly in Latin America (Adams, 1970; Press, 1969; Salovesh, 1978; Wolf, 1956) and Southeast Asia (Geertz, 1960) and sometimes in Africa (Silver, 1979), the Arctic (Paine, 1971), and the United States (Hannerz, 1974).

In anthropological literature, the term *culture broker* has been applied to a variety of roles that link various sections of society: teachers, religious and political leaders, artists, public health physicians, and agricultural extension agents. For example, Adams (1970) notes that in Guatemala, as in many other Latin American countries, the male school teacher is a cultural representative of the national system working in a culture different from that in which he is used to operating. Although the teacher translates information from the national system to the local community, he usually has no power of his own. Adams also notes that the same may be said for the public health physician and the agricultural extension agent. Adams defines the culture broker as an individual from one level who lives or operates among individuals of another level. Whatever influence he or she may have on the other level depends basically not on the power the broker can wield but on personal skill and personal influence. Culture brokers are usually sponsored through upper-level decisions and act at lower levels. Their tasks are seldom of high priority, however, because the failure in performance of their duties is not a threat to the position of the individuals sponsoring them at the national level.

Essential to the functioning of the broker is the broker's marginal status (Press, 1969). From his study of a Yucatan peasant community, Press suggests that role ambiguity serves as a crucial mechanism in the genesis of the broker role. During the development of the innovative role, ambiguity allows novel behavior while retarding negative sanction. In this study, Press described the manner in which culture brokers arise, receive permission to innovate, and create a role in which innovative behavior becomes an expectation.

As cited by Whitten and Wolfe (1973), Boissevian conceptualized brokers as dealing through interpersonal linkages by transforming and using interpersonal relations for some perceived advantage. In the process, they affect social relationships. These brokers transmit, direct, filter, receive, code, decode, and interpret messages. Such strategically placed persons may turn their skills as brokers into personal power, manipulating networks to their own advantage.

Similarly, Wolf (1956), Press (1969), Salovesh (1978), and Silver (1979) all discuss the notion that it is to the benefit of a person in a permanent culture broker role to deliberately leave tensions unresolved or perhaps even increase them in order to maintain the continuing need for a buffering agent. Wolf (1956) contends that the position of these brokers is an exposed one because, Janus-like, they face two directions at once. They must serve some of the interests of the groups operating on both the community and the national levels, and they must cope with the conflicts raised by the collision of these interests. Permanent brokers, however, cannot afford to totally resolve conflicts, because by doing so they would abolish their usefulness to others.

Weidman (1973, 1975, 1982) and Sussex and Weidman (1975) developed the concept of culture broker in the health care delivery system. The culture broker role, according to Weidman (1973), is that of an intermediary, and this could be applied whenever there is a need to recognize the existence of separate cultural or subcultural traditions and to acknowledge an individual's role in establishing meaningful linkages between them. As Weidman conceived the role, however, the culture broker was an anthropologist who was placed in a health care setting and would be emulated by health care professionals. She views the culture broker as having the responsibility of linking, negotiating, and meshing aspects of two health culture systems that confront each other the moment the physician and patient meet.

There is an important distinction between Culture Brokerage as the full-time role covered by Weidman and as a nursing intervention (Tripp-Reimer & Brink, 1985). As a full-time role, the concept had its origins in political anthropology. There the broker needed to maintain distance, barriers, and tensions between groups. Otherwise, the broker's role would end; that is, if brokerage is too successful, the broker is out of a job. Although Culture Brokerage in both anthropology and nursing mandates action (Chrisman, 1982; Press, 1969), it is the therapeutic mandate of nursing that drives nursing's definition of Culture Brokerage. When Culture Brokerage is used as a nursing intervention, it is one possible intervention among many, and as such is not a full-time role. There is no utility to maintaining barriers between the patient and the health care system. Successful Culture Brokerage is an advantage in that it produces an environment in which the nurse and other health professionals can move on to new and more health-oriented interventions after the broker role has been fulfilled.

Culture Brokerage can be of particular utility when a nurse is confronted with a situation involving ethical issues. Ethics evolve from the values and mores held by a society (Holleran, 1990) and differ crossculturally. Furthermore, health care professionals cannot automatically assume that a particular patient or ethnic group subscribes to bioethics, "a field whose origins lie in the branches of Western (primarily Anglo-American) philosophy and law that give primacy to the individual and emphasize individual rights, self-determination, and privacy" (Muller, 1994, p. 450). Different cultures have varying approaches to such topics as autonomy, individual versus societal rights, the right to die, disclosure, reproductive freedom, and other concepts of ethical concern (Gruzalski & Nelson, 1982; McCloskey & Grace, 1990; Pellegrino, Mazzarella & Corsi, 1992). The moral decision making of people and groups is contextualized within their cultural systems, and to be an effective culture broker in a situation involving an ethical dilemma, the nurse should be familiar with the concept of moral pluralism, "the idea that the views held by a group of people, however defined, of what is good and bad, right and wrong may legitimately differ from those held by other groups and further, that the differences often derive from a variation in the cultural values, customs, norms, and the 'worldview' of the groups whose morals are being compared" (Murray, 1992, p. 36).

Beyond being familiar with the concept of moral pluralism, the nurse should be cognizant of the utility of the concept and work within it to mediate and negotiate toward a resolution that is satisfactory to the groups involved in the situation. A perspective of interest to nursing is that espoused by Pellegrino (1992) in calling for metacultural ethics, which can transcend culture by emphasizing the dignity of the human person and the inalienable position of what it means to be a human being. This is similar to Tripp-Reimer and Fox's (1990) cautionary note on categorization and differentiation that can preclude the delivery of holistic and humanistic care.

Within nursing, Culture Brokerage has been described in almost every case example involving nurse–client interactions when the nurse is from one culture or ethnic group and the client is from another. However, rarely have the descriptions labeled the intervention as Culture Brokerage, more often using the terms *negotiation* or *mediation*. Barbee (1987) reports the results of a qualitative study of the primary role of nurses in Botswana and describes how nurses broker between traditional and biomedical beliefs. Jezewski (1990) discusses culture brokering in migrant farm worker health care and identifies nurses as the health professionals most often involved in the brokering role. Subsequently, Jezewski (1995) depicted a multistaged grounded theory of Culture Brokerage as conflict resolution. Chalanda (1995) addressed conceptual issues in multicultural nursing, and Banoub-Baddour and Laryea (1992) used Culture Brokerage as a strategy in assessing and managing cancer pain in preschool children.

INTERVENTION TECHNIQUES

Culture Brokerage was adopted as a nursing intervention by the NIC in 1992 and preserved in the expanded and revised second edition (McCloskey & Bulechek, 1996). The intervention includes a list of nursing activities designed to achieve patient outcomes in keeping with the NIC definition of the intervention. (See Table 40–1 for NIC definition and activities.) There are several techniques that fit under the rubric of Culture Brokerage.

One strategy of Culture Brokerage is to treat cultural assessment as a process rather than simply a content area (Tripp-Reimer, Brink & Saunders, 1984). Culture Brokerage requires a clinically appropriate cultural assessment of the patient (whether individual or group) that elicits several basic data sets by using the patient as a cultural informant who is more knowledgeable about the culture than is the health professional. The health professional, therefore, uses the patient as the resource for cultural data. The nurse enters into the clinical interview with an eye toward gaining an increased understanding of the culture from which the patient comes, in addition to learning the patient's health history and eliciting a description of symptoms. The first phase of cultural assessment consists of collecting three sets of data: (1) background information including ethnicity, degree of ethnic affiliation, language preference, religion, and patterns of decision making; (2) problem-specific information including the patient's definition of the problem and treatment beliefs and preferences; (3) intervention-specific data including an assessment of the cultural appropriateness of the standard recommended therapy, patient and family plans for self-care, and need for family involvement in continued care. In the second phase of cultural assessment, the nurse compares the patient data with comparable information derived from standards of practice from the nursing profession or agency policy. The nurse then mediates between the patient and the nursing protocols or agency policies. One book, *Community, Culture, and Care: A Cross Cultural Guide for Health Workers* (Brownlee, 1978), is devoted to the process of practical assessments in situations demanding Culture Brokerage. Brownlee states that she wrote the book to "provide a readily accessible and practically oriented guide for health workers and students on what they need to learn about their own culture and organization and the culture around them, why the information is important and how to go about gathering it" (p. vi). Each chapter deals with three aspects of assessment: (1) what to find out, (2) why it is important, and (3) how to do it. Because of the sheer practicality of the volume, its simplicity of language, and its almost outline format, Brownlee's book continues to provide the most comprehensive approach to cultural assessment.

The intervention technique of *negotiation* is described by Katon and Kleinman (1981) as used for clinical interviews between the health professional and the patient. They define negotiation as a "bilateral arrangement in which the two principal parties attempt to work out a solution. . . . The goal is to reduce conflict in a way that promotes cooperation" (pp. 262, 276). Negotiation, as an intervention strategy for Culture Brokerage, is used when a conceptual difference exists between the patient and the nurse. When conflicts or discrepancies arise between clients and health professionals, the following model of negotiation is offered:

1. The health professional asks questions to find out how the patient explains the illness or health problem.
2. The health professional then clearly and fully presents (in lay terms) an explanation of the disorder, including the recommended treatment, and invites questions from patient and family, to which full explanations are given. The point here is to work within the patient's frame of reference and level of understanding.
3. A working alliance is possible when the patient's personal explanation of the illness either agrees with or shifts to the health professional's model, or if the recommendations of the health professional shift more toward the patient's expectations of treatment.
4. At times, discrepancies remain. When this occurs, the health professional can openly acknowledge and clarify conflict. The health professional is ethically entitled to provide references and data to support his or her position but should also allow the patient and the patient's family to provide references and data to argue their position. The health professional continues to elicit the patient's explanatory model until understanding is reached.
5. At this juncture, either the professional or the patient will change sides to arrive at a mutually desired treatment.
6. When a conflict cannot be resolved, the health professional should attempt to arrive at an acceptable compromise of treatment based on biomedical knowledge, knowledge of the patient's point of view, and ethical standards.
7. When all else fails, the health professional needs to recognize that the role is to provide expert advice and rationale for the treatment recommendations but that it is the patient (or patient's family) who is the final decision maker in the situation. If a complete stalemate is reached, the health professional is responsible for offering a referral to another person. Finally, the patient may seek advice from another health provider without fear of reprisal by the system.
8. Throughout this process, each negotiation involves an ongoing monitoring of the agreement and of each party's participation in the agreement (Katon & Kleinman, 1981).

The concept of negotiation in Culture Brokerage is based on the idea that health professionals and patients should meet and interact with each other as equals in an attempt to achieve an outcome satisfactory to both parties in the interaction. In order to achieve this goal, power must shift from residing almost solely with the clinician to an aspect shared with the patient or patient's family. Only by doing this first step can the nursing intervention of Culture Brokerage be successful. Negotiation of treatment plans for patients should include investigation into whether the patient's health beliefs and practices are helpful (adaptive), neither helpful nor harmful (neutral), or harmful (maladaptive), with the goal of incorporation of helpful or adaptive beliefs and practices, accommodation of neutral beliefs and practices, and repatterning of harmful or maladaptive beliefs and practices (Jackson, 1993; Leininger, 1984; Tripp-Reimer et al., 1984).

A third strategy of the Culture Brokerage intervention is the therapeutic use of time (Zola, 1981). Clients and their families need time to absorb information. Time, therefore, needs to be set aside, specifically, for the processing of information between the history, the physical examination, and the diagnosis; between the diagnosis and the treatment alternatives; and between the treatment alternatives and the decision by the patient or family to accept or reject the information provided. Instant decisions in health-illness situations deprive clients of the right to work through decision making at their own pace. Concomitant with the client's decision making is the encouragement and presence of significant others during all phases of the health encounter. "What patients are responding to when they do not cooperate is not the medical treatment but how they are treated, not how they regard their required medical regimen but how they themselves are regarded" (Zola, 1981, p. 250).

Health professionals need to be aware that interactions with clients of different cultures or ethnic groups will take more time and that an important skill of the professional is to appear relaxed and unhurried. Longer appointment periods can be scheduled to allow for the time it will take for translation, for discussion and clarification of concepts, for explanation of the diagnosis, for negotiation of a treatment regimen, and for socialization to the health care delivery system (Harwood, 1981). Culture Brokerage takes time. Even when the client is of the same culture as the health professional, the same process of negotiation needs to take place, and time must be given to the process. Many times health professionals forget that they represent the "health culture" with its jargon and belief systems, whereas the client represents the "lay culture" with all its belief systems (Brink & Saunders, 1976). Just because two people speak English and grew up in the United States does not automatically translate into clear communication.

The client expects the health professional to be knowledgeable about the illness, its symptoms, and its cure, and to care for the patient as a person, not as a case. These characteristics are demonstrated by the practitioner's ability to use nontechnical language, to explain the symptoms of the illness that the patient is experiencing rather than the biomedical causes (or the pathology), and to explain the relationship between the symptoms, the diagnosis, and the treatment plan with the prediction of the outcome. This is, of course, done in a professional manner, which is projected by careful listening, politeness, warmth, and an unhurried manner (Harwood, 1981). The importance of patience and an unhurried manner has been explicated in discussions of cultural awareness in the context of terminal illness (Pickett, 1993), the process of intercultural communication (Nance, 1995), and elicitation of health beliefs (Jackson, 1993).

A fourth strategy of Culture Brokerage involves the use of a translator for the client for whom English is not the preferred language. In this case, either the translator or the nurse serves as broker and creates the link between the two parties. Again, taking time, offering an appearance of being unhurried, and selecting a place that is comfortable to the client are all brokerage techniques. Although the translator may assist in translating from one language to another, the nurse is still responsible for determining the meaning of the words and their emotional impact on the situation. Two articles address the complexity of translation in the communication process. Coler (1994) points out that problems in communication often begin when translation is done as a word-for-word process without considering possible culture-bound interpretations and perceptions, and Nance (1995) discusses the theory that the communication process is transactional, and as such is not only message transfer but also the creation of meaning.

As was noted earlier, Culture Brokerage does not involve simply a one-way interaction in which the health professional learns to adapt and translate the patient's needs and meanings; Culture Brokerage may be directed toward health professionals as well. There are times when the nurse will "broker" between patients and other health professionals. At these times, the same strategies apply to the health professional as to the patient. One key to assisting the health professional to work with a patient of another culture is for the nurse to translate what the patient means in terminology readily understood by the health professional. Whereas patients may need lay terms to understand, the health professional sometimes needs professional language in order to make sense of an interaction.

One example of a brokerage tool used in clinical nursing education was developed by the School of Medicine at the University of Miami in an inservice training program (Scott, 1983). A chart composed of two axes is given to the students. On the vertical axis are five categories of data: (1) symptoms that identify the disease, (2) causes of the disease, (3) labels for the disease, (4) perception of bodily function when the disease is present, and (5) ways of preventing, curing, and treating the disease. On the horizontal axis, there are two categories: (1) the traditional folk beliefs of the patient or client group and (2) the orthodox or Western biomedical beliefs about the disease. The chart is used in a group work session in which a group of students is assigned a particular disease, such as diabetes, and is then asked to fill in all areas of the chart. The chart easily identifies the patient's idea of illness and contrasts it with the professional's concept. In this way, areas of cultural conflict are immediately apparent. The same sort of Culture Brokerage tool could be developed for graduate programs in nursing, particularly in nurse practitioner programs, in order to "translate" culture content into the frame of reference of the student.

ASSOCIATED NURSING DIAGNOSES
■

Because culture pervades all domains of life, there are no nursing diagnoses that specifically indicate the intervention of Culture Brokerage. That is, virtually any behavioral category of nursing diagnosis may have a culturally based etiology and need Culture Brokerage. Some suggested nursing diagnoses that may call for this intervention are Impaired Verbal Communication, Anxiety, Noncompliance, Ineffective Coping, Fear, Altered Health Maintenance, Knowledge Deficit, Altered Nutrition, Altered Parenting, Powerlessness, disturbance in self concept, Social Isolation, Spiritual Distress, and Impaired Social Interaction. Frequently, it is the diagnosis of Noncompliance that triggers the identification of the need for Culture Brokerage. It may be only when the patient is noncompliant that health professionals become aware that there is a problem that cannot be solved in the usual way. Culture Brokerage is a time-consuming intervention and is not usually chosen when there is little time to spare. Only when there is a disruption of the routines of the health professionals and their work becomes impaired or inefficient does the need for further assessment and different intervention strategies become apparent. At this time, the intervention of Culture Brokerage may be the most appropriate. Geissler (1991b) suggests that *nonadherence* would be a more culturally relevant diagnosis, being less value laden.

However, it is important to recognize that nursing diagnoses from the North American Nursing Diagnosis Association (NANDA) have been criticized as being ethnocentric and offering little guidance in caring for culturally diverse clients. Geissler (1991a) particularly cited problems with the diagnoses of Impaired Verbal Communication, Impaired Social Interaction, and Noncompliance. For example, language differences may result in a diagnosis of Impaired Verbal Communication; the consequent brokerage intervention would be to find methods or individuals for translating information between practitioner and client. Geissler clearly points out that the difficulty is not impaired verbal communication. Because both the nurse and the client are fluent in their respective languages, the real difficulty is a barrier to mutual understanding.

ASSOCIATED NURSING OUTCOMES

As was true of nursing diagnoses, there are no nursing outcomes that specifically flow from the intervention Culture Brokerage. Virtually any behavioral category of nursing outcome may derive from Culture Brokerage. Most typically, however, the associated outcomes come from the following broad categories of the Nursing Outcomes Classification (NOC) in the following decreasing order: Health Attitudes, Knowledge, and Behavior; Perceived Well-Being, Psychological, and Cognitive Status; Social and Role Status; Family Caregiver Status; and Safety Status. Physical Functional Status and Physiological Status are the outcomes least likely to be targeted areas of outcomes for the intervention Culture Brokerage. Although research has not yet been conducted in this area, the following specific nursing outcomes would be commonly expected as goals of this intervention: Health Seeking Behavior: adherence and compliance; Knowledge (All); Health Beliefs (All); Well-Being; Identity; Hope; Symptom Control Behavior; Health Orientation; Spiritual Well-Being; Grief Resolution; Participation: Health Care Decisions; Decision Making; Coping; Social Support; Health Promoting Behavior; and Health Seeking Behavior.

A frequent outcome of Culture Brokerage is adherence, which means that the client follows a prescribed treatment regimen. Adherence can be enhanced by enlisting the family or significant others to reinforce the treatment regimen; including the most influential member of the family in the treatment plan; discontinuing the treatment when the symptoms have gone or explaining why treatment should continue; using the client's preferred methods of treatment when they are not directly contradictory to the treatment needed; and placing treatment in the setting where it is most wanted—home or hospital.

Harwood (1981) has a series of suggestions that health professionals can use to promote adherence:

1. For most lay persons (non–health professionals), relief of pain or a decrease or cessation of specific symptoms generally indicates the person is cured. Discuss with patient whether treatment is necessary beyond relief of symptoms and if so, explain why.
2. Discuss in depth those symptoms that appear to be most anxiety provoking for the client or the client's family, especially with regard to cause, severity, and ways in which treatment will affect them.
3. Determine which forms of medical treatment are most anxiety provoking for the patient and family.
4. Discuss with the patient and family alternative ways of fulfilling the sick person's responsibilities while the individual is sick.
5. Discuss any limitations on valued activities resulting from medical treatment, and help patients devise ways of coping with them (Harwood, 1981, pp. 492–495).

CASE STUDIES

Case Study 1

One of the authors was called in for a consultation on an inpatient acute care unit. The nursing staff stated that too many visitors were in the room at one time and that this was against the hospital policy. In assessing the situation, the culture broker established the environmental parameters of the situation by determining whether or not there was any contraindication to nursing care by having a large number of people in the room at one time. The social environment was also assessed in relation to whether or not the patient had a roommate and whether this was causing a problem. On establishing that the large number of visitors was not of health significance but was simply violating a hospital rule, the nurse consultant suggested that the patient be allowed to have the visitors. Although the patient and patient's family were not adhering to a hospital rule, the nonadherence was not a true problem but simply an infraction of a nonfunctional rule. The culture broker translated to the nursing staff the social needs of the patient (who was Amish) during hospitalization to show that these needs took precedence over a general rule that did not apply to a particular situation. In this case, the nurse consultant was a culture broker to the staff and not to the patient.

Case Study 2

A nurse in a large western city was doing a home visit to find out why a child was not attending school. The child was in a special education program for the mentally retarded. The mother was Native American and had, until recently, lived on a reservation. During the interview, the nurse discovered that the child had refused to return to school and that the mother had not insisted. The nurse understood that many Native Americans contend that children have the right to make their own decisions for themselves. It was up to the nurse to explain the school system, the beliefs about truancy, and the benefits of the special education program. Once the mother was convinced, the nurse then enticed the child back to school. The original nursing diagnosis that triggered the "clinical negotiation" strategy of the Culture Brokerage intervention was Noncompliance. The action was to translate the new urban environmental requirements to the mother and to counsel her on survival strategies. The second aspect of the intervention was for the nurse to disregard her personal beliefs about how much autonomy a child should have as she talked to the child in the child's terms and at the child's level of understanding. Once the nurse accepted the fact that the child had the final decision-making power about going to school, the nurse was able to adapt her clinical strategies to those of a different belief system.

SUMMARY

Culture Brokerage is commonly triggered by the nursing diagnosis of Noncompliance or nonadherance. The first step in brokering is conducting a cultural assessment. The cultural assessment is valuable in yielding data that assist the nurse in targeting and adapting the intervention to obtain optimal outcomes. Constant clarification of each party's positions, repeated checking of perceptions, and ongoing monitoring of each party's participation in the negotiation are essential actions in the brokering process. Initiating this intervention, the nurse then moves into an unhurried time strategy and assumes that flexibility of beliefs and values is needed, because differences will probably exist in these areas. The nurse may find that the patient needs to be allowed to retain a belief rather than abandon it. At other times, just listening is enough. Finally, there are times when the staff must be taught to accept the patient's position and allow the patient to dictate a style of health care more in keeping with that of the patient's beliefs and values.

References

Adams, R. (1970). Brokers and career mobility systems in the structure of complex societies. *Southwestern Journal of Anthropology, 26*, 315–327.

Banoub-Baddour, S., and Laryea, M. (1992). Culture brokering: The essence of nursing care for preschool children suffering from cancer-related pain. *Canadian Oncology Nursing Journal, 2*(4), 132–136.

Barbee, E. L. (1987). Tensions in the brokerage role: Nurses in Botswana. *Western Journal of Nursing Research, 9*, 244–256.

Brink, P. J., and Saunders, J. (1976). Culture shock: Theoretical and applied. In P. Brink (Ed.), *Transcultural nursing: A book of readings* (pp. 126–138). Englewood Cliffs, NJ: Prentice-Hall.

Brownlee, A. T. (1978). *Community, culture, and care: A cross cultural guide for health workers.* St. Louis: C. V. Mosby.

Chalanda, M. (1995). Brokerage in multicultural nursing. *International Nursing Review, 42*(1), 19–22.

Chrisman, N. J. (1982). Anthropology in nursing: An exploration of adaptation. In N. J. Chrisman and T. W. Maretzki (Eds.), *Clinically applied anthropology* (pp. 35–59). Dordecht, Holland: D. Reidel Publishing.

Coler, M. S. (1994). Achieving linguistic clarity: A model to aid translations. *Nursing Diagnoses, 5*(3), 102–105.

Cross, T. L., Bazron, B. J., Dennis, K. W., and Isaacs, M. R. (1989). *Towards a culturally competent system of care: A monograph on effective services for minority children who are severely emotionally disturbed.* Washington, DC: Child and Adolescent Service System Program (CASSP), CASSP Technical Assistance Center, Georgetown University Child Development Center.

DeSantis, L. (1994). Making anthropology clinically relevant to nursing. *Journal of Advanced Nursing, 20*, 707–715.

Eisenberg, L. (1977). Disease and illness: Distinction between popular and professional ideas of sickness. *Culture, Medicine and Psychiatry, 1*, 9–23.

Geertz, C. (1960). The Javanese Kijaji: The changing role of a culture broker. *Comparative studies in Society and History: An International Quarterly, 2*, 228–249.

Geissler, E. M. (1991a). Nursing diagnoses of culturally diverse patients. *International Nursing Review, 38*(5), 150–152.

Geissler, E. M. (1991b). Transcultural nursing and nursing diagnoses. *Nursing and Health Care, 12*(4), 190–192, 203.

Gruzalski, B., and Nelson, C. (1982). *Value conflicts in health care delivery.* Cambridge, MA: Ballinger Publishing.

Hannerz, U. (1974). Ethnicity and opportunity in urban America. In A. Cohen (Ed.), *Urban ethnicity* (pp. 37–76). New York: Tavistock.

Harwood, A. (1981). Guidelines for culturally appropriate health care. In A. Harwood (Ed.), *Ethnicity and medical care* (pp. 482–507). Cambridge, MA: Harvard University Press.

Holleran, C. A. (1990). What are the ethical issues from a worldwide viewpoint. In J. C. McCloskey and H. K. Grace (Eds.), *Current issues in nursing.* St. Louis: C. V. Mosby.

Jackson, L. E. (1993). Understanding, eliciting, and negotiating clients' multicultural health beliefs. *Nurse Practitioner, 18*(4), 30–32, 37–43.

Jezewski, M. A. (1990). Culture brokering in migrant farmworker health care. *Western Journal of Nursing Research, 12*, 497–513.

Jezewski, M. A. (1995). Evolution of a grounded theory: Conflict resolution through cultural brokering. *Advances in Nursing Science, 17*(3), 14–30.

Katon, W., and Kleinman, A. (1981). Doctor-patient negotiation and other social science strategies in patient care. In L. Eisenberg and A. Kleinman (Eds.), *The relevance of social science for medicine* (pp. 253–279). Boston: D. Reidal Publishing.

Kleinman, A., Eisenberg, M., and Good, B. (1978). Culture, illness, and care. *Annals of Internal Medicine, 88*, 251–258.

Leininger, M. M. (1984). Southern rural black and white American lifeways with focus on care and health phenomena. In M. M. Leininger (Ed.), *Care: The essence of nursing and health* (pp. 133–159). Thorofare, NJ: Slack.

Lenburg, C. B., Lipson, J. G., Demi, A. S., Blaney, D. R., Stern, P. N., Schultz, P. R., and Gage, L. (1995). *Promoting cultural competence in and through nursing education: A critical review and comprehensive plan for action.* Washington, DC: American Academy of Nursing.

McCloskey, J. C., and Bulechek, G. M. (1996). *Nursing interventions classification (NIC)* (2nd ed.). St. Louis: Mosby–Year Book.

McCloskey, J. C., and Grace, H. K. (Eds.). (1990). *Current issues in nursing.* St. Louis: C. V. Mosby.

Meleis, A. I., Isenberg, M., Loerner, J. E., Lacey, B., and Stern, P. N. (1995). *Diversity, marginalization, and culturally competent health care: Issues in knowledge development.* Washington, DC: American Academy of Nursing.

Muller, J. H. (1994). Anthropology, bioethics, and medicine: A provocative trilogy. *Medical Anthropology Quarterly, 8*, 448–467.

Murray, R. F., Jr. (1992). Minority perspectives on biomedical ethics. In E. Pellegrino, P. Mazzarella, and P. Corsi (Eds.), *Transcultural dimensions in medical ethics* (pp. 35–42). Frederick, MD: University Publishing Group.

Nance, T. A. (1995). Intercultural communication: Finding common ground. *Journal of Obstetric and Gynecological Neonatal Nursing, 24*, 249–255.

Paine, R. (1971). A theory of patronage and brokerage. In R. Paine (Ed.), *Patrons and brokers in the east Arctic* (Newfoundland Social and Economic Papers #2). Toronto, Canada: University of Toronto Press.

Pellegrino, E. D. (1992). Prologue: Intersections of western biomedical ethics and world culture. In E. Pellegrino, P. Mazzarella, and P. Corsi (Eds.), *Transcultural dimensions in medical ethics* (pp. 13–19). Frederick, MD: University Publishing Group.

Pellegrino, E. D., Mazzarella, P., and Corsi, P. (1992). *Transcultural dimensions in medical ethics.* Frederick, MD: University Publishing Group.

Pickett, M. (1993). Cultural awareness in the context of terminal illness. *Cancer Nursing, 16*(2), 102–106.

Press, I. (1969). Ambiguity and innovation: Implications for the genesis of the culture broker. *American Anthropologist, 71*, 205–217.

Salovesh, M. (1978). When brokers go broke: Implications of role failure and culture brokerage. In R. Holloman and S. Arutiunov (Eds.), *Perspective on ethnicity* (pp. 351–371). The Hague, Netherlands: Mouton.

Scott, C. S. (1983). A technique for teaching transculturally oriented health care. *Medical Anthropology Quarterly, 14*(3), 7.

Silver, H. (1979). Beauty and the "I" of the beholder: Identity, aesthetics, and social change among the Ashanti. *Journal of Anthropological Research, 35,* 191–207.

Sussex, J., and Weidman, H. (1975). Toward responsiveness in mental health care. *Psychiatric Annals, 5,* 306–311.

Tripp-Reimer, T. (1984). Reconceptualizing the construct of health: Integrating emic and etic perspectives. *Research in Nursing and Health, 7,* 101–109.

Tripp-Reimer, T., and Brink, P. (1985). Culture brokerage. In G. M. Bulechek and J. McCloskey (Eds.), *Nursing interventions: Treatments for nursing* (pp. 352–364). Philadelphia: W. B. Saunders.

Tripp-Reimer, T., Brink, P., and Saunders, J. (1984). Cultural assessment: Content and process. *Nursing outlook, 32*(2), 78–82.

Tripp-Reimer, T., and Fox, S. (1990). Beyond the concept of culture: Or, how knowing the cultural formula does not predict clinical success. In J. C. McCloskey and H. K. Grace (Eds.), *Current issues in nursing* (pp. 542–546). St. Louis: C. V. Mosby.

Weidman, H. (1973, March). *Implications of the culture broker concept for the delivery of health care.* Paper presented at the annual meeting of the Southern Anthropological Society, Wrightsville Beach, NC.

Weidman, H. (1975). Concepts as strategies for change. *Psychiatric Annals, 5,* 312–314.

Weidman, H. (1982). Research strategies, structural alterations and clinically applied anthropology. In N. Chrisman and T. Maretzki (Eds.), *Clinically applied anthropology: Anthropologists in health science settings* (pp. 201–241). Boston: D. Reidel Publishing.

Whitten, N., and Wolfe, A. (1973). Network analysis. In J. Honigman (Ed.), *Handbook of social and cultural anthropology* (pp. 717–746). Chicago: Rand McNally.

Wolf, E. (1956). Aspects of group relations in a complex society: Mexico. *American Anthropologist, 58,* 1065–1078.

Zola, I. K. (1981). Structural constraints in the doctor-patient relationship: The case of non-compliance. In L. Eisenberg and A. Kleinman (Eds.), *The relevance of social science for medicine* (pp. 241–252). Boston: D. Reidel Publishing.

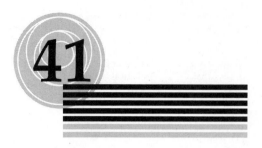

Visitation Facilitation

Jeanette Marie Daly

Visitation Facilitation is described in the Nursing Interventions Classification (NIC) as "promoting beneficial visits by family and friends" (McCloskey & Bulechek, 1996, p. 594). An intervention as defined in the NIC is "any treatment, based upon clinical judgment and knowledge, that a nurse performs to enhance patient/client outcomes" (McCloskey & Bulechek, 1996, p. xvii). Thus, Visitation Facilitation is a treatment performed by a nurse to enhance the Nursing Outcomes Classification (NOC) patient outcomes of Comfort Level, Energy Conservation, and Rest (Johnson & Maas, 1997). Visitation Facilitation (Table 41–1) is an intervention with activities that nurses can use in all specialties and in all settings. The concept is broad so that it can be used with the strictest visitation policy as well as with the least restrictive policy.

The individual nurse activities that compose Visitation Facilitation, performed on behalf of patients and their families, are not new but have changed over time. During the 15th century, in Florence, Italy, there were 35 hospitals that were generously supported and elegantly constructed. Visitation was described as the following: "Many ladies took turns to visit the hospitals and tend the sick, keeping their faces veiled, so that no one knows who they were; each remains a few days and then returns home, another taking her place" (Kalisch & Kalisch, 1978, p. 12). During that time period, persons did not want to be associated with hospitals and individuals who were ill. In the late 1800s, people were fearful of hospitals and frequently refused to go to the hospital. As a result, when surgery was required, all the needed surgical equipment was carried to the patient's home. The surgical nurse would usually go to the home a few hours before the operation to scrub everything. The kitchen table was used for the surgical procedure. "Occasionally members of the family helped. It was

Table 41–1   Visitation Facilitation

DEFINITION: Promoting beneficial visits by family and friends.

ACTIVITIES:

Determine patient's preferences for visitation

Determine need for limited visitation, such as too many visitors, patient's being impatient or tired, or physical status

Determine need for enhanced visitation

Identify specific problems with visits, if any

Discuss visiting policy with family members/significant others

Discuss policy for overnight stay of family members/significant others

Discuss family's understanding of patient's condition

Negotiate family/significant others' responsibilities and activities to assist patient, such as feeding

Establish optimal times for family/significant others to visit patient

Provide rationale for limited visiting time

Evaluate periodically with both the family and the patient whether visitation practices are meeting the needs of the patient/family, and revise accordingly

Inform visitors what they may expect to see and hear before their first hospital visitation, as appropriate

Encourage the family member to use touch, as well as verbal communication, as appropriate

Provide a chair at the bedside

Be flexible with visitation while facilitating periods of rest

Monitor patient's response to family visitation

Facilitate visitation of children, as appropriate

Screen visitors, especially children, for communicable diseases before visitation

Clarify the meaning of what the family member perceived during the visit

Provide support and care for family members after visitation, as needed

Provide family with unit telephone number to call when they go home

Inform family that a nurse will call at home if significant change in patient status occurs

Source: McCloskey, J. C., and Bulechek, G. M. (Eds.). (1996). *Nursing interventions classification (NIC)* (2nd ed.). St. Louis: Mosby–Year Book.

better to keep them occupied and away from interfering with our surgical supplies" (Kalisch & Kalisch, 1978, p. 172).

With this same philosophy of including the family but in a different era, the hospice manifests the concept of Visitation Facilitation. Hospice programs make it possible for terminally ill patients to have open visitation privileges. Family and friends are encouraged to be at the bedside providing physical and emotional support. A hospice differs from other types of health care programs in that it offers comfort-oriented care rather than curative treatment, emphasizing quality of life rather than length of life. Patients and families are a vital part of the decision-making process, which includes Visitation Facilitation (Iowa City Hospice, 1997).

LITERATURE REVIEW

There is a body of literature on the psychological care of patients and families in the hospital setting and especially in the critical care areas. The common themes are patients' opinions on visits, families' needs to visit, nurses' opinions on visits, policies regarding frequency and length of visits, and ethical and legal issues.

Patients' Opinions on Visits

Patients resoundingly report that visits are helpful, reassuring, and very important. Patients state that contact with their family is not tiring and helps them cope with their illness. Numerous studies indicate that patients prefer flexible visiting practices (Boykoff, 1986; Halm & Titler, 1990; Simpson, 1991, 1993; Titler & Walsh, 1992).

The routine for visiting a person in a health care institution is to enter the facility, find the location of the room, enter the room, and visit the person. But many variables can impinge on this typical visitation. When a relative is located in an area where visitation is restricted, the routine of visiting a patient is different. Restricted visitation can be found in many critical care areas. The visitor must gain access to the patient and may confront a variety of stressful situations. Attempting to communicate with the patient or simply being there with the patient is a matter that may be impeded by the illness, environment, and technology.

Clarke (1995), using grounded theory methodology, described the process of family members' visits to the intensive care unit (ICU). By interviewing and observing eight patients, four stages were identified: getting into the unit, getting past fears and anxieties, attempting communication with the patient, and being there with the patient.

Critical care patients have favored less frequent but longer visits with fewer visitors, realizing that their health needs are important (Halm & Titler, 1990; Simpson, 1991, 1993). This group of patients has been generally opposed to having a visitor in the room while a procedure is being performed. They also prefer not to have visits from children younger than age 12 (Makielski et al., 1986). Halm and Titler (1990) reported that 50% of patients wanted their family to visit more often, with 65% of the 77 patients desiring two to six visits per day. Simpson (1991, 1993) found that most patients wanted only two to three visitors at a time. Surgical intensive care patients wanted open visiting hours, and patients older than age 65 wanted unlimited length of visiting time.

Families' Perceptions

Visits from family members are important. When family members come for a visit, they need to be reassured, comforted, and supported. Quinn, Redmond, and Begley (1996a) found that the most important need for the family was to know they would be called at home concerning any changes in the patient's condition. Family members wanted to be called and be available in any emergency. Health care professionals need to call the family when a deviation occurs in the patient's behavior.

Visiting the patient is a high priority for the family member (Stillwell, 1984), and flexibility during the visitation is beneficial (Freismuth, 1986). Flexible standards should apply to the number of visits, the length of the visit, the time of day of the visit, and the age of the visitor. Flexibility can meet the working and extended family members' needs while reducing their stress and anxiety. Another serendipitously added benefit is the family's and patient's satisfaction with the health care stay.

A new phenomenon is occurring, "family systems nursing," which is nursing practice targeting the family as a unit when a nursing intervention is implemented (Johnson et al., 1995). This concept is applicable for Visitation Facilitation. A family member's illness disrupts the role function of the family. Home routines are disrupted, family members attempt to expand their normal family roles, and the balance is difficult. The researchers mentioned earlier found common themes that occur in families with an ill member: pulling together, fragmentation of families, increased dependence and independence, increased responsibilities, and change in routine and feelings. These findings influence the visitation process and influence nurses' opinions about visits.

Nurses' Opinions on Visits

Nurses play a pivotal role in regulating facility visiting policies. They can implement the visiting policy strictly, leniently, or not at all. Nurses' opinions on visitation vary depending on the clinical setting. Critical care nurses seem most concerned that visitors may tire their patients and delay the healing process. They are strong advocates for their patients' welfare and believe that family visits interfere with patient care (Lazure, 1997). Another point of view, however, is that of the nurses belonging to the Emergency Nurses Association (ENA), who "approved a resolution endorsing family presence during invasive procedures and resuscitation" (Eichhorn, Meyers, Mitchell, & Guzzetta, 1996, p. 61). These two diverse opinions about family visits may indicate that visitation policies should differ by setting and situation.

Nurses' perceptions of patient visitation needs differ from those of the families and patients. Halm and Titler (1990) found that almost all the physicians and nurses rated restricted visiting as slightly important or not important to the patient's recovery. They also feared that unlimited visitation might be detrimental to the patient's health. Other studies have noted that critical care staff consider family visitation a major stressor to their work and an impediment to the process (Cassem & Hackett, 1971; Hickey & Lewandowski, 1988).

Early research regarding Visitation Facilitation addressed such issues as length of the visit and frequency of the visit. The current trend is toward open visiting hours. This brings about the same visitation problems for nurses but on a continuous basis. Concerns about adequate rest and increased nursing stress when families are especially demanding are still evident in the literature. Assessing the patient's verbal and nonverbal cues provides information to help the nursing staff promote and control visitations.

Nurses are advocates for patients during the Visitation Facilitation intervention. Patients should be empowered to assess their own energy level and preferences for visitation. Nurses support patients by assisting them to think about the type of visitor and visit they prefer (Lazure, 1997).

Visitation Policies

Surveys of intensive care units reveal a wide variety of restrictions on frequency of visits, length of time per visit, number of visitors, and minimum age requirements (Kirchhoff, 1982; Stockdale & Hughes, 1988; Youngner, Coulton, Welton, Juknialis & Jackson, 1984). Consensus on the ideal visiting policy has not been found.

Scope of nursing practice varies regarding the visitation process. Whitis (1994) found that 86% of 125 hospitals surveyed have open visiting hours for pediatric patients; that is, visits are allowed 24 hours a day. Visitation in critical care units is usually restricted to 5 to 10 minutes hourly. Stockdale and Hughes (1988) noted that 73% of ICUs restrict visitation frequency.

Overall, hospital visitation policies vary but are similar regarding visiting by children. Children younger than age 12 usually are not allowed to visit in the critical care areas (Makielski et al., 1986). Whitis (1994) found that 64% of 125 randomly selected hospitals did not allow children younger than age 12 or 14 to visit. This is congruent with the survey results of Poster and Betz (1987), who found that many hospitals still restrict patient visitation by children.

Although the American Academy of Pediatrics issued a position statement in 1971 allowing visitation of hospitalized children by other children, these suggestions are not followed in practice. The basic suggestion was to encourage peers and siblings to visit to facilitate the developmental needs of the hospitalized child. Research has demonstrated that this practice does not increase infection rates (Umphenour, 1980). Although child visitation is encouraged and has been demonstrated not to promote infection, the practice is discouraged by nurses (Umphenour, 1980).

Ethical and Legal Issues of Visitation

Many ethical and legal issues can arise concerning patient visitation. Some of the main issues are patient safety and well-being, nurses' responsibility and accountability, and assault and battery.

Health care institution rules, policies, and procedures are established to promote consistency while providing for the welfare of employees, patients, and visitors. When following an institution's rules, nurses must be aware of violations to the principle of *primum non nocere*—that is, to avoid harming a patient (Veach & Fry, 1987). For example, a coronary care unit has a visitation policy of 15 minutes every two hours. A patient who is generally afraid, tense, and tearful becomes less stressed when visited by his or her significant other. A racing pulse rate decreases, and heart rhythm returns to normal sinus rhythm. This patient is harmed by the implementation of the visitation policy. Subjective and objective data must be considered regarding harm to a patient, and deviation from the rules must be undertaken when appropriate.

Nurses must be accountable for their actions and responsible for the duties they perform. "Accountability refers to being answerable to someone for something one has done, while responsibility refers to the carrying out of duties associated with a particular role assumed by the nurse" (Constantino, 1995, p. 156). If nurses deviate from the institution's rules, they must be able to explain their actions to peers and supervisors. Their actions must be based on sound rationale.

The logical decision in the example just given would be to allow the significant other to visit longer than the policy allows. Each situation has to be considered carefully for Visitation Facilitation. When nurses and visitors are unable to agree on rules for visitation, neutral parties not attached to the situation should review the problems. Referring any difficulties to an ethics committee would be appropriate.

Visitation Facilitation Intervention

The NIC intervention Visitation Facilitation lists the activities nurses perform to promote beneficial visits to a patient by family and friends. The resounding theme found throughout the intervention is a focus on the family and significant others. Some of the specific activities listed in the NIC are (1) determine need for limited visitation, such as too many visitors, patient's being impatient or tired, or physical status; (2) determine need for enhanced visitation; (3) identify specific problems with visits, if any; (4) discuss visiting policy with family members and significant others; and (5) discuss family's understanding of patient's condition. (See Table 41–1 for the complete intervention.)

After review of the literature, additional activities will be recommended to the Iowa Intervention Project for inclusion in the intervention Visitation Facilitation. The suggestions will expand the activities of the intervention. Some of the suggestions for new activities are (1) consider the telephone as a visitor, (2) note patient's verbal and nonverbal cues regarding the visitation, (3) provide bedrooms for relatives close to the unit as appropriate, and (4) provide a reclining chair for the visitor. (See Table 41–2 for a list of suggested additional activities for inclusion in the intervention.)

Visitation Facilitation has been linked to various nursing diagnoses. The NIC provides a list of all North American Nursing Diagnosis Association (NANDA) nursing diagnoses, with suggested interventions for each diagnosis (McCloskey & Bulechek, 1996; NANDA, 1994). The intervention Visitation Facilitation has been linked to the following nursing diagnoses: Altered Family Processes, Anxiety, Decreased Cardiac Output, Diversional Activity Deficit, Parental Role Conflict, Relocation Stress Syndrome, Risk for Loneliness, and Social Isolation. For only one of the nursing diagnoses, Risk for Loneliness, is the intervention Visitation Facilitation highly emphasized for problem resolution.

Table 41–2   List of Additional Activities for Visitation Facilitation Nursing Intervention

Consider the telephone as a visitor

Note patient's verbal and nonverbal cues regarding the visitation

Provide bedrooms for relatives close to the unit, as appropriate

Provide a reclining chair for the visitors

Establish flexible, patient-centered visiting policies

Suggest family members take turns staying overnight to prevent fatigue

Assist family members to find adequate lodging and meals

Inform family of legislation that provides the right to 12 weeks' unpaid leave of absence from work

Answer questions honestly

Give explanations of care in terms that visitors can understand

Convey feelings of acceptance to the visitors

Explain procedures being done

Assist family members to see the physician

Arrange animal visitation, as appropriate

Discuss death with family members, as appropriate

Consider legal and ethical implications regarding patient and family visitation rights

Table 41–3   Sample Care Plan for Case Study 2

Nursing Diagnosis	Outcome	Intervention
Anticipatory Grieving (related to son in emergency room, as manifested by expression of distress at potential loss)	Grief Resolution (adjustment to actual or impending loss)	Visitation Facilitation (promoting beneficial visits by family and friends)
	Social Support (perceived availability and actual provision of reliable assistance from others)	Grief Work Facilitation (assistance with the resolution of a significant loss)
	Loneliness (the extent of emotional, social, or existential isolation responses)	

CASE STUDIES

Case Study 1

BW, a patient with dementia, was admitted to the skilled unit in a long-term care facility following hospitalization for a fall. In the hospital, he had been restrained and was prevented from getting out of bed independently. At the nursing home, he was not restrained, and 48 hours after admission he fell and fractured his hip. This occurred during the night. He was returned to the hospital, but, as surgical intervention was not possible, he came back to the nursing home. His family was very upset and wanted to visit the nursing home at any time to be able to check on him. Visiting hours were 9 AM to 7 PM. The director of nursing invited the family to visit at any hour of the day, explaining that at 9 PM the front doors were locked but that they could ring the doorbell for entry. They were also invited to spend the night if they so desired. In addition to extending visiting hours, a body alarm was used to identify when BW was leaving his bed, and staff more closely monitored him. The family members visited frequently, and their visits were helpful to the staff in monitoring BW and assisting him in adjusting to the new environment.

One of the activities the director of nursing implemented was determining the need for enhanced visitation. Other activities were used, such as discussing the policy for visitation and overnight stay. As you will note, not all the activi-

ties for the intervention are appropriate in each situation. Activities are completed when they are appropriate for the situation.

Case Study 2

A 6-month-old infant was brought to the emergency room in critical condition with a life-threatening cardiac anomaly. A full code was initiated to resuscitate the infant. The mother wanted to stay in the emergency room with her baby. The physician asked that the mother be escorted from the emergency room. The nurse allowed the mother to stay based on knowledge of the legal and ethical implications regarding patient and family visitation rights during an emergency.

The infant died, and the nurse prepared the infant for his mother's visit. She arranged a quiet, secluded area with a rocking chair; she encouraged the mother to hold her infant and begin the grieving process. The nurse used many of the Visitation Facilitation activities; she encouraged the family member to use touch, provided a chair, and offered support and care for the family member. Another possible activity is discussing death with the family member; this should be included in the activities of this intervention. A sample care plan demonstrating the use of the intervention Visitation Facilitation can be found in Table 41–3, in which a NANDA diagnosis and NIC interventions and NOC outcomes are used.

Conclusion

■

Visitation Facilitation is an intervention whose activities focus on family members, significant others, and the patient. Appropriate consideration of family members and use of visits can benefit nursing practice and patient care. It is obvious that one rule should not be applied to all patients. Each patient is a unique individual with varying needs. Each visitor is a unique individual with other needs. The nurse judges these needs and implements Visitation Facilitation according to the situation.

References

Boykoff, S. L. (1986). Visitation needs reported by patients with cardiac disease on their families. *Heart and Lung, 15*, 573–578.

Cassem, N., and Hackett, T. (1971). Psychiatric consultation in a coronary care unit. *Annals of Internal Medicine, 75*, 9–14.

Clarke, S. P. (1995). Increasing the quality of family visits to the ICU. *Dimensions of Critical Care Nursing, 14*, 200–212.

Constantino, R. E. (1995). Escorting the family out of the ICU: Ethical and legal issues. *Dimensions of Critical Care Nursing, 14*, 154–158.

Eichhorn, D. J., Meyers, T. A., Mitchell, T. G., and Guzzetta, C. E. (1996). Opening the doors: Family presence during resuscitation. *Journal of Cardiovascular Nursing, 10*(4), 59–70.

Freismuth, C. (1986). Meeting the needs of families of critically ill patients: A comparison of visiting policies in the intensive care setting. *Heart and Lung, 15*, 309–310.

Halm, M. A., and Titler, M. G. (1990). Appropriateness of critical care visitation: Perceptions of patients, families, nurses, and physicians. *Journal of Nursing Quality Assurance, 5*, 25–37.

Hickey, M., and Lewandowski, L. (1988). Critical care nurses' role with families: A descriptive study. *Heart and Lung, 17*, 670–676.

Iowa City Hospice. (1997). *Hospice patient family handbook*. Iowa City, IA: Author.

Johnson, M., and Maas, M. (Eds.). (1997). *Nursing outcomes classification (NOC)*. St. Louis: Mosby–Year Book.

Johnson, S. K., Craft, M., Titler, M., Halm, M., Kleiber, C., Montgomery, L., Megivern, K., Nicholson, A., and Buckwalter, K. (1995). Perceived changes in adult family members' roles and responsibilities during critical illness. *Image, 27*, 238–243.

Kalisch, P. A., and Kalisch, B. (1978). *The advance of American nursing*. Boston: Little, Brown.

Kirchhoff, K. T. (1982). Visiting policies for patients with myocardial infarction: A national survey. *Heart and Lung, 11*, 571–576.

Lazure, L. L. A. (1997). Strategies to increase patient control of visiting. *Dimensions of Critical Care Nursing, 16*(1), 11–19.

Makielski, M., Winet, E., Kaufman, M., Gerbasich, K., Meert, S., and Gaibraith, B. (1986). The effects of open visitation on the stress and perceptions of cardiac care patients. *Heart and Lung, 15*, 312–313.

McCloskey, J. C., and Bulechek, G. M. (1996). *Nursing interventions classification (NIC)* (2nd ed.). St. Louis: Mosby–Year Book.

North American Nursing Diagnosis Association. (1994). *Nursing diagnoses: Definitions and classification 1995–1996*. Philadelphia: Author.

Poster, E. D., and Betz, C. L. (1987). Survey of sibling and peer visitation policies in southern California hospitals. *Children's Health Care, 15*(3), 166–171.

Quinn, S., Redmond, K., and Begley, C. (1996a). The needs of relatives visiting adult critical care units as perceived by relatives and nurses. Part 1. *Intensive and Critical Care Nursing, 12*(3), 168–172.

Quinn, S., Redmond, K., and Begley, C. (1996b). The needs of relatives visiting adult critical care units as perceived by relatives and nurses. Part 2. *Intensive and Critical Care Nursing, 12*(4), 239–245.

Simpson, T. (1991). Critical care patients perceptions of visits. *Heart and Lung, 20*, 681–688.

Simpson, T. (1993). Visit preferences of middle aged versus older critically ill patients. *American Journal of Critical Care, 2*, 339–345.

Stillwell, S. B. (1984). Importance of visiting needs as perceived by family members of patients in the intensive care unit. *Heart and Lung, 13*, 238–242.

Stockdale, L. L., and Hughes, I. P. (1988). Critical care unit visiting policies: A survey. *Focus on Critical Care, 15*(6), 45–48.

Titler, M. G., and Walsh, S. M. (1992). Visiting critically ill adults: Strategies for practice. *Critical Care Nursing Clinics of North America, 4*, 623–632.

Umphenour, J. K. (1980). Bacterial colonization in neonates with sibling visitation. *Journal of Obstetric and Gynecological Nursing, 9*(2), 73–75.

Veach, R., and Fry, S. (1987). *Case studies in nursing ethics*. Philadelphia: J. B. Lippincott.

Whitis, G. (1994). Visiting hospitalized patients. *Journal of Advanced Nursing, 19*, 85–88.

Younger, S. J., Coulton, C., Welton, R., Juknialis, B., and Jackson, D. L. (1984). ICU visiting policies. *Critical Care Medicine, 12*, 606–608.

Sustenance Support

Juanita K. Hunter

Organized nursing has its roots in the provision of health care to the poor and to those discriminated against and powerless to advocate on their own behalf. The nursing role evolved from a core concern for meeting the basic needs of these same individuals, families, and groups. Those basic health care needs are often intertwined with issues of food, shelter, and clothing. Throughout organized nursing's history, nurses have quietly assumed the responsibility for assisting their clients to secure the goods and services that promote healing, a return to a healthy state, and maintenance of health. In so doing, nursing has also addressed individual, community, and system barriers to the provision of basic and holistic health care.

Community health nursing is most often identified as that specialty area of nursing that encompasses a broad base of services for individual clients, groups, and communities (Deal, 1994). The very essence of the role of the public health nurse developed from an assertion that public health was a social activity designed to build a program of community service. The establishment of the Nurses' Settlement in New York City by Lillian Wald in 1893 is a prime example (Kalisch & Kalisch, 1995). Its emphasis on environment, health promotion, and disease prevention continues today as the underpinning of community health nursing.

Most health care professionals are unaware of the environmental health and protection issues, which include areas of clean water, safe food, and housing (Kotchian, 1995). The concept of coordinating all aspects of the physical, social, psychological, and environmental factors affecting a client's health care plan has not been embraced by all nurses (Smith & Maurer, 1995).

The implementation of nursing activities that address the basic need of sustenance has not received much attention. Often, little thought is given to the specific activities that are undertaken on the client's behalf. Clients are referred to other providers, and the nurse fails to document the steps of the nursing process that were initiated, the referrals that were made, or the coordination efforts that follow. Those activities are thus absent from the documented nurse's role.

LITERATURE RELATED TO THE INTERVENTION

The Nursing Interventions Classification (NIC) intervention of Sustenance Support is described in Table 42–1. It is defined as "helping a needy individual/family to locate food, clothing, or shelter" and includes such activities as providing information about available resources, assisting individuals to make application for financial aid, and securing food and clothing for clients. The underpinnings of nurses providing sustenance can be traced to the Old Testament (Bullough & Bullough, 1978). The evolution of the practice of nursing reflects the religious influences of Christianity and the charity and charitable organizations recognized in Jewish and canon laws. Those Jewish laws spearheaded charitable societies for clothing the poor, visiting the sick, sheltering the aged, and offering assistance to prisoners, among many other activities (Bullough & Bullough, 1978). Charity was one of the leading virtues of Christianity, and Jesus set an example of concern for the poor and sick that could not be ignored. It was from religious orders that the first nurses evolved.

Once the scientific method was embraced, nursing utilized information from many different disciplines to build a foundation for practice: sociology, psychol-

Table 42–1 Sustenance Support

DEFINITION: Helping a needy individual/family to locate food, clothing, or shelter.

ACTIVITIES:

Inform individual/families about how to access local food pantries and free lunch programs, as appropriate

Inform individual/families about how to access low rent housing and subsidy programs, as appropriate

Inform individual/families of available emergency housing shelter programs, as appropriate

Arrange transportation to emergency housing shelter, as appropriate

Discuss with the individual/families available job service agencies, as appropriate

Arrange for individual/families transportation to job services, if necessary

Inform individual/families of agency providing clothing assistance, as appropriate

Arrange transportation to agency providing clothing assistance, as necessary

Inform individual/families of agency programs for support, such as Red Cross and Salvation Army, as appropriate

Discuss with the individual/families financial aid support available

Assist individual/families to complete forms for assistance, such as housing and financial aid

Inform individual/families of available free health clinics

Assist individual/families to reach free health clinics

Inform individual/families of eligibility requirements for food stamps

Inform individual/families of available schools and/or day care centers, as appropriate

Source: McCloskey, J. C., and Bulechek, G. M. (Eds.). (1996). *Nursing interventions classification (NIC)* (2nd ed., p. 540). St. Louis: Mosby–Year Book.

ogy, anthropology, and all the natural sciences. Theories or paradigms from other disciplines have provided the basis for nursing theories (Chitty, 1997; Kozier, Erb, & Blais, 1997). Some examples include systems theory, developmental theory, needs theory, interpersonal theory, and existentialist philosophy (O'Bryan-Doheny, Cook, & Stopper, 1997). These theories and viewpoints are all included in the idea of the intervention of Sustenance Support (Alligood & Marriner-Tomey, 1997; Isenberg, 1997).

It is clear from the writings of Florence Nightingale that nursing was conceptualized as a holistic practice. She outlined five essential points as guidelines for securing the health of households and promoting health. They are (1) pure air, (2) pure water, (3) efficient drainage, (4) cleanliness, and (5) light (Stanhope & Lancaster, 1996). In her book *Notes on Nursing*, originally published in 1860, Nightingale instructed nurses to "put the patient in the best condition for nature to act upon him" (Nightingale, 1966, p. 133). Person, health, and environment are concepts on which most nursing theories have been developed (Catalano, 1996).

Maslow's (1968) theory of hierarchal needs was one of the key foundations for the development of nursing theories. Nursing theorists further refined the five Maslow categories of physiological, safety and security, love and belonging, self-esteem, and self-actualization needs with activities of aid and support. A brief review of four of the most discussed nursing theories demonstrates that they provide descriptions of how to help patients become comfortable, how to deliver treatment with the least damage, and how to enhance high-level wellness (Meleis, 1997).

For example, Henderson's definition of nursing states that "the unique function of the nurse is to assist the individual, sick or well, in the performance of those activities contributing to health or its recovery (or to a peaceful death) that he would perform unaided if he had the necessary strength, will or knowledge. And to do this in such a way as to help him gain independence as rapidly as possible" (Furukawa & Howe, 1990, p. 66). The role of the nurse in this theory is one of prime helper and member of an interdisciplinary health team, and the nurse will substitute for whatever the client lacks.

Henderson (1966) identified 14 components that constitute basic nursing care. They include assisting the individual with breathing normally; eating and drinking adequately; eliminating body waste; moving and maintaining desirable postures; sleeping and resting; selecting suitable clothes; maintaining body temperature; keeping the body clean, well groomed, and protected; avoiding dangers in the environment; communicating with others in expressing emotions, needs, fears, or opinions; worshipping according to one's faith; working with a sense of accomplishment; participating in various forms of recreation; learning, discovering, or satisfying the curiosity that leads to normal development and health; and using available facilities.

Henderson (1966) focused on the individual person and on human needs, with care of both ill and well individuals. Of particular relevance to the intervention of Sustenance Support, the goal of nursing in the Henderson theory was completeness or wholeness and independence of the client to perform daily activities.

The works of other nursing theorists also support the basis for the intervention. Nightingale focused on the environmental factors that support this specific nursing intervention. Roy's adaptation model (Roy & Andrews, 1991) focuses on the human adaptive system to a constantly changing environment. Orem's (1991) model addresses the individual needing assistance with self-care activities, which may focus on food and other environmental factors that relate to shelter and clothing. King's (1992) goal attainment model emphasizes the nurse's primary functions of caring for individuals and meeting their basic needs (Nunnery, 1997).

Supporting documentation was also found in a few articles that addressed the nurse's role in this area. For example, a relationship between the message of an artist, George Frederic Watts, and starvation highlighted the complex issues of the problem of nutritional deficit and the role of the nurse in meeting this need of clients (Iveson, 1982). In a study of Orem-based nursing care designed to support nutritional self-care, it was found that men and women responded to the nursing care by consuming less total fat and saturated fat compared with controls (Onyango, Tucker, & Eisemon, 1994). Although poor nutrition is often related to female-headed households, McGarrity and Knox (1995), in a study of de facto female headship in Kenya, found that children of female heads consumed a greater variety of foods than children in male-headed households.

Many studies have been devoted to the exploration of and relationship between homelessness and mental illness. Little is known about the mental, physical, and social deprivation that often accompanies this phenomenon. Wagner and Menke (1991a) found in a study of 76 homeless school-age children that more than 40% were depressed and in need of psychiatric referral. Other authors have documented that as many as 50% of homeless children are depressed (Bassuk & Rubin, 1987; Wagner & Menke, 1991a). These data have implications for nursing activities, which will be discussed later.

FOOD, CLOTHING, AND SHELTER

The intervention Sustenance Support is targeted to helping a needy person to locate food, clothing, and shelter. The model developed by the American Family Inns (Fig. 42–1) was developed to assist homeless families to meet their multiple and interconnected needs. This model is also appropriate for other low-income and poor individuals and families. Although the American Family Inn program is initiated in a residential setting, components of the model are applicable to any provider or setting addressing food, clothing, and shelter for clients.

Food

Access to food is facilitated by the nurse with a variety of activities. In a well-child or prenatal clinic, the nurse is keenly aware of the need to ensure sufficient nutrients for the newborn of the pregnant or lactating mother (Burcher, Larson, Nelson, & Lenihan, 1993). Results of a study of anemia in a Head Start population suggests that this problem is increasing among low-income families (Esielionis, Williams, & Yarandi, 1993). The food culture of poor and ethnic groups may contribute to their nutritional risk (Nelson et al, 1993). The federal government supplements the budget of low-income families with food stamps that extend their food budget. Nurses participate in qualifying families for this benefit. In other settings, such as community or school clinics, a nurse may determine that a child is at nutritional risk and assist with a referral for the free lunch program.

The nurse may also provide the family with a listing of local churches and food banks that give bags of food to needy families and identify neighborhood dining sites for the family that are free or have a minimal fee. Many very poor and near homeless families use such facilities, which helps them remain adequately fed. Gelber, Stein, & Neumann (1995) demonstrated that persons with access to free food sources were less undernourished than those without those resources. A family living on a limited income may be helped by a referral

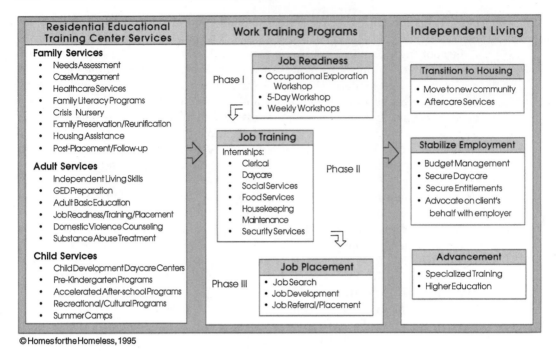

© Homes for the Homeless, 1995

Figure 42–I   The American Family Inn—"Main Street." (From Homes for the Homeless, Inc., New York, NY, January 1995, p. 5. Reprinted with permission.)

to a nutritionist in a neighborhood clinic who will review budgeting and food buying practices and provide tips for meal planning.

Elders are often at nutritional risk. They are prone to nutritional risk owing to limited income, social isolation, and physical or psychological changes that often accompany the aging or disease process. The nurse may encounter these individuals in community clinics or senior citizen centers, through home visiting, or in an inpatient setting. The nurse should assess the needs of the client and suggest several activities that may address the situation. For example, Meals on Wheels is a program that provides home-delivered meals for low-income elderly clients on a sliding-fee scale. This program has been most successful in meeting the nutritional needs of the frail elderly, those recovering from serious illnesses, and others who may be unable to prepare meals as a result of disabilities. In addition, this program is implemented by volunteers who provide the very important function of meeting the socialization needs of this group on a daily basis. Also, city and federal funding has supported dining sites in urban areas where senior citizens may secure a hot lunch for a nominal fee. Local churches and soup kitchens may also provide a hot meal during the day.

Clothing

Clothing is considered essential for a client's well-being, in addition to meeting society's expectations for public decency. Nurses know that individuals who are victims of violence, accidents, or psychological impairment may enter the health care system inappropriately clothed and vulnerable to infections, frostbite, or even death because of exposure to the elements. Women often flee from abusive situations to safe houses in the middle of winter with only the clothing on their body. For homeless clients, lack of funds to purchase clothing adequate for the season is an additional need to their lack of housing.

Nurses must first assess the client's particular situation to determine a problem. For example, a child is brought to the emergency room dressed in a diaper and a sweater when the temperature is below freezing. The nurse should sensitively ask questions about the parent's living status and any concerns the parent may have about the child's dress. If appropriate, the nurse then initiates activities by making referrals to sites where clothing is given away free of charge or where clothing may be purchased at a nominal fee.

It may be necessary to discuss transportation arrangements in order for the parent to follow through on the suggestions. Most homeless shelters (e.g., city mission) have some free clothing available for their residents. You should keep in mind that clients who are referred to traditional sites, such as the Salvation Army or the Goodwill, will be expected to pay a nominal fee for the clothing, and some individuals may not have that minimum amount.

Shelter

The activities outlined in this intervention to assist individuals and families in obtaining food, shelter, and clothing imply that nurses have the necessary information to provide to their clients. The nurse should work to empower the client to avoid increasing client victimization. Each locality will differ in relation to unrestricted, affordable, and appropriate housing. The nurse should be aware of those housing agencies in the community that assist individuals to secure safe, affordable housing. Some communities have a community services handbook that lists agencies by the services provided. Community health nurses assess environmental conditions within a client's home as well as outside and make recommendations for modifications if needed.

Community health nurses are often in contact with housing agencies when concerns related to client safety or appropriate level of care for the client arise. For example, if a high-risk infant is living in an apartment with insufficient heat or with infestation, the community health nurse may contact the landlord or make a referral to the city or county environmental department. The community health nurse may also contact all providers assisting the individual or family and set up a multidisciplinary conference to discuss the specifics of the situation and to formulate a coordinated plan of care.

In a hospital situation, a discharge planning nurse will become actively involved in determining appropriate arrangements for housing for the client when limitations exist because of new diagnoses or changes in health status. Major modifications may be required in the home before the client can be safely discharged to that environment.

Local social service agencies may provide clients with listings of low-income apartments. Public housing is available in most large urban areas; however, there may be a waiting list. For example, housing is available for handicapped individuals and senior citizens and transitional units are available for homeless individuals. Social workers are usually helpful in assisting clients in this area.

In communities where there is a sizeable homeless population, nurses working in homeless shelters may be more actively involved in assisting clients with securing housing. Clients are often referred to homeless shelters from social service agencies, churches, and health care facilities when suitable housing in the community cannot be obtained readily. Nurses who work in these settings may discuss housing needs with their clients as a part of the nursing history before care is provided.

Access to resources for shelter can also be obtained from the American Hotel & Motel Association, 1201 New York Avenue NW, Suite 600, Washington, DC 20036 (202-289-3100). Another potential contact person is the president of the nearest chapter of the Cornell Society of Hotelmen. These names and addresses may be obtained from the Office of Alumni Affairs, School of Hotel Administration, Cornell University (607-255-3565). Examples of the kinds of assistance your community may be able to offer are (1) obtaining furniture, fixtures, and equipment; (2) obtaining bedding (mattresses, sheets, towels); (3) obtaining laundry machines; and (4) obtaining security and safety systems (Hales, Eyster, & Ford, 1993). See Table 42–2 for additional resources.

Table 42–2   National Resources on Food, Shelter, and Clothing

Anybody looking for services in the immediate area is instructed to first contact the local **Mayor's office** or **public school** (which is required through the McKinney Act's Education for Homeless Children and Youth Program to maintain such information). One might try the local Housing and Urban Development (HUD), Health and Human Services (HHS), or Federal Emergency Management Agency (FEMA) representative.

The following national agencies offer services in many, if not most, regions; a call to information will get you a listing:

Salvation Army
Red Cross
United Way
Catholic Charities
YMCA
YWCA

The following national organizations provide information and advocacy assistance:

National Coalition for the Homeless
1612 K Street NW, #1004
Washington, DC 20006
(202) 775-1322

National Alliance to End Homelessness
1518 K Street NW, Suite 206
Washington, DC 20005
(202) 638-1526

National Low Income Housing Coalition
1012 14th Street NW, Suite 1200
Washington, DC 20005
(202) 662-1530

Housing Assistance Council
1025 Vermont Avenue NW, Suite 606
Washington, DC 20005
(202) 842-8600

National Network of Runaway and Youth Services
1319 F Street NW, Suite 401
Washington, DC 20004
(202) 783-7949

World Hunger Year
505 Eighth Avenue, 21st Floor
New York, NY 10018-6582
(212) 629-8850

Source: Homes for the Homeless, 36 Cooper Square, 6th Floor, New York, NY 10003.

INFORMATION SHARING

Many of the activities included in the Sustenance Support intervention list include the action verbs inform, assist, and arrange. The goal is to advocate for the client and to empower him or her. The nursing role in implementing these activities may be patient education, providing information, or taking action on behalf of the client. McCloskey, Bulechek, Moorhead, and Daly (1996) describe and discuss the two roles of caregiver and integrator, or direct and indirect caregiver. These outlined activities also overlap, primarily with the traditional social worker role.

For example, in the Nursing Center for the Homeless in Buffalo, New York, a social worker was part of the multidisciplinary team, which used a case management model in providing services to the homeless in several shelters (Hunter, 1993). After the nurse identified through initial interviews with clients that housing needs were the primary concern of most clients, referrals were made to the social worker for the information needed to begin the housing search. Information regarding how to apply for social services was also provided by the shelter intake staff person or the other social workers assigned to the shelter (Hunter, 1993).

If the nurse is working in a setting where he or she is the sole provider, it will be necessary to have information readily available to share with clients about housing, food, and clothing resources. The telephone book is a good place to start for the nurse beginning to assist clients in these areas. Local social service, community health, and other social agencies also have resource information and brochures to share with individuals and families. It is important for the nurse to remember that the client in need of food, clothing, and shelter is most likely in crisis related to his or her circumstances.

Providing information that is obsolete or sending a client to an agency that no longer exists is not helpful. The nurse should confirm with the agency that the service is available and, to the extent possible, determine that the client is eligible for the service before making that referral. The nurse should determine whether the appropriate approach is to give the information to the client and allow him or her to follow through or whether it is more appropriate to actively become the advocate on behalf of the client (Cohen, 1989).

There are specific situations where this determination will be important in the development of rapport with the client. The circumstances that the client is experiencing are extremely stressful; therefore, when working with homeless clients and those who are in crisis, information must be presented simply, and directions should be written on one slip or card that the client can fold and easily carry. Avoiding these pitfalls of overload and multiple expectations will alleviate the common belief that these clients lack motivation. Life circumstances make food, clothing, and shelter priority concerns. Thus, when setting priorities, the activities that have the greatest potential for meeting these needs are undertaken first. In these situations, one can observe the demonstration of Maslow's hierarchy of needs. Further, nurses must consider access to and cost of transportation when recommending that the client take action.

SELF-HELP AND REFERRAL

Self-help strategies have been widely used in psychiatric settings and with substance abuse clients. Little is known about the use of this strategy with low-income and homeless clients. The Nursing Center for the Homeless in Buffalo,

New York, initiated a weekly support group with homeless women in a shelter. The purpose of this group was to facilitate communication with the women to assess their immediate needs and to identify those women who were in need of psychiatric–mental health counseling or referral. The results of this activity demonstrated that these women were fearful and mistrusting and that many were unable to identify a plan for themselves that would address their homelessness. Hastings-Vertino (1992) used Yalon's listing of factors intrinsic to the therapeutic process to develop a tool to study the relationship of these factors to outcomes of a support group. She found the tools useful in rating these therapeutic factors in a group session.

In a related study, researchers examined the self-help strategies of poor households assisting friends and relatives to keep them from living on the streets or becoming homeless. These doubled-up families, as they are described, were included in a household study in the state of Washington, with a result that 59% of the sample of 277 reported sheltering homeless friends or relatives. The authors conclude that the doubled-up homeless population is greater than the sheltered homeless population and that self-help plays a key role in reducing homelessness (Marin & Vacha, 1994).

It was previously mentioned that a large number of homeless children have been determined to be depressed and in need of psychiatric referral. Nurses working with homeless families are in a key position to implement a variety of activities to assist in accurate identification of these children, to assess the children for potential self-destructive behavior, and to refer the children to mental health and social welfare agencies. In addition, the nurse should address the physical needs of food and shelter, assist in management of emotional distress of the family, and help nurture hope (Wagner & Menke, 1991b). All these activities require some social system advocacy and possibly crisis intervention (Wagner & Menke, 1991a).

IDENTIFICATION OF ASSOCIATED NURSING DIAGNOSES

The nursing intervention Sustenance Support is related to several North American Nursing Diagnosis Association (NANDA) diagnoses. They include the following:

Community Coping, Ineffective
Family Processes, Altered
Fear
Health Maintenance, Altered
Hopelessness
Individual Coping, Ineffective
Individual, Management of Therapeutic Regimen, Ineffective
Infection, Risk for
Knowledge Deficit (Specify)
Noncompliance (Specify)
Nutrition: Less Than Body Requirements, Altered
Powerlessness
Protection, Altered
Self Care Deficit: Dressing/Grooming
Self Esteem, Chronic Low
Skin Integrity, Impaired
Skin Integrity, Risk for Impaired

Sleep Pattern Disturbance
Social Interaction, Impaired
Social Isolation
Spiritual Distress

It is clear from this list that the intervention Sustenance Support is an integral part of multiple activities related to these specific nursing diagnoses. The appropriate client groups include those from across the life span—infants, children, adolescents, pregnant women, families, the elderly, the mentally ill, substance abusers, and victims of domestic violence. It is worth noting that these groups are those most often found in homeless shelters. Although the reasons for the homelessness may be many and varied, the nursing diagnoses and activities related to the intervention Sustenance Support are similar to those needed by this group. However, it suggests that NANDA consider a new diagnosis such as basic needs, compromised. The nursing-sensitive outcomes of Caregiver Well-Being, Comfort Level, Coping, Decision Making, Hope, Knowledge: Health Behaviors, and Nutritional Status are examples of outcomes that relate to Sustenance Support (Johnson & Maas, 1997).

CASE STUDIES

Case Study 1

Background

S is a 43-year-old single woman who lives alone in a one-bedroom subsidized apartment. She was admitted to a community health agency with a diagnosis of leg ulcers and an order for twice-a-day dressing change. On initial assessment, the community health nurse determined that S was living on a very limited budget and was ineligible to receive social services financial benefits. She was receiving Medicaid benefits, and this was the source of payment for the nursing visits. S lived in a small second-floor apartment and had no means of transportation. Because of the limited mobility of the client (she weighed 302 pounds) and the presence of leg ulcers, S was essentially homebound. The leg wounds had copious amounts of drainage, requiring frequent changes of S's slacks, which she wore mostly for warmth. She owned only two pairs of pants and did not have a washing machine in her apartment. One activity that the primary nurse initiated was to conduct a clothing drive within the agency. All agency staff were asked to donate one item of clothing for this client.

Questions to be answered by the nurse

1. What are the nursing diagnoses? What are the desired outcomes?
2. What are the activities to carry out the

intervention of Sustenance Support for this individual?
3. What referrals are indicated?

Case Study 2

Background

RS is a 34-year-old single mother with a 5-year-old boy, an 8-year-old girl, and a 9-year-old boy. She has lived at a religious-supported homeless shelter in western New York for 2 months. Before that time, she lived in a public-supported homeless shelter for 2 months. The reason for the homelessness is that RS was evicted from her apartment. Her husband, the father of the three children, is in Pennsylvania living on Supplemental Security Income (SSI) because of a psychiatric diagnosis. He cannot stand the noise or bother of the children, so he moved back to Pennsylvania to be with his family about 8 months ago. RS appears limited in her intelligence and speaks very basic English. She does not grasp complex ideas regarding her situation and feels that "it will get better some day." She applied for housing at Buffalo Municipal Housing Authority but was turned down because she was ineligible (reason unknown).

RS found an apartment, but the landlord would not take the Department of Social Services' statement for a security deposit. She is also pregnant by a married man who will not leave his wife for her. She is due to deliver in 4 months and has no friends or relatives in New York State with whom to leave the children while she is in the hospital. RS has had to cancel two sonogram tests because the children have been sick both times and the shelter does not provide babysitting services. She feels the shelter "provides a roof over her head and food in her children's stomachs." One of the children has a birth defect, another is developmentally delayed, and the third is very aggressive with children and adults.

The staff at the shelter state that the children are wild and out of hand. RS states that she really has little patience and little control. She feels she cannot give her children anything else, so she can at least give in to them when they want something—usually candy, subs, Big Macs, soda, or junk food. They do not ask for toys.

RS has overextended her stay at the shelter. Her 30 days are exhausted, but she cannot find anywhere to live, and the longer she cannot find a place, the more decline is seen in her children's behavior. She also interviewed at the YWCA live-in program about 3 weeks ago but has heard nothing. The Nursing Center refers RS to the emergency room of the local hospital when one of her children sustains a head laceration after an altercation with another child in the shelter.

Questions to be answered by the triage nurse

1. What are nursing diagnoses? What are the desired outcomes?
2. What are the activities to carry out the intervention of Sustenance Support for this family?
3. What referrals are indicated?

SUMMARY

Today, nursing finds itself in a position whereby cost implications often dictate the nursing care provided, and all aspects of a client care plan must be documented and justified to meet reimbursement demands. These current pressures constrain implementation of the holistic and broader dimensions of the nursing process. Generally, most nurses still remain most committed to those who cannot provide for themselves—for example infants and children, low-income single mothers, the disabled, the homeless, the mentally ill, and the elderly. For all these groups, lack of food, clothing, and shelter is often a problem that must be addressed in the course of implementing a plan of care. Sustenance Support is therefore an integral component of the nursing process.

References

Alligood, M. R., and Marriner-Tomey, A. (Eds.). (1977). *Nursing theory: Utilization and application.* St. Louis: Mosby–Year Book.

Bassuk, E., and Rubin, L. (1987). Homeless children: A neglected population. *American Journal of Orthopsychiatry, 57,* 279–286.

Bullough, V., and Bullough, B. (1978). *The care of the sick: The emergence of modern nursing.* Prodist, NY: Watson Publishing International.

Burcher, P. A., Larson, L. C., Nelson, M. D., and Lenihan, A. J. (1993). Prenatal WIC participation can reduce low birthweight and newborn medical costs: A cost-benefit analysis of WIC participation in North Carolina. *Journal of the American Dietetic Association, 93*(2), 163–166.

Catalano, J. T. (1996). *Contemporary professional nursing.* Philadelphia: F. A. Davis.

Chitty, K. K. (1997). *Professional nursing concepts and challenges* (2nd ed.). Philadelphia: W. B. Saunders.

Cohen, M. B. (1989). Social work practice with homeless mentally ill people: Engaging the client. *Social Work, 34*(6), 505–509.

Deal, L. W. (1994). The effectiveness of community health nursing interventions: A literature review. *Public Health Nursing, 11,* 315–322.

Esielionis Francis, E., Williams, D., and Yarandi, H. (1993). Anemia as an indicator of nutrition in children enrolled in a Head Start program. *Journal of Pediatric Health Care, 7*(4), 156–160.

Furukawa, C. Y., and Howe, J. K. (1990). Virginia Henderson. In J. B. George (Ed.), *Nursing theories—the base for professional practice* (3rd ed., chap. 5, 61–78). Stamford, CT: Appleton & Lange.

Gelberg, L., Stein, J. A., and Neumann, C. G. (1995). Determinants of undernutrition among homeless adults. *Public Health Reports, 110,* 448–454.

Hales, A., Eyster, J., and Ford, J. (1993). The homeless: Help from hotels and restaurants. *Nursing Management, 24*(7), 108–112.

Hastings-Vertino, K., Getty, C., and Wooldridge, P. (1996). Development of a tool to measure therapeutic factors in group process. *Archives of Psychiatric Nursing, 10,* 221–228.

Hastings-Vertino, K. A. (1992). *Depression and social sup-*

port in unemployed persons with work related injuries. Unpublished master's thesis, State University of New York at Buffalo, Buffalo.

Henderson, V. (1966). *The nature of nursing.* New York: Macmillan Publishing.

Henderson, V. (1978). The concept of nursing. *Journal of Advanced Nursing, 3,* 16–17.

Hunter, J. K. (1987–1993). *A center for homeless persons in Buffalo, N.Y.* [Final Report]. DHHS, Division of Nursing Grant D106000-95.

Isenberg, M. (1997). Nursing models and their use in practice. In Oermann, M. H. (Ed). *Professional nursing practice.* Stamford, CT: Appleton & Lange.

Iveson, J. (September 22, 1982). Satisfy basic needs first. *Nursing Mirror,* 31.

Johnson, M., and Maas, M. (1997). *Nursing outcomes classification (NOC).* St. Louis: Mosby–Year Book.

Kalisch, P. A., and Kalisch, B. J. (1995). *The advance of American nursing* (3rd ed.). Philadelphia: J. B. Lippincott.

King, I. M. (1992). King's theory of goal attainment. *Nursing Science, 5,* 19–25.

Kotchian, S. B. (1995). Environmental health services are prerequisites to health care. *Community Health, 18*(3), 45–53.

Kozier, B., Erb, G., and Blais, K. (1997). *Professional nursing practice concepts and perspectives* (3rd ed.). Menlo Park, CA: Addison-Wesley.

Marin, M. V., and Vacha, E. F. (1994). Self-help strategies and resources among people at risk of homelessness: Empirical findings and social services policy. *Social Work, 39,* 649–657.

Maslow, A. (1968). *Toward a psychology of being* (2nd ed.). New York: D. Van Nostrand.

McCloskey, J. C., and Bulechek, G. M. (Eds.). (1996). *Nursing interventions classification* (NIC) (2nd ed.). St. Louis: Mosby–Year Book.

McCloskey, J. C., Bulechek, G. M., Moorhead, S., and Daly, J. (1996). Nurse's use and delegation of indirect care interventions. *Nursing Economics, 14* (1), 22–33.

McGarrity, C., and Knox, B. (1995). Socio-economic determinants of dietary habits. *Social Sciences in Health: International Journal of Research and Practice, 1* (2), 94–106.

Meleis, A. I. (1997). *Theoretical nursing: Development and progress* (3rd ed.) p. 187. Philadelphia: J. B. Lippincott.

Nelson, M., Bowser, R., Jackson, M., Lugton, B., Murray-Bachmann, R., Wolman, P., and Karp, R. (1993). Problem of changing food habits: Reaching disadvantaged families through their own food cultures. In R. J. Karp (Ed.), *Malnourished children in the United States: Caught in the cycle of poverty* (Chap. 19, 194–211). New York: Springer Publishing.

Nightingale, F. (1966). *Notes on nursing: What it is and what it is not.* Philadelphia: J. B. Lippincott.

Nunnery, R. K. (1997). *Advancing your career: Concepts of professional nursing.* Philadelphia: F. A. Davis.

O'Bryan-Doheny, M., Benson Cook, C., and Stopper, M. C. (1997). *The discipline of nursing: An introduction* (4th ed.). Stamford, CT: Appleton & Lange.

Onyango, A., Tucker, K., and Eisemon, T. (1994). Household headship and child nutrition: A case study in Western Kenya. *Social Science and Medicine, 39,* 1633–1639.

Orem, D. E. (1991). *Nursing: Concepts of practice.* St. Louis: Mosby–Year Book.

Roy, C., and Andrews, H. A. (1991). *The Roy adaptation model: The definitive statement.* Norwalk, CT: Appleton & Lange.

Smith, C. M., and Maurer, F. A. (1995). *Community health nursing theory and practice.* Philadelphia: W. B. Saunders.

Stanhope, M., and Lancaster, J. (1996). *Community health nursing: Promoting health of aggregates, families, and individuals* (4th ed.). St. Louis: Mosby.

Wagner, J., and Menke, E. (1991a). The depression of homeless children: A focus for nursing intervention. *Issues in Pediatric Nursing, 14,* 17–29.

Wagner, J., and Menke, E. (1991b). *Homeless children and their mothers. Final report to Ohio Department of Mental Health.* Columbus, OH: Ohio State University.

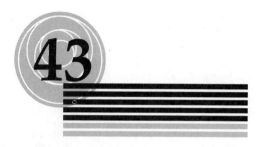

Telephone Consultation

Sheila A. Haas and Ida A. Androwich

Telephone nursing practice is rapidly evolving and becoming a major dimension of nursing roles both in ambulatory care settings (Cooley, Lin, & Hunter, 1994; Haas & Hackbarth, 1995; Haas, Hackbarth, Kavanagh, & Vlasses, 1995; Hackbarth, Haas & Kavanagh, & Vlasses, 1995) and in the hospital (Beckie, 1989; Bowman, Howden, Allen, Webster, & Thompson, 1994). The penetration of managed care throughout the health care market has markedly increased the search for cost-effective practice refinements that will maintain quality and consumer satisfaction yet reduce costly provider time. One such refinement involves the substitution of the telephone for a face-to-face encounter in diagnosis; prescription of care alternatives for patients; and teaching, support, surveillance, and follow-up of patients after surgery, treatment, or hospitalization. *Demand management* is a term currently used that subsumes telephone practice. Demand management is defined as "techniques to achieve an appropriate and desired balance of health care resources and service utilization" (Alliance for Health Care Strategy and Marketing, 1995).

Although use of the telephone for scheduling appointments and calling for advice is common in a fee-for-service environment, in the past patients were, more often than not, asked to come in to the physician's office for a visit, where a diagnosis was made. As early as 1975, Murphy and Dineen describe nursing by telephone in a health maintenance organization (HMO). In the past, most surgery and treatments frequently required hospitalization, and hospital stays were longer. Hospital stays began to shorten under diagnosis-related group (DRG) prospective payment and have become increasingly shorter under managed care capitation arrangements. Today, surgeries and procedures once done in the hospital are now done in an ambulatory care setting. Consequently, patients' learning needs are often assessed over the telephone before treatment, patients may be taught by phone, and they often receive follow-up telephone calls when they are discharged early from the hospital or ambulatory care setting.

In managed care, the focus on use of a primary care provider as a gatekeeper has increased the use of the telephone to provide diagnosis and treatment plans over the telephone so that the patient does not have to visit a provider. This is usually satisfying to the patient and cost-effective for the provider, who saves the time and the cost of a visit when working under a capitated payment system. Managed care organizations use telephone triage to determine the urgency of clients' complaints and to both route patients to the appropriate provider and provide authorization for care. Use of telephone advice services and "after hours" call-in services (Anders, 1997), where nurses answer patient questions on a toll-free line, has become popular and is a marketing tool for competing health care organizations. In the past, little telephone consultation was done by nurses; now, in any surgical area or area where chronically ill patients receive care, nurses find themselves on the telephone doing teaching, surveillance, support, advice, and follow-up. Emergency department (ED) nurses receive telephone triage calls and often advise patients to come into the ED (Wheeler, 1989). Telephone advice, teaching, and triage have been common in pediatric office practice for many years (Fosarelli, 1983; Goodman & Perrin, 1978; Greenlick, 1973; Perrin, 1978; Poole, Schmitt, Carruth, Peterson-Smith, & Slusarski, 1993; Strain, 1971; Strasser, Levy, Lamb, & Rosecrans, 1979).

Although patient encounters via telephone are far more common today, they are not less challenging. A telephone nursing encounter is far more complex than a face-to-face encounter with a patient or family member. Telephone encounters require expert communication skills on the part of the provider. Telephone assessment is limited to information and respenses elicited from the patient because no physical assessment or visual cues are available. In essence, the nurse is doing an assessment with a blindfold on, hands tied behind the back, and nose pinched. In addition, the time for the telephone encounter is very limited, and there is little time for "second" thoughts. Telephone triage nurses can do as many as 80 calls in an 8-hour period, or one every 6 minutes (Wheeler & Windt, 1993).

The increase in health care organization mergers has led to the development of complex integrated delivery systems. This, along with the increased use of the telephone as a diagnostic device and treatment coordination tool, has also given rise to concerns about standardizing telephone practice in all its forms. There are now computerized and hard copy telephone guidelines for telephone triage, telephone advice, and telephone teaching (Simonsen, 1996; Smith, Burcham, Chase, & Bashore, 1993). The American Academy of Ambulatory Care Nursing (AAACN) Telephone Nursing Practice Administration and Practice Standards were released in early 1997. These standards are a "work in progress." They acknowledge that "definition of practice standards will help define clear responsibilities and accountabilities for both clinical practitioners and administrators responsible for providing telephone care" (AAACN, 1997, p. 10). The challenge in writing telephone practice standards has been to limit the standards to those that can be applied across a variety of practice settings. The AAACN telephone practice standards include standards addressing structure and organization of telephone nursing, staffing competency, use of the nursing process in telephone nursing practice, continuity of care, ethics and patient rights, environment, research, and quality management.

Another issue regarding telephone practice interventions involves the appropriate and necessary documentation of the telephone encounter. It is easy to document a telephone encounter when the patient's chart is readily available. This is not the case in many situations, particularly in ambulatory care or in the ED. Few ambulatory care settings have online access to their patients' medical records, and none has a fully integrated electronic patient record. Therefore, documentation policies and procedures have been evolving.

ISSUES WITH TELEPHONE CONSULTATION

Telephone Consultation is now expanding and will continue to expand as a major dimension in the roles of nurses working in ambulatory care (Haas & Hackbarth, 1995; Hackbarth et al. 1995. There are three major areas where issues arise with telephone nursing practice. First are issues with cost-effectiveness; these involve issues with quality of care, patient satisfaction, and risk management. Second are issues with nursing workload management, and third are issues related to standardized language.

Cost-Effectiveness Issues

There are many goals for Telephone Consultation in a managed care environment, such as (1) reducing unnecessary visits to health care providers in the office or emergency department, (2) directing patients to primary care providers or preferred provider organizations, (3) standardizing health information for consistency and risk management purposes, (4) enhancing patient ability to make informed and appropriate health care decisions, and (5) assisting patients in determining appropriate self-care (Matherly & Hodges, 1992).

As stated previously, patients are often very satisfied with the opportunity to call and consult with a nurse about health care concerns. One study actually found that patients ask nurses questions that they are too embarrassed to ask the doctor (Murphy & Dineen, 1975). Patients are also often satisfied with diagnosis and treatment prescribed over the telephone, because they do not have the inconvenience of going in for an office visit. Anders (1997) recounts that every dollar spent in telephone triage is two dollars saved on ED charges. HMOs have tapped into the telephone triage concept (Janowski, 1995), recognizing its potential for cost-effectiveness.

However, there are potential quality issues regarding accurate diagnosis and prescription of treatment and consistency of diagnosis and treatment between telephone encounters with the same patient or across multiple patients. These are both potential quality and risk management issues. Another risk management issue involves consistent and thorough documentation of each telephone encounter in a readily retrievable format.

Stock (1995) delineates some of the risks of telephone triage: Telephone triage involves great risks from a legal and risk management perspective. Few, if any established standards of practice exist for telephone triage with methods of telephone triage ranging from receptionists, medical assistants, or licensed practical or vocational nurses giving information and advice without the benefit of written guidelines or protocols and then passing a message on later to a physician, resulting in a significant delay in care, to sophisticated computer systems simultaneously either recording or prompting documentation of client calls and allowing advice to be dispatched immediately (p. 20).

Professional nursing has strongly stated that only professional nurses have the necessary preparation and skills for telephone nursing interventions, such as telephone triage, teaching, advice, and consultation (AAACN/American Nurses Association [ANA] Task Force, 1997). Sadly, the reality in many settings is that telephone interventions may fall to anyone who answers a patient telephone call. Unless ambulatory care receptionists or schedulers have a prescribed series of questions to ask a patient who is calling for an appointment, schedulers can be doing triage by default at great risk to the patient, the providers, and the organization. If the scheduler does not ascertain whether the patient has an immediate problem and schedules a visit for a later date, there can be an unnecessary, and perhaps harmful, delay in diagnosis and treatment.

Telephone nursing is a dimension of the professional nurse role in ambulatory care (AAACN/ANA Task Force, 1997; Haas & Hackbarth, 1995; Hackbarth et al., 1995; Matherly & Hodges, 1992). "Telephone triage is a nursing function that incorporates the five components of the nursing process. . . . As such, telephone triage nurses are accountable for the advice and care they recommend to clients" (Packard & Scott, 1990). Yet many nurses are performing telephone nursing practice without structured education or training; without protocols, procedures, or standards; and without standardized documentation protocols (Stock, 1995).

> Unfortunately, advice or information given to callers in the current system may be inconsistent, and the degree of advice may vary according to the educational or experience level of the health care staff rendering the advice. This approach offers little means of legal protection for the health care professional or his or her employer (Stock, 1995, p. 20).

Katz (1990) used a cause-and-effect diagram to demonstrate the complexity of telephone interventions (Fig. 43–1). Katz's diagram developed six major variables (patient, type of call, skill and preparation of staff, constraints of the

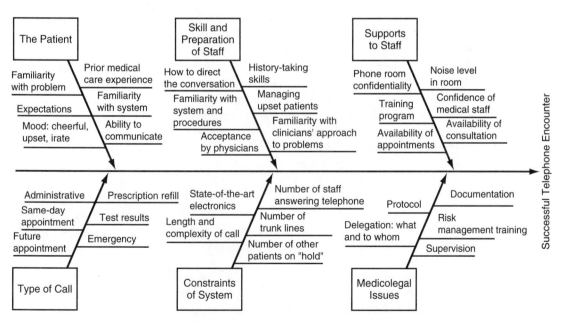

Figure 43–1. Ishikawa cause-and-effect diagram. Fishbone diagram illustrating the interplay of variables or inputs that determine a desired outcome. (From Katz: *Telephone medicine: Triage and training*, F. A. Davis Company, Philadelphia, PA © 1990. Previously published by Slack, Inc., Thorofare, NJ.)

system, supports to staff, and medicolegal issues) that explain a desired outcome in a telephone encounter.

Little cost-effectiveness research has been done. Bedleck (1996) reported patients, family, and physician satisfaction with telephone responsiveness of nurses as well as a decrease in ED visits and length of stay for the patient population managed. Mazurek (1996) reported that the Henry Ford Health System experienced referral savings of $1,355,550 on ED visits that were referred to urgent care or primary care. She concluded that "nurse-driven telemanagement services are cost-effective and improve utilization management" (p. 11). There is a need for identification of effectiveness indicators in addition to cost and satisfaction. Effectiveness indicators should be imbedded in documentation systems so that data are easily retrievable.

Workload Issues

Nurses are spending increasing amounts of time in telephone encounters with patients, whether the nurses are working in ambulatory care settings or in the hospital. Telephone encounters engender workload issues as well as the issues already discussed regarding levels and preparation of nursing personnel who are doing telephone encounters. Therefore, it is necessary to completely capture the breadth and depth of aspects of telephone nursing practice as discrete nursing interventions. Telephone nursing practice must be well delineated so that appropriate professional nursing personnel are selected and educated to do telephone nursing practice and so that the content of telephone nursing practice can be developed for education, setting of standards, and evaluation purposes. Finally, clear delineation of telephone nursing practice interventions is needed to demonstrate the level of complexity of telephone nursing practice and the time needed to do such practice (Nelson, 1991). Delineation of telephone nursing interventions will also assist in development of this component of nursing intensity, especially in ambulatory care nursing.

Research needs to be conducted regarding the competencies necessary for effective telephone nursing practice. When telephone nursing practice competencies are delineated, research needs to be done on the most effective means of educating both practicing nurses and student nurses regarding these competencies. There is interest in certification in telephone nursing practice. If this gains momentum, a core curriculum in telephone nursing practice must be developed.

Proposed telephone interventions speak to maintaining patient confidentiality. Use of the telephone or other telecommunication systems exproses patients and providers to increased opportunities for breaks in confidentiality. The proposed telephone Nursing Interventions Classification (NIC) interventions also speak to identification of persons other than the patient who can be given telephone information on the patient's behalf. Patient perceptions of confidentiality should be researched.

Telephone nurse productivity must also be researched. Research questions that describe frequency of common telephone nursing interventions and their relationship to both positive outcomes and negative outcomes such as delayed treatment, escalation of problems or complications, and fragmentation of care must be studied. Use of the NIC and the Nursing Outcomes Classification (NOC) with their coding systems will expedite such work and allow comparisons to be made between and within settings.

Standardized Language Issues

Currently, of the five standardized languages in nursing recognized by the American Nurses Association (ANA), only three deal with nursing interventions. The Saba Home Health Care Classification (Saba, 1992) and the Omaha System (Martin & Sheet, 1992) do not have telephone nursing interventions delineated specifically. However, the Saba system has modifiers to describe activities related to broad nursing actions such as teaching or referral. The NIC has only one telephone intervention, Telephone Consultation (Table 43–1). The definition of Telephone Consultation is very broad: "Exchanging information, providing health education and advice, managing symptoms, or doing triage over the

Table 43–1 Telephone Consultation

DEFINITION: Exchanging information, providing health education and advice, managing symptoms, or doing triage over the telephone.

ACTIVITIES:

Identify purpose of the call

Calm caller by giving simple instructions for action, as needed

Obtain information related to the purpose of the call, as necessary (e.g., nature of crisis, medical diagnoses, past health history, and current treatment regimen)

Identify concerns about health status

Obtain data related to effectiveness of treatment

Determine whether concerns require medical evaluation

Provide first aid instructions or emergency directions for crises (e.g., CPR instructions and birthing)

Stay on the line while contacting emergency services

Provide clear directions for transport to the hospital, as needed

Provide instruction on how to access needed care, if concerns are acute

Provide information about treatment regimen and resultant self-care responsibilities, as necessary, according to scope of practice and established protocols

Provide information about prescribed therapies and medications, as appropriate

Provide information about health promotion/health education, as appropriate

Identify actual/potential problems related to implementing self-care

Facilitate problem solving about self-care regimen

Make recommendations about regimen changes, as appropriate

Consult with physician about changes in the treatment regimen, as necessary

Provide instructions about preparation for planned diagnostic tests/medical procedures

Notify patient of test results, as indicated

Assist with prescription refills, according to established protocols

Answer questions

Provide emotional support, as needed

Maintain confidentiality, as indicated

Provide information about community resources, educational programs, support groups, and self-help groups, as indicated

Establish a time and date for follow-up care, including further telephone consultation

Determine how patient or family member can be reached for a return telephone call, as appropriate

Record any advice, instructions, or other information given to patient

Follow up by calling the client back, if uncomfortable with the communication

Source: McCloskey, J. C., and Bulechek, G. M. (1996). *Nursing interventions classification (NIC)* (2nd ed.). St. Louis, Mosby–Year Book.

telephone" (McCloskey & Bulecheck, 1996, p. 560). This chapter proposes that providing health education, exchanging information (consultation) and advice, managing symptoms (follow-up), and performing triage are discrete NIC telephone practice interventions, each with a set of unique activities. In addition, two other telephone nursing practice interventions are proposed: telephone surveillance and telephone support.

The authors used the current NIC Telephone Consultation intervention depicted in Table 43–1 as well as current literature to initially develop six discrete telephone nursing practice interventions: telephone triage, telephone teaching, telephone advice/consultation, telephone follow-up, telephone support, and telephone surveillance.

Each of these proposed NIC telephone interventions was submitted to the American Academy of Ambulatory Care Nursing (AAACN) Telephone Nursing Practice (TPN) Special Interest Group (SIG) '97–'98 Steering Committee and to two other experts who could serve as an expert panel for evaluation and feedback. Specifically, the experts were sent the NIC Telephone Consultation intervention (McCloskey & Bulechek, 1996), an overview of the NIC, and the proposed NIC telephone interventions and were asked to evaluate the definitions of each proposed intervention, as well as the activities listed for each intervention. The SIG members were also asked to critique the proposed activities under each intervention and to add or delete activities and give a rationale for each activity added or deleted. Nine of the 10 experts responded with feedback on the proposed telephone nursing practice interventions.

In the development of these proposed NIC telephone interventions, the authors tried to think futuristically. Today, we think of telephone encounters as one-to-one experiences; however, there can easily be one or more nurses in an encounter with one or more patients or a patient and family members in a conference call format. Today, we also think of telephone practice as synchronous with an immediate interaction; however, voice mail and E-mail are making asynchronous interactions common. One expert panelist summarized this issue well:

> Implicit in all interventions is a dyadic encounter: one nurse–one patient, talking together at a single point in time, yet telecommunications technology supports a one-to-many model of interaction. Furthermore, telecommunications technology supports both synchronous as well as asynchronous communication. It is possible that additional nursing skills and critical judgment about the nature and timing of the communications should be reflected in the activities. It is likely that, as technology provides new communication methods, new activities and strategies for the effective use of these methods will need to be developed. (P. F. Brennan, personal communication, June 11, 1997).

The six proposed telephone nursing interventions—telephone triage, telephone teaching, telephone advice/consultation, telephone follow-up, telephone support, and telephone surveillance—were submitted to the Iowa Intervention Project–NIC Review Committee for consideration and eventual approval. The NIC Review Committee suggested that the original NIC Telephone Consultation intervention (See Table 43–1) be retained and that the activities specific to telephone support and telephone teaching be added to it. The NIC Review Committee felt that teaching and support were part of consultation and difficult to separate. The definition of Telephone Consultation was also altered to include the fact that either the patient and family or the nurse could initiate the call. The proposed revised intervention Telephone Consultation is in Table 43–2. The NIC Review Committee also suggested modifications to the other proposed telephone interventions. The revised interventions are triage: telephone (Table

Table 43–2   Telephone Consultation (Proposed Revision)

DEFINITION: A nurse- or patient-initiated phone encounter where the nurse elicits patient concerns, listens, and provides support, information, or teaching about a health problem, health promotion, or disease prevention in response to patient stated concerns.

ACTIVITIES:

Identify self with name and credentials, organization; let caller know if call is being recorded (e.g., for quality monitoring)

Inform patient about call process and obtain consent

Consider cultural, socioeconomic barriers to patient's response

Obtain information related to purpose of the call (e.g., medical diagnoses if any, past health history, and current treatment regimen)

Identify patient concerns about health status

Establish level of caller's knowledge and source of that knowledge

Determine patient's ability to understand telephone teaching/instructions (presence of hearing deficits, confusion)

Provide means of overcoming any identified barrier to learning or use of support system(s)

Identify degree of family support

Inquire about related complaints/symptoms (according to standard protocol, if available)

Obtain data related to effectiveness of current treatment(s), if any, by consulting and citing approved references as sources (e.g., "American Red Cross suggests . . .")

Determine psychological response to situation and availability of support system(s)

Determine safety risk to caller and/or others

Determine whether concerns require further evaluation (use standard protocol)

Provide clear instruction on how to access needed care, if concerns are acute

Provide information about treatment regimen and resultant self-care responsibilities as necessary according to scope of practice and established guidelines

Provide information about prescribed therapies and medications, as appropriate

Provide information about health promotion/health education, as appropriate

Identify actual/potential problems related to implementation of self-care regimen

Make recommendations about regimen changes as appropriate (using established guidelines, if available)

Consult with physician/primary care provider about changes in the treatment regimen, as necessary

Provide information about community resources, educational programs, support groups, and self-help groups as indicated

Provide services in a caring and supportive manner

Involve family/significant others in the care and planning

Answer questions, determine caller's understanding of information provided

Maintain confidentiality, as indicated

Document any assessments, advice, instructions, or other information given to patient according to specified guidelines

Follow guidelines for investigating or reporting suspected child, geriatric, or spousal abuse situations

Follow up to determine disposition, document disposition, and patient's intended action(s)

Determine need and establish time intervals for further, intermittent assessment

Determine how patient or family member can be reached for a return telephone call, as appropriate

Document permission for return call and identify persons able to receive call information

Discuss and resolve problem calls with supervisory/collegial help

Table 43–3 Triage: Telephone (Proposed Intervention)

DEFINITION: A patient-initiated telephone encounter requiring the professional nurse to determine the nature and urgency of a problem(s) and to provide directions for the level of care required.

ACTIVITIES:

Identify self with name and credentials, organization; let caller know if call is being recorded (e.g., for quality monitoring)

Direct, facilitate, and calm caller by giving simple instructions for action as needed

Display willingness to help (e.g., "How may I help?")

Obtain information about purpose of the call (e.g., nature of crisis, symptoms, medical diagnosis, past health history, and current treatment regimen)

Consider cultural, socioeconomic barriers to patient's response

Identify patient's concerns about health status. Whenever possible, speak directly to the patient

Prioritize reported symptoms, determining those with highest possible risk first

Use standardized symptom-based guidelines to identify and evaluate significant data and classify urgency of symptoms, as available

Inquire about related complaints/symptoms (according to standard guidelines, if available)

Obtain data related to effectiveness of current treatment(s), if any

Determine whether concerns require further evaluation (use standard guidelines, if available)

Provide first aid instructions or emergency directions for crises (e.g., CPR instructions or birthing) using standard guidelines

Stay on the line while contacting emergency services, according to organization's protocol

Provide clear directions for transport to the hospital, as needed

Advise patient on options for referral and/or intervention

Provide clear instruction on how to access needed care, if concerns are acute

Provide information about treatment regimen and resultant self-care responsibilities as necessary, according to scope of practice and established guidelines

Confirm patient's understanding of advice or directions through verbalization

Determine need and establish time intervals for further, intermittent assessment

Document any assessments, advice, instructions, or other information given to patient according to specified guidelines

Determine how patient or family member can be reached for return telephone calls as appropriate

Document permission for return call and identify persons able to receive call information

Follow up, as necessary, to determine disposition, document disposition, and patient's intended action

Maintain confidentiality, as indicated

Discuss and resolve problem calls with supervisory/collegial help

43–3), telephone follow-up (Table 43–4), and surveillance: telephone (Table 43–5). These revisions will appear in the third edition of NIC.

NURSING DIAGNOSES, OUTCOMES, AND TYPICAL PATIENT POPULATIONS ASSOCIATED WITH PROPOSED TELEPHONE INTERVENTIONS

Given the nature of telephone interventions, there are many nursing diagnoses that could be associated with each and every one of the proposed interventions (NANDA, 1994). Table 43–6 was created to demonstrate this phenomenon. Also, any patient could initiate any one of the telephone interventions, or nurses could initiate telephone interventions with a broad array of patient populations, such

Table 43–4 Telephone Follow-Up (Proposed Intervention)

DEFINITION: A nurse-initiated phone encounter where the nurse provides results of testing or evaluates response to previous treatment or examination and assesses potential for problems as a result of previous treatment or testing.

ACTIVITIES:

Identify self with name and credentials, organization; let caller know if call is being recorded (e.g., for quality monitoring)

Inform patient about call process and obtain consent

Determine that you are actually speaking to the patient or, if someone else, that you have the patient's permission to give information to them

Notify patient of test results, as indicated (positive results, such as biopsy results, should not be given over the phone by the nurse)

Use intermediary services such as language relay services, TTY/TDD (for hearing impaired), or emerging telecommunication technologies such as computer networks or visual displays, as appropriate

Assist with prescription refills, according to established guidelines

Answer questions

Provide information about community resources, educational programs, support groups, and self-help groups as indicated

Establish a time and date for follow-up care or referral appointment

Provide information about treatment regimen and resultant self-care responsibilities as necessary, according to scope of practice and established guidelines

Maintain confidentiality, as indicated

Document any assessments, advice, instructions, or other information given to patient according to specified guidelines

Determine how patient or family member can be reached for a return telephone call, as appropriate

Document permission for return call and identify persons able to receive call

---

as pre- or postsurgical patients, high-risk obstetrics patients, and frail elderly patients. However, parents are usually the callers for the pediatric population, and caregivers are often the callers or callees for patients with chronic illnesses or those on surveillance devices.

Similarly, there is a broad array of potential nursing outcomes that could be associated with any one of the telephone interventions, depending on the nursing diagnosis or diagnoses made during the telephone encounter. Table 43–7 was created to show potential nursing outcomes from the NOC (Johnson & Maas, 1997) that could result from telephone interventions.

The two case studies that follow were developed to show how a nurse can implement one of the proposed telephone interventions with a patient-initiated telephone encounter (surveillance: telephone, see Table 43–5) and a nurse-initiated encounter (triage: telephone, see Table 43–3).

CASE STUDIES

Case Study I

Mary Stewart, BSN, is employed as a care coordinator at the Hudson Medical Center. She works primarily with the elderly congestive heart failure (CHF) patient population. One of her responsibilities is to monitor those CHF patients who are receiving home care services. Hudson Home Care uses HANC (Home Assisted Nursing Care) by Health Tech Service Corporation. HANC may be termed a *cognitive robot* and is capable of assisting patients in the home with dispensing medications and monitoring vital signs (blood pressure, temperature, and pulse) or can be used as a memory device to remind patients of activi-

Table 43–5 Surveillance: Telephone (Proposed Intervention)

DEFINITION: Purposeful and ongoing acquisition of patient data via electronic modalities from distant locations, as well as interpretation and synthesis of patient data for clinical decision making with individuals or population.

ACTIVITIES:

Identify self with name and credentials, organization; let caller know if call is being recorded (e.g., for quality monitoring)

Inform patient about call process and obtain consent

Determine patient's health risk(s), as appropriate

Obtain information about normal patient behavior and routine

Identify or aggregate data that have programmatic or population implications

Establish the frequency of data collection and interpretation, as indicated by status of the patient

Monitor incoming data for validity and reliability

Interpret results of diagnostic indicators such as vital signs, glucose readings, EKGs

Collaborate/consult with physician resources as necessary

Explain test results and interventions to patient and family

Monitor comfort level, and take appropriate action

Monitor coping strategies and actions used by patient and family

Initiate skin surveillance in high-risk patient

Monitor for potential problems based on current status (i.e., infection, fluid and electrolyte balance, tissue perfusion, nutrition and elimination)

Troubleshoot equipment and systems to enhance acquisition of reliable patient data

Coordinate placement/replacement/set-up of equipment/supplies

Compare current status with previous status to detect improvements or deterioration in patient's condition

Initiate and/or change medical treatment to maintain patient parameter with the limits ordered by the physician using established guidelines

Facilitate acquisition of interdisciplinary services (e.g., pastoral services) as appropriate

Prioritize actions based on patient status

Analyze physician orders in conjunction with patient status to ensure safety of the patient

Obtain consultation from appropriate health care worker to initiate new treatment or change existing treatments

Advocate for patient's welfare, as necessary

Main confidentiality, as indicated

Determine need and establish time intervals for further, intermittent assessment

Document assessments, advice, instructions, or other information given to patient according to specified guidelines

Determine how patient or family member can be reached for return telephone calls as appropriate

Document permission for return call and identify person(s) able to receive call

---

ties, or a patient education device that can guide the patient through any self-administered procedure. HANC can also be used to take electrocardiograms (EKGs) or test blood glucose levels and as an infusion pump, scale, pulse oximeter, and spirometer. The nurse at the central station is able to view the patient, because HANC provides for two-way direct observation. HANC has the capacity to monitor the blood oxygen levels of home care patients. Once Mary reads and evaluates the pulse oximeter results, she will use established guidelines to adjust the oxygen dose appropriately to maintain adequate blood oxygen levels.

Today, Mary is concerned about Mr. F, an 81-year-old man who has had CHF for 20 years. Because of severe arthritis and residual right-sided weakness that has limited his mobility, as well as a recent bout of pneumonia, Mr. F has been receiving home care services and uses HANC to monitor his weight, EKGs, and oxygen levels. His oxygen dosage has been adjusted three times in the past 2 weeks, and Mary is planning to call him to evaluate potential causes of this recent fluctuation.

Table 43–6   Proposed Telephone Interventions and Associated NANDA Nursing Diagnoses

Proposed Telephone Interventions—Key:

1 Telephone Consultation
2 Telephone Follow-Up
3 Surveillance: Telephone
4 Triage: Telephone

Examples of NANDA nursing diagnoses that can be linked to proposed telephone interventions include the following:

Adjustment, Impaired	1
Anxiety	1
Breastfeeding, Ineffective	1
Breathing Pattern, Ineffective	1, 3
Caregiver Role Strain	1
Caregiver Role Strain, Risk for	1
Community Coping, Ineffective	4
Community, Management of Therapeutic Regimen, Ineffective	3
Decisional Conflict	1
Family Coping: Disabling, Ineffective	1, 2
Family, Management of Therapeutic Regimen, Ineffective	1, 2, 4
Fear	1, 2
Grieving, Anticipatory	1, 3
Health Seeking Behaviors	1, 3
Individual Coping, Ineffective	1, 2
Individual, Management of Therapeutic Regimen, Ineffective	1, 2, 3, 4
Infection, Risk for	3
Injury, Risk for	3
Knowledge Deficit	1
Parenting, Altered, Risk for	1, 2, 4

Source: North American Nursing Diagnosis Association. (1994). *NANDA nursing diagnosis: definition and classification 1995–1996.* Philadelphia: Author.

As part of the surveillance: telephone intervention, Mary will ascertain that the incoming data from HANC are reliable and valid by having the home health care nurse do a concurrent pulse oximeter reading with her portable pulse oximeter. The home care nurse will also recalibrate HANC according to manufacturer's specifications, if necessary. When Mary speaks with Mr. F, she will assess his mobility level and daily routines to look for any recent changes that could explain his newly fluctuating oxygen saturation. Because his daughter has been heavily involved in his care, and because Mr. F has indicated his desire to have his daughter participate, Mary will set up a three-way conference call. Before the call, she will have consulted with the pharmacist and the physician to determine how Mr. F's current respiratory infection and antibiotics therapy may be affecting his oxygenation status. During the conference call, Mary will discuss a plan for ongoing monitoring of Mr. F's oxygenation status, to which Mr. F and his daughter will agree. Once this has been negotiated, along with timing and indications for future calls, Mary will document the surveillance encounter.

Case Study 2

Later that day, around 7:00 PM, Julie Grant, BSN, a nurse in the medicine clinic at Hudson, receives a frantic call from Martha Williams, the visiting sister of H, age 47, a diabetic. It appears that Martha, who lives out of state, has been visiting her brother, and they had been planning to go out for a late lunch. While she was getting ready, H was resting and now seems unable to get up and is talking incoherently. He is "sweating and

Table 43–7 Proposed Telephone Interventions and Associated NOC Outcomes

Proposed Telephone Interventions—Key:

1 Telephone Consultation
2 Telephone Follow-Up
3 Surveillance: Telephone
4 Triage: Telephone

Examples of NOC outcomes that can be linked to proposed telephone interventions include the following:

Acceptance: Health Status	1
Adherence Behavior	1
Anxiety Control	1
All "Caregiver" outcomes (e.g., Caregiver Emotional Health, Caregiver Performance: Direct Care)	1
Compliance Behavior	1
Coping	1, 2
Decision Making	1, 4
All "Health" outcomes (e.g., Health Beliefs: Perceived Control, Health Beliefs: Perceived Resources)	1
Hope	1
Information Processing	1
All "Knowledge" outcomes (e.g., Knowledge: Health Behaviors, Knowledge: Infection Control)	1, 4
All "Nutritional Status" outcomes (e.g., Nutritional Status: Energy, Nutritional Status: Body Mass)	1
Pain Control Behavior	1, 2, 4
Participation: Health Care Decisions	1, 2, 4
Quality of Life	1
Risk Control	3, 4
Risk Detection	3, 4
Role Performance	1
All "Safety" outcomes (e.g., Safety Behavior: Fall Prevention, Safety Behavior: Home Physical Environment)	1
All "Self-Care" outcomes (e.g., Self-Care: Hygiene, Self-Care: Parenteral Medication)	1, 4
Social Support	1
Spiritual Well-Being	1
Suicide Self-Restraint	4
Well-Being	1, 2

Source: Johnson, M., and Maas, M. (Eds). (1997). *Nursing outcomes classification (NOC).* St. Louis: Mosby–Year Book.

sluggish." Julie ascertains that when H picked Martha up at the airport at 9:00 AM he mentioned that he did not eat breakfast but did take his neutral protamine Hagedorn (NPH) insulin at 7:00 AM, the usual time. He was able to tell Martha to call the clinic, and Martha thought that he was asking for a glass of orange juice. She wanted instructions as to how to proceed with his care. Because Julie knew H, who not infrequently had insulin reactions when routine meal-times were delayed, she decided that the reaction could be managed at home. She calmed Martha, further assessed H's condition, and instructed Martha to give H some orange juice. Because Martha now appeared quite calm, Julie judged her able to carry out the instructions and report appropriately. Julie instructed Martha on how to complete a blood glucose level check, and H's blood glucose level was 62. In 20 minutes, it had risen to 112. Julie instructed Martha further and made an appointment for H for later that afternoon at the clinic. Julie documented the call fully and made a note on the chart to advise H to keep some high-glucose tablets on hand for emergencies.

It is important to consider the nursing diagnoses that might drive the selection of a specific telephone intervention. Using the North American Nursing Diagnosis Association (NANDA)–NIC linkage list in the second edition of the NIC as a guide, Table 43–6 demonstrates some suggestions for potential linkages. (This is not intended to be a comprehensive list of all possible nursing diagnoses but will serve as an example.)

CONCLUSION

The telephone nursing practice interventions presented in this chapter have been resubmitted to the Iowa Intervention Project–NIC Review Committee for evaluation, and it is to be hoped that they will be approved for use in the near future. Because of space constraints, reference lists for each proposed intervention are not included in this chapter, but they will be attached to each telephone intervention when submitted for evaluation.

One goal of this chapter is to demonstrate the responsiveness of the NIC to modification based on evolving practice. Another goal is to demonstrate how NIC interventions can be instrumental in setting standards and training and evaluating professional nurses, as well as identifying potential risk management issues and research questions and attending to nursing intensity and workload issues.

Finally, the use of an expert panel to refine six proposed telephone interventions was demonstrated. The expert panel was consulted so that confidence in the content and discriminate validity of each proposed telephone intervention could be demonstrated given the number of proposed telephone interventions in the chapter and the fact that telephone nursing practice is rapidly evolving.

Acknowledgments

The authors would like to acknowledge the contributions of the following members of the American Academy of Ambulatory Care Nursing Telephone Nursing Practice Special Interest Group Steering Committee: Kathleen Blanchfield, PhD, RN; Marie DesChamps, RNC, CNA, BA; Leslie Hes, MN, RN; Patricia Reisinger, MS, RN; Lisa Schwarzentraub, BSN, RN; Carol Stock, JD, NM, RN; and Charlene Williams, BSN, CDE, RN, C. The two other experts consulted were Sandi Dahl, BSN, MA, RN, C, Helix TeleHealth Center, Baltimore, and Patricia Flatley Brennan, PhD, RN, FAAN, FACMI, Moehlman Bascom Professor, School of Nursing and College of Engineering, University of Wisconsin–Madison.

References

Alliance for Health Care Strategy and Marketing. (1995). *Trend Watch, 5*(2), 3–5.

American Academy of Ambulatory Care Nursing. (1997). *Telephone nursing practice administration and practice standards.* Pitman, NJ: Anthony J. Jannetti.

American Academy of Ambulatory Care Nursing/ American Nurses Association Task Force. (1997). *Nursing in ambulatory care: The future is here.* Washington, DC: American Nurses Publishing.

Anders, G. (1997, February 4). Telephone triage: How nurses take calls and control the care of patients from afar. *The Wall Street Journal,* A1, A6.

Beckie, T. (1989). A supportive-educative telephone program: Impact on knowledge and anxiety after coronary artery bypass graft surgery. *Heart and Lung, 18*(1), 46–55.

Bedleck, A. K. (1996). Innovations in ambulatory care: A new approach to primary nursing. *AAACN Viewpoint, 18*(1), 10.

Bowman, G. S., Howden, J., Allen, S., Webster, R. A., and Thompson, D. R. (1994). A telephone survey of medical patients 1 week after discharge from hospital. *Journal of Clinical Nursing, 3,* 369–373.

Cooley, M. E., Lin, E. M., and Hunter, S. W. (1994). The ambulatory oncology nurse's role. *Seminars in Oncology Nursing, 10,* 245–253.

Fosarelli, P. (1983). The telephone in pediatric medicine. *Clinical Pediatrics, 22,* 293–296.

Goodman, H. C., and Perrin, E. C. (1978). Evening telephone call management by nurse practitioners and physicians. *Nursing Research, 27,* 233–236.

Greenlick, M. (1973). Determinants of medical utilization: The role of the telephone in total medical care. *Medical Care, 11,* 121–134.

Haas, S., and Hackbarth, D. (1995). Dimensions of the staff nurse role in ambulatory care: Part III—Using research data to design new models of nursing care delivery. *Nursing Economics, 13,* 230–241.

Haas, S., Hackbarth, D., Kavanagh, J., and Vlasses, F. (1995). Dimensions of the staff nurse role in ambulatory care: Part II—Comparison of role dimensions in four ambulatory settings. *Nursing Economics, 13,* 152–165.

Hackbarth, D., Haas, S., Kavanagh, J., and Vlasses, F. (1995). Dimensions of the staff nurse role in ambulatory care: Part I—Methodology and analysis of data on current staff nurse practice. *Nursing Economics, 13,* 89–98.

Janowski, M. (1995). Is telephone triage calling you? *American Journal of Nursing, 95*(1), 59–62.

Johnson, M., and Maas, M. (Eds.). (1997). *Nursing outcomes classification (NOC).* St. Louis: Mosby–Year Book.

Katz, H. P. (1990). *Telephone medicine, triage and training: A handbook for primary care health professionals.* Philadelphia: F. A. Davis.

Martin, K. S., and Sheet, M. J. (1992). *The Omaha System: Applications for community health nursing.* Philadelphia: W. B. Saunders.

Matherly, S., and Hodges, S. (1992). *Telephone nursing: The process.* Englewood, CA: Center for Research in Ambulatory Health Administration.

Mazurek, P. (1996). Automated support to telephone triage: Applications and outcomes. *AACN Viewpoint, 18*(2), 10–11.

McCloskey, J. C., and Bulechek, G. M. (Eds.). (1996). *Nursing interventions classification (NIC)* (2nd ed.). St. Louis: Mosby–Year Book.

Murphy D., and Dineen, E. (1975). Nursing by telephone. *American Journal of Nursing, 75,* 1137–1139.

Nelson, W. B. (1991). Communications: Distributing on-cology outpatient telephone calls. *Nursing Management, 22*(10), 40–44.

North American Nursing Diagnosis Association. (1994). *NANDA nursing diagnosis: Definition and classification 1995–1996.* Philadelphia: Author.

Packard, A., and Scott, M. (1990). *Telephone assessment and protocols for nursing practice.* Philadelphia: W. B. Saunders.

Perrin, E. (1978). Telephone management of acute pediatric illnesses. *New England Journal of Medicine, 298,* 13–135.

Poole, S. G., Schmitt, B. D., Carruth, T., Peterson-Smith, A., and Slusarski, M. (1993). After-hours telephone coverage: The application of an area-wide telephone triage and advice system for pediatric practices. *Pediatrics, 92,* 670–679.

Saba, V. K. (1992). The classification of home health care nursing diagnoses and interventions. *Caring, 11*(3), 50–57.

Simonsen, S. (1996). *Telephone health assessment: Guidelines for practice.* St. Louis: C. V. Mosby.

Smith, C. W., Burcham, L., Chase, J. A., and Bashore, P. A. (Eds.). (1993). *Telephone triage: A manual for orthopaedic nurses.* Pitman, NJ: Anthony J. Jannetti.

Stock, C. M. (1995). Standardization of telephone triage: Is it time? *Journal of Nursing Law, 2*(2), 19–25.

Strain, J. (1971). The preparation, utilization, and evaluation of a registered nurse trained to give telephone advice in a private pediatric office. *Pediatrics, 47,* 1051–1055.

Strasser, P., Levy, J., Lamb, G. A., and Rosecrans, J. (1979). Controlled clinical trial of pediatric telephone protocols. *Pediatrics, 64,* 553–557.

Wheeler, S. Q. (1989). ED telephone triage: Lessons learned from unusual calls. *Journal of Emergency Nursing. 15,* 481–487.

Wheeler, S. Q., and Windt, J. H. (Eds.). (1993). *Telephone triage: Theory, practice, and protocol development.* Albany, NY: Delmar Publishers.

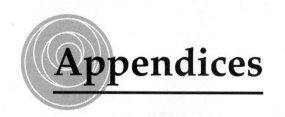

Appendices

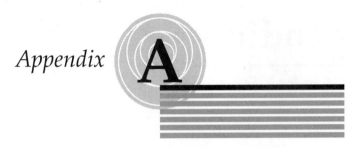

Appendix

North American Nursing Diagnosis Association (NANDA) Diagnosis Labels and Definitions, 1997–1998

Activity Intolerance   A state in which an individual has insufficient physiological or psychological energy to endure or complete required or desired daily activities.

Activity Intolerance, Risk for   A state in which an individual is at risk of experiencing insufficient physiological or psychological energy to endure or complete required or desired daily activities.

Adjustment, Impaired   The state in which the individual is unable to modify his/her lifestyle/behavior in a manner consistent with a change in health status.

Airway Clearance, Ineffective   A state in which an individual is unable to clear secretions or obstructions from the respiratory tract to maintain airway patency.

Anxiety   A vague, uneasy feeling whose source is often nonspecific or unknown to the individual.

Aspiration, Risk for   The state in which an individual is at risk for entry of gastrointestinal secretions, oropharyngeal secretion, or solids or fluids into tracheobronchial passages.

Body Image Disturbance   Disruption in the way one perceives one's body image.

Body Temperature, Risk for Altered   The state in which an individual is at risk for failure to maintain body temperature within normal range.

Breastfeeding, Effective   The state in which a mother-infant dyad/family exhibits adequate proficiency and satisfaction with breastfeeding process.

Breastfeeding, Ineffective The state in which a mother, infant, or child experiences dissatisfaction or difficulty with the breastfeeding process.

Breastfeeding, Interrupted A break in the continuity of the breastfeeding process as a result of inability or inadvisability to put baby to breast for feeding.

Breathing Pattern, Ineffective The state in which an individual's inhalation and/or exhalation pattern does not enable adequate pulmonary inflation or emptying.

Cardiac Output, Decreased A state in which the blood pumped by an individual's heart is sufficiently reduced that it is inadequate to meet the needs of the body's tissues.

Caregiver Role Strain A caregiver's felt difficulty in performing the family caregiver role.

Caregiver Role Strain, Risk for A caregiver is vulnerable for felt difficulty in performing the family caregiver role.

Communication, Impaired Verbal The state in which an individual experiences a decreased or absent ability to use or understand language in human interaction.

Community Coping, Ineffective A pattern of community activities for adaptation and problem solving that is unsatisfactory for meeting the demands or needs of the community.

Community Coping, Potential for Enhanced A pattern of community activities for adaptation and problem solving that is satisfactory for meeting the demands or needs of the community but can be improved for management of current and future problems/stressors.

Community, Management of Therapeutic Regimen, Ineffective A pattern of regulating and integrating into community processes programs for treatment of illness and the sequelae of illness that are unsatisfactory for meeting health-related goals.

Confusion, Acute The abrupt onset of a cluster of global, transient changes and disturbances in attention, cognition, psychomotor activity, level of consciousness, and/or sleep/wake cycle.

Confusion, Chronic An irreversible, long-standing and/or progressive deterioration of intellect and personality characterized by decreased ability to interpret environmental stimuli and decreased capacity for intellectual thought processes and manifested by disturbances of memory, orientation, and behavior.

Constipation A state in which an individual experiences a change in normal bowel habits characterized by a decrease in frequency and/or passage of hard, dry stools.

Constipation, Colonic The state in which an individual's pattern of elimination is characterized by hard, dry stool which results from a delay in passage of food residue.

Constipation, Perceived The state in which an individual makes a self-diagnosis of constipation and ensures a daily bowel movement through abuse of laxatives, enemas, and suppositories.

Decisional Conflict (Specify) The state of uncertainty about course of action to be taken when choice among competing actions involves risk, loss, or challenge to personal life values.

Defensive Coping   The state in which an individual repeatedly projects falsely positive self evaluation based on a self protective pattern which defends against underlying perceived threats to positive self regard.

Denial, Ineffective   The state of a conscious or unconscious attempt to disavow the knowledge or meaning of an event to reduce anxiety/fear to the detriment of health.

Diarrhea   A state in which an individual experiences a change in normal bowel habits characterized by the frequent passage of loose, fluid, unformed stools.

Disuse Syndrome, Risk for   A state in which an individual is at risk for deterioration of body systems as the result of prescribed or unavoidable musculoskeletal inactivity.

Diversional Activity Deficit   The state in which an individual experiences a decreased stimulation from (or interest or engagement in) recreational or leisure activities.

Dysreflexia   The state in which an individual with a spinal cord injury at T7 or above experiences a life threatening, uninhabited sympathetic response of the nervous system to a noxious stimulus.

Energy Field Disturbance   A disruption in the flow of energy surrounding a person's being which results in a disharmony of the body, mind, and/or spirit.

Environmental Interpretation Syndrome, Impaired   Consistent lack of orientation to person, place, time or circumstances over more than 3 to 6 months necessitating a protective environment.

Family Coping: Compromised, Ineffective   A usually supportive primary person (family member or close friend) is providing insufficient, ineffective, or compromised support, conform, assistance, or encouragement which may be needed by the client to manage or master adaptive tasks related to his or her health challenge.

Family Coping: Disabling, Ineffective   Behavior of significant person (family member or other primary person) that disables his or her own capacities and the capacity to effectively address tasks essential to either person's adaptation to the health challenge.

Family Coping: Potential for Growth   Effective managing of adaptive tasks by family member involved with the health challenge, who now is exhibiting desire and readiness for enhanced health and growth in regard to self and in relation to the client.

Family, Management of Therapeutic Regimen, Ineffective   A pattern of regulating and integrating into family processes a program for treatment of illness and the sequelae of illness that is unsatisfactory for meeting specific health goals.

Family Processes, Altered   The state in which a family that normally functions effectively experiences a dysfunction.

Family Process, Altered: Alcoholism   The state in which the psychosocial, spiritual, and physiological functions of the family unit are chronically disorganized, leading to conflict, denial of problems, resistance to change, ineffective problem-solving, and a series of self-perpetuating crises.

Fatigue   An overwhelming sustained sense of exhaustion and decreased capacity for physical and mental work.

Fear   Feeling of dread related to an identifiable source which the person validates.

Fluid Volume Deficit   The state in which an individual experiences vascular, cellular, or intracellular dehydration.

Fluid Volume Deficit, Risk For   The state in which an individual is at risk of experiencing vascular, cellular, or intracellular dehydration.

Fluid Volume Excess   The state in which an individual experiences increased fluid retention and edema.

Gas Exchange, Impaired   The state in which an individual experiences a decreased passage of oxygen and/or carbon dioxide between the alveoli of the lungs and the vascular system.

Grieving, Anticipatory   Intellectual and emotional responses and behaviors by which individuals work through the process of modifying self-concept based on the perception of potential loss.

Grieving, Dysfunctional   Extended, unsuccessful use of intellectual and emotional responses by which individuals attempt to work through the process of modifying self-concept based upon the perception of loss.

Growth and Development, Altered   The state in which an individual demonstrates deviations in norms from his/her age-group.

Health Maintenance, Altered   Inability to identify, manage, and/or seek out help to maintain health.

Health Seeking Behaviors (Specify)   A state in which an individual in stable health is actively seeking ways to alter personal health habits and/or the environment to move toward a higher level of health.

Home Maintenance Management, Impaired   Inability to independently maintain a safe growth-promoting immediate environment.

Hopelessness   A subjective state in which an individual sees limited or no alternatives or personal choices available and is unable to mobilize energy on own behalf.

Hyperthermia   A state in which an individual's body temperature is elevated above his/her normal range.

Hypothermia   The state in which an individual's body temperature is reduced below normal range.

Incontinence, Bowel   A state in which an individual experiences a change in normal bowel habits characterized by involuntary passage of stool.

Incontinence, Functional   The state in which an individual experiences an involuntary, unpredictable passage of urine.

Incontinence, Reflex   The state in which an individual experiences an involuntary loss of urine, occurring at somewhat predictable intervals when a specific bladder volume is reached.

Incontinence, Stress   The state in which an individual experiences a loss of urine of less than 50 mL occurring with increased abdominal pressure.

Incontinence, Total   The state in which an individual experiences a continuous and unpredictable loss of urine.

Incontinence, Urge The state in which an individual experiences passage of urine occurring soon after a strong sense of urgency to void.

Individual Coping, Ineffective Impairment of adaptive behaviors and problem-solving abilities of a person in meeting life's demands and roles.

Individual, Management of Therapeutic Regimen, Effective A pattern of regulating and integrating into daily living a program for treatment of illness and its sequelae that is satisfactory for meeting specific health goals.

Individual, Management of Therapeutic Regimen, Ineffective A pattern of regulating and integrating into daily living a program for treatment of illness and the sequelae of illness that is unsatisfactory for meeting specific health goals.

Infant Behavior, Disorganized Alteration in integration and modulation of the physiological and behavioral systems of functioning (i.e. autonomic, motor, state, organizational, self-regulatory, and attentional-interactional systems).

Infant Behavior, Potential for Enhanced, Organized A pattern of modulation of the physiologic and behavioral systems of functioning of an infant (i.e. autonomic, motor, state, organizational, self-regulatory, and attentional-interactional systems) that is satisfactory but that can be improved, resulting in higher levels of integration in response to environmental stimuli.

Infant Behavior, Risk for Disorganized Risk for alteration in integration and modulation of the physiological and behavioral systems of functioning (i.e. autonomic, motor, state, organizational, self-regulatory, and attentional-interactional systems).

Infant Feeding Pattern, Ineffective A state in which an infant demonstrates an impaired ability to suck or coordinate the suck-swallow response.

Infection, Risk for The state in which an individual is at increased risk for being invaded by pathogenic organisms.

Injury, Risk for A state in which an individual is at risk of injury as a result of environmental conditions interacting with the individual's adaptive and defensive resources.

Intracranial Adaptive Capacity, Decreased A clinical state in which intracranial fluid dynamic mechanisms that normally compensate for increases in intracranial volumes are compromised, resulting in repeated disproportionate increases in intracranial pressure (ICP) in response to a variety of noxious and non-noxious stimuli.

Knowledge Deficit (Specify) Absence or deficiency of cognitive information related to specific topic.

Loneliness, Risk for A subjective state in which an individual is at risk of experiencing vague dysphoria.

Memory, Impaired The state in which an individual experiences the inability to remember or recall bits of information or behavioral skills. Impaired memory may be attributed to pathophysiological or situational causes that are either temporary or permanent.

Noncompliance (Specify) A person's informed decision not to adhere to a therapeutic recommendation.

Nutrition: Less Than Body Requirements, Altered The state in which an individual experiences an intake of nutrients insufficient to meet metabolic needs.

Nutrition: More Than Body Requirements, Altered The state in which an individual is experiencing an intake of nutrients which exceeds metabolic needs.

Nutrition: Potential for More Than Body Requirements, Altered The state in which an individual is at risk of experiencing an intake of nutrients which exceeds metabolic needs.

Oral Mucous Membrane, Altered The state in which an individual experiences disruptions in the tissue layers of the oral cavity.

Pain A state in which an individual experiences and reports the presence of severe discomfort or an uncomfortable sensation.

Pain, Chronic A state in which an individual experiences pain that continues for more than 6 months in duration.

Parental Role Conflict The state in which a parent experiences role confusion and conflict in response to crisis.

Parent/Infant/Child Attachment, Risk for Altered Disruption of the interactive process between parent/significant other and infant that fosters the development of a protective and nurturing reciprocal relationship.

Parenting, Altered The state in which a nurturing figure(s) experiences an inability to create an environment which promotes the optimum growth and development of another human being.

Parenting, Risk for Altered The state in which a nurturing figure(s) is at risk to experience an inability to create an environment which promotes the optimum growth and development of another human being.

Perioperative Positioning Injury, Risk for The state in which the client is at risk for injury as a result of the environmental conditions found in the perioperative setting.

Peripheral Neurovascular Dysfunction, Risk for The state in which an individual is at risk of experiencing a disruption in circulation, sensation, or motion of an extremity.

Personal Identity Disturbance Inability to distinguish between self and non-self.

Physical Mobility, Impaired The state in which an individual experiences a limitation of ability for independent physical movement.

Poisoning, Risk for Accentuated risk of accidental exposure to, or ingestion of, drugs or dangerous products in doses sufficient to cause poisoning.

Post-Trauma Response The state in which an individual experiences a sustained painful response to an overwhelming traumatic event(s).

Powerlessness Perception that one's own action will not significantly affect an outcome; a perceived lack of control over a current situation or immediate happening.

Protection, Altered The state in which an individual experiences a decrease in the ability to guard the self from internal or external threats such as illness or injury.

Rape-Trauma Syndrome Forced, violent sexual penetration against the victim's will and consent. The trauma syndrome that develops from this attack or attempted attack includes an acute phase of disorganization of the victim's lifestyle and a long-term process of reorganization of lifestyle.

Rape-Trauma Syndrome: Compound Reaction Forced, violent sexual penetration against the victim's will and consent. The trauma syndrome that develops from this attack or attempted attack includes an acute phase of disorganization of the victim's lifestyle and a long-term process of reorganization of lifestyle.

Rape-Trauma Syndrome: Silent Reaction Forced, violent sexual penetration against the victim's will and consent. The trauma syndrome that develops from this attack or attempted attack includes an acute phase of disorganization of the victim's lifestyle and a long-term process or reorganization of lifestyle.

Relocation Stress Syndrome Physiological and/or psychosocial disturbances as a result of transfer from one environment to another.

Role Performance, Altered Disruption in the way one perceives one's role performance.

Self Care Deficit: Bathing/Hygiene A state in which the individual experiences an impaired ability to perform or complete bathing/hygiene activities for oneself.

Self Care Deficit: Dressing/Grooming A state in which the individual experiences an impaired ability to perform or complete dressing and grooming activities for oneself.

Self Care Deficit: Feeding A state in which the individual experiences an impaired ability to perform or complete feeding activities for oneself.

Self Care Deficit: Toileting A state in which the individual experiences an impaired ability to perform or complete toileting activities for oneself.

Self Esteem, Chronic Low Long standing negative self evaluation/feelings about self or self capabilities.

Self Esteem Disturbance Negative self evaluation/feelings about self or self capabilities, which may be directly or indirectly expressed.

Self Esteem, Situational Low Negative self evaluation/feelings about self which develop in response to a loss or change in an individual who previously had a positive self evaluation.

Self Mutilation, Risk for A state in which the individual is at risk to perform an act upon the self to injure, not kill, which produces tissue damage and tension relief.

Sensory/Perceptual Alterations: Auditory A state in which the individual experiences a change in the amount or patterning of oncoming stimuli accompanied by a diminished, exaggerated, distorted, or impaired response to such stimuli.

Sensory/Perceptual Alterations: Gustatory A state in which the individual experiences a change in the amount or patterning of oncoming stimuli accompanied by a diminished, exaggerated, distorted, or impaired response to such stimuli.

Sensory/Perceptual Alterations: Kinesthetic A state in which the individual experiences a change in the amount or patterning of oncoming stimuli accompanied by a diminished, exaggerated, distorted, or impaired response to such stimuli.

Sensory/Perceptual Alterations: Olfactory A state in which the individual experiences a change in the amount or patterning of oncoming stimuli accompanied by a diminished, exaggerated, distorted, or impaired response to such stimuli.

Sensory/Perceptual Alterations: Tactile A state in which the individual experiences a change in the amount or patterning of oncoming stimuli accompanied by a diminished, exaggerated, distorted, or impaired response to such stimuli.

Sensory/Perceptual Alterations: Visual A state in which the individual experiences a change in the amount or patterning of oncoming stimuli accompanied by a diminished, exaggerated, distorted, or impaired response to such stimuli.

Sexual Dysfunction The state in which the individual experiences a change in sexual function that is viewed as unsatisfying, unrewarding, inadequate.

Sexuality Patterns, Altered The state in which the individual expresses concern regarding his/her sexuality.

Skin Integrity, Impaired A state in which the individual's skin is adversely altered.

Skin Integrity, Risk for Impaired A state in which the individual's skin is at risk for being adversely altered.

Sleep Pattern Disturbance Disruption of sleep time causes discomfort or interferes with desired lifestyle.

Social Interaction, Impaired A state in which the individual participates in an insufficient or excessive quantity or ineffective quality of social exchange.

Social Isolation Aloneness experienced by the individual and perceived as imposed by others and as a negative or threatened state.

Spiritual Distress Disruption in the life principle which pervades a person's entire being and which integrates and transcends one's biological and psychosocial nature.

Spiritual Well-Being, Potential for Enhanced Spiritual well-being is the process of an individual's developing/unfolding of mystery through harmonious interconnectedness that springs from inner strengths.

Suffocation, Risk for Accentuated risk of accidental suffocation (inadequate air available for inhalation).

Swallowing, Impaired The state in which the individual has decreased ability to voluntarily pass fluids and/or solids from the mouth to the stomach.

Thermoregulation, Ineffective The state in which the individual's temperature fluctuates between hypothermia and hyperthermia.

Thought Processes, Altered A state in which the individual experiences a disruption in cognitive operations and activities.

Tissue Integrity, Impaired A state in which the individual experiences damage to mucous membrane, corneal, integumentary, or subcutaneous tissue.

Tissue Perfusion, Altered: Cardiopulmonary The state in which the individual experiences a decrease in nutrition and oxygenation at the cellular level due to a deficit in capillary blood supply.

Tissue Perfusion, Altered: Cerebral The state in which the individual experiences a decrease in nutrition and oxygenation at the cellular level due to a deficit in capillary blood supply.

Tissue Perfusion, Altered: Gastrointestinal The state in which the individual experiences a decrease in nutrition and oxygenation at the cellular level due to a deficit in capillary blood supply.

Tissue Perfusion, Altered: Peripheral The state in which an individual experiences a decrease in nutrition and oxygenation at the cellular level due to a deficit in capillary blood supply.

Tissue Perfusion, Altered: Renal A state in which an individual experiences a decrease in nutrition and oxygenation at the cellular level due to a deficit in capillary blood supply.

Trauma, Risk for Accentuated risk of accidental tissue injury, e.g. wound, burn, fracture.

Unilateral Neglect A state in which an individual is perceptually unaware of, and inattentive to, one side of the body.

Urinary Elimination, Altered The state in which an individual experiences a disturbance in urine elimination.

Urinary Retention The state in which the individual experiences incomplete emptying of the bladder.

Ventilation, Inability to Sustain Spontaneous A state in which the response pattern of decreased energy reserves results in an individual's inability to maintain breathing adequate to support life.

Ventilatory Weaning Response, Dysfunctional A state in which a patient cannot adjust to lowered levels of mechanical ventilator support, which interrupts and prolongs the weaning process.

Violence, High Risk for: Self-Directed or Directed at Others A state in which an individual experiences behaviors that can be physically harmful either to the self or others.

Source: North American Nursing Diagnosis Association. (1996). *NANDA nursing diagnoses: Definitions and classification 1997–1998.* Philadelphia: Author.

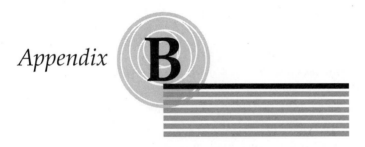

Appendix

Nursing Interventions Classification (NIC) Intervention Labels and Definitions, 2nd Edition, 1996

Abuse Protection Identification of high-risk dependent relationships and actions to prevent further infliction of physical or emotional harm

Abuse Protection: Child Identification of high-risk, dependent-child relationships and actions to prevent possible or further infliction of physical, sexual, or emotional harm or neglect of basic necessities of life

Abuse Protection: Elder Identification of high-risk, dependent elder relationships and actions to prevent possible or further infliction of physical, sexual, or emotional harm; neglect of basic necessities of life; or exploitation

Acid-Base Management Promotion of acid-base balance and prevention of complications resulting from acid-base imbalance

Acid-Base Management: Metabolic Acidosis Promotion of acid-base balance and prevention of complications resulting from serum HCO_3 levels lower than desired

Acid-Base Management: Metabolic Alkalosis Promotion of acid-base balance and prevention of complications resulting from serum HCO_3 levels higher than desired

Acid-Base Management: Respiratory Acidosis Promotion of acid-base balance and prevention of complications resulting from serum pCO_2 levels higher than desired

Acid-Base Management: Respiratory Alkalosis Promotion of acid-base balance and prevention of complications resulting from serum pCO_2 levels lower than desired

Acid-Base Monitoring   Collection and analysis of patient data to regulate acid-base balance

Active Listening   Attending closely to and attaching significance to a patient's verbal and nonverbal messages

Activity Therapy   Prescription of and assistance with specific physical, cognitive, social, and spiritual activities to increase the range, frequency, or duration of an individual's (or group's) activity

Acupressure   Application of firm, sustained pressure to special points on the body to decrease pain, produce relaxation, and prevent or reduce nausea

Admission Care   Facilitating entry of a patient into a health care facility

Airway Insertion and Stabilization   Insertion or assisting with insertion and stabilization of an artificial airway

Airway Management   Facilitation of patency of air passages

Airway Suctioning   Removal of airway secretions by inserting a suction catheter into the patient's oral airway and/or trachea

Allergy Management   Identification, treatment, and prevention of allergic responses to food, medications, insect bites, contrast material, blood, or other substances

Amnioinfusion   Infusion of fluid into the uterus during labor to relieve umbilical cord compression or to dilute meconium-stained fluid

Amputation Care   Promotion of physical and psychological healing after amputation of a body part

Analgesic Administration   Use of pharmacologic agents to reduce or eliminate pain

Analgesic Administration: Intraspinal   Administration of pharmacologic agents into the epidural or intrathecal space to reduce or eliminate pain

Anesthesia Administration   Preparation for and administration of anesthetic agents and monitoring of patient responsiveness during administration

Anger Control Assistance   Facilitation of the expression of anger in an adaptive nonviolent manner

Animal-Assisted Therapy   Purposeful use of animals to provide affection, attention, diversion, and relaxation

Anticipatory Guidance   Preparation of patient for an anticipated developmental and/or situational crisis

Anxiety Reduction   Minimizing apprehension, dread, foreboding, or uneasiness related to an unidentified source of anticipated danger

Area Restriction   Limitation of patient mobility to a specified area for purposes of safety or behavior management

Art Therapy   Facilitation of communication through drawings or other art forms

Artificial Airway Management   Maintenance of endotracheal and tracheostomy tubes and preventing complications associated with their use

Aspiration Precautions   Prevention or minimization of risk factors in the patient at risk for aspiration

Assertiveness Training Assistance with the effective expression of feelings, needs, and ideas while respecting the rights of others

Attachment Promotion Facilitation of the development of the parent-infant relationship

Autogenic Training Assisting with self-suggestions about feelings of heaviness and warmth for the purpose of inducing relaxation

Autotransfusion Collecting and reinfusing blood which has been lost intraoperatively or postoperatively from clean wounds

Bathing Cleaning of the body for the purposes of relaxation, cleanliness, and healing

Bed Rest Care Promotion of comfort and safety and prevention of complications for a patient unable to get out of bed

Bedside Laboratory Testing Performance of laboratory tests at the bedside or point of care

Behavior Management Helping a patient to manage negative behavior

Behavior Management: Overactivity/Inattention Provision of a therapeutic milieu which safely accommodates the patient's attention deficit and/or overactivity while promoting optimal function

Behavior Management: Self-Harm Assisting the patient to decrease or eliminate self-multilating or self-abusive behaviors

Behavior Management: Sexual Delineation and prevention of socially unacceptable sexual behaviors

Behavior Modification Promotion of a behavior change

Behavior Modification: Social Skills Assisting the patient to develop or improve interpersonal social skills

Bibliotherapy Use of literature to enhance the expression of feelings and the gaining of insight

Biofeedback Assisting the patient to modify a body function using feedback from instrumentation

Birthing Delivery of a baby

Bladder Irrigation Instillation of a solution into the bladder to provide cleansing or medication

Bleeding Precautions Reduction of stimuli that may induce bleeding or hemorrhage in at risk patients

Bleeding Reduction Limitation of the loss of blood volume during an episode of bleeding

Bleeding Reduction: Antepartum Uterus Limitation of the amount of blood loss from the pregnant uterus during third trimester of pregnancy

Bleeding Reduction: Gastrointestinal Limitation of the amount of blood loss from the upper and lower gastrointestinal tract and related complications

Bleeding Reduction: Nasal Limitation of the amount of blood loss from the nasal cavity

Bleeding Reduction: Postpartum Uterus Limitation of the amount of blood loss from the postpartum uterus

Bleeding Reduction: Wound Limitation of the blood loss from a wound that may be a result of trauma, incisions, or placement of a tube or catheter

Blood Products Administration Administration of blood or blood products and monitoring of patient's response

Body Image Enhancement Improving a patient's conscious and unconscious perceptions and attitudes toward his/her body

Body Mechanics Promotion Facilitating the use of posture and movement in daily activities to prevent fatigue and musculoskeletal strain or injury

Bottle Feeding Preparation and administration of fluids to an infant via a bottle

Bowel Incontinence Care Promotion of bowel continence and maintenance of perianal skin integrity

Bowel Incontinence Care: Encopresis Promotion of bowel continence in children

Bowel Irrigation Instillation of a substance into the lower gastrointestinal tract

Bowel Management Establishment and maintenance of a regular pattern of bowel elimination

Bowel Training Assisting the patient to train the bowel to evacuate at specific intervals

Breastfeeding Assistance Preparing a new mother to breastfeed her infant

Calming Technique Reducing anxiety in patient experiencing acute distress

Cardiac Care Limitation of complications resulting from an imbalance between myocardial oxygen supply and demand for a patient with symptoms of impaired cardiac function

Cardiac Care: Acute Limitation of complications for a patient recently experiencing an episode of an imbalance between myocardial oxygen supply and demand resulting in impaired cardiac function

Cardiac Care: Rehabilitative Promotion of maximum functional activity level for a patient who has suffered an episode of impaired cardiac function which resulted from an imbalance between myocardial oxygen supply and demand

Cardiac Precautions Prevention of an acute episode of impaired cardiac function by minimizing myocardial oxygen consumption or increasing myocardial oxygen supply

Caregiver Support Provision of the necessary information, advocacy, and support to facilitate primary patient care by someone other than a health care professional

Cast Care: Maintenance Care of a cast after the drying period

Cast Care: Wet Care of a new cast during the drying period

Cerebral Edema Management Limitation of secondary cerebral injury resulting from swelling of brain tissue

Cerebral Perfusion Promotion Promotion of adequate perfusion and limitation of complications for a patient experiencing or at risk for inadequate cerebral perfusion

Cesarean Section Care Preparation and support of patient delivering a baby by cesarean section

Chemotherapy Management   Assisting the patient and family to understand the action and minimize side effects of antineoplastic agents

Chest Physiotherapy   Assisting the patient to move airway secretions from peripheral airways to more central airways for expectoration and/or suctioning

Childbirth Preparation   Providing information and support to facilitate childbirth and to enhance the ability of an individual to develop and perform the role of parent

Circulatory Care   Promotion of arterial and venous circulation

Circulatory Care: Mechanical Assist Device   Temporary support of the circulation through the use of mechanical devices or pumps

Circulatory Precautions   Protection of a localized area with limited perfusion

Code Management   Coordination of emergency measures to sustain life

Cognitive Restructuring   Challenging a patient to alter distorted thought patterns and view self and the world more realistically

Cognitive Stimulation   Promotion of awareness and comprehension of surroundings by utilization of planned stimuli

Communication Enhancement: Hearing Deficit   Assistance in accepting and learning alternate methods for living with diminished hearing

Communication Enhancement: Speech Deficit   Assistance in accepting and learning alternate methods for living with impaired speech

Communication Enhancement: Visual Deficit   Assistance in accepting and learning alternate methods for living with diminished vision

Complex Relationship Building   Establishing a therapeutic relationship with a patient who has difficulty interacting with others

Conscious Sedation   Administration of sedatives, monitoring of the patient's response, and provision of necessary physiological support during a diagnostic or therapeutic procedure

Constipation/Impaction Management   Prevention and alleviation of constipation/impaction

Contact Lens Care   Prevention of eye injury and lens damage by proper use of contact lenses

Controlled Substance Checking   Promoting appropriate use and maintaining security of controlled substances

Coping Enhancement   Assisting a patient to adapt to perceived stressors, changes, or threats which interfere with meeting life demands and roles

Cough Enhancement   Promotion of deep inhalation by the patient with subsequent generation of high intrathoracic pressures and compression of underlying lung parenchyma for the forceful expulsion of air

Counseling   Use of an interactive helping process focusing on the needs, problems, or feelings of the patient and significant others to enhance or support coping, problem-solving, and interpersonal relationships

Crisis Intervention   Use of short-term counseling to help the patient cope with a crisis and resume a state of functioning comparable to or better than the precrisis state

Critical Path Development   Constructing and using a timed sequence of patient care activities to enhance desired patient outcomes in a cost efficient manner

Culture Brokerage   Bridging, negotiating, or linking the orthodox health care system with a patient and family of a different culture

Cutaneous Stimulation   Stimulation of the skin and underlying tissues for the purpose of decreasing undesirable signs and symptoms such as pain, muscle spasm, or inflammation

Decision-Making Support   Providing information and support for a patient who is making a decision regarding health care

Delegation   Transfer of responsibility for the performance of patient care while retaining accountability for the outcome

Delirium Management   Provision of a safe and therapeutic environment for the patient who is experiencing an acute confusional state

Delusion Management   Promoting the comfort, safety, and reality orientation of a patient experiencing false, fixed beliefs that have little or no basis in reality

Dementia Management   Provision of a modified environment for the patient who is experiencing a chronic confusional state

Developmental Enhancement   Facilitating or teaching parents/caregivers to facilitate the optimal gross motor, fine motor, language, cognitive, social and emotional growth of preschool and school-aged children

Diarrhea Management   Prevention and alleviation of diarrhea

Diet Staging   Instituting required diet restrictions with subsequent progression of diet as tolerated

Discharge Planning   Preparation for moving a patient from one level of care to another within or outside the current health care agency

Distraction   Purposeful focusing of attention away from undesirable sensations

Documentation   Recording of pertinent patient data in a clinical record

Dressing   Choosing, putting on, and removing clothes for a person who cannot do this for self

Dying Care   Promotion of physical comfort and psychological peace in the final phase of life

Dysreflexia Management   Prevention and elimination of stimuli which cause hyperactive reflexes and inappropriate autonomic responses in a patient with cervical or high thoracic cord lesion

Dysrhythmia Management   Preventing, recognizing, and facilitating treatment of abnormal cardiac rhythms

Ear Care   Prevention or minimization of threats to ear or hearing

Eating Disorders Management   Prevention and treatment of severe diet restriction and overexercising or binging and purging of food and fluids

Electrolyte Management   Promotion of electrolyte balance and prevention of complications resulting from abnormal or undesired serum electrolyte levels

Electrolyte Management: Hypercalcemia   Promotion of calcium balance and prevention of complications resulting from serum calcium levels higher than desired

Electrolyte Management: Hyperkalemia Promotion of potassium balance and prevention of complications resulting from serum potassium levels higher than desired

Electrolyte Management: Hypermagnesemia Promotion of magnesium balance and prevention of complications resulting from serum magnesium levels higher than desired

Electrolyte Management: Hypernatremia Promotion of sodium balance and prevention of complications resulting from serum sodium levels higher than desired

Electrolyte Management: Hyperphosphatemia Promotion of phosphate balance and prevention of complications resulting from serum phosphate levels higher than desired

Electrolyte Management: Hypocalcemia Promotion of calcium balance and prevention of complications resulting from serum calcium levels lower than desired

Electrolyte Management: Hypokalemia Promotion of potassium balance and prevention of complications resulting from serum potassium levels lower than desired

Electrolyte Management: Hypomagnesemia Promotion of magnesium balance and prevention of complications resulting from serum magnesium levels lower than desired

Electrolyte Management: Hyponatremia Promotion of sodium balance and prevention of complications resulting from serum sodium levels lower than desired

Electrolyte Management: Hypophosphatemia Promotion of phosphate balance and prevention of complications resulting from serum phosphate levels lower than desired

Electrolyte Monitoring Collection and analysis of patient data to regulate electrolyte balance

Electronic Fetal Monitoring: Antepartum Electronic evaluation of fetal heart rate response to movement, external stimuli, or uterine contractions during antepartal testing

Electronic Fetal Monitoring: Intrapartum Electronic evaluation of fetal heart rate response to uterine contractions during intrapartal care

Elopement Precautions Minimizing the risk of a patient leaving a treatment setting without authorization when departure presents a threat to the safety of patient or others

Embolus Care: Peripheral Limitation of complications for a patient experiencing, or at risk for, occlusion of peripheral circulation

Embolus Care: Pulmonary Limitation of complications for a patient experiencing, or at risk for, occlusion of pulmonary circulation

Embolus Precautions Reduction of the risk of an embolus in a patient with thrombi or at risk for developing thrombus formation

Emergency Care Providing life-saving measures in life-threatening situations

Emergency Cart Checking Systematic review of the contents of an emergency cart at established time intervals

Emotional Support Provision of reassurance, acceptance, and encouragement during times of stress

Endotracheal Extubation Purposeful removal of the endotracheal tube from the nasopharyngeal or oropharyngeal airway

Energy Management Regulating energy use to treat or prevent fatigue and optimize function

Enteral Tube Feeding Delivering nutrients and water through a gastrointestinal tube

Environmental Management Manipulation of the patient's surroundings for therapeutic benefit

Environmental Management: Attachment Process Manipulation of the patient's surroundings to facilitate the development of the parent-infant relationship

Environmental Management: Comfort Manipulation of the patient's surroundings for promotion of optimal comfort

Environmental Management: Community Monitoring and influencing of the physical, social, cultural, economic, and political conditions that affect the health of groups and communities

Environmental Management: Safety Monitoring and manipulation of the physical environment to promote safety

Environmental Management: Violence Prevention Monitoring and manipulation of the physical environment to decrease the potential for violent behavior directed toward self, others, or environment

Environmental Management: Worker Safety Monitoring and manipulating of the worksite environment to promote safety and health of workers

Examination Assistance Providing assistance to the patient and another health care provider during a procedure or exam

Exercise Promotion Facilitation of regular physical exercise to maintain or advance to a higher level of fitness and health

Exercise Promotion: Stretching Facilitation of systematic slow-stretch-hold muscle exercises to induce relaxation, prepare muscles/joints for more vigorous exercise, or to increase or maintain body flexibility

Exercise Therapy: Ambulation Promotion and assistance with walking to maintain or restore autonomic and voluntary body functions during treatment and recovery from illness or injury

Exercise Therapy: Balance Use of specific activities, postures, and movements to maintain, enhance, or restore balance

Exercise Therapy: Joint Mobility Use of active or passive body movement to maintain or restore joint flexibility

Exercise Therapy: Muscle Control Use of specific activity or exercise protocols to enhance or restore controlled body movement

Eye Care Prevention or minimization of threats to eye or visual integrity

Fall Prevention Instituting special precautions with patient at risk for injury from falling

Family Integrity Promotion Promotion of family cohesion and unity

Family Integrity Promotion: Childbearing Family   Facilitation of the growth of individuals or families who are adding an infant to the family unit

Family Involvement   Facilitating family participation in the emotional and physical care of the patient

Family Mobilization   Utilization of family strengths to influence patient's health in a positive direction

Family Planning: Contraception   Facilitation of pregnancy prevention by providing information about the physiology of reproduction and methods to control conception

Family Planning: Infertility   Management, education, and support of the patient and significant other undergoing evaluation and treatment for infertility

Family Planning: Unplanned Pregnancy   Facilitation of decision-making regarding pregnancy outcome

Family Process Maintenance   Minimization of family process disruption effects

Family Support   Promotion of family values, interests and goals

Family Therapy   Assisting family members to move their family toward a more productive way of living

Feeding   Providing nutritional intake for patient who is unable to feed self

Fertility Preservation   Providing information, counseling, and treatment that facilitate reproductive health and the ability to conceive

Fever Treatment   Management of a patient with hyperpyrexia caused by nonenvironmental factors

Fire Setting Precautions   Prevention of fire setting behaviors

First Aid   Providing initial care of a minor injury

Flatulence Reduction   Prevention of flatus formation and facilitation of passage of excessive gas

Fluid Management   Promotion of fluid balance and prevention of complications resulting from abnormal or undesired fluid levels

Fluid Monitoring   Collection and analysis of patient data to regulate fluid balance

Fluid Resuscitation   Administering prescribed intravenous fluids rapidly

Fluid/Electrolyte Management   Regulation and prevention of complications from altered fluid and/or electrolyte levels

Foot Care   Cleansing and inspecting the feet for the purposes of relaxation, cleanliness, and healthy skin

Gastrointestinal Intubation   Insertion of a tube into the gastrointestinal tract

Genetic Counseling   Use of an interactive helping process focusing on the prevention of a genetic disorder or on the ability to cope with a family member who has a genetic disorder

Grief Work Facilitation   Assistance with the resolution of a significant loss

Grief Work Facilitation: Perinatal Death   Assistance with the resolution of a perinatal loss

Guilt Work Facilitation   Helping another to cope with painful feelings of responsibility, actual or perceived

Hair Care   Promotion of neat, clean, attractive hair

Hallucination Management   Promoting the safety, comfort, and reality orientation of a patient experiencing hallucinations

Health Care Information Exchange   Providing patient care information to health professionals in other agencies

Health Education   Developing and providing instruction and learning experiences to facilitate voluntary adaptation of behavior conducive to health in individuals, families, groups, or communities

Health Policy Monitoring   Surveillance and influence of government and organization regulations, rules, and standards that affect nursing systems and practices to ensure quality care of patients

Health Screening   Detecting health risks or problems by means of history, examination, and other procedures

Health System Guidance   Facilitating a patient's location and use of appropriate health services

Heat Exposure Treatment   Management of patient overcome by heat due to excessive environmental heat exposure

Heat/Cold Application   Stimulation of the skin and underlying tissues with heat or cold for the purpose of decreasing pain, muscle spasms, or inflammation

Hemodialysis Therapy   Management of extracorporeal passage of the patient's blood through a dialyzer

Hemodynamic Regulation   Optimization of heart rate, preload, afterload, and contractility

Hemorrhage Control   Reduction or elimination of rapid and excessive blood loss

High-Risk Pregnancy Care   Identification and management of a high-risk pregnancy to promote healthy outcomes for mother and baby

Home Maintenance Assistance   Helping the patient/family to maintain the home as a clean, safe, and pleasant place to live

Hope Instillation   Facilitation of the development of a positive outlook in a given situation

Humor   Facilitating the patient to perceive, appreciate, and express what is funny, amusing, or ludicrous in order to establish relationships, relieve tension, release anger, facilitate learning, or cope with painful feelings

Hyperglycemia Management   Preventing and treating above normal blood glucose levels

Hypervolemia Management   Reduction in extracellular and/or intracellular fluid volume and prevention of complications in a patient who is fluid overloaded

Hypnosis   Assisting a patient to induce an altered state of consciousness to create an acute awareness and a directed focus experience

Hypoglycemia Management   Preventing and treating below normal blood glucose levels

Hypothermia Treatment   Rewarming and surveillance of a patient whose core body temperature is below 35° C

Hypovolemia Management Expansion of intravascular fluid volume in a patient who is volume depleted

Immunization/Vaccination Administration Provision of immunizations for prevention of communicable disease

Impulse Control Training Assisting the patient to mediate impulsive behavior through application of problem solving strategies to social and interpersonal situations

Incident Reporting Written and verbal reporting of any event in the process of patient care that is inconsistent with desired patient outcomes or routine operations of the healthcare facility

Incision Site Care Cleansing, monitoring, and promotion of healing in a wound that is closed with sutures, clips, or staples

Infant Care Provision of developmentally appropriate family-centered care to the child under 1 year of age

Infection Control Minimizing the acquisition and transmission of infectious agents

Infection Control: Intraoperative Preventing nosocomial infection in the operating room

Infection Protection Prevention and early detection of infection in a patient at risk

Insurance Authorization Assisting the patient and provider to secure payment for health services or equipment from a third party

Intracranial Pressure (ICP) Monitoring Measurement and interpretation of patient data to regulate intracranial pressure

Intrapartal Care Monitoring and management of stages one and two of the birth process

Intrapartal Care: High-Risk Delivery Assisting vaginal birth of multiple or malpositioned fetuses

Intravenous (IV) Insertion Insertion of a needle into a peripheral vein for the purpose of administering fluids, blood, or medications

Intravenous (IV) Therapy Administration and monitoring of intravenous fluids and medications

Invasive Hemodynamic Monitoring Measurement and interpretation of invasive hemodynamic parameters to determine cardiovascular function and regulate therapy as appropriate

Kangaroo Care Promoting closeness between parent and physiologically stable preterm infant by preparing the parent and providing the environment for skin-to-skin contact

Labor Induction Initiation or augmentation of labor by mechanical or pharmacological methods

Labor Suppression Controlling uterine contractions prior to 37 weeks of gestation to prevent preterm birth

Laboratory Data Interpretation Critical analysis of patient laboratory data in order to assist with clinical decision-making

Lactation Counseling Use of an interactive helping process to assist in maintenance of successful breastfeeding

Lactation Suppression Facilitating the cessation of milk production and minimizing breast engorgement after giving birth

Laser Precautions Limiting the risk of injury to the patient related to use of a laser

Latex Precautions Reducing the risk of systemic reaction to latex

Learning Facilitation Promoting the ability to process and comprehend information

Learning Readiness Enhancement Improving the ability and willingness to receive information

Leech Therapy Application of medicinal leeches to help drain replanted or transplanted tissue engorged with venous blood

Limit Setting Establishing the parameters of desirable and acceptable patient behavior

Malignant Hyperthermia Precautions Prevention or reduction of hypermetabolic response to pharmacological agents used during surgery

Mechanical Ventilation Use of an artificial device to assist a patient to breathe

Mechanical Ventilatory Weaning Assisting the patient to breathe without the aid of a mechanical ventilator

Medication Administration Preparing, giving, and evaluating the effectiveness of prescription and nonprescription drugs

Medication Administration: Enteral Delivering medications through an intestinal tube

Medication Administration: Interpleural Administration of medication through an interpleural catheter for reduction of pain

Medication Administration: Intraosseous Insertion of a needle through the bone cortex into the medullary cavity for the purpose of short-term, emergency administration of fluid, blood, or medication

Medication Administration: Oral Preparing and giving medications by mouth and monitoring patient responsiveness

Medication Administration: Parenteral Preparing and giving medications via the intravenous, intramuscular, intradermal, and/or subcutaneous route

Medication Administration: Topical Preparing and applying medications to the skin and mucous membranes

Medication Administration: Ventricular Reservoir Administration and monitoring of medication through an indwelling catheter into the lateral ventricle

Medication Management Facilitation of safe and effective use of prescription and over-the-counter drugs

Medication Prescribing Prescribing medication for a health problem

Meditation Altering the patient's level of awareness by focusing specifically on an image or thought

Memory Training Facilitation of memory

Milieu Therapy Use of people, resources, and events in the patient's immediate environment to promote optimal psychosocial functioning

Mood Management Providing for safety and stabilization of a patient who is experiencing dysfunctional mood

Multidisciplinary Care Conference   Planning and evaluating patient care with health professionals from other disciplines

Music Therapy   Using music to help achieve a specific change in behavior or feeling

Mutual Goal Setting   Collaborating with patient to identify and prioritize care goals, then developing a plan for achieving those goals through the construction and use of goal attainment scaling

Nail Care   Promotion of clean, neat, attractive nails and prevention of skin lesions related to improper care of nails

Neurologic Monitoring   Collection and analysis of patient data to prevent or minimize neurological complications

Newborn Care   Management of neonate during the transition to extrauterine life and subsequent period of stabilization

Newborn Monitoring   Measurement and interpretation of physiologic status of the neonate the first 24 hours after delivery

Nonnutritive Sucking   Provision of sucking opportunities for infant who is gavage fed or who can receive nothing by mouth

Normalization Promotion   Assisting parents and other family members of children with chronic illnesses or disabilities in providing normal life experiences for their children and families

Nutrition Management   Assisting with or providing a balanced dietary intake of foods and fluids

Nutrition Therapy   Administration of food and fluids to support metabolic processes of a patient who is malnourished or at high risk for becoming malnourished

Nutritional Counseling   Use of an interactive helping process focusing on the need for diet modification

Nutritional Monitoring   Collection and analysis of patient data to prevent or minimize malnourishment

Oral Health Maintenance   Maintenance and promotion of oral hygiene and dental health for the patient at risk for developing oral or dental lesions

Oral Health Promotion   Promotion of oral hygiene and dental care for a patient with normal oral and dental health

Oral Health Restoration   Promotion of healing for a patient who has an oral mucosa or dental lesion

Order Transcription   Transferring information from order sheets to the nursing patient care planning and documentation system

Organ Procurement   Guiding families through the donation process to ensure timely retrieval of vital organs and tissue for transplant

Ostomy Care   Maintenance of elimination through a stoma and care of surrounding tissue

Oxygen Therapy   Administration of oxygen and monitoring of its effectiveness

Pain Management   Alleviation of pain or a reduction in pain to a level of comfort that is acceptable to the patient

Parent Education: Adolescent Assisting parents to understand and help their adolescent children

Parent Education: Childbearing Family Preparing another to perform the role of parent

Parent Education: Childrearing Family Assisting parents to understand and promote the physical, psychological, and social growth and development of their toddler, preschool, or school-aged child/children

Pass Facilitation Arranging a leave for a patient from a health care facility

Patient Contracting Negotiating an agreement with a patient which reinforces a specific behavior change

Patient Controlled Analgesia (PCA) Assistance Facilitating patient control of analgesic administration and regulation

Patient Rights Protection Protection of health care rights of a patient, especially a minor, incapacitated, or incompetent patient unable to make decisions

Peer Review Systematic evaluation of a peer's performance compared with professional standards of practice

Pelvic Floor Exercise Strengthening the pubococcygeal muscles through voluntary, repetitive contraction to decrease stress or urge incontinence

Perineal Care Maintenance of perineal skin integrity and relief of perineal discomfort

Peripheral Sensation Management Prevention or minimization of injury or discomfort in the patient with altered sensation

Peripherally Inserted Central (PIC) Catheter Care Insertion and maintenance of a peripherally inserted central catheter

Peritoneal Dialysis Therapy Administration and monitoring of dialysis solution into and out of the peritoneal cavity

Phlebotomy: Arterial Blood Sample Obtaining a blood sample from an uncannulated artery to assess oxygen and carbon dioxide levels and acid-base balance

Phlebotomy: Blood Unit Acquisition Procuring blood and products from donors

Phlebotomy: Venous Blood Sample Removal of a sample of venous blood from an uncannulated vein

Phototherapy: Neonate Use of light therapy to reduce bilirubin levels in newborn infants

Physical Restraint Application, monitoring, and removal of mechanical restraining devices or manual restraints which are used to limit physical mobility of a patient

Physician Support Collaborating with physicians to provide quality patient care

Play Therapy Purposeful use of toys or other equipment to assist a patient in communicating his/her perception of the world and to help in mastering the environment

Pneumatic Tourniquet Precautions Applying a pneumatic tourniquet while minimizing the potential for patient injury from use of the device

Positioning   Moving the patient or a body part to provide comfort, reduce the risk of skin breakdown, promote skin integrity, and/or promote healing

Positioning: Intraoperative   Moving the patient or body part to promote surgical exposure while reducing the risk of discomfort and complications

Positioning: Neurologic   Achievement of optimal, appropriate body alignment for the patient experiencing or at risk for spinal cord injury or vertebrae irritability

Positioning: Wheelchair   Placement of a patient in a properly selected wheelchair to enhance comfort, promote skin integrity, and foster independence

Postanesthesia Care   Monitoring and management of the patient who has recently undergone general or regional anesthesia

Postmortem Care   Providing physical care of the body of an expired patient and support for the family viewing the body

Postpartal Care   Monitoring and management of the patient who has recently given birth

Preceptor: Employee   Assisting and supporting a new or transferred employee through a planned orientation to a specific clinical area

Preceptor: Student   Assisting and supporting learning experiences for a student

Preconception Counseling   Screening and counseling done before pregnancy to avoid or decrease the risk for birth defects

Pregnancy Termination Care   Management of the physical and psychological needs of the woman undergoing a spontaneous or elective abortion

Prenatal Care   Monitoring and management of patient during pregnancy to prevent complications of pregnancy and promote a healthy outcome for both mother and infant

Preoperative Coordination   Facilitating preadmission diagnostic testing and preparation of the surgical patient

Preparatory Sensory Information   Describing both the subjective and objective physical sensations associated with an upcoming stressful health care procedure/treatment

Presence   Being with another during times of need

Pressure Management   Minimizing pressure to body parts

Pressure Ulcer Care   Facilitation of healing in pressure ulcers

Pressure Ulcer Prevention   Prevention of pressure ulcers for a patient at high risk for developing them

Product Evaluation   Determining the effectiveness of new products or equipment

Progressive Muscle Relaxation   Facilitating the tensing and releasing of successive muscle groups while attending to the resulting differences in sensation

Prosthesis Care   Care of a removable appliance worn by a patient and the prevention of complications associated with its use

Quality Monitoring   Systematic collection and analysis of an organization's quality indicators for the purpose of improving patient care

Radiation Therapy Management   Assisting the patient to understand and minimize the side effects of radiation treatments

Rape-Trauma Treatment   Provision of emotional and physical support immediately following an alleged rape

Reality Orientation   Promotion of patient's awareness of personal identity, time, and environment

Recreation Therapy   Purposeful use of recreation to promote relaxation and enhancement of social skills

Rectal Prolapse Management   Prevention and/or manual reduction of rectal prolapse

Referral   Arrangement for services by another care provider or agency

Reminiscence Therapy   Using the recall of past events, feelings, and thoughts to facilitate adaptation to present circumstances

Reproductive Technology Management   Assisting a patient through the steps of complex infertility treatment

Research Data Collection   Assisting a researcher to collect patient data

Respiratory Monitoring   Collection and analysis of patient data to ensure airway patency and adequate gas exchange

Respite Care   Provision of short-term care to provide relief for family caregiver

Resuscitation   Administering emergency measures to sustain life

Resuscitation: Fetus   Administering emergency measures to improve placental perfusion or correct fetal acid-base status

Resuscitation: Neonate   Administering emergency measures to support newborn adaptation to extrauterine life

Risk Identification   Analysis of potential risk factors, determination of health risks, and prioritization of risk reduction strategies for an individual or group

Risk Identification: Childbearing Family   Identification of an individual or family likely to experience difficulties in parenting and prioritization of strategies to prevent parenting problems

Role Enhancement   Assisting a patient, significant other, and/or family to improve relationships by clarifying and supplementing specific role behaviors

Seclusion   Solitary containment in a fully protective environment with close surveillance by nursing staff for purposes of safety or behavior management

Security Enhancement   Intensifying a patient's sense of physical and psychological safety

Seizure Management   Care of a patient during a seizure and the postictal state

Seizure Precautions   Prevention or minimization of potential injuries sustained by a patient with a known seizure disorder

Self-Awareness Enhancement   Assisting a patient to explore and understand his/her thoughts, feelings, motivations, and behaviors

Self-Care Assistance   Assisting another to perform activities of daily living

Self-Care Assistance: Bathing/Hygiene   Assisting patient to perform personal hygiene

Self-Care Assistance: Dressing/Grooming   Assisting patient with clothes and makeup

Self-Care Assistance: Feeding   Assisting a person to eat

Self-Care Assistance: Toileting   Assisting another with elimination

Self-Esteem Enhancement   Assisting a patient to increase his/her personal judgment of self worth

Self-Modification Assistance   Reinforcement of self-directed change initiated by the patient to achieve personally important goals

Self-Responsibility Facilitation   Encouraging a patient to assume more responsibility for own behavior

Sexual Counseling   Use of an interactive helping process focusing on the need to make adjustments in sexual practice or to enhance coping with a sexual event/disorder

Shift Report   Exchanging essential patient care information with other nursing staff at change of shift

Shock Management   Facilitation of the delivery of oxygen and nutrients to systemic tissue with removal of cellular waste products in a patient with severely altered tissue perfusion

Shock Management: Cardiac   Promotion of adequate tissue perfusion for a patient with severely compromised pumping function of the heart

Shock Management: Vasogenic   Promotion of adequate tissue perfusion for a patient with severe loss of vascular tone

Shock Management: Volume   Promotion of adequate tissue perfusion for a patient with severely compromised intravascular volume

Shock Prevention   Detecting and treating a patient at risk for impending shock

Sibling Support   Assisting a sibling to cope with a brother's or sister's illness

Simple Guided Imagery   Purposeful use of imagination to achieve relaxation and/or direct attention away from undesirable sensations

Simple Massage   Stimulation of the skin and underlying tissues with varying degrees of hand pressure to decrease pain, produce relaxation, and/or improve circulation

Simple Relaxation Therapy   Use of techniques to encourage and elicit relaxation for the purpose of decreasing undesirable signs and symptoms such as pain, muscle tension, or anxiety

Skin Care: Topical Treatments   Application of topical substances or manipulation of devices to promote skin integrity and minimize skin breakdown

Skin Surveillance   Collection and analysis of patient data to maintain skin and mucous membrane integrity

Sleep Enhancement   Facilitation of regular sleep/wake cycles

Smoking Cessation Assistance   Helping a patient to stop smoking

Socialization Enhancement   Facilitation of another person's ability to interact with others

Specimen Management   Obtaining, preparing, and preserving a specimen for a laboratory test

Spiritual Support   Assisting the patient to feel balance and connection with a greater power

Splinting   Stabilization, immobilization, and/or protection of an injured body part with a supportive appliance

Staff Supervision Facilitating the delivery of high quality patient care by others

Subarachnoid Hemorrhage Precautions Reduction of internal and external stimuli or stressors to minimize risk of rebleeding prior to aneurysm surgery

Substance Use Prevention Prevention of an alcoholic or drug use lifestyle

Substance Use Treatment Supportive care of patient/family members with physical and psychosocial problems associated with the use of alcohol or drugs

Substance Use Treatment: Alcohol Withdrawal Care of the patient experiencing sudden cessation of alcohol consumption

Substance Use Treatment: Drug Withdrawal Care of a patient experiencing drug detoxification

Substance Use Treatment: Overdose Monitoring, treatment, and emotional support of a patient who has ingested prescription or over-the-counter drugs beyond the therapeutic range

Suicide Prevention Reducing risk of self-inflicted harm for a patient in crisis or severe depression

Supply Management Ensuring acquisition and maintenance of appropriate items for providing patient care

Support Group Use of a group environment to provide emotional support and health-related information for members

Support System Enhancement Facilitation of support to patient by family, friends, and community

Surgical Assistance Assisting the surgeon/dentist with operative procedures and care of the surgical patient

Surgical Precautions Minimizing the potential for iatrogenic injury to the patient related to a surgical procedure

Surgical Preparation Providing care to a patient immediately prior to surgery and verification of required procedures/tests and documentation in the clinical record

Surveillance Purposeful and ongoing acquisition, interpretation, and synthesis of patient data for clinical decision-making

Surveillance: Late Pregnancy Purposeful and ongoing acquisition, interpretation, and synthesis of maternal-fetal data for treatment, observation, or admission

Surveillance: Safety Purposeful and ongoing collection and analysis of information about the patient and the environment for use in promoting and maintaining patient safety

Sustenance Support Helping a needy individual/family to locate food, clothing, or shelter

Suturing Approximating edges of a wound using sterile suture material and a needle

Swallowing Therapy Facilitating swallowing and preventing complications of impaired swallowing

Teaching: Disease Process Assisting the patient to understand information related to a specific disease process

Teaching: Group   Development, implementation, and evaluation of a patient teaching program for a group of individuals experiencing the same health condition

Teaching: Individual   Planning, implementation, and evaluation of a teaching program designed to address a patient's particular needs

Teaching: Infant Care   Instruction on nurturing and physical care needed during the first year of life

Teaching: Preoperative   Assisting a patient to understand and mentally prepare for surgery and the postoperative recovery period

Teaching: Prescribed Activity/Exercise   Preparing a patient to achieve and/or maintain a prescribed level of activity

Teaching: Prescribed Diet   Preparing a patient to correctly follow a prescribed diet

Teaching: Prescribed Medication   Preparing a patient to safely take prescribed medications and monitor for their effects

Teaching: Procedure/Treatment   Preparing a patient to understand and mentally prpare for a prescribed procedure or treatment

Teaching: Psychomotor Skill   Preparing a patient to perform a psychomotor skill

Teaching: Safe Sex   Providing instruction concerning sexual protection during sexual activity

Teaching: Sexuality   Assisting individuals to understand physical and psychosocial dimensions of sexual growth and development

Technology Management   Use of technical equipment and devices to monitor patient condition or sustain life

Telephone Consultation   Exchanging information, providing health education and advice, managing symptoms, or doing triage over the telephone

Temperature Regulation   Attaining and/or maintaining body temperature within a normal range

Temperature Regulation: Intraoperative   Attaining and/or maintaining desired intraoperative body temperature

Therapeutic Touch   Directing one's own interpersonal energy to flow through the hands to help or heal another

Therapy Group   Application of psychotherapeutic techniques to a group, including the utilization of interactions between members of the group

Total Parenteral Nutrition (TPN) Administration   Preparation and delivery of nutrients intravenously and monitoring of patient responsiveness

Touch   Providing comfort and communication through purposeful tactile contact

Traction/Immobilization Care   Management of a patient who has traction and/or a stabilizing device to immobilize and stabilize a body part

Transcutaneous Electrical Nerve Stimulation (TENS)   Stimulation of skin and underlying tissues with controlled, low-voltage electrical vibration via electrodes

Transport   Moving a patient from one location to another

Triage Establishing priorities of patient care for urgent treatment while allocating scarce resources

Truth Telling Use of whole truth, partial truth, or decision delay to promote the patient's self-determination and well-being

Tube Care Management of a patient with an external drainage device exiting the body

Tube Care: Chest Management of a patient with an external water-seal drainage device exiting the chest cavity

Tube Care: Gastrointestinal Management of a patient with a gastrointestinal tube

Tube Care: Umbilical Line Management of a newborn with an umbilical catheter

Tube Care: Urinary Management of a patient with urinary drainage equipment

Tube Care: Ventriculostomy/Lumbar Drain Management of a patient with an external cerebrospinal fluid drainage system

Ultrasonography: Limited Obstetric Performance of ultrasound exams to determine ovarian, uterine, or fetal status

Unilateral Neglect Management Protecting and safely reintegrating the affected part of the body while helping the patient adapt to disturbed perceptual abilities

Urinary Bladder Training Improving bladder function for those with urge incontinence by increasing the bladder's ability to hold urine and the patient's ability to suppress urination

Urinary Catheterization Insertion of a catheter into the bladder for temporary or permanent drainage of urine

Urinary Catheterization: Intermittent Regular periodic use of a catheter to empty the bladder

Urinary Elimination Management Maintenance of an optimum urinary elimination pattern

Urinary Habit Training Establishing a predictable pattern of bladder emptying to prevent incontinence for persons with limited cognitive ability who have urge, stress, or functional incontinence

Urinary Incontinence Care Assistance in promoting continence and maintaining perineal skin integrity

Urinary Incontinence Care: Enuresis Promotion of urinary continence in children

Urinary Retention Care Assistance in relieving bladder distention

Values Clarification Assisting another to clarify her/his own values in order to facilitate effective decision-making

Venous Access Devices (VAD) Maintenance Management of the patient with prolonged venous access via tunneled, non-tunneled catheters, and implanted ports

Ventilation Assistance Promotion of an optimal spontaneous breathing pattern that maximizes oxygen and carbon dioxide exchange in the lungs

Visitation Facilitation Promoting beneficial visits by family and friends

Vital Signs Monitoring   Collection and analysis of cardiovascular, respiratory, and body temperature data to determine and prevent complications

Weight Gain Assistance   Facilitating gain of body weight

Weight Management   Facilitating maintenance of optimal body weight and percent body fat

Weight Reduction Assistance   Facilitating loss of weight and/or body fat

Wound Care   Prevention of wound complications and promotion of wound healing

Wound Care: Closed Drainage   Maintenance of a pressure drainage system at the wound site

Wound Irrigation   Flushing of an open wound to cleanse and remove debris and excessive drainage

Source: McCloskey, J. C., and Bulechek, G. M. (Eds.) (1996). *Nursing interventions classification (NIC)* (2nd ed.). St. Louis: Mosby–Year Book.

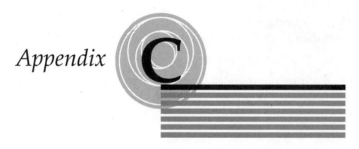

Nursing Outcomes Classification (NOC) Outcome Labels and Definitions, 1997

Abuse Cessation   Evidence that the victim is no longer abused

Abuse Protection   Protection of self or dependent others from abuse

Abuse Recovery: Emotional   Healing of psychological injuries due to abuse

Abuse Recovery: Financial   Regaining monetary and legal control or benefits following financial exploitation

Abuse Recovery: Physical   Healing of physical injuries due to abuse

Abuse Recovery: Sexual   Healing following sexual abuse or exploitation

Abusive Behavior Self-Control   Management of own behaviors to avoid abuse and neglect of dependents or significant others

Acceptance: Health Status   Reconciliation to health circumstances

Adherence Behavior   Self-initiated action taken to promote wellness, recovery, and rehabilitation

Aggression Control   Ability to restrain assaultive, combative or destructive behavior toward others

Ambulation: Walking   Ability to walk from place to place

Ambulation: Wheelchair   Ability to move from place to place in a wheelchair

Anxiety Control   Ability to eliminate or reduce feelings of apprehension and tension from an unidentifiable source

Balance   Ability to maintain body equilibrium

Blood Transfusion Reaction Control   Extent to which complications of blood transfusions are minimized

Body Image Positive perception of own appearance and body functions

Body Positioning: Self-Initiated Ability to change own body positions

Bone Healing The extent to which cells and tissues have regenerated following bone injury

Bowel Continence Control of passage of stool from the bowel

Bowel Elimination Ability of the gastrointestinal tract to form and evacuate stool effectively

Breastfeeding Establishment: Infant Proper attachment of an infant to and sucking from the mother's breast for nourishment during the first 2–3 weeks

Breastfeeding Establishment: Maternal Maternal establishment of proper attachment of an infant to and sucking from the breast for nourishment during the first 2–3 weeks

Breastfeeding Maintenance Continued nourishment of an infant through breastfeeding

Breastfeeding Weaning Process leading to the eventual discontinuation of breastfeeding

Cardiac Pump Effectiveness Extent to which blood is ejected from the left ventricle per minute to support systemic perfusion pressure

Caregiver Adaptation to Patient Institutionalization Family caregiver adaptation of role when the care recipient is transferred outside the home

Caregiver Emotional Health Feelings, attitudes and emotions of a family care provider while caring for a member or significant other over an extended period of time

Caregiver Home Care Readiness Preparedness to assume responsibility for the health care of a family member or significant other in the home

Caregiver Lifestyle Disruption Disturbances in the lifestyle of a family member due to caregiving

Caregiver-Patient Relationship Positive interactions and connections between the caregiver and care recipient

Caregiver Performance: Direct Care Provision by family care provider of appropriate personal and health care for a family member or significant other

Caregiver Performance: Indirect Care Arrangement and oversight of appropriate care for a family member or significant other by family care provider

Caregiver Physical Health Physical well-being of a family care provider while caring for a family member or significant other over an extended period of time

Caregiver Stressors The extent of biopsychosocial pressure on a family care provider caring for a family member or significant other over an extended period of time

Caregiver Well-Being Primary care provider's satisfaction with health and life circumstances

Caregiving Endurance Potential Factors that promote family care provider continuance over an extended period of time

Child Adaptation to Hospitalization Child's adaptive response to hospitalization

Child Development: 2 Months Milestones of physical, cognitive and psychosocial progression by two months of age

Child Development: 4 Months Milestones of physical, cognitive and psychosocial progression by four months of age

Child Development: 6 Months Milestones of physical, cognitive and psychosocial progression by six months of age

Child Development: 12 Months Milestones of physical, cognitive and psychosocial progression by twelve months of age

Child Development: 2 Years Milestones of physical, cognitive and psychosocial progression by two years of age

Child Development: 3 Years Milestones of physical, cognitive, and psychosocial progression by three years of age

Child Development: 4 Years Milestones of physical, cognitive and psychosocial progression by four years of age

Child Development: 5 Years Milestones of physical, cognitive and psychosocial progression by five years of age

Child Development: Middle Childhood (6–11 Years) Milestones of physical, cognitive and psychosocial progression between six and eleven years of age

Child Development: Adolescence (12–17 Years) Milestones of physical, cognitive and psychosocial progression between twelve and seventeen years of age

Circulation Status Extent to which blood flows unobstructed, unidirectionally, and at an appropriate pressure through large vessels of the systemic and pulmonary circuits

Cognitive Ability Ability to execute complex mental processes

Cognitive Orientation Ability to identify person, place, and time

Comfort Level Feelings of physical and psychological ease

Communication Ability Ability to receive, interpret, and express spoken, written and non-verbal messages

Communication: Expressive Ability Ability to express and interpret verbal and/or non-verbal messages

Communication: Receptive Ability Ability to receive and interpret verbal and/or non-verbal messages

Compliance Behavior Actions taken on the basis of professional advice to promote wellness, recovery, and rehabilitation

Concentration Ability to focus on a specific stimulus

Coping Actions to manage stressors that tax an individual's resources

Decision Making Ability to choose between two or more alternatives

Dignified Dying Maintaining personal control and comfort with the approaching end of life

Distorted Thought Control Ability to self-restrain disruption in perception, thought processes, and thought content

Electrolyte & Acid/Base Balance Balance of the electrolytes and non-electrolytes in the intracellular and extracellular compartments of the body

Endurance Extent that energy enables a person's activity

Energy Conservation   Extent of active management of energy to initiate and sustain activity

Fear Control   Ability to eliminate or reduce disabling feelings of alarm aroused by an identifiable source

Fluid Balance   Balance of water in the intracellular and extracellular compartments of the body

Grief Resolution   Adjustment to actual or impending loss

Growth   A normal increase in body size and weight

Health Beliefs   Personal convictions that influence health behaviors

Health Beliefs: Perceived Ability to Perform   Personal conviction that one can carry out a given health behavior

Health Beliefs: Perceived Control   Personal conviction that one can influence a health outcome

Health Beliefs: Perceived Resources   Personal conviction that one has adequate means to carry out a health behavior

Health Beliefs: Perceived Threat   Personal conviction that a health problem is serious and has potential negative consequences for lifestyle

Health Orientation   Personal view of health and health behaviors as priorities

Health Promoting Behavior   Actions to sustain or increase wellness

Health Seeking Behavior   Actions to promote optimal wellness, recovery, and rehabilitation

Hope   Presence of internal state of optimism that is personally satisfying and life-supporting

Hydration   Amount of water in the intracellular and extracellular compartments of the body

Identity   Ability to distinguish between self and non-self and to characterize one's essence

Immobility Consequences: Physiological   Compromise in physiological functioning due to impaired physical mobility

Immobility Consequences: Psycho-Cognitive   Extent of compromise in psychocognitive functioning due to impaired physical mobility

Immune Hypersensitivity Control   Extent to which inappropriate immune responses are suppressed

Immune Status   Adequacy of natural and acquired appropriately-targeted resistance to internal and external antigens

Immunization Behavior   Actions to obtain immunity from a preventable communicable disease

Impulse Control   Ability to self-restrain compulsive or impulsive behaviors

Infection Status   Presence and extent of infection

Information Processing   Ability to acquire, organize, and use information

Joint Movement: Active   Range of motion of joints with self-initiated movement

Joint Movement: Passive   Range of motion of joints with assisted movement

Knowledge: Breastfeeding   Extent of understanding conveyed about lactation and nourishment of infant through breastfeeding

Knowledge: Child Safety   Extent of understanding conveyed about safely caring for a child

Knowledge: Diet   Extent of understanding conveyed about diet

Knowledge: Disease Process   Extent of understanding conveyed about a specific disease process

Knowledge: Energy Conservation   Extent of understanding conveyed about energy conservation techniques

Knowledge: Health Behaviors   Extent of understanding conveyed about the promotion and protection of health

Knowledge: Health Resources   Extent of understanding conveyed about healthcare resources

Knowledge: Infection Control   Extent of understanding conveyed about prevention and control of infection

Knowledge: Medication   Extent of understanding conveyed about the safe use of medication

Knowledge: Personal Safety   Extent of understanding conveyed about preventing unintentional injuries

Knowledge: Prescribed Activity   Extent of understanding conveyed about prescribed activity and exercise

Knowledge: Substance Use Control   Extent of understanding conveyed about managing substance use safely

Knowledge: Treatment Procedure(s)   Extent of understanding conveyed about procedure(s) required as part of a treatment regimen

Knowledge: Treatment Regimen   Extent of understanding conveyed about a specific treatment regimen

Leisure Participation   Use of restful or relaxing activities as needed to promote well-being

Loneliness   The extent of emotional, social or existential isolation response

Memory   Ability to cognitively retrieve and report previously stored information

Mobility Level   Ability to move purposefully

Mood Equilibrium   Appropriate adjustment of prevailing emotional tone in response to circumstances

Muscle Function   Adequacy of muscle contraction needed for movement

Neglect Recovery   Healing following the cessation of substandard care

Neurological Status   Extent to which the peripheral and central nervous systems receive, process, and respond to internal and external stimuli

Neurological Status: Autonomic   Extent to which the autonomic nervous system coordinates visceral function

Neurological Status: Central Motor Control   Extent to which skeletal muscle activity (body movement) is coordinated by the central nervous system

Neurological Status: Consciousness   Extent to which an individual arouses, orients, and attends to the environment

Neurological Status: Cranial Sensory/Motor Function   Extent to which cranial nerves convey sensory and motor information

Neurological Status: Spinal Sensory/Motor Function Extent to which spinal nerves convey sensory and motor information

Nutritional Status Extent to which nutrients are available to meet metabolic needs

Nutritional Status: Biochemical Measures Body fluid components and chemical indices of nutritional status

Nutritional Status: Body Mass Congruence of body weight, muscle, and fat to height, frame, and gender

Nutritional Status: Energy Extent to which nutrients provide cellular energy

Nutritional Status: Food & Fluid Intake Amount of food and fluid taken into the body over a 24 hour period

Nutritional Status: Nutrient Intake Adequacy of nutrients taken into the body

Oral Health Condition of the mouth, teeth, gums, and tongue

Pain Control Behavior Personal actions to control pain

Pain: Disruptive Effects Observed or reported disruptive effects of pain on emotions and behavior

Pain Level Amount of reported or demonstrated pain

Parent-Infant Attachment Behaviors which demonstrate an enduring affectionate bond between a parent and infant

Parenting Provision of an environment that promotes optimum growth and development of dependent children

Parenting: Social Safety Parental actions to avoid social relationships that might cause harm or injury

Participation: Health Care Decisions Personal involvement in selecting and evaluating health care options

Physical Aging Status Physical changes that commonly occur with adult aging

Physical Maturation: Female Normal physical changes in the female that occur with the transition from childhood to adulthood

Physical Maturation: Male Normal physical changes in the male that occur with the transition from childhood to adulthood

Play Participation Use of activities as needed for enjoyment, entertainment, and development by children

Psychosocial Adjustment: Life Change Psychosocial adaptation of an individual to a life change

Quality of Life An individual's expressed satisfaction with current life circumstances

Respiratory Status: Gas Exchange Alveolar exchange of CO_2 or O_2 to maintain arterial blood gas concentrations

Respiratory Status: Ventilation Movement of air in and out of the lungs

Rest Extent and pattern of diminished activity for mental and physical rejuvenation

Risk Control Actions to eliminate or reduce actual, personal, and modifiable health

Risk Control: Alcohol Use   Actions to eliminate or reduce alcohol use that poses a threat to health

Risk Control: Drug Use   Actions to eliminate or reduce drug use that poses a threat to health

Risk Control: Sexually Transmitted Diseases (STD)   Actions to eliminate or reduce behaviors associated with sexually transmitted disease

Risk Control: Tobacco Use   Actions to eliminate or reduce tobacco use

Risk Control: Unintended Pregnancy   Actions to reduce the possibility of unintended pregnancy

Risk Detection   Actions taken to identify personal health threats

Role Performance   Congruence of an individual's role behavior with role expectations

Safety Behavior: Fall Prevention   Individual or caregiver actions to minimize risk factors that might precipitate falls

Safety Behavior: Home Physical Environment   Individual or caregiver actions to minimize environmental factors that might cause physical harm or injury in the home

Safety Behavior: Personal   Individual or caregiver efforts to control behaviors that might cause physical injury

Safety Status: Falls Occurrence   Number of falls in the past week

Safety Status: Physical Injury   Severity of injuries from accidents and trauma

Self-Care: Activities of Daily Living (ADL)   Ability to perform the most basic physical tasks and personal care activities

Self-Care: Bathing   Ability to cleanse own body

Self-Care: Dressing   Ability to dress self

Self-Care: Eating   Ability to prepare and ingest food

Self-Care: Grooming   Ability to maintain kempt appearance

Self-Care: Hygiene   Ability to maintain own hygiene

Self-Care: Instrumental Activities of Daily Living (IADL)   Ability to perform activities needed to function in the home or community

Self-Care: Non-Parenteral Medication   Ability to administer oral and topical medications to meet therapeutic goals

Self-Care: Oral Hygiene   Ability to care for own mouth and teeth

Self-Care: Parenteral Medication   Ability to administer parenteral medications to meet therapeutic goals

Self-Care: Toileting   Ability to toilet self

Self-Esteem   Personal judgement of self-worth

Self-Mutilation Restraint   Ability to refrain from intentional self-inflicted injury (non-lethal)

Sleep   Extent and pattern of sleep for mental and physical rejuvenation

Social Interaction Skills   An individual's use of effective interaction behaviors

Social Involvement   Frequency of an individual's social interactions with persons, groups, or organizations

Social Support   Perceived availability and actual provision of reliable assistance from other persons

Spiritual Well-Being   Personal expressions of connectedness with self, others, higher power, all life, nature and the universe that transcend and empower the self

Substance Addiction Consequences   Compromise in health status and social functioning due to substance addiction

Suicide Self-Restraint   Ability to refrain from gestures and attempts at killing self

Symptom Control Behavior   Personal actions to minimize perceived adverse changes in physical and emotional functioning

Symptom Severity   Extent of perceived adverse changes in physical, emotional, and social functioning

Thermoregulation   Balance among heat production, heat gain, and heat loss

Thermoregulation: Neonate   Balance among heat production, heat gain, and heat loss during the neonatal period

Tissue Integrity: Skin & Mucous Membranes   Structural intactness and normal physiological function of skin and mucous membranes

Tissue Perfusion: Abdominal Organs   Extent to which blood flows through the small vessels of the abdominal viscera and maintains organ function

Tissue Perfusion: Cardiac   Extent to which blood flows through the coronary vasculature and maintains heart function

Tissue Perfusion: Cerebral   Extent to which blood flows through the cerebral vasculature and maintains brain function

Tissue Perfusion: Peripheral   Extent to which blood flows through the small vessels of the extremities and maintains tissue function

Tissue Perfusion: Pulmonary   Extent to which blood flows through intact pulmonary vasculature with appropriate pressure and volume perfusing alveoli/capillary unit

Transfer Performance   Ability to change body locations

Treatment Behavior: Illness or Injury   Personal actions to palliate or eliminate pathology

Urinary Continence   Control of the elimination of urine

Urinary Elimination   Ability of the urinary system to filter wastes, conserve solutes, and to collect and discharge urine in a healthy pattern

Vital Signs Status   Temperature, pulse, respiration, and blood pressure within expected range for the individual

Well-Being   An individual's expressed satisfaction with health status

Will to Live   Desire, determination, and effort to survive

Wound Healing: Primary Intention   The extent to which cells and tissues have regenerated following intentional closure

Wound Healing: Secondary Intention   The extent to which cells and tissues in an open wound have regenerated

Source: Johnson, M., and Maas, M. (Eds.) (1997). *Nursing outcomes classification (NOC).* St. Louis: Mosby–Year Book.

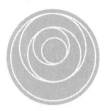

Index

Note: Page numbers in *italics* indicate figures; those followed by t indicate tables; those followed by b indicate boxes.

ISBN 0-7216-7724-X

90038

9 780721 677248